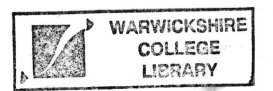

CURRENT THERAPY IN EQUINE MEDICINE
4

**N. EDWARD ROBINSON, B. Vet. Med., Ph.D., M.R.C.V.S.,
Docteur Honoris Causa (Liège)**

Matilda R. Wilson Professor of Large Animal Clinical Sciences
Michigan State University College of Veterinary Medicine
East Lansing, Michigan

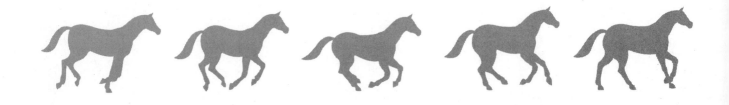

PHILADELPHIA   LONDON   TORONTO   MONTREAL   SYDNEY   TOKYO

CURRENT THERAPY IN EQUINE MEDICINE

4

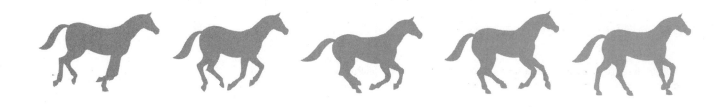

W.B. SAUNDERS COMPANY A Division of Harcourt Brace & Company

W.B. SAUNDERS COMPANY
A Division of Harcourt Brace & Company

The Curtis Center
Independence Square West
Philadelphia, Pennsylvania 19106

CURRENT THERAPY IN EQUINE MEDICINE 4   ISBN 0–7216–2633–5

Printed in the United States of America.

Last digit is the print number: 9   8   7   6   5   4   3   2   1

Current Therapy in Equine Medicine

DEDICATION

To our clients, whose love and admiration for their horses makes them demand the best of medical care.

CONTRIBUTORS

JENNIFER G. ADAMS, B.S., D.V.M.

Assistant Professor, Oregon State University, College of Veterinary Medicine, Corvallis, Oregon.

Thrombocytopenia

MONICA ALEMAN, M.V.Z.

Resident, Large Animal Medicine, Equine Emphasis, School of Veterinary Medicine, University of California at Davis, Davis, California.

Subcutaneous Abscesses Caused by Corynebacterium pseudotuberculosis

DONNA WALTON ANGARANO, D.V.M., Dipl. A.C.V.D.

Professor of Dermatology, Department of Small Animal Surgery and Medicine, College of Veterinary Medicine, Auburn University, Auburn, Alabama.

Dermatologic Conditions Associated With Oral Lesions

E. MURL BAILEY, Jr., D.V.M., Ph.D, Dipl. A.B.V.T.

Professor of Toxicology, Department of Veterinary Physiology and Pharmacology, College of Veterinary Medicine, Texas A&M University, College Station, Texas.

Industrial Toxicants; Appendix 4: Antidotes for Common Poisons

BARRY A. BALL, D.V.M., Ph.D.

Associate Professor of Theriogenology, College of Veterinary Medicine, Cornell University, Ithaca, New York.

Early Pregnancy Loss in Mares: Applications for Progestin Therapy

JANE A. BARBER, D.V.M., M.S.

Veterinary Medical Associate, Theriogenology Division, Department of Clinical and Population Sciences, College of Veterinary Medicine, University of Minnesota, St. Paul, Minnesota.

Diseases of the Ovary; Perinatal Behavior of the Mare and Foal

ALISTAIR R. S. BARR, M.A., Vet. M.S., Ph.D., D.V.R., D.E.C., Dipl. E.C.V.S.

Lecturer in Equine Orthopedics, Department of Clinical Veterinary Science, School of Veterinary Science, University of Bristol, Langford, Bristol, England.

Deep Digital Flexor Tendinitis; Noninfectious Conditions of the Digital Flexor Tendon Sheath

DAVID BARTRAM, B.V.Sc., D.V.A., M.R.C.V.S.

Greenwood, Ellis and Partners, Newmarket, Suffolk, England.

Postanesthetic Myopathy

S. ANNE BASKETT, D.M.V.

Clinical Resident, Large Animal Surgery, Department of Large Animal Medicine, College of Veterinary Medicine, University of Georgia, Athens, Georgia.

Musculoskeletal Injuries in the Eventing Horse; Salivary Gland Disease

ANDREW P. BATHE, M.A., Vet. M.B., Cert. E.S. (Orth.), M.R.C.V.S.

Equine Surgeon, Gibsons Veterinary Hospital, Oakham, Rutland, England.

Penetrating Injuries of the Foot

GARY M. BAXTER, V.M.D., M.S.

Associate Professor of Surgery, Department of Clinical Sciences, Veterinary Teaching Hospital, Colorado State University, Fort Collins, Colorado.

Laminitis

WILLIAM V. BERNARD, D.V.M., Dipl. A.C.V.I.M.

Internist, Rood and Riddle Equine Hospital, Lexington, Kentucky.

Botulism; Hypoxic Ischemic Encephalopathy

KAREN M. BLUMENSHINE, D.V.M., R.D.M.S., R.D.C.S.

Santa Barbara Equine Practice, Santa Barbara, California.

Soft Tissue Injuries of the Hock

LINDA L. BLYTHE, D.V.M., Ph.D.

Interim Assistant Dean and Professor of Veterinary Neurology, College of Veterinary Medicine, Oregon State University, Corvallis, Oregon.

Degenerative Myeloencephalopathy; Peripheral Neuropathy; Temporohyoid Osteoarthropathy (Middle Ear Disease)

THOMAS C. BOHANON, D.V.M., M.S.
Staff Surgeon, Littleton Large Animal Clinic, Littleton, Colorado.
Pain Associated With the Distal Tarsal Joints of the Hock

GEORGE BOHART, D.V.M.
Instructor, Department of Large Animal Clinical Sciences, College of Veterinary Medicine, Michigan State University, East Lansing, Michigan.
Anesthesia of Horses in the Field

JOHN D. BONAGURA, D.V.M., M.S., Dipl. A.C.V.I.M.
Gilbreath McLorn Professor of Veterinary Cardiology, Department of Veterinary Medicine and Surgery, University of Missouri, Columbia, Missouri.
Diagnosis of Cardiac Arrhythmias

PHILIP BOYDELL, B. Vet. Med., M.R.C.V.S.
Head of Ophthalmology, Animal Medical Centre Referral Services, Manchester, England.
Cataract; Periocular Disease

JAMES P. BRENDEMUEHL, D.V.M., Ph.D.
Assistant Professor, Department of Large Animal Services, Tuskegee University School of Veterinary Medicine, Tuskegee, Alabama.
Reproductive Aspects of Fescue Toxicosis

LESLIE H. BREUER, Jr., Ph.D.
Consultant, L. H. Breuer & Associates, East Alton, Illinois.
Selecting and Utilizing Manufactured Feeds

DUANE F. BROBST, D.V.M., Ph.D.
Emeritus Professor of Clinical Pathology, Washington State University College of Veterinary Medicine, Pullman, Washington.
Normal Clinical Pathology Data

DENNIS E. BROOKS, D.V.M., Ph.D.
Associate Professor of Ophthalmology, Ophthalmology Service Chief, College of Veterinary Medicine, University of Florida, Gainesville, Florida.
Glaucoma; Ocular Problems in the Foal; The Prepurchase Ophthalmic Examination

CHRISTOPHER M. BROWN, B.V.Sc., Ph.D., M.R.C.V.S.
Professor and Department Executive Officer, Department of Veterinary Clinical Sciences, and Director, Veterinary Teaching Hospital, College of Veterinary Medicine, Iowa State University, Ames, Iowa.
Polyuria

JANA L. CARGILE, D.V.M., Ph.D., Dipl. A.C.V.I.M.
Associate Veterinarian, Equine Medical Associates, Glencoe, Missouri.
Medical Management of Colic

ELIZABETH A. CARR, D.V.M., Dipl. A.C.V.I.M.
Postgraduate Researcher, Department of Veterinary Surgery and Radiology, School of Veterinary Medicine, University of California at Davis, Davis, California.
Examination of the Urinary System

DAN CARTER, D.V.M.
Resident, College of Veterinary Medicine, Auburn University, Auburn University, Alabama.
Topical Therapy

G. KENT CARTER, D.V.M., M.S., Dipl. A.C.V.I.M.
Associate Professor, Department of Large Animal Medicine and Surgery, College of Veterinary Medicine, Texas A&M University, College Station, Texas.
Bacterial Pleuropneumonia

EDUOARD CAUVIN, D.V.M, M.V.M., Cert V.R., M.R.C.V.S.
Resident in Diagnostic Imaging, Department of Veterinary Clinical Studies, Royal (Dick) School of Veterinary Studies, University of Edinburgh, Easter Bush, Roslin, Midlothian, Scotland.
Techniques for Examination of the Oral Cavity

M. KEITH CHAFFIN, D.V.M., M.S., Dipl. A.C.V.I.M.
Assistant Professor, Department of Large Animal Medicine and Surgery, College of Veterinary Medicine, Texas A&M University, College Station, Texas.
Bacterial Pleuropneumonia

CEDRIC C-H. CHAN, B.V.Sc., Cert. E.S.(O.), M.R.C.V.S.
Resident in Equine Surgery, Department of Veterinary Surgery, Glasgow University Veterinary School, Bearsden, Glasgow, Scotland.
Congenital Abnormalities of the Mouth and Associated Structures

CAROL K. CLARK, D.V.M.
College of Veterinary Medicine, University of Florida, Gainesville, Florida.
Ocular Problems in the Foal

NOAH D. COHEN, V.M.D., M.P.H., Ph.D., Dipl. A.C.V.I.M.
Assistant Professor of Equine Medicine, Department of Large Animal Medicine and Surgery, College of Veterinary Medicine, Texas A & M University, College Station, Texas.
Diarrheal Diseases of Foals

ROBERT J. COLEMAN, B.Sc., M.Sc.
Provincial Horse Specialist, Alberta Agriculture Food and Rural Development, Animal Industry Division, Horse Industry Section, Edmonton, Alberta, Canada.
Feeds and Feeding in the Northwestern United States and Western Canada

CHRYSANN COLLATOS, B.A., V.M.D., Ph.D.

Practitioner and Owner, High Desert Veterinary Service, Reno, Nevada.

Blood Loss Anemia; Blood and Blood Component Therapy; Anemia Resulting from Inadequate Erythropoiesis; Hemostatic Dysfunction

TIMOTHY CORDES, D.V.M.

Senior Staff Veterinarian, Equine Diseases, United States Department of Agriculture, Riverdale, Maryland.

Quarantine Considerations and Medical Management of Horses During International Shipment

A. MORRIE CRAIG, Ph.D.

Professor, College of Veterinary Medicine, Oregon State University, Corvallis, Oregon.

Degenerative Myeloencephalopathy

ANN A. CULLINANE, M.V.B., Ph.D., M.R.C.V.S.

Head of Virology, Irish Equine Centre, Johnstown, Naas, County Kildare, Ireland.

Viral Respiratory Disease

JOHN F. CUMMINGS, D.V.M., Ph.D.

Professor, Department of Anatomy, New York State College of Veterinary Medicine, Cornell University, Ithaca, New York.

Equine Motor Neuron Disease

TIM J. CUTLER, M.V.B., M.R.C.V.S.

Resident, Department of Large Animal Clinical Sciences, College of Veterinary Medicine, University of Florida, Gainesville, Florida.

Equine Herpesvirus-1 Myeloencephalitis

ROBIN M. DABAREINER, D.V.M., M.S.

Clinical Instructor of Equine Surgery, Marion duPont Scott Equine Medical Center, Virginia-Maryland Regional College of Veterinary Medicine, Virginia Tech and University of Maryland, Blacksburg, Virginia.

Peritonitis in Horses

PETER F. DAELS, D.V.M., Ph.D.

Assistant Professor of Theriogenology, College of Veterinary Medicine, Cornell University, Ithaca, New York.

Early Pregnancy Loss in Mares: Applications for Progestin Therapy

JULIE M. DELGER, D.V.M., Dipl. A.C.V.D.

Owner, South Carolina Dermatology Referral Service, Columbia, South Carolina.

Pruritic Dermatoses

FREDERIK J. DERKSEN, D.V.M., Ph.D., Dipl. A.C.V.I.M.

Professor and Chair, Department of Large Animal Clinical Sciences, College of Veterinary Medicine, Michigan State University, East Lansing, Michigan.

Inhalation Therapy for the Treatment of Lower Airway Disease

THOMAS J. DIVERS, D.V.M., Dipl. A.C.V.I.M.

Associate Professor of Medicine, Veterinary Teaching Hospital, College of Veterinary Medicine, Cornell University, Ithaca, New York.

Equine Hepatic Disorders; Equine Motor Neuron Disease

PADRAIC M. DIXON, M.V.B., Ph.D., M.R.C.V.S.

Senior Lecturer, Department of Veterinary Clinical Studies, Royal (Dick) School of Veterinary Studies, University of Edinburgh, Easter Bush, Roslin, Midlothian, Scotland.

Dental Disease

NORM G. DUCHARME, D.M.V., M.Sc., Dipl. A.C.V.S.

Professor of Surgery, Equine Hospital; Head, Equine and Farm Animal Hospitals, College of Veterinary Medicine, Cornell University, Ithaca, New York.

Intermittent Dorsal Displacement of the Soft Palate

DAVID DUGDALE, M.A., Vet. M.B., M.R.C.V.S.

Greenwood, Ellis and Partners, Newmarket, Suffolk, England.

Intermittent Upward Fixation of the Patella and Disorders of the Patellar Ligaments

NOËL DYBDAL, D.V.M., Ph.D.

Scientist and Veterinary Pathologist, Genentech, Inc., South San Francisco, California.

Pituitary Pars Intermedia Dysfunction (Equine Cushing's-like Disease)

SUE J. DYSON, M.A., Vet. M.B., Ph.D.

Equine Centre, Animal Health Trust, Snailwell Road, Newmarket, Suffolk, England.

Muscular Disorders; Aortoiliacofemoral Thrombosis; Problems Associated With the Neck: Neck Pain and Stiffness, Abnormal Posture, and Forelimb Gait Abnormalities; Proximal Metacarpal or Metatarsal Pain; Soft Injuries of the Hock; The Diffusely Filled Limb

LUCY M. EDENS, D.V.M., M.S., Dipl. A.C.V.I.M.

Assistant Professor, Large Animal Internal Medicine, Department of Large Animal Clinical Science, College of Veterinary Medicine, University of Florida, Gainesville, Florida.

Abdominal Hemorrhage; Medical Management of Colic; Umbilical Disorders

WILLIAM C. EDWARDS, D.V.M., M.S.

Director and Toxicologist, Oklahoma Animal Disease Diagnostic Laboratory, Oklahoma State University, Stillwater, Oklahoma.

Medicolegal Investigation of the Sudden or Unexpected Equine Death: Toxicologic Implications

DAVID ELLIS, B. Vet. Med., D.E.O., F.R.C.V.S.

Partner, Greenwood, Ellis and Partners, Newmarket, Suffolk, England.

Flexural Deformities

MELVYN L. FAHNING, D.V.M., Ph.D.

Professor and Head, Division of Theriogenology, Department of Population and Clinical Sciences, College of Veterinary Medicine, University of Minnesota, St. Paul, Minnesota.

Dystocia; Retained Fetal Membranes

CLARA FENGER, D.V.M., Ph.D., Dipl. A.C.V.I.M.

Equine Internal Medicine Consulting, Lexington, Kentucky.

Equine Protozoal Myeloencephalitis

DAVID E. FREEMAN, M.V.B., Ph.D., Dipl. A.C.V.S.

Assistant Professor, College of Veterinary Medicine, University of Illinois, Urbana, Illinois.

Hemorrhage From the Upper Respiratory Tract

MARTIN FURR, D.V.M., Dipl. A.C.V.I.M.

Associate Professor, Marion duPont Scott Equine Medical Center, Virginia-Maryland Regional College of Veterinary Medicine, Virginia Tech and University of Maryland, Blacksburg, Virginia.

Evaluation of Colic in the Neonatal Foal

FRANCIS D. GALEY, D.V.M., Ph.D., Dipl. A.B.V.T.

Associate Professor of Clinical Diagnostic Veterinary Toxicology, California Veterinary Diagnostic Laboratory System–Toxicology Laboratory, School of Veterinary Medicine, University of California at Davis, Davis, California.

Diagnostic Toxicology

TAM GARLAND, B.S., D.V.M., Ph.D., Dipl. A.B.V.T.

Research Associate, Department of Veterinary Physiology and Pharmacology, College of Veterinary Medicine, Texas A & M University, College Station, Texas.

Industrial Toxicants; Appendix 4: Antidotes for Common Poisons

RAYMOND J. GEOR, B.V.Sc., M.V.Sc., Dipl. A.C.V.I.M.

Associate Professor, Large Animal Medicine, Department of Clinical Studies, and Clinician, Veterinary Teaching Hospital, Ontario Veterinary College, University of Guelph, Guelph, Ontario, Canada.

Acute Renal Failure; Aminoglycoside Dosing

STEEVE GIGUERE, D.M.V.

Graduate Research Assistant, Department of Pathobiology, Ontario Veterinary College, University of Guelph, Guelph, Ontario, Canada.

Vasculitis

CAROL L. GILLIS, D.V.M., Ph.D.

Lecturer, Department of Surgical and Radiological Sciences, School of Veterinary Medicine, University of California at Davis, Davis, California.

Biceps Brachii Tendinitis and Bicipital (Intertubercular) Bursitis; Soft Tissue Swelling on the Dorsal Aspect of the Carpus

J. A. GRAY, B.Sc.

Graduate Student, Newmarket, England.

Biochemical Bone Markers

ELEANOR M. GREEN, D.V.M., Dipl. A.C.V.I.M., Dipl. A.B.V.P.

Professor and Chair, Department of Large Animal Clinical Sciences, College of Veterinary Medicine, University of Florida, Gainesville, Florida.

Fescue Toxicosis

PETER GREEN, B.V.Sc., M.R.C.V.S.

Fellowes Farm Equine Clinic, Abbotts Ripton, Huntingdon, Cambridgeshire, England.

Laceration or Rupture of the Digital Flexor Tendons

SHERRIL L. GREEN, D.V.M., Ph.D.

Assistant Professor, Department of Comparative Medicine, Stanford University School of Medicine, Stanford, California.

Rabies

TIMOTHY R. C. GREET, B.V.M.S., M.V.M., Cert. E.O., D.E.S.T.S., Dipl. E.C.V.S., F.R.C.V.S.

Surgeon, Rossdale and Partners, Beaufort Cottage Stables, Newmarket, Suffolk, England.

Penetrating Injuries of the Foot; Fractures of the Lower and Upper Jaws

RICHARD P. HACKETT, D.V.M., M.S., Dipl. A.C.V.S.

Associate Professor of Surgery, Equine Hospital, College of Veterinary Medicine, Cornell University, Ithaca, New York.

Intermittent Dorsal Displacement of the Soft Palate

JOHN C. HALIBURTON, D.V.M., Ph.D.

Head, Diagnostic Toxicology, Texas Veterinary Medical Diagnostic Laboratory, Amarillo, Texas.

Medicolegal Investigation of the Sudden or Unexpected Equine Death: Toxicologic Implications

R. REID HANSON, D.V.M., Dipl. A.C.V.S.

Assistant Professor of Equine Surgery, Department of Large Animal Surgery and Medicine, College of Veterinary Medicine, Auburn University, Auburn, Alabama.

Cryotherapy for Equine Skin Conditions

JOANNE HARDY, D.V.M., M.S., Dipl. A.C.V.S.

Instructor, Department of Veterinary Clinical Sciences, College of Veterinary Medicine, The Ohio State University, Columbus, Ohio.

Disorders of the Proximal Sesamoid Bones

JOYCE C. HARMAN, D.V.M., M.R.C.V.S.

Harmony Equine Clinic, Washington, VA.

Complementary (Alternative) Therapies for Poor Performance, Back Problems, and Lameness

PAT HARRIS, R.A., Vet. M.B., Ph.D., M.R.C.V.S.

The Walthar Centre for Animal Nutrition, Waltham-on-the-Wolds, Leicestershire, England.

Biochemical Bone Markers; Muscular Disorders; Equine Rhabdomyolysis Syndrome; Feeds and Feeding in the United Kingdom

SEBASTIAN E. HEATH, B.Sc., Vet. M.B., M. Vet. Sci., M.P.V.M.

Assistant Professor, School of Veterinary Medicine, Purdue University, West Lafayette, Indiana.

Planning for the Care of Horses in Disasters

KENNETH W. HINCHCLIFF, B.V.Sc., M.S., Ph.D.

Associate Professor, Department of Veterinary Clinical Sciences, College of Veterinary Medicine, The Ohio State University, Columbus, Ohio.

Nonsteroidal Anti-inflammatory Drugs

MELISSA TROGDON HINES, D.V.M., Ph.D.

Associate Professor, Department of Veterinary Clinical Sciences, College of Veterinary Medicine, Washington State University, Pullman, Washington.

Immunodeficiencies of Foals

KATRIN HINRICHS, D.V.M., Ph.D.

Associate Professor and Head, Section of Theriogenology, School of Veterinary Medicine, Tufts University, North Grafton, Massachusetts.

Assisted Reproductive Techniques in the Mare

HAROLD F. HINTZ, B.S., Ph.D.

Professor, Animal Nutrition, College of Veterinary Medicine, Cornell University, Ithaca, New York.

Feeds and Feeding in the Northeastern United States

DAVID R. HODGSON, B.V.Sc., Ph.D., Dipl. A.C.V.I.M.

Associate Professor, Department of Animal Health, University of Sydney, and Director, Rural Veterinary Center, Camden, New South Wales, Australia.

Acute Equine Respiratory Syndrome

JENNIFER L. HODGSON, B.V.Sc., Ph.D., Dipl. A.C.V.I.M.

Lecturer, Department of Animal Health, University of Sydney, and Clinical Pathologist, Rural Veterinary Centre, Camden, New South Wales, Australia.

Acute Equine Respiratory Syndrome

ROBERT J. HUNT, D.V.M., M.S., Dipl. A.C.V.S.

Hagyard-Davidson-McGee Associates, PSC, Lexington, Kentucky.

Noninfectious Musculoskeletal Disorders of Foals

BRAD R. JACKMAN, D.V.M., M.S., Dipl. A.C.V.S.

Staff Surgeon, Pioneer Equine Hospital, Inc., Oakdale, California.

Dysuria

HEATHER JAQUAY, B.S.

Farm Store Specialist, Cargill-Nutrena, Hamilton, New York.

Feeds and Feeding in the Northeastern United States

K. ANN JEGLUM, V.M.D.

Adjunct Associate Professor of Medical Oncology, School of Veterinary Medicine, University of Pennsylvania and The Wistar Institute, Philadelphia, Pennsylvania. Owner and Director, Veterinary Oncology Services and Research Center, West Chester, Pennsylvania.

Melanomas

BILL JOHNSON, D.V.M.

Associate Professor of Clinical Diagnostic Pathology, California Veterinary Diagnostic Laboratory System, School of Veterinary Medicine, University of California at Davis, Davis, California.

Forensic Necropsy of the Horse

R. GARETH JONES, B.V.Sc., Cert. V. Ophthal., M.R.C.V.S.

Partner, The Park Veterinary Group, Leicester, England.

Ocular Trauma

TINA KEMPER, D.V.M., Dipl. A.C.V.I.M.

Internist, Equine Hospital, Yorba Linda, California.

Smoke Inhalation

A. BRUCE KING, D.V.M.

Private Veterinary Practitioner, Ponti Veterinary Hospital, Otis Orchards, Washington.

Chronic Renal Failure

KEVIN KISTHARDT, D.V.M.

Resident, Department of Internal Medicine, College of Veterinary Medicine, Auburn University, Auburn, Alabama.

Pastern Dermatitis

THOMAS R. KLEI, B.S., Ph.D.

Boyd Professor, Parasitology and Veterinary Science, Department of Veterinary Microbiology and Parasitology, School of Veterinary Medicine, Louisiana State University, Baton Rouge, Louisiana.

Parasite Control Programs

DEREK C. KNOTTENBELT, B.V.M., D.V.M.

Senior Lecturer, Department of Veterinary Clinical Studies, University of Liverpool, Leahurst, England.

Medical Disorders of the Mouth

JEFF C. H. KO, D.V.M., M.S., Dipl. A.C.V.A.

Assistant Professor of Anesthesiology, Department of Large Animal Clinical Sciences, College of Veterinary Medicine, University of Florida, Gainesville, Florida.

Sedation and Anesthesia in Foals

NORBERT KOPF, Dr. Med. Vet., Univ.-Dos.

University Lecturer, Veterinärmedifiuiscke Universität Wien, and Veterinarian, Tierklinik, Breitensee, Vienna, Austria.

Rectal Examination of the Colic Patient

ANNE M. KOTERBA, D.V.M., Ph.D., Dipl. A.C.V.I.M.

Courtesy Associate Professor in Large Animal Medicine and Neonatology, College of Veterinary Medicine, University of Florida, Gainesville, Florida.

Prematurity

JEFFREY LAKRITZ, D.V.M., Ph.D.

Postgraduate Researcher, Department of Anatomy, Physiology, and Cell Biology, School of Veterinary Medicine, University of California at Davis, Davis, California.

Bronchointerstitial Pneumonia and Acute Respiratory Distress

SHEILA LAVERTY, M.V.B., M.R.C.V.S., Dipl. A.C.V.S.

Associate Professor, Département de Sciences Cliniques, Faculté de Médecine Vétérinaire, Université de Montréal, St.-Hyacinthe, Québec, Canada.

Thoracic Trauma; Sinusitis

JEAN-PIERRE LAVOIE, D.M.V., Dipl. A.C.V.I.M.

Associate Professor of Equine Medicine, Département de Sciences Cliniques, Faculté de Médecine Vétérinaire, Université de Montréal, St.-Hyacinthe, Québec, Canada.

Chronic Obstructive Pulmonary Disease; Lung Abscesses in Mature Horses

LAURIE LAWRENCE, D.V.M.

Department of Animal Sciences, University of Kentucky, Lexington, Kentucky.

Section 15: Nutrition

GUY D. LESTER, B.V.M.S., Ph.D., Dipl. A.C.V.I.M.

Assistant Professor, College of Veterinary Medicine, University of Florida, Gainesville, Florida.

Neonatal Pulmonary Disease; Prematurity

JEANNE LÖFSTEDT, B.V.Sc., M.S.

Associate Professor, Health Management, Atlantic Veterinary College, University of Prince Edward Island, Charlottetown, Prince Edward Island, Canada.

Diagnostic Approach to Anemia

CHARLES C. LOVE, D.V.M., Ph.D.

Veterinarian, Florissant, Missouri.

Reproductive Diseases in the Stallion

JOHN MacDONALD, D.V.M., Dipl. A.C.V.D.

Associate Professor, Department of Small Animal Surgery and Medicine, College of Veterinary Medicine, Auburn University, Auburn, Alabama.

Topical Therapy

ROBERT J. MacKAY, B.V.Sc., Ph.D.

Associate Professor of Equine Medicine, College of Veterinary Medicine, University of Florida, Gainesville, Florida.

Cauda Equina Syndrome; Equine Herpesvirus-1 Myeloencephalitis

SCOTT MADILL, B.V.Sc., D.V.Sc.

Graduate Student, Department of Clinical and Population Sciences, College of Veterinary Medicine, University of Minnesota, St. Paul, Minnesota.

Breeding Soundness Examination of the Mare

JOHN B. MADISON, V.M.D.

Associate Professor of Surgery, Department of Large Animal Clinical Sciences, University of Florida, Gainesville, Florida.

Infectious Orthopedic Disease in Foals

T. S. MAIR, B.V.Sc., Ph.D., M.R.C.V.S.

Partner, Bell Equine Veterinary Clinic, Mereworth, Maidstone, Kent, England.

Hypertrophic Osteopathy

MARCEL MARCOUX, D.M.V., M.Sc.

Professor and Clinician, Département de Sciences Cliniques, Faculté de Médecine Vétérinaire, Université de Montréal, St.-Hyacinthe, Québec, Canada.

Tracheal Collapse

DAN MARKS, V.M.D.

Santa Fe, New Mexico.

Back Pain

CELIA M. MARR, B.V.M.S., M.V.M., Ph.D., M.R.C.V.S.

Cardiologist and General Practitioners, Valley Equine Hospital, Lambourn, United Kingdom.

Treatment of Cardiac Arrhythmias and Cardiac Failure

ANDREW G. MATTHEWS, B.V.M.&S., Ph.D., F.R.C.V.S.

Honorary Lecturer, University of Glasgow, Glasgow, Scotland. Honorary Fellow, University of Edinburgh, Edinburgh, Scotland. Partner, McKenzie, Bryson and Marshall, Veterinary Surgeons, Kilmarnock, Ayrshire, Scotland.

The Cornea

ABBY D. MAXSON, M.S., V.M.D., Dipl. A.C.V.I.M.

Assistant Professor of Medicine in the George D. Widener Hospital, New Bolton Center, School of Veterinary Medicine, University of Pennsylvania, Kennett Square, Pennsylvania.

Congenital Cardiac Disease

JILL JOHNSON McCLURE, D.V.M., M.S., Dipl. A.C.V.I.M., Dipl. A.B.V.P.

Professor of Equine Medicine, School of Veterinary Medicine, Louisiana State University, Baton Rouge, Louisiana.

Neonatal Isoerythrolysis

ANDREW M. McDIARMID, B.V.M.&S., M.R.C.V.S.

Lecturer in Large Animal Surgery, Royal (Dick) School of Veterinary Studies, University of Edinburgh, Easter Bush, Roslin, Midlothian, Scotland.

Desmitis of the Accessory Ligament of the Deep Digital Flexor Tendon

NAT T. MESSER IV, B.S., D.V.M., Dipl. A.B.V.P.

Associate Professor of Equine Medicine and Surgery, University of Missouri, Columbia, Missouri.

Thyroid Disease (Dysfunction)

ELSPETH MILNE, B.V.M.&S., Ph.D., M.R.C.V.S.

Veterinary Investigation Officer, Scottish Agricultural College Veterinary Services, St. Mary's Industrial Estate, Dumfries, Dumfriesshire, Scotland.

Differential Diagnosis of Dysphagia; Grass Sickness

RICHARD MITCHELL, D.V.M.

Fairfield Equine Associates, Munro, Connecticut.

Quarantine Considerations and Medical Management of Horses During International Shipment

LAURIE A. MITTEN, D.V.M., M.S., Dipl. A.C.V.I.M.

Resident, Department of Veterinary Clinical Sciences, College of Veterinary Medicine, The Ohio State University, Columbus, Ohio.

Nonsteroidal Antiinflammatory Drugs

HUSSNI O. MOHAMMED, B.V.Sc., M.V.Sc., D.P.V.M., Ph.D.

Associate Professor of Epidemiology, Department of Clinical Sciences, New York State College of Veterinary Medicine, Cornell University, Ithaca, New York.

Equine Motor Neuron Disease

BONNIE RUSH MOORE, D.V.M., M.S.

Assistant Professor, College of Veterinary Medicine, Kansas State University, Manhattan, Kansas.

Central Nervous System Trauma; Cervical Stenotic Myelopathy

JAMES N. MOORE, D.V.M., Ph.D.

Professor, Departments of Large Animal Medicine and Physiology and Pharmacology, College of Veterinary Medicine, University of Georgia, Athens, Georgia.

Medical Vs. Surgical Treatment of Horses With Colic

GRAHAM MUNROE, B.V.Sc. (Hons.), Ph.D., Cert. E.O., D.E.S.M., F.R.C.V.S.

Senior Lecturer in Large Animal Surgery, Department of Veterinary Clinical Studies, Royal (Dick) School of Veterinary Studies, University of Edinburgh, Easter Bush, Roslin, Midlothian, Scotland.

Techniques for Examination of the Oral Cavity; Congenital Abnormalities of the Mouth and Associated Structures; Congenital Ocular Disease

MIKE MURPHY, D.V.M., Ph.D., Dipl. A.B.V.T.

Associate Professor, Department of Veterinary Diagnostic Medicine, College of Veterinary Medicine, University of Minnesota, St. Paul, Minnesota.

Toxic Plants

MICHAEL J. MURRAY, D.V.M., M.S., Dipl. A.C.V.I.M.

Associate Professor and Adelaide C. Riggs Chair in Equine Medicine, Marion duPont Scott Equine Medical Center, Virginia-Maryland Regional College of Veterinary Medicine, Virginia Tech and University of Maryland, Blacksburg, Virginia.

Acute Colitis; Diagnostic Procedures for Evaluation of the Gastrointestinal Tract; Gastroduodenal Ulceration

JOE NEWTON, D.V.M., Ph.D.

Associate Professor, Department of Pathobiology, College of Veterinary Medicine, Auburn University, Auburn, Alabama.

Pythiosis

EDGAR A. OTT, B.S., M.S., Ph.D.

Professor of Equine Nutrition, Animal Science Department, University of Florida, Gainesville, Florida.

Feeds and Feeding in the Southern United States

LUISITO S. PABLO, D.V.M., M.S., Dipl. A.C.V.A.

Assistant Professor of Anesthesiology, Department of Large Animal Clinical Science, College of Veterinary Medicine, University of Florida, Gainesville, Florida.

Sedation and Anesthesia in Foals

SCOTT E. PALMER, V.M.D.

President and Staff Surgeon, New Jersey Equine Clinic, Clarksburg, New Jersey.

Splints, Fractures of the Second and Fourth Metacarpal/Metatarsal Bones, and Associated Suspensory Ligament Desmitis

MARY ROSE PARADIS, D.V.M., M.S.

Associate Professor of Large Animal Medicine, School of Veterinary Medicine, Tufts University, North Grafton, Massachusetts.

Neonatal Septicemia

ERIC J. PARENTE, D.V.M.

Assistant Professor of Sports Medicine, New Bolton Center, School of Veterinary Medicine, University of Pennsylvania, Kennett Square, Pennsylvania.

Diagnostic Techniques for Upper Airway Diseases; Soft Tissue Collapse of the Upper Airway

ANDREW H. PARKS, M.A., Vet. M.B.

Associate Professor, Department of Large Animal Medicine, College of Veterinary Medicine, University of Georgia, Athens, Georgia.

Hoof Cracks and Hoof Wall Avulsions; Hoof Imbalance and Lameness; Salivary Gland Disease

BRUCE W. PARRY, B.V.Sc., Ph.D., Dipl. A.C.V.P.

Senior Lecturer, Department of Veterinary Science; Director, Department of Veterinary Clinic and Hospital, The University of Melbourne, Werribee, Victoria, Australia.

Normal Clinical Pathology Data

JOHN R. PASCOE, B.V.Sc., Ph.D., Dipl. A.C.V.S.

Associate Dean of Academic Programs and Professor of Surgery, Department of Surgical and Radiological Sciences, School of Veterinary Medicine, University of California at Davis, Davis, California.

Exercise-Induced Pulmonary Hemorrhage; Sinusitis

SUE PATERSON, M.A., Vet. M.B., D.V.D., Dipl. E.C.V.D., M.R.C.V.S.

Consultant Veterinary Dermatologist, Animal Medical Centre Referral Service, Chorlton, Manchester, England.

Periocular Disease

MARK W. PATTESON, M.A., Vet. M.B., Ph.D., D.V.C., Cert. V.R., M.R.C.V.S.

Recognised Teacher, Department of Clinical Veterinary Science, School of Veterinary Science, University of Bristol, Langford, Avon, England. Private Practitioner, Vale Veterinary Group, Bushy Farm Equine Clinic, Breadstone, Berkeley, Gloucestershire, England.

Acquired Cardiac Disease

ERWIN G. PEARSON, D.V.M., M.S.

Professor of Large Animal Medicine, College of Veterinary Medicine, Oregon State University, Corvallis, Oregon.

Pyrrolizidine Alkaloid Toxicosis

TIM J. PHILLIPS, B. Vet. Med., D.E.S.T.S., Cert E.P., Cert. E.D., D.E.C.V.S., M.R.C.V.S.

The Equine Veterinary Hospital, Liphook, England.

Infection of the Digital Flexor Tendon Sheath

PETER W. PHYSICK-SHEARD, B.V.Sc., M.Sc., F.R.C.V.S.

Associate Professor, Large Animal Medicine and Equine Health Management, Departments of Clinical Studies and Population Medicine, and Clinician, Large Animal Division, Veterinary Teaching Hospital, Ontario Veterinary College, University of Guelph, Guelph, Ontario, Canada.

Diagnostic Techniques in Equine Cardiology

ROB PILSWORTH, M.A., Vet. M.B., B.Sc., Cert. V.R., M.R.C.V.S.

Partner, Rossdale and Partners, Beaufort Cottage Stables, Newmarket, Suffolk, England.

Stress Fractures

R. SCOTT PIRIE, B.V.M. & S., Cert. E.P., Cert. E.M.V.

Lecturer in Equine Medicine, Royal (Dick) School of Veterinary Studies, University of Edinburgh, Easter Bush, Roslin, Midlothian, Scotland.

Neoplasia of the Mouth and Surrounding Structures

DAVID PLATT, B.V.Sc., Ph.D., C.V.R., D.E.O., F.R.C.V.S., R.C.V.S., Dipl. Equine Surgery

Lecturerer in Equine Surgery, Royal Veterinary College, University of London, North Mymms, Hatfield, Hertfordshire, England.

Carpal Canal Syndrome

R. SCOTT PLEASANT, D.V.M., M.S., Dipl. A.C.V.S.

Assistant Professor, Department of Large Animal Clinical Sciences, Virginia-Maryland Regional College of Veterinary Medicine, Virginia Tech and University of Maryland, Blacksburg, Virginia.

Interpretation of Local Analgesic Techniques in the Foot Region; Proximal and Distal Interphalangeal Joint Pain

KONSTANZE H. PLUMLEE, D.V.M., M.S.

Diagnostic Toxicologist, California Veterinary Diagnostic Laboratory System, School of Veterinary Medicine, University of California at Davis, Davis, California.

Mycotoxins

JOHN F. PRESCOTT, M.A., Vet. M.B., Ph.D.

Professor, Department of Pathobiology, Ontario Veterinary College, University of Guelph, Guelph, Ontario, Canada.

Antimicrobial Drug Selection for Lower Airway Infection

JOHN K. PRINGLE, D.V.M., D.V.Sc.

Associate Professor, Large Animal Medicine, Atlantic Veterinary College, University of Prince Edward Island, Charlottetown, Prince Edward Island, Canada.

Congenital Disorders of the Urinary Tract; Miscellaneous Disorders of the Urinary Tract

MERL F. RAISBECK, D.V.M., M.S., Ph.D.

Professor of Veterinary Toxicology, Department of Veterinary Sciences, University of Wyoming, Laramie, Wyoming.

Feed-Associated Poisoning; Fescue Toxicosis

JOHN REAGOR, Ph.D.

Head, Toxicology Department, Texas Veterinary Medical Diagnostic Laboratory, Texas A&M University, College Station, Texas.

Toxic Plants

VIRGINIA B. REEF, D.V.M., Dipl. A.C.V.I.M.

Professor of Medicine in the George D. Widener Hospital, and Director of Large Animal Cardiology and Ultrasonography, New Bolton Center, School of Veterinary Medicine, University of Pennsylvania, Kennett Square, Pennsylvania.

Electrocardiography and Echocardiography in the Exercising Horse

JILL D. RICHARDSON, M.A., M.Sc., Vet. M.B., C.V.R., F.R.C.V.S.

Assistant in Practice, Endell Veterinary Group, Salisbury, Wiltshire, England.

Aging of the Horse by Dentition

CHRISTOPHER M. RIGGS, B.Sc., B.V.Sc., Ph.D., Cert. E.O., M.R.C.V.S.

Lecturer in Equine Orthopaedics, Division of Equine Studies, Faculty of Veterinary Science, University of Liverpool, Leahurst, Neston, South Wirral, England.

Implications of Bone Adaptation in the Thoroughbred Racehorse

N. EDWARD ROBINSON, B. Vet. Med., Ph.D., M.R.C.V.S.

Matilda R. Wilson Professor, Department of Large Animal Clinical Sciences, College of Veterinary Medicine, Michigan State University, East Lansing, Michigan.

Requirements for Interstate Shipment of Horses; Appendix 1: Table of Drugs: Approximate Doses

JOSE M. ROMERO, Licenciado En Veterinara

Major, Spanish Army, Madrid, Spain.

The Diffusely Filled Limb

ELIZABETH M. SANTSCHI, D.V.M.

Assistant Professor of Large Animal Surgery, College of Veterinary Medicine, University of Minnesota, St. Paul, Minnesota.

Prepartum Conditions

JOHN W. SCHLIPF, Jr., D.V.M., M.S.

Equine Internist, Equine Services Surgical Hospital, Simpsonville, Kentucky.

Dermatologic Conditions Associated With Crusts and Scales

L. MICHAEL SCHMALL, D.V.M., M.S.

Associate Professor Department of Veterinary Clinical Sciences, College of Veterinary Medicine, The Ohio State University, Columbus, Ohio.

Fluid and Electrolyte Therapy; Immunizations

DAVID A. SCHNEIDER, D.V.M.

Resident, Large Animal Medicine, and Graduate Student, Physiology and Pharmacology, Department of Large Animal Medicine, College of Veterinary Medicine, University of Georgia, Athens, Georgia.

Lymphoproliferative and Myeloproliferative Disorders

HAROLD C. SCHOTT II, D.V.M., Ph.D.

Assistant Professor, Department of Large Animal Clinical Sciences, Michigan State University, East Lansing, Michigan.

Chronic Renal Failure; Congenital Disorders of the Urinary Tract; Miscellaneous Disorders of the Urinary Tract; Dysuria; Hematuria

JOHN SCHUMACHER, D.V.M., M.S.

Professor, Department of Large Animal Medicine and Surgery, College of Veterinary Medicine, Auburn University, Auburn, Alabama.

Pythiosis

HOWARD J. SEEHERMAN, Ph.D., V.M.D.

Assistant Professor, Large Animal Section, School of Veterinary Medicine, Tufts University, North Grafton, Massachusetts. Senior Scientist, Genetics Institute, Andover, Massachusetts.

Left Recurrent Laryngeal Neuropathy

DEBRA C. SELLON, D.V.M., Ph.D.

Assistant Professor of Equine Medicine, College of Veterinary Medicine, North Carolina State University, Raleigh, North Carolina.

Hemolytic Anemia

MIKE SHEPHERD, B.V.Sc., M.R.C.V.S.

Assistant, Rossdale and Partners, Beaufort Cottage Stables, Newmarket, Suffolk, England.

Stress Fractures

PAUL SIROIS, M.S.

Forage Laboratory Manager, North East Dairy Herd Improvement Association, Ithaca, New York.

Feeds and Feeding in the Northeastern United States

ROGER K. W. SMITH, M.A., Vet. M.S., Cert. E.O., M.R.C.V.S.

Lecturer in Equine Surgery, Department of Farm Animal and Equine Medicine and Surgery, The Royal Veterinary College, University of London, London, England.

Soft Tissue Injuries of the Pastern

BRUCE A. SOMERVILLE, D.M.V.

Resident, Large Animal Medicine, Equine Emphasis, School of Veterinary Medicine, University of California at Davis, Davis, California.

Subcutaneous Abscesses Caused by Corynebacterium pseudotuberculosis

MICHAEL S. SPENSLEY

Manager of Clinical Development, Solvay Animal Health, Inc., Mendota Heights, Minnesota.

Dystocia; Retained Fetal Membranes

SHARON J. SPIER, D.V.M., Ph.D., Dipl. A.C.V.I.M.

Assistant Professor, Department of Medicine and Epidemiology, School of Veterinary Medicine, University of California at Davis, Davis, California.

Subcutaneous Abscesses Caused by Corynebacterium pseudotuberculosis

BERNHARD M. SPIESS, Dr. Med. Vet., Dr. Habil.

Associate Professor of Veterinary and Comparative Ophthalmology, Department of Surgery, School of Veterinary Medicine, Zurich, Switzerland.

Equine Recurrent Uveitis

CORINNE R. SWEENEY, D.V.M.

Associate Professor of Medicine, New Bolton Center, School of Veterinary Medicine, University of Pennsylvania, Kennett Square, Pennsylvania.

Fungal Diseases of the Lower Respiratory Tract

FRANK G. R. TAYLOR, B.V.Sc., Ph.D., M.R.C.V.S.

Senior Lecturer in Equine Medicine, Department of Clinical Veterinary Science, School of Veterinary Science, University of Bristol, Langford, North Somerset, England.

Differential Diagnosis of Dependent Edema

ALAIN P. THÉON, Doct. Vét., M.S.

Associate Professor, Department of Surgical and Radiological Sciences, School of Veterinary Medicine, University of California at Davis, Davis, California.

Cisplatin Treatment for Cutaneous Tumors

J. MATTHEW J. TONG, B.V.Sc., M.R.C.V.S.

Fellowes Farm Equine Clinic, Abbots Ripton, Huntingdon, England.

Laceration or Rupture of the Digital Flexor Tendons

W. HENRY TREMAINE, B. Vet. Med., Cert. E.S.

Resident in Large Animal Surgery, Royal (Dick) School of Veterinary Studies, University of Edinburgh, Easter Bush, Roslin, Midlothian, Scotland.

Neoplasia of the Mouth and Surrounding Structures

MATS H. T. TROEDSSON, D.V.M., Ph.D.

Assistant Professor, Department of Clinical and Population Sciences, College of Veterinary Medicine, University of Minnesota, St. Paul, Minnesota.

Breeding Soundness Examination of the Mare; Diseases of the External Genitalia; Dystocia; Retained Fetal Membranes; Abortion; Diseases of the Ovary; Diseases of the Uterus

ERIC TULLENERS, D.V.M., Dipl. A.C.V.S.

Lawrence Baker Sheppard Associate Professor of Surgery, New Bolton Center, School of Veterinary Medicine, University of Pennsylvania, Kennett Square, Pennsylvania.

Epiglottitis; Soft Palate Ulceration

DICKSON D. VARNER, D.V.M., M.S., Dipl. A.C.T.

Associate Professor, Department of Large Animal Medicine and Surgery, College of Veterinary Medicine, Texas A&M University, College Station, Texas.

Care of Stallion Semen

NICHOLAS J. VATISTAS, D.V.M., Dipl. A.C.V.S.

Lecturer, Department of Surgical and Radiological Sciences, School of Veterinary Medicine, University of California at Davis, Davis, California.

Biceps Brachii Tendinitis and Bicipital (Intertubercular) Bursitis; Soft Tissue Swelling on the Dorsal Aspect of the Carpus

LAURENT VIEL, D.V.M., M.Sc. Ph.D.

Associate Professor, Department of Clinical Studies, Ontario Veterinary College, University of Guelph, Guelph, Ontario, Canada.

Lower Airway Inflammation in Young Performance Horses

SALLY VIVRETTE, D.V.M., Ph.D.

Assistant Professor, Food Animal and Equine Medicine, School of Veterinary Medicine, North Carolina State University, Raleigh, North Carolina.

Parturition and Postpartum Complications

ANDRÉ VRINS, D.M.V.

Equine Internal Medicine, Faculté de Médecine Vétérinaire, Université de Montréal, St.-Hyacinthe, Québec, Canada.

Equine Interstitial Pneumonia

ROBERT D. WALKER, M.S., Ph.D.

Professor, Department of Microbiology, and Section Chief, Bacteriology/Mycology Section, College of Veterinary Medicine, Michigan State University, East Lansing, Michigan.

New Perspectives on Antimicrobial Chemotherapy

JOHN P. WALMSLEY, M.A., Vet. M.B., Cert. E.O., Dipl. E.C.V.S., M.R.C.V.S.

Senior Partner, Walmsley, Mantell, Summerhays, Duncan & Phillips, The Equine Veterinary Hospital, Liphook, Hampshire, England.

Cruciate, Meniscal, and Meniscal Ligamental Injuries; Injuries to the Lips and Mouth

BARBARA J. WATROUS, D.V.M., Dipl. A.C.V.R.

Professor of Radiology, College of Veterinary Medicine, Oregon State University, Corvallis, Oregon.

Temporohyoid Osteoarthropathy (Middle Ear Disease)

JOHANNA L. WATSON, D.V.M., Ph.D.

Lecturer, Department of Medicine and Epidemiology, School of Veterinary Medicine, University of California at Davis, Davis, California.

Summer Pasture–Associated Obstructive Pulmonary Disease

PETER M. WEBBON, B. Vet. Med., D.V.R., Ph.D., M.R.C.V.S.

Senior Lecturer in Equine Medicine, Department of Farm Animal and Equine Medicine and Surgery, The Royal Veterinary College, University of London, London, England.

Soft Tissue Injuries of the Pastern

NATHANIEL A. WHITE II, D.V.M., M.S.

Theodora Ayer Randolph Professor of Surgery, Marion duPont Scott Equine Medical Center, Virginia-Maryland Regional College of Veterinary Medicine, Virginia Tech and University of Maryland, Blacksburg, Virginia.

Risk Factors Associated With Colic

DAVID L. WILLIAMS, M.A., Vet. M.B., Cert. V. Ophthal., Ph.D., M.R.C.V.S.

Research Ophthalmologist, Animal Health Trust, Newmarket, Suffolk, England.

Ocular Pharmacology and Therapeutics

M. AMY WILLIAMS, D.V.M., M.S., Dipl. A.B.V.P., Dipl. A.C.V.I.M.

Associate Professor, Department of Large Animal Surgery and Medicine, College of Veterinary Medicine, Auburn University, Auburn, Alabama.

Papillomatosis: Warts and Aural Plaques

LISA WILLIAMSON, M.S., D.V.M., Dipl. A.C.V.I.M.

Assistant Professor, Large Animal Medicine Department, University of Georgia College of Veterinary Medicine, Athens, Georgia.

Medical Management of Eventing Horses

DAVID G. WILSON, D.V.M.

Clinical Associate Professor, Department of Surgical Sciences, and Chief of Staff, Large Animal Services, Veterinary Medical Teaching Hospital, School of Veterinary Medicine, University of Wisconsin at Madison, Madison, Wisconsin.

Equine Canker

W. DAVID WILSON, B.V.M.S., M.S., M.R.C.V.S.

Professor, Department of Medicine and Epidemiology, and Director, Center for Equine Health and Performance, School of Veterinary Medicine, University of California at Davis, Davis, California.

Foal Pneumonia; Bronchointerstitial Pneumonia and Acute Respiratory Distress

LEILA WORTH, V.M.D., Ph.D.

New Bolton Center, School of Veterinary Medicine, University of Pennsylvania, Kennett Square, Pennsylvania.

Aortoiliacofemoral Thrombosis

ANTHONY A. YU, B.Sc., D.V.M., M.S.

Veterinary Dermatologist and Owner, Animal Allergy and Skin Clinic of Oregon, Portland, Oregon.

Dermatologic Conditions Associated With Abnormal Pigmentation

Current Therapy in Equine Medicine

PREFACE

Preparing a new edition of *Current Therapy in Equine Medicine* every 4 to 5 years provides me with an opportunity to review the recent advances in equine practice. Past editions of this book have described improvements in the diagnosis and treatment of colic, the advances in neonatal medicine, and the developing specialty of sports medicine. The big advance that has changed equine medicine over the past 5 years is the increasing availability to the practicing veterinarian of equipment for diagnostic imaging. This technology is being used on almost all organ systems but particularly on the reproductive, musculoskeletal, and cardiovascular systems.

This edition follows the same format as for earlier editions. The book is designed to be a handy reference for the busy equine practitioner and the general large animal veterinarian who treats horses. The book generally assumes that a tentative diagnosis has been made and therefore provides information on tests to confirm the diagnosis and on therapy. The latter is emphasized, so that the practitioner will find details of equipment, dosages, and treatment schedules. Each edition of *Current Therapy in Equine Medicine* emphasizes different material, and the reader should refer therefore to earlier editions either if a topic is not covered in this book or for the opinion of a different clinician.

Current Therapy in Equine Medicine 4 includes a greatly expanded section on musculoskeletal problems that can be treated medically, a new section on the mouth, and expanded sections on foal, urinary, and respiratory diseases. As in past editions, editors who are specialists suggested content of sections, selected authors, and reviewed manuscripts for the accuracy of information. To these editors and to the authors, I offer my sincerest thanks. They worked on and adhered to short deadlines so that a short production time ensured that the book offers the latest information. I also want to thank Victoria and Thoralf Hoelzer-Maddox, who tracked the flow of manuscripts, checked references, and assisted with proofing; Cathy Carroll and the staff of W.B. Saunders Co., who produced the text with their usual attention to quality; and my family, who accept the evening hours that I spend editing and proofing.

It is always gratifying to hear that practitioners appreciate the practical nature of this book. I hope that you will find *Current Therapy in Equine Medicine 4* as useful as earlier editions.

N. EDWARD ROBINSON

Current Therapy in Equine Medicine

NOTICE

Equine medicine practice is an ever-changing field. Standard safety precautions must be followed, but as new research and clinical experience grow, changes in treatment and drug therapy become necessary or appropriate. The authors and editors of this work have carefully checked the generic and trade drug names and verified drug dosages to ensure that dosage information is precise and in accord with standards accepted at the time of publication. Readers are advised, however, to check the product information currently provided by the manufacturer of each drug to be administered to be certain that changes have not been made in the recommended dose or in the contraindications for administration. This is of particular importance in regard to new or infrequently used drugs. Recommended dosages for animals are sometimes based on adjustments in the dosages that would be suitable for humans. Some of the drugs mentioned here have been given experimentally by the authors. Others have been used in dosages greater than those recommended by the manufacturer. In these kinds of cases, the authors have reported on their own considerable experience. It is the responsibility of those administering a drug, relying on their professional skill and experience, to determine the dosages, the best treatment for the patient, and whether the benefits of giving a drug justify the attendant risk. The editors cannot be responsible for misuse or misapplication of the material in this work.

THE PUBLISHER

Current Therapy in Equine Medicine

CONTENTS

Section 2   THE MOUTH
Edited by Graham Munroe

Section 3   THE GASTROINTESTINAL SYSTEM
Edited by Michael J. Murray

Section 4   THE CARDIOVASCULAR SYSTEM
Edited by Mark W. Patteson

Section 9   THE RESPIRATORY SYSTEM
Edited by Jean-Pierre Lavoie

Section 10   THE URINARY SYSTEM
Edited by Harold C. Schott II

THE MUSCULOSKELETAL SYSTEM

Edited by Sue J. Dyson

Problems Associated With the Neck: Neck Pain and Stiffness, Abnormal Posture, and Forelimb Gait Abnormalities

SUE J. DYSON
Newmarket, England

The purpose of this section is to discuss abnormal neck shape, abnormalities of neck posture observed when the horse is either at rest or moving, pain and stiffness of the neck, and forelimb lameness associated with primary abnormalities of the neck. Neurologic conditions associated with compression of the cervical spinal cord are not considered unless they are transient and are the result of acute trauma of the neck.

Head and neck carriage depend in part on conformation, such as the way the neck "comes out" of the shoulder, and the shape of the neck, the latter also being influenced by the way in which the horse works. If a horse carries its head and neck high with the head somewhat extended, the ventral "strap" muscles tend to be overdeveloped, resulting in a ewe-neck conformation. Many horses turn more easily to the right than to the left, or vice versa, and the muscles on the side of the neck, especially dorsocranially, develop asymmetrically. This is particularly obvious if the neck is viewed from above. If a horse is excessively thin, the cervical vertebrae become prominent and the caudal dorsal neck region becomes dorsally concave. In a fit, well-muscled horse this region is dorsally convex, especially if the horse works regularly "on the bit" (i.e., with the poll flexed so that the front of the head is approximately vertical). Most stallions have a prominent dorsal convexity to the neck region, resulting in a "cresty" appearance. An excessively fat horse may have adipose deposits throughout the body, including the neck region, and these can be misinterpreted as abnormal neck swellings.

CLINICAL EXAMINATION

When a horse is presented with an abnormal neck or head posture, the entire horse should be clinically evaluated because signs of posture abnormalities may reflect a primary lesion elsewhere. Abnormal neck or head posture may be associated with vestibular disease, fracture of the dorsal spinous processes of the cranial thoracic vertebrae, mediastinal or cranial thoracic abscess, or a systemic disease such as tetanus. Detailed examination of the neck should include:

1. Assessment of neck conformation, shape and posture at rest and of the position of the head relative to the neck and trunk

2. Examination for patchy sweating, suggestive of local nerve damage

3. Simultaneous palpation of the left and right sides of the neck to assess symmetry and the presence of abnormal

1

swellings or depressions, and to identify muscle pain, abnormal tenseness, or fasciculation

4. Independent deep palpation of the left and right sides of the neck to identify pain

5. Assessment of lateral and dorsoventral neck flexibility. It is helpful to hold a bowl of food by each shoulder of the horse in turn to assess lateral flexibility. Observing the horse graze is useful to assess ventral mobility of the neck.

6. Assessment of the consistency and patency of the jugular veins

7. Assessment of skin sensation and local reflexes such as the cervicofacial reflex and the thoracolaryngeal reflex

8. Observation of the moving horse to assess neck posture and the presence of either lameness or gait abnormalities of neurologic origin. Forelimb lameness is occasionally associated with a primary cervical lesion, usually but not invariably together with other clinical signs referable to the neck.

Additional diagnostic tests include radiography, nuclear scintigraphy, ultrasonography, hematology and serum biochemistry, tuberculosis testing, measurement of *Brucella* titers, and bone biopsy.

OCCIPITOATLANTOAXIAL MALFORMATION

Occipitoatlantoaxial malformation (OAAM) is the most common congenital abnormality of the cervical vertebrae. It is a congenital abnormality of any breed, but it appears to be heritable in Arabs. Clinical signs are usually recognized within the first few months of life and include an abnormal neck shape in the poll region, with prominence of either the left or right side and/or scoliosis, which is best appreciated when the neck is viewed from above. The head and neck may appear unusually extended. Soft tissue swelling or detectable pain is unusual. Movement of the poll region may be abnormally limited, and audible clicks may or may not be noted as the neck moves. The gait should be assessed for neurologic abnormalities, the result of compression of the spinal cord, which merit a hopeless prognosis. However, in many cases of OAAM there are no associated neurologic signs. Diagnosis is confirmed by radiography. Both lateral and ventrodorsal views should be obtained to gain maximal information about the bony abnormalities, which may include fusion of the atlas to the occiput, atlantoaxial luxation, and abnormal shapes of both the atlas and axis, frequently asymmetrical.

There is no treatment. Prognosis for athletic function is determined by the degree of neck stiffness. Because of the heritable nature of this condition in Arabs, breeding of affected horses is inadvisable.

OTHER CONGENITAL ABNORMALITIES

Congenital torticollis is seen occasionally resulting from malformation of more caudal cervical vertebrae. Acquired torticollis is comparatively rare. Vertebral body fusion is usually seen in association with a meningomyelocoele, resulting in neurologic abnormalities.

SUBLUXATION OF THE FIRST AND SECOND CERVICAL VERTEBRAE

Subluxation of the first and second cervical vertebrae is unusual and is associated with damage to the ventral longitudinal ligaments between the two vertebrae or occurs as a consequence of a fracture of the odontoid peg or dens. No breed or gender predilection exists. It is likely that trauma is the underlying cause, although there may be no recent history of such.

An affected horse usually presents with a stiff neck and a tendency for the head and neck to be somewhat extended. It may be difficult to differentiate between neck pain and stiffness. An audible clicking may emanate from the region and, occasionally, abnormal movement between the vertebrae can be appreciated. Because of the relatively wide sagittal diameter of the vertebral canal at the affected site, compression of the cervical spinal cord and ataxia are rare. If neurologic gait abnormalities are present, they are frequently associated with displacement of the fractured odontoid peg.

Diagnosis is based on radiographic examination using lateral views in both natural (neutral) and extended positions. Radiologic abnormalities may include:

1. Abnormal position of the odontoid peg, resulting in narrowing of the space between it and the dorsal lamina of the vertebral arch of the first cervical vertebra. In a study of yearling Thoroughbreds, the mean minimum sagittal diameter was 34 mm, and the least was 26 mm.

2. Abnormal orientation of the first two cervical vertebrae

3. Abnormal shape of the odontoid peg because of secondary new bone formation

4. Alteration in the shape of the facet joints between the first two cervical vertebrae

5. Narrowing of the distance between the vertebral arches of the first two cervical vertebrae in the extended but not in the neutral positions

6. Fracture of the odontoid peg.

Fractures of the odontoid peg in foals have been successfully treated by surgical stabilization, although there is a dearth of long-term follow-up information. No reports of treatment of subluxation are available in adult horses. The prognosis for return to full athletic function with conservative management is poor.

FRACTURES OF THE CERVICAL VERTEBRAE

Fractures of the cervical vertebrae are usually the result of trauma, from the horse rearing up and falling over backwards or sideways, the horse pulling back when tied, or a fall sustained while jumping, especially at speed. Consequently, clinical signs are generally sudden in onset and include holding the neck in an abnormally low and extended position, neck stiffness, a focal or more diffuse area of pain, with or without localized or more diffuse soft tissue swelling, and muscle guarding. Crepitus is sometimes audible and palpable. The horse may be unable to lower its head to the ground or may do so by pronounced straddling of the forelimbs. Hindlimb and forelimb ataxia may be present, which can be either transient and self-resolving or persistent. Patchy sweating and localized muscle atrophy may develop. Occasionally there is unilateral or bilateral forelimb lameness.

Diagnosis is confirmed by radiographic examination. Most fractures are detectable in lateral projections, although ventrodorsal views may give additional information about the extent of the fracture, especially those involving the atlas and axis. Recognizing that multiple fractures may occur concurrently, radiographs must be interpreted with care, and physes and separate centers of ossification must be carefully distinguished from fractures. Soft tissue mineralization dorsal to the atlas, caudal to the occiput, is sometimes seen as a radiologic abnormality in the absence of clinical signs and therefore may be an incidental abnormality of no clinical significance.

The prognosis depends on the site and configuration of the fracture, the degree of displacement, and the likelihood of permanent compression of the spinal cord, either by a displaced fracture or by subsequent callus formation. The latter may be difficult to predict in the acute stage.

Fractures of the first two cervical vertebrae, especially through the physis between the center of ossification of the odontoid and the body of the axis, are particularly common in young foals. Provided that there is no evidence of ataxia, the prognosis for complete recovery is fair. Usually no treatment is required other than confinement to a small stall. If ataxia persists for more than a few days without improvement, the prognosis is guarded and surgical stabilization could be considered.

Fractures of the cervical vertebrae of adults commonly involve the body or arch of the midcervical vertebrae (C3 to C6), or the facet joints of the caudal cervical vertebrae (C5 to C7). Associated ataxia due to local hemorrhage and edema usually resolves within several days; persistence of ataxia is a poor prognostic indicator. Most fractures heal by formation of a callus that may subsequently impinge on the spinal cord, resulting in ataxia. Fracture of a vertebral body may also damage the adjacent intervertebral disk and associated ligaments, resulting in disc protrusion into the vertebral canal, compression of the spinal cord, and ataxia.

Many fractures of the cervical vertebral bodies and of the synovial articular facet joints heal spontaneously, at least by fibrous union. Horses may be able to return to athletic function, albeit with some degree of neck stiffness. In the acute stage the horse should be confined to a stall. Although analgesics may be necessary to control severe pain, they should be used judiciously or the horse may move its neck excessively. The position of the manger and water bucket should be adjusted so that the horse can eat and drink from normal head height. Preferably, the hay should be fed loose at head height. If a haynet is used, hay should be well shaken out, not packed tightly, and the holes of the net should be large to allow easy extraction of hay. The haynet should be hung at head height. The horse should not be tied up during the convalescent period in case it pulls back. It is helpful to reappraise the horse clinically and radiographically at 6- to 8-week intervals to assess progress. Maximal clinical improvement is often not apparent until 6 to 9 months after the injury.

MYELOMA

Myeloma is a myeloproliferative disorder that can cause pain and radiolucent lesions in any bone. Myeloma involving the cervical vertebrae has been observed in horses of a wide range of ages and breeds. Clinical signs include intermittent fever of unknown origin, severe neck pain and stiffness, intermittent forelimb lameness variable in degree, weight loss, and in some cases a variety of other abnormalities. Diagnosis is based on hematology testing, radiography, and bone biopsy results. Hematologic abnormalities include anemia, leukocytosis, neutrophilia, and lymphocytosis. Total protein concentration is markedly elevated. Protein electrophoresis shows a monoclonal peak in the gamma region. Radiographic evaluation of affected bones reveals clearly demarcated lucent zones, usually without a sclerotic rim. Bone biopsy is useful to confirm the diagnosis. There is no treatment and the prognosis is hopeless.

VERTEBRAL OSTEOMYELITIS

Cervical vertebral osteomyelitis usually occurs as a consequence of a systemic disease such as *Rhodococcus equi* infection in foals, *Streptococcus equi* infection (strangles), tuberculosis, or brucellosis. Clinical signs may include intermittent pyrexia, neck stiffness and pain, an abnormal head and neck position, and weight loss with or without a depressed appetite. Generally, leukocytosis, neutrophilia, and hyperfibrinogenemia are present. Radiographic examination of the cervical vertebrae may reveal focal radiolucent zones of varying size, sometimes with surrounding sclerosis, in one or more vertebrae. Other diagnostic tests that may be helpful include bone biopsy, tuberculosis skin testing, and measurement of *Brucella* titers. Aggressive appropriate antimicrobial therapy may result in some amelioration of clinical signs, but the prognosis must be guarded.

OTHER LUCENT ZONES IN THE CERVICAL VERTEBRAE

Occasionally single or multiple well-circumscribed radiolucent areas are identified in one or more adjacent cervical vertebrae associated with profound neck pain, with or without forelimb lameness. Clinical signs are usually acute in onset. These lesions have not been proved as the result of either osteomyelitis or myeloma. A definitive diagnosis can only be reached by either bone biopsy or postmortem evaluation, and although obvious lesions may be found, their etiology may remain unknown.

(approximately 1 L) to dilute the irritant drug, combined with local anesthetic (e.g., mepivacaine 2%, 10 to 20 ml, without epinephrine) to reduce pain. Periodic hot packing seems to help relieve the clinical signs. Generally, no further treatment is required. If initially untreated, and local tissue necrosis supervenes, skin slough is almost inevitable. Consideration should be given to systemic prophylactic antimicrobial therapy.

Supplemental Readings

Butler JA, Colles CM, Dyson SJ, Kold SF, Poulos PW: The spine. *In* Clinical Radiology of the Horse, ed 1. Oxford, Blackwell Scientific Publications, 1993, pp 355–398.
Ricardi G, Dyson SJ: Forelimb lameness associated with radiographic abnormalities of the cervical vertebrae. Equine Vet J 25:422–426, 1993.
Whitwell KE, Dyson S: Interpreting radiographs 8: Equine cervical vertebrae. Equine Vet J 19:8–14, 1987.

Back Pain

DAN MARKS
Santa Fe, New Mexico

For the purposes of this chapter, back pain is regarded as either primary spinal pain (i.e., related to the thoracolumbar vertebrae and their associated ligaments) or primary soft tissue pain from the skin or epaxial muscles. Pain emanating from the sacroiliac region is also addressed. Neurologic conditions such as spinal cord or nerve root compression frequently seen in humans are not a part of the syndrome in horses and are not considered here. The underlying origin of the problem must be resolved to effect a requisite result; therefore, an accurate diagnosis is essential. Therapy usually requires a combination of medical treatment and management. Throughout the text the first thoracic vertebra to the sixth lumbar vertebra are referred to as T1 to L6.

RECOGNITION

The initial diagnostic step is the recognition that a painful back problem exists. When the pain is severe, this is obvious. In more subtle cases, it is only of significance at the extremes of athletic performance, such as when jumping, when racing, or with extreme collection, and may not affect ordinary gaits. There may be coexisting lameness. This makes recognition dependent upon a careful history, examination, and response to therapy. The veterinarian's familiarity with the particular sport is often quite helpful. Because poor riding technique can also induce back pain, cooperation with a skilled, sensitive rider can be helpful.

HISTORY

Some back problems are manifested after overexertion, a fall, or being cast, but most develop insidiously with no specific traumatic incident. The majority of horses are presented with a complaint of loss of performance that developed gradually and is accentuated by increased stress. Frequently, there is a change in behavior, evidenced by discomfort from grooming or being "scraped off" over the back, saddling, or even being blanketed. Additional discomfort is apparent when the horse is urinating, holding the hind legs up for the farrier, being mounted ("coldback"), or getting up from recumbency. The horse may show reluctance to lie down, or one that previously enjoyed rolling may no longer roll. The horse can undergo a personality change, appear unhappy in the stall, and resent being caught. An astute horseman probably suspects a back problem. When ridden, the horse may be "nappy," may grind its teeth, continually look back, ring its tail or carry it to one side, kick out, or sulk to signify discomfort. The horse assumes a constrained carriage with its head and neck elevated, and the hind legs do not engage under the horse. A sensitive rider can feel a loss of elasticity; the back feels stiff, and there is a lack of propulsive thrust.

If changing the saddle or adding pads improves the performance, back soreness of some type is likely. The source may simply be a poorly fitting saddle, or pain may be related to the thoracolumbar spine.

Bearing in mind that back pain frequently coexists with bilateral hindlimb lameness, the anamnesis should be directed toward any response to intra-articular medication or systemic nonsteroidal anti-inflammatory drugs (NSAIDs). Phenylbutazone and flunixin are generally much more effective for joint or foot problems than for thoracolumbar pain.

More back problems exist in racehorses than is generally recognized. Affected horses tend to be slow out of the starting gate, are unable to fully extend their stride, and experience inordinate fatigue. Dirt tracks that break away from the propulsive forces of the hind legs (cuppy) and especially overly dry wood-chip tracks accentuate the problem and can, by themselves, cause epaxial and gluteal myositis. Usually affected horses race better on the flat than over fences. If horses are trained with a heart rate monitor, the rider may notice an elevated heart rate, which is merely a reflection of pain.

Because of the exactitude of dressage and the necessity for bilateral symmetry, back pain is especially deleterious to performance. Dressage horses experience difficulty with increasing collection. The swing or undulation of the back, which is necessary for all correct movements, is lost. Transitions tend to be rough. Lateral movements such as zigzag half pass at the trot may show irregularity. A tendency to run off in the extended canter may be apparent. With slow, progressive, classical training, the likelihood of back problems is lessened, but accelerated dressage training stresses the back more.

Show jumping seems to be the most severe stressor for the back. Problems are first evidenced by the horse hitting rails behind, especially over oxers. Horses with back pain have difficulty going from extreme ventroflexion of the back at the apogee of the jump to maximal dorsiflexion in the landing ("the hind end doesn't follow through," "loses its bascule," "jumps flat"); some horses trail their hind legs. Frequently there is a loss of propulsive thrust ("feels weak off the ground"). The horse may experience difficulty maintaining impulsion while shortening its stride and, therefore, tight distances to a wide jump are more difficult. Kicking up after a jump or on course can also signify back discomfort. Expressions of anxiety such as rushing or refusing can also occur.

None of these signs is pathognomonic for back pain and all can be caused by other physical problems or simply by unartful riding. Inability to ride effectively such as restricting movement with the hand in an attempt to work the horse on the bit without generating sufficient hindlimb impulsion can produce signs that mimic those of primary back pain. This problem is seen particularly in horses ridden by low-grade dressage riders.

CLINICAL EXAMINATION

Initial observation begins with an appraisal of the horse's conformation and stance. Dorsal spinous impingement occurs more commonly in short-backed horses, whereas long backs incur more supraspinous ligament and lumbar muscle strains. However, this generalization has many exceptions. Although asymmetrical tuber sacrale suggest sacroiliac subluxation or previous pelvic fracture, they may not be a source of discomfort. Disuse atrophy of the longissimus dorsi muscles suggests back pain, whereas that of the trapezius suggests a poorly fitting saddle. Gluteal atrophy is frequent with sacroiliac soreness. Kyphosis ("roach back") may denote back pain, but is usually caused by bilateral stifle soreness, or may be a normal conformational variation. A history of a change in stance is meaningful. Young horses with congenital lordosis ("sway back") frequently suffer back pain in their first 2 or 3 years of training; many of their backs stabilize and are pain free thereafter. Scoliosis can be discerned by viewing the horse from above, and although usually spastic in origin, it may be congenital.

A visual examination of the back and girth path discloses skin lesions such as rubs, ringworm, parasitic lesions, and sarcoids. Eosinophilic nodular dermatoses are the most common cause of round, firm, pain-free, nonpruritic nodules in the skin. The hair over the lesions is normal. Such lesions are frequently located in the saddle or girth region and are from 0.5 to 5 cm across. Because they are asymptomatic, treatment is not usually warranted. When the cosmetic appearance justifies treatment, intralesional triamcinolone (1–3 mg per site) is frequently effective. It is sometimes necessary to repeat the treatment after 2 weeks.

The total dose of triamcinolone at any one treatment should not exceed 18 mg because of the danger of steroid-induced laminitis. There is a tendency for these lesions to return the next summer. Older calcified lesions require surgical excision by unroofing and slightly cratering the nodule.

White hairs usually result from a badly fitting saddle or too tight a roller. If the problem has been corrected, this is of no clinical significance. Hair worn off under the rear of one or both panels may signify a poorly fitting saddle, but with back pain and muscle splinting, even well-fitting saddles rub the hair excessively. This excessive hair loss may be unilateral or bilateral, depending on which muscles tighten.

Palpation of the neck at times reveals secondary soreness. The mouth is examined because dental or biting problems that induce a constrained head carriage can induce or exaggerate back problems. If this is suspected, the horse should be ridden in a hackamore for a week to see if the signs regress.

Palpation of the back begins by gently running the hand over the dorsal midline from the withers to the tail. This reassures and relaxes the horse, which is essential for this examination, and the examiner can detect increased heat, swelling, scars, or bony enlargements. Edema on the midline or over a tuber sacrale is noteworthy. The muscles on both sides are similarly examined by light pressure and then firmer digital pressure. The degree of muscular soreness is evaluated by the change in compliance, the muscle tightening, or the horse's withdrawal from the pressure. The dorsal spines from withers to tail are next palpated using firm digital pressure while moving caudally. Obviously sensitive areas are skipped and palpated last to avoid apprehensive guarding. If the horse has been in work and shows a painful response to palpation on the midline, there is always a soreness of the adjacent epaxial muscles usually beginning about 4 cm caudal to the spinal pain.

With experience, a distinction between normal reflex withdrawal and a painful response is usually possible. Usually, thoracolumbar pain also elicits an associated reaction over the dorsal processes of the sacrum. Cranial thoracic pain causes sensitivity over the cranial sacrum, whereas more caudal thoracic or lumbar pain evinces sensitivity along the caudal sacral midline.

The horse is made to repeatedly cycle its back through utmost flexion (ventroflexion, roaching) and extension (dorsiflexion, dipping) of its spine. Ventroflexion is accomplished by firm digital pressure over the sacrum, or squeezing the tailhead, or by pushing up on the abdomen and dorsiflexion by digital pressure over the longissimus muscles. Signs of back muscle spasm or of resentment, excessive evasion, or an unwillingness to flex and extend probably signify pain from thoracolumbar movement. Much variation occurs in the natural flexibility of the spine between individuals; therefore, range of motion is difficult to judge. Lateral flexibility is evaluated by running a ballpoint pen caudally along each epaxial muscle. If the horse repeatedly cycles its back with no significant discomfort, the likelihood of serious spinal disease is minimal.

A rectal examination is performed if a recent injury suggests a pelvic fracture or psoas muscle strain. Usually rectal examination is not indicated.

The horse is next observed in hand. It is walked in tight circles in both directions to ascertain lateral flexibility and evidence of neurologic signs. It is backed up. The horse is trotted to detect lameness. Flexion and manipulative tests are performed, with particular attention directed to the hocks. Uncomplicated back disease does not elicit a dramatic response to a hock flexion test, and rarely do thoracolumbar problems cause frank lameness, but rather they manifest an unevenness, decreased hind leg protraction, stiffness, and a lack of impulsion. Therefore, conspicuous lameness should be suspected as originating in the limbs and must be thoroughly investigated. Only by eliminating this possibility can the lameness be ascribed to a back problem. Front leg lameness also affects the back by causing an overloading of the back and hind legs, and there have been cases of symmetrical, bilateral, front leg lameness that mimic back soreness (e.g., reluctance to work on the bit). Such causes of back pain are apparent only after desensitizing the lame legs.

Pre- and post-exercise serum creatine phosphokinase levels are evaluated if the history suggests an exertional myopathy. The horse is lunged at the trot and canter, and it is observed for flexibility of the back, smoothness, and impulsion of the gaits. Severe cases of thoracolumbar pain exhibit a rigid back with the neck elevated and the hind legs not engaging ("inverted"). Less painful cases may affect only the carriage under the rider's weight or may not be evident at ordinary gaits at all.

The horse's regular saddle is checked for a broken tree. If several horses on which a certain saddle is used are sore in the same place, the saddle is the likely culprit. The horse is saddled and the fit carefully checked. Some back problems are simply bruising from an ill-fitting saddle, but with any back problem it is important that the fit of the saddle be optimal. The horse's response to saddling and mounting is noted. The horse is then observed at the trot and canter including circles and ideally performing the athletic activity that had been affected. Deterioration of the gaits under the rider's weight is strongly suggestive of back soreness, but because hindlimb problems are often exaggerated by the rider's weight, it is not pathognomonic. Although back pain can cause the horse to cross-canter ("disunited"), this is more likely to be brought about by a hind leg lameness, or in some cases cross-cantering is simply a habit. Having the rider post hard rather than standing in the stirrups often accentuates back pain. Usually the discomfort is reflected in a change in the horse's facial expression, elevation of the neck, and generalized stiffness. If the horse raises its head in time with a posting trot (mimicking a lameness), but not with the rider standing in the stirrups, back pain in the caudal thoracocranial lumbar region is likely. With spinal pain between T7 and T13 there is a restriction of scapular rotation, which can be more apparent at a medium canter than the trot. Because the rider's weight is especially concentrated between T12 and T15, lesions in this region tend to lead to evasions such as sulkiness, rearing, head throwing, and difficulty in backing up. More caudal lesions tend to cause stiffness and a reduced amplitude of hind leg stride. Sometimes only certain movements such as lateral work or a tight canter circle in one direction demonstrate the problem. After riding, the back is again palpated. An increase in reactivity indicates a more serious problem and a poorer prognosis than one that warms out of the sensitivity.

Local anesthesia can be used diagnostically by injecting between the dorsal processes in the palpably painful areas or in those that show radiographic lesions. Seven milliliters of local anesthetic is deposited per site using the technique described later under Impingement of the Dorsal Spinous Processes. The horse is ridden again after 10 minutes. A positive response is a dramatic decrease in signs, although a complete resolution is not always obtained.

The diagnosis of fractures, spondylosis, degenerative joint disease (DJD) of the articular facet joints, dorsal spinous impingement, and avulsion of the dorsal spinous ligament is aided by radiographic examination. Ultrasonography has been used to examine the supraspinous ligament and is well suited if a fracture of the ilium is suspected. Nuclear scintigraphy is helpful for detecting pelvic fractures and some sacroiliac joint disease, and for confirming the significance of subtle radiographic abnormalities (e.g., enlargements and irregularities of outline of an articular facet joint typical of degenerative joint disease). Thermography localizes more superficial lesions, but the large surrounding muscle mass prevents detection of deep heat.

SADDLE BRUISING

A poorly fitted saddle or one with a broken tree can cause bruising of the skin and deeper structures. Because the shape of the back changes as the horse loses weight and gets fitter, a saddle that fit well a few months previously may no longer do so. The panels of an English saddle should be symmetrical and have even contact over a maximal area with no pressure points. Under no circumstances should there be contact with the horse's midline. Some riders position the saddle too far forward, and clinicians can aid the fit by moving the saddle back several centimeters. Western and endurance saddles depend on the tree fitting the back exactly. If the tree is insufficiently curved to conform to the back, it concentrates pressure at the ends, and if too long for the horse, can dig in just behind the scapula. A dry spot under the saddle after riding is indicative of excessive pressure and must be addressed immediately. Swelling and digital sensitivity require careful examination to detect areas where the saddle exerts inordinate pressure. The skin is best evaluated a few hours after removing the saddle, because it is easier to feel the skin when the hair is dry, and it takes some time for edema to become manifest. Chronic pressure can cause hair to turn white. If this is corrected the hair may grow in normally at the next coat change, but with more severe damage to the follicles the color change is permanent. The recent introduction of a computerized saddle pad* to measure pressures holds promise in fitting saddles.

Treatment

The therapy for acute injury includes rest until all sensitivity resolves. Ultrasound therapy is beneficial to reduce the swelling, as are aluminum- or lead acetate–based astringent lotions. The obvious solution is to change or restuff

---

*Equitech, Woodside, CA

the saddle so that the weight of the rider is evenly supported over a maximal area of the horse's back with no pressure points. Using pads is a poorer substitute, and this must be done appropriately. If, for example, the saddle is too narrow and is pinching the withers, adding a pad only exaggerates the problem.

EPAXIAL MUSCLE STRAIN

Myositis of the epaxial muscles is diagnosed by palpable muscle soreness in the absence of dorsal midline sensitivity. The horse may be reluctant to vigorously cycle its back but will do so if gently encouraged. Generally, mild exercise reduces soreness.

If overexertion such as too much work in cuppy going is the cause, the solution is reduced exercise or changing the going. Muscle soreness resulting from spinal pain or hind leg lameness resolves if the primary problem is corrected. When perfect resolution of the primary problem is not feasible, treatment of the ongoing muscle soreness is indicated. Faradic stimulation, moist heat, massage, and especially ultrasound therapy all tend to relieve mild muscle soreness. NSAIDs, especially naproxen (4–8 mg/kg p.o. s.i.d. or b.i.d.) and/or a course of muscle relaxants (e.g., methocarbamol 9.4 mg/kg IV s.i.d. for 3 days), facilitate recovery. Some horses with chronic low-grade myositis benefit from daily oral potassium supplementation (30 g potassium acetate in the feed b.i.d.).

Acute muscle spasm can be relieved by chiropractic manipulation. In addition, the injection of trigger points, by use of a 22-gauge 3.7-cm needle, with 2 to 3 ml of a mixture of five parts of bupivacaine 0.5%* and one part of isoflupredone acetate† 2 mg per ml provides immediate relief. The injection of 2 ml of 2% iodine in oil at multiple sites within the sore muscle, to cause a so-called internal blister, followed by 4 to 6 days of mild exercise effects a profound improvement in most cases.

Exertional rhabdomyolysis ("tying-up") is a separate condition, but it aggravates back problems. Therefore, this too must be addressed (see page 115). If there has been obvious muscle tearing as the result of a fall, the lesion is initially treated with ice and requires at least 5 weeks of rest and a very judicious return to work.

IMPINGEMENT (OVERRIDING) OF THE DORSAL SPINOUS PROCESSES ("KISSING SPINES")

The most common causes of serious spinal pain are impingement of the dorsal processes and strain of the supraspinous and interspinous ligaments. These conditions are most commonly found in jumpers but occur in all horses. It is interesting to note that "kissing spines" have been found in *Equus occidentalis* that lived some 20,000 years before horses were domesticated. Significant pain on palpation of the dorsal midline is typical. If the horse has

been in work, the longissimus muscles are also sensitive to palpation. Edema on the midline suggests damage to the supraspinous ligament. The horse resents continual cycling of its back. Radiographs may support the diagnosis by demonstrating an avulsion by the supraspinous ligament seen as a radiodense thin strip separated from the dorsal surface of the spinous processes or a peaked outline as the result of new bone formation from a healed lesion. Impingement lesions are evidenced by marked sclerotic and lytic changes along the vertical edges of the spinous processes. Cyst-like radiolucencies larger than 5 mm in diameter are especially significant. Because many clinically normal horses have some radiographic changes, only the severe lesions are diagnostically significant. It is also possible to have ligamentous strain with no radiologic findings. Diagnostic ultrasound has been advocated to visualize the supraspinous ligament and surrounding soft tissue, and scintigraphy demonstrates bony activity. Local anesthesia confirms the diagnosis of impinging dorsal spinous processes.

Conventional needle acupuncture, injection of the acupuncture points, or laser stimulation of the points is frequently helpful. The lack of side effects or contraindications recommends acupuncture as an exclusive or adjunctive therapy in most or all cases of chronic back pain. Weekly treatments can take up to 5 to 8 weeks to be effective. The reader is referred to the publication by A. Klide for more details on the procedure. The interval between treatments is then increased or treatment stopped as required. Nonsteroidal anti-inflammatory drugs such as phenylbutazone and flunixin have only limited effect on the spinal pain, but naproxen (4–8 mg/kg p.o. b.i.d.) relieves the associated muscle soreness.

In clinically severe cases, the treatment of choice is interspinous injection of corticosteroids. The painful areas are determined before tranquilizing the horse. The dorsal midline is scrubbed and swabbed with alcohol. Needles (21-gauge 5-cm) are placed on the midline and directed downward between the involved dorsal spines. Making the horse ventroflex its back opens the interspaces and facilitates placement. The needles are inserted to their full depth and 3 to 8 ml of a mixture of one part methylprednisolone acetate* (40 mg/ml), two parts isoflupredone acetate† (2 mg/ml), and three parts serapin‡ is injected while withdrawing the needle. Serapin is an aqueous solution from the pitcher plant (Sarraniaceae). It selectively blocks C fibers carrying pain sensation in peripheral nerves. Infrequently the curvature of the vertebra and the narrow interspace make needle placement impossible. In such cases, the injection is made laterally through the epaxial muscle and the site is located by walking the needle off the process until the interspace is felt. The horse is not ridden for 3 days, but turning out, lunging, or leading the horse from another horse ("ponying") is acceptable. Normal work is then resumed and the back is re-evaluated in 10 to 14 days. An area that is still sensitive may be reinjected. Usually a good clinical response occurs within 10 days, but occasionally it takes up to 3 weeks to see a significant

*Marcaine, Winthrop Pharmaceuticals, New York, NY
†Predef 2X, The Upjohn Company, Kalamazoo, MI

*Depo-Medrol, The Upjohn Company, Kalamazoo, MI
†Predef 2X, The Upjohn Company, Kalamazoo, MI
‡Serapin, High Chemical, Levittown, PA

improvement. This treatment is repeated whenever soreness reappears. Repeated treatments tend to last longer, and many horses require only one or two treatments yearly. This is generally supplemented by acupuncture and occasionally with specific treatment for the epaxial muscle soreness.

Subacute or chronic supraspinous ligament sprain has been successfully treated using daily therapeutic ultrasound at a setting of 0.75 watts/cm^2 for 8 to 15 minutes, depending upon the length of the painful area.

A surgical technique for resection of one or more of the impinging spinous processes was first proposed in 1968. The results on high-level show jumpers have been generally disappointing, but there has been an occasional success. A long convalescence is required. In the author's opinion, surgery is indicated only when all else has failed, the impingement is limited to three processes or fewer, and the signs dramatically improve with local anesthesia.

FRACTURED WITHERS

Fractures of the dorsal spinous processes of T4 to T9 are common as a result of falling over backward. The withers are swollen and sensitive to palpation, and the horse may be reluctant to raise its head and neck. The gait is restricted and the feet are placed on the midline ("base-narrow"). Radiography confirms the diagnosis. However, the normal radiopaque caps (i.e., separate centers of ossification) on these vertebrae should not be mistaken for fractures. Usually these fractures respond well to rest and the horse suffers no long-term athletic impairment. The resulting distortion of the withers may necessitate a specially fitted saddle.

VERTEBRAL BODY FRACTURES

Fractures of the thoracic or lumbar vertebrae are usually a result of a violent fall or of being cast. Compression fractures of the bodies usually occur in the region of T11 to T14 as the result of extreme muscular contraction. They usually cause spinal cord compression with ataxia and sometimes paralysis; euthanasia is required. Compression fractures are occasionally an incidental finding at postmortem examination in cases of electrocution. Fractures of the sacrum have been reported associated with neurologic signs from cauda equina damage.

OTHER VERTEBRAL PROBLEMS

Arthritis of the interneural joints, stress fractures of the vertebral lamina, and ventral spondylosis are diagnoses that can be inferred only clinically and are not easily separated from one another. Usually, performance-limiting back pain is reported. Cycling the back causes discomfort and is sometimes so excruciating that the horse may refuse to bend its back at all. Local anesthesia between the dorsal processes has no effect. Radiography or nuclear scintigraphy is required for diagnosis. Marked spondylosis is charac-

terized radiographically as remodeling and osteophyte formation of the ventral aspect of the vertebral body. It is occasionally seen as an incidental radiographic abnormality. Therefore, nuclear scintigraphy is helpful to confirm the significance of the lesion. Very high quality nuclear scans, preferably obtained under general anesthesia, are also useful to identify abnormalities of the articular facets.

Clinically, mildly affected cases may respond to NSAIDs and a course of acupuncture treatments. More severe cases are not sufficiently responsive, and affected horses should be turned out for 6 to 12 months in hope of a bony union.

SACROILIAC PAIN

Problems in this area have been postulated to result from arthrosis and instability of the sacroiliac joint, desmitis and elongation of the ligaments of this joint, fractures of the ilium, arthrosis of the lumbosacral joint, and strain of the lumbosacral ligaments. Stress fractures of the ilium are usually observed in younger horses doing fast work and occur in the region of the sacroiliac joint. Clinically they are manifested as low-grade lameness with the affected leg being placed close to the midline ("plaiting"). The muscles over the area are tender to palpation. If the fracture becomes complete, severe lameness and pain on pressure over the tubera coxae result. Crepitus is sometimes present. Surprisingly, the acute signs of muscle soreness improve in a few days, and the horse then simply exhibits the gait abnormalities described earlier. The tuber sacrale on the affected side is quite sensitive to downward pressure and can be depressed. This is the opposite of that which is expected with an elongation of the cranial ligaments of the sacroiliac joint. The diagnosis is established ultrasonagraphically by visualizing the ilium. The horse is rested for 3 months. Provided that the fracture does not involve the sacroiliac joint, the prognosis is quite good, even if there is remaining asymmetry of the tubera sacrale. Bilateral fractures, although rare, carry a grave prognosis.

A poorly understood but reasonably well-defined clinical syndrome is characterized by pain elicited when pressure is exerted over the dorsal lumbosacral space and by squeezing lateral to the tubera sacrale. On rare occasions, there is subcutaneous pitting edema over a tuber sacrale. This usually does not cause severe lameness, but is manifested by reduced protraction and sometimes toe dragging of one or both hind legs. This can also be apparent during reining back. In severe cases, the horse may prefer to canter rather than trot. The rider reports a loss of impulsion and, if jumping, difficulty with spread fences ("loss of scope"). Dressage horses experience the leg on the affected side "jumping short" in the one tempi changes. Local anesthesia can aid the diagnosis. A 20-gauge 8.7-cm needle is inserted on the midline between the last lumbar and first sacral vertebra, and 15 ml of local anesthetic is fanned out at 20°. It is directed ventrocaudolaterally toward the affected side. This frequently ameliorates the signs. Administration of NSAIDs decreases the signs, but their continued use may mask a progression. In mild cases, injection of the lumbosacral area as described earlier, but using 20 ml of corticosteroids mixed with serapin remedies the problem. In severe cases, or those unresponsive to initial treatment, the horse should be rested for at least 3 months after all signs have resolved. Attempting to keep the horse in work can lead to a chronic condition that apparently resolves with rest only to return with work. As with thoracolumbar disease, good muscle development and elimination of excessive fatigue are helpful. Acupuncture is indicated for chronic cases. The injection of a sclerosing agent* has been advocated.

Some horses with a history of sacroiliac pain have an exaggerated rolling motion of the pelvis when viewed from behind; this may conceivably be due to excessive laxity of the ligaments supporting the joint.

It has been suggested that a prominent tuber sacrale ("hunter's or jumper's bump") is always pathologic, resulting from muscle atrophy or skeletal damage. However, many clinically normal horses with no history of an associated problem have this "jumper's bump" and perform at a very high level. Furthermore, the condition seems to run in certain blood lines.

COEXISTING HIND-LEG LAMENESS

Many horses with back disease also have coexistent hind-limb lameness, the most common being bilateral arthritis of the distal tarsal joints. Of course, pure back pain can exist without any hind-leg lameness and vice versa. However, a relationship seems to exist between the two in that each can exacerbate the other. If both back pain and hind-leg lameness are prominent, both are treated. If the back pain seems mild compared with the lameness, the latter is treated, and frequently the back pain disappears. The corollary also appears true; the successful treatment of significant back pain with mild coexistent hindlimb lameness can result in resolution of the lameness. In the author's opinion, serious tarsitis is best treated by injecting both distal joints (centrodistal and tarsometatarsal) with corticosteroids, which can be supplemented with hyaluronic acid or polysulfated glycoaminoglycan.†

MISCELLANEOUS

Horses with reduced performance and soreness in the caudal lumbar epaxial muscles and the tongue of the medial gluteal muscle usually benefit from estrone sulfate (0.1 mg/kg IM every 4–14 days as indicated). It is speculated that the action is caused by relaxation of the pelvic ligaments.

Infrequently, ovarian pain just preceding ovulation can cause apparent back pain or signs of low-grade colic. This pain remits after ovulation ends, which can be expedited by administration of chorionic gonadotropin.

MANAGEMENT

Many horses with chronic back problems are athletically useful only if the veterinarian and horseman cooperate in

the horse's management. A stiff rider, riding too long, or doing too much sitting trot on an improperly conditioned horse, or any combination of these can lead to back soreness. Riders who do not sit well may encourage horses with extreme back movement to protect themselves, leading to soreness. These riders must evaluate themselves frankly and minimize the amount of sitting trot and strive to improve their equitation. Overly tight side reins or over-checks can induce back soreness.

A horse with back soreness of acute onset or history of a recent, precipitating, traumatic etiology should be rested until all soreness disappears. The horse should be returned to full work gradually while continually being monitored for recurrence of signs of pain. Most of these horses do not develop any chronic back problems. A significant percentage of chronic back problems also are cured by a protracted rest of 4 to 12 months, and this should be attempted if time permits. However, horses with serious kissing spines usually become pain free with rest, only to relapse with work.

Cold-back takes several forms, ranging from stiffening or dipping the back when mounted to bucking or almost going down behind. Cold-back seems to be related to discomfort from the initial weight of the rider on the back or from the tightening of the girth with pressure on the ventrum. The latter type has at times been responsive to chiropractic manipulation to stretch and relax the deep pectoral muscles. If horses exhibit a cold-back, it may well signify an underlying problem, but some horses that have only a cold-back and no other signs or performance deficit can be managed by lunging before riding or gradually tightening the girth. A strategy that is sometimes effective is to gradually tighten the girth and walk the horse in hand until the girth is one or two holes overtight and then loosen it to normal before mounting.

The rider should be sensitive to the horse's back and allow frequent rest periods during which the horse can relax and stretch its neck. Excessive fatigue should be avoided. Developing the back, gluteal, and abdominal muscles by proper dressage and graduated exercise is very profitable. Weak muscles lead to spasm and pain. The exercise familiar to dressage riders as "long and low" is useful for pre- and post-exercise stretching and strengthening. The horse must be kept very active so that the hind legs really engage and round the back. Proper lunging with a chambon can achieve a similar effect and is very useful for warming up horses with pain between T9 and T13. Ample warm-up is essential. Racehorses benefit from ponying for 30 minutes prior to a race or work, and jumpers can be schooled several hours before competition and then lunged immediately before the class and shown with a minimum of warm-up jumps. The back should be carefully examined after stressful work and the time between competitions influenced by the time the signs resolve. Horse owners must keep the horse's back warm and avoid chills by using adequate blanketing, quarter sheets, infrared heat lamps, and warming liniments before exercise.

The riding surface can play a critical role. Cuppy going, deep mud, or slippery surfaces tend to aggravate back soreness. Horses must have adequate traction devices be-

*P2G, Martindale Pharmaceuticals, Romford, Essex, England
†Adequan, Luipold Pharmaceutical, Shirley, NY

hind to prevent slipping. Racehorses do better on turf than on dirt tracks.

The farrier should avoid radically lowering the hind heels. This in itself can induce back pain. Raising the hind heels 3 to 6° benefits some, but can cause horses to move closer behind and can lead to interfering. It can be worthwhile to experiment with egg bar shoes behind. They prevent the heels from lowering into the ground and extend the ground surface caudally.

Hills exacerbate back problems, and going downhill can cause obvious pain. Hills should be avoided when the back is painful and then used prudently if required for the horse's conditioning. The same applies to bank jumps.

Swimming demands a lordotic posture and usually exacerbates back problems. It should be avoided. Jumping is probably the most stressful athletic endeavor for backs. Downgrading the size of the jumps may, for example, allow a Grand Prix horse to do well in speed or junior competitions. In some cases, a horse may not be capable of competitive dressage or jumping, but is pain free when used for hacking. The veterinarian should try to ensure that the horse is not subjected to an activity causing back pain that may escape the owner's recognition.

CONCLUSION

The recognition, diagnosis, treatment, and management of back pain in horses are in their infancy, but new awareness and imaging techniques are adding to our knowledge. Study and documentation help to develop a more scientific approach. Although many back problems are incurable, a combination of management and therapeutic techniques can enable a high degree of athletic performance from some and a useful, if somewhat athletically limited, career for others.

Supplemental Readings

Harman JC: Practical use of a computerized saddle pressure measuring device to determine the effects of saddle pads on the horse's back. J Equine Vet Sci 14(11):606–611, 1994.

Jeffcott LB: Disorders of the thoracolumbar spine of the horse. A survey of 443 cases. Equine Vet J 12(4):197–210, 1980.

Jeffcott LB, Dalin G, Ekman S, Olsson S-E: Sacroiliac lesions as a cause of chronic poor performance in competitive horses. Equine Vet J 17(2):111–118, 1985.

Klide AM, Benson MB: Methods of stimulating acupuncture points for treatment of chronic back pain in horses. J Am Vet Med Assoc 195:1375–1379, 1989.

Pilsworth RC, Shepherd MC, Herinckx BMB, Holmes MA: Fracture of the wing of the ilium, adjacent to the sacroiliac joint, in Thoroughbred racehorses. Equine Vet J 26(2):94–99, 1994.

Biceps Brachii Tendinitis and Bicipital (Intertubercular) Bursitis

CAROL L. GILLIS
Davis, California

NICHOLAS J. VATISTAS
Davis, California

The soft tissues of the cranial aspect of the shoulder are an infrequent site for equine lameness. Three percent of cases examined by the Large Animal Ultrasound Service of the University of California are diagnosed with biceps brachii tendinitis or bicipital bursitis. The biceps tendon is a dense, short, and predominantly fibrocartilaginous structure palpable over the cranial aspect of the point of the shoulder. The biceps tendon provides attachment for the biceps muscle to the supraglenoid tubercle. A tendinous band of tissue passes through the middle of the biceps muscle and divides distally to insert onto the radial tuberosity, medial collateral ligament of the elbow, and tendon of the extensor carpi radialis. The action of the bicipital tendon is facilitated by the bicipital or intertubercular bursa, which is interposed between the tendon and underlying bicipital groove of the proximal aspect of the humerus. The bicipital bursa in domestic species extends from the groove to the cranial aspect of the bicipital tendon.

CLINICAL SIGNS

Lameness caused by inflammation and damage to or infection of the bicipital tendon and associated bursa is often severe. Athletic horses of all types are affected, including racehorses (Thoroughbreds, Quarterhorses, and Standardbreds), show jumpers, and western competition horses. Causes of noninfectious tendinitis or bursitis include an overuse injury to the tendon, which may include the bursa, or direct trauma to the affected shoulder. The resulting lameness usually responds to rest and stall confinement, only to return once work is resumed. Lameness is pronounced at the trot, with a shortened cranial phase to the stride. Other clinical signs may include resentment of flexion and/or extension of the shoulder and pain on palpation of the affected structure. Effusion into the bicipital bursa is rarely palpable owing to the large brachiocephalicus muscle overlying the biceps brachii tendon and the bursa.

Radiography of the area in a standing horse is generally unrewarding, because only mediolateral and craniomedial-caudolateral oblique radiographs of the proximal aspect of the humerus are possible. Radiographs should, however, be obtained to identify areas of roughening and demineralization on the tubercles of the humerus. A cranioproximal-craniodistal (skyline) projection of the flexed scapulohumeral joint may also be useful, because lesions of the tubercles of the proximal humerus not observed with the standard views may become apparent.

Ultrasonography is the diagnostic method of choice. A 7.5-MHz transducer provides the most detailed image of the area, although occasionally with heavily muscled horses a 5.0-MHz transducer is required to reach adequate depth of field. An area over the point of the shoulder is clipped or shaved, gel is applied, and the biceps brachii tendon is imaged in transverse and longitudinal planes. The tendon is a bilobate structure at the level of the point of the shoulder, with the narrowest point between the lobes superficial to the intermediate tubercle of the humerus. The lateral head is teardrop-shaped, whereas the medial head is an elongated rectangle.

To reduce artifact and to measure accurately tendon size, it is helpful to obtain images of the lateral and medial heads of the biceps brachii tendon separately. The lateral head is generally 100 mm^2 larger in cross-sectional area than the medial head. The biceps tendon normally has a slightly uneven echogenicity. A linear fiber pattern is normal for the longitudinal view. The bicipital bursa lies between the biceps brachii tendon and the humeral tubercles, extending around the lateral and medial borders of the tendon. Normally, no fluid is imaged superficial to the biceps tendon. Between the tendon and the humerus the bursa is normally filled with anechoic fluid, measuring 3 mm or less from superficial to deep.

Ultrasonographic changes observed in the presence of biceps brachii tendinitis include enlargement of one or both heads in comparison with the opposite limb, hypoechogenicity, either generalized or focal, including core lesions, and deterioration of the fiber pattern on longitudinal view. Chronic tendinitis may result in ectopic calcification of a previous tendon lesion; this can be seen ultrasonographically as an echogenic body within the tendon, which casts an acoustic shadow. It is common to find tendinitis as well as bursitis (Fig. 1), although one condition can develop in the absence of the other. Signs of bursitis include effusion, which is seen as an increase in space between the tendon and the humerus (Fig. 2), and occasionally as fluid superficial to the tendon as the bursal sac distends. An increase in echogenicity of the bursal fluid may be seen, either of uniform echogenicity as a result of hemorrhage, or as echogenic masses floating in the bursal fluid associated with fibrin production. In chronic cases, adhesions may be seen between the tendon and the bursal lining adjacent to the humerus.

Ultrasonography is also useful to guide needle placement for aspiration of bursal fluid and to administer either diagnostic nerve blocks or medication into the bicipital bursa. A transverse view of the bursa is maintained while a 6.3-cm (2.5-inch) 18-gauge needle is inserted 3.5 cm distal and

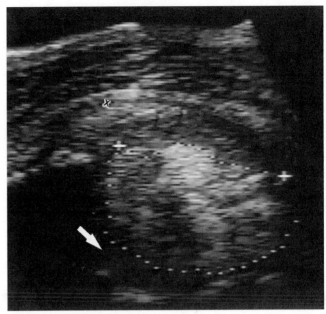

Figure 1. A cross-sectional ultrasonographic image of the biceps brachii tendon and bicipital bursa. The crosses indicate the borders of the bursa superficial to the tendon. The echoic fluid within the bursa represents a hematoma from a kick sustained 2 weeks before examination. The hypoechoic regions within the outlined lateral head of the biceps tendon represent tendinitis. The arrow indicates the hypoechoic fluid deep in the bursa deep to the biceps tendon.

7 cm caudal to the cranial prominence of the lateral humeral tubercle and directed mediad and proximad. The needle can be seen as a very echoic thin white line, and penetration of the bursa can be verified. Aspiration or injection can be visualized. Occasionally, the bursa is penetrated shallow rather than deep to the biceps tendon. Injections can be effectively made at this site because fluid can be seen ultrasonographically to enter the bursa, but

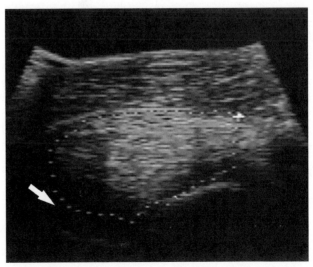

Figure 2. A cross-sectional ultrasonographic image of the biceps brachii tendon and bicipital bursa. No fluid is seen in the bursa superficial to the tendon. The arrow indicates anechoic fluid in the bursa between the tendon and the humerus. The lateral head of the biceps brachii tendon is outlined. The tendon is of normal size and echogenicity.

aspiration may be unproductive unless distension of the bursa is marked, probably resulting from the very thin bursal membrane and the overlying muscle, which allow the membrane to be pulled into the needle tip when suction is applied. Aspirated bursal fluid may be submitted for cytology and culture testing to differentiate inflammation from sepsis. Five to 10 ml of local anesthetic solution may be injected into the bursa to confirm the source of pain.

Infectious bursitis may occur following a blow or a penetrating wound over the point of the shoulder. Although synovial fluid aspirated from an infected bicipital bursa often has a white blood cell count higher than 30,000/mm³ and a total protein level higher than 3.0 g/dl, lower values have been found in more chronic cases. Additional synovial fluid should be collected for culture and sensitivity testing. Serum titers to *Brucella abortus* of more than 40 IU/ml have been reported in horses with septic bicipital bursitis. In view of the zoonotic nature of the organism, titers to *B. abortus* should be obtained from all horses suspected of having an infected bicipital bursa.

TREATMENT

Medical therapy for biceps brachii tendinitis includes initial anti-inflammatory medication such as phenylbutazone (1 g p.o. b.i.d. for 3 weeks) and cold therapy, usually 15 minutes of cold water b.i.d. Topical application of dimethyl sulfoxide may be helpful to reduce inflammation. Injection of hyaluronic acid (20–50 mg, varying with brand, or one intra-articular dose) into the bicipital bursa in acute cases reduces inflammation associated with tendinitis and helps to prevent adhesions. Physical therapy consists of stall rest with hand walking, beginning at 15 minutes twice daily and gradually increasing to 45 to 60 minutes per day, over a 3-month period. Ultrasonographic examinations are indicated every 60 to 90 days to monitor tendon healing and dictate increasing exercise levels. Biceps brachii tendinitis requires a 6- to 9-month healing period before the horse can be expected to return to full work. If an early diagnosis can be made, the prognosis for return to full use is fair. Chronic cases have a poor prognosis for return to full work owing to permanent enlargement of the tendon within the confined space between the brachiocephalicus muscle and the humerus, and to loss of gliding of the tendon over the humeral tubercles.

Medical therapy for aseptic bicipital bursitis is similar to that for tendinitis except that in the absence of tendinitis, injection of 100 mg of a corticosteroid such as methylprednisolone acetate into the bursa is useful to reduce inflammation. Physical therapy for bursitis is the same as that for tendinitis. Ultrasonographic examination at 60 days is indicated to assess resolution of bursitis; if bursal fluid is reduced to 3 mm and is anechoic, training can be resumed. Prognosis for return to full use is fair to good for acute cases.

Treatment of septic synovial structures is based on elimination of the causative organism and removal of the deleterious inflammatory mediators. Treatment with antimicrobials and through-and-through lavage should be reserved for those horses diagnosed within 24 to 48 hours. Most horses with septic bicipital bursitis are diagnosed weeks or months following the inciting incident, and in these cases, surgical intervention has been employed with favorable results. An incision is made through the skin and brachiocephalicus muscle, in the direction of its fibers. An enlarged and discolored bicipital bursa is visualized and incised. The bursa is entered and a subtotal synovectomy performed. A suction drain may be placed, the incision closed, and the horse placed on broad-spectrum antimicrobials. Horses may remain lame for 3 to 4 months following surgery, possibly because of the formation of adhesions. The use of controlled exercise on a gradually increasing scale of intensity and the administration of nonsteroidal anti-inflammatory drugs has produced favorable results. Hyaluronic acid has been used to prevent adhesions in the digital flexor tendon sheath of the horse and may be beneficial following surgery for septic bicipital bursitis. Following surgery, horses have recovered completely and have even returned to racing, even when treatment was delayed for several months.

Supplemental Readings

Crabill MR, Chaffin KM, Schmitz DG: Ultrasonographic morphology of the bicipital tendon and bursa in clinically normal Quarter Horses. Am J Vet Res 56(1):5–10, 1995.

Dyson SJ, Dik KJ: Miscellaneous conditions of tendons, tendon sheaths and ligaments. Vet Clin North Am Equine Pract 11(2):315–337, 1995.

Gaughan EM, Nixon AJ, Krook LP, Yeager AE, Mann KE, Mohammed H, Bartel DL: Effects of sodium hyaluronate on tendon healing and adhesion formation in horses. Am J Vet Res 52:764–773, 1991.

Grant BD, Peterson PR, Bohn A, Rantanen NW: Diagnosis and surgical treatment of traumatic bicipital bursitis in the horse. Proc 38th Annu Conv Am Assoc Equine Pract 349–355, 1992.

Schneider RK, Bramlage LR, Mecklenburg LM, Moore RM, Gabel AA: Open drainage, intra-articular and systemic antibiotics in the treatment of septic arthritis/tenosynovitis in horses. Equine Vet J 24:443–449, 1992.

Soft Tissue Swellings on the Dorsal Aspect of the Carpus

CAROL L. GILLIS

NICHOLAS J. VATISTAS
Davis, California

The carpal extensor tendons include the extensor carpi radialis, the common digital extensor, the lateral digital extensor, and the extensor carpi obliquus. Each tendon is surrounded by a synovial sheath from just proximal to several centimeters distal to the carpus. Tendinitis and synovitis can occur separately or together, depending on the inciting cause. Distension of the extensor tendon sheaths, damage to one or more extensor tendons, or effusion into the antebrachiocarpal or middle carpal joints results in swelling on the dorsal aspect of the carpus. Hygroma, an acquired subcutaneous bursa, over the dorsal aspect of the carpus may result from a hematoma or seroma, from a fall or blow to the dorsum of the carpus, or from herniation of the sheath of one of the extensor tendons following trauma. Cellulitis occurring over the dorsal aspect of the carpus presents as diffuse swelling. Each of these conditions requires an accurate diagnosis to provide appropriate treatment and prognosis.

EXTENSOR TENDINITIS

Tendinitis of the extensor tendons may result from trauma such as a fall or hitting a jump. The extensor tendons are not primary load-bearing structures, and are not under prolonged strain during work as are the flexor tendons; thus, overuse tendinitis is rarely encountered. The clinical signs of extensor tendinitis include swelling of the affected tendon and pain on palpation, if the condition is acute. Lameness, if any, is transient, seldom lasting more than 3 to 5 days following injury. Ultrasonographic examination reveals an increase in tendon size (cross-sectional area) at the damaged site, a loss of echogenicity, sometimes including a core lesion, and deterioration of normal fiber pattern.

Treatment should include an initial course of anti-inflammatory medication such as phenylbutazone (1 g p.o. b.i.d. for 3 weeks), cold therapy such as 15 minutes of hosing twice daily, and stall rest with limited hand walking, starting at 15 minutes per day and increasing over 60 days to 45 minutes per day. Ultrasonographic re-evaluation should reveal a decrease toward normal cross-sectional area (40–50 mm^2), increasing echogenicity of a core lesion, and improvement of fiber pattern. Exercise can gradually be increased. Four to 6 months of rehabilitation are usually required before the horse has healed sufficiently to return to full use. The prognosis for return to full work is good.

RUPTURE OF THE COMMON DIGITAL EXTENSOR TENDON

Rupture of the common digital extensor tendons may occur in neonatal foals. The condition is usually bilateral and may be accompanied by other birth defects, such as flexural deformities. Swelling occurs over the dorsolateral aspect of the carpus. When the foal walks, it may knuckle over at the fetlock owing to lack of extensor function. The ruptured ends of the tendon can be palpated, unless swelling of the sheath is too great.

Ultrasonographic examination provides a definitive diagnosis. The separated tendon ends can easily be visualized within the distended tendon sheath. Treatment consists of stall rest and application of full limb bandages to support the carpus and protect the dorsal surface of the fetlock from abrasion. The progress of tendon repair can be monitored ultrasonographically. Prognosis for full recovery from this condition is good.

Adult horses may sever extensor tendons as part of lacerations on the dorsum of the carpus. The separated ends may be seen within the wound bed, or may be palpated during exploration of the wound. Treatment of the lacerated extensor tendon is the same as for neonates. Management of the wound consists of debridement and lavage with 0.1% povidone-iodine solution followed by systemic administration of an antimicrobial such as trimethoprim/sulfa (3–5 mg [trimethoprim]/kg p.o. b.i.d.). Treatment of sheath sepsis is discussed later in the chapter. Prognosis for recovery following extensor tendon laceration is good, provided that wound infection is controlled. Ultrasonography can be used to monitor tendon healing and to dictate exercise level during the recovery period.

ASEPTIC TENOSYNOVITIS

Aseptic synovitis of an extensor tendon sheath (tenosynovitis) may occur in conjunction with tendinitis or may develop as a primary condition following trauma, such as a blow to the dorsal aspect of the carpus or a fall onto the carpus. A fluctuant swelling is limited to the extent of the affected sheath. Lameness is mild or absent; however, flexion of the carpus may cause discomfort. Ultrasonography is useful to define the type of synovitis; hemorrhage is seen as swirling hypoechogenic material, whereas serum and fibrin are seen as anechoic fluid containing floating masses (Fig. 1). Medical therapy is similar to treatment for

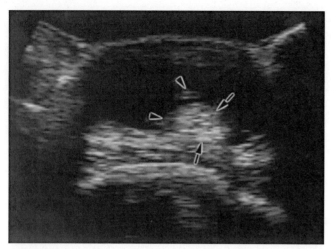

Figure 1. Cross-sectional ultrasonographic image of the common digital extensor tendon and its sheath at the level of the distal radius. The sheath is distended with fluid, seen as black (anechoic) on this image. Arrows indicate the common digital extensor tendon. Arrowheads indicate fibrin on the surface of the tendon.

tendinitis. Intrathecal injection of hyaluronic acid can reduce inflammation and may inhibit proliferation of the synovial lining of the sheath. A full limb bandage to place light compression over the carpus is useful to reduce swelling in cases of a few days' duration, as is the use of an oral combination of a diuretic and a corticosteroid (for example, trichlormethiazide 200 mg with dexamethasone 5 mg b.i.d. for 1 day, then s.i.d. for 3 days). Four to 6 weeks of rest is required to resolve active synovitis. Even after inflammation subsides, the sheath may remain distended. Ultrasonographic examination reveals anechoic fluid with little or no synovial proliferation. As long as synovial proliferation is not evident, the sheath swelling can be regarded as a blemish rather than a cause of unsoundness.

HYGROMA

The clinical presentation of a hygroma, or acquired subcutaneous bursa, is a diffuse swelling over the dorsum of the carpus. The swelling is usually cool and nonpainful to either palpation or carpal flexion. Diagnosis by ultrasonography and treatment are the same as for synovitis. It is important to treat synovitis/hygroma as early as possible; a delay of several days increases the likelihood of chronic sheath distension or persistence of the acquired bursa. Surgical excision of chronic hygromas can yield good results; however, 4 to 6 weeks of confinement and bandaging is required to allow the surgical repair to heal. Tenoscopy of extensor tendon sheaths may be useful to debride adhesions and flush inflammatory products from the sheath in persistent cases.

SEPTIC SYNOVITIS

Septic synovitis may be caused by a penetrating wound or by extension of infection from an adjacent structure (Fig. 2). Signs of septic tenosynovitis are lameness, acute and turgid swelling, and pain on carpal flexion. Aspiration

of sheath fluid for cytology and culture testing provides a definitive diagnosis. A total protein level higher than 3.0 g/dl and a total white cell count higher than 30,000/mm³ are indicative of infection. Incubation of aspirated fluid in a blood culture medium enhances retrieval of causative organisms; however, a negative culture result does not preclude infection. Treatment should consist of lavage of the sheath, preferably with 4 to 5 L of a balanced polyionic solution such as lactated Ringer's solution, and systemic broad-spectrum antibiotics. Until culture results become available, initial antimicrobial therapy may consist of potassium penicillin (20,000 IU/kg IV q.i.d.) and gentamicin sulfate at either 2.2. mg/kg (IV t.i.d.) or 6.6 mg/kg (IM or IV s.i.d.). In the field, procaine penicillin G (40,000 IU/kg IM s.i.d.) may be employed in lieu of potassium penicillin in situations in which multiple intravenous injections are not possible. However, procaine penicillin G may not achieve the serum concentrations attained following intravenous administration of potassium penicillin. Antimicrobial therapy should be adjusted according to culture results and should continue until clinical signs of pain and swelling have subsided and synovial white blood cell count is less than 30,000/mm³. Lavage may be repeated several times on an every-other-day schedule to reduce bacterial concentration and remove inflammatory products. Tenoscopy of the extensor sheath may be useful in chronic cases to remove proliferative synovia, break down adhesions, and flush out inflammatory mediators. Prognosis depends on duration of infection before initiation of treatment, ranging from fair in the first 48 hours to poor as the infection becomes chronic. Consequently, if penetration of a tendon sheath is suspected, aspiration of a fluid sample from a remote site of the sheath should be performed as soon as possible and early aggressive treatment initiated to increase the likelihood of a successful outcome.

CARPAL JOINT CAPSULE DISTENSION

Distension of a carpal joint capsule may be the result of primary synovitis, degenerative joint disease, hemarthrosis,

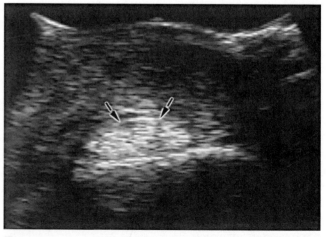

Figure 2. Cross-sectional ultrasonographic image of the common digital extensor tendon and its sheath at the level of the distal radius. The common digital extensor tendon is enlarged and mottled, as indicated by arrows. The sheath is distended with echogenic fluid.

or sepsis. Distension of the antebrachiocarpal or middle carpal joints produces swelling at the corresponding level on the dorsal face of the carpus. Application of digital pressure to the palmar pouch of the affected joint should exacerbate dorsal distension. Degree of lameness and of pain on carpal flexion depends on the inciting cause, ranging from mild to moderate for synovitis, to severe for joint hemarthrosis and sepsis. Standard radiographic views should be obtained to determine the presence and extent of bone involvement. Ultrasonographic examination helps to differentiate joint capsule distension from tendon sheath distension and to characterize the joint fluid. Anechoic fluid is usually seen with mild synovitis and degenerative joint disease. Evenly echogenic swirling fluid is suggestive of hemorrhage; these patients may have acute pain. The presence of echogenic masses or strands signals the presence of fibrin. Definitive diagnosis and treatment are the same as for sheath synovitis. Prognosis depends upon the underlying cause, the duration of the condition before treatment, and the extent of degenerative joint disease.

CELLULITIS

Cellulitis over the dorsum of the carpus may result from a wound, from extension from another site, or from bacteremia. Diffuse fluctuant to firm swelling, moderate to severe lameness, and pain on carpal flexion are present. Ultrasonography can be used to rule out involvement of deep structures and to locate any discrete area, such as an abscess, for aspiration and culture. Treatment for cellulitis includes the same antimicrobial therapy used for septic synovitis pending culture results, in conjunction with heat therapy (hot water and Epsom salt soaks or nitrofurazone sweats) to relieve tissue edema. Abscesses should be drained and flushed with a 0.1% povidone-iodine solution. Prognosis for cellulitis depends on the causative organism and on early appropriate therapy. If the infection can be eliminated, no permanent gait deficit should result, although the involved subcutaneous tissue may remain permanently thickened.

Supplemental Readings

Belknap JK, Baxter GM, Nickels FA: Extensor tendon lacerations in horses: 50 cases (1982–1988). J Am Vet Med Assoc 203:428–431, 1993.
Dyson SJ, Dik KJ: Miscellaneous conditions of tendons, tendon sheaths and ligaments. Vet Clin North Am Equine Pract 11:315–337, 1995.
Honnas CM, Schumaker J, Cohen ND, Watkins JP, Taylor TS: Septic tenosynovitis in horses: 25 cases (1983–1989). J Am Vet Med Assoc 199:1616–1622, 1991.
McIlwraith CW: Diseases of joints, tendon, ligaments and related structures. In Stashak TS (ed): Adams' Lameness in Horses, 4th ed. Philadelphia, Lea & Febiger, 1987, pp 339–485.

Carpal Canal Syndrome

DAVID PLATT
North Mymms, England

The carpal canal is a complex anatomic structure, the boundaries of which are formed by the palmar ligaments of the carpus, the axial surface of the accessory carpal bone, and the thick fascia of the palmar carpal retinaculum. The retinaculum stretches from the accessory carpal bone to the medial collateral ligament and proximal extremity of the second metacarpal bone. The canal is lined by synovial membrane and the carpal synovial sheath, which produces the synovial fluid that bathes the deep and superficial digital flexor tendons, as they course through the carpal tunnel. Encapsulated within the palmar carpal retinacular fascia lie the lateral palmar artery, vein, and nerve; the radial artery; and the medial palmar vein. The medial palmar artery and nerve lie within the carpal tunnel and are associated with the medial aspect of the flexor tendons. The term *carpal canal syndrome* can be defined as any pathology of the anatomic structures in the palmar aspect of the carpus causing distortion of the carpal canal lumen and resulting in compression of the soft tissue structures lying within the canal. Enlargement of the structures within the canal, or reduction in the size of the lumen of the carpal canal, resulting from injury of surrounding structures, such as chronic fibrosis of the palmar carpal retinaculum, can cause pain. Analogies can be drawn between carpal canal syndrome and annular ligament constriction of the fetlock.

CLINICAL SIGNS

Clinical signs of lameness associated with carpal canal syndrome cover a spectrum ranging from acute-onset, very severe lameness to insidious, gradually progressive chronic lameness, and signs reflect the pathology involved. Lameness caused by pain associated with the carpal tendon sheath is almost always associated with palpable effusion of the carpal synovial sheath. Such effusion can be variable and can be identified as a swelling on the caudolateral aspect of the distal radius, between the tendons of the lateral digital extensor and the ulnaris lateralis, or on the caudomedial aspect, between the flexor carpi ulnaris and flexor carpi radialis. In addition, if carpal sheath effusion is severe, fluid swelling may be palpated palmarodistally around the flexor tendons in the proximal metacarpal region. Heat, restricted flexibility, pain on carpal flexion, and lameness are signs associated with acute inflammatory conditions. Fibrous thickening of the carpal retinaculum, restricted flexibility, reduced pulse amplitude in the peripheral limb during carpal flexion, and intermittent lameness of variable severity are identified in cases when chronic fibrosis of the palmar retinaculum is the underlying etiology. Radiography and ultrasonography are valuable diagnostic aids to determine the underlying pathology responsible for the development of pain associated with the carpal canal.

PRIMARY CARPAL TENDON SHEATH SYNOVITIS

Idiopathic inflammation of the carpal synovial sheath is an infrequently diagnosed condition, which may represent subtle damage to intrasynovial structures. It is difficult to conceive how the synovial membrane of the carpal tunnel becomes irritated or inflamed as a primary event without damage to other carpal structures, when it is anatomically so well protected. The refinement of ultrasonographic equipment and techniques, however, has improved our ability to evaluate the individual structures within the carpal tunnel. The result will undoubtedly be identification of more specific lesions.

In the absence of identifiable tendinous or ligamentous pathology, treatment of inflammation of the carpal sheath remains symptomatic and should include hydrotherapy, topical administration of dimethyl sulfoxide (DMSO), bandaging, systemic nonsteroidal anti-inflammatory drugs (NSAIDs) (phenylbutazone 4–8 mg/kg per day), and stall rest for approximately 4 weeks. Administration of intrathecal hyaluronan (20 mg high molecular weight hyaluronan) and/or corticosteroids (10 mg triamcinolone acetonide) should be considered in more severe cases.

INTRATHECAL TENDON PATHOLOGY

Acute carpal canal syndrome is often associated with pathology of the flexor tendons within the carpal synovial sheath. These injuries predominantly involve strains of the superficial digital flexor tendon, although deep digital flexor tendon pathology is occasionally identified. Tendinous injury within the carpal canal may represent the proximal limit of damage in the mid-metacarpal region of the limb, or less frequently the lesion is restricted to the carpal canal. Superficial digital flexor tendon (SDFT) lesions that occur in the mid-metacarpal region and extend proximally into the carpal canal are associated with only mild distension of the carpal synovial sheath, whereas lesions restricted to the carpal sheath generally have greater distension and more severe lameness.

Ultrasonographic evaluation is essential to define the nature of the fibrillar damage and to monitor rate of healing of the tendinous injury. The fibrillar disruption is most commonly restricted predominantly to the central fibers of the SDFT. Muscular tissue within the digital flexor tendons should not be confused with a lesion; comparison with the contralateral limb may be useful.

Treatment of tendon injuries within the carpal synovial sheath initially involves strict stall rest during the 3 to 4 weeks of the acute inflammatory phase. Hydrotherapy, ice packing, topical DMSO, and bandaging are beneficial during this initial period and should be combined with systemic NSAIDs (phenylbutazone 4–8 mg/kg per day). Intrathecal injection of hyaluronan (20 mg high molecular weight hyaluronan [MW >3000]) into the synovial sheath during the acute period may be beneficial in suppressing the inflammatory response and may reduce the risk of developing intrasynovial adhesions. Intrasynovial corticosteroids are contraindicated in the presence of tendon disruption. Following the period of initial confinement, controlled ascending hand walking exercise encourages axial alignment of collagen during the early repair phase and should be undertaken before a period of prolonged pasture rest. The prognosis for tendinous lesions within the carpal synovial sheath is very guarded, however, because the lesions tend to persist or progress ultrasonographically, and lameness frequently recurs on return to work.

A less commonly diagnosed condition affecting the SDFT or deep digital flexor tendon (DDFT) is a partial or complete avulsion of the musculotendinous junction, within the proximal limit of the carpal synovial sheath. Avulsion injuries produce a very severe lameness, with massive effusion and hemorrhage into the carpal sheath. This lesion is seen in horses that jump at racing speeds (steeple chasing) and appears to be a specific catastrophic overload injury. The prognosis for an athletic career following this type of injury is hopeless and warrants euthanasia in animals with no potential for breeding. Extended stall rest of 8 to 12 weeks followed by an ascending exercise rehabilitation program is indicated for animals that are to be salvaged.

Intrathecal Infection

Septic tenosynovitis resulting from penetrating wounds to the carpal tendon sheath, in common with infection of any synovial structure, carries a guarded prognosis. It is associated with obvious distension of the sheath and severe lameness. Positive contrast radiography can be extremely useful in determining communication between a traumatic wound and the carpal synovial sheath. Analysis of an aseptically harvested synovial fluid sample is a valuable aid in diagnosis of established sepsis. Moderate elevation of total protein content indicates nonseptic inflammation (20–25 g/L), whereas septic tenosynovitis stimulates an intense inflammatory response and severe elevation of total protein content (>35 g/L). Increase in leukocyte numbers above 10,000 cells/mm³ consisting predominantly of neutrophils supports a diagnosis of infection. Bacteriologic culture from harvested synovial fluid is definitive for sepsis, but culture amplification techniques are required to maximize the frequency of positive cultures.

Treatment of septic tenosynovitis, in common with other traumatically damaged synovial structures, should involve debridement, extensive intrasynovial lavage using isotonic saline, and administration of appropriate intravenous broad-spectrum antibiotics (e.g., penicillin G sodium [30,000 IU/kg t.i.d.] and gentamicin [2.2 mg/kg t.i.d.]) and NSAIDs (phenylbutazone 4–8 mg/kg per day) as soon after injury as possible. The use of tenoscopic techniques, to visualize the intrasynovial lumen for partial synovectomy and removal of established fibrinous material, can significantly improve the response to therapy. The prognosis for successful resolution of an established septic tenosynovitis is extremely guarded and demonstrates the need for early diagnosis and aggressive therapy.

FRACTURES OF THE ACCESSORY CARPAL BONE

The axial border of the accessory carpal bone forms the lateral wall of the carpal canal. Fracture of the accessory carpal bone is the most common cause of chronic inflammation of the carpal sheath. Such injuries range from small chip fractures to extensive comminuted fractures, producing variable trauma to tissues adjacent to the carpal canal and may, depending upon fracture conformation, enter directly into the carpal sheath. The most common fracture configuration is a sagittal fracture through the body of the bone. Although many sagittal fractures heal by fibrous union with complete resolution of lameness, conservative or surgical management of these or other fractures may result in long-standing inflammation adjacent to the carpal canal. The inflammation can result in secondary fibrosis and thickening of the palmar carpal retinaculum. Chronic fibrosis of the carpal retinaculum, or the development of intraluminal callus, may cause narrowing of the canal lumen, resulting in pressure on the flexor tendons, which occasionally can be the cause of chronic lameness. Rarely, such chronic fibrosis may result in stenosis and constriction of the vessels and nerves lying within the retinacular fascia, resulting in a reduced blood flow to the distal limb and aberrant neurologic transmission in the palmar nerves. If animals that have suffered a fracture of the accessory carpal bone remain lame for longer than 6 to 8 months, carpal canal syndrome should be suspected.

Surgical treatment of chronic fibrosis of the palmar carpal retinaculum may be indicated in selected cases and involves a linear or elliptical desmotomy of the retinacular fascia, on the palmaromedial aspect of the carpus, to relieve the restrictive canal compression. Fractures entering the carpal sheath can act as sites for the development of intraluminal adhesions, between the canal synovium and the ensheathed flexor tendons. Ultrasonographic identification of such intraluminal adhesions, following healing of an accessory carpal bone fracture, is justification for tenoscopic resection followed by early physiotherapy, to attempt to prevent the reformation of restrictive adhesions.

SOLITARY OSTEOCHONDROMA

Solitary osteochondroma is a rare form of space-occupying mass, which is identified on the caudodistal aspect of the radius and is almost always associated with the caudal aspect of the radial metaphysis. This lesion is characterized by a bony protuberance that is continuous with the cortex of the bone. The mass slowly enlarges by endochondral ossification in a manner similar to growth within the epiphysis of a growing foal. Most osteochondromas have been reported to become clinically significant in animals of 5 years or older, suggesting that the neoplasm develops from physeal stem cells unresponsive to the cellular signaling that regulates closure of the distal radial physis. No evidence exists for a hereditary basis to this condition. Diagnosis is based on identification of swelling at the caudodistal aspect of the radius, pain on carpal flexion, and lameness. Radiographic examination reveals a bony lesion at the level of the distal radial metaphysis that can be variable in size and shape and may be smooth or irregular in outline. The treatment of choice is surgical excision; treatment carries an excellent functional and cosmetic prognosis, with complete resolution of the distended carpal sheath.

Supplemental Readings

Barr ARS, Sinnott MJA, Denny HR: Fractures of the accessory carpal bone in the horse. Equine Vet J 126:432, 1990.

Brokken TD: Acute carpal canal injury in the Thoroughbred. Proc 34th Annu Conv Am Assoc Equine Pract, 1988, pp 389–392.

Ghoshal N: Equine heart and arteries. In Getty R (ed): Sisson and Grossman's The Anatomy of the Domestic Animal, ed 5. Philadelphia, WB Saunders, 1975, pp 554–618.

Held JP, Patton CS, Shires M: Solitary osteochondroma of the radius in three horses. J Am Vet Med Assoc 193:563–564, 1988.

McIlwraith CW, Turner AS: Surgical relief of carpal canal syndrome. In McIlwraith CW, Turner AS (eds): Equine Surgery Advanced Techniques. Philadelphia, Lea & Febiger, 1987, pp 176–178.

Mackay-Smith MP, Cushing LS, Leslie JA: Carpal canal syndrome in horses. J Am Vet Med Assoc 160:993–997, 1972.

Flexural Deformities

DAVID ELLIS
Newmarket, England

Flexural deformities, congenital or acquired, are also known as hyperflexions or, less accurately, as contractures. They are common in all breeds of horses and donkeys and mostly affect the distal limb joints.

CONGENITAL FLEXURAL DEFORMITIES

Congenital flexural deformities are characterized by abnormal flexion with reduced or absent extension of a distal limb joint. The agonist/antagonist imbalance is rapidly self-correcting after birth, provided that the foal can stand on its feet without knuckling over. Some authors have associated congenital flexural deformities with nutritional disorders in the pregnant mare. In mares that have produced foals with severe or multiple deformities, there may be changes in the allantois suggestive of pressure molding and reduced placental fluid volume during late gestation. Congenital flexural deformities are rare in surviving twins or other premature or dysmature foals. The author has known some mares that have produced more than one affected foal, but the hereditary nature of the condition cannot be proven. The etiology of the majority of cases is unknown.

Congenital flexural deformities involve the fetlock, distal interphalangeal, and carpal joints, in descending order of incidence. Quite often several of these joints are affected in the same foal. Deformities of the metacarpophalangeal and metatarsophalangeal joints are often bilateral but are rarely symmetrical or quadrilateral. Flexure of the fetlock may be accompanied by angular deformity, usually varal. Flexures of the distal interphalangeal joint are mostly bilateral. They are very rare in the hindlimb.

Most of the milder flexural deformities self-correct during the first 24 to 48 hours, particularly if the foal is allowed limited exercise on a good surface, such as grass or a well-trodden straw bed. If the foal cannot stand or walk without knuckling, support is necessary and is best achieved by applying a shaped fiberglass gutter splint to the front of the distal limb, which has been well bandaged into a cylindrical shape using gamgee tissue, cotton, or orthopedic foam material. The splint is removed after 24 to 48 hours and all but the most severe cases are able to walk without knuckling. The bandaging remains as support for a further 2 to 3 days, and exercise is controlled so that the foal does not become too tired or run in deep bedding. Even the most severe fetlock flexure can respond to careful repeated splinting. Specialized splints are available but they must be used carefully and with adequate padding to prevent pressure sores. The application, under general anesthesia, of a cast that can be left in situ or split lateromedially and used as a splint is also a possible line of treatment. Physiotherapy in the form of regular manual extension of the distal limb is helpful in all cases and may be sufficient to correct borderline cases.

Occasionally, a foal with congenital flexure of the distal interphalangeal joint is slow to adopt a normal posture with its heel on the ground. Stable rest and corrective hoof trimming, lowering the heels, may be successful. Application of a grass tip or plastic shoe or building up the toe with acrylic have all been used successfully. If all fails by 6 weeks of age, ultimately inferior check ligament desmotomy may be necessary. The author has been unsuccessful in using high-dose oxytetracycline (20 mg/kg IV) and has never had to contemplate surgery in the neonatal period. If surgery is thought necessary for a newborn foal with flexural deformities, the author's experience is that euthanasia is more likely to be appropriate.

The author has encountered a rare case of quadrilateral flexural deformity of the distal limbs accompanied by hypoplasia of the phalanges.

Flexural deformity of the carpus is always bilateral and can be severe enough to cause dystocia. Affected animals have been called "contracted foals," and the carpal flexure frequently occurs in conjunction with other deformities or malformations such as scoliosis, torticollis, eventration, other flexural or angular deformities, rhinocampylus, ruptured bladder, anencephaly, scrotal hernia, and others. Such multiple defects can occur in foals from mares of all ages and occasionally more than once from the same mare.

Because of the likelihood of other deformities, a foal born with carpal flexure must be examined carefully before treatment is instituted. If it is unable to stand and particularly if the angle of maximal extension is no straighter than 135°, euthanasia is often the wisest course. Such cases have arthrogryposis and, even if every flexor structure proximal and distal to the carpus is severed, little extension will be achieved. Forced extension of the carpus under general anesthesia ruptures the palmar joint capsules and ligaments. This approach has been attempted with and without section of the palmar joint capsules. It can be considered only a salvage procedure. The discovery of other malformations can reinforce the wisdom of euthanasia.

Foals with a mild carpal flexure may be able to stand for short periods before tiring and respond well to regular manual extension every 3 to 4 hours. Exercise is valuable but periods must be limited, starting at half an hour morning and afternoon in a cage or yard. As the foal strengthens, it tolerates longer exercise, but care must be taken not to let it overtire or run in a large paddock until it can cope without weakening. It may take 4 to 6 weeks before a foal can lead a normal life. Surgical section of the ulnaris lateralis and flexor carpi ulnaris attachments to the proximal margin of the accessory carpal bone has been suggested for the foal that still stands markedly over at the knee by 1 month of age. The author has not yet found this procedure necessary.

If the foal cannot stand without knuckling forward, support must be applied to the front of the limb. The foal with mild carpal flexure accompanied by distal limb flexure may respond well to splint support of the fetlock and phalanges only. If the foal is unable to maintain the carpus in extension sufficient to stand, either splints or casts must be applied from elbows to feet. Splints have the advantage of not requiring general anesthesia for their application and of being easy to change. Fortunately the modern synthetic casting materials are strong and light enough for young foals to manage, although some help to rise from recumbency may be necessary in the early stages. If an affected foal is unable to stand within 72 hours of birth despite good nursing and support, euthanasia is justified.

A foal born with a mild flexural deformity of forelimbs whose condition suddenly worsens with knuckling forward on the carpus is most likely to have ruptured the common digital extensor tendon on the dorsal aspect of the carpus. This injury is usually bilateral and is accompanied by swelling of the tendon sheath, within which the separated ends of the ruptured tendon can often be palpated. Some such foals can stand and tolerate limited exercise without tiring and knuckling forward and require only controlled exercise for the following 4 to 6 weeks. The animal that knuckles forward requires support on the dorsum of the limb. The application of fiberglass casts, from elbows to feet for 3 to 4 weeks, is usually sufficient. Although the residual conformation of the young animal will be good, tendon sheath swelling on the front of the knee may take several months to disappear. The author has observed only one foal that failed to respond to casting. In this foal, the distal end of the ruptured tendon had curled distally through 180°, thus preventing healing. Ultrasound examination before and after casting can help clinicians identify such a rare occurrence, and surgery is indicated.

Congenital flexures, with arthrogryposis, have been seen

in tarsocrural joints, and the foals were destroyed. Flexures of more proximal joints have been noted in aborted fetuses.

ACQUIRED FLEXURAL DEFORMITIES

It has long been recognized that the normal foal, yearling, or immature horse or donkey may develop a flexural deformity of the distal limb during growth. Unless deformities result from a specific lameness or injury, acquired flexural deformities occur at anatomically distinct sites at certain ages. Distal interphalangeal joint flexure occurs in foals (1–6 months old) and fetlock flexure in older foals (3 months of age and older), yearlings, or 2-year-olds. The pathogenesis and etiology of acquired flexural deformities are complex and incompletely understood. It is not unreasonable to suggest that they are an off-loading phenomenon resulting from skeletal pain, but many cases of flexural deformity of the fetlock joint, or particularly the distal interphalangeal joint, arise with no lameness or apparent cause.

The suggested disparity in growth between bone and musculotendinous units does not explain the frequently unilateral flexure of the distal interphalangeal joint in young foals or its extreme rarity in the hind leg. No proof of copper deficiency has been demonstrated to occur in foals, but some clinicians have claimed good responses from supplementation. Likewise, high doses of tetracyclines or single injections of phenylbutazone have their advocates. Lack of exercise and walking on hard ground have also been suggested as causes. Stable rest is usually successful in correcting deformities, particularly in the young foal.

Acquired distal interphalangeal flexures are considered to be diseases of opulence caused by overfeeding, particularly protein or carbohydrate, or by grazing young stock on recently fertilized or young (less than 7-year-old) pasture. The author believes these anecdotal reasons to be more valid than most and that heredity may play a predisposing part.

Acquired Flexure of the Distal Interphalangeal Joint

Acquired flexure of the distal interphalangeal joint can occur in foals as young as 10 to 14 days of age but is more commonly encountered between 1 and 4 months of age. Almost invariably it involves forelimbs and may be uni- or bilateral. The foal must be inspected on a hard level surface to detect the early flexure. The deformity is characterized by the foal walking on its toe with the heel raised off the ground and may be sudden in onset. Within a few days a normal foal may acquire a nearly vertical dorsal wall of the hoof. The dorsal coronet becomes more prominent and the contour of the dorsal hoof wall concave. The foal stands more upright on its pastern and may overextend its carpus. Affected foals are usually in good or heavy bodily condition and otherwise healthy. Ultimately the unworn heels grow long and the foot adopts a boxy shape.

Early diagnosis is invariably rewarded by successful conservative treatment with a rapid recovery. The foal should be rested in the stable until normal conformation is restored. For the mild case, 2 to 3 weeks may suffice. Only

the least affected case can successfully have its heels lowered and be allowed to stay out at grass 24 hours per day. Even the severe case with the dorsal hoof wall slightly beyond the vertical responds to corrective hoof trimming and rest. The heels are rasped down until the horn is soft every 10 days, and the foal is given at least 6 to 8 weeks' stable rest. The mare's rations should be reduced and the foal's access to her feed prevented. If the toe is worn, a grass tip, a steel or plastic shoe, or an acrylic filler can be applied. Although this may protect the toe, it can make regular lowering of the heels more difficult to achieve, which is crucial to the successful treatment of flexure of the distal interphalangeal joint. Nonsteroidal anti-inflammatory drugs (NSAIDs) are not used on these foals in case such treatment causes gastric or duodenal ulcers.

The foal that is 3 months or older may improve rapidly if it is weaned. The weanling should remain confined and be fed limited amounts of good hay (clover or alfalfa hay can be used) and a mineral and vitamin mix ensuring a positive (>2:1) calcium:phosphate balance.

The author has had no success giving high doses of oxytetracycline. If the flexure is long-standing when diagnosed, conservative measures are still worth trying for 4 to 6 weeks. However, the foal that does not respond to rigorous conservative efforts should undergo surgical section of the accessory ligament of the deep digital flexor tendon (DDFT). Results have been good for animals in which the dorsal hoof wall is less than, or no more than slightly over, the vertical. It is important for the foal to be hand walked from the day after surgery. Improvement is immediately obvious and continues over the ensuing month. Shoes are not usually necessary, but phenylbutazone may be required in the first 10 to 14 days. If NSAID treatment is given to a foal under 6 months of age, simultaneous antiulcer treatment is advisable. Carprofen (0.7 mg/kg IV) is safer than other NSAIDs. Some thickening may persist at the surgical site, but the prognosis for an athletic career is good. The foal with the dorsal hoof wall well over the vertical requires section of the DDFT, and the procedure must be regarded as salvage surgery. Even if the residual conformation is good, the prognosis for a demanding athletic career is poor. Regular corrective hoof trimming to lower the heels is essential postoperative care following either surgery.

Flexural deformity of the distal interphalangeal joint can be accompanied by lameness that may be primary or secondary to the flexure. The author has seen flexural deformity develop following proximal sesamoid fracture, septic arthritis, or osteochondritis dissecans (OCD) of the shoulder. The only deformity encountered in a hindlimb followed a chronic stifle lameness.

Lameness as a consequence of the flexure mostly results from excess wear on the toe, which can lead to infection and abscess formation along the white line or to sandcrack. Erosion of the toe of the distal phalanx has been seen in chronically affected animals. Radiographically the bone may exhibit a roughened and blunted tip or the toe may be turned upward like a Turkish slipper. These bony changes need not compromise a horse's athletic career, provided that a reasonable shape and angle are restored to the hoof walls.

Although the "pull" of the DDFT is similar to that which occurs in laminitis, divergence of the dorsal hoof wall from the dorsal cortex of the third phalanx is uncommon. The chronically affected animal that has not regained a normal conformation has a narrow hoof with thin upright walls. The heels are long and narrow and may be sheared. There may be a dropped sole dorsal to the frog. Nailing and keeping shoes on such feet can be very difficult, and adhesive shoes are a real benefit. Grooving the quarters of such feet in older foals or young yearlings may help to broaden the heels.

The young horse that retains a clubfooted conformation may subluxate the ipsilateral proximal interphalangeal joint dorsally. Although this gives the appearance of a ringbone, degenerative joint disease is rarely present, and such cases are usually sound athletes. Rare individuals have been encountered that, during surgical or conservative treatment for acquired flexural deformity in forelimbs, have developed degenerative joint disease in the proximal interphalangeal joints of the hindlimbs. Some of these joints have been found to have subchondral bone cysts in the distal first phalanx.

Older horses may develop flexural deformity of the distal interphalangeal joint following chronic lameness. The upright boxy foot used to be considered an important feature of chronic navicular disease. Recent investigations have clarified some of the changes occurring in the heel area of the hoof, so that the blanket diagnosis of "navicular" is less commonly thrust onto the animal afflicted with a lameness that is abolished by a low palmar digital nerve block.

Off-loading after a serious injury, such as suspensory disruption, comminuted fracture of the first phalanx, or other serious fracture may also result in a boxy foot. Marked elevation of the heels following severance of a flexor tendon can result in permanent flexure if the heels are not lowered early enough in the recovery period.

Certain breeds of horse or pony, and especially donkeys, regularly have narrow boxy feet with a hoof-pastern axis suggestive of a flexural deformity. Some Thoroughbred sires are noted for producing stock with narrow feet or foals that acquire flexural deformity. The author has been surprised at the long-term athletic soundness of horses with boxy feet and believes this conformation defect to be a lesser evil than broad feet with shallow collapsed heels.

Acquired Flexural Deformity of the Fetlock Joint

This deformity is considered to have been acquired if the foal, yearling, or horse knuckles forward involuntarily at the fetlock when it should be bearing weight with the joint extended. The sole of the foot remains flat on the ground, and only in long-standing cases does the hoof acquire an upright and boxy shape. The flexure is usually bilateral and symmetrical and can affect fore-, hind-, or all four limbs. It occurs most commonly in the older foal or yearling and can be evident when the horse is standing or in motion.

The knuckling seen in the forward leg when grazing should not be considered abnormal. The most commonly encountered cases of this flexure are seen in weanling foals, 6 to 9 months old, that are prepared and offered at auction sales. These foals have been fed high-energy diets and given extra walking exercise on a firm surface. They knuckle forward on their hind fetlocks during the weight-bearing phase when walking but usually extend the joint just before the limb is advanced for the next stride. These foals recover normal conformation and gait following rest and reduction of the energy content of their diet.

Flexural deformity of the fetlock is probably an off-loading response to chronic skeletal pain originating there or more proximally in the limbs. It can occur in association with physitis in the distal metacarpus or metatarsus in foals 2 to 6 months old. It is seen most commonly in the young animal with physitis in the distal radius or tibia, which may affect foals from 7 to 9 months old, yearlings, or 2-year-olds. It is most likely to occur in the spring of the yearling year. In addition, it often accompanies OCD in the femoro-patellar or fetlock joints. The author recently encountered it in the forelimbs of a yearling that had recovered from distal radial physitis but that was found at postmortem examination to have osteochondrosis lesions in the articular facets of the fourth, fifth, and sixth cervical vertebrae and the hocks.

The affected animal that is identified early in the progress of the deformity responds well to rest and analgesic treatment. The energy level of the diet should be reduced to maintenance level or less and a positive calcium:phosphate balance must be ensured. It is paramount that the animal be examined thoroughly to discover osteochondrosis or physitis lesions so that they may be treated appropriately. Hoof care is a very difficult but important aspect of treatment. Normal hoof shape must be restored, but prevention of knuckling by shoeing is difficult to achieve. A shoe that raises the heel and lengthens the toe can encourage the pastern and fetlock to extend. The chronically affected animal may improve gradually, taking several months (1 year in one case seen by the author) to stop knuckling the fetlocks forward; such animals usually acquire a hyperextension of the carpus.

Surgical treatment may be considered if no underlying cause, such as OCD, is treatable and if there is no response to at least 6 weeks of conservative measures. If palpation reveals that the superficial flexor tendon is under most tension, desmotomy of the superior check ligament should be successful. This technique is less satisfactory if the superficial and deep digital flexors are involved. Simultaneous inferior check ligament desmotomy is then recommended. Controlled exercise, including walking backward, and shoeing as described earlier are important measures to be undertaken in the immediate postoperative period. Concurrent NSAID treatment is essential. Section of the superficial flexor tendon or the suspensory ligament has been attempted but is cosmetically less satisfactory and is likely to affect the pastern axis. Generally, surgery is a less satisfactory solution to flexure of the fetlock than is inferior check ligament desmotomy for flexure of the distal interphalangeal joint.

Flexural deformity of the metacarpophalangeal joint has been documented in an adult horse that was found to have traumatically induced adhesions between the inferior check ligament and the superficial flexor tendon. Some flexure of the distal interphalangeal joint was also present. Surgical freeing of the adhesions and surgical shoeing provided a good response. Such cases are unusual, but thorough examination, including ultrasonography, is essential to their correct diagnosis and successful treatment.

Suggested Readings

Embertson RM: Congenital abnormalities of tendons and ligaments. Vet Clin North Am Eq Pract 10(3):351–364, 1994.

Fackelman GE: Equine flexural deformities of developmental origin. Proc 26th Ann Conv Am Assoc Equine Pract 26:97–105, 1980.

Wagner PC: Flexural deformity of the distal interphalangeal joint (contracture of the deep digital flexor tendon). *In* White NA, Moore JN (eds): Current Practice of Equine Surgery. Philadelphia, JB Lippincott, 1994, pp 472–475.

Wagner PC: Flexural deformity of the metacarpophalangeal joint (contracture of the superficial digital flexor tendon). *In* White NA, Moore JN (eds): Current Practice of Equine Surgery. Philadelphia, JB Lippincott, 1994, pp 476–480.

Wagner PC: Flexural deformity of the carpus. *In* White NA, Moore JN (eds): Current Practice of Equine Surgery. Philadelphia, JB Lippincott, 1994, pp 480–482.

The Diffusely Filled Limb

JOSE M. ROMERO
Madrid, Spain

SUE J. DYSON
Newmarket, England

A diffusely filled limb is a common clinical presentation. Knowledge of the common causes facilitates accurate diagnosis, although in some acute cases, symptomatic therapy resolves the problem without the need to determine the underlying cause. The clinician must determine from the initial clinical evaluation if further diagnostic tests are required or whether symptomatic treatment will suffice. In some circumstances, symptomatic therapy may be applied for several days and then the situation is reappraised, because accurate diagnosis may be easier with some reduction in swelling. In acute cases associated with lameness, or in chronic cases, additional diagnostic tests such as ultrasonography and radiography may be indicated initially, to accurately determine the diagnosis, most appropriate treatment, and prognosis.

Diffuse filling of the limb may be the result of a number of causes:

1. Inflammation due to local infection, trauma, cellulitis, lymphangitis, dermatitis, photosensitization
2. Noninflammatory edema due to impaired lymphatic flow, increased venous pressure, immune-mediated vasculitis, or systemic disease (e.g., equine viral arteritis)
3. Fluctuant fluid accumulation due to a hematoma, seroma, abscess, or synovial distension
4. Bony enlargements and secondary soft tissue reaction
5. Soft tissue masses including granulation tissue or scars and tumors
6. Enlargement of specific soft tissue structures including the superficial (SDFT) and deep (DDFT) digital flexor tendons, the accessory ligament of the DDFT (ALDDFT), the suspensory ligament (SL), and the digital flexor tendon sheath.

DIAGNOSIS

Diagnosis is based on history and clinical examination, response to symptomatic therapy, and the results of radiographic and ultrasonographic examinations and other ancillary tests. The history should establish how many horses are involved, which limbs are affected, the color of the limbs, the environment in which the horse is kept, the duration of clinical signs, the response to previous therapy, and other concomitant clinical signs suggestive of systemic disease.

Table 1 summarizes the clinical features of a variety of causes of filled legs. The whole horse should be appraised in the clinical examination because a systemic disease, such as equine viral arteritis (*Current Therapy in Equine Medicine* 2, page 313, and 3, page 511) or purpura hemorrhagica (*Current Therapy in Equine Medicine* 2, page 312, and 3, page 164) may be the underlying cause. Temperature, pulse, and respiratory values should be measured. All four limbs should be evaluated, paying particular attention to the extent of swelling (pastern, metacarpus/metatarsus, carpus/tarsus, or further proximal); its position (symmetrically around the limb or asymmetrically, localized on the lateral, medial, dorsal, or palmar/plantar aspects); the firmness of the swelling (hard, possibly bony, firm, or soft); whether the swelling fluctuates or pits on pressure; and reaction to palpation of the swollen area and specific related structures. The presence of heat should be noted, bearing in mind that clipped areas are usually warmer and the limb must be carefully examined to detect skin lesions including puncture wounds, abrasions, an open wound, or serum oozing. The horse should be evaluated at the walk and the trot to detect lameness.

MUD FEVER OR CRACKED HEELS

Mud fever and *cracked heels* (see also page 398) are synonymous terms for a bacterial folliculitis, which primarily affects the palmar/plantar aspect of the pastern. The infection may extend into the subcutis. Many bacteria have been implicated, including *Dermatophilus congolensis*, *Staphylococcus* species, *Corynebacterium*, and β-hemolytic streptococci. Usually only one horse is affected, but certain soil types and weather conditions may predispose horses in an

TABLE 1. DIFFERENTIAL DIAGNOSIS OF CAUSES OF A DIFFUSELY FILLED LIMB

Cause	Extent of Soft Tissue Swelling	Distribution	Consistency	Heat	Pain on Palpation	Lameness	Pyrexia	Diagnostic Aids
Mud fever/cracked heels	Pastern, fetlock, distal metacarpus/metatarsus	Symmetrical	Soft	Yes	Yes	Yes +→++	No	Response to treatment
Cellulitis	Variable	Symmetrical	Soft	Yes	Yes	Yes +→+++	Yes/no	Hematology, ultrasonography, response to treatment
Lymphangitis	Entire limb to elbow or stifle	Symmetrical	Soft	Yes/no	Yes/no	Yes +→++++	Yes/no	Hematology, ultrasonography, response to treatment
Purpura hemorrhagica	Entire limbs to elbow and stifle	Symmetrical	Soft	Yes	Yes	Stiffness	Yes	Hematology, skin biopsy
Subsolar abscess	Metacarpus/metatarsus distally	Symmetrical	Soft	Yes	No	Yes ++→++++	Yes/no	Exploration of foot
Hemorrhage	Metacarpus/metatarsus	Symmetrical or asymmetrical	Soft	Yes	Yes	Yes ++→+++	No	Ultrasonography
Tight bandage	Palmar/plantar metacarpus/metatarsus	Symmetrical	Soft	Yes	Yes	No	No	Ultrasonography, response to treatment
Idiopathic infection of SDFT/DDFT	Metacarpus/metatarsus distally	Symmetrical	Soft	Yes	Yes	Yes +++	No	Ultrasonography
Cold edema	Metacarpus/metatarsus distally	Symmetrical	Soft	No	No	Yes	No	Response to treatment
Suspensory desmitis and fractured MC/MTII/IV	Metacarpus/metatarsus	Symmetrical or asymmetrical	Soft	Yes	Yes	Yes +→++	No	Ultrasonography, radiography
Rupture of SDFT	Metacarpus distally	Symmetrical	Soft	Yes	Yes	Yes +++	No	Posture
Hypertrophic osteopathy	Variable	Symmetrical usually	Soft/firm	Yes	Yes	Stiffness	Yes/no	Radiography
Localized trauma	Variable	Asymmetrical	Soft	Yes	Yes	Yes/no	No	Response to treatment, radiography
Equine viral arteritis	Metacarpus/metatarsus distally	Symmetrical	Soft	Yes	Yes/no	Stiffness/no	Yes	Serology

+ = mild; ++ = moderate; +++ = severe

area so that several horses managed similarly may have clinical signs. Horses with long hair coats that are kept in damp conditions are particularly susceptible. Washing the legs after work and not drying them or using over-reach boots that traumatize the skin may also predispose horses to the condition.

Clinical Signs

One or more limbs may be affected, sometimes all four. The affected pastern is usually diffusely firmly filled on the palmar/plantar aspects; swelling may extend proximal to the fetlock. Crusty skin lesions may exude serum-like material. In several cases, there are deep fissures in the thickened skin. Progressive hair loss may be present. Usually the limb exhibits localized heat, and pain is induced by either localized pressure or flexion of the distal limb joints. Lameness varies from mild stiffness to more severe lameness, if there is associated cellulitis.

Treatment

The affected limb should be clipped to above the proximal extent of the lesions. The crusty skin lesions may be very painful, so it may be helpful both to sedate the horse and to wash the limb first with warm water and antiseptic soap, which will soften the crusts and allow their removal. This is done using a gloved fingernail and may induce bleeding.

Povidone-iodine shampoo is applied with warm water and left in situ for 7 minutes before being rinsed off. After careful drying, an antibiotic-corticosteroid cream or nitrofurazone is applied. In severe cases, a dry bandage should be applied, which includes the bulbs of the heel and the back of the shoe, to prevent the bandage from riding up. The bandage minimizes irritation from the bedding. The horse should be stabled if at all possible. Systemic antimicrobial drugs (e.g., procaine-penicillin [20,000 IU/kg IM b.i.d.] or trimethoprim sulfur [15 mg/kg b.i.d.]) should be used for 3 to 5 days in severe cases. In competition horses, gentamicin (6.6 mg/kg s.i.d.) may be preferable to procaine penicillin because of its shorter elimination time.

The limbs should be re-treated daily by washing, crust removal, and repeated topical treatments for several days, and then every 2 to 3 days thereafter, until the lesions resolve. Premature cessation of treatment tends to result in recurrence; therefore, treatment should continue until skin defects have healed, there are no crusts, and swelling is gone. Light work, avoiding mud and wet environments, can continue and may help to resolve the swelling. Mild lesions can successfully be treated within 3 to 4 days, whereas chronic severe cases may take several weeks. Prognosis is generally good, although with chronic severe lesions, prolonged treatment is required.

Prevention

Early detection of lesions is important, and this may be facilitated by keeping the distal limb clipped. Clipping also permits more thorough washing and drying.

CELLULITIS

Cellulitis is an infection that spreads through the tissue planes and can be caused by a variety of organisms including *Staphylococcus* species, *Streptococcus* species, *Corynebacterium*, and *Clostridium* species. Bacteria usually gain entry through a skin defect and may multiply and spread rapidly.

Clinical Signs

Usually only one limb is affected, especially hindlimbs. The wound may be difficult to identify, even after clipping the hair. Very extensive soft tissue swelling is present, which develops rapidly and may spread proximal to the carpus or tarsus. The swelling is often greatest on the side of the wound. The swelling is firm, hot, and painful to palpation. Lameness may be severe. Rectal temperature is often elevated, and the horse may be depressed and anorexic in severe cases. As the condition progresses, there may be oozing of serous exudate through the skin.

Treatment

The area of the wound should be identified, clipped, and cleaned, as should areas of exudation. One of the following broad-spectrum systemic antimicrobial treatment regimens should be administered: sodium penicillin G (50,000 iu/kg IV q.i.d.) and gentamicin (6 mg/kg s.i.d.); sodium penicillin G (50,000 IU/kg IV q.i.d.) and trimethoprim/sulfa (15 mg/kg b.i.d.); tetracycline (5 mg/kg IV s.i.d.); procaine penicillin G (20,000 IU/kg IM b.i.d.) and gentamicin (6 mg/kg s.i.d.); or procaine penicillin G (20,000 IU/kg IM b.i.d.) and trimethoprim/sulfa (15 mg/kg b.i.d.). Support therapy should include nonsteroidal anti-inflammatory drugs (NSAIDs) (e.g., phenylbutazone 3 mg/kg b.i.d., flunixin meglumine 1 mg/kg s.i.d., ketoprofen 2 mg/kg s.i.d.). Treatment also includes exercise such as hand walking several times daily to promote edema reabsorption, as soon as the horse can walk without undue discomfort; warm water hosing and washing with chlorhexidine or povidone-iodine shampoo to clean the area and promote circulation; bandaging the affected and contralateral limb; and careful monitoring to identify secondary bacteremia or laminitis.

Prognosis

Clinical improvement is generally seen within 24 to 48 hours of initiating treatment. Early aggressive therapy is required. Prolonged clinical signs may lead to fibrosis and chronic thickening, or lymphangitis.

LYMPHANGITIS

Lymphangitis is a severe form of cellulitis, with inflammation of the lymphatic vessels and peripheral lymph nodes. The precise pathogenesis is very poorly understood. Ulcerated nodules may develop in some cases associated with infection with *Corynebacterium pseudotuberculosis* infection (see page 393). Chronic lymphangitis results in permanent diffuse enlargement of the limb and/or a tendency for re-exacerbation of clinical signs following innocuous cuts and grazes. Ulcerative lymphangitis due to *Corynebacterium pseudotuberculosis* can affect more than one limb and may be an endemic problem in some farms, affecting several horses. Other cases of lymphangitis are usually sporadic and commonly affect a single hindlimb.

Swelling may extend from the stifle distally, and its extent produces severe hindlimb stiffness. Serum may ooze out through the skin in severe cases.

Treatment

Treatment is aimed at reducing soft tissue swelling, promoting vascular and lymphatic circulation, and eliminating infection. Hydrotherapy, massage, and bandaging may help to reduce soft tissue swelling. Forced exercise should also help to reduce swelling and promote circulation. Systemic corticosteroids seem to be beneficial (e.g., dexamethasone IV 0.04 mg/kg s.i.d., then reducing to 0.02 mg/kg s.i.d. for not longer than 5 days). Prolonged antimicrobial therapy (minimum 4 weeks) is essential, and this poses a dilemma between cost, ease of administration, and efficacy. It is often not possible to culture the infecting organism, and thus broad-spectrum combinations as discussed under cellulitis are indicated. Erythromycin (10 mg/kg IV or 25 mg/kg p.o.) may be more effective in treatment of *C. pseudotuberculosis* infection. With early, aggressive, prolonged therapy, clinical signs may resolve, but there is a relatively high rate of recurrence.

COLD EDEMA

Cold edema describes swelling of the distal limbs, especially the hindlimbs, due to nonpainful edema. The edema disappears with exercise. It is a very common condition of unknown etiology, occurring particularly in stabled horses. It may be due to accumulation of fluid in the interstitial space associated with poor lymphatic circulation.

The condition usually is bilaterally symmetrical, involving both hindlimbs and sometimes also the forelimbs. The filling usually involves the distal metatarsus, fetlock, and pastern, but may extend further proximally. The edema is soft and nonpainful and pits on pressure, and it is not associated with lameness; therefore, treatment is not required.

Regular exercise prevents the condition to some extent. Stable bandages should be applied.

SUBSOLAR ABSCESS

Diffuse filling of the distal limb is a common feature associated with subsolar abscess.

Clinical Signs

Usually, moderate to severe lameness is present, which is of greater severity than would be expected with tendinitis. Limb filling is restricted to the lame limb. The swollen limb is usually hot and may be painful. The digital vessels are enlarged and the pulse amplitude in the digital arteries is increased. The horse may be febrile. The foot may be warm. Usually, pain can be elicited by pressure and/or compression applied to the foot with hoof testers.

Treatment

The shoe should be removed. Having established a focus of pain using hoof testers, the sole should be pared with a hoof knife to establish drainage of pus. If the foot is very hard, it may be impossible to locate a focus of pain. In such cases, the foot should be soaked and poulticed for several days to soften the horn, and then re-explored. Once drainage is established, daily soaking and poulticing are useful until no further pus is obtained. Local application of metronidazole may accelerate resolution of infection. Systemic antimicrobial drugs are not usually used, because they may suppress infection without eliminating it totally.

The distal limb swelling usually dissipates rapidly after establishment of drainage. When infection is resolved, the exposed solar tissues need to dry and harden.

HEMORRHAGE

Hemorrhage from a traumatized blood vessel can result in the rapid development of diffuse filling of the limb and moderate to severe lameness. The degree of soft tissue swelling may make it difficult to accurately palpate the tendons and ligaments.

Clinical Signs

Diffuse soft tissue swelling, which may be fluctuant, is present along with heat and pain on palpation over a rather diffuse area. Lameness is invariably present. The area should be examined carefully for the possible presence of a skin wound, which may predispose to infection. Diagnostic ultrasonography is invaluable for excluding other causes of swelling and confirming the diagnosis.

Treatment

Cold therapy may be useful in the very acute stage, but application of a modified Robert Jones bandage left in situ for several days is probably the best treatment. If a hematoma persists, massaging heparinoid ointment and dimethyl sulfoxide (DMSO) topically, several times daily, may facilitate its resorption, which may take from 2 to 14 days.

TIGHT BANDAGE

Pressure from an overly tight bandage, or a bandage with inadequate and/or uneven padding, may result in local or diffuse swelling, especially on the palmar aspect of the limb. The extent of the swelling may make it difficult to properly evaluate the SDFT and differentiate it from tendinitis. Diagnostic ultrasonography is useful to determine the nature of the swelling. However, aggressive local cooling therapy usually results in resolution of swelling within 24 to 48 hours. The tendons should be carefully reappraised after dissipation of the swelling.

IDIOPATHIC INFECTION OF THE SUPERFICIAL OR DEEP DIGITAL FLEXOR TENDON

Infection of a tendon may develop as a result of a wound, but it occasionally occurs with no history of trauma and no detectable skin lesion. A variety of bacteria have been cultured, including coagulase-positive *Staphylococcus*. Once established within a tendon, infection spreads rapidly, resulting in widespread destruction of the tendon substance.

Clinical Signs

Although swelling may initially be localized to the primary focus of infection, with spread of infection, soft swelling rapidly involves the entire metacarpus or metatarsus. There is heat, pain on pressure, and very severe lameness. Rectal temperature is usually normal. Diagnosis is based on the clinical signs and diagnostic ultrasonography. Infection within a tendon is characterized by an anechoic central core lesion in the tendon, which spreads rapidly. The degree of lameness is far greater than would be anticipated in aseptic tendinitis.

Treatment

Early diagnosis is essential for successful treatment, because infection spreads so rapidly and its effect is so destructive. Aggressive systemic antimicrobial therapy has not been successful in the author's (SJD) experience in cases presented more than 48 hours after the onset of clinical signs. Early surgical debridement, combined with broad-spectrum antimicrobial treatment with crystalline penicillin and gentamicin, is most likely to be successful, but based on the author's (SJD) experience to date, a guarded prognosis is warranted.

SUSPENSORY LIGAMENT DESMITIS

Mild cases of suspensory desmitis are usually associated with swelling clearly localized to the SL. However, with severe desmitis, in conjunction with a fracture of the distal one third of the second and/or fourth metacarpal or metatarsal bone, swelling is extensive and diffuse. The latter injuries are particularly common in steeplechasers and Standardbreds, and only these are discussed further here.

Clinical Signs

Diffuse soft tissue swelling is found principally on the medial and lateral aspects of the limb. In the acute stage, the degree of swelling may prohibit accurate evaluation of the SL and small metacarpal bones. Pain is present on palpation along with localized heat. Lameness is usually moderate. Distal limb flexion may be resented and may accentuate lameness. Diagnosis may be suspected based on the clinical signs and confirmed ultrasonographically and radiographically.

Treatment

Initial therapy is aimed at reducing inflammation and pain and includes local hydrotherapy, pressure bandaging, and systemic administration of nonsteroidal anti-inflammatory drugs (e.g., phenylbutazone 3 mg/kg IV b.i.d.) and confinement to stall rest. Prognosis is ultimately dependent on the degree of suspensory desmitis. Although some fractures of the second and fourth metacarpal bones heal, surgical removal is usually advocated. To date, there have been no effective treatments to accelerate or improve healing of the SL, although early trials with β-aproprionitrile-fumarate (BAPTEN) indicate that this drug may be beneficial. Severe SL lesions are associated with a high incidence of recurrent injury, regardless of the method of management and duration of rest.

Other causes of a diffusely filled limb include rupture of the SDFT (see page 34) and hypertrophic pulmonary osteoarthropathy (see page 129).

Supplemental Readings

Barbet JL, Baxter GM, McMullan WC: Diseases of the skin. *In* Colahan PT, Mayhew IG, Merritt AM, Moore JN (eds): Equine Medicine and Surgery, ed 4. Goleta, CA, American Veterinary Publications, 1991, pp 1569–1734.
Brown CM: Limb and ventral edema. *In* Problems in Equine Medicine. Philadelphia, Lea & Febiger, 1989, pp 138–149.
Cohen M: Ulcerative lymphangitis. *In* Robinson NE (ed): Current Therapy in Equine Medicine, ed 2. Philadelphia, WB Saunders, 1983, pp 31–32.

Desmitis of the Accessory Ligament of the Deep Digital Flexor Tendon

ANDREW M. McDIARMID
Edinburgh, Scotland

The accessory ligament of the deep digital flexor tendon (ALDDFT) is also called the inferior check ligament, subcarpal check ligament, distal check ligament, carpal check ligament, and the tendinous head of the deep digital flexor tendon (DDFT). Desmitis of the ALDDFT is a relatively common cause of forelimb lameness. The incidence of forelimb ALDDFT desmitis appears greatest in older horses, with most cases occurring in animals over 9 years of age. The majority of affected animals are involved in athletic work, particularly some form of jumping. A higher frequency of ALDDFT desmitis has been noted in ponies, and it has been claimed to be the most common tendon and ligament injury in draft horses. Desmitis of the hindlimb ALDDFT occurs less frequently and appears to carry a better prognosis for future soundness.

The ALDDFT originates as a continuation of the palmar carpal ligament and combines with the DDFT in the mid-metacarpus. The ligament has an elongated V shape, with a broader and thicker origin, narrowing distally. It is bordered on its dorsal aspect by the third interosseous muscle (suspensory ligament) and on the palmar aspect for most of its length, before joining the DDFT, by the dorsal compartment of the carpal sheath. The ALDDFT is believed to provide stability for the carpus during limb extension, whereas during the weightbearing phase of the stride it relieves some of the tensile load of the DDFT. Ultrasonographically the ALDDFT is normally the most echodense of the tendinous structures in the palmar metacarpus.

PATHOGENESIS

Although considerable work has been conducted into tendinitis of the superficial digital flexor tendon (SDFT), limited research into the etiology of ALDDFT desmitis has been performed. It is generally accepted that SDFT injuries usually result from repeated submaximal damage that weakens the overall tendon before the occurrence of clinical "breakdown." This theory is supported by postmortem evidence that collagen fiber degeneration is present in many clinically normal tendons. It has been suggested that there may be an age-related degeneration in the ALDDFT, and recent in vitro work confirms that ligament rupture occurs at lower forces in older horses. It was also found that the in vitro force required for the first evidence of fibrillar failure was lower in older horses. Changes in collagen "crimp" formation, reduction in cell populations, changes in tenocyte nuclei, and areas of chrondroid metaplasia develop within the SDFT and DDFT with age. It has been speculated that these changes may result in a reduction in the tensile strength of the SDFT, and a similar situation *may* occur within the ALDDFT.

The ultrasonographic presence of concurrent abnormalities within the DDFT may suggest that following ALDDFT desmitis an increased load, in particular hyperextension, may be placed on the DDFT. The development of SDFT tendinitis following ALDDFT desmitis is difficult to explain with the current knowledge of tendon biomechanics; however, the fact that the ALDDFT provides some stability to the carpus when the limb is in extension may result in increased loading on the SDFT following ALDDFT damage.

Many chronic cases of ALDDFT desmitis remain permanently lame despite good clinical and ultrasonographic evidence of healing. The reason for persistent lameness is unclear but may be the result of development of adhesions, predominantly from the ALDDFT onto the abaxial margins of the SDFT (Fig. 1), that result in circumferential compression of the DDFT and carpal sheath. The presence of such adhesions can also explain the development of a broken forward hoof pastern axis in many chronic cases.

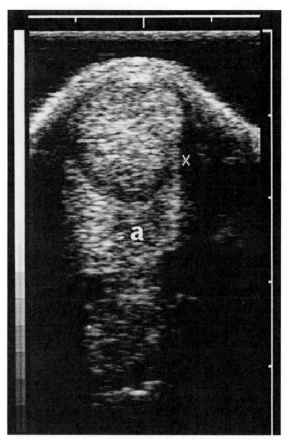

Figure 1. Transverse ultrasonogram obtained approximately 7 cm distal to the accessory carpal bone, 8 months following the onset of acute ALDDFT desmitis. An irregular area of decreased echogenicity is still present within the ALDDFT (a). Adhesion formation between the medial aspect of the ALDDFT and SDFT is indicated by the cursor (x). Note the presence of anechoic fluid within the dorsal pouch of the carpal sheath and the apparent lack of adhesion formation across the sheath.

CLINICAL SIGNS

Typically horses or ponies with ALDDFT desmitis have a history of acute-onset lameness, often occurring during or shortly after exercise. The author has, however, observed a few horses and ponies older than 12 years of age that developed ALDDFT desmitis after several days of complete rest while at pasture.

With acute ALDDFT desmitis, there is considerable swelling of the ALDDFT and surrounding soft tissues. Periligamentous hemorrhage may also occur and the resultant proximopalmar metacarpal swelling may lead the owner to suspect that the horse has simply sustained a traumatic injury to the limb and thus immediate veterinary advice may not be sought. The degree of swelling may make differentiation between the DDFT and ALDDFT difficult; however, after initial resolution of the swelling, it is normally possible to detect heat, pain, and swelling in the ALDDFT. The most swollen area usually corresponds with the site of maximal damage found ultrasonographically.

Ultrasonographic examination should be conducted on all cases of ALDDFT desmitis to determine the degree and extent of ligament damage (Figs. 2, 3). If ALDDFT desmitis is not recognized and the animal resumes work

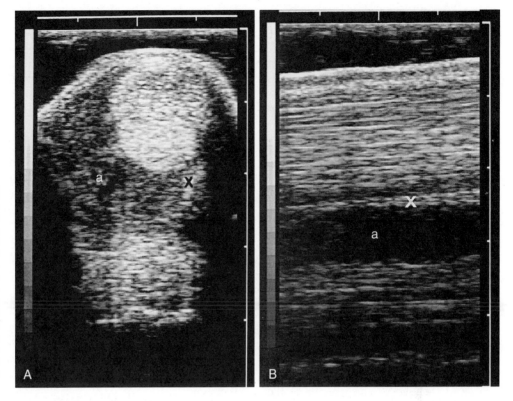

Figure 2. Ultrasonograms obtained approximately 9 cm distal to the distal border of the accessory carpal bone in a horse with acute ALDDFT desmitis. (*A*) Transverse view demonstrating total lack of any echogenicity within almost the entire cross-sectional area of the ALDDFT; the lateral aspect appears to be wrapping around the DDFT toward the abaxial margins of the SDFT (a). A small area of healthy ALDDFT is present on the medial aspect (X). (*B*) Longitudinal scan of the same area showing a total lack of linear echoes (a) within the affected area of the ALDDFT.

when the lameness has resolved, usually after a few weeks, further desmitis is very likely.

Chronic desmitis of the ALDDFT is not uncommon. This can occur after repeated episodes of ALDDFT desmitis, following chronic SDFT tendinitis, especially in older horses, or following injury to the ALDDFT of the contralateral limb. Chronic cases of ALDDFT desmitis may remain permanently lame and can develop postural changes in the limb. The horse may stand with the heel of the affected limb slightly elevated, can develop a broken for-

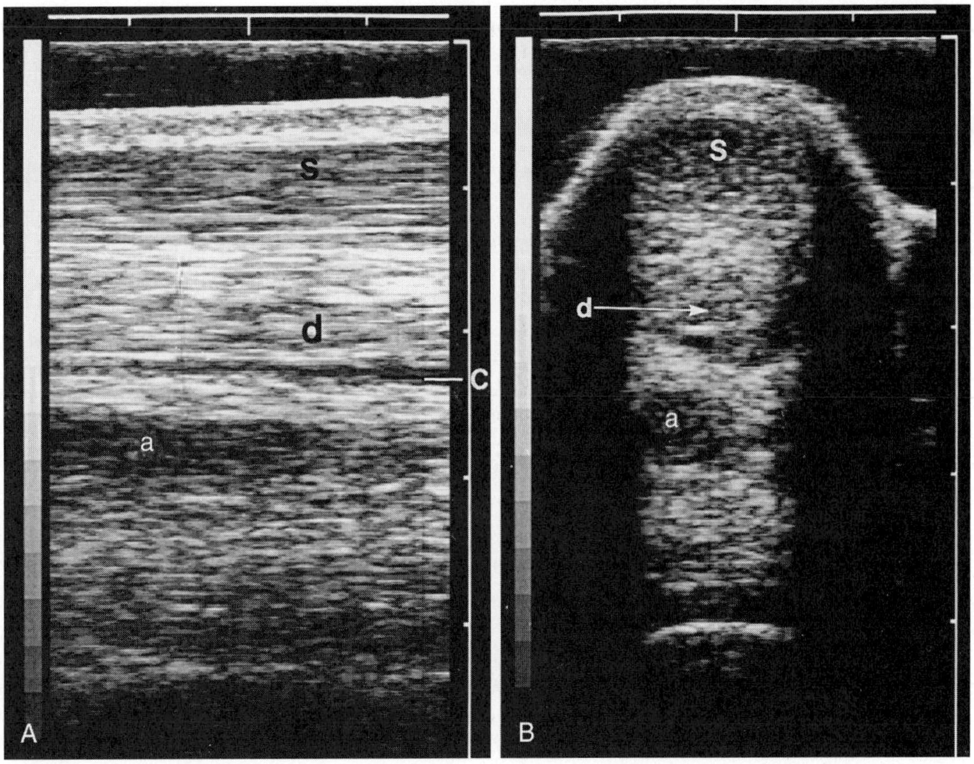

Figure 3. Ultrasonograms obtained approximately 9 cm distal to the distal margin of the accessory carpal bone 3 weeks following the development of acute ALDDFT desmitis. (*A*) Longitudinal ultrasonogram demonstrating very little fibril alignment within the area of the ALDDFT damage (a). Fibrillar disruption is also present within the palmar aspect of the SDFT (s) and the dorsal aspect of the DDFT (d). Note the anechoic line of fluid (c) within the carpal sheath. (*B*) Transverse ultrasonogram demonstrating a focal area of decreased echogenicity within the dorsolateral aspect of the ALDDFT (a), the dorsal aspect of the DDFT (d), and the palmar aspect of the SDFT (s).

ward hoof pastern axis, and may develop a flexural deformity of the metacarpophalangeal joint. The latter condition can develop over a relatively short period of time (a few weeks) and is often associated with concurrent SDFT tendinitis. In most, if not all, of these cases, there is extensive adhesion formation, and differentiation between the two flexor tendons and ALDDFT by palpation is almost impossible.

ULTRASONOGRAPHIC EXAMINATION

Ultrasonographic examination of the ALDDFT is carried out from the palmar aspect of the metacarpus, and the structures should be evaluated in both transverse and longitudinal planes (see Fig. 2). In addition, oblique palmaromedial-dorsolateral and/or palmarolateral-dorsomedial views can be useful to observe the nature and extent of adhesion formation. In acute desmitis, frequently there is a reduction in the echogenicity of the entire lateromedial cross-sectional area of the ALDDFT (see Fig. 2A). This area of decreased echogenicity often occupies much of the proximodistal length of the ligament, and more than 75% of its length may be involved (see Fig. 2B). In many of these cases, the ALDDFT also shows considerable enlargement around the margins of the carpal sheath, toward the abaxial surface of the SDFT. The margins of the ALDDFT are often poorly defined. Alternatively, there may be smaller focal areas of decreased echogenicity (see Fig. 3). The affected area can be in a central (core) or marginal area of the ALDDFT and tends to occupy less proximodistal length than the former type of abnormality.

In cases of acute ALDDFT desmitis, ultrasonographic abnormalities within the flexor tendons may also be detected. A typical lesion is a small focal area of decreased echogenicity within the dorsal aspect of the DDFT (see Fig. 3). Focal and diffuse areas of decreased echogenicity within the SDFT may also be found (see Fig. 3). In three published reports on desmitis of the ALDDFT the incidence of coexisting flexor tendon ultrasonographic abnormalities was 33%, 37%, and 90%. Cases of ALDDFT desmitis should be ultrasonographically re-evaluated at 2- to 3-month intervals (see Fig. 3). Features that indicate healing is progressing are an increased echogenicity within the affected area, longitudinal images demonstrating the presence of parallel "fibril" alignment, and showing these "fibrils" becoming longer and more organized in outline.

Differential diagnosis for acute ALDDFT desmitis is carpal sheath distension, DDFT tendinitis, some acute cases of desmitis of the proximal one third of the third interosseous muscle ("high suspensory desmitis"), and periligamentous hemorrhage. In the latter condition the affected horse may present with acute-onset severe lameness with considerable swelling in the region of the ALDDFT. Tendinitis of the DDFT in the proximal and mid-metacarpus is very rare.

TREATMENT

Treatment for the inflammatory phase of ALDDFT desmitis is similar to that for SDFT tendinitis. One of the most important aspects of the treatment of ALDDFT desmitis is

reduction of adhesion formation. Prompt aggressive treatment in the first 48 hours following the development of desmitis is probably the single most important factor in preventing adhesions. Reduction of the acute inflammatory response during this period is accomplished with a combination of local and systemic anti-inflammatory treatments. The local treatment should include cold water hydrotherapy and/or ice packs applied around the ALDDFT for 20 to 30 minutes several times per day. A pressure bandage should be applied between these treatments. More prolonged application of cold should be avoided because it induces reflex vasodilation. Systemic administration of anti-inflammatory medication should also be conducted in the acute stage. Nonsteroidal anti-inflammatory drugs (NSAIDs) (phenylbutazone 2.2 mg/kg b.i.d. or flunixin meglumine 1.1 mg/kg b.i.d. for 5–7 days) are most widely used. Corticosteroids are potent anti-inflammatory drugs and decrease inflammation, edema, and adhesion formation; however, they inhibit fibroplasia as well as collagen and glycosaminoglycan synthesis. As a consequence only short-acting corticosteroid preparations (e.g., 0.06 mg/kg betamethasone) should be used and limited to the acute inflammatory phase (i.e., the first 3–4 days after injury). Intraligamentous injections of corticosteroids should be avoided because they may induce fibrocyte death, dystrophic calcification, and collagen fiber necrosis. Additional care should be taken when administering corticosteroids to ponies because of their susceptibility to laminitis.

Following resolution of the inflammatory stage, typically after 7 to 10 days, several medical treatments can be used. Polysulfated glycosaminoglycan (PSGAG) has been successfully used in the treatment of ALDDFT desmitis. PSGAG decreases inflammation, inhibits collagenase activity and macrophage activation, and improves the orientation of the healing collagen fibrils. PSGAG also induces faster resolution of SDFT core lesions and can be used intramuscularly or intralesionally. The author favors intramuscular administration (500 mg every 4 days for 4–7 treatments). Because most ALDDFT lesions involve such a large percentage of the ALDDFT, intralesional injections are less satisfactory in the treatment of ALDDFT desmitis than in a focal SDFT core lesion.

Sodium hyaluronate (HA) is not widely used in the treatment of acute tendinitis or ALDDFT desmitis, although there are good theoretical reasons for its use in the late acute and early repair phases of ligament healing. HA is thought to be important in the initiation of angiogenesis and in the invasion and differentiation of fibroblasts. In cases of tenosynovitis or tendonosynovitis within the digital sheath, intrasynovial use of HA is also known to reduce adhesion formation. The use of HA within the carpal sheath may decrease adhesion formation in cases of ALDDFT desmitis; however, because most adhesions appear to develop around the carpal sheath, the use of HA into the carpal sheath may be of limited value.

Therapeutic ultrasound produces alterations in blood flow, may facilitate fibroplasia and collagen production, and is reported to reduce adhesion formation. The author recommends the use of therapeutic ultrasound for all early cases of ALDDFT desmitis to help reduce inflammation and adhesion formation. At approximately 5 to 7 days following the development of desmitis, a 7- to 10-day ultrasound course is started (pulsed 0.3 watts/cm² for 8–10 minutes twice daily). Ultrasound therapy may be detrimental if used in the inflammatory stage because it may increase edema and hematoma formation, and, because many acute cases of ALDDFT are associated with considerable hemorrhage, it should be used only at a very low wattage (pulsed 0.1 watts/cm²), if at all, at this early stage.

Soft and cold lasers have been used for many years in both human sports medicine and equine work. Their use in the treatment of ALDDFT desmitis has not yet been critically evaluated. The alleged therapeutic effects of cold lasers that may benefit ALDDFT healing are increased protein and collagen production, fibroblast proliferation, and pain relief. The use of electromagnetic therapy in the treatment of ALDDFT desmitis is of no advantage over therapeutic ultrasound. Counterirritation (e.g., blistering and firing) is contraindicated in the treatment of ALDDFT desmitis because of its tendency to induce further desmitis and greater adhesion formation.

Two very important aspects of treatment are rest from athletic work and a controlled exercise program of increasing intensity. Stall rest for at least 10 to 12 weeks is essential in the acute phase of ALDDFT healing. Following resolution of maximal lameness, usually 5 to 7 days after the onset of desmitis, controlled walking should be encouraged, initially 5 to 10 minutes twice daily and increased to approximately 20 minutes twice daily by week 6. After 12 weeks, the exercise can be further increased but, because of stabling costs, some horses may have to be turned out to grass at this stage. If possible this turn out should be controlled, and the use, for several weeks, of a large indoor enclosure or very small paddock is preferable before turn out. The controlled exercise program should be determined by the ultrasonographic appearance at follow-up examinations.

A common cause of recurrent ALDDFT desmitis is the reintroduction of the animal into work too quickly. In general, horses with ALDDFT desmitis require at least 6 months' rest from full athletic work, and sometimes up to 15 months' rest. Work should be reintroduced only when the ultrasonographic appearance of affected ALDDFT has returned to a uniform echogenicity similar to that of the contralateral limb. Following resumption of normal work, some horses develop a degree of heat in the region of the ALDDFT. Ultrasonographic examination should be conducted at this stage to eliminate the possibility of recurrent desmitis. Often this is not present and the heat is assumed to be due to adhesion breakdown.

In chronic cases of ALDDFT desmitis that remain lame as a result of either adhesion formation or the development of a flexural deformity of the metacarpophalangeal joint, desmotomy of the ALDDFT can be undertaken. The surgery can be particularly frustrating because the landmarks of the palmar metacarpal tendinous structures are lost as a consequence of extensive adhesion formation, and great care should be taken not to transect the DDFT. The use of intraoperative ultrasonography may aid the surgery. Although the flexural deformity may resolve, the prognosis for future soundness following surgery in these cases is poor.

PROGNOSIS

The prognosis for ALDDFT desmitis–affected horses returning to the same level of work undertaken before the injury is guarded. Recurrent desmitis and SDFT desmitis commonly occur, and desmitis may also develop in the contralateral limb. Following recurrent ALDDFT desmitis, the development of a metacarpophalangeal joint flexural deformity in older animals can occur. In a high percentage of ALDDFT desmitis cases, a thickening of the ALDDFT remains, despite the fact that the animal is sound. Because ALDDFT desmitis often affects older horses, many are retired or used as breeding animals.

Supplemental Readings

Becker CK, Savelberg HHCM, Barneveld A: *In vitro* mechanical properties of the accessory ligament of the deep digital flexor tendon in horses in relation to age. Equine Vet J 26:454–459, 1994.

Dyson SJ: Desmitis of the accessory ligament of the deep digital flexor tendon: 27 cases (1986–1990). Equine Vet J 23:438–444, 1991.

McDiarmid AM: Eighteen cases of desmitis of the accessory ligament of the deep digital flexor tendon. Equine Vet Ed 6:49–56, 1994.

Silver LA, Brown PM, Goodship AE (eds): Biochemistry and pathology of tendon injury and healing. Equine Vet J 1[Suppl]:5–22, 1983.

van den Belt AJM, Becker CK, Dik KJ: Desmitis of the accessory ligament of the deep digital flexor tendon in the horse: Clinical and ultrasonographic features, a report of 24 cases. J Vet Med Series A 40(7):492–500, 1993.

Webbon PM: A histological study of macroscopically normal equine digital flexor tendons. Equine Vet J 10:253–259, 1978.

Deep Digital Flexor Tendinitis

ALISTAIR R. S. BARR
Bristol, England

Characterization of injuries to the tendons and ligaments on the palmar/plantar aspect of equine distal limbs has become more accurate over the last 10 years, with the advent of ultrasonographic imaging. Diagnostic ultrasound has confirmed observations from earlier postmortem surveys suggesting that strain injuries to the deep digital flexor tendon (DDFT) are relatively uncommon, compared with injuries to the superficial digital flexor tendon (SDFT), accessory ligament of the deep digital flexor tendon (ALDDFT), or suspensory ligament (SL). In particular, ultrasonography has revealed that horses with marked swelling of the SDFT in the metacarpal region usually have a normal DDFT lying beneath and that concurrent injury of the SDFT and DDFT is unusual. In this situation the SDFT often spreads around the DDFT medially, making the latter difficult to assess by palpation alone. In a postmortem survey of 589 tendons from 206 horses, a total of 34 DDFT abnormalities were found, compared with 105 SDFT abnormalities. Most of the DDFT abnormalities (23 tendons) were described as "degenerative changes in the distal phalangeal region," and 21 of these 23 lesions were found in the forelimb. All but one of these lesions continued no further proximally than the proximal interphalangeal joint. Such distal lesions of the DDFT, as it crosses the flexor cortex of the navicular bone, are usually considered to be a component of the navicular disease syndrome. Unfortunately, the DDFT is difficult to image satisfactorily at this distal site using currently available ultrasonographic equipment, and there is little documentation of these particular lesions in vivo. In the same postmortem survey "stress-induced DDFT injuries" were seen in only six tendons. Of these six injuries, four were at the level of the proximal sesamoid bones and two were in the phalangeal region. Deep digital flexor (DDF) tendinitis has also been recognized in a small number of horses in association with desmitis of the ALDDFT, with focal areas of decreased echogenicity in the dorsal aspect of the DDFT in the proximal half of the metacarpus.

In the majority of cases of ultrasonographically confirmed DDF tendinitis seen by the author, the lesion has occurred at, or just above, the level of the metacarpophalangeal joint, within the digital flexor tendon sheath (DFTS).

CLINICAL FINDINGS

History

DDFT sprain injuries within the DFTS are seen predominantly in middle-aged and older horses used for competition activities, hunting, and general-purpose riding. An even distribution of injuries occurs between fore- and hindlimbs, which is in marked contrast to other palmar metapodial soft tissue injuries, where the forelimb is more commonly affected. No apparent asymmetry exists in the left/right distribution of the injuries. Affected animals usually have a history of a sudden onset of mild to moderate lameness associated with filling of the digital sheath. In a minority of animals, there may be a history of a preceding chronic mild lameness, which has become worse recently.

Clinical Signs

Most horses have mild to moderate unilateral lameness (1/2–2° on a scale of 0–4°) at the trot in a straight line on a firm surface. The lameness is exacerbated by flexion of the distal limb joints in approximately half the cases. Distension of the DFTS is usually present, varying from mild to severe, and increased skin surface temperature over the DFTS may be present in acute cases. The DDFT is occasionally thickened and painful on palpation, particularly with the limb flexed and non-weightbearing; however,

it is often difficult to appreciate enlargement of the DDFT within a distended digital sheath. Thickening of the palmar/plantar annular ligament and resentment of flexion of the affected distal limb are also sometimes seen.

DIAGNOSIS

Intrasynovial analgesia of the DFTS consistently improves the degree of lameness. Regional analgesia of the palmar/plantar and palmar/plantar metacarpal/metatarsal nerves proximal to the fetlock (four-point block) also produces a significant improvement; however, there is a less consistent response to abaxial sesamoid nerve block.

Ultrasonographically most cases have small, distinct, often circular, focal hypoechoic areas within the deep digital flexor tendon in the distal metacarpus/metatarsus usually within the digital sheath proximal to the proximal sesamoid bones (Fig. 1). These hypoechoic areas tend to be localized and extend only a short distance proximodistally—usually less than 1 cm. The lesions are therefore focal rather than true "core" lesions, as understood for the SDFT, and are easy to miss if the DDFT is not carefully examined throughout the digital sheath. Horses presented with persistent lameness associated with distension of the DFTS should therefore have repeated ultrasonographic examinations, if DDFT lesions are not seen on initial examination. Less frequent findings are enlargement of the DDFT and irregularity of its border. All cases have an increase in the amount of fluid in the DFTS. Echogenic material within the tendon sheath around or adjacent to the flexor tendons is seen in a minority of cases and may represent adhesion formation.

DDF tendinitis may be seen concurrently with clinical and ultrasonographic evidence of thickening of the annular

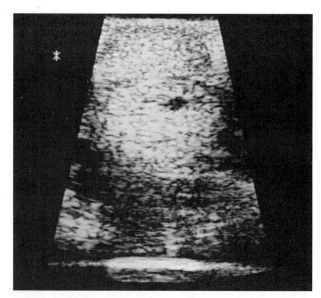

Figure 1. Transverse ultrasonographic scan of the plantar aspect of the distal left metatarsus (4 cm proximal to the metatarsophalangeal joint) of a 12-year-old Thoroughbred gelding used for advanced eventing. The image was made 8 days after a sudden-onset left hindlimb lameness associated with distension of the DFTS. A circular 4-mm-diameter hypoechoic lesion is present within the substance of the DDFT.

ligament. The nature of the relationship between desmitis of the annular ligament and tendinitis of the DDFT within the digital sheath remains unclear; however, horses presenting with clinical signs of annular ligament syndrome should have a careful ultrasonographic examination to exclude the possibility of a concurrent DDFT injury, which may adversely affect the prognosis. A small number of horses have also been seen with enlargement of the DFTS, echodense material within the sheath, and hypoechoic lesions in the DDFT, in addition to osteomyelitis of the proximal sesamoid bones. The possibility of concurrent proximal sesamoid bone disease should therefore also be kept in mind in formulating a diagnosis.

TREATMENT

Management

The basis of treatment is a period of stall rest and controlled exercise of progressively increasing intensity. The precise regimen used for each horse needs to be tailored to its individual injury and regular clinical and ultrasonographic re-evaluations of the progress of healing. Ideally, re-evaluations should be performed at 2-month intervals. The overall duration of rest and controlled exercise may vary from 2 to 12 months, depending on clinical response; however, most horses should not be allowed free exercise at pasture for at least 6 months. Affected horses should be completely stall rested until signs of acute inflammation have subsided. Thereafter, a typical program may involve 8 weeks of walking exercise in hand for 20 minutes twice daily, 8 weeks of ridden walking exercise for 20 minutes twice daily, 12 weeks of ridden walking and short periods of slow trotting for 30 minutes twice daily, and 12 weeks of ridden exercise with increasing duration and speed of trotting.

Medical Treatment

The exercise program may be supplemented, particularly in the acute stage, by various forms of medical therapy including systemic nonsteroidal anti-inflammatory drugs such as flunixin meglumine (1.1 mg/kg s.i.d.), phenylbutazone (2.2 mg/kg b.i.d.), or ketoprofen (2.2 mg/kg s.i.d.); intrasynovial sodium hyaluronate (20 mg into the DFTS); systemic (500 mg IM q4 days on up to seven occasions) or intralesional (50 mg) polysulfated glycosaminoglycan; or intrasynovial, low-dose, short-acting corticosteroids such as betamethasone (10 mg into the DFTS).

Surgical Treatment

Horses with clinical and/or ultrasonographic abnormalities of the palmar/plantar annular ligament may be treated surgically by performing a palmar/plantar annular ligament (PAL) desmotomy. Splitting of core lesions of the DDFT may be beneficial, although, at present, there are no documented results available to assess the efficacy of this procedure.

PROGNOSIS

The degree of lameness and DFTS swelling generally improves with stall rest, and the ultrasonographically apparent lesions reduce in size. However, exacerbation of the clinical signs and ultrasonographic lesions is common when affected horses are allowed free exercise at pasture or returned to athletic work. Ultrasonographically the lesions in the DDFT tend to persist and may be still visible up to 2 years after the initial injury.

Of 24 cases in one series, only seven made a full recovery and returned to their intended athletic activity. Ultrasonographically, the DDFT had returned to normal in two of these seven horses, the lesion was still visible in two horses at the time of last examination, and the long-term ultrasonographic outcome was unknown in three horses. Of five horses that received intrasynovial medication, two made a full recovery. Of eight horses that had PAL desmotomies only two made full recoveries. Thus, neither intrasynovial medication nor PAL desmotomy appeared to improve the prognosis in horses with DDFT injuries. Fifteen of the 24 horses experienced recurrent or persistent lameness leading to retirement from athletic activity, or destruction on economic grounds. DDFT lesions within the digital sheath therefore appear to be persistent and the overall prognosis is guarded.

Supplemental Readings

Barr ARS, Dyson SJ, Barr FJ, O'Brien JK: Tendonitis of the deep digital flexor tendon associated with tenosynovitis of the digital sheath in the horse. Equine Vet J 27S:348–355, 1995.
Dyson S: Desmitis of the accessory ligament of the deep digital flexor tendon: 27 cases (1986–1990). Equine Vet J 23:438–444, 1991.
Webbon P: A post mortem study of equine digital flexor tendons. Equine Vet J 9:61–67, 1977.

Laceration or Rupture of the Digital Flexor Tendons

PETER GREEN

J. MATTHEW J. TONG
Abbots Ripton, England

Disruption of the direct action of the flexor muscles upon the distal limb may occur either as the result of a laceration through the skin or because of rupture of the muscle/tendon unit, under conditions of overload. Flexor lacerations that are sustained by horses at rest or in the paddock, when the palmar or plantar aspects of the limbs are injured by sharp objects or as the result of a kick, exhibit different tendon pathology from those sustained at speed during racing or during strenuous work. Sharp incisions in resting horses may give rise to clean, single-site sectioning of the flexor tendons with or without gross contamination, whereas lacerations caused by limb interference or crashing falls in galloping horses result in frayed and significantly disrupted tendon ends, with considerable concomitant peritendinous tissue damage. Rupture of the flexor tendons without laceration must be considered as the extreme manifestation of the syndrome of exercise-induced tendon strain, and is most likely to occur in horses that have previously suffered episodes of tendinitis. In these cases, the tendon often has failed at the interface between normal tendon tissue and the disorganized scarring, where the previous episodes have healed. Ruptures and lacerations during exertion are normally accompanied by massive local tissue reaction, hemorrhage, and exudation, involving the tendon itself and the paratenon or sheath, according to the site of the trauma. Sharp lacerations at rest may occur with less local reaction. In all cases, the principal purpose of emergency therapy must be to limit this peritendinous and intratendinous inflammation and to immobilize the distal limb. Lacerations are also subject to contamination, which progresses to infection within 8 hours. Subsequent therapy is aimed at restoring the functional integrity of the tendon and permitting normal loading of the limb during exercise, without restriction of joint movement.

ASSESSMENT OF RUPTURES AND LACERATIONS

Because the normal weightbearing conformation of the distal limb depends upon the integrity of the flexor tendons, changes in conformation can serve as a guide to the structures involved in tendon trauma. Hyperextension ("dropping") of the fetlock, with normal foot placement, indicates superficial digital flexor tendon (SDFT) separa-tion. Hyperextension of the fetlock, with distal interphalangeal extension, resulting in a dropped fetlock and elevation of the toe, indicates SDFT and deep digital flexor tendon (DDFT) severance. Normal fetlock conformation with toe elevation suggests DDFT failure alone, in which case the lesion is likely to be in the region of the pastern, where the DDFT continues distad to the divided SDFT insertions. Complete collapse of the distal limb, with the fetlock on the ground, indicates severe trauma to both SDFT and DDFT, with failure of the suspensory structures, usually suspensory ligament severance.

Flexor tendon rupture or laceration is not always immediately accompanied by severe lameness, and the practitioner who inspects horses coming off the race track or pulling up after strenuous competitions should pay careful attention to the symmetry of limb extension during weightbearing. Cases may be detected before trainers or owners are alerted by the lameness, which may take up to 30 minutes to become apparent.

Examination of acute flexor tendon injuries should include meticulous palpation of the tendons, in both flexion and normal weightbearing. Lacerations may be obvious, with a large wound on the palmar/plantar aspect of the limb, above or below the fetlock, and exposure of traumatized tendon, but severe tendon lacerations may underlie minor wounds. In the authors' experience, large skin flaps are less likely to be associated with tendon severances than short horizontal wounds with minimal hemorrhage. For this reason, all wounds on the palmar/plantar aspect of the limbs should be suspected of tendon involvement until they are carefully examined. With both lacerations and possible ruptures, the tendons should be carefully palpated as the distal limb is repeatedly flexed and extended to assess the edges and borders of the tendon as it glides through the paratenon or sheath. Skin wounds may not be in direct alignment with an underlying tendon laceration. Palpation of the tendon as it moves through the tissues assists in detection of tendon damage, which may be several centimeters away from the skin aperture. If the laceration was sustained during fast work, the lacerations of skin, sheath, and tendon may be aligned only when the distal limb is maximally flexed. For detailed assessment of structures involved in such lacerations, the area should be closely clipped, aseptically prepared (see under Emergency Treatment, later) and manually explored with gloved fingers. Horses usually do not resent gentle digital exploration of these wounds. Partial tendon lacerations are not accompanied by changes in weightbearing conformation, but must be aggressively treated to achieve good repair in the long term.

The neurovascular bundles should always be assessed by direct digital palpation, exploration, and assessment of the pulse amplitude distal to the laceration. This is especially important in cases of laceration of the pastern. Other structures that may be involved in lacerations at the level of the cannon include synovial sheaths, suspensory ligament, splint bones, proximal sesamoids, and periosteum. Wounds with tendon laceration distal to the fetlock may also affect collateral joint ligaments, synovial joint capsules, distal sesamoidean ligaments, and lateral cartilages, as well as the phalangeal bones themselves.

Flexor tendon ruptures without skin penetration usually involve the SDFT and are most often encountered in steeplechasers and hurdlers. Two sites appear predisposed to overload rupture during racing; the majority of cases occur at the proximal limit of the digital sheath in the distal third of the metacarpus. Thickening or scarring from previous episodes of tendinitis may be obvious. Initial lameness may be mild, but hyperextension of the fetlock is obvious and, in the acute phase, within 30 minutes of the injury, the rupture may be visible as a depression or notch on the palmar contour of the metacarpus, giving the limb an hourglass appearance. Palpation at this stage is very profitable; with the limb flexed, an index finger or thumb placed firmly across the palmar aspect of the tendons at the site of the suspected rupture clearly encounters the palmar surface of the DDFT. The ends of the tendon may be indistinct. After 30 minutes the SDFT deficit will be filled with exudate and hemorrhage, making the palpation less definitive, and lameness will be more severe.

The second site for overload failure of the SDFT is at the aponeurosis of the SDFT muscle bellies with the tendon at the level of the distal caudal radius. The authors have seen several such cases in steeplechasing Thoroughbreds. Affected horses pull up with obvious hyperextension of the fetlock, but unlike ruptures in the region of the metacarpus, these horses are acutely and severely lame, with signs of great pain, including sweating and pawing of the affected limb. Diagnosis is difficult, because palpation of the tendons distal to the carpus reveals no abnormalities, and there is little initial swelling at the site of the rupture. Differential diagnosis includes non-displaced fractures of the distal radius, carpal fractures, and non-displaced proximal metacarpal fractures. The tendency of the fetlock to sink when attempts are made to bear weight, in the absence of palpable tendon damage, should suggest the possibility of this injury. Tendon rupture due to overload is extremely rare in the hindlimbs.

EMERGENCY TREATMENT WITHIN 12 HOURS OF INJURY

During the acute insult phase of tendon injury (Table 1), the mechanical disruption of the tendon is quickly followed by hemorrhage, edema, local tissue anoxia, and liberation of inflammatory mediators from the damaged cells. The eventual quality of the repair of the tendon

TABLE 1. EMERGENCY TREATMENT OF FLEXOR TENDON RUPTURES AND LACERATIONS

Goal	Treatment
Examination	Palpation, exploration, assessment of conformation
Reduce contamination of lacerations	Clip, shave, manual removal of gross contamination; lavage with 0.2% povidone-iodine at 10 psi
	Application of powder aerosol of bacitracin, polymyxin, neomycin (1:15:50 IU)
Local anti-inflammatory measures	Ice-cold therapy in 30-min cycles repeated three times using ice packs, water frozen in polystyrene cups, Koolpacks, etc.
	Apply topical NSAID gel (piroxicam 0.5%, felbinac 3.17%)
Immobilization	Firm high-volume dressing (cotton tissue, gauze, bandages) from foot to carpus/tarsus + dorsal splint, board splint, Kimzey, Monkey splint, etc.
Systemic anti-inflammatory treatment	IV dexamethasone 0.1 mg/kg IV body weight + IV NSAID (phenylbutazone 4.4 mg/kg or flunixin 1.1 mg/kg)
Systemic antibiosis for lacerations	IV sodium penicillin 50,000 IU/kg and gentamicin 4 mg/kg pending wound culture

greatly benefits from the salvage of as many of the intrinsic tenocytes of the tendon as possible. Emergency treatment of both lacerations and ruptures must therefore be aimed at reducing the release and the effect of the degradative enzymes, free radicals, and inflammatory mediators at the local level. Hemorrhage and edema must be minimized by the intensive use of local cooling agents in regular cycles with pressure bandaging and limb support (see Table 1). Topical nonsteroidal anti-inflammatory drugs (NSAIDs) such as piroxicam or felbinac are applied under firm dressings. Systemic anti-inflammatory therapy should include a single large dose of dexamethasone (0.1 mg/kg IV) and systemic NSAIDs such as flunixin meglumine (1.1 mg/kg). The use of heel wedges to reduce tendon loading represents a misunderstanding of tendon mechanics; elevation of the heel without immobilization of the fetlock simply induces a distal interphalangeal rotation and overloads the SDFT (Fig. 1). Emergency support must include rigid splinting of the distal limb with the dorsal surfaces of all bones in alignment (Fig. 2). Proprietary emergency splints are excellent for this purpose.

In the case of lacerations, contamination should be removed before infection becomes established. This is best achieved by vigorous emergency lavage and irrigation of the wound with large volumes of sterile isotonic fluid, after careful clipping or shaving. Pressures of about 10 psi can be achieved with a hand-held domestic garden sprayer, which can be filled with a solution of povidone-iodine at a maximum rate of 2 ml/L (0.2%), or chlorhexidine (0.5%). Greater pressures carry the risk of driving contamination inwards, and greater solution strengths may be cytotoxic. The wound should be treated in the field with a high-dose combination antibiotic powder aerosol, which innoculates broad-spectrum antibacterial treatment into the wound. Intravenous antibiosis is essential (see Table 1) and sterile

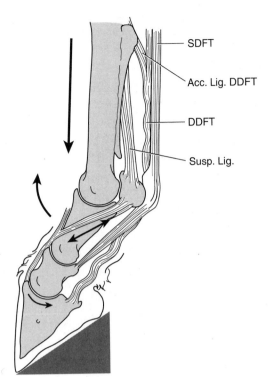

Figure 1. Wedging of the heel induces a distal interphalangeal (DIP) rotation and overloads the SDFT and suspensory ligament.

TABLE 2. MIDTERM MANAGEMENT OF FLEXOR TENDON LACERATIONS AND RUPTURES

Goal	Treatment
Full evaluation	
1. Ruptures	Palpation, ultrasound imaging
2. Lacerations	Exploration and debridement under general anesthesia
	Further lavage with 0.2% povidone-iodine or 0.5% chlorhexidine at 10 psi
	Assess level of contamination/infection; wound swabs + culture
Surgical tendon repair	1. Immediate surgical apposition of severed tendon ends
	or
	2. Immediate partial synovectomy to cause "washboard sheath" production
	or
	3. Delayed repair after course of antibiotics, insertion of wound drains, daily dressing changes and splinting Dexamethasone by mouth 1 mg/50 kg pending repair
Immobilization	Resin or fiberglass cast applied over cotton gauze and sterile dressings
	Stall rest
	Cast change at 3 weeks under sedation or general anesthesia
	Cast removal at 6 weeks
Anti-inflammatory/analgesic therapy	Phenylbutazone 4.4 mg/kg or flunixin 1.1 mg/kg by mouth from day 1
	Discontinue dexamethasone after surgical repair
	IM polysulfated glycosaminoglycans every 3 days for up to 7 doses
Antibiotic therapy	Systemic antibiosis indicated by wound culture; continue for 5 days post-surgery

dressings must be applied. Closure of lacerations and suturing of the severed tendons should not be the immediate goal of emergency therapy in the field. Following initial irrigation and cleansing, the acute inflammation of the laceration should be treated in the same way as a rupture.

MIDTERM MANAGEMENT

Tendon Ruptures

After appropriate emergency treatment and transportation of the horse to the clinic or home stable, detailed assessment of the tendons should be performed by ultrasonographic imaging (Table 2). Completely ruptured tendons offer little prospect of surgical repair because the ends of the tendon are usually massively disrupted. Ruptures within the digital sheath may benefit from exposure to nonsynovial peritendinous tissue, and a partial synovectomy may be indicated. During the induction phase of tendon repair, when the blood clot in the tendon deficit reorganizes into fibroblastic proliferation, granulation tissue production, and tropocollagen deposition, treatment is aimed at immobilization of the tendon system and encouragement of maximal vascularization. This is best achieved by splinting or casting the limb and confining the horse in a small box stall. Forelimbs should be cast with the distal limb in normal weightbearing conformation, because casting in flexion may leave long-term flexural deformities. The reciprocal linkage of the hindlimb means that hindlimb casts are best applied with the distal limb in slight flexion. Concurrent administration of nonsteroidal anti-inflamma-

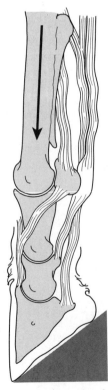

Figure 2. Heel support plus splinting in dorsal alignment is necessary to relieve tension on all flexor structures.

tory drugs limits undesirable ongoing inflammation. A course of polysulfated glycosaminoglycans may improve the quality of the collagen deposition (see Table 2). Casts should be changed at 3 weeks and replaced with firm dressings after 6 weeks.

Tendon Lacerations

Flexor tendon lacerations almost invariably warrant exploration and debridement under general anesthesia. The decision whether to proceed with an immediate attempt at repair, or attempt delayed primary repair at a later date, depends upon the level of contamination and the delay between injury and surgery. If infection is established, radical excision of septic tissues and further lavage are indicated, followed by wound management, which should include drains, regular dressing changes, and splinting. Bacteriologic culture test results indicate appropriate antibiosis, which may be combined with ongoing administration of low-dose oral dexamethasone (see Table 2) to limit fibrosis during the initial prerepair period. Immobilizing the limb with a proprietary splint has the advantage of allowing daily or twice-daily dressing changes. The attempts at surgical reconstruction of the tendon must await the control of the sepsis. Dexamethasone should not be continued after the repair, but antibiotics should continue for 5 further days to cover the inevitable foreign body response to the implanted sutures.

Lacerations in the area of the paratenon may heal with conservative management, and partial flexor tendon lacerations do not benefit from tendon suturing. Total severances within the digital sheath, either above or below the fetlock, do not heal without surgical repair, which should include partial synovectomy and the creating of "washboard sheaths." Details of surgical techniques are given in appropriate surgical texts; monofilament nylon is the repair material of choice and the suture pattern depends upon the structures involved. Locking loops have been very effective in SDFT repair, and pulley loops work well in the more cylindric DDFT. Once elimination of sepsis and surgical repair have been achieved, casting and management should proceed as for ruptured tendons described earlier. The temptation to cast flexor lacerations of the pastern in a flexed position must be resisted because subsequent extension of the pastern will be prohibited (see Table 2). Some separation of tendon ends under limb extension is inevitable, even in a cast.

LONG-TERM MANAGEMENT

Casting of the limb must not be prolonged for more than 6 weeks to avoid the formation of large disorganized scars and adhesions to the peritendinous tissues (Table 3). Cast changing and removal is rendered easier by the use of the alpha$_2$-agonist sedatives, in combination with an opiate (e.g., romifidine 80 µg/kg plus butorphanol 20 µg/kg IV). Once the cast is finally removed, the limb should be firmly dressed for another 3 weeks, with daily application of topical NSAIDs at the site of injury, combined with gentle walking (see Table 3). Lacerations of the DDFT alone are supported at this stage by surgical shoes with extended branches or trailers; special shoes have little to offer SDFT

TABLE 3. LONG-TERM MANAGEMENT OF FLEXOR TENDON RUPTURES AND LACERATIONS

Goal	Treatment
Reassessment	Remove cast
	Ultrasonographic imaging + palpation of tendons
Provide support while limiting adhesions and reducing scar formation	Replace cast with firm soft dressings
	Local application of NSAIDs (piroxicam gel 0.5% or felbinac foam 3.17% t.i.d. for 6 weeks)
	DDFT severances: shoe with extended branch shoes
Remobilize tendon within peritendinous tissue	Controlled walking exercise (in hand) from cast removal 10 minutes b.i.d. for 1 week (after application of local NSAIDs) (support dressings as horse stands in box)
	10 minutes t.i.d. for 3 weeks (after application of local NSAIDs) (replace dressings with firm stable bandages after 4 weeks from cast removal)
	Increase controlled walking for up to 30 minutes b.i.d. for a further 5–6 weeks
	From 10 weeks after cast removal surgical shoes may be discontinued and the horse turned into a small pen with up to 1 hour twice-daily walking
Reassessment	Ultrasonographic evaluation every 3 weeks
	Full pasture liberty when lesion is uniformly echogenic at approximately 16–20 weeks after cast removal

injuries. The regimen for controlled exercise is given in Table 3. Assessment of the quality of the repair is difficult at this stage, because ultrasonographic images reveal massive and apparently disorganized proliferation of tissues at the level of the injury, but 3-weekly assessment helps monitor healing and reorganization. Controlled walking should be continued for at least 10 weeks before the horse is allowed out into a small pen and given prolonged controlled walking; the use of horse-walking machines at this stage is very beneficial. Local NSAIDs should be used to encourage remodeling and tissue mobility for 6 weeks after cast removal. Full pasture liberty should not be permitted for at least 4 to 5 months after cast removal, when the repair tissue is uniformly echogenic, and return to work should not occur within 10 months of the original injury (see Table 3).

PROGNOSIS

Ruptures or contaminated severances of the SDFT alone or together with DDFT carry a poor prognosis for return to competitive work; at best, affected horses may be salvaged for light work, hacking, or breeding. Simple clean severances of the SDFT may respond favorably to repair and the horse may return to extensive work such as hunting or showjumping, but return to racing is unlikely. Partial lacerations of the flexor tendons, if they are intensively treated, may offer a good prognosis for return to the original level of athletic ability. Three principal factors account for failure of cases selected for therapy. Infection may become established within the laceration, because of inappropriate attempts at early closure or because of ineffective initial debridement and lavage coupled with poor antibiotic selection. Nonunion of ruptured or severed tendon ends may result if separation has occurred within the synovial regions that have not been subject to partial synovectomy. In these cases, massive proliferation of synovium and granulation tissue may occur, with persistent discharge from a synovial sinus. The successful repair of the tendon may be ruined by persistent flexural deformities induced by casting the limb in flexion and by prolonging the cast support for too long.

Supplemental Readings

Bertone AL: Tendon lacerations. Vet Clin North Am Equine Pract 11(2):293–314, 1995.
Dyson SJ, Denoix J-M: Tendon, tendon sheath and ligament injuries in the pastern. Vet Clin North Am Equine Pract 11(3):217–233, 1995.
Stashak TS: Management of wounds associated with tendons, paratendons and tendon sheaths. In Equine Wound Management. Philadelphia, Lea & Febiger, 1991, pp 238–257.
Watkins JP: Treatment principles of tendon disorders. In Auer JA (ed): Equine Surgery. Philadelphia, WB Saunders, 1992, pp 916–924.

Proximal Metacarpal or Metatarsal Pain

SUE J. DYSON
Newmarket, England

Lameness associated with pain originating from the proximal metacarpal or metatarsal regions can be the result of a variety of conditions. Because clinical signs other than lameness may be subtle, transient, or absent, local anesthesia is often required to identify the source of pain.

INTERPRETING THE RESPONSE TO LOCAL ANESTHESIA

The principal sensory innervation of the proximal metacarpal region is via the palmar and palmar metacarpal nerves. In the hindlimb, innervation is via the plantar or plantar metatarsal nerves. Ideally, the fetlock and more distal limb should first be excluded as potential sources of pain by perineural analgesia of the palmar/plantar nerves at the mid-cannon and the palmar metacarpal/plantar metatarsal nerves distal to the end of the second and fourth metacarpal/metatarsal bones. In the hindlimb, the dorsal metatarsal nerves should also be anesthetized. It must be borne in mind that local anesthetic solution may diffuse proximally and partially alleviate pain from the proximal metacarpal or metatarsal area, resulting in improvement in lameness.

Perineural analgesia of the palmar metacarpal/plantar metatarsal nerves distal to the carpus/tarsus generally results in substantial improvement of lameness associated with proximal suspensory desmitis, an avulsion fracture of the third metacarpal/metatarsal bone at the origin of the suspensory ligament, or a stress or fatigue fracture of the proximal palmar aspect of the third metacarpal bone. The effect may be due to perineural analgesia itself or to local diffusion of the anesthetic solution. False-positive results may arise from inadvertent deposition of local anesthetic solution into the palmar/plantar outpouchings of the middle carpal/tarsometatarsal joint capsules and alleviation of pain from these joints. False-negative results may be due to injection into the carpal or tarsal sheaths, or more proximal entry of nerve fibers into the painful structure. Perineural analgesia of the ulnar or tibial nerves should substantially improve lameness associated with proximal suspensory desmitis in those horses that fail to respond to subcarpal or subtarsal analgesia, without influencing carpal or tarsal joint pain.

Perineural analgesia of either the medial or lateral palmar metacarpal/metatarsal nerve alone should not substantially influence lameness associated with proximal suspensory desmitis unless an excessive volume of local anesthetic solution is used and pain is alleviated by local diffusion of the anesthetic solution. However, pain associated with a "splint" should be diminished. Perineural analgesia of the palmar or plantar nerves alone should not influence pain associated with proximal suspensory desmitis, an avulsion fracture of the third metacarpal/metatarsal at the origin of the suspensory ligament, or a palmar cortical fatigue fracture, but pain associated with the superficial or deep digital flexor tendons should be reduced.

Therefore, in the differentiation of causes of proximal metacarpal or metatarsal pain it can be very useful to perform separately perineural analgesia of the palmar metacarpal/plantar metatarsal nerves and the palmar/plantar nerves. Given the very close relationship between the palmar metacarpal/plantar metatarsal nerves and the middle carpal/tarsometatarsal joint capsules, the effects of intra-articular and perineural analgesia should be compared. When interpreting the response to intra-articular analgesia it is important to be aware that local anesthetic solution may leak backwards from the palmar/plantar injection sites of the middle carpal/tarsometatarsal joints, which inadvertently may result in perineural analgesia of the palmar metacarpal/plantar metatarsal nerves. The dorsal approach to the middle carpal joint is therefore preferred. Some palmar cortical fatigue fractures extend proximally into the carpometacarpal joint, and lameness is improved by intra-articular analgesia of the middle carpal joint. The clinician should also be aware of paradoxical results; for example, an Arab endurance horse that sustained a sagittal fracture of the third carpal bone and rupture of the medial palmar intercarpal ligament had greater improvement in lameness after perineural analgesia of the palmar metacarpal nerves at subcarpal level, compared with the response to intra-articular analgesia of the middle carpal joint.

PROXIMAL SUSPENSORY DESMITIS

Proximal suspensory desmitis is used to describe lesions of the suspensory ligament confined to the proximal third of the metacarpal or metatarsal region. Avulsion fractures of the third metacarpal or metatarsal bone at the origin of the suspensory ligament are considered to be a separate but allied condition. A fatigue fracture of the palmar cortex of the third metacarpal bone is thought to be an unrelated condition.

Clinical Signs

Proximally, suspensory desmitis occurs in both forelimbs and hindlimbs in horses of all ages and from all disciplines. In forelimbs, during the acute phase, lameness is usually sudden in onset and varies from mild to moderate in degree and often resolves rapidly with rest, but recurs if work is resumed prematurely. There may be slight localized heat, distension of the medial palmar vein, and slight pain when pressure is applied over the proximal aspect of the suspensory ligament. Rarely is local swelling appreciated in the acute phase. The pain is usually less than that associated with either an avulsion fracture of the third metacarpal bone at the origin of the suspensory ligament or a palmar cortical fatigue fracture. In more chronic cases, forelimb lameness tends to be more consistent both within and between examinations. In bilateral cases, the forelimb stride is shortened and trainers may complain of "loss of action." Lameness is often worse when the horse works in a circle with the lame limb on the outside, especially on a soft surface. Careful palpation may reveal slight rounding of the margins of the suspensory ligament at the most proximal level at which they can be palpated, but other localizing signs are frequently absent.

Hindlimb cases are sometimes more insidious in onset, and lameness is often moderate to severe when first recognized. Severely lame horses move with profound asymmetry of the hindquarters, a markedly irregular rhythm, and often a toe drag. Bilateral hindlimb cases may present with poor hindlimb impulsion. In mildly lame horses, lameness may appear more obvious when the horse is ridden. Carpal flexion rarely influences lameness associated with forelimb proximal suspensory desmitis, whereas hock flexion may accentuate lameness in a hindlimb. Fetlock flexion often exaggerates lameness in both forelimbs and hindlimbs.

Forelimb proximal suspensory desmitis is often seen in association with poor foot balance, and a causal relationship may exist. It may also be seen in conjunction with other concurrent causes of lameness such as palmar foot pain; therefore, the combination of distal limb nerve blocks and subcarpal analgesia is important to identify both sources of pain. A causal relationship appears to exist between straight hock conformation and/or hyperextension of the metatarsophalangeal joints and the development of hindlimb proximal suspensory desmitis. Progressive hyperextension of the metatarsophalangeal joint has also been observed as a sequel to hindlimb proximal suspensory desmitis.

Response to Local Anesthesia

Forelimb lameness associated with proximal suspensory desmitis alone is usually improved, although it is rarely alleviated fully by perineural analgesia of the palmar metacarpal nerves. An ulnar nerve block produces a similar or greater improvement in lameness. Lameness is usually not influenced by intra-articular analgesia of the middle carpal joint, provided that a dorsal approach is used. There is a higher incidence of false-negative responses to perineural analgesia of the plantar metatarsal nerves in the hindlimb, but lameness is generally substantially improved by a tibial nerve block. Intra-articular analgesia of the tarsometatarsal joint results in improvement in lameness associated with hindlimb proximal suspensory desmitis in a small proportion of cases.

Ultrasonography

Definitive diagnosis of proximal suspensory desmitis is made by ultrasonographic examination. In view of the considerable variation between horses in the ultrasonographic appearance of the proximal aspect of the suspensory ligament, comparison between contralateral limbs is very important. In most normal horses there is bilateral symmetry between the proximal suspensory ligaments of both the forelimbs and hindlimbs, but hypoechoic areas mimicking lesions are common incidental findings. In the hindlimb, imaging artifacts caused by local blood vessels and the base (head) of the fourth metatarsal bone may compromise interpretation. Air introduced during local analgesia may also confuse interpretation, and if in doubt the horse should be reassessed 24 hours later. Each limb should be viewed in both transverse and sagittal planes. Care should be taken, especially in longitudinal images, not to confuse off-normal incidence artifacts as lesions, particularly at the origin of the suspensory ligament. Abnormalities consistent with proximal suspensory desmitis include one or more of the following:

1. Enlargement of the suspensory ligament
2. Localized well-circumscribed or more diffuse areas of reduced echogenicity
3. Diffuse decrease in echogenicity of the entire cross section of the suspensory ligament
4. Loss of definition of one or more of the margins of the suspensory ligament, especially the dorsal margin
5. Hyperechogenic foci
6. Irregularities of the palmar/plantar cortex of the third metacarpal/metatarsal bone (entheseophyte formation).

The optimal time to examine the suspensory ligament ultrasonographically after the first recognition of lameness is still unknown. Some lesions are readily apparent within

24 hours, whereas some are more obvious 7 to 10 days later. In bilaterally lame horses, structural abnormalities of the suspensory ligament cannot always be identified in the less lame limb. In a small proportion of horses the only discernible abnormality is enlargement of the suspensory ligament.

Radiography

Radiographic examination is performed to identify secondary radiologic abnormalities and to exclude other potential causes of lameness. Secondary radiologic abnormalities are best identified in lateromedial and dorsopalmar/dorsoplantar projections. They include thickening of the palmar/plantar cortex of the third metacarpal/metatarsal bone, sclerosis of subchondral trabeculae and entheseophyte formation, and occasionally radiolucent areas. Comparison with the contralateral limb is useful. Radiologic abnormalities are identified more commonly in hindlimbs than forelimbs, and probably reflect the chronicity of the injury, possibly subclinically. Ultrasonography is a more sensitive indicator of entheseophyte formation than is radiography.

Nuclear Scintigraphy

Few good correlative studies have been made between the ultrasonographic findings associated with proximal suspensory desmitis and the results of nuclear scintigraphic examination. The nuclear scintigraphic findings are rather nonspecific and include increased uptake of technetium (Tc 99m) in the region of the proximal palmar/plantar aspect of the third metacarpal/metatarsal bone.

Treatment

The response to treatment of proximal suspensory desmitis is considerably better in the fore- than the hindlimbs. This may be the result of different biomechanical forces, chronicity of the injury when first recognized, and severity of the injury. In the forelimb, most horses respond well to stall rest and a controlled ascending walking exercise program, combined with corrective trimming and shoeing to restore appropriate foot balance and to provide ample palmar support by the use, for example, of egg bar shoes. In acute cases, lameness usually resolves within 7 to 10 days but is slower to disappear in more chronic cases. Usually, progressive in-filling of lesions is seen ultrasonographically, although enlargement of the ligament may persist. Some lesions fill in to some extent but remain less echogenic than the surrounding ligament. The speed of resolution of lesions is usually proportional to the duration of lameness before initiation of rest. The average convalescence time is 3 months. Premature resumption of work tends to result in recurrent lameness, although some acute injuries have resolved satisfactorily within 6 weeks. Provided that there is no detectable entheseophyte formation, most cases do not recur. The use of internal blisters has been described but generally the author has not found this necessary. A small proportion of cases do experience recurrent lameness; these are usually chronic at the time of first recognition and are associated with entheseophyte formation. They have proved difficult to manage successfully on a long-term basis.

In the hindlimb, the success rate of treatment is compar-atively low, especially in horses with conformational abnormalities of the hindlimbs. The greatest success has been achieved in cases in which the lameness was less than 4 weeks in duration before recognition. Horses have been treated by stall rest, controlled walking, and egg bar shoes. Local injections of corticosteroids, a glycosaminoglycan polysulfate, sodium hyaluronate, and homeopathic remedies do not appear to have materially influenced the outcome. In the cases that have been successfully managed, the lameness has resolved rapidly, within 4 weeks, and there has been progressive improvement in the ultrasonographic appearance of the suspensory ligament. Persistence of lameness is a very poor prognostic indicator. Recent postmortem data suggest that enlargement of the suspensory ligament may result in compression of and secondary damage to the plantar metatarsal nerves, and thus very aggressive anti-inflammatory therapy and strict box rest in the acute phase may be beneficial. Tibial neurectomy has successfully relieved lameness in a small number of horses with chronic unresponsive lameness associated with proximal suspensory desmitis, with no untoward sequelae to date.

AVULSION FRACTURE OF THE THIRD METACARPAL/METATARSAL BONE AT THE ORIGIN OF THE SUSPENSORY LIGAMENT

Avulsion fractures of the third metacarpal/metatarsal bone at the origin of the suspensory ligament occur in both forelimbs and hindlimbs, more commonly in forelimbs. This is usually but not invariably a unilateral injury, which occurs in all types of horses, young (6 years of age or less) racehorses (Thoroughbreds and Standardbreds) predominating. It is considered to be a distinct but allied condition to proximal suspensory desmitis.

Clinical Signs

Usually there is an acute onset of moderate to severe lameness, which is associated with a marked pain response to pressure applied over the proximal suspensory ligament. Lameness in forelimbs and the response to palpation in both forelimbs and hindlimbs tend to be greater than those associated with proximal suspensory desmitis alone. Lameness tends to be worse on hard ground, but may be accentuated on a circle with the lame forelimb on the outside. There may be localized heat and edema in the acute phase. Foot imbalance may be a predisposing factor.

Response to Local Anesthesia

Lameness is usually improved by subcarpal or subtarsal analgesia of the palmar metacarpal or plantar metatarsal nerves. This may be the effect of local diffusion of anesthetic solution. Only rarely are ulnar or tibial nerve blocks required.

Ultrasonography

Ultrasonography may be more sensitive than radiography in the detection of acute, small avulsed fragments, especially if they are minimally displaced. They are most readily detected in longitudinal images of the palmar/plantar cortex of the third metacarpal/metatarsal bone and are seen as a discontinuity in the bone outline. Ultrasonography is certainly more sensitive than radiography in detecting callus formation in the healing phase. There is usually a localized hypoechoic defect in the suspensory ligament at the site of the avulsion.

Radiography

Dorsopalmar/dorsoplantar or slightly oblique dorsopalmar/dorsoplantar views are best for radiographic detection of an avulsion fracture. The radiologic appearance is usually of a crescent-shaped horizontal radiolucent line that may occur in the center of the bone or more toward either the medial or lateral aspect. Occasionally, a "punched-out" radiopaque fragment can be seen.

Nuclear Scintigraphy

Nuclear scintigraphy examination should not be necessary to diagnose this condition, but an avulsion fracture will result in focal increased uptake of Tc 99m in the palmar/plantar cortex of the third metacarpal/metatarsal bone.

Treatment

Stall rest is the only treatment required. Lameness is generally slow to resolve. Monitoring of healing is most accurately done ultrasonographically. A convalescent period of from 3 to 6 months is usually necessary. Once moderate callus formation is detectable ultrasonographically, walking exercise may commence. The majority of horses make a complete recovery, and the incidence of reinjury is low.

PALMAR CORTICAL FATIGUE OR STRESS FRACTURES OF THE THIRD METACARPAL BONE

Palmar cortical fatigue fractures have also been called incomplete longitudinal fractures of the third metacarpal bone. They have only been recognized in forelimbs and occur predominantly in young horses undergoing an increase in work intensity. They occur both unilaterally and bilaterally and are unrelated to injuries of the suspensory ligament.

Clinical Signs

Lameness or "loss of action" is usually sudden in onset, improves somewhat with rest, and deteriorates with work. Lameness is worst on hard ground and varies from mild to moderate in degree between horses. During an examination period, the lameness tends to deteriorate the farther the horse trots, decreases after the horse is walked and turned around, and then deteriorates again as the horse trots farther. Usually there is no detectable heat or swelling, although occasionally distension of the middle carpal joint capsule is observed. The response to firm palpation over the proximal suspensory ligament is variable. Distal limb flexion usually does not alter the lameness.

Response to Local Anesthesia

Lameness is usually substantially improved by perineural analgesia of the palmar metacarpal nerves distal to the carpus, or the effect of local diffusion of anesthetic solution. Intra-articular analgesia of the middle carpal joint has improved lameness in horses in which the fracture has been seen radiologically to extend close to the carpometacarpal joint.

Ultrasonography

No ultrasonographic abnormalities of either the palmar cortex of the third metacarpal bone or the suspensory ligament have been identified by the author.

Radiography

Almost invariably there is diffuse sclerosis of the proximomedial aspect of the third metacarpal bone seen in a dorsopalmar projection. In some horses this is the only detectable radiologic abnormality, especially in the less lame limb of a bilaterally lame horse. Often there is a longitudinally orientated radiolucent line, within the sclerotic region, extending a variable distance proximodistally. Occasionally this lucent line extends as far proximally as the carpometacarpal joint or as far distally as the principal nutrient foramen.

Treatment

Lameness usually resolves within 7 to 14 days of initiation of box rest. Horses are confined to box rest for 2 months and then start walking exercise, slowly resuming normal work after 3 months. At 3 months after injury, the radiolucent lines are no longer detectable, although some sclerosis persists. This sclerosis becomes inapparent by 12 months after injury. The incidence of reinjury is exceedingly low.

DEGENERATIVE JOINT DISEASE OF THE CARPOMETACARPAL JOINT

Degenerative joint disease of the carpometacarpal joint is a relatively unusual condition and is characterized radiologically by narrowing of the joint space (usually more on one side than the other) and small subchondral lucent zones and new bone formation on the most narrowed side of the joint, extending distally along the proximal metaphysis of the small metacarpal bone. The etiology of the condition is unknown. This condition is important in the differential diagnosis of proximal metacarpal pain because the moderate unilateral lameness is improved in most horses by perineural analgesia of the palmar metacarpal nerves distal to the carpus. Generally, no localizing clinical signs are apparent. No ultrasonographic abnormalities have been identified. The author has no experience with the results of nuclear scintigraphy. Neither rest nor intra-articular medication with sodium hyaluronan, glycosaminoglycan polysulfates, or corticosteroids has resulted in long-term remission of lameness.

OSSEOUS CYST-LIKE LESIONS OF THE SECOND AND FOURTH CARPAL BONES

Osseous cyst-like lesions of the second and fourth carpal bones are radiologic findings of uncertain clinical significance. These lesions can be seen in normal horses. Although they are often bilaterally symmetrical, lameness associated with pain localized to the proximal metacarpus may be unilateral. These radiologic abnormalities of the second and fourth carpal bones are seen most commonly in association with the presence of either a first or fifth carpal bone, respectively. A concurrent lucent zone also may be present in the base of the second or fourth metacarpal bone. The radiologic appearance of the lesions does not change with time. The author considers that these radiologic observations are generally not of clinical significance, but has not had the opportunity to use nuclear scintigraphy to examine a horse with proximal metacarpal pain and no other identifiable cause of lameness.

SUPERFICIAL DIGITAL FLEXOR TENDINITIS RESTRICTED TO THE PROXIMAL METACARPAL OR METATARSAL REGION

Localized superficial digital flexor tendinitis restricted to the proximal metacarpus or metatarsus occasionally occurs in horses of all ages and disciplines, although in the author's experience the incidence appears to be greatest in the forelimbs of old dressage horses. There is generally localized "thickening" although definitive enlargement of the superficial digital flexor tendon may be difficult to assess by palpation. There may be slight peritendinous edema and heat and slight pain on palpation. If the lesion extends proximally there may be distension of the carpal sheath (see page 17). There is usually mild lameness, which is worse on soft ground. Lameness is not influenced by palmar metacarpal/plantar metatarsal nerve blocks distal to the carpus/tarsus but is improved by palmar/plantar nerve blocks. Diagnosis is confirmed ultrasonographically by identification of an enlarged tendon, with either a central hypoechoic area or a diffuse reduction in echogenicity. Treatment with rest alone has resulted in rapid resolution of lameness in the hindlimbs of young Thoroughbred racehorses, with resolution of the lesion ultrasonographically

and successful return to work within 6 months of injury. The success of treatment of proximal forelimb injuries has been more variable with particularly poor results in older horses. Lesions have been slow to resolve ultrasonographically and hypoechoic defects have often persisted long-term, with recurrent lameness on return to work. Tendon splitting or local injection of sodium hyaluronan or glycosaminoglycan polysulfate has not appeared to influence the long-term outcome. Treatment with β-aminoproprionitrile fumarate* may offer the best prognosis.

DEEP DIGITAL FLEXOR TENDINITIS

Deep digital flexor tendinitis restricted to the proximal metacarpus has not been recognized by the author or described in the literature except in conjunction with desmitis of its accessory ligament (see page 27), but it has been seen in the proximal metatarsus in young Thoroughbreds in racehorse training. There is diffuse filling of the proximal metatarsus, localized heat and slight pain associated with mild to moderate lameness. Lameness is improved by perineural analgesia of the plantar nerves. Diagnosis is made by ultrasonography. Abnormalities include enlargement of the deep digital flexor tendon, poor definition of the margins, and a localized or more diffuse reduction in echogenicity. The response to conservative treatment by stall rest for 2 months has been good and the incidence of recurrent injury low.

Supplemental Readings

Dyson S: Problems encountered in equine lameness diagnosis with special reference to local analgesic techniques, radiology and ultrasonography. Newmarket, England, R & W Publications Ltd, 1995.

Dyson S, Arthur M, Palmer S, Richardson D: Suspensory ligament desmitis. Vet Clin North Am Equine Pract 11(2):177–215, 1995.

Palmer SE, Genovese R, Longo KL, Goodman N, Dyson S: Practical management of superficial digital flexor tendinitis in the performance horse. Vet Clin North Am Equine Pract 10(2):425–481, 1994.

*Bapten, Alaco Inc., Tucson, AZ

Noninfectious Conditions of the Digital Flexor Tendon Sheath

ALISTAIR R. S. BARR
Bristol, England

TENOSYNOVITIS

Tenosynovitis refers to inflammation of the synovial lining of a tendon sheath. This usually results in distension of the sheath with excess synovial fluid and hence a visible and palpable, often fluctuant, swelling. In the case of the digital flexor tendon sheath (DFTS) this is usually most apparent on either side of the superficial and deep digital flexor tendons for approximately 8 cm proximal to the metacarpo/metatarsophalangeal joint. Smaller lateral and medial swellings are sometimes also apparent just distal to the metacarpo/metatarsophalangeal joint. At the level of the metacarpo/metatarsophalangeal joint itself, the DFTS is constrained by an annular ligament. On the palmar/plantar aspect of the digit, the DFTS is constrained by digital annular ligaments. Nonseptic inflammation of the DFTS may be primary and associated with overstretching of the sheath or, less commonly, direct blunt trauma. Inflammation also may be the result of conditions of the contained flexor tendons or the annular ligament.

Benign (Idiopathic) Tenosynovitis

Many horses have bilaterally symmetrical, mild to moderate distension of the DFTS over a prolonged period of time, without associated evidence of pain or lameness. This is particularly common in the hindlimbs. The condition, known colloquially as *wind-galls*, is usually of no functional significance, and treatment is therefore unnecessary.

Acute Tenosynovitis

Acute tenosynovitis may be the result of overstretching of the tendon sheath, most likely as a consequence of hyperextension of the metacarpo/metatarsophalangeal joint, or direct trauma. There may be accompanying damage to the digital flexor tendons within the sheath.

Clinical Signs

Acute tenosynovitis is characterized by the rapid and recent onset of DFTS distension, accompanied by local signs of increased skin surface temperature, pain on palpation or metacarpo/metatarsophalangeal joint flexion, and varying degrees of lameness. Ultrasonographic scanning confirms the presence of an increased volume of fluid within the DFTS and may show additional digital flexor tendon damage, if this is present as a complicating feature.

Treatment

Treatment involves prevention of further mechanical damage by initial stall rest and support bandaging; local anti-inflammatory treatment with cold water or ice; systemic nonsteroidal anti-inflammatory drugs such as flunixin meglumine (1.1 mg/kg s.i.d.), phenylbutazone (2.2 mg/kg b.i.d.), or ketoprofen (2.2 mg/kg s.i.d.); intrasynovial sodium hyaluronate (20 mg into the DFTS); systemic (500 mg IM q4 days up to 7 occasions) or intrasynovial (250 mg into the DFTS) polysulfated glycosaminoglycan; or intrasynovial, low-dose, short-acting corticosteroids such as betamethasone (10 mg into the DFTS). Intrasynovial treatments should be preceded by drainage of excess synovial fluid from the sheath and followed by support bandaging, to try to limit recurrence of the swelling. Once the acute signs of inflammation have subsided, the horse should be put onto a program of controlled exercise of gradually increasing intensity. Most uncomplicated cases of acute tenosynovitis resolve satisfactorily within 2 to 6 weeks.

Chronic Tenosynovitis

Chronic tenosynovitis may be a sequel to acute tenosynovitis or a more insidious result of chronic repetitive trauma. It may be complicated by coexistent lesions including adhesions within the DFTS, tendon sprain injuries, synovial masses, and desmitis of the annular ligament.

Clinical Signs

Chronic tenosynovitis is characterized by persistent DFTS distension with associated lameness, which is usually mild to moderate in severity. The lameness should demonstrably improve in response to intrasynovial analgesia of the DFTS. Ultrasonographic scanning confirms the presence of an increased volume of fluid within the DFTS and often shows additional features, including thickening of the synovial lining of the DFTS, adhesion formation, synovial masses, digital flexor tendon damage, or thickening of the annular ligament. Particular care should be taken when scanning the DFTS to check for small core lesions in the deep digital flexor tendon (DDFT), which appear to substantially reduce the prognosis for return to athletic activity.

Treatment

Simple cases of chronic tenosynovitis of the DFTS may respond to a program of rest and controlled exercise of gradually increasing intensity, coupled with medical therapy as outlined for acute tenosynovitis. More complex cases with adhesions, synovial masses, or annular ligament constriction are usually candidates for surgical treatment. Surgery may be performed by open incision into the DFTS or endoscopically, and may involve various combinations of resection of adhesions, removal of synovial masses, sectioning of the annular ligament, and in some cases splitting of core lesions within the digital flexor tendons, depending on the lesions present in individual cases. Postoperatively intrasynovial sodium hyaluronate (20 mg) injected into the DFTS may help to reduce further adhesion formation. A specific program of progressively increasing walking exercise should be instituted as soon as the surgical wounds have healed satisfactorily, to further hinder the development of adhesions. The timing of return to work varies according to the lesion from 3 months with uncomplicated annular ligament thickening to 6 to 12 months for horses with DDFT core lesions.

ANNULAR LIGAMENT SYNDROME

The metacarpo/metatarsophalangeal annular ligament of the DFTS extends transversely across the caudal aspect of the sheath between the proximal sesamoid bones. It creates, with the intersesamoidean ligament, a relatively indistensible canal through which pass the superficial and deep digital flexor tendons. There is a normal attachment between the annular ligament and the palmar surface of the SDF tendon, through which the tendon receives part of its blood supply.

Annular ligament syndrome refers to the situation where there is constriction of the digital flexor tendons within the DFTS, on the palmar/plantar aspect of the metacarpo/metatarsophalangeal joint as a result of thickening (i.e., desmitis) of the annular ligament itself, or swelling of the tissues within the DFTS, including the synovial lining of the sheath or the digital flexor tendons themselves.

Clinical Signs

The condition may be seen in all types of horse, including ponies, and may affect either a forelimb or a hindlimb. Affected horses present with persistent, usually mild to moderate lameness associated with distension of the DFTS. There is often a shortened caudal phase to the stride on the affected limb, which is particularly noticeable at the walk. The constriction caused by the annular ligament may be visible as an indentation in the palmar/plantar outline of the limb at the level of the metacarpo/metatarsophalangeal joint in some horses, whereas in others and particularly in ponies, the thickened annular ligament presents as a firm swelling at the same level.

Ultrasonographic scanning usually reveals thickening of the annular ligament, which may be compared with the normal contralateral limb if there is doubt. Care should be taken to check carefully for the other lesions described earlier that may be associated with chronic tenosynovitis of the DFTS, because their presence affects treatment and prognosis.

Treatment

Medical therapy is usually unrewarding in horses with established DFTS constriction at the level of the annular ligament. Surgical division of the ligament carries a good prognosis in uncomplicated cases. Surgery may be performed by open incision into the DFTS or endoscopically.

The digital sheath appears to be particularly prone to iatrogenic infection, and rigid aseptic technique should always be adhered to when performing annular ligament desmotomy, despite the apparent simplicity of the surgery. An endoscopic technique employing a specifically designed slotted cannula to guard and guide a knife blade has been described and has potential advantages in terms of minimizing surgical trauma and reducing the risks of infection and wound dehiscence.

As outlined earlier for the surgical management of chronic tenosynovitis in general, postoperative treatment with intrasynovial sodium hyaluronate (20 mg) injected into the DFTS and a specific program of progressively increasing walking exercise help to reduce adhesion formation. Uncomplicated, surgically treated cases can usually return to work approximately 3 months postoperatively. The prognosis in these horses is good; however, extensive adhesions or concomitant DDFT injuries worsen the prognosis.

TENDINITIS WITHIN THE DFTS

Tendinitis of the superficial digital flexor tendon (SDFT) most commonly affects the tendon throughout most of the metacarpal region, with an extensive core or diffuse lesion. If this damage extends into the DFTS, it may be associated with tenosynovitis and possible annular ligament syndrome. Treatment is usually as for SDFT tendinitis in general, with initial complete rest and local and systemic anti-inflammatory treatment and later a specific program of controlled exercise of progressively increasing intensity. Associated acute or chronic tenosynovitis and/or annular ligament syndrome are treated as outlined earlier. The prognosis for SDFT injuries does not appear to be radically altered by the fact that they extend into the region of the digital sheath. DDF tendinitis is much less common, but when it does occur it is often seen as a very focal lesion within the DDFT at, or most commonly just above, the level of the metacarpo/metatarsophalangeal joint. Fore- or hindlimbs may be affected, and the condition may present as an acute or chronic tenosynovitis of the digital sheath. Concomitant annular ligament thickening may be present in up to one third of cases. The prognosis for DDFT injuries within the digital sheath is generally poor, with only a minority of horses ultimately able to return to sustained athletic activity.

Supplemental Readings

Dik KJ, Van Den Belt AJM, Keg PR: Ultrasonographic evaluation of fetlock annular ligament constriction in the horse. Equine Vet J 23:285–288, 1991.

Genovese RL, Rantanen NW, Hauser ML, Simpson BS: Diagnostic ultrasonography of equine limbs. Vet Clin North Am Equine Pract 2:145–226, 1986.

Gerring EL, Webbon PM: Fetlock annular ligament desmotomy: A report of 24 cases. Equine Vet J 16:113–116, 1984.

Nixon AJ, Sams AE, Ducharme NG: Endoscopically assisted annular ligament release in horses. Vet Surg 22(6):501–507, 1993.

Reef VB, Martin BB, Elser A: Types of tendon and ligament injuries detected with diagnostic ultrasound: Description and followup. Proc 35th Annu Conv Am Assoc Equine Pract 1988, pp 245–248.

Splints, Fractures of the Second and Fourth Metacarpal/Metatarsal Bones, and Associated Suspensory Ligament Desmitis

SCOTT E. PALMER
Clarksburg, New Jersey

Injuries of the small, second and fourth, metacarpal/metatarsal bones and the suspensory ligament are extremely common in the performance horse. Acute periosteal proliferative reactions known as *splints* often cause lameness in young horses but may not be clinically significant in mature animals. Fractures of the proximal portion of the small metacarpal/metatarsal bones are usually the result of external trauma and are often contaminated. Fractures of the distal portion of these bones are usually associated with suspensory ligament desmitis and are caused by the stresses of athletic training and competition. Injury of these structures can destabilize and eventually lead to degenerative changes of the fetlock joint. The prognosis and management of these injuries depend upon whether the injury is acute or chronic at the time of presentation, and vary with the extent of injury and number of components of the suspensory apparatus that are involved.

SPLINTS

Clinical Signs and Diagnosis

Splints, a proliferative periostitis of the second and fourth metacarpal/metatarsal bones, are most commonly seen in the forelimbs of young horses, but may also occur in the hindlimbs. Because of anatomic considerations, the second metacarpal bone is most commonly involved. Periostitis produces a proliferative exostosis or callus, as a response to sprain of the interosseous ligament, external trauma, or fracture of the small metacarpal/metatarsal bones. *Blind splints* represent trauma to the interosseous ligament that is unaccompanied by a bony callus. Horses with active splints usually have localized soft tissue swelling, and they resent palpation of the proximal and medial aspect of the small metacarpal/metatarsal bones when the limb is held in flexion.

Radiographic signs of splints include thickening of the diaphysis of the small metacarpal/metatarsal bones and periosteal proliferative changes in the vicinity of the interosseous ligament. It is important to recognize that splints are not always a cause of lameness. In many cases, splints simply represent a historic record of the stress of training early in a horse's career and are a cosmetic lesion. Scintigraphic imaging using technetium 99m bound to methylene diphosphonate can help to distinguish metabolically active from healed lesions. Phase 3 bone scans are generally performed 2 hours after radiopharmaceutical injection, allowing the isotope to clear vascular and extracellular fluid spaces. Increased uptake of the radiopharmaceutical preparation in the area of a splint at that time indicates increased metabolic and vascular activity associated with an active lesion. The relative contribution of splints to a current lameness may also be determined by use of local anesthesia.

Treatment and Prognosis

Simply discontinuing training for 30 to 60 days eliminates lameness associated with most uncomplicated splints. Medical therapy is primarily directed at reducing the time of inactivity and keeping affected horses in a relatively active training program. Treatment of acute splints should include both systemic anti-inflammatory medication and topical physical therapy to reduce swelling and pain associated with the injury. Physical therapy may include daily cold water or ice application and whirlpool treatments. Acute splints may also be treated by subcutaneous injection with corticosteroids such as isoflupredone acetate (10 mg) and compression bandaging. Additionally, horses may be referred to veterinarians licensed to handle nuclear medicine materials for interstitial implant radiotherapy to desensitize the area. Appropriate isolation of the horse should be enforced when using radioactive implants. Cryosurgical therapy also eliminates the local pain associated with splints, although focal necrosis and secondary granulation tissue formation of the overlying skin may require additional medical treatment and cause a cosmetic blemish.

Chronic splints are rarely a cause of lameness in older performance horses and should be confirmed as a cause of lameness by use of local anesthesia before treatment. Chronic splints that are associated with clinical signs of acute inflammation are treated with systemic anti-inflammatory medication such as phenylbutazone (4.4 mg/kg IV or p.o. b.i.d.) in conjunction with topical application of dimethyl sulfoxide (DMSO) gel or solution. Those cases not accompanied by inflammatory signs are treated by counterirritation, including liniments, blisters, and pin firing. Selection of specific counterirritant therapy is made on an individual basis, usually with regard to the degree of

45

lameness and type of training program. Liniments and mild blisters are preferred in the treatment of Thoroughbred and Standardbred racehorses, if the horse is sound enough to be kept in training. Pin firing is usually reserved for those cases in which the horse is taken out of training for 30 to 60 days. It is important to acquire a good history of previous treatment before using pin firing, because recent use of corticosteroids may complicate the healing process of pin firing and increase the risk of infection.

Impingement of a splint on the suspensory ligament is diagnosed by palpation with the limb held in flexion of a pronounced axial callus, with tenderness of the adjacent portion of the suspensory ligament. In such cases or when the splint becomes a cause of interference, surgery may be considered to remove the exostosis. Although this procedure is successful in most cases, new bone growth that can exceed that of the original callus may develop postoperatively at the surgery site. Owners interested in the cosmetic outcome of this procedure should be advised of this potential complication before surgery. Meticulous hemostasis, elimination of dead space, use of a Penrose drain, and compression bandages postoperatively help to minimize the development of a postoperative callus. Splints that are caused by interference can be successfully treated only by eliminating the underlying cause of the interference. Although the prognosis for treatment of splints is good in most instances, cases in which poor conformation, such as a base-narrow, toe-out conformation, is a primary cause of interference have a guarded to poor long-term prognosis.

FRACTURES OF THE SMALL METACARPAL/METATARSAL BONES

Clinical Signs and Diagnosis

Acute fractures of the small metacarpal/metatarsal bones are characterized by localized heat, pain and swelling, and varying degrees of lameness. Lameness may be increased following passive flexion of the fetlock joint. Thorough palpation of the small metacarpal/metatarsal bones is conducted first with the limb in a normal standing position while the suspensory ligament is under tension and, second, with the limb flexed from the carpus to relax the suspensory ligament and flexor tendons, allowing complete digital examination of the medial aspect of the small metacarpal/metatarsal bones, as well as the origin, body, and branches of the suspensory ligament. Radiographic examination typically reveals a transverse fracture line through the diaphysis of the small metacarpal/metatarsal bone. Incomplete fractures are frequently associated with periosteal proliferative changes or thickening of the diaphysis of the small metacarpal/metatarsal bones. In some cases, the distal portion of the bone may deviate abaxially at an acute angle, in association with thickening and fiber disruption of the suspensory ligament.

Treatment and Prognosis

Treatment of acute fractures of the second or fourth metacarpal/metatarsal bones initially involves reduction of associated soft tissue inflammation. Systemic and topical therapy is the same as that for acute splints and usually eliminates local edema within 7 to 10 days. Once the acute inflammation has resolved, fractures involving the distal segment of these bones are best treated by removal of the fractured portion in conjunction with removal of exostoses that may be present. In the racehorse, nonsurgical management of distal fractures often leads to delayed union or nonunion, with a protracted healing phase that most trainers find unacceptable. Treatment of associated suspensory ligament desmitis should be administered as necessary. Fractures of the proximal portions of the second and fourth metacarpal/metatarsal bones are often successfully treated with stall rest and compression bandaging. Such fractures should be radiographically monitored during a healing interval that averages 4 to 6 months. In some cases, internal fixation may be required. Although some surgeons recommend screw fixation of the proximal segment of the small metacarpal/metatarsal bones to the third metacarpal/metatarsal bone when more than the distal one half or two thirds of those bones is removed, this author has not found this practice to be gratifying. Removal of the entire small metacarpal/metatarsal bone has been reported, but removal may be associated with residual lameness, particularly in the case of fractures of the second metacarpal/metatarsal bone. In this author's opinion, fractures of the proximal segment of these bones are best treated with nonsurgical management or by internal fixation techniques, such as Association for the Study of Internal Fixation (ASIF) finger plates, that provide for retention of the distal portion of the bone whenever possible.

Contaminated, comminuted, and compound fractures of the small metacarpal/metatarsal bones should be treated with systemic antimicrobial drugs, based upon results of culture and sensitivity testing, anti-inflammatory medication, and compression bandaging. In light of potential septic arthritis of the carpometacarpal or tarsometatarsal joints in these cases, therapeutic levels of appropriate antimicrobial medication should be administered for approximately 6 weeks. Debridement and removal of sequestered fragments may speed resolution of these cases.

Chronic fractures of the second or fourth metacarpal/metatarsal bones that are healing well, with minimal callus, and are not associated with lameness may be managed conservatively. Fractures that are associated with soft tissue inflammation and represent a confirmed cause of lameness are best treated by systemic and/or local anti-inflammatory medication and physical therapy as for acute fractures. In cases when the fracture is unstable or the callus is impinging upon the body of the suspensory ligament, surgery to remove the fractured distal segment and its associated callus is indicated, just as in the case of acute fractures.

Postoperative management of splint fractures typically includes 2 to 4 weeks of stall rest, followed by 4 to 6 weeks of walking in hand. A follow-up ultrasonographic examination of the associated suspensory ligament should be performed at the end of this walking period and before a return to active training. Because this type of injury can be associated with contralateral suspensory ligament injury, ultrasonographic evaluation of the contralateral limb may be indicated in some cases. The length of time spent out of training is a function of the degree of associated suspensory ligament trauma. Rehabilitation of these horses is the same as that described for suspensory ligament desmitis.

The prognosis for treatment of fractures of the small metacarpal/metatarsal bones depends upon the presence and degree of suspensory ligament injury. The prognosis for athletic activity is good, provided that there is limited associated suspensory ligament involvement. The prognosis worsens according to the extent and chronicity of suspensory ligament damage.

SUSPENSORY LIGAMENT DESMITIS

Clinical Signs and Diagnosis

Injury of the suspensory ligament is characterized by inflammation and thickening of the body or branches of the ligament and decreased range of motion of the fetlock joint in chronic cases. If the support of the fetlock joint is compromised by injury of the suspensory apparatus, unphysiologic loading and degenerative changes can occur within that joint. Suspensory ligament injuries may be evaluated by applying digital pressure to an apparently painful region of the suspensory ligament for 1 minute, then jogging the horse to see if the lameness is aggravated. Because fractures of the small metacarpal/metatarsal bones and the proximal sesamoid bones often accompany injury of the body or branches of the suspensory ligament, radiographic assessment of these structures should be a routine part of the diagnostic evaluation of suspensory ligament injury.

Ultrasonographic evaluation of the suspensory ligament is best accomplished with a 7.5-MHz transducer. Although a standoff is not required to evaluate the body, it may be helpful to evaluate the branches of the suspensory ligament. Sonographic evidence of suspensory ligament injury may include enlargement, core lesions, fluid infiltration, or diffuse fiber disruption. Lesions of the suspensory ligament should be imaged in both the transverse and longitudinal plane to accurately define the limits of the lesion and to minimize the chance of erroneous interpretation. Lesions may be graded as type 1 to 4, according to the same standards published for classification of tendon injuries (see *Current Therapy in Equine Medicine 3*, pages 140–143). Although many lesions of the suspensory ligament are easily imaged, ultrasonographic evidence of fiber disruption at the junction of the body and branches of the suspensory ligament or at the insertion onto the abaxial borders of the proximal sesamoid bones may be difficult to detect. In cases when injury to these sites is suspected on the basis of clinical signs such as localized pain or swelling, the contralateral limb should be examined ultrasonographically for comparison. Acute lesions should have a follow-up scan performed 10 to 14 days after the start of anti-inflammatory therapy to more accurately assess the degree of fiber disruption.

Nuclear scintigraphy may also be useful for diagnostic evaluation of suspensory ligament injury. The soft tissue phase (phase 2) of the examination is performed within 20 minutes of radiopharmaceutical injection while the isotope is distributed within the capillary bed and extracellular fluid. Localized increased uptake of the isotope in the area of the suspensory ligament at that time is characteristic of suspensory ligament desmitis. This can be of particular importance when evaluating lesions of the proximal portion of the suspensory ligament, because local anesthesia in that area can yield inconclusive and confusing findings.

Treatment and Prognosis

Treatment of acute injury of the suspensory ligament involves use of physical therapy such as application of cold water and ice and whirlpool treatments, compression bandaging, and nonsteroidal anti-inflammatory medication such as phenylbutazone (4.4 mg/kg IV or p.o. b.i.d.). Gelatin-impregnated bandages* soaked in ice water before application are helpful to reduce acute inflammation and support injured tissues. The affected limb may be soaked in a tub of ice water with the bandage in place the day following bandage application. The gelatin bandage should be replaced on alternate days and hydrotherapy continued until the inflammation subsides. Treatment of suspensory ligament injuries during the subacute or chronic phase may involve use of systemic nonsteroidal anti-inflammatory medication as described earlier; local subcutaneous injection of corticosteroids (10 mg isoflupredone acetate); counterirritation with liniments, leg paints, or blisters; and controlled exercise monitored by ultrasonographic evaluation. Specific treatment selection is based upon the degree of inflammation and lameness that may be present and the type and schedule of athletic activity. Core lesions of the suspensory ligament may be split under ultrasonographic guidance to evacuate the hematoma and promote linear fiber arrangement during the healing process. Therapeutic trimming for suspensory ligament injury includes shortening the toe and correcting medial to lateral or dorsal to palmar/plantar imbalance of the digit. Toe grabs and heel caulks should be eliminated, and shoes should have a rolled toe to ease breakover when possible. Bilateral suspensory ligament desmitis is common in all performance breeds because affected horses shift weight between contralateral limbs to compensate for the primary injury. For this reason, support wraps on both the involved and contralateral limbs should be worn during competition.

Ultrasonographic monitoring of healing suspensory ligament injuries is critical to the successful management of these cases. Ultrasonographic evaluation enables the clinician to periodically evaluate the resolution of fiber disruption and suggest a controlled exercise program based upon the degree of uniform echogenicity and linear arrangement of fibers rather than a clinical impression based upon palpation or clinical signs. Training decisions based upon ultrasonographic data reduce the likelihood of reinjury of the suspensory ligament when the horse is returned to active training.

Rehabilitation programs for performance horses with injuries of the suspensory ligament vary considerably according to the breed and degree of injury of the involved tissues. Nevertheless, it is important in all cases to incorporate appropriate recovery intervals within periods of increasing load. On a weekly basis, the schedule should include alternating days of work and rest. The rest day

---

*Gelocast, Beiersdorf, Norwalk, CT

represents relatively light exercise compared with the work day. In the early stages of rehabilitation, rest may mean stall confinement, whereas later in the program a rest day may include swimming, jogging, or even light cantering. On a monthly basis, the work level should gradually increase during the first 3 weeks, then drop back down to the level of week 2 during the final week of the month. The pattern of reducing the level of training in the fourth week back to the level of the second week continues until normal training levels are achieved. Throughout a horse's athletic career, periods of "active rest" should be incorporated into the training program to prevent reinjury.

The prognosis for treatment of suspensory ligament injuries is determined largely by the degree of fiber disruption. As a general rule, Standardbred racehorses are better able to train successfully with chronic injuries of the suspensory ligament than are Thoroughbreds. The reason for this is unclear, but it may be related to the type of training and competition that is unique to this breed, or the increased percentage of muscle fibers present in the suspensory ligament of Standardbreds compared with Thoroughbreds. Although there appears to be significant case to case variation, the author's experience suggests that fiber disruption of the branches of the suspensory ligament suggests a poorer prognosis for future athletic performance than does injury of the body of the suspensory ligament. In general, the more proximal the lesion, the better the prognosis.

Supplemental Readings

Du Preez P: Fractures of the small metacarpal and metatarsal bones (splint bones). Equine Vet Ed 6(5):279–283, 1994.

Dyson SJ, Arthur R, Palmer SE, Richardson D: Suspensory ligament desmitis. Vet Clin North Am Equine Pract 11(2):177–215, 1995.

Hardy J: Sesamoiditis and suspensory desmitis. In Robinson NE (ed): Current Therapy in Equine Medicine 3. Philadelphia, WB Saunders, 1992, pp 140–143.

Lamb CR, Koblik PD: Scintigraphic evaluation of skeletal disease and its application to the horse. Vet Radiol 29(1):16–27, 1988.

Peloso JG, Mundy GD, Cohen ND: Prevalence of, and factors associated with, musculoskeletal racing injuries of Thoroughbreds. J Am Vet Med Assoc 204(4):620–626, 1994.

Ray C, Baxter GM: Splint bone injuries in horses. Comp Cont Ed Pract Vet 17(5):723–731, 1995.

Stashak TS: Lameness. In Adams' Lameness in Horses, 4th ed. Philadelphia, Lea & Febiger, 1987, pp 486–785.

Infection of Digital Flexor Tendon Sheath

TIM J. PHILLIPS
Liphook, England

Infection of the digital flexor tendon sheath results almost invariably from a traumatic penetration. Injuries occur with similar frequencies in fore- and hindlimbs and range from extensive lacerations to small punctures, the point of entry of which may not be obvious by the time of presentation. Typical histories include pitch fork wounding, wire wounds, collisions with sharp objects, or interference injuries. The latter result from the hind feet in the case of forelimbs or from other horses' hooves in the case of hindlimbs. Tendon sheath sepsis resulting from bacteremia has been reported in foals, but is rare compared with the incidence of "joint-ill." The digital flexor tendon sheath sleeves the two flexor tendons and is closely related to a number of other structures, including the suspensory ligament, the proximal sesamoid bones and their ligaments, synovial cavities of the fetlock and interphalangeal joints plus the navicular bursa, and the palmar/plantar and palmar/plantar digital neurovascular bundles. Consequently, there is a high propensity for injury to soft and osseous tissues in association with digital tendon sheath sepsis, and this can have significant bearing on the prognosis of the case. It therefore behooves the clinician to make a comprehensive examination before deciding on the treatment regimen.

DIAGNOSIS

Clinical signs usually have an acute onset. Synovial sepsis of any kind is characteristically very painful, and thus severe lameness can be expected, frequently to the extent that the horse is reluctant to bring the heels of the foot of the affected limb to the ground. Drainage of synovial fluid through an open wound may lead to less pain than might be expected because of the relative lack of distension of the fibrous sheath capsule. However, the soft tissue trauma that typically attends sheath penetrations usually accounts for marked discomfort in any case. Digital pressure applied to intrasynovial structures through the wall of the tendon sheath, or fetlock flexion, are resented by the horse.

Swellings and heat develop, which are localized to the distal limb with their epicenters tending toward the palmar/plantar aspect. Swellings develop intra- or extrathecally. The digital flexor tendon sheath distends in regions where it is not constrained by dense retinacular tissue. Sheath effusions can therefore be palpated as outpouchings occurring (1) proximal to the palmar/plantar annular ligament, medial and lateral to the deep digital flexor tendon; (2) between the palmar/plantar annular ligament and the proximal digital annular ligament, as small medial and lateral pouches on the palmar/plantar aspect of the distal fetlock; (3) collateral to the fetlock plate, as palmarolateral and palmaromedial swellings just below the fetlock level; and (4) distal to the fetlock plate, as a palmar/plantar swelling in the distal pastern. Sites 1 and 4 produce the most readily apparent distensions. In some cases, detection of these synovial outpouchings may be obscured by a more diffuse interstitial cellulitis. If tendon sheath penetration is suspected, but not apparent, it is worthwhile to closely clip the distal limb to inspect the skin for small marks. Clipping is also a necessary prelude to treatment of cases involving overt wounds.

If it is not immediately obvious that a laceration has penetrated the wall of the tendon sheath, passive manipulation of the limb may re-establish leakage of synovium through a track that has become occluded. Failing this, palpation with a blunt probe is indicated, after analgesic and aseptic preparation of the site. If doubt persists, the injection into the sheath of a sterile saline solution through a portal distant to the site of injury may result in a flow of fluid out of the wound, confirming communication with the sheath cavity. Similarly a retrograde radiographic contrast study can be performed using 5 to 10 ml iohexol (300 mg iodine/ml).

Infection of the tendon sheath can be confirmed by laboratory analysis of a synovial aspirate. Any of the sheath outpouchings can provide a suitable site of access to the synovial cavity; however, the proximal pouch is frequently lined by a mass of proliferative and hyperemic synovial membrane, which may obstruct the bore of a needle or may result in substantial hemorrhagic artifact in the sample. The most convenient site for collection is therefore the distal pouch.

The palmar/plantar aspect of the pastern of the affected limb is prepared for an aseptic procedure. An assistant raises the limb off the ground and holds the foot in an extended position, thus maximizing the presentation of the site to the operator. A bleb of local anesthetic solution is placed subcutaneously in the midline directly over the palpable bulge of the distal pouch. A sterile hypodermic needle (18-, 19-, or 20-g, 2.5 or 3.75 cm) is then inserted perpendicularly through the skin into the sheath. Fluid usually flows spontaneously and can be drawn into a syringe, before distribution is made into culture broth bottles or anticoagulant containers. Sometimes flow can be encouraged by "milking" fluid from proximal to distal or by flexing the fetlock passively. Fluid analysis should include at the minimum evaluation of gross appearance and protein content, plus total and differential white cell counts. A Gram's stain can also be useful in guiding antibiotic selection, before culture and sensitivity results become available. The appearance of infected synovial fluid changes with the chronicity of the process. Initially, slightly discolored, thin fluid is produced and this progressively becomes sanguinous to xanthochromic, more turbid with the accumulation of white cells and ultimately flocculent with fibrinous debris. A protein content of greater than 30 g/L is suspicious for infection; greater than 40 g/L is virtually pathognomonic. This value is accompanied by massive white cell infiltration, with total counts ranging from 10 to more than 100×10^9/L. Neutrophils predominate in proportions

greater than 90% and in the active stages of infection many will appear degenerate.

Ultrasonography, using a 7.5-MHz linear scanner, is another means of assessing cases. It is possible to predict infection from the appearance of large quantities of synovial fluid with swirling echogenic particles. However, the procedure often causes discomfort and may be difficult to complete because of lack of patient cooperation. Radiography is indicated to rule in or out concurrent osseous damage, particularly involving the proximal sesamoid bones.

TREATMENT

Infection within a digital flexor tendon represents a clinical emergency. Treatment involves a multivalent approach aimed at debulking the sources of contaminating pathogens, lavaging fluid containing inflammatory mediators and degradative enzymes, administering antibacterial and anti-inflammatory medications, employing physiotherapeutic techniques, and, possibly, giving drugs used to enhance the physiologic repair processes or to inhibit adhesion formation.

Surgery, to a greater or lesser extent, is an integral part of the management. In acute stages, copious lavage of the sheath may suffice. Portals for ingress (14- to 16-g needles), and egress (16- to 18-g needles), should be as distant from each other as possible. Several liters of sterile polyionic solution should be instilled under pressure for through-and-through lavage. Intermittently the egress port should be occluded to distend and irrigate the sheath and thus maximize the debriding effect. Lavage may need to be repeated at 24-, 48-, or 72-hour intervals, depending on response. However, as the infective process progresses, organisms locate in synovial membrane and fibrinopurulent aggregates accumulate, thus defeating the simple lavage technique.

As a general rule, infections beyond 24 hours' duration do not respond to irrigation alone. One alternative is the use of tenoscopy to facilitate the removal of debris and proliferative synovial membrane. However, the degree of difficulty is greater than in analogous arthroscopic procedures, and frequently it is preferable to expose the contents of the sheath, via an incision in the proximal pouch possibly including an annular desmotomy, plus a separate exposure of the distal pouch. Such access allows for performance of radical synovectomy and debridement, which are indicated if success is to be achieved. Insertion of indwelling lavage systems or drains is recommended by some, but their efficacy is frequently thwarted by blockage, dislodging, or potentiation of inflammation, and they are no substitute for a comprehensive surgical procedure in the first instance.

Considering the circumstances under which penetrations occur, bacterial contaminants are likely to comprise mixed species including anaerobes. Although culture and sensitivity testing is ideal, negative results are not uncommon and antibiosis must at least begin on an empirical basis. Broad-spectrum bactericidal drugs are indicated, and a combination of soluble penicillin G (20–40,000 IU/kg IV t.i.d.) plus an aminoglycoside (e.g., gentamicin sulfate, 6.6 mg/kg IV s.i.d. or in three divided doses) is the therapy of choice in most clinics. Metronidazole can be administered orally to combat penicillin-resistant anaerobes, such as *Bacteroides fragilis*. Intrasynovial administration of gentamicin sulfate, either by direct instillation of 100 to 200 mg or by implanting a chain of polymethylmethacrylate beads, each containing 7.5 mg gentamicin, into the proximal sheath is currently enjoying favor in many clinics. Administration of antibiotics into a limb vein distal to a tourniquet can also be considered as a technique to maximize drug concentrations at the site of the pathologic process.

Nonsteroidal anti-inflammatory drugs (NSAIDs) are prescribed both for their analgesic and beneficial anti-inflammatory effects. Phenylbutazone (2.2 mg/kg IV or p.o. b.i.d.) remains the choice for reliable efficacy. A caveat should be considered in that the pain of synovial sepsis is highly susceptible to the analgesic effects of NSAIDs, and a good response does not necessarily equate to a resolution of the infection. The drug should be regularly withdrawn so that signs can be properly monitored and assessment of other parameters (such as sequential synovial fluid analyses) can run hand in hand with treatment. Adding 400 mg dimethyl sulfoxide (DMSO) to the last 2 L of a lavage solution provides another pharmacologic means of counteracting the inflammatory cascade. In addition, 100 mg of high-molecular-weight sodium hyaluronate may be another adjunct to the anti-inflammatory therapy, particularly with a view to minimizing adhesion formation. However, recommendations on the optimal time or frequency of treatment are presently subjective. Deciding when to stop parenteral antibiotic and anti-inflammatory therapy can be a difficult judgment. Therapy for several weeks is sometimes necessary. As a rule of thumb, antibiotics can be withdrawn after signs of ongoing inflammation such as heat, cellulitis, gross exudate, and profound neutrophilia in the synovial fluid have been absent for several days, independent of NSAID administration. Analgesics are often needed for longer periods.

Beyond the treatment aimed specifically at the septic tenosynovitis, further surgical procedures may be warranted to benefit the other consequences of the wound. In particular, lacerations or severance of one or both flexor tendons and the straight sesamiodean ligament distally are relatively common complications. Primary repair of these is often contraindicated in an infected environment, or because of the chronicity of the presentation, but debridement at least is needed. Cases involving fracture of the proximal sesamoid bones may require curettage, and the possibility of extension of infection into the fetlock joint should not be overlooked.

Postoperatively, the mechanical environment provided for the limb becomes an important consideration. Counterpressure bandaging is invariably helpful in the short term because it aids analgesia. The advantage of bandages is the relative ease of regular reinspections of the site and drain management. However, tendon injuries involving substantial tissue deficits make half-limb casting mandatory, perhaps for several weeks. In cases in which acute septic tenosynovitis occurs in isolation, phased mobilization reduces the opportunity for adhesion formation and probably favors the restoration of normal synovial fluid production. However, the coexistence of a severe tendon injury may preclude such therapy.

PROGNOSIS

The prognosis for infected tendon sheaths depends on the virulence and chronicity of the infection, the extent of damage to associated tissues, and financial constraints imposed upon what nearly always amounts to very expensive treatment regimens. Some cases, for instance those with both flexor tendons severed, justify euthanasia. By contrast, a simple puncture wound into the sheath of a hindleg, presented within a few hours of occurrence, represents an eminently treatable scenario, carrying a good prognosis for a full recovery. Often a less than satisfactory outcome results, in which the sepsis has been controlled but return to soundness is prevented by the limited quality of repair to tendinous tissue, or by the development of a secondary complaint, such as annular ligament constriction. The keys to success lie in the early presentation of the case plus a thorough evaluation so that a reasonable prediction of outcome can be made at the outset.

Supplemental Reading

Nixon AJ: Septic tenosynovitis. *In* White NA, Moore JN (eds): Current Practice of Equine Surgery. Philadelphia, JB Lippincott, 1990, pp 451–455.

Disorders of the Proximal Sesamoid Bones

JOANNE HARDY
Columbus, Ohio

The two proximal sesamoid bones are situated palmar (plantar) to the distal metacarpus (metatarsus). They are associated with the fetlock joint by their articular surfaces, which conform to the distal end of the third metacarpal (metatarsal) bone, and the suspensory apparatus through ligamentous attachments. The palmar (plantar) surfaces of the proximal sesamoid bones also provide a gliding surface for the deep digital flexor tendon. The lateral and medial branches of the suspensory ligament, the palmar annular ligament, and the distal sesamoidean ligaments attach to the proximal sesamoid bones and may be involved with sesamoid bone injuries.

SESAMOID FRACTURES

Sesamoid fractures are common injuries of racehorses, but they also occur with lesser frequency in horses used in other disciplines. They typically occur during high-speed training or racing and are usually an acute, single-event injury. Sesamoid fractures may be classified into apical, midbody, basilar, axial or sagittal, and abaxial types. Sagittal or axial fractures usually accompany condylar fractures of the distal metacarpus (metatarsus).

Diagnosis

Horses with a sesamoid fracture usually have an acute, severe lameness after high-speed training or racing. With apical sesamoid fractures, the lameness may be delayed for a few hours, whereas midbody or large basilar fractures are immediately painful. Small basilar fragments are not associated with severe lameness, and clinical signs are similar to those of small osteochondral fragments of the fetlock joint. Edema of the suspensory ligament branch and fetlock joint effusion are often present owing to the close anatomic relationship of these structures. These local signs may resolve with rest and bandaging, particularly with apical sesamoid fractures. Deep palpation of the affected sesamoid bone and flexion of the fetlock joint elicit a painful response. Relief of the lameness is achieved with regional anesthesia of the palmar (plantar) nerves.

The diagnosis is confirmed radiographically. Occasionally, transverse non-displaced fractures may be difficult to demonstrate, or to differentiate from linear radiolucent changes in the sesamoid bone. Axial fractures are best demonstrated using a 125° dorsopalmar projection. Ultrasonographic evaluation of the suspensory and distal sesamoidean ligaments should be performed to evaluate the degree of accompanying desmitis, because suspensory or distal sesamoidean desmitis may be the limiting factor to recovery.

Treatment

Apical, midbody, and basilar sesamoid fractures are amenable to surgical treatment. Surgical removal of apical fractures is recommended to minimize chronic suspensory ligament irritation and can be performed through an arthrotomy or arthroscopic approach. The prognosis for return to the previous level of performance is excellent, provided that there is little or no suspensory ligament desmitis. Midbody and large basilar fragments are under tension during the healing phase and therefore usually undergo displacement and heal with a fibrous union. To improve the quality of healing and obtain a more solid bony union, several surgical techniques have been described, which include lag screw fixation, circumferential wiring, autogenous bone grafting, and a combination of internal fixation and bone grafting. Internal fixation techniques are currently thought to improve outcome. The technique used is dependent on the surgeon's preference. Small basilar osteochondral fragments may be removed through an arthrotomy or by arthroscopic technique.

Prognosis

Horses with apical and small basilar fragments have an excellent prognosis for recovery after fragment removal, provided that there is minimal injury to the suspensory or distal sesamoidean ligaments. Abaxial basilar sesamoid fractures are more likely to be associated with distal sesamoidean desmitis. Horses treated by surgical fixation of midbody or large basilar fragments have a guarded prognosis for return to athletic soundness; horses usually perform at a lower level than before the injury.

SESAMOIDITIS

Sesamoiditis is defined as a local inflammation of the proximal sesamoid bones at the site of ligament attachment, the entheses, which usually affects the attachment of the suspensory ligament on the abaxial surface of the proximal sesamoid bones. Occasionally, an enthesopathy of the attachment of the distal sesamoidean ligament onto the base of the sesamoid bone may be observed. Osteoarthritis of the fetlock joint may result in osteophyte formation at the apical and basilar aspects of the sesamoid bones, which should not be confused with sesamoiditis. Sesamoiditis develops in performance animals, particularly racehorses, and is a performance-limiting injury.

Diagnosis

Lameness caused by sesamoiditis is most evident during periods of hard training or racing, and it subsides with rest.

The lameness is mild (grade 1 to 2 on a scale of 5), but may be more severe the day after training. It is accentuated by fetlock flexion. Thickening of the soft tissues may be apparent around the fetlock, and the horse shows a tendency to hold the fetlock in an upright position. Fetlock joint effusion is absent. Intra-articular anesthesia of the fetlock joint does not improve the lameness, but perineural analgesia of the medial and lateral palmar nerves usually results in obvious improvement.

Radiographic lesions observed with sesamoiditis include lytic and proliferative changes on the abaxial surface of the sesamoid bones at the suspensory ligament insertion. The primary radiographic lesion of sesamoiditis is enlarged linear defects (sometimes referred to as *vascular channels*) measuring 2 mm or more in diameter, which are ill-defined and often have a club-shaped appearance (Fig. 1). These findings have consistently been associated with lameness in a horse in training. In the chronic stage, osseous proliferation may also be observed on the abaxial surface of the proximal sesamoid bones.

In normal horses in training, one or two lytic linear defects less than 1 mm wide are often seen on the abaxial surface of the sesamoid bones, without clinical signs. The number of these linear defects may rise with increased bone remodeling in response to training. Horses affected with other suspensory apparatus injuries, including suspensory desmitis and flexor tendinitis, as well as sesamoid fractures, may also have secondary changes in the sesamoid bones. The presence of three or more well-defined linear defects measuring 1 mm or less in diameter should be considered a reflection of increased bone metabolism resulting from training or inflammatory changes in adjacent structures. It is not diagnostic of sesamoid disease. If such changes are present in association with lameness, the soft tissue structures of the suspensory apparatus should be assessed.

Treatment

Therapy for sesamoiditis is not rewarding. Most horses become sound with rest, only to have recurrence of lameness with speed work. Extended rest periods of 6 to 12 months are advocated. Systemic therapy with nonsteroidal anti-inflammatory drugs (NSAIDs) such as phenylbutazone (4.4 mg/kg s.i.d.) or flunixin meglumine (1.1 mg/kg s.i.d. or b.i.d.) is helpful to control the lameness, particularly after training sessions. Topical therapy including bandaging, administration of dimethyl sulfoxide, and topical sweat bandages is helpful to control the edema and inflammatory reaction. Pin firing and cryosurgery have been recommended with anecdotal success but have not been objectively investigated. Careful trimming and shoeing should provide adequate medial to lateral hoof balance and should minimize stress on the suspensory apparatus. A shorter toe eases breakover, as does removal of toe grabs. The angle of the hoof wall should be parallel to the pastern axis. Excessive heel height increases strain on the suspensory apparatus, but an excessively short heel has the same effect during the breakover phase of the stride at speed. Adjustments in the training schedule, to emphasize extended work periods at lower speeds, may be helpful. Some horses may be able to perform satisfactorily at lower performance levels, if they are given adequate management.

INFECTIOUS OSTEITIS

Infectious osteitis of the proximal sesamoid bones is caused by direct inoculation from a puncture wound or from extension of infection from an adjacent structure. Septic tenosynovitis of the digital flexor tendon sheath, ligamentous infection of a branch of the suspensory ligament from a puncture wound, and septic arthritis of the fetlock joint have all been reported in association with infectious osteitis of the proximal sesamoid bones. Infection of the tendon sheath or joint fetlock may result from puncture wounds, lacerations, hematogenous spread, or injections into these synovial structures.

Diagnosis

The history is of acute, subacute, or chronic lameness of the affected limb. Infectious osteitis of a proximal sesamoid bone should also be suspected in horses with septic tenosynovitis of the digital flexor tendon sheath that suffer recurrent lameness. Pain occurs on both flexion of the fetlock and palpation of the proximal sesamoids; pain also occurs from soft tissue swelling of the fetlock area and

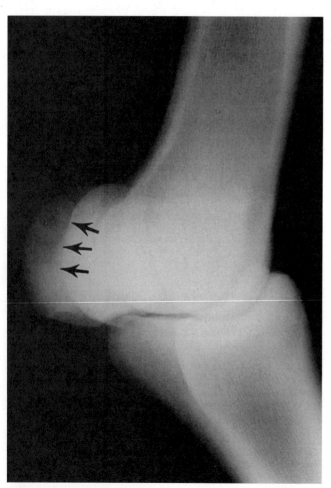

Figure 1. Severe sesamoiditis (*arrows*) of a proximal sesamoid bone. Note the large lytic club-shaped defects on the abaxial surface of the affected sesamoid bone.

tendon sheath effusion. Fetlock joint effusion may also be present. Lameness varies from grade 3 to 5 on a scale of 5. Synoviocentesis of the fetlock joint or digital tendon sheath may reveal inflammation or the result may be consistent with sepsis, but test results may also be normal if the septic process is confined to the sesamoid bone. Synovial fluid should be evaluated cytologically and cultured aerobically and anaerobically.

Radiography reveals lysis at the site of infection (Fig. 2); however, these lesions may not be visible in the acute stages. Radiographic re-evaluation at weekly intervals is therefore recommended. Ultrasonography is useful to detect lesions within the tendon, tendon sheath effusion, flocculent material within the tendon sheath fluid, or an irregular border of the proximal sesamoid bones. Scintigraphy reveals increased uptake in the bone phase in the affected fetlock and is useful to detect early changes. The use of computed tomography, although not widely available, enhances the ability to detect early changes in the sesamoid bone.

Treatment

Aggressive long-term therapy is indicated for infectious osteitis. Adjacent affected structures, such as the digital flexor tendon sheath and fetlock joint should also be treated with local lavage, long-term effective drainage, and systemic and local antibiotic therapy. Common isolates from septic tenosynovitis include *Staphylococcus* species if infection follows an injection or surgery, whereas Enterobacteriaceae and anaerobes are more common following penetrating wounds. Broad-spectrum antibiotic coverage effective against gram-positive and gram-negative organisms should be administered until results of culture and sensitivity tests are available. Based on recent reports of organisms isolated from infected joints or tendon sheaths, the combination of a cephalosporin such as cefazolin (15 mg/kg IV or IM t.i.d.) and amikacin (7.5 mg/kg t.i.d. or 22.5 mg/kg IV or IM s.i.d.) provides the best coverage for treatment of septic tenosynovitis. Alternatively, penicillin K (20,000 IU/kg IV q.i.d.) and gentamicin (2.2 mg/kg IV t.i.d. or 6.6 mg/kg IV s.i.d.) can be used. Local injection of antibiotics in the tendon sheath is recommended daily until clinical signs and synovial fluid analysis show improvement. An aminoglycoside such as amikacin (250 mg) or gentamicin (100 to 200 mg) is recommended for that purpose. Systemic analgesics such as phenylbutazone (4.4 mg/kg s.i.d. or b.i.d.; do not administer maximum dose for more than 4 days) should be administered as needed to improve use of the limb and minimize complications of non-weightbearing lameness. Bandaging is indicated to protect draining tracts, but further immobilization is usually not recommended because it may impede drainage and cause early sealing over of the draining port. Poor blood supply to the proximal sesamoid bones, and therefore poor penetration of antibiotics, warrants early, aggressive curettage of bony lesions for resolution of the infection. Curettage of the sesamoid bone can usually be performed by a lateral or medial longitudinal approach through the flexor tendon sheath, followed by reflection of the deep digital flexor tendon.

Prognosis

The prognosis for sesamoid bone infectious osteitis is at best guarded. Treatment of these lesions requires aggressive medical and surgical long-term therapy, and is expensive. In addition, involvement of the tendon sheath or fetlock joint further complicates treatment. Potential complications include laminitis of the contralateral limb, tendon contracture of the affected limb, annular ligament constriction, nonresolution of the infection, spread to adjacent structures, and pathologic fracture of the affected sesamoid bone.

DESMITIS OF THE BRANCHES OF THE SUSPENSORY LIGAMENT

Injuries to the suspensory ligament occur at the origin, body, medial and lateral branches, or insertion into the proximal sesamoid bone. This section describes injuries to the suspensory branches at their attachment onto the proximal sesamoid bones. The suspensory ligament branches act to stabilize the proximal sesamoid bones against the distal metacarpus (metatarsus) during weightbearing, and to limit abaxial movement of the fetlock during asymmetrical weightbearing. Injury to the suspensory branches is caused by excessive or asymmetrical weightbearing on the fetlock joint. This may also result in sesamoid or splint bone injury. It is a common injury of performance horses, particularly racehorses.

Diagnosis

Injury to the branches of the suspensory ligament results in moderate to severe lameness in the acute stage. Standardbred horses are often affected in both forelimbs and

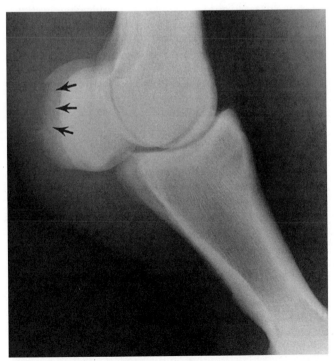

Figure 2. Lateral to medial projection of the metacarpophalangeal joint of a horse with septic tenosynovitis of 2 weeks' duration. Note the severe lysis on the abaxial surface of the sesamoid bone *(arrows)*, which is consistent with osteitis.

hindlimbs, whereas Thoroughbred horses are more commonly affected in the forelimbs. A painful swelling may be apparent over the affected area. However, swelling subsides with a few days of local therapy, making palpation an unreliable tool for diagnosis. Small tears may not be associated with local swelling, but continued training results in worsening of the tear and acute clinical signs. Damage of the suspensory insertion into the sesamoid bones may result in periarticular edema and pain on fetlock flexion.

Cytologic evaluation of the joint fluid may indicate traumatic inflammation, but intra-articular anesthesia of the fetlock usually does not relieve the lameness. Radiographs should be obtained to assess the integrity of the sesamoid bones and splint bones. Ultrasonographic examination of the suspensory ligament is the most useful technique to assess the presence and severity of suspensory damage, and provides a basis for monitoring healing. A 7.5-MHz transducer is used, with and without a standoff. The entire suspensory ligament should be examined. Accurate assessment of the injury includes measurement of the cross-sectional area of both the lesion and the affected suspensory branch and the length of damaged fibers, and evaluation of axial fiber alignment in longitudinal section. Lesions are graded on a scale of one to four: type 1 lesions are mostly echogenic; type 2 lesions are half echogenic and half anechoic; type 3 lesions are mostly anechoic; type 4 lesions are totally anechoic and represent the most highly pathologic state.

Treatment

The initial goal of therapy is to decrease the inflammatory reaction. Systemic anti-inflammatory agents such as phenylbutazone (4.4 mg/kg s.i.d.) and flunixin meglumine (1.1 mg/kg s.i.d. or b.i.d) may be used. Local therapy may include ice packs and bandaging.

Surgical therapy of suspensory desmitis includes ligament splitting. Ligament splitting has been used with success when a core lesion can be demonstrated in the branch of the suspensory ligament and may help vascularize the damaged area. In horses with distal splint fractures, surgical removal is suggested if the suspensory ligament injury is resolving with therapy and is not expected to severely limit the horse's performance.

In cases in which severe damage has resulted in loss of fetlock joint support, splinting for 6 to 8 months, until scar tissue is strong enough to support the fetlock, has been used. Alternatively, fetlock joint arthrodesis has been used successfully. Laminitis of the opposing limb is a frequent complication in these cases, and thus functional weightbearing should be provided as soon as possible.

In all cases, ultrasonographic re-evaluation is important to monitor the degree and quality of healing before return to exercise. Resolution of lameness and improved external appearance of the suspensory ligament may give a false impression of adequate healing. Early return to work often results in recurrence of the injury, often with additional damage.

COMPLETE DISRUPTION OF THE SUSPENSORY APPARATUS

Complete disruption of the suspensory apparatus, also known as breakdown, is a severe injury most frequently encountered in the forelimb of the Thoroughbred racehorse. The injury occurs at the end of a race and may be the result of muscular fatigue.

Diagnosis

When complete disruption of the suspensory ligament occurs, there is loss of support to the fetlock joint. In these cases, failure of the suspensory ligament is often accompanied by fracture of the proximal sesamoid bones. Severe soft tissue damage is generally present, which may include thrombosis of the palmar digital arteries, severe skin abrasion of the palmar aspect of the pastern, or deep digital flexor laceration.

Treatment

The goal of treatment of breakdown injuries is to salvage the horse for pasture soundness or breeding purposes. When acute disruption of the suspensory ligament is diagnosed, adequate limb support should be provided as soon as possible to prevent stretching and thrombosis of the palmar arteries. Thrombosis of the palmar arteries may result in loss of the hoof wall. Fetlock joint support can be provided with a board splint or a Kimzey apparatus. Additional therapies that may be considered in the acute stages include anti-inflammatory agents, such as phenylbutazone (2.2–4.4 mg/kg s.i.d. to b.i.d.), anti-thrombotic therapy such as aspirin (15 mg/kg p.o. on alternate days), and broad-spectrum antibiotics such as penicillin K (20,000 IU/kg IV q.i.d.) and gentamicin (2.2 mg/kg IV t.i.d. or 6.6 mg/kg IV or IM s.i.d.). Complete suspensory disruption can be managed with fetlock joint support for 6 to 8 months. However, laminitis of the supporting limb is a common complication in these cases. Surgical arthrodesis of the metacarpophalangeal joint provides an earlier return to functional weightbearing, thereby decreasing complications and morbidity.

DESMITIS OF THE DISTAL SESAMOIDEAN LIGAMENTS

Inflammation of the distal sesamoidean ligaments can occur at their origin, in the main body of the ligaments, or at their insertion. Inflammation of the origin of the ligament is often accompanied by fracture of the base of the sesamoid bone. Desmitis of the distal sesamoidean ligaments is most common in horses working over fences, particularly 3-day event and steeplechase horses. It is also a common injury of polo ponies. Horses with a long upright pastern and low heel conformation may also be predisposed to this type of injury, as well as injury to the navicular area. Although this condition may be primary, it is also observed accompanying other conditions of the suspensory apparatus such as suspensory desmitis or sesamoiditis.

Diagnosis

In the acute phase, edema and pain in the palmar or plantar aspect of the pastern may be observed. In chronic cases, thickening can be appreciated on palpation over the affected area, and digital pressure results in increased lameness.

Although clinical signs and palpation often serve to direct

the clinician toward the problem area, diagnostic infiltration may be used, particularly in cases where multiple problems are present. The region distal to the affected area should be desensitized first, if indicated, to rule out lameness originating in the foot or distal interphalangeal joint. Radiographically, periosteal proliferation may be present in the area of attachment of the affected ligament. Ultrasonography of the palmar or plantar aspect of the pastern is helpful to evaluate the extent of the injury and its severity.

Treatment

Rest and anti-inflammatory therapy are recommended for treatment of distal sesamoidean ligament injuries. Small avulsion fractures from the base of the sesamoid bone may benefit from removal. Close attention to shoeing and hoof angle should be accorded to minimize stress on the ligaments. Because this injury is often associated with multiple problems, a guarded prognosis is usually warranted. When basilar avulsion fractures are present, a return to a high level of performance is unlikely.

Supplemental Readings

Denoix J-M, Crevier N, Azevdedo C: Ultrasound examination of the pastern in horses. Proc 37th Annu Conv Am Assoc Equine Pract, 1991, pp 363–380.

Hardy J, Marcoux M, Breton L: Clinical relevance of radiographic findings in proximal sesamoid bones of two-year-old Standardbreds in their first year of race training. J Am Vet Med Assoc 198:2089–2094, 1991.

Henninger RW, Bramlage LR, Schneider RK, Gabel AA: Lag screw and cancellous bone graft fixation of transverse proximal sesamoid bone fractures in horses: 25 cases (1983–1989). J Am Vet Med Assoc 199:606–612, 1991.

Martin BB Jr, Nunamaker DM, Evans LH, Orsini J, Palmer SE: Circumferential wiring of mid-body and large basilar fractures of the proximal sesamoid bone in 15 horses. Vet Surg 20:9–14, 1991.

Parente EJ, Richardson DW, Spencer P: Basal sesamoidean fractures in horses: 57 cases (1980–1991). J Am Vet Med Assoc 202:1293–1297, 1993.

Proximal and Distal Interphalangeal Joint Pain

R. SCOTT PLEASANT
Blacksburg, Virginia

Lameness originating from the interphalangeal joints may have many causes. This section focuses on diagnosis and management of degenerative joint disease, pain with no radiographic abnormalities, and osteochondrosis.

PROXIMAL INTERPHALANGEAL JOINT

Degenerative Joint Disease

Degenerative joint disease (DJD) of the proximal interphalangeal joint occurs most commonly in horses that make quick turns and abrupt stops, such as western performance horses, polo ponies, and jumpers. A high incidence has also been noted in draft horses and in Tennessee Walking Horses. In most instances the problem appears to be the result of chronic "use trauma" to the articular cartilage and soft tissue support structures of the proximal interphalangeal joint and/or acute trauma. Other possible inciting causes are intra-articular fractures of the proximal or middle phalanx; poor distal limb conformation, which results in abnormal joint loading, joint subluxation, or joint luxation; septic arthritis; and osteochondrosis (see later).

Clinical Signs

DJD of the proximal interphalangeal joint may occur in either the forelimbs or the hindlimbs, but is more common in the forelimbs. The condition is often bilateral, but lameness usually predominates in one limb. Affected horses are usually more lame when worked on hard ground or in circles, and flexion and rotation of the digits often elicit pain. Some horses may show sensitivity to digital pressure over the pastern region, and periarticular thickening may be noted in more advanced cases. Lameness is usually greatly reduced by analgesia of the palmar (plantar) nerves at the level of the proximal sesamoid bones and may be partially improved, or sometimes completely alleviated, by analgesia of the palmar (plantar) digital nerves, presumably owing to proximal diffusion of local anesthetic solution.

Radiography

Definitive diagnosis is based on radiographic findings compatible with DJD including osteophytosis, periosteal new bone growth, narrowing of the joint space, and changes in subchondral bone. Although enthesopathy may be seen in association with DJD, it is not necessarily synonymous with it.

Narrowing of the joint space may represent direct evidence of cartilage loss; care must be taken when using this finding as the sole criterion for diagnosis. The width of the normal joint space varies with the joint, the age of the animal, and the variation in the loading of the joint. If a horse is not standing squarely when a radiograph is obtained, marked changes in the degree of loading of the articular cartilage may occur and the joint space may appear artificially narrow. Assessment of the adjacent joints can help to identify false narrowing of the joint space in unevenly loaded joints. If uneven loading of the joint is suspected, a second radiograph should be obtained after repositioning the horse. During the early stages of DJD, osteophytes and enthesophytes appear radiographically as small, fluffy, indistinct deposits of new bone and require careful radiographic examination for identification. Later in the disease process, osteophytes and enthesophytes become more heavily mineralized, which allows for easier detection. Flexed oblique radiographic views are particularly useful for detecting modeling changes of the dorsal aspects of both the proximal interphalangeal and distal interphalangeal joints.

Treatment

The method of treatment for DJD of the proximal interphalangeal joint depends on the extent of joint disease, the intended use of the horse, and economic considerations. Treatment of early DJD is aimed at halting or reducing the rate of joint destruction. Rest or discontinuation of work is important to allow acute inflammation to subside and restoration of soft tissue function. The amount of rest required varies with each case and may range from a few weeks to several months. Nonsteroidal anti-inflammatory drugs (NSAIDs) such as phenylbutazone (4–8 mg/kg per day) are useful in providing anti-inflammatory and analgesic effects to acutely inflamed joints. These drugs may also be used in lower dosages as needed, to help to maintain soundness. Systemic or intra-articular medication with agents such as hyaluronic acid and polysulfated glycosaminoglycans is valuable in diminishing the inflammatory response in both the synovium and the cartilage and in restoring the normal joint environment. In established DJD, these medications often require frequent administration, and cost may prohibit their use. Intra-articular corticosteroids can provide potent anti-inflammatory and analgesic effects, but the fear of steroid arthropathy has limited their use in recent years. However, studies suggest that when used at an appropriate dose and frequency, intra-articular corticosteroids can provide significant anti-inflammatory and chondroprotective effects, without deleterious side effects. Although specific dose and administration frequency recommendations cannot be made with certainty, intra-articular administration of 15 to 30 mg betamethasone may prove useful in the management of DJD of the proximal interphalangeal joint. Existing hoof imbalances should be corrected. The feet should be trimmed to establish a proper hoof-pastern axis (i.e., the dorsal surface of the hoof wall should be parallel to the dorsal surface of the pastern) and the hoof shod with squared or rockered toe shoes to ease breakover. The use of a full pad or rim pad between the shoe and foot may also be beneficial. In most instances, management of early DJD of the proximal interphalangeal joint also necessitates reduction in work loads and expectations for the horse.

Unfortunately, DJD of the proximal interphalangeal joint often progresses to the point where it can no longer be managed conservatively, and affected horses must be retired. An alternative to retirement is surgical arthrodesis of the proximal interphalangeal joint. The elimination of joint movement eliminates the associated pain. From reported cases, a return to full use can be expected in approximately 60% of surgically treated cases. The success rate tends to be better for pastern arthrodesis of the hindlimb compared with the forelimb. A 1-year convalescence after arthrodesis should be expected.

Lameness With No Radiographic Abnormalities

In some horses the site of lameness may be localized to the digital region by analgesia of the palmar (plantar) digital nerves at the level of the proximal sesamoid bones, but subsequent radiographs of the area fail to demonstrate a lesion. In these cases, the cause of lameness may be further localized by performing distal interphalangeal joint and proximal interphalangeal joint blocks.

The site of injection into the proximal interphalangeal joint is on the dorsal surface of the digit, 1 cm distal to the lateral distal eminence of the proximal phalanx and 2 to 3 cm lateral to the midline. A 2.5- to 3.8-cm 20-gauge needle is directed medially and inward to enter the joint beneath the common digital extensor tendon and 5 ml of local anesthetic solution is injected. The dorsal pouch of the proximal interphalangeal joint is relatively large and is usually easy to enter, particularly for clinicians with an appreciation of the local anatomy. Intra-articular analgesia of the proximal interphalangeal joint should have a pronounced effect on pain associated with the synovial membrane, but may have an inconsistent effect on pain associated with the joint capsule, collateral ligaments, and subchondral bone; therefore, in the presence of advanced radiologic abnormalities intra-articular analgesia may not relieve the lameness.

Treatment

Recognition of proximal interphalangeal joint inflammation or injury before radiographic changes have occurred is ideal. Early institution of appropriate therapy should reduce the likelihood of DJD. The most important therapy is rest to allow acute inflammation to subside. NSAIDs such as phenylbutazone (4–8 mg/kg per day) may hasten resolution of clinical signs. Foot imbalance should be corrected by appropriate trimming. The feet should be trimmed so that the dorsal surface of the hoof is parallel to the dorsal aspect of the pastern. Squared or rockered toe shoes ease breakover, and the use of full or rim pads may help reduce concussion. Polysulfated glycosaminoglycans administered intramuscularly, or hyaluronic acid administered intravenously, may also be beneficial. Exercise can usually be resumed in 2 to 4 weeks if lameness has resolved. Training schedules may need to be adjusted to reduce the amount and level of work to prevent recurrence. If lameness persists, low-dose intra-articular administration of corticosteroids (15 to 30 mg betamethasone) can be very valuable in reducing joint inflammation with minimal risk of side effects. Intra-articular administration of medications, such as hyaluronic acid and polysulfated glycosaminoglycans, is probably most efficacious before radiographic evidence of joint disease has occurred and is indicated if performance declines or lameness recurs. These products may also be administered prophylactically, at biweekly or monthly intervals, after the horse has returned to work. Duration of response is difficult to predict and is probably related to the stage of the disease when the problem was diagnosed, underlying conformational abnormalities, and the type and level of the work that the horse is expected to perform. Early diagnosis and aggressive treatment, in the absence of conformational abnormalities, merit the best prognosis.

Osteochondrosis

In young horses, DJD of the proximal interphalangeal joint is occasionally seen as a sequela to osteochondrosis. Affected horses are presented for lameness and often have pronounced periarticular thickening. The condition occurs more commonly in the hindlimbs than the forelimbs and can be bilateral. The disorder is unique in that by the time lameness is identified, there are often obvious degenerative changes within the joint. Typical radiographic findings include single or multiple subchondral cyst-like lesions in the distal end of the proximal phalanx, narrowing of the joint space, and osteophyte and enthesophyte formation. Conservative management of the condition is usually unrewarding, and surgical arthrodesis of the joint is often employed in an attempt to achieve serviceability.

DISTAL INTERPHALANGEAL JOINT

Degenerative Joint Disease

Degenerative joint disease of the distal interphalangeal joint is seen occasionally in all breeds and types of horses. As with DJD of the proximal interphalangeal joint, the condition appears to be most commonly the result of chronic "use trauma." Other possible causes of DJD of the distal interphalangeal joint are intra-articular fractures of the distal phalanx, middle phalanx, or navicular bone; joint subluxation or luxation; and septic arthritis.

The "use trauma" form of the disease occurs almost exclusively in the forelimbs and is often bilateral. Affected horses are usually more lame when worked in circles or on hard ground. Flexion of the digits is usually resented by the horse and exacerbates the lameness. In some instances there may be palpable distension of the distal interphalangeal joint capsule, dorsal to the coronary band. In advanced cases distortion of the distal dorsal pastern region and dorsal hoof wall may be observed, which is a condition known as *buttress foot*. Occasionally, pain to deep digital pressure over the distal interphalangeal joint is present.

Perineural analgesia of the palmar (plantar) digital nerves may improve the horse's gait, but analgesia of the palmar (plantar) nerves at the level of the proximal sesamoid bones is sometimes required to eliminate the lameness completely. Radiographically, the first lesions recognized are usually proliferative and lytic changes of the extensor process of the distal phalanx and distal dorsal and distal palmar aspects of the middle phalanx. In some instances discrete osseous opacities may be seen just proximal to the extensor process of the distal phalanx. These changes are often very subtle and require careful radiographic examination for identification. Flexed oblique radiographic views are particularly useful. In advanced cases these changes are more pronounced and there may also be evidence of narrowing of the joint space. Care must be taken not to interpret the eminences at the attachment of the collateral ligaments on the medial and lateral aspects

of the middle phalanx as signs of DJD. It is also important to realize that the presence of radiographic abnormalities does not necessarily imply current distal interphalangeal joint pain. The radiographic changes should always be interpreted in light of the clinical findings.

Treatment

Treatment of DJD of the distal interphalangeal joint is directed at stopping or slowing the rate of joint degeneration (see Degenerative Joint Disease of the Proximal Interphalangeal Joint). Initially, rest is important to reduce concomitant synovitis. NSAIDs such as phenylbutazone (4–8 mg/kg per day) may also be used initially to help reduce inflammation, and then repeated as needed to help maintain soundness. Systemic and intra-articular medication with drugs such as hyaluronic acid and polysulfated glycosaminoglycans is valuable, but frequent administration is usually required and cost may prohibit their use in some cases. Intra-articular corticosteroids can provide potent analgesic and anti-inflammatory effects, but low doses (15 to 30 mg betamethasone) should be used to minimize the risk of steroid arthropathy. Pre-existing hoof imbalances should be corrected and the horse shod with squared or rockered toes to ease breakover. Use of a full pad or rim pad may also provide some relief. A reduction in work load and expectations is usually necessary for the horse to be useful. Management of advanced DJD of the distal interphalangeal joint is difficult, and because surgical arthrodesis is not a viable option, most horses are retired. Low-dose phenylbutazone therapy may be required to keep horses comfortable.

Lameness With No Radiographic Abnormalities

In recent years distal interphalangeal joint pain has been suggested to be a significant cause of lameness in horses. This idea was based on the finding that many horses in which lameness was localized to the foot region with perineural analgesia also responded to intra-articular analgesia of the distal interphalangeal joint. It was assumed that intra-articular analgesia of the distal interphalangeal joint was specific for pain arising from the joint. In many instances no radiographic abnormalities of the distal interphalangeal joints were detected.

However, the specificity of intra-articular analgesia of the distal interphalangeal joint has been recently refuted. Clinical and experimental studies have shown that injection of local anesthetic solution into the distal interphalangeal joint can alleviate lameness associated with the navicular bone, navicular bursa, and related structures. In light of this information, it is likely that primary distal interphalangeal joint pain has been overrated. Scintigraphic examination may aid in the differentiation of pain associated with the distal interphalangeal joint and navicular apparatus when clinical and radiographic findings are inconclusive.

Realistically, differentiation between the two problems when radiographic abnormalities are not present may not be of great importance because the treatment is similar for both. Initial therapy should be as aggressive as finances allow to reduce the likelihood of irreversible pathologic changes occurring. Rest or cessation of work is important to allow acute inflammation associated with synovitis, bursitis, or bone remodeling to subside. Exercise can usually be resumed in 2 to 4 weeks. Horses should be gradually returned to work, and training schedules may need to be adjusted to reduce the amount and level of work to prevent recurrence. NSAIDs may also be used to help resolve acute inflammation. Systemic administration of hyaluronic acid and polysulfated glycosaminoglycans is valuable in reducing the inflammatory response in both the synovium and cartilage of the distal interphalangeal joint and the navicular bursa. These products may also be used prophylactically after the horse has returned to work. Low-dose intra-synovial (intra-articular and/or intra-bursal) corticosteroids may provide potent analgesic and anti-inflammatory effects with minimal risk of deleterious side effects. Isoxsuprine hydrochloride can be administered (0.6–1.2 mg/kg p.o. b.i.d.) in an attempt to improve subchondral bone microcirculation. Pre-existing hoof problems such as medial to lateral imbalances or broken hoof pastern axes should be corrected and the horses shod with squared or rockered toe shoes to ease breakover. Alternatively the horse may be shod with a wide web, lightweight shoe such as one of aluminum. The shoes should be set full and long to allow for hoof expansion and to provide palmar support. Full pads or rim pads may be used to reduce concussion.

Osteochondrosis

Osteochondrosis of the distal interphalangeal joint may be manifested as an osteochondral fragment off the extensor process or as a solitary subchondral bone cyst in the distal phalanx. Osteochondral fragments off the extensor process are often seen as incidental findings, although they may be associated with lameness. These fragments may be difficult to distinguish from extensor process fractures, but they are usually self-limiting and respond to conservative management. The fragments may be removed arthroscopically if persistent lameness occurs.

Subchondral bone cysts in the distal phalanx are seen most commonly in mature horses. The condition occurs almost exclusively in the forelimbs and is usually associated with lameness of sudden onset. The lameness usually is reduced greatly with perineural analgesia of the palmar digital nerves or intra-articular analgesia of the distal interphalangeal joint. Repeated radiographic examinations have revealed that some cysts may enlarge and others may resolve.

Conservative treatment with rest, NSAIDs, or intra-articular medications should be attempted initially. If lameness persists, surgical enucleation and curettage of the cyst via a distal-to-proximal approach may be attempted. Alternatively, the horse may be retired.

Supplemental Readings

Dyson SJ, Kidd L: A comparison of responses to analgesia of the navicular bursa and intra-articular analgesia of the distal interphalangeal joint in 59 horses. Equine Vet J 25:93–98, 1993.
McIlwraith CW, Goodman NL: Conditions of the interphalangeal joints. Vet Clin North Am Equine Pract 5(1):161–178, 1989.
Nixon AJ: Intra-articular medication. *In* Robinson NE (ed): Current Therapy in Equine Medicine, ed 3. Philadelphia, WB Saunders, 1992, pp 127–131.
Richardson DW: Degenerative joint disease. *In* Robinson NE (ed): Current Therapy in Equine Medicine, ed 3. Philadelphia, WB Saunders, 1992, pp 137–140.
Schmotzer WB, Trim KI: Local anesthetic techniques for diagnosis of lameness. Vet Clin North Am Equine Pract 6(3):705–725, 1990.
Widmer WR, Blevins WE: Radiographic evaluation of degenerative joint disease in horses: Interpretive principles. Comp Cont Ed Pract Vet 16:907–917, 1994.

Interpretation of Local Analgesic Techniques in the Foot Region

R. SCOTT PLEASANT
Blacksburg, Virginia

Diagnosis and treatment of lameness is an important part of an equine practitioner's work. Effective treatment is generally dependent on achieving an accurate diagnosis. In many instances, physical examination of the lame horse does not result in a definitive diagnosis, and it is necessary to use local analgesia to identify the source of the lameness. Techniques for induction of analgesia are an important and sometimes vital part of a lameness investigation. However, there are some instances when these procedures yield unexpected results or results that are difficult to interpret. Experience has made it clear that these techniques are not as precise as once thought, especially in the foot region. To properly interpret the results of local analgesia in this region, the clinician must have a thorough knowledge of the neuroanatomy and understand the limitations of each technique. The results should always be interpreted in light of historic and clinical abnormalities and findings on other diagnostic procedures such as radiography, scintigraphy, or ultrasonography.

PALMAR (PLANTAR) DIGITAL NERVE BLOCK

The palmar digital nerve block is probably the most commonly performed nerve block in the horse. The palmar

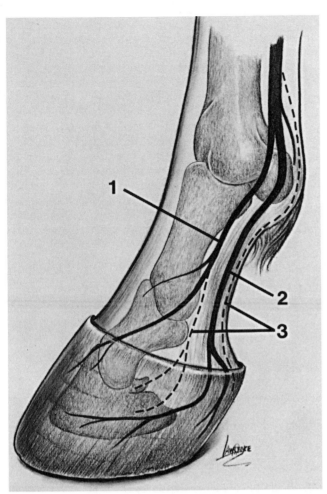

Figure 1. Example of nerve supply to the foot. (1) Dorsal branch of palmar digital nerve; (2) palmar digital nerve; (3) possible variant nerve branches.

interphalangeal joint, which is presumably the result of proximal diffusion of local anesthetic solution.

Occasionally, it may be difficult to assess whether adequate desensitization has occurred. Traditionally, the absence of skin sensation distal to a local block has been used as an indicator of successful local analgesia. However, cutaneous desensitization is not always synonymous with loss of deep sensation and vice versa. Nerve distribution to the digit of the horse is complex and variable. In some individuals, variant nerve branches may transmit deep sensation from the palmar aspect of the foot (see Fig. 1). If these variant branches escape anesthesia with a routine palmar digital nerve block, there may be cutaneous desensitization without relief of lameness, despite the lameness originating in the palmar aspect of the foot. In other individuals, variant nerve branches that provide cutaneous sensation may occur. If these nerve branches escape anesthesia with a routine palmar digital nerve block, cutaneous sensation may persist despite adequate analgesia of deep structures. Thus, to test the effectiveness of a palmar digital nerve block, both cutaneous and deep sensation need to be evaluated. Cutaneous and deep sensation in the heel bulb region should be checked with a blunt object. The pressure is applied gently at first, and then firmly to assess deep sensation. Deep sensation should also be checked with hoof tester pressure over the frog and heels. Regardless of the result, the effect on pre-existing lameness should be evaluated. Occasionally, despite alleviation of lameness, a positive response to hoof testers and cutaneous sensation apparently persists.

Another problem that may be encountered when interpreting the response to a palmar digital nerve block is deciding whether sufficient improvement has occurred. This is especially true in horses that are only slightly lame. It is important to observe these horses moving under the conditions in which the lameness is most obvious (e.g., on hard surfaces, on a lunge line, under tack). Sufficient time should be spent observing the horse before performing the nerve block to ensure that the lameness does not spontaneously improve with work. In conditions that cause severe pain, such as a subsolar abscess, laminitis, or fracture of the navicular bone or distal phalanx, lameness may improve only slightly with local anesthesia. Conditions that cause less severe pain usually demonstrate marked improvement. In the author's experience, complete abolition of lameness only occurs with conditions that cause mild pain. Lamenesses associated with mechanical impairment of motion such as that caused by adhesions between the navicular bone and the deep digital flexor tendon may only show partial improvement. In some horses, lameness may be improved dramatically when they exercise in straight lines, but still may be detectable during exercise on a circle. This may be the result of an incomplete block, inability to desensitize the area fully, or occasionally a remote second source of pain. If lameness obviously persists during exercise in straight lines but is improved during exercise on a circle, this usually reflects more than one source of pain. It is also important to recognize that local anesthetic solution may diffuse proximally; thus, pain associated with the proximal interphalangeal joint may be partially alleviated.

digital nerves are usually anesthetized in the midpastern region, anywhere from just proximal to the cartilages of the foot (i.e., the lateral cartilages of the distal phalanx) to just proximal to the pastern joint. Theoretically, when both the medial and lateral nerves are blocked, the palmar half of the foot is anesthetized. A positive response is indicated by resolution or a marked reduction in the lameness.

In most horses, this technique is reasonably easy to perform and interpretation is straightforward. However, in some instances the entire foot can be anesthetized following a palmar digital nerve block, leading to confusion or an erroneous diagnosis. This is usually the result of the dorsal branches of the palmar digital nerves becoming anesthetized during the procedure (Fig. 1). Thus, it is very important to always evaluate the limitations of desensitization by checking sensation on the dorsal surface of the pastern area and by applying hoof testers to the dorsal sole region. The likelihood of inadvertently blocking the dorsal branches of the palmar digital nerves can be reduced by blocking the nerves as distal as possible with judicious amounts (1.5 to 2.0 ml) of anesthetic solution. Even then, despite persistence of cutaneous sensation on the dorsal aspect of the coronary band, there may be improvement in lameness associated with pain arising from the proximal

UNILATERAL (MEDIAL OR LATERAL) PALMAR DIGITAL NERVE BLOCK

Perineural analgesia of either the medial or lateral palmar digital nerve may be very useful to differentiate pain arising from the navicular bone and associated structures, the distal interphalangeal joint, a unilateral bruise (corn), focal laminar tearing, or a fracture of palmar process of the distal phalanx. When pain is arising from the navicular bone or related structures or the distal interphalangeal joint, a unilateral nerve block may alleviate lameness but rarely totally, especially if the horse is reappraised during exercise both in straight lines and circles.

DISTAL INTERPHALANGEAL JOINT BLOCK

Distal interphalangeal joint pain has been reported to be a significant cause of lameness in horses. It has been recommended that if a horse responds to a palmar digital nerve block, intra-articular analgesia of the distal interphalangeal joint be performed after analgesia of the palmar digital nerves resolves. It is suggested that a positive response to intra-articular analgesia of the distal interphalangeal joint indicates pain arising from the joint.

However, the specificity of intra-articular analgesia of the distal interphalangeal joint has recently been refuted. Clinical and experimental investigations have demonstrated that injection of local anesthetic solution into the distal interphalangeal joint can alleviate lameness associated with pain arising from the navicular bone, navicular bursa, and related structures. The majority of horses demonstrate improvement within 5 minutes of anesthetic administration. These findings are supported by immunocytochemical and dye distribution studies, which suggest that the sensory nerves innervating the navicular bone are desensitized by injections of anesthetic solution into the distal interphalangeal joint, and that there may be an indirect and potentially functional communication between the distal interphalangeal joint and the navicular bursa.

It should also be noted that the proximal palmar pouch of the distal interphalangeal joint lies in very close proximity to the palmar digital nerves as they course along the medial aspects of the lateral cartilages, making it possible that anesthetic diffusion could block nerve conduction at this level. If this were to occur, administration of anesthetic solution into the distal interphalangeal joint could improve lamenesses associated with the palmar processes of the distal phalanx, the digital cushion, the frog, the sole, and the hoof wall. Given all of this information, the question arises: How often does primary distal interphalangeal joint pain occur and how can it be confirmed?

ANALGESIA OF THE NAVICULAR BURSA

It has also been proposed that lameness identified in the palmar aspect of the foot be further localized by anesthetic administration into the navicular bursa. However, it is uncertain whether the injected anesthetic solution remains within the navicular bursa. It is highly probable that there is some diffusion of anesthetic into the distal interphalangeal joint. Furthermore, as with the proximal palmar pouch of the distal interphalangeal joint, diffusion of anesthetic from the proximal cul-de-sac of the navicular bursa could anesthetize the palmar digital nerves as they course along the medial aspects of the lateral cartilages. Injection into the navicular bursa can also be somewhat difficult, and a common mistake is to inadvertently inject into the distal interphalangeal joint. Radiographic control is recommended to ensure accurate injection. Nonetheless, this technique can be useful for confirming pain associated with the navicular bone and related structures, especially in association with subtle or absent radiologic abnormalities.

PALMAR (PLANTAR) ABAXIAL SESAMOID NERVE BLOCK

The palmar (plantar) nerves may be blocked at the level of the proximal sesamoid bones, resulting theoretically in complete desensitization of the foot and thus alleviation of lameness associated with foot pain. However, in the presence of severe pain associated with a subsolar abscess or laminitis, improvement may only be mild. For example, although the horse may turn better, lameness may persist virtually unchanged when the horse is walked or trotted in straight lines. Palmar (abaxial sesamoid) nerve blocks may also improve lameness associated with degenerative joint disease of the proximal interphalangeal joint, injuries of the palmar soft tissue structures of the pastern such as the digital flexor tendons or the distal sesamoidean ligaments, incomplete sagittal fracture of the proximal phalanx, proximal sesamoid fractures, fetlock joint pain, and digital flexor tendon sheath pain.

SUMMARY

This discussion is not intended to discourage the use of local analgesic techniques in the foot region but to make the reader aware of some of the difficulties in interpreting the response to these techniques. It is clear that there is considerable overlap between these techniques. However, it may be that specific problems show a differential response to each technique. For example, a horse with synovitis of the distal interphalangeal joint may demonstrate partial improvement after a palmar digital nerve block or analgesia of the navicular bursa, but there may be a greater response to intra-articular analgesia of the distal interphalangeal joint. Further studies are needed to determine if this is the case.

Supplemental Readings

Bowker RM, Rockershousen SJ, Vex KB, Sonea IM, Caron JP, Kotyk R: Immunocytochemical and dye distribution studies of nerves potentially desensitized by injections into the distal interphalangeal joint or the navicular bursa of horses. J Am Vet Med Assoc 203:1708-1714, 1993.

Dyson S: Problems associated with the interpretation of the results of regional and intra-articular anaesthesia in the horse. Vet Rec 118:419-422, 1986.

Dyson SJ, Kidd L: A comparison of responses to analgesia of the navicular bursa and intra-articular analgesia of the distal interphalangeal joint in 59 horses. Equine Vet J 25:93-98, 1993.

Pleasant RS, Moll HD, Ley WB, Lessard P: Effect of intra-articular anesthesia of the distal interphalangeal joint on lameness associated with amphotericin-induced equine navicular bursitis [abstract]. Vet Surg 22:395, 1993.

Schmotzer WB, Trim KI: Local anesthetic techniques for diagnosis of lameness. Vet Clin North Am Equine Pract 6(3):705-728, 1990.

Stashak TS: Diagnosis of lameness. In Stashak TS (ed): Adams' Lameness in Horses, ed 4. Philadelphia, Lea & Febiger, 1987, pp 100-156.

Wright IM: A study of 118 cases of navicular disease: Clinical features. Equine Vet J 25:488-492, 1993.

Soft Tissue Injuries of the Pastern

ROGER K.W. SMITH

PETER M. WEBBON
North Mymms, England

Soft tissue injuries of the palmar* pastern are relatively common. They produce a variable degree of lameness and swelling that is frequently the result of nonspecific edema or fibrosis, making diagnosis by palpation difficult. Diagnostic local anesthesia is often unrewarding, serving only to confirm that the pain emanates from the pastern. It may also be unreliable in differentiating intrasynovial and extrasynovial lesions, because digital sheath pain due to both adhesions and sepsis is not entirely eliminated by intrasynovial anesthesia. Diagnosis therefore depends on a combination of palpation, the observation of postural changes, synoviocentesis with or without intrasynovial anesthesia, radiography, and ultrasonography (Tables 1 and 2).

DIAGNOSTIC PROCEDURES

Synoviocentesis

Many pastern injuries involve the digital flexor tendon sheath, so that synoviocentesis, analysis of synovial fluid, and the injection of local anesthetic and/or contrast agent is frequently performed. The site in the proximal sheath between the flexor tendons and the suspensory ligament branches is notoriously difficult for obtaining samples even in distended sheaths, because of the presence of synovial plica. A superior site is immediately distal to the proximal digital annular ligament and into the synovial pouch, which can be palpated when distended. Care has to be taken to avoid damaging the deep digital flexor tendon (DDFT) and to ensure aseptic technique, because of the proximity of a potentially dirty foot. The local anesthetic agent and/or contrast material can also act as a negative contrast agent for ultrasonographic examination, although ideally an ultrasonographic examination should be performed before injection. Care should be taken to avoid introducing air into the digital sheath during injection.

Radiographic Examination

Soft tissue injuries in the pastern region may be accompanied by bony lesions, and thus radiographic examination is important. Four views are routinely obtained: lateromedial, dorso-15°-proximal-palmarodistal oblique (with the cassette held at the same angle along the palmar aspect of the pastern), and two oblique views, centered on the pastern region. Common findings are avulsion fractures and enthesiophytosis. Further oblique projections such as dorsolateroproximal-palmaromediodistal obliques and a careful ultrasonographic examination can be used to diagnose the origin of the avulsed fragments. Enthesiophytosis at the insertion sites of the oblique (middle) distal sesamoidean ligaments (ODSL) is a consequence of chronic inflammation at the insertion of these ligaments, but it is usually not a cause of lameness.

Ultrasonography

Ultrasonography of the pastern region is technically more demanding than that of the metacarpal region, but good diagnostic images can be obtained with a little practice. It is easier to perform the ultrasonographic examination after the radiographic appraisal, allowing the soft tissue components to be "superimposed" on the known bony pathology. A linear probe cannot be used to scan an area farther distal than the proximal interphalangeal joint in the normal weightbearing position, but caudal placement of the limb allows imaging of the more distal structures. The manipulation of a sector probe in this region is difficult because the handle frequently contacts the ground. This problem can be alleviated by placing the foot on a block, but even weightbearing between limbs for evaluation of tendon cross-sectional area is then more difficult. A sector probe, however, does allow scanning distal to the proximal interphalangeal joint, by placing the probe between the bulbs of the heel. Longitudinal views can occasionally be easier to obtain with a sector probe, although small linear (rectal) probes fit longitudinally within the pastern region,

---

*For palmar also read plantar unless stated otherwise.

TABLE 1. CLINICAL SIGNS ASSOCIATED WITH SOFT TISSUE INJURIES OF THE PASTERN

Condition	Lameness	Posture	Palpation Findings	Primary Diagnostic Tests
Injuries Not Associated With Percutaneous Injury				
Aseptic digital sheath tenosynovitis	Absent (in idiopathic form) Mild to severe	Unaltered	Swollen sheath +/− pain over sheath	Ultrasonography Digital sheath synoviocentesis
SDFT tendinitis	Moderate to severe Persists for longer than in metacarpal SDFT tendinitis	Sinking of fetlock when limb loaded (if severe)	Thickened pastern Pain over proximal palmar pastern (proximal to bifurcation) and palmarolateral and palmaromedial distal pastern (branches)	Ultrasonography
DDFT tendinitis	Persistent, severe	Unaltered Upward moving toe if ruptured	Pain over DDFT Digital sheath effusion Thickened pastern	Ultrasonography
Distal sesamoidean ligament desmitis	Moderate to severe	Unaltered Dorsal subluxation of PIP joint and sinking of fetlock if severe	Thickened pastern +/− pain in proximal pastern region	Radiography Ultrasonography
Digital annular ligament pathology	?Variable Severe with avulsion fracture	Unaltered	Thickened pastern Pain over palmarolateral and palmaromedial aspects of proximal first phalanx	Radiography Ultrasonography
Percutaneous Soft Tissue Injuries				
Penetrating injuries	Mild to severe depending on tendon damage and presence of sepsis	Unaltered	+/− visible wound Thickened pastern Digital sheath effusion Pain localized over tendon damage or generalized over whole of digital sheath if septic	Radiography Ultrasonography Digital sheath synoviocentesis
Tendon lacerations	Moderate to severe	SDFT branch only—unaltered SDFT proximal to bifurcation or both branches only (unusual)—sinking of fetlock only when limb fully loaded DDFT—upward moving toe DSL—sinking of fetlock +/− subluxation of PIP joint	Wound Open digital sheath Tendon ends palpable	Ultrasonography proximal and distal to wound
Heel lacerations	None or mild (can be severe immediately after injury, but this often resolves quickly)	Unaltered	Wound +/− disrupted coronary band	Digital sheath synoviocentesis and contrast study Surgical exploration

TABLE 2. ULTRASONOGRAPHIC CHANGES ASSOCIATED WITH SOFT TISSUE INJURIES OF THE PASTERN

Tendon/Ligament Affected	Summary of Pertinent Ultrasonographic Findings
Injuries Not Involving Percutaneous Injury	
Aseptic digital sheath tenosynovitis	Primary cause (if present)—e.g., tendinitis
	Digital sheath effusion (anechoic)—best identified proximal to metacarpophalangeal joint and in midline distal to digital annular ligaments
	+/− thickened subcutaneous tissues +/− digital annular ligaments if chronic
	+/− thickened digital sheath wall—best identified proximal to proximal sesamoid bones
	+/− echogenic bodies within sheath (adhesions)—also manifest as uneven or indistinct surface of flexor tendons but beware of confusing with epitenon inflammation. Do not mistake synovial plica between digital sheath wall and DDFT in proximal digital sheath for adhesions
	Mineralization of digital sheath wall if chronic (hyperechoic foci with acoustic shadowing)
	+/− digital annular ligament thickening
Superficial digital flexor tendon (SDFT) tendinitis	*Proximal to bifurcation*
	Thickened SDFT with reduced and heterogenous echogenicity
	Loss of longitudinal striated pattern
	Digital sheath effusion
	Thickened subcutaneous tissues +/− digital annular ligaments
	SDFT branches
	Enlarged SDFT branch with variable amounts of central or peripheral hypoechogenicity. Size of branch increases in proximodistal fashion in normal horse. Therefore, compare size of branch with contra-axial and contralateral branches (but beware of bilateral injury) and other tendons/ligaments in pastern
	+/− digital sheath effusion
	Thickened subcutaneous tissues +/− digital annular ligaments
	Loss of longitudinal striated pattern (difficult to assess because of obliquity)
Deep digital flexor tendon (DDFT) tendinitis	Enlarged heterogenous DDFT. Often multiple hypoechoic fissures. Lesion often centered on metacarpophalangeal joint region and restricted to the digital sheath (in forelimb)
	Loss of longitudinal striated pattern
	+/− intratendinous mineralization if chronic
	Digital sheath effusion
	Thickened subcutaneous tissues +/− digital annular ligaments
	OR: Focal, hypoechoic lesions proximal to metacarpophalangeal joint
	OR: +/− mild enlargement in distal pastern region (navicular disease)
Distal sesamoidean ligament (DSL) desmitis	Enlarged, hypoechoic and heterogenous DSL
	Thickened subcutaneous tissues +/− digital annular ligaments
	Entheseophytosis at insertion points (irregular and thickened bone-surface echo at point of insertion; often other soft tissue pathology [if active])
	+/− avulsion fragments (difficult to identify at base of proximal sesamoid bones because of angle of probe to bone surface)
Digital annular ligament pathology	Thickened subcutaneous tissues
	Thickened digital annular ligaments (best identified on palmarolateral and palmaromedial aspects)
	OR: Avulsion fractures at insertion points
Percutaneous Injuries	
Penetrating wounds	+/− digital sheath effusion
	+/− DDFT (and SDFT) damage—varies from shallow surface defects to deeper lesions (beware of normal midline depression in DDFT)
	+/− digital sheath sepsis (hypoechoic thickened digital sheath wall, digital sheath effusion of variable echogenicity, flocculent material within sheath, edematous subcutaneous tissues, air within sheath)
	+/− adhesions
	+/− foreign bodies
	Hypoechoic tract should be identified and followed to its limit to identify all pathology including foreign material, which tends to reside at limit of tract
	+/− septic tendinitis (rapidly progressive over days) hypoechoic/anechoic lesion with minimal tendon enlargement, "erosive"
	?"Aseptic degeneration" of tendon can occur over weeks/months
Tendon lacerations	Little use at laceration site because of large wound
	Proximal and distal examination can demonstrate extent of tendon damage
	Uniaxial SDFT branch laceration can result in lateral (for medial branch laceration) or medial (for lateral branch laceration) displacement of the SDFT at the level of the metacarpophalangeal joint
Heel lacerations	Ultrasonography of little use
	+/− digital sheath effusion

especially if the probe is rotated so that the lead leaves the probe proximally rather than distally.

The procedure for scanning the pastern region varies, but the authors' technique with a linear probe is first to obtain three transverse and one longitudinal views from the palmar aspect of the limb (Fig. 1). Two additional transverse levels or zones distally have been described for the sector probe. Because many of the soft tissue structures run obliquely across the pastern, it is vital that the probe be moved subsequently to the palmarolateral and palmaro-

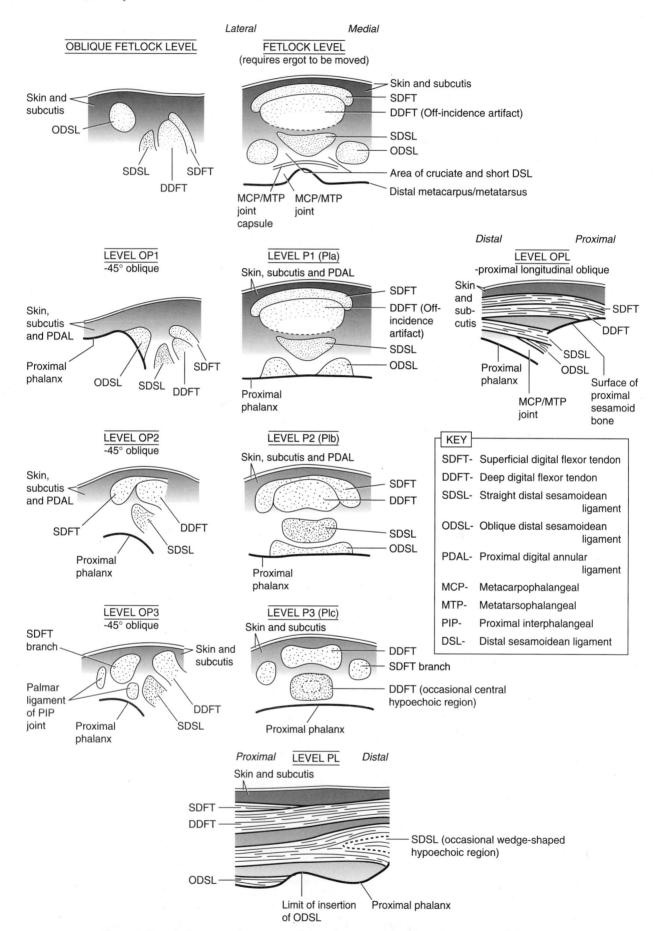

Figure 1. Normal ultrasonographic anatomy of the soft tissues on the palmar/plantar aspect of the pastern.

medial aspects of the limb to evaluate adequately the ODSL proximally and the branches of the superficial digital flexor tendon (SDFT) distally (see Fig. 1).

In the proximal pastern region, the orientation of the probe with respect to the DDFT invariably gives rise to an anechoic region on the dorsal aspect of the DDFT. This is artifactual and should not be confused with a lesion. At the distal insertion of the straight distal sesamoidean ligament (SDSL), onto the middle scutum on the palmar aspect of the proximal interphalangeal joint, a normal, central, hypoechoic region frequently can be identified. In the longitudinal views, it is wedge-shaped with the apex pointing proximally. It does not normally extend farther proximally than the distal limit of insertion of the ODSL.

SOFT TISSUE INJURIES NOT ASSOCIATED WITH PERCUTANEOUS INJURY

Aseptic Tenosynovitis of the Digital Sheath

Etiology

Aseptic tenosynovitis of the digital sheath can be primary or secondary, acute or chronic. Primary causes include overextension injury of the distal limb, local trauma, or idiopathic. Secondary tenosynovitis is associated with tendinitis within the tendon sheath, palmar and/or digital annular ligament constriction, disruption of adhesions within the sheath, and sympathetic effusion with adjacent but not confluent septic foci.

Clinical Signs and Diagnosis

Idiopathic tenosynovitis ("wind-galls") rarely causes lameness, whereas acute primary tenosynovitis often produces moderate to severe lameness. Secondary and chronic tenosynovitis result in variable lameness depending on the primary cause and the presence of adhesions, respectively.

The clinical diagnosis of tenosynovitis is usually easy. Synoviocentesis differentiates sepsis from asepsis, but ultrasonography is useful to identify a primary cause and the presence of adhesions and palmar and/or digital annular ligament thickening. Other ultrasonographic findings include the presence of a hypoechogenic effusion within the sheath, a thickened synovial membrane, and a variable amount of subcutaneous fibrosis. In addition to adhesions, chronic cases may occasionally have mineralization of the digital sheath wall, manifested ultrasonographically as hyperechoic foci with acoustic shadowing. Adhesions can be overdiagnosed. Confident diagnosis can be made by identification of separate echogenic bodies. These may be recognized best in the presence of effusion, or by the injection of fluid such as local anesthetic into the sheath as a negative contrast agent. A less reliable sign is loss of clarity of the DDFT margins, especially in the absence of effusion, because it may represent inflammation of the epitenon. The full length of the sheath should be examined ultrasonographically. In the proximal sheath, the normal synovial reflections (plica), which join the lateral and medial borders of the DDFT to the digital sheath wall, must not be confused with adhesions but can provide a useful assessment of the thickness of the synovial membrane. At the same level, dorsal to the DDFT, the full digital sheath wall thickness can be seen as single or twin parallel thin lines that thicken and become confluent with tenosynovitis, especially when it is chronic.

Treatment and Prognosis

Treatment of acute tenosynovitis should include immediate rest and anti-inflammatory therapy involving application of cold, bandaging, and the use of anti-inflammatory drugs. Phenylbutazone (2 mg/kg q12h p.o.) can be used to provide analgesia. Short-acting corticosteroids, for example betamethasone, can be administered systemically (0.04–0.08 mg/kg) or into the tendon sheath (4 mg) provided that there is no possibility of the sheath being infected. Sodium hyaluronate (20 mg) can also be injected into the sheath, although the danger of provoking a "flare" in the digital sheath is more common in acutely inflamed sheaths. Most cases of acute tenosynovitis resolve with rest and analgesia, but early treatment reduces the chances of adhesions. Lavage of the sheath, under sedation or general anesthesia, is usually restricted to cases with severe tenosynovitis or hemorrhage or sepsis within the sheath. General anesthesia allows a more complete lavage and concurrent tenoscopic evaluation of the sheath. Chronic tenosynovitis can be treated palliatively with methylprednisolone acetate (80 mg intrasynovially). Adhesiolysis performed by tenoscopy, or via an open technique, is still controversial as a treatment of chronic tenosynovitis.

Strict rest should be continued until the acute inflammation has disappeared. Repeated injections of sodium hyaluronate at weekly intervals, if there are no financial restraints, are recommended. An exercise regimen of progressively increasing intensity can be started as soon as the horse becomes sound.

The prognosis for tenosynovitis is related to the primary cause and the presence of adhesions, which cause a mechanical lameness and may tear, provoking further tenosynovitis. Uncomplicated, primary, acute tenosynovitis has a favorable prognosis if it is treated early and no adhesions form, but there is some evidence that chronic tenosynovitis can damage the flexor tendons in the long term. Serial ultrasonography is therefore useful to monitor the state of the sheath and tendons.

Superficial Digital Flexor Tendinitis

Etiology

Tendinitis of the SDFT in the pastern region is less common than in the metacarpal region, usually occurring secondarily to previous metacarpal SDFT tendinitis, or concurrently with severe tendinitis, which also involves the metacarpal region of the SDFT. In the hindlimb it is more common to find it as a primary injury.

Clinical Signs and Diagnosis

The lameness is often severe in the acute stages, with improvement as the acute inflammation subsides, but tendinitis in this region tends to result in a longer lasting lameness than in the metacarpal region. Nonspecific subcutaneous thickening is present, especially on the palmar aspect proximally and palmarolateral and palmaromedial aspect distally, where a pain response may sometimes also be evident. A digital sheath effusion often is present.

Diagnosis is best achieved using ultrasonography. If the SDFT proximal to its bifurcation is affected it is thickened and hypoechogenic, whereas normally it is a thin structure at this level. This needs to be differentiated from thickening of the digital sheath wall, the digital annular ligaments, and the subcutaneous tissues. If the branches are affected, they are enlarged, with variable degrees of central and peripheral hypoechogenicity. The branches should be examined with the probe on the palmarolateral and palmaromedial aspects of the pastern. Enlargement can be difficult to assess, because the branches increase in size as they approach their insertion. Careful comparison with the other branch on the same limb and the branches on the contralateral limb at the same level should be made, although the veterinarian must be aware of the possibility of biaxial and bilateral injuries.

Treatment and Prognosis

Early treatment is anti-inflammatory with rest, cold application, and bandaging. The intratendinous injection of polysulfated glycosaminoglycans is a possible therapy in those acute or subacute cases with an obvious central hypoechoic region, although this treatment remains unproven. Injection of 250 mg should be made into the hypoechoic regions in several sites, using aseptic technique and the same 23-gauge 1.2-cm needle, to avoid the loss of most of the agent in multiple needle hubs. An early return to walking exercise is recommended, as soon as the acute inflammatory phase has passed. The rate of increase in work is dictated by the rate of healing, monitored ultrasonographically. The horse may not return to work for several months depending on the severity of the initial injury.

The prognosis for this injury is guarded because of its association with metacarpal tendinitis, even if none can be identified clinically. Hindlimb SDFT tendinitis has a better prognosis than that in the forelimb.

Deep Digital Flexor Tendinitis

Etiology

Tendinitis of the DDFT in the pastern is a rare injury with a different etiology from SDFT tendinitis. It arises primarily from overextension of the distal interphalangeal joint and/or the metacarpophalangeal joint. Commonly this occurs with fixation of the foot with the horse's body moving over it. Often the provoking incident is unnoticed. Mucoid, calcifying, or fibrous central lesions may be associated with the "tendinous form of navicular disease" and are occasionally palpable. However, it is difficult to scan with ultrasound sufficiently distally to identify the more severe changes overlying the navicular bone.

Clinical Signs and Diagnosis

Tendinitis of the DDFT tends to produce severe lameness that persists. Injuries are often centered at the metacarpophalangeal joint and are either partial ruptures, which provoke numerous fibrous adhesions, or total ruptures, which never heal. Pain is usually pronounced over the affected tendon, and there is an accompanying tenosynovitis. Confirmation of injury is made ultrasonographically.

The damage to this tendon is usually severe, with considerable enlargement and multiple hypoechoic foci or fissures within the body of the tendon, often extending into the pastern region. More focal lesions within the digital sheath proximal to the metacarpophalangeal joint have been described as a cause of chronic lameness (see page 43). The etiology of these lesions is unclear.

Treatment and Prognosis

Treatment of this condition is frequently unrewarding and is largely restricted to first-aid anti-inflammatory treatment and rest. Casting may be indicated in the acute stages, to prevent continuing injury to the tendon. The prognosis is poor, because lameness is persistent and often associated with the production of extensive adhesions within the sheath.

Distal Sesamoidean Ligament Desmitis

Etiology

The etiology of distal sesamoidean ligament (DSL) desmitis is similar to that of suspensory branch desmitis, and the conditions can coexist. Overextension of the metacarpophalangeal joint is the initiating trauma, but degenerative changes may predispose the ligaments to injury. Ultrasonography has revealed that many cases that previously have been diagnosed as DSL desmitis are either SDFT branch tendinitis or digital sheath lesions.

Clinical Signs and Diagnosis

Lameness is usually moderate to severe. The palmar pastern region is swollen. The short DSL and cruciate DSL cannot be accurately delineated ultrasonographically from the fibrous joint capsule of the palmar pouch of the metacarpophalangeal joint. The short DSL lies dorsal to the ODSL, and the cruciate DSL can be found dorsal to the SDSL in the midline. They can be more consistently identified if the ergot is moved proximally and the probe is placed over the palmar aspect of the metacarpophalangeal joint. However, there are no reports of injuries to these ligaments, and the authors have not recognized damage to these structures.

Severe disruption of these ligaments can remove the palmar support to both the metacarpophalangeal and the proximal interphalangeal joints, which results in sinking of the fetlock or subluxation of the proximal interphalangeal joint. The latter is seen as a "ring-bone"-like swelling on the dorsal aspect of the pastern, clicking of the proximal interphalangeal joint during walking, or an uneven joint space dorsopalmarly in lateromedial radiographs.

The ODSL lie on the palmarolateral and palmaromedial aspects of the proximal pastern and run distally and toward the midline. Oblique views are therefore necessary to examine them. They are discrete oval structures immediately distal to the proximal sesamoid bones but become triangular distally and lie adjacent to the palmar surface of the first phalanx. They decrease in size distally, as they insert on the palmar aspect of the first phalanx in a V-shaped area. Injury is manifested by enlargement, alterations in internal echogenicity, and periligamentous fibrosis. Enthesiophytosis or avulsion fragments can frequently be identified at their insertion, which may or may not be the cause of lameness. Uniaxial enlargement without reduced echogenicity has been identified in horses with pronounced valgus deformity of the metacarpophalangeal joint. This is assumed to be an adaptive response and not necessarily a cause of lameness.

The SDSL can be visualized from the palmar aspect of the pastern as the most echogenic structure in the pastern region. It is triangular proximally, becomes reniform in the midpastern and, before insertion on the middle scutum on the palmar aspect of the proximal interphalangeal joint, is square. In longitudinal views, it enlarges in a proximodistal direction, but there is usually a space between the SDSL and the DDFT and between the SDSL and the palmar aspect of the proximal phalanx distal to the insertion of the ODSL. Injury to this ligament results in obliteration of these spaces and alteration in the normal striated pattern of the ligament. In the transverse views, there is enlargement, extensive periligamentous fibrosis, and focal or diffuse reduction in the internal echogenicity of the ligament. Care should be taken not to confuse the central hypoechoic region close to its insertion as a lesion.

Radiography occasionally demonstrates osseous bodies on the palmar aspect of the pastern. These fragments can be identified ultrasonographically as intraligament calcification, avulsion fractures, or enthesiophytosis.

Treatment and Prognosis

Treatment is rest, anti-inflammatory therapy in the acute phase, and an exercise program that increases in intensity over several months. Horses with severe damage with subluxation of the proximal interphalangeal joint or sinking of the fetlock benefit from 6 to 8 weeks in a distal limb cast and may require arthrodesis of the proximal interphalangeal joint. A successful return to work following arthrodesis depends on the healing of the DSL lesions.

The prognosis for these injuries is guarded. Recurrence is said to be very common, although no large series based on accurate ultrasonographic diagnosis has been published.

Digital Annular Ligament Disease

Etiology

In the authors' opinion, thickening of the digital annular ligaments is usually the result of other soft tissue disease of the region such as tendinitis or digital sheath distension. Primary desmitis of the ligaments has been described as giving rise to a condition similar to palmar annular ligament syndrome. Avulsion of the insertion of the proximal digital annular ligament has been recognized. Its etiology is speculative but may be a consequence of rapid increase in tension in the digital flexor tendons associated with metacarpophalangeal joint overextension and interphalangeal joint flexion, giving a bowstring effect.

Clinical Signs and Diagnosis

The only clinical sign of primary thickening of these ligaments is swelling, and it still remains to be shown if this change can be the cause of lameness. Ultrasonographically, the proximal digital annular ligaments can be identified on the palmarolateral and palmaromedial aspects of the proximal pastern region where they are more discrete structures, lying immediately deep to the subcutaneous tissues. They merge with the digital sheath wall in the midline, which makes their definition difficult at this site unless they are enlarged. Avulsion fractures are identified radiographically as bony fragments on the palmarolateral or palmaromedial aspect of the proximal aspect of the proximal phalanx, about 1 to 2 cm below the joint margin. They can be confirmed as avulsion fractures with ultrasonography. Avulsion fractures with no concurrent ligament damage have been recognized recently by the authors in a small number of cases, all presenting with acute onset of severe lameness.

Treatment and Prognosis

Treatment is directed at the primary problem, if one can be identified. The ligaments can be transected surgically if primary thickening is thought to be producing a constrictive effect, although the veterinarian should always be conscious that other undetected lesions could be the primary problem. Avulsion fractures are treated with rest in a stall and nonsteroidal anti-inflammatory drugs (e.g., phenylbutazone [2 mg/kg p.o. b.i.d.]) until the acute signs of lameness and local pain have resolved, when the horse can be turned out in a small paddock. The prognosis is good after a total of 3 to 6 months' rest.

Too few cases have been seen to give an accurate assessment of prognosis. However, the one reported case that was treated by surgical transection returned to work. Avulsion fractures have a good prognosis after a period of rest.

PERCUTANEOUS SOFT TISSUE INJURIES

Open wounds in the pastern region are common. Exploration and debridement of the wound are more important than systemic antibacterial therapy. Nonetheless, after appropriate local treatment, the majority of horses should be given a course of an antibacterial agent. This may range from 3 to 5 days of penicillin intramuscularly (IM) for a contaminated superficial wound, to a 2- to 3-week course of a broad-spectrum antimicrobial such as trimethoprim-potentiated sulfonamide or combination of agents (e.g., penicillin and gentamicin) when there is gross contamination or synovial sheath involvement.

Penetrating Injuries to the Palmar Pastern

Penetrating injuries to the pastern are extremely common but frequently misdiagnosed. The skin wounds may be small and belie the seriousness of the damage to the underlying soft tissues. As a result, serious injury can be overlooked, and delayed appropriate treatment results in an unfavorable prognosis. Consequently, horses with such injuries should be examined ultrasonographically at the first consultation.

Clinical Signs and Diagnosis

Penetration of the skin and the digital sheath initially produces only transient lameness. In contrast, penetration of a tendon or ligament produces more severe, persistent lameness and a painful focus on palpation. After 24 to 48 hours, if infection becomes established, more severe lameness develops and pain and swelling become more generalized throughout the region.

The area should be carefully inspected, and penetrating wounds should be followed to their limit ultrasonographically, to identify foreign material, which is obvious as bright hyperechoic foci casting an acoustic shadow or reverberation artifact in the case of metal or gas. Careful examination of all of the structures in the pastern, in at least two views, helps to identify subcutaneous abscessation, digital sheath penetration, and flexor tendon damage. In many cases, only the surface of the DDFT is damaged. This can be easily missed ultrasonographically, especially because the DDFT has a normal midline depression in the midpastern and distal pastern regions, which can be mistaken for a surface defect. It is important to identify these injuries, because they will be sites of subsequent adhesion formation.

Ultrasonographic examination can lead to a suspicion of sepsis of either the digital sheath or tendon. The former is recognized as a thickened and edematous synovial membrane, digital sheath effusion, which may contain flocculent material, edematous subcutaneous tissues, or air within the sheath. Septic tendinitis appears as hypoechoic defects within a mildly enlarged tendon. Re-examination after a few days reveals rapid progression of the lesion, unlike a strain injury. Septic tendinitis occurring within the digital sheath is also usually associated with digital sheath sepsis.

If digital sheath violation is suspected based on either clinical or ultrasonographic examination results, digital sheath synoviocentesis is indicated to confirm or exclude sheath sepsis.

Treatment and Prognosis

Cases in which the digital sheath has not been entered require local debridement of the wound, if present, and systemic antibacterial treatment. Injection of sodium hyaluronate into the sheath is recommended in an attempt to limit adhesion formation if there is evidence of trauma to the sheath or tendons. Those cases that do not have digital sheath or tendon sepsis, but significant tendon damage, can have slow, progressive degeneration of tendon tissue around the injury over 1 to 2 months ("aseptic degeneration"). Surgical debridement of these areas should be considered to limit adhesion formation. Tenoscopic debridement is the treatment of choice, because it is associated with minimal morbidity of the digital sheath and therefore reduces the risk of subsequent adhesions.

If there is established sepsis in the subcutaneous tissues, digital sheath, or tendon, surgery is recommended. If the wound is open, exploration and debridement can be performed through the wound, but if the wound has healed, tenoscopy is the surgical method of choice. Debridement of the infected area and lavage of the digital sheath must be performed at the earliest opportunity. If there is considerable damage to the tendons and sheath, the limb can be cast postoperatively for 2 to 6 weeks.

Those cases without sepsis have a fair prognosis for a full return to work, although this is dependent on the extent of the damage and the formation of adhesions within the sheath. Cases of uncomplicated digital sheath sepsis have a good prognosis if treatment is started within 24 hours. Those cases with established sepsis have poorer prognoses, although even those with combined sheath and tendon sepsis can become sound enough to perform low levels of exercise satisfactorily.

Tendon Lacerations in the Pastern Region

Clinical Signs and Diagnosis

Wire and sharp objects such as glass can result in tendon laceration rather than simple penetration. Lameness is severe and often involves an alteration in foot, pastern, or fetlock conformation, depending on the structure lacerated and the extent of the laceration. Partial laceration causes few conformational changes. Complete laceration of the SDFT branches, which is rare, results in sinking of the fetlock only when the limb is loaded. Complete laceration of the DDFT produces an upward-moving toe when the limb is loaded and can result in subluxation of the distal interphalangeal joint, if chronic. If the DSL are lacerated in conjunction with either of the above, there is further sinking of the fetlock, with or without subluxation of the proximal interphalangeal joint. The latter can also be provoked if the laceration extends into the palmar ligaments of this joint. Any laceration to the palmar aspect of the pastern is highly likely to enter the digital sheath, and synovial fluid may be seen leaking from the wound.

Diagnosis is based on the clinical signs and careful exploration of the wound, which is usually performed under general anesthesia. Ultrasonography has limited use, because the large wound that usually accompanies these injuries allows direct visualization of the damaged tendons and can prevent good contact with the probe. However, ultrasonography can be useful to assess the degree of damage to the tendons proximal and distal to the wound. Complete laceration of only one SDFT branch can result in displacement of the SDFT to the contralateral side farther proximally.

Treatment and Prognosis

The wound and tendon ends must be debrided and the digital sheath lavaged. The severed tendon ends should be sutured, preferably using three-loop pulley or interlocking loop suture patterns of monofilament absorbable suture material such as polydioxanone (PDS). Many partial lacerations do not require suturing to maintain the integrity of the tendon, but suturing is still recommended within a sheath because tendon ends heal poorly within a synovial cavity.

These injuries result in damage to both the digital sheath and the tendons, and thus adhesions are a common sequela. Consequently, these injuries carry a poor prognosis.

Heel Lacerations

Clinical Signs and Diagnosis

Lacerations involving the heel bulbs, hoof wall, and the deeper soft tissues of the pastern are a common occurrence in equine practice, either as a result of wire wounds or entrapment of the foot. They are frequently severely contaminated and contused and may contain foreign bodies. It is important to establish the extent of the damage. Radiography should detect bony lesions and the presence of radiopaque foreign bodies within the hoof capsule. Water-soluble ionic contrast agents (e.g., 15 ml of Urografin 310 or 370° diluted 1:1 with sterile saline) can be injected into the digital sheath proximally to illustrate communication with the wound. Ultrasonography has little use in this region, because a large wound is usually present and the hoof is often involved.

Treatment and Prognosis

Conservative management of these cases is frequently disappointing, with scar tissue distorting the affected heel. Surgical debridement under general anesthesia is the treatment of choice, with a careful search for foreign bodies. This is particularly important if the laceration has involved a radiolucent material, such as wood, and the laceration has extended into the hoof capsule where foreign bodies can remain hidden. The debrided wound is then closed partially or fully, whichever is possible, using tension-spreading suture patterns such as vertical mattress sutures, and the distal limb is placed in a cast for 3 to 4 weeks. This produces a good cosmetic effect in uncomplicated cases. If the digital sheath is involved, it should be lavaged. Disruption of the coronary band should be debrided carefully and the two edges of the coronary band apposed surgically to minimize the ensuing hoof wall defect. If the wound cannot be debrided fully, delayed closure can be

_____

Schering Health Care Ltd; Burgess Hill, West Sussex, UK

performed with the wound managed conservatively for 3 to 5 days before undergoing surgical closure and casting. In the absence of digital sheath involvement, the prognosis is good. Owners should be warned of possible hoof wall deficits if the coronary band has been damaged.

Supplemental Readings

Baxter GM: Retrospective study of lower limb wounds involving tendons, tendon sheaths or joints in horses. Proc 33rd Annu Meet Am Assoc Equine Pract, 1987, pp 715–728.

Denoix J-M, Crevier N, Azevedo C: Ultrasound examination of the pastern in horses. Proc 37th Annu Meet Am Assoc Equine Pract, 1991, pp 363–380.

Dyson SJ, Denoix J-M: Tendon, tendon sheath and ligament injuries in the pastern. Vet Clin North Am Equine Pract 11:217–233, 1995.

Hago BED, Vaughan LC: Radiographic anatomy of tendon sheaths and bursae in the horse. Equine Vet J 18:102–106, 1986.

Moyer W: Distal sesamoidean desmitis. Proc 28th Annu Meet Am Assoc Equine Pract, 1982, pp 245–251.

Nixon AJ: Endoscopy of the digital flexor tendon sheath in horses. Vet Surg 19:266–271, 1990.

Redding WR: Evaluation of the equine digital flexor tendon sheath using diagnostic ultrasound and contrast radiography. Vet Radiol Ultrasound 35:42–48, 1994.

Stashak TS: Management of lacerations and avulsion injuries of the foot and pastern region and hoof wall cracks. Vet Clin North Am Equine Pract 5:195–220, 1989.

Weaver JCB, Stover SM, O'Brien TR: Radiographic anatomy of soft tissue attachments in the equine metacarpophalangeal and proximal phalangeal region. Equine Vet J 24:310–315, 1992.

_____

Penetrating Injuries of the Foot

ANDREW P. BATHE
Oakham, England

TIMOTHY R. C. GREET
Newmarket, England

Penetrating injuries of the foot are a common problem in equine practice. The majority of wounds tend to be superficial and respond well to treatment. Deeper penetrations can lead to more serious sequelae, which may have a hopeless prognosis without prompt diagnosis and treatment. Injuries to the middle third of the frog are the most damaging, because of the underlying deep digital flexor tendon, navicular bone and bursa, impar ligament, distal interphalangeal joint, and digital tendon sheath. Deep injuries adjacent to this region may involve the distal phalanx, digital cushion, or collateral cartilages. Fracture, osteomyelitis, and synovial sepsis are all possible sequelae. It is therefore essential to determine accurately the site, direction, and depth of penetration, because accurate diagnosis and rapid treatment give the best chance of a successful outcome, especially if the navicular bursa is involved.

DIAGNOSTIC PROCEDURES

History

The history may range from the immediate detection of a penetration of the foot to unexplained lameness. In an acute injury, as much information as possible should be obtained regarding the anatomic location, depth and direction of penetration, and nature of the object causing the penetration. Leaving a foreign body in situ until a veterinarian has examined the injury can facilitate accurate assessment of structures involved but increases the risk of further trauma. Horses with deep penetrations may develop severe lameness immediately after puncture; in other cases sepsis may lead to the development of lameness some days later. A more thorough history is necessary with chronic lesions, including the duration of the problem and response to treatment. In all cases, tetanus antitoxin should be administered if there is any doubt as to the tetanus immunity of the animal.

Clinical Examination

Horses with penetrating injuries of the foot often "point" the foot forward. The foot may be placed preferentially to protect specific areas of pain; for instance, a heel injury may lead to a toe-first foot placement. Lameness is generally evident when the horse walks and is exacerbated by trotting on a firm surface. The degree of lameness depends on the nature and time course of the injury. Synovial sepsis often produces a very severe persistent lameness. Deep infections such as septic osteitis of the distal phalanx or a digital cushion abscess may present minimal lameness if there is free drainage. Typically, the degree of lameness increases if there is obstruction of drainage and subsequent pressure build-up, such as in a simple subsolar abscess.

The digital pulse amplitude is usually increased, and evaluation of its symmetry may assist in localizing the lesion to the medial or lateral side. Swelling of the distal limb is common, and some cases develop cellulitis, which can preclude accurate palpation. The digital sheath and distal interphalangeal joint capsule should be palpated for distension. The coronary band and heels should be carefully evaluated for evidence of tracking infection, revealed as areas of softening or a discharging sinus.

The solar surface must be carefully examined, which may necessitate shoe removal. A foreign body penetrating the hoof should be left in place and the foot should be radiographed immediately. Digital palpation of the solar area may identify areas of warmth or pain. It is preferable to reserve the use of hoof testers until the end of the foot examination, because the horse may be less cooperative after induction of severe pain. Carefully paring the solar area allows detection of any tracts. These can be especially difficult to detect in the frog, because the relatively soft horn tends to collapse around the tract once the penetrating object is removed. The frog should therefore be cut back to fresh tissue. Suspicious tracts should be probed with a narrow, blunt, sterile instrument to determine their depth and direction. The surrounding horn can then be pared away to explore the sensitive structures for foreign material or pus.

If the horse is very lame and uncooperative, thorough examination is often facilitated by sedation with detomidine and butorphanol. Regional analgesia may be necessary for examination of the sensitive regions of the foot. If there is profuse hemorrhage, a simple tourniquet of elastic cohesive bandage material placed tightly around the fetlock improves visualization and decreases blood loss.

Radiographic Examination

A radiographic examination is recommended to identify radiodense foreign bodies, osseous sepsis, gas shadows associated with areas of infection (Fig. 1), and other abnormalities such as fractures or subluxation of the distal interphalangeal joint. Careful foot preparation and packing help to minimize radiographic artifacts, facilitating interpretation. Lateromedial and dorsoproximal-palmarodistal oblique ("upright pedal" view of the distal phalanx) plain radiographic projections of the foot should be obtained as an absolute minimum. It is preferable to obtain multiple ra-

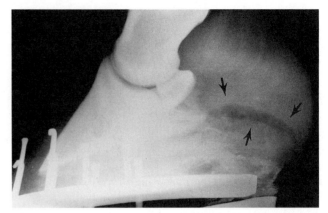

Figure 1. Plain lateromedial radiograph of a foot with a puncture wound in the frog region of 2 weeks' duration. Arrows indicate gas shadow in digital cushion region. Gas and pus were subsequently drained from this region.

diographic views, including dorsopalmar (standing), dorsoproximal-palmarodistal oblique ("upright pedal" view for the navicular bone), and palmaroproximal-palmarodistal oblique ("flexor view") projections. The latter projection is especially valuable for detecting lesions on the flexor cortex of the navicular bone, and is extremely useful in detecting the early radiologic signs of osteomyelitis (Fig. 2). Septic osteitis of the distal phalanx usually appears as lysis without periosteal reaction, and there may be sequestration. Exposure factors may be varied to assess soft tissue structures and bone detail. Lesion-oriented oblique views can be obtained as indicated by each individual case. Serial radiographic examinations may be necessary because osseous changes due to sepsis may take 2 weeks or more to appear.

If the penetrating object is still present, at least two perpendicular projections should be obtained to appreciate accurately its anatomic location. If the penetrating object is not present, a sterile malleable metallic probe should be introduced carefully and radiographs obtained. A liquid radiopaque contrast medium° may be introduced via a catheter. Contrast filling of a synovial structure is definite evidence of penetration, and sepsis should be presumed.

°*Conray, Mallinckrodt, Northants, UK*

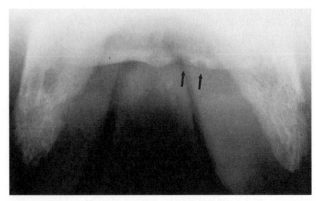

Figure 2. Palmaroproximal-palmarodistal oblique radiograph of navicular bone. A radiolucent area on the sagittal ridge has resulted from osteomyelitis. This was not evident on any other projection.

Some tracts are better identified with probes, whereas in others a contrast medium offers more information. Synovial involvement cannot be ruled out by use of these radiographic techniques because penetration does not always result in a persistent tract. Some tracts, especially chronic ones, are very difficult to follow. In other cases, infection adjacent to a synovial cavity may erode through, causing a delayed synovial sepsis.

Further Diagnostic Techniques

Regional analgesia may be helpful to confirm the foot as the source of pain. However, it should be noted that pain in horses with severe foot lameness is often refractory to local analgesia. Thus, a negative or poor response to a nerve block does not rule out foot pain. Some of the more invasive techniques described later may be more easily performed under general anesthesia.

Synoviocentesis is usually necessary to confirm the presence of synovial sepsis and should be carried out as deemed appropriate by clinical evaluation. Radiography may be necessary to ensure accurate needle placement in the navicular bursa. It is important to avoid conducting synoviocentesis through an area of infection because of the risk of synovial contamination.

Synovial fluid samples can usually be collected, but with more difficulty in chronic cases in which fibrin and synovial membrane hypertrophy tend to block the needle. Samples should be submitted for white blood cell count and differential, cytologic examination, protein concentration determination, and bacteriology examination. The leukocyte count is the most useful parameter and in established sepsis is usually greater than 10×10^9/L, with neutrophils predominating. Occasionally, the leukocyte count may be lower in the presence of sepsis, especially with recent contamination. The leukocyte count may be elevated, but to a lesser degree, by infection and inflammation adjacent to the synovial cavity. In such less clear-cut cases, protein concentration determination and cytologic examination are beneficial. The success rate for bacterial culture, useful in ensuring appropriate antibiosis, is greatly enhanced if samples are placed immediately into a broth culture medium.[*]

Distending the synovial cavity with sterile saline or a polyionic solution may cause detectable leakage if there is a penetration. A more accurate form of assessment is a positive contrast study (Fig. 3), using a sterile water-soluble iodine preparation.[†] This may be more precise than fistulography, because many tracts are too narrow for the easy passage of a catheter.

Ultrasonographic examination may be beneficial in the assessment of soft tissue swellings in the coronary band, tendon, and tendon sheath regions, although this is a difficult area for accurate interpretation. Experiences in our clinic with gamma scintigraphy after the intravenous injection of radiolabeled leukocytes have shown that this can be a very sensitive means of diagnosing occult sepsis.

MANAGEMENT OF SUPERFICIAL PENETRATIONS

The majority of superficial penetrations set up a subsolar or submural abscess, which responds well to removal of

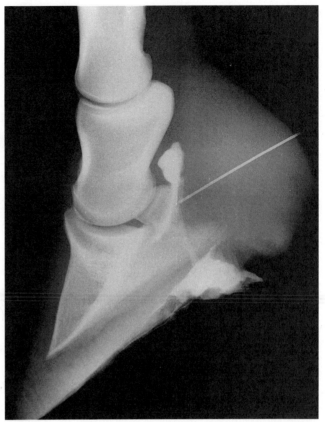

Figure 3. Lateromedial radiograph of foot after injection of contrast medium into navicular bursa. The contrast medium is seen to leave the bursa along a sinus tract. (From Smith RKW, Schramme MC: The use of contrast agents in the diagnosis of penetrating wounds of the foot in five cases. Equine Vet Educ 4:177–182, 1992.)

the overlying hard horn. A large hole encourages free drainage, but the aggressive management of a smaller hole can lead to quicker healing, which is an important consideration in competition horses. Infections of the white line due to a horseshoe nail being driven deep to the stratum corneum often drain adequately once the nail is removed. Dilute hydrogen peroxide is a useful lavage solution because of its mechanical cleansing activity. Clinical experience suggests that topical metronidazole is also extremely effective in these sites. Systemic antibiotics are generally considered unnecessary. Soaking the foot in a warm hypertonic solution of sodium chloride, or magnesium sulphate, helps draw septic fluids out of the soft tissues. Poulticing by applying a hot wet dressing[*] to the foot is most beneficial in softening hard horn before paring and in helping to bring a developing abscess to a head. Care must be taken not to oversoften the hoof with repeated poulticing. Superficial penetrations sometimes resolve quicker if they are allowed to develop a small abscess, which is then drained, rather than being pared repeatedly in the early stages.

Once drainage is established, the wound should be packed or covered with povidone-iodine–soaked swabs and a waterproof bandage applied. Stall rest on clean bedding is recommended to reduce the risk of contamination. Non-

[*]*Bloodgrow, Medical Wire and Equipment Co., Wilts, UK*
[†]*Hypaque meglumine 60%, Winthrop Pharmaceuticals, New York, NY*

[*]*Animalintex, Robinson Animal Healthcare, Chesterfield, UK*

steroidal anti-inflammatory drugs are beneficial because inflammation often persists even after resolution of infection. Once the wound is granulating and nonexudative it may be packed with a bacteriostatic filler.*

MANAGEMENT OF DEEP PENETRATIONS

Detailed discussion of surgical procedures for deep penetrations or extensive hoof injuries is beyond the scope of this text, and the reader is referred to the reading list. These injuries require local treatment as well as systemic medical treatment. Broad-spectrum systemic antibiosis, such as a combination of penicillin (20–40,000 IU/kg IV t.i.d.) and gentamicin (2.2 mg/kg IV t.i.d.), is generally preferred for deep penetrations. Other antibiotics that have proved useful in these generally mixed infections include ceftiofur (2.2 mg/kg IM b.i.d.), oxytetracycline (2.6 mg/kg IV b.i.d.), and metronidazole (22 mg/kg p.o. b.i.d.). Nonsteroidal anti-inflammatory drugs are beneficial on humane grounds; they also reduce the risk of a weightbearing laminitis in the contralateral limb. They may potentially interfere with the assessment of the response to treatment, but the lameness is usually so severe that this should not be a major concern.

Surgical procedures can be performed either with the horse under general anesthesia or with the horse standing. In the latter situation, treatment is facilitated by sedation, local analgesia, and a tourniquet. Acute deep penetrations of the soft tissue structures or distal phalanx can be treated by conservative conical debridement of the tract, accompanied by lavage and systemic antibiotics. More established infections require a greater degree of exposure and debridement but still carry a generally good prognosis.

Sepsis involving the navicular bone, bursa, and/or distal interphalangeal joint requires rapid radical surgical intervention. The navicular bursa is debrided and drained by an approach through the frog, digital cushion, and deep digital flexor tendon (i.e., the "streetnail operation"). Even with intensive postoperative management and prolonged convalescence, the prognosis is often poor. In some cases the primary infection cannot be controlled, whereas in

---

Keratex Hoof Putty, EPC, Somerset, UK

TABLE 1.   DURATION OF TREATMENT AND OUTCOME FOR PENETRATING INJURIES OF THE FOOT

	Approximate Duration of Treatment	Prognosis
Subsolar abscess	Days	Excellent
Septic osteitis of the distal phalanx	Weeks	Very good
Acute septic navicular bursitis	Weeks	Poor
Chronic septic navicular bursitis	Months	Very poor

others, necrotic tendinitis or severe fibrous adhesions develop. Septic arthritis of the distal interphalangeal joint often follows penetrations through the navicular bursa and impar ligament. Treatment is by through-and-through lavage, which may have to be repeated on several occasions.

Treatment plate shoes are easily made by securing an aluminum plate to the ground surface of a bar shoe with bolts or studs. This greatly simplifies the postoperative management of solar defects, because it is easy to maintain and change the protective packing. Wedging the heels in cases of septic navicular bursitis often enables the horse to stand more comfortably, and a useful rule of thumb is to shoe the horse to maintain the position in which it prefers to hold its affected foot.

PROGNOSIS

The prognosis for return to full athletic function is directly related to the severity of the injury and its chronicity. A summary of likely duration of treatment and outcome is provided in Table 1.

Supplemental Readings

DeBowes RM, Yovich JV: Penetrating wounds, abscesses, gravel, and bruising of the equine foot. Vet Clin North Am Equine Pract 5(1):179–194, 1989.

Richardson GL, Pascoe JR, Meagher D: Puncture wounds of the foot in horses: Diagnosis and treatment. Comp Cont Ed Pract Vet 8:S379–S387, 1986.

Steckel RR: Puncture wounds, abscesses, thrush, and canker. In Robinson NE (ed): Current Therapy in Equine Medicine, ed 2. Philadelphia, WB Saunders, 1987, pp 266–272.

Hoof Cracks and Hoof Wall Avulsions

ANDREW H. PARKS
Athens, Georgia

HOOF CRACKS

Hoof cracks are longitudinal defects in the hoof wall that parallel the direction of hoof growth. Several characteristics are used to categorize hoof cracks:

1. The location (i.e., at the toe, quarter, heel, or bar)
2. The origin (i.e., at the coronary band or ground surface)
3. Their length, complete or incomplete
4. Their depth; superficial cracks are confined to the stratum medium, whereas deep cracks extend to the corium.

Many conditions cause hoof cracks. A condition that damages the biomechanical properties of the hoof wall, increases overall stresses to the hoof wall, or concentrates stress locally increases the likelihood that the hoof wall deforms or fractures. The biomechanical properties of the hoof wall are altered by changes in hydration and pre-existing disease. Although stiffness and yield stress decrease with increasing moisture content, resistance to fracture is greatest at intermediate hydration. Therefore, very dry or moist environmental conditions facilitate formation of hoof cracks. Fracture toughness of the dorsal hoof wall is uniform except at its distal margin, where it decreases by 50%. This fact correlates well with the clinical observation that distal hoof cracks are common in horses with overgrown hooves. The hoof wall structure is weakened in chronic laminitis by the abnormal formation of the keratinized tissues by the damaged laminae. Previous trauma and infection also weaken the hoof wall. The overall stresses on the horse's hoof are increased by repetitive work on hard surfaces. Local concentration of stress owing to foot imbalance, or the addition of calks to shoes, increases shear stresses, thereby enhancing the likelihood of fractures of the hoof wall.

Clinical Signs

Many cracks probably start within the stratum medium of the hoof wall. By the time hoof cracks are clinically evident, they have usually broken through the external surface, so that their location and length is obvious. In contrast, bar cracks may not be evident without close inspection. Application of hoof testers to suspicious lines or fissures may elicit a withdrawal response or may demonstrate instability of the hoof wall, thereby confirming the presence of a hoof crack. Response to hoof testers may also indicate the approximate location of clinically significant occult cracks. The outward appearance of a crack is often deceptive, because a narrow fissure may hide a wider defect in the stratum medium. Most hoof cracks are narrow, unless hoof wall has been lost owing to wear at the ground surface. However, the width of a crack associated with a coronary band injury depends on the width of the coronary band defect. Hemorrhage or purulent exudate in a crack indicates trauma to the corium and infection, respectively.

Midsagittal toe cracks are usually superficial and are often associated with a flattening or slight concavity of the dorsal hoof wall. Quarter cracks and heel cracks are more likely to be deep, and consequently are more likely to cause lameness than are toe cracks.

Hoof cracks need not result in lameness, unless either instability causes pinching of the laminar corium or the affected tissue is infected. Application of hoof testers and a uniaxial palmar digital or abaxial sesamoid nerve block confirms the crack as the source of a horse's lameness.

Treatment

The objectives of treatment are to resolve infection, allow epidermal defects to heal, prevent the crack from propagating farther, and stabilize the crack to allow it to grow out. The specific treatment of the crack depends upon the nature of the crack, the thickness of the hoof wall, the experience of the farrier and veterinarian, the type of work for which the horse is intended, and the time available for rest.

When foot imbalance contributes to the cause of the hoof crack, normal balance should be restored. Foot imbalance not associated with displacement of the coronary band is corrected readily, by trimming the foot appropriately. Superficial toe cracks can be treated simply by re-establishing foot balance and shoeing. More complicated cracks may require additional forms of therapy. If there is proximal displacement of the coronary band, the imbalance cannot be corrected immediately by trimming, because the coronary band has to descend. Therefore, it is best to correct the imbalance before proceeding with further repair of the crack. Otherwise the persistent instability, caused by the imbalance, will contribute to failure of the crack repair, or the repair may impede descent of the coronary band to its normal position.

Various methods have been used to stabilize hoof cracks: grooving the hoof wall isolates a crack; bridging sutures reduce tension across a crack; filling the crack counteracts compression across the crack; and rigidly bridging the crack reduces both tension and compression. To prevent propagation of a crack effectively by grooving the hoof wall, the groove must be at least as deep as the crack. Horizontal grooves are positioned at the distal end of proximal cracks, or at the proximal end of distal cracks. Alternatively, a proximal crack can be isolated between two oblique

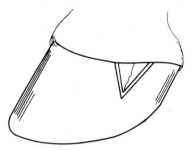

Figure 1. Isolation of a proximal hoof crack with two grooves forming a V.

grooves that form a V (Fig. 1). To add stability to the hoof wall adjacent to distal toe cracks, clips may be drawn up from the shoe approximately 2 cm on either side of the crack.

All cracks that are infected or require stabilization with prosthetic hoof material must be explored with a small motorized burr or router bit. Infected cracks should be debrided and wrapped with a topical antiseptic, such as povidone-iodine, until all infection has cleared and the wound has completely epithelialized. Only then should the hoof crack repair be completed.

Deep or painful cracks require further stabilization. Various rapid-setting synthetic polymers, including acrylics and epoxy resins, have been used as prosthetic hoof materials. These synthetic polymers are used with or without the support of implants, which include wire or synthetic multifilament sutures, sheet metal screws, woven fiberglass, and metal plates. The crack is first prepared to accept the prosthetic hoof material, then bridged with implants if required, and last, the prosthetic hoof material is applied.

The margins of the crack are undermined to aid retention of the polymers within the defect. Horizontal notches, made at intervals along the margins of the crack, prevent slippage of the composite along the axis of the defect. The hoof surface is sanded and thoroughly cleaned with acetone to ensure that the polymers will adhere to the hoof.

Wire or synthetic sutures are threaded through holes drilled in the hoof wall. These holes can usually be drilled perpendicular to the crack from either side, and the sutures are placed in horizontal mattress or bootlace patterns (Fig. 2). Stents formed from small metal plates, with holes drilled to accommodate the sutures, decrease the tendency for the sutures to pull through the hoof wall. Alternatively, for cracks that involve the distal hoof wall, four holes are

drilled proximally from the ground surface of the wall, just outside the white line, to exit the wall in a staggered fashion, approximately 12 and 15 mm from each side of the defect; the holes most distant to the defect exit the wall near the most proximal extent of the defect, whereas the two inner holes exit the wall approximately halfway up the defect. A single multifilament synthetic suture is then threaded through the four holes in a near-far far-near pattern (Fig. 3). Sutures applied to toe cracks should be tied while the horse is bearing weight on the foot. Sutures applied to quarter or heel cracks should be tied with the foot off the ground. Application of cyanoacrylate adhesive to knots prevents slippage of synthetic fiber sutures while the repair is completed. Sheet metal screws are used to anchor figure-of-eight wire sutures, or woven fiberglass. The screws must have their points ground off before they are placed into holes predrilled with a motorized burr. The screws must not be placed so deep that they impinge on the corium; this can be difficult to judge where the wall is thin. Hoof cracks repaired with implants are stronger than those without implants, but a portion of the hoof wall may be lost if the repair pulls away from the hoof wall.

The epoxy or acrylic is poured into a pocket that has been built up around the hoof crack with aluminum foil or polyester film. Narrow defects are filled with the synthetic polymer alone. Larger defects caused by hoof wall loss are filled with several layers of woven fiberglass cut to size and sandwiched between layers of the synthetic polymer. After the defect is filled, the bridging materials are incorporated into the repair to provide additional stability and give the repair a smooth surface. Some of the polymers set to a hard brittle finish that is prone to fracture, which necessitates replacement of the repair. Other polymers are rubberized to prevent fracturing of the repair.

A technique for patching infected cracks that allows for drainage beneath the repair has been described for horses that are expected to perform before the infection has resolved. The crack is explored and prepared as previously described. The hoof wall defect is plugged with water-soluble clay along which a rigid drain is placed so that the drain exits the proximal aspect of the final repair. The hoof crack is bridged with woven fiberglass and an acrylic or epoxy patch. After the repair material has set, the clay is flushed from beneath the repair. The crack is then lavaged and medicated through the drain until the crack has healed.

The foot is shod to protect the repair and provide stability. "Floating" the hoof on one or both sides of the crack is not recommended because it may induce further instability,

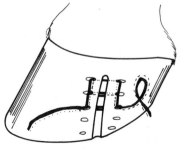

Figure 2. Application of a bootlace suture to a crack. Note that the holes are drilled perpendicular to the direction of the hoof crack.

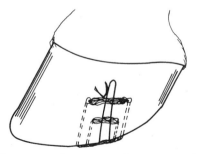

Figure 3. A far-near near-far suture used to repair cracks that involve the ground surface of the wall.

unless floating the hoof is required to restore normal balance. Some clinicians prefer to shoe the horse before repairing the crack to avoid disrupting the repair. Others prefer to have good exposure at the ground surface of the wall during the repair process, and therefore apply the shoe afterwards. An open shoe may be used with toe cracks, but all others require a bar shoe. Nails can be driven through rubberized polymers but not through brittle polymers because they are liable to fracture. As the foot grows, the hoof repair moves distally. When the horse is reshod, the distal margin of the patch must be filed even with the new level of the hoof wall; rubberized polymers tolerate filing better than more brittle polymers. For obvious reasons, it is important that the farrier be aware of the presence of metallic implants in the hoof crack repair.

Horses with refractory cracks at the heel or quarter have been treated by complete resection of the wall of the affected heel. This radical procedure is reserved for the most difficult cases. A longitudinal full-thickness cut is made through the hoof wall immediately dorsal to the crack. This cut should extend from the proximal margin of the crack, often the coronary band, to the ground surface. A second longitudinal cut may be necessary palmar/plantar to the crack. A groove is then made in the white line below the affected area. If the hoof crack does not extend to the coronary band, a horizontal groove is cut into the wall at the proximal limit of the hoof to be removed. The wall at the heel is then grasped with a pair of hoof pullers and the affected heel is elevated and removed. The defect is bandaged with an antiseptic dressing and the foot shod with a heart bar or full-support shoe. The bandages are changed until the defect is completely epithelialized, and the method of shoeing is maintained until the defect has grown out.

The prognosis for superficial cracks that do not involve the coronary band is good. Although treatment of horses with deep cracks that are infected or long-standing is often successful, a guarded prognosis should be given. Hoof cracks that involve a defect in the coronary band may be impossible to eliminate, necessitating constant management by trimming and shoeing.

Prevention

Prevention of recurrence of hoof cracks involves identifying and then eliminating the cause. In some instances the cause is obvious. For example, minor imbalances or poor shoeing are readily corrected. Extremely wet or dry environmental conditions are easy to identify, although the moisture content of the hoof wall itself is difficult to assess. Hoof wall hydration can be crudely regulated by changing the environmental conditions; a horse with excessively moist hooves can be placed in a well-drained stall and bedded on kiln-dried shavings. Conversely, hoof dressings can be applied to excessively dry hooves. In other circumstances the cause is identifiable, but it is not simple to eliminate or the treatment is not compatible with the horse's intended use. For example, the changes to the epidermal and dermal lamellae after laminitis are not reversible, although the problem may be managed by appropriate trimming and shoeing. In addition, a racehorse with a quarter crack could be treated easily if the horse is rested or exercised on a different surface, but these changes are not often feasible. The cause for the crack may remain obscure.

HOOF WALL AVULSIONS

Traumatic injuries to the foot can result in avulsion of hoof wall, the heels and quarters being most commonly affected. The avulsion may be complete or partial; in the latter instance, at least one border of the avulsed hoof wall remains attached to the foot. The injury can also involve the integument of the pastern proximal to the coronary band, and the sole and frog of the hoof. Depending on the depth of the injury, structures within the hoof and pastern region can also be involved, and are often the determining factors in prognosis and treatment. These structures include the middle and distal phalanges, navicular bone, the distal interphalangeal joint, navicular bursa, deep digital flexor tendon and sheath, and collateral ligaments.

Clinical Signs

The degree of lameness in affected horses is highly variable. If the palmar digital nerves have been transected, the lameness may be mild. In contrast, the lameness can be severe if infection is present within one of the synovial structures. Examination of the wound may be difficult if the horse is agitated and the wound is heavily soiled. Severe bleeding from a severed palmar digital vessel can precipitate hypotensive shock and hinder inspection of the wound. If the horse is in shock, hemorrhage must be controlled by pressure wraps and appropriate systemic therapy instituted before inspection of the wound can continue. Sedation and regional local anesthesia facilitate clipping the pastern area, cleansing with antiseptics, control of hemorrhage, and inspection of the wound. Ligation of a single palmar digital vessel can usually be performed without compromising the vascularity of the foot as a whole.

The extent of hoof wall loss is obvious. The position and extent of attachment of partial avulsions to the hoof are important factors in determining the method of treatment. The involvement of deeper structures is not always visually obvious, although the location of the injury indicates which structures may be involved. The edges of bone and cartilage may be palpated beneath the avulsed tissue. Excessive laxity on manipulation of the digit suggests damage to the collateral ligaments of the distal interphalangeal joint. Synovial structures may be aspirated and lavaged from a site distant to the wound. Although synovial fluid is rarely obtained by aspiration, if that structure is involved, the presence of lavage fluid in the wound confirms its involvement. Where possible, the vascular integrity of all damaged structures should be assessed by observing them for hemorrhage and tissue color. Radiographs indicate the presence of fractures, luxations, or partial loss of the distal phalanx and navicular bone.

Horses with chronic hoof wall avulsions usually present because of persistent lameness, failure of the wound to heal, or the growth of a horny spur after an incomplete avulsion. The degree of lameness is variable, but is more likely to be mild to moderate. Failure of a wound to heal necessitates inspection of the wound to determine the cause. Osteitis or sequestration of the distal phalanx or the presence of a foreign body should be suspected, although in some hoof injuries the rate of healing of the granulation bed decreases owing to a less than optimal environment at the wound surface. Horny spurs can contribute to lameness if they are not stable, because they may pinch the underlying corium.

Treatment

Treatment of horses with acute hoof wall avulsions can be subdivided into general wound management, management of involved deeper structures, and management of the hoof wall defects. Surgical debridement and reconstruction are best performed with the horse under general anesthesia.

The foot must be prepared for exploration and surgery. After the pastern area is clipped and the hoof wall is lightly rasped to remove contamination, the hoof is aseptically prepared with povidone-iodine and rinsed with sterile saline. After exploration of the wound, it is thoroughly lavaged and debrided. Areas of questionable viability may be left and observed, particularly if they are adjacent to the distal interphalangeal joint, navicular bursa, or tendon sheath, to avoid iatrogenic involvement of these structures. The wound is dressed with topical antiseptics, and bandaged or cast. Frequent dressing changes are required until all surfaces are granulating, and the wound is kept bandaged or enclosed within a cast until it has completely epithelialized. The horse is treated with antibiotics until all exposed surfaces are covered in healthy granulation tissue. For superficial wounds, procaine penicillin G (22,000 IU/kg IM b.i.d.) or trimethoprim sulfadiazine (18–30 mg/kg p.o. b.i.d.) is usually sufficient. If involvement of the deeper structures within the foot is suspected, it is advisable to treat the horse with potassium penicillin (22,000 IU/kg IV q.i.d.) and gentamicin sulfate (2.2 mg/kg IV t.i.d.).

Management of deep injuries of the foot is directed at the specific structures involved. It is often difficult to appreciate the depth of tendon or ligamentous necrosis; all obviously devitalized tissue is removed, and further debridement may be necessary later as the full extent of the injury becomes apparent. Fracture fragments are removed, and areas of septic osteitis curetted. Damaged collateral ligaments necessitate stabilizing the foot with a half-limb cast. Shoeing the foot with an extended heel, when possible, provides support when the deep digital flexor tendon is damaged. Involved synovial structures are repeatedly lavaged through the wound if the defect is large, or from a site distant to the wound if the defect is small, until the infection appears to resolve. Systemic antibiotics are usually continued for 2 or more weeks after the opening into the synovial structure has closed.

Hoof wall defects must heal by secondary intention. Because the margins of the wound are splinted by the remaining hoof, wound contraction does not occur. Therefore, the wound must heal by granulation and epithelialization. All healthy structures within the foot form granulation tissue, although the rate at which they do so differs; bone, ligament, and tendon form granulation tissue slower than corium. Epithelialization of the defect occurs from all adjacent margins, including the coronary, laminar, solar, and cuneate epithelium, and the integument of the pastern. The nature of the wall after the injury depends on the origin of the epithelial tissue in the defect. Epithelium that migrates over the wall from the adjacent laminae, frog, and sole, keratinizes and forms hoof that is thinner and less resilient than normal wall. If the coronary band proximal to the defect is intact, a new wall grows distally to displace the keratinized epithelium derived from the dorsal, palmar, and distal margins of the wound. When the coronary epithelium is absent at the proximal aspect of the injury, epithelium from the integument proximal to the wound can grow down to occupy part of the defect, or the laminar epithelium can grow proximal to the level of the coronary band. Consequently, the integument of the pastern merges into the newly keratinized laminar epithelium. Despite the absence of a normal wall, the newly generated wall is often functional.

Specific treatment of horses with acute hoof wall avulsions can be further subdivided by the nature of the avulsion. Horses with complete avulsions are simplest to treat because decisions about which hoof tissues to resect are usually redundant and no reconstruction is possible. The defect is handled as an open wound and allowed to heal by secondary intention over several months.

Horses with incomplete avulsions not involving the coronary band are treated by resecting the avulsed tissue, usually at its proximal margin. The hoof wall is cut with an oscillating saw, or motorized burr, at the proximal limit of the separated hoof. This procedure prevents adjacent hoof wall from being damaged as the avulsed hoof is removed. The residual defect is handled as previously described.

Incomplete avulsions that involve the coronary band must be assessed to determine the area of attachment and viability of the coronary tissues. If the coronary band is obviously avascular and the surrounding tissues are grossly contaminated or infected, all avulsed tissue is removed. This procedure converts the injury to a complete avulsion, after which it is managed as such. When the hoof wall including the coronary band has been separated at the heel or quarter and is still well vascularized by its attachment to the tissues of the pastern, the hoof wall immediately distal to the coronary band is resected and the coronary band may be sutured in place. To permit placement of sutures, the coronary band, the adjacent hoof wall, and any hoof remaining attached to the coronary band must be thinned down, with a motorized burr or router bit, to the very pale inner layers of the stratum medium. The distal hoof wall defect is then managed as an open wound. Casting the distal limb helps to maintain the coronary band in position as it heals.

Even if there was no loss of underlying tissues at the time of the original injury, extensive demineralization of the distal phalanx adjacent to the injured area is common. If a portion of the distal phalanx is missing and a normal hoof wall is present, a large wedge of weaker keratinized tissue will fill the defect between the wall and sole. If the wall adjacent to the defect in the distal phalanx has not formed from the coronary band, the new modified wall is likely to follow the contour of the defect. In any of these scenarios, a bar shoe is often necessary to stabilize the foot and protect new weaker hoof. Prosthetic hoof materials can be used to fill hoof wall defects.

Chronic wounds that fail to heal may simply require superficial debridement and improvement of the surface environment for healing to progress. Alternatively, debridement of deeper structures may be necessary. Horny spurs resulting from incomplete avulsions that have healed in a displaced position may be resected and attempts made to reposition the coronary band. After the spur is removed, the wedge of tissue underlying the coronary band is resected so that the coronary band can be repositioned, with or without sutures. The distal limb is then cast.

Prognosis

The prognosis is dependent on the structures involved, their vascular integrity, and the degree of contamination or infection present. Unfortunately, the vascular integrity of these structures may be uncertain at the time of the original injury. Therefore, it can be impossible to give the owners an accurate prognosis at the beginning of treatment. Despite this, if the coronary band is intact and no damage to underlying structures has occurred, the prognosis for future use and even cosmetic appearance is fair. If there is severe instability of the foot, or infection of the deeper structures of the foot, the prognosis for survival is guarded to poor.

Supplemental Readings

Moyer W, Sigafoos RD: A Guide to Equine Hoof Wall Repair. Trenton, NJ, Veterinary Learning Systems Inc., 1993.
Nickels FA: Hoof cracks. *In* Robinson NE (ed): Current Therapy in Equine Medicine, ed 2. Philadelphia, WB Saunders, 1987, pp 272–275.
Nickels FA: Hoof lacerations and avulsions. *In* Robinson NE (ed): Current Therapy in Equine Medicine, ed 2. Philadelphia, WB Saunders, 1987, pp 275–277.
Pollitt CC: Color Atlas of the Horse's Foot. Philadelphia, Mosby-Wolfe, 1995, pp 141–147.
Stashak TS: Management of lacerations and avulsion injuries of the foot and pastern region and hoof wall cracks. Vet Clin North Am Equine Pract 5(1):195–220, 1989.

Hoof Imbalance and Lameness

ANDREW H. PARKS
Athens, Georgia

Hoof imbalance has long been considered a cause of lameness in horses, and it has been assumed that balanced feet allow a horse to remain in work. Interestingly, feral horses wear their feet differently than do shod horses; their toes and heels are shorter, the ground surface of the wall is not level, and the frog is fuller. It is highly unlikely that imbalance is common among this group of horses. The majority of shod horses are not considered to be imbalanced or lame. However, many horses that are considered to be imbalanced by existing definitions are not lame. Conversely, other horses with a foot-related lameness respond to minor corrections of imbalance. Therefore, an accurate, universally applicable definition of hoof balance is lacking. Current theories of hoof balance are based mostly on theoretical reasoning and practical experience, but also on an emerging body of applied research.

ANATOMIC AND BIOMECHANICAL CONSIDERATIONS

Several anatomic and biomechanical parameters are important in understanding theories of hoof balance. For simplicity, the following discussion refers to the fore feet unless otherwise stated, but similar principles apply to the hind feet. On firm flat surfaces, the horse's weight is borne by the hoof wall and bars and a thin margin of the adjacent sole. The hoof wall is longest and thickest at the toe and shortest and thinnest at the heel. The slope of the hoof wall indicates the acuteness of the angle the hoof makes with the ground. The slope of the dorsal hoof wall varies considerably between horses, but the median lies between 50 and 54° in the fore feet and 53 and 57° in the hind feet. These angles should coincide with the slope of the dorsal margin of the pastern. The relationship between the slope of the hoof and the slope of the pastern is termed the *foot-pastern axis*. The slope and length of medial and lateral walls are usually nearly symmetrical; the medial wall may be slightly steeper and shorter than the lateral wall. In classical descriptions, the slope of the heel equals the slope of the toe; however, this is seldom the case in shod horses. The heel is usually at a more acute angle to the ground than is the toe.

When viewed from the dorsal surface of the foot, an imaginary line drawn between any two comparable points on the medial and lateral aspects of the coronary band should be parallel to the ground. The foot should appear centered on the pastern. The height of the coronary band at any point on its circumference is the vertical distance between that point and the ground. When viewed from the lateral or medial aspect, the coronary band should form an almost straight line that slopes distopalmarly and drops off at the heels. When viewed from the solar surface of the foot, the wall should be arranged symmetrically around the frog. The frog width should be two thirds of its length. Left and right hooves should form a matched pair.

The hoof wall and sole have different physical characteristics and growth patterns. The physical appearance of the hoof wall is retained as the wall projects distal to its laminar origins, although its fracture toughness decreases at its distal margin. In contrast, the sole maintains a constant thickness of healthy resilient sole below which its appearance changes as it loses resilience, dries out, and exfoliates. The inner surface of the wall is supported by the distal phalanx through the sensitive laminae and by the sole through its attachment at the white line. As the wall projects below the healthy resilient sole, its support decreases where it is attached to exfoliating sole. Ultimately, the wall receives no inner support where it is free of solar attachment.

At rest, a horse is estimated to bear between 28 and 33% of its weight on each forelimb. In contrast, all of a horse's weight accelerating toward the ground is borne on one hoof at a canter. Therefore, the stresses applied to any point of the hoof wall are functions of the horse's weight, the size of its hoof, and the gait. Small feet have been defined as those with weight-to-surface area greater than 2.28×10^3 kg/m². The body weight is transferred to the hoof through the skeletal system. Although the exact center of vertical forces transmitted through the metacarpus is unknown, it is likely to be slightly dorsomedial to the geometric center of the bone. For the purposes of this discussion, the geometric center will be used. The position of the resultant hoof reaction force, representing the summation of instantaneous vertical forces between the hoof and the ground, during full weightbearing is palmar to the geometric center of the foot, in the dorsal third of the frog. When a horse is in motion, the position of the resultant hoof reaction force changes with the phase of stride. The horizontal distance between the position of the resultant hoof reaction force and the geometric center of the metacarpus will be called *load distance* (modified from Snow and Birdsall) for the purposes of this discussion. The importance of the load distance is reflected in descriptions of the normal conformational relationships between the metacarpus, pastern, and foot. In these descriptions, a vertical line bisecting the metacarpal region should brush the palmar surface of the heels. Alternatively, a vertical line dropped from the geometric center of the metacarpal bone should touch the heels at the ground surface. Although stated differently, these two descriptions define a similar anatomic relationship. If the foot is positioned farther forward than indicated by these descriptions, the stresses in the flexor structures increase, the position of the resultant hoof reaction force moves palmarly, or a combination of the two occurs. Conversely, if the foot is farther back, the stresses in the flexor structures decrease, or the resultant hoof reaction force is located farther dorsally.

It is the function of the hoof to transmit forces from the skeletal structures to the ground and provide traction for locomotion. The stresses applied to any portion of the wall are dependent on the proximity of that portion to the resultant hoof reaction force, and the magnitude of that force. How the wall resists these stresses and bending moments depends upon the thickness and mechanical properties of the hoof and the length and slope of the wall.

Several kinetic and kinematic studies have examined the relationship between hoof conformation and joint angulation, at rest and in motion, stride temporal relationships, and hoof ground force interactions. Raising the horse's heels decreases hyperextension of the distal and proximal interphalangeal joint and increases hyperextension of the metacarpophalangeal joints. These angular changes cause the tension in the deep digital flexor tendon to decrease. It is likely that the position of the resultant hoof reaction force must move dorsally, or the load distance decreases, or a combination of the two occurs. Evidence on the effect of elevating the heel on the superficial flexor tendon and suspensory ligament is conflicting; one report states that neither changes, and another states that tension decreases in the superficial flexor tendon and increases in the suspensory ligament. Lowering the heels has the opposite effect to raising them. Angulation of the dorsal hoof wall also affects the pattern of foot fall; horses with acute angulation of the hoof caused by long toes show an increased frequency of toe-first landings. Interestingly, both increasing and decreasing hoof angle away from a straight foot-pastern axis increases the total impulse (area under the force-time curve) on the foot at the walk, trot, and canter. These data suggest that the proprioceptive reflexes are oriented toward optimal placement of the distal phalanx at the beginning of the stride, and support the concept that a straight foot-pastern axis is the most biomechanically favorable conformation for the foot. Deliberately creating medial and lateral imbalance increases the tendency for foot fall to occur on the longer wall or at the toe. Decreasing angulation of the hoof and increasing hoof length both decrease the speed of breakover, but neither increases stride length.° Flat-footed landings are more likely to occur at faster gaits.

MEDIOLATERAL BALANCE

When reading the literature about equine locomotion, one commonly encounters two definitions for mediolateral balance: static and dynamic balance. Static balance is achieved when the plane of the sole of the foot and an imaginary line connecting any two comparable points on the medial and lateral coronary band are perpendicular to the axis of the metacarpus. Consequently, static balance is determined by anatomic examination of the foot. Dynamic balance is determined by observing the manner in which the horse's feet land at a walk or trot; dynamic balance is achieved when medial and lateral heels land simultaneously.

The traditional way to determine static balance is to view the plane of the sole of the foot in relation to the longitudinal axis of the metacarpus with the limb off the ground. The metacarpus is held parallel to the ground and the pastern and foot are allowed to passively extend. This practice is effective as long as the axis of the limb is perpendicular to the ground and the axis of the pastern is the same as the axis of the metacarpus. However, when the limb is viewed in this manner, the metacarpophalangeal joint is not as extended as it is when the limb is bearing weight. Therefore, if the pastern axis is deviated away from the axis of the metacarpus and the metacarpophalangeal joint is in partial extension, it can be argued reasonably that the plane of the sole of the foot will not be perpendicular to the axis of the metacarpus. If the foot is toed out, the lateral wall will appear longer than the medial wall. If the foot is toed in, the medial wall will appear longer than the lateral wall. This argument is borne out by clinical observation. A T-square can be used to increase the accuracy of this visual estimate of balance.

°*Olin Balch, personal communication, 1996.*

Another variation for measuring static balance is by assessing the contour of the coronary band. The wall length is measured at several points around the circumference of the foot; the wall length is plotted graphically against the position around the contour of the coronary band. With the toe at the center of the plot, the graph should be approximately symmetrical, allowing for slight discrepancies in slopes of the lateral and medial walls. Deviations from this symmetrical plot are indicative of areas of excesses or deficiencies in wall length.

Mediolateral balance has also been measured radiographically. The horse's foot is positioned on a block containing an embedded linear radiopaque marker oriented perpendicular to the axial plane of the foot. A dorsopalmar radiograph is then made and examined to determine the distances between the medial and lateral solar margins of the third phalanx and the radiographic marker. The foot is said to be balanced if these two distances are equal. If the foot is imbalanced, the medial and lateral widths of the phalangeal and metacarpophalangeal joints may be unequal. Some caution should be exercised in interpreting these results. If the radiopaque marker is not perpendicular to the primary beam, the distal phalanx may appear artificially angled. If the horse is not bearing weight evenly on the foot, the distal phalanx may appear artificially sloped and the joint spaces artificially uneven.

Dynamic balance is achieved by ensuring simultaneous landing of both heels. There are two drawbacks to the use of this method. First, the time interval between ground contact of the medial and lateral heels is so short that it is difficult to detect at a walk, and it is not detectable at the trot unless the discrepancy is moderate to severe. Therefore, unless high-speed video recording equipment is used, preferably in conjunction with controlled exercise on a treadmill, simultaneous landing of the heels cannot accurately be assessed. Second, the assertion that both heels should land simultaneously is not true for the majority of horses. From the results of a limited study it appears that the majority of horses land on the lateral aspect of the foot first, but any portion of the foot may land first.

In some horses attainment of static and dynamic balance yields the same result. In other horses, one method may produce superior results, and in other horses a compromise or intermediate method may be required for optimal performance.

Mediolateral imbalance is usually caused iatrogenically by trimming so that the medial and lateral aspects of the coronary band are at unequal distances above the ground surface of the foot. This may involve an entire side of the hoof or a smaller portion of the wall. The foot may be deliberately imbalanced to improve the appearance of a horse with either a toed-out or toed-in conformation. Imbalances may also be created unintentionally by inappropriate application of the methods used to determine balance. Mediolateral imbalance is sometimes deliberately created in foals to correct developmental varus and valgus deformities; however, it is more appropriate to level the foot rather than deliberately create an imbalance.

Effects of Mediolateral Imbalance

The effects of mediolateral imbalance are often subtle and are easiest to explain by considering a hypothetical horse in which a gross mediolateral imbalance is deliberately created. If we assume that the lateral wall is trimmed shorter than the medial wall, several immediate sequelae are apparent when the foot is viewed from the dorsal surface: the coronary band is no longer parallel to the ground, but slopes distolaterally; the axial plane of the foot appears rotated medially compared with the axial plane of the pastern; the angle between the lateral wall and the ground is more obtuse, whereas the angle of the medial wall is more acute; and the distal phalanx may appear displaced laterally on the pastern axis. If a dorsopalmar radiograph is examined, the solar margin of the distal phalanx is no longer parallel to the ground but slopes in the same direction as the coronary band; the phalangeal joints appear compressed medially and distracted laterally.

With time, partial or complete compensation for distal phalanx displacement may occur. The medial solar margin of the distal phalanx descends, rendering the solar margin of the distal phalanx more nearly parallel with the ground. Because the length of the wall has not changed since the imbalance was created, the wall has migrated proximally in relation to the distal phalanx. In addition, the toe may rotate back out laterally, the angles of the medial and lateral walls return toward normal, and the axial plane of the foot aligns with that of the pastern. Hoof growth may be retarded, with growth rings being closer together on the medial side of the foot. The medial wall flares, whereas the lateral wall becomes underrun. Finally, the shape of the distal phalanx may also change.

A specific example of mediolateral imbalance is the sheared heel syndrome. This syndrome arises when one heel is left longer than the other when the hoof is trimmed. The long heel then bears a disproportionate amount of the initial impact force at the beginning of the stride, thereby displacing the coronary band on that side of the heel proximally. The affected wall becomes steeper, and a deep central sulcus may develop. In contrast to the effects of generalized lengthening of the one wall, a flare develops between the opposite toe and quarter.

Lameness Associated With Mediolateral Imbalance

Clinical causes of lameness that accompany mediolateral imbalance include joint effusion of the distal interphalangeal, proximal interphalangeal, and metacarpophalangeal joints; sheared heels; and hoof cracks. The precise reasons that mediolateral imbalance causes these problems are unknown. However, it is likely that the torque applied to the joints and the compression of one side and the distraction of the other side of the joint resulting from a mediolateral tilt of the distal phalanx cause synovitis and joint effusion. The eventual result is degenerative joint disease. Therefore, it is not surprising that many horses with mediolateral imbalance become sound with intra-articular anesthesia.

Vertical shear stresses associated with vertical displacement of the coronary band and horizontal compressive and distracting forces associated with loss of the convexity of the outer hoof wall are the likely causes of hoof cracks that occur in horses with mediolateral imbalance.

Horses with sheared heels often have a deep central sulcus. The elongated heel lands prematurely at the beginning of the stride, causing the opposing surfaces within the sulcus to become abraded and painful from the constant shearing. The premature landing of the elongated heel may also cause other inapparent painful injuries, such as bruising of the corium.

Frequently, the secondary signs are diagnosed and treated, and the precipitating mediolateral imbalance remains unidentified. Unfortunately, failure to treat the mediolateral imbalance leads to recurrence of the secondary clinical signs.

CORRECTIVE TRIMMING AND SHOEING

The objectives of corrective trimming and shoeing for mediolateral imbalance are to restore the ground surface of the foot to balance and restore the normal symmetry of the coronary band. If normal symmetry of the coronary band is present, no specific adjustments need be made. The correct length of the foot is determined and the hoof is trimmed accordingly. Although this removes areas of excessive length, areas where the wall is deficient are not addressed. These latter areas may be filled with a leather shim or an acrylic patch. The shim must be applied under a shoe. Acrylic patches do not require application of a shoe, but they last longer with the added protection.

There are two approaches to correction of proximal displacement of the coronary band. In the first approach, the foot is trimmed to its correct length. The ground surface of the hoof is then "floated" in areas that correspond to areas of proximal displacement of the coronary band. The hoof is usually shod with a bar shoe to increase stability. If the coronary band is displaced proximally at the heels, further support is attained with either a heart bar or egg bar/heart bar shoe. The floated areas should migrate distally until they contact the shoe. The foot may also be poulticed or soaked to encourage the softened hoof wall to migrate distally and the contour of the coronary band to return to normal. Poultices must be used cautiously to avoid excessive weakening of the hoof. In the second technique, the foot is soaked and/or poulticed before a shoe is applied to encourage the return of the coronary band contour to normal. The horse is stall rested during treatment. Once the normal contour has returned, the foot can be trimmed and shod as if there were no displacement of the coronary band.

A flare of the medial or lateral wall should be removed. If the horse is to be shod, the shoe should be fitted to the estimated natural shape of the foot and not to the acquired shape of the foot; therefore, the shoe fits tightly against the quarter that has had a flare removed, and it protrudes beyond the wall at the underrun quarter.

DORSOPALMAR IMBALANCE

Classically, a horse is said to be in dorsopalmar balance when the foot-pastern axis is straight. The foot-pastern axis is "broken back" when the slope of the hoof exceeds that of the pastern, and "broken forward" when the slope of the pastern exceeds that of the foot. However, the foot length and load distance are also very important.

Visual estimation of the correct foot-pastern axis is simple if the horse's distal limb is viewed from the side with the horse standing square on firm level ground. It is far more difficult to approximate optimal wall length at the toe. Hoof length has been related to the horse's weight, as previously mentioned, but this is only a rough guideline. An alternative is to determine the optimal thickness of the sole and trim the wall accordingly. This is an equally difficult technique and is based on the assumption that the physical characteristics of the sole change as it exfoliates; exfoliating sole is removed until the more resilient underlying sole is exposed. Unfortunately, there are no reliable anatomic landmarks by which to accurately judge correct hoof wall length or sole thickness. Lateromedial radiographic views of the foot are helpful only in determining the angle of the solar surface of the distal phalanx to the ground, alignment of the phalanges, and the length of hoof distal to the distal phalanx.

Load distance is a function of the slope and length of the hoof, and the slope and length of the pastern. The slope and length of the foot can be altered by trimming, the angle of the pastern is altered marginally by changes in the hoof angle, and the length of the pastern is genetically determined and unalterable. Therefore, load distance is not altered directly but changes as a consequence of adjustments in hoof length and angle.

Dorsopalmar imbalance is often deliberately induced in race horses when owners adhere to the erroneous belief that a long-toe, low-heel conformation increases stride length. Once underrun heels have developed, they are often allowed to persist because farriers and veterinarians are reluctant to shorten the heel. This hesitancy to remove heel is based on a commonly held belief that, once shortened, heels are notoriously difficult to grow out again. Unfortunately, if the heels are underrun, they cannot grow back at the proper angle until they have been shortened. It is feasible that Thoroughbred horses have a genetic tendency toward this conformation.

As mediolateral imbalance dictates the mediolateral distribution of stresses on the hoof, so does dorsopalmar balance determine the distribution of stresses in a dorsopalmar direction. Broken forward foot-pastern axes are not as commonly encountered as broken back foot-pastern axes. A broken back foot-pastern axis increases the slope of the dorsal and palmar walls of the hoof, and increases the tension in the deep digital flexor tendon. Increased tension in the deep digital flexor tendon increases the pressure on the navicular bone and bursa. The decrease in hoof angle associated with a broken back foot-pastern axis causes a slight increase in the angle of the pastern, which probably is accompanied by movement of the resultant hoof reaction force palmarly, or an increase in load distance, or a combination of the two.

Elongation of the hoof wall increases both the length of the poorly supported wall distal to the sole and the summed peak forces on the foot. The greater the length of unsupported wall and the greater its slope, the larger the bending moment applied to it by vertically acting forces. The greater the bending moment, the more likely the wall is to deform. The wall at the heels and bars is more likely to deform than the wall at the toe, because the wall in the former areas is thinner and is closer to the resultant hoof reaction force. Therefore, collapse of the heels is most likely to occur in horses with a broken back foot-pastern axis, a long hoof, and a long pastern.

Lameness Associated With Dorsopalmar Imbalance

Navicular disease, underrun heels, and hoof cracks are the most commonly cited causes of lameness associated with a broken back foot-pastern axis. Horses with navicular disease and underrun heels commonly have a residual lameness after the foot has been desensitized. This lameness, which is abolished with subcarpal or middle carpal joint anesthesia, is probably a result of changes in gait caused by compensating for heel pain. Although the response to anesthesia implicates the proximal suspensory ligament, it is often normal on ultrasound testing. Solar bruising is also reported as a secondary source of lameness caused by compensation for heel pain. Prolonged heel pain often leads to changes in hoof conformation, which leaves the heels elongated, narrower, and closer together. Consequently, the frog atrophies and becomes narrow, and the central sulcus of the frog extends proximal to the coronary band. Severely narrowed heels associated with a deep central cleft may become ulcerated and painful to digital palpation. The delayed breakover with a long sloping toe also predisposes the horse to overreaching injuries.

Broken forward foot-pastern axis most commonly occurs in horses with flexural deformities of the distal interphalangeal joint. Foot soreness in these horses is caused by solar bruising around the dorsal margin of the distal phalanx.

Other problems not traditionally considered to be imbalances but that do involve hoof length or slope of the dorsal hoof wall include excessive shortening of the foot and "dubbing the toe." Trimming the foot too short causes excessive pressure on the solar corium and results in lameness. Dubbing, or excessive thinning of the dorsal wall with a rasp, puts more of the dorsal margin of the sole in contact with the shoe, also causing bruising; the technique may destabilize the distal phalanx.

Corrective Trimming and Shoeing

The objectives in correcting dorsopalmar imbalance are to restore the foot to optimal length, ensure that the foot-pastern axis is straight, and thereby prevent excessive load distance. The correct length of the foot at the toe is estimated and the hoof trimmed. The heels are then trimmed so that the foot-pastern axis is straight. This is often not possible if the heels were originally very short or underrun. An egg bar shoe is commonly used in this situation, until the heels have grown. Less commonly, a wedge pad is used temporarily to restore the foot-pastern axis to normal. If excessive load distance cannot be redressed by correction of the wall length and foot-pastern axis, the dorsal wall may be thinned and an egg bar shoe set back well under the heels to move the ground contact palmarly. Several methods have been used to encourage the heels to spread, including egg bar shoes, slippering the heels of the shoes, grooving the heels, and application of springs. Heart bar/egg bar shoes, also called full-support shoes, have been used to encourage heel growth, particularly if the heels are floated.

When all deliberate efforts to improve either mediolateral or dorsopalmar balance fail, removing a horse's shoes and turning the horse out to pasture for 6 months may be effective in improving lameness resulting from foot conformation. Owners should be warned that the physical appearance of the foot will deteriorate over the first 2 to 3 months. At the opposite extreme, the foot balance of a sound horse that is apparently imbalanced should be adjusted only with great caution.

Traditionally, farriery has been an art, but it is emerging as a science. Theories of balance, including those expressed here, will be affirmed or refuted, new theories will be proposed, and discrepancies and contradictions between current theories and practices will be resolved as scientific methods are applied to the art of trimming and shoeing horses.

Supplemental Readings

Balch O, White K, Butler D: Factors involved in the balancing of equine hooves. J Am Vet Med Assoc 198:1980–1989, 1991.

Balch OK, Ratzlaff MH, Hyde ML, White KK: Locomotor effects of hoof angle and mediolateral balance of horses exercising on a high-speed treadmill: preliminary results. Proc 37th Annu Conv Am Assoc Equine Pract, 1991, pp 687–705.

Page B, Anderson GF: Diagonal imbalance of the equine foot: a cause of lameness. Proc 38th Annu Conv Am Assoc Equine Pract, 1992, pp 413–417.

Seeherman HJ, Morris E, O'Callaghan MW: Comprehensive clinical evaluation of performance. In Auer JA (ed): Equine Surgery. Philadelphia, WB Saunders, 1992, pp 1133–1173.

Snow VE, Birdsall DP: Specific parameters used to evaluate hoof balance and support. Proc 36th Annu Conv Am Assoc Equine Pract, 1990, pp 299–311.

Turner TA: The use of hoof measurements for the objective assessment of hoof balance. Proc 38th Annu Conv Am Assoc Equine Pract, 1992, pp 389–395.

Intermittent Upward Fixation of the Patella and Disorders of the Patellar Ligaments

DAVID DUGDALE
Newmarket, England

INTERMITTENT UPWARD FIXATION OF THE PATELLA

When a horse extends its hindlimbs, the patella rides to the top of the femoral trochlea, and the fibrocartilaginous medial patellar ligament hooks over the medial ridge of the trochlea. This locking mechanism allows the horse to rest its hindlimbs. When the horse needs to flex the stifle, the quadriceps femoris muscle first contracts to lift the patella clear of the notch, then relaxes to allow it to slide down the trochlea. Any factor that interferes with the coordination of the releasing process leads to the patella being locked in position and an inability to flex the stifle. This is called *upward fixation of the patella* and is usually intermittent.

Etiology

The degree of locking of the patella is governed both by the conformation of the hindlimb and the size of the retropatellar fat pad. An excessively straight hind leg predisposes to intermittent upward fixation of the patella, as does loss of the retropatellar fat pad, which follows loss of bodily condition. A third suggested etiology is that upward fixation of the patella is caused by poor coordination between the flexor and extensor muscles of the stifle.

Intermittent upward fixation of the patella is therefore commonly seen in young animals in poor bodily condition, before they have started training. It is also seen in horses previously in exercise, which are then confined to a stable for a period of rest. These animals experience both a loss of bodily condition and a loss of muscle tone and coordination. For example, intermittent upward fixation of the patella has been noted following fracture of the ilial shaft of the pelvis. Intermittent upward fixation of the patella is more common in pony breeds than in Thoroughbreds, and Shetland ponies are most commonly affected. A hereditary predisposition has been suggested in some breeds.

Clinical Signs

Clinical signs are extremely variable both in severity and frequency. In animals with complete upward fixation of the patella, the clinical signs are caused by a sudden inability of the animal to flex its hindlimb. This results in the leg pointing backwards in extreme extension. The fetlock is still able to flex and the front of the hoof wall may become excessively worn. Locking can occur at any pace but usually occurs at the walk or trot. It is usually noticed when the animal moves off from a standstill or turns in the stable.

The duration of locking can vary from momentary, followed by immediate release, to several minutes, or even permanent upward fixation. The intervals between locking vary enormously but the condition generally recurs. Intermittent upward fixation of the patella is mostly bilateral, although it may affect one leg more than the other.

Diagnosis

Unless the upward fixation is frequent or permanent, an affected animal may appear normal when examined. A diagnosis is based on obtaining a clear history. Turning, backing, slowly walking, and repeatedly stopping and starting the animal may elicit the characteristic signs. Locking may be provoked by manually pushing the patella over the top of the femoral trochlea and walking the animal forward. Walking the affected horse up and down a slope can exaggerate the condition. Affected animals are often reluctant to extend the hindlimbs fully, giving the impression of a restricted hindlimb action.

If upward fixation is apparently permanent, care should be taken to differentiate this condition from luxation of the coxofemoral joint, the clinical signs of which are superficially similar. With luxation of the coxofemoral joint, the limb appears to be fixed in extension, but in contrast to upward fixation of the patella, the limb is not extended caudally.

Some animals exhibit a partial locking. Although there is no obvious upward fixation of the patella, the leg snaps into flexion accompanied by an audible click. This is most noticeable when the animal is turned in a short circle with the affected limb on the inside; this condition should not be confused with stringhalt. In some chronic cases of intermittent upward fixation of the patella, gonitis may be present with distension and thickening of the femoropatellar joint capsule.

Subtle delayed release of the patella is sometimes seen. The patella appears to move in a jerky fashion especially as the horse decelerates. This can cause low-grade discomfort and loss of performance. The clinical signs may be accentuated when the horse is tired or if it is worked in deep, holding going. Care should be taken to differentiate this condition from low-grade hindlimb ataxia.

Treatment

In young animals starting exercise for the first time, the combination of increased exercise and increased feeding leads to an increase in the retropatellar fat pad and improves muscle tone and coordination. These factors generally lead to a rapid resolution of the condition. In animals

82

with intermittent upward fixation of the patella that need to remain confined to their stables for other reasons, bedding the animal on deep litter allows the hind toe to sink into the bedding and makes locking less likely. A shoe with a raised heel also makes locking less likely, until exercise can be resumed. Raised-heel shoes also help in horses that are being exercised and exhibit mild signs of intermittent upward fixation of the patella.

It is rare for conservative methods to fail in young Thoroughbreds. However, if conservative methods do fail, or the upward fixation is prolonged, surgical section of the medial patellar ligament should be carried out. This is a straightforward procedure. It is carried out in the standing sedated animal under local anesthesia, using a curved bistoury, through a stab incision. Both stifles should be operated on simultaneously, because even if the problem appears unilateral, the other stifle may become affected at a later time. When the medial patellar ligament has been sectioned the locked stifle releases dramatically, and it should no longer be possible manually to lock the patella proximally. The animal should be confined to a stable for 4 weeks, followed by an exercise program of increasing intensity.

In a small number of cases, fragmentation and chondromalacia of the distal patella have been described as complications following medial patellar ligament desmotomy. Degeneration of the articular cartilage occurs at the apex of the patella as a result of repetitive trauma, and this leads to hindlimb stiffness and synovial effusion. It is thought to develop because the patella is slightly malaligned following section of the medial patellar ligament. However, if surgery is reserved for cases that resist vigorous conservative measures, and for animals severely affected, this is an acceptable risk. Sectioning of the medial patellar ligament should not be carried out unless a clear diagnosis has been made.

An alternative treatment for horses with intermittent upward fixation of the patella in the absence of palpable swelling of the femoropatellar joint capsule is the injection of counterirritants into the middle and medial patellar ligaments in multiple sites. This is performed in the standing sedated horse. Commonly used irritants contain iodine, and this leads to a thickening of the middle and medial patellar ligaments, making upward fixation less likely. Although widely practiced in North America, it is rarely carried out in the United Kingdom.

If the patella is locked in position and resistant to unlocking, the horse should be stood with the weight on the affected limb. With the limb in this position the palm of the hand is placed on the distolateral edge of the patella, and firm pressure is applied proximomedially. This generally releases the patella, although persistence may be required. If unlocking is especially difficult, a rope should be placed around the hind pastern of the affected leg and the limb drawn forward as far as possible, before applying pressure to the patella. Following release, the horse should be walked for 5 to 10 minutes, because locking can recur rapidly.

LUXATION OF THE PATELLA

Patellar luxation and subluxation are rare occurrences. They are either congenital or acquired as a result of trauma

in older animals. Unilateral lateral luxation is the most common.

Etiology

Congenital luxation is the result of hypoplasia of the lateral trochlear ridge of the distal femur, or hypoplasia of the ligamentous supporting structures. It can be unilateral or bilateral. Luxation can also occur in older foals as a result of defective development of the lateral trochlear ridge, following severe osteochondrosis. In older horses, luxation or subluxation usually follows trauma. Distal luxation of the patella has been described, which is the result of tearing of the insertion of the quadriceps femoris from the proximal patella.

Clinical Signs

When complete congenital displacement of both patellas occurs, the foal is unable to stand, and it assumes a crouched position. The hips, stifles, and hocks are in extreme flexion, and the patella can be palpated laterally. Manual repositioning of the patella allows the foal to bear weight until luxation recurs. Post-traumatic luxation in adult animals also is manifested as an inability to bear weight on the limb.

Diagnosis

Radiographs of the stifles should be obtained to assess concomitant bony damage or degenerative changes within the joint. A cranioproximal/craniodistal oblique (sky-line) view of the patella is helpful to show the degree of displacement. Care must be taken in young foals not to overdiagnose osteochondrosis of the proximal trochlear ridges because an irregular outline is normal in young foals as a result of incomplete ossification.

Treatment

Animals with congenital lateral luxation of the patella do not respond to conservative treatment. Surgical treatment involves the release of the retinaculum on the lateral aspect of the stifle and imbrication of the medial aspect of the joint. This stabilizes the patella in the patellar groove and allows weightbearing. Once the patella is in its correct position, pressure exerted by the patella deepens the intertrochlear groove with time and allows formation of a normal stifle joint. With bilateral patellar luxation in a foal, surgery should be done on both stifles at the same time, otherwise excessive weightbearing by the corrected limb leads to breakdown of the surgical fixation.

Traumatic luxations in the absence of bony damage in adult animals can be reduced manually. This should be carried out in the standing sedated animal if possible. Once the patella is back in the trochlear groove, the damaged periarticular soft tissue structures are allowed to heal by fibrosis. The animal should be cross-tied in a stall for the first 3 to 4 weeks to minimize the risk of the luxation recurring, followed by a further 3 to 4 weeks of stable rest. If general anesthesia and surgical repair are necessary, there is a likelihood of luxation recurring during recovery from anesthesia.

Prognosis

In foals, the degree of bony damage and trochlear ridge hyopoplasia should be assessed carefully, before surgery is undertaken. If luxation is not associated with bony damage, a fair prognosis for future athletic performance can be given following surgery. If luxation is associated with severe osteochondrosis, leading to the loss of the lateral trochlear ridge of the femur, surgery is not indicated, and euthanasia should be considered. In adult animals, traumatic luxations without any bony damage carry a fair prognosis, and a full return to soundness can be expected. If the luxation is associated with fracture of the patella, the severity of the patella damage limits the prognosis.

SPRAIN OF THE PATELLAR LIGAMENTS

The medial, middle, and lateral patellar ligaments are effectively a continuation of the quadriceps femoris muscle, and they insert on the proximal tibia. Sprain or tearing of these ligaments is not well documented, but since the advent of diagnostic ultrasonography a small number of cases have been identified. Sprain of the middle patellar ligament has been characterized by mild lameness associated with low-grade effusion into the femoropatellar joint. Focal hypoechoic defects have been identified ultrasono-

graphically in the middle patellar ligament. Box rest and controlled exercise for 2 to 3 months has resulted in resolution of lameness and restoration of normal echogenicity. Partial tearing of the proximal attachment of the middle patellar ligament has also been seen and resulted in moderate lameness and an abnormal movement of the patella. Conservative treatment was unsuccessful. The outcome of surgical treatment by medial patellar ligament desmotomy is not yet known. Complete tearing of the middle patellar ligament results in an inability or an unwillingness to extend the stifle and in severe lameness. The prognosis is hopeless. Complete tears of the middle and medial patellar ligaments have also been seen.

Supplemental Readings

Auer JA: Diseases of the stifle. In Colahan PT, Mayhew IG, Merritt AM, Moore JN (eds): Equine Medicine and Surgery, 4th ed. Goleta, CA, American Veterinary Publications, 1991, pp 1488–1493.
Stashak TS: Lameness. In Stashak TS (ed): Adams' Lameness in Horses, 4th ed. Philadelphia, Lea & Febiger, 1987, pp 486–785.
Turner AS, McIlwraith CW: Medial patellar desmotomy. In Turner AS, McIlwraith CW (eds): Techniques in Large Animal Surgery. Philadelphia, Lea & Febiger, 1982, pp 133–135.
Wyn-Jones G: Equine Lameness. Oxford, Blackwell Scientific Publications, 1988.

Cruciate, Meniscal, and Meniscal Ligamental Injuries

JOHN P. WALMSLEY
Liphook, England

Cruciate ligament injuries are usually associated with acute and often severe traumatic episodes like jumping, road accidents, or falls when loading. The cranial cruciate ligament (CRCL) is under tension during extension of the femorotibial joint and is most likely to be injured when the joint is in hyperextension. It can also be damaged if the joint is hyperflexed with concurrent inward rotation of the tibia. Injuries to the caudal cruciate ligament (CACL) are rarer and follow rupture of the CRCL. Either ligament can be damaged by direct trauma to the stifle. Midbody lesions are the most common in the CRCL. Avulsions of its origin in the central fossa of the tibial plateau and the medial intercondylar eminence of the tibia occur, and they may also be seen at its insertion in the lateral aspect of the intercondylar fossa of the femur. Many of these injuries are accompanied by lesions in other structures of the stifle including the collateral ligaments, the menisci and their ligaments, and the joint surfaces and bony prominences such as the intercondylar eminence of the tibia. Seven percent of stifle lamenesses are due to CRCL injuries, but there are fewer reports of CACL injuries. This author has

recorded varying degrees of desmitis in 26 cranial cruciate and two caudal cruciate ligaments in 168 horses examined arthroscopically for stifle lameness.

Meniscal and meniscal ligamental injuries are less well documented and are probably underdiagnosed. Acute meniscal injuries in the dog are caused by a combination of weightbearing (i.e., crushing), tibial rotation, and flexion or extension of the stifle. Internal rotation affects the medial meniscus and external the lateral, whereas the cranial horn is damaged during extension and the caudal during flexion. The crushing forces split the fibers vertically. Degenerative changes are usually horizontal cleavage lesions, and this also pertains to humans. It is possible that these pathogeneses are relevant to the horse. In a survey by this author the incidence of meniscal tears was 21 in 168 horses examined arthroscopically for stifle lameness. Fraying of the axial edge of the meniscal ligaments without signs of meniscal lesions is much more common (35% in the above series) and may be a chronic wear lesion and not necessarily significant as a cause of lameness. Tearing of the meniscal ligaments also occurs frequently in association with meniscal injury.

INJURIES TO THE CRUCIATE LIGAMENTS

Clinical Signs

Acute injuries of the cruciate ligaments are usually manifested by severe lameness of sudden onset following a fall, an awkward movement during exercise, or a direct trauma to the stifle. The horse resents manipulation of the limb, making the cruciate draw test very difficult to perform, and flexion of the limb often makes the horse non-weightbearing. The femoropatellar joint and the medial or more rarely the lateral femorotibial joints may be distended. Crepitus in the joint may be detected in some cases.

Chronic cruciate ligamental injuries are manifested less obviously as a seat of pain in the stifle, especially if the ligament is only sprained. Usually a history is given of acute onset of lameness. Joint distension is variable and may not be present in the milder cases. The intensity of lameness depends on the severity of the injury and its chronicity. Lameness is exacerbated by flexion of the limb.

Diagnosis

If there is no history of direct trauma to the stifle, or obvious distension of femoropatellar or femorotibial joints, and no crepitus or pain on palpation, diagnostic anesthesia may be necessary to establish the seat of pain. The cruciate draw test may have a positive result, although it is often difficult to perform, especially in acute cases. It is hard to demonstrate joint laxity in the standing horse. In many cases the median septum between the femorotibial joints is destroyed, and there is often increased communication with the femoropatellar compartment. This means that intra-articular anesthesia of any compartment of the stifle may abolish or at least improve the lameness, and this should be borne in mind when attributing significance to anesthesia of the individual compartments of the joint.

In cases of midbody cruciate lesions, radiographic examination may be unrewarding. Avulsion fractures involving the CRCL or the CACL are best seen radiographically on the caudocranial and flexed lateromedial views as changes in the outline of the intercondylar fossa of the femur or fragments off the intercondylar eminence of the tibia. Bone fragments off the intercondylar eminence of the tibia are not necessarily associated with cruciate injuries. In chronic cases, proliferative new bone may develop cranial to the intercondylar eminence of the tibia, but this can also be a feature following tearing of the cranial meniscal ligaments; thus new bone development is not specific to cruciate lesions. Osseous cyst-like lesions are occasionally encountered adjacent to the insertion of the CRCL distal to the intercondylar eminence of the tibia. Concurrent collateral ligament damage may result in a widened femorotibial joint space on a stressed caudocranial view. In chronic cases there can be remodeling of the insertions of the collateral ligaments, particularly on the medial aspect of the medial condyle of the tibia. Some chronic cases with secondary involvement of joint surfaces have degenerative changes in the tibial plateau and femoral condyles. Contrast radiography and ultrasonography have limited diagnostic value for cruciate injuries. Ultrasonographic imaging is incomplete and can be difficult to interpret.

Arthroscopy is currently the most informative diagnostic procedure for determining which tissues are involved and the extent of the lesions. The cranial approach, between the middle and medial patellar ligaments, into the medial femorotibial joint, with the stifle in 90° flexion, allows reasonable access to the cranial and middle parts of the CRCL and the proximal CACL. The lateral approach, between the lateral patellar ligament and the long digital extensor tendon of origin, gives a more restricted view. Another approach uses a longer telescope from the femoropatellar compartment. Using the medial approach, the medial femorotibial joint can be examined. The CACL, medial intercondylar eminence of the tibia, medial femoral condyle, and medial meniscus with its cranial ligament are seen. The normal CRCL lies under the median septum. The median septum is often broken down when there is a femorotibial joint injury, allowing a direct view of the lateral femorotibial joint. In the presence of acute desmitis, hemorrhage and fibrin must be cleared before the CRCL can be assessed. Having examined the medial femorotibial joint, the telescope is replaced with a blunt obturator and pushed through the median septum into the lateral femorotibial joint. The CRCL can then be viewed more clearly lying axial to the lateral femoral condyle (Fig. 1A). The CACL cannot be seen in this joint. The tibial insertion of the CACL can be seen through a caudal approach to the medial femorotibial joint.

In cases of acute severe desmitis or rupture of the CRCL, once the hemorrhage and fibrin have been cleared, the ligament appears as a mass of disorganized tissue, the normal configuration of which is difficult to distinguish. In less severe acute injuries, hemorrhagic areas and torn ligamental tissue are seen on the surface of the CRCL (Fig. 1B). Careful probing is usually necessary to explore the extent of the injury. Avulsion fractures of the intercondylar eminence of the tibia can be viewed in the medial femorotibial joint. When the injury is more chronic, there may be varying amounts of fibrinous adhesions over the ligament and median septum, and the septum may be broken down. Occasionally there is merely a mild fibrinous deposit or discoloration on the surface of the ligament, and in other horses the CRCL fibers appear to be abnormally separated longitudinally. The significance of these mild chronic changes is uncertain. In the author's experience they are often associated with lameness. Concurrent injury to the menisci and their ligaments or to articular cartilage may be observed.

Treatment

If mild cruciate desmitis is suspected, the horse should receive stall rest and nonsteroidal anti-inflammatory medication, such as phenylbutazone (2 mg/kg p.o. b.i.d. for 1 week; then 1 mg/kg the second week). It is safer not to turn out the horse, but to start a controlled exercise program after 4 to 6 weeks and monitor progress. If there is no improvement or for more serious cases, an arthroscopic investigation is indicated. The arthroscopic examination establishes the severity of the injury and the structures affected. While the horse is anesthetized, laxity in the femorotibial joints can be assessed. Debridement of loose and inflamed tissue and lavage of the joint should assist the healing process. Avulsion fracture fragments can be

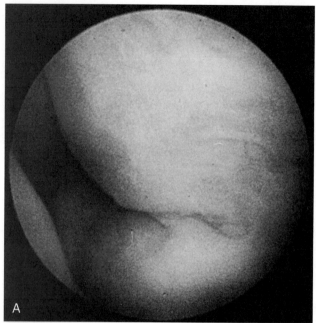

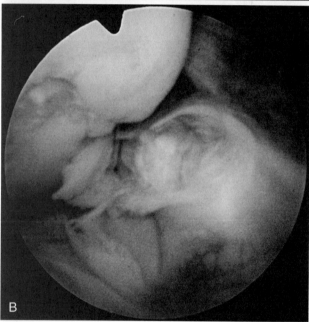

Figure 1. (*A*) An arthroscopic view of a normal right cranial cruciate ligament viewed in the lateral femorotibial joint. The lateral femoral condyle is on the left of the picture and the median septum on the right. (*B*) An arthroscopic view of a torn right cranial cruciate ligament. The lateral femoral condyle has an articular defect and is on the left of the picture above the cranial ligament of the lateral meniscus that is torn. The median septum is on the right.

dissected off the tibia and removed. This author has treated one case by arthroscopic internal fixation using an AO/ASIF cortical screw. A careful search for concurrent joint damage should be made because such damage significantly affects the prognosis. No technique has yet been established for the repair of complete ruptures of the CRCL in the horse. Postoperatively, a controlled exercise program, following 4 to 6 weeks of stable rest, should be maintained for several months. Early pasture turn out increases the possibility of reinjury.

Prognosis

The prognosis for a cruciate injury in horses is guarded and worse when multiple structures are involved. Those with severe injuries rarely achieve athletic use. Some cases in which avulsion fragments have been treated have resumed normal work, but developing degenerative joint disease sometimes causes a recurrence of lameness.

INJURIES TO THE MENISCI AND MENISCAL LIGAMENTS

Clinical Signs

Most meniscal injuries have a history of acute onset and an initial moderately severe lameness. The acute phase usually settles into a persistent low-grade lameness. More severe cases have distension of the femoropatellar or medial femorotibial joints. Concurrent injury to other structures in the femorotibial joints, typically the CRCL and the medial collateral ligament, exacerbate the clinical signs. Thickening over the medial aspect of the medial femorotibial joint may be palpable in chronic cases of medial meniscal injury, particularly if the medial collateral ligament is also damaged.

Diagnosis

Meniscal injury is very difficult to diagnose definitively in a clinical investigation. A distended medial femorotibial joint may be seen but is not pathognomonic for meniscal lesions. Lameness usually worsens with exercise and is exacerbated by flexion of the limb. Intra-articular anesthesia of the femorotibial joints improve lameness, but may not completely abolish it, presumably because of a mechanical component in the lameness. Experience is needed to detect meniscal lesions ultrasonographically, and not all of the menisci and their ligaments can be imaged. Radiographically, lesions are not likely to be found in the acute case, although a narrowing of the joint space may be demonstrable if the horse will bear weight on the affected limb. Chronic cases may have proliferative new bone on the cranial aspect of the medial intercondylar eminence of the tibia, but this may also be seen in cruciate injuries (see earlier). The diseased tissues, more commonly in the cranial aspect of the joint, become mineralized in some more severe cases, and degenerative joint disease in the femorotibial joints is sometimes manifest. Contrast radiography is unrewarding.

Arthroscopic investigation is currently the most accurate diagnostic tool for diagnosing meniscal injuries. The cranial poles of the menisci (Fig. 2A) can be viewed through the cranial portals (see earlier for cruciate ligaments) and their caudal edges through the caudal portals, but most of the meniscal body cannot be seen. Medial meniscal tears are more common than lateral meniscal tears. Complete tears usually have considerable disruption of the cranial ligament, and loose torn meniscal tissue is seen protruding from between the femur and tibia in the axial part of the joint (Fig. 2B). The morphology of meniscal tears in horses is not well documented, partly because of poor arthroscopic access. Longitudinal tears of the cranial pole seem to be the most common and may be analogous to bucket handle

copy. Degenerative meniscal disease, developing with age, may occur in horses, but is rarely diagnosed ante mortem owing to the inaccessibility of the meniscal body.

The cranial ligaments of the medial and lateral menisci (Fig. 3A) may have lesions without apparent concurrent meniscal damage. Fraying of the axial edge is relatively common but its significance is uncertain. Disruption of the ligaments may be seen (Fig. 3B) and appears to cause lameness. Longitudinal tears also occur, generally about 1.5 cm from the axial edge, and are usually associated with

Figure 2. *(A)* An arthroscopic view of the cranial pole of a normal right medial meniscus lying beneath the medial femoral condyle. *(B)* An arthroscopic view of a torn right medial meniscus. The cranial pole of the meniscus has been extruded cranially from under the medial femoral condyle.

tears in humans, although in many cases the cranial, axial part is torn off the rest of the meniscus. In chronic cases, articular cartilage of the medial femoral or tibial condyles adjacent to the lesion in the meniscus often has signs of degenerative change. Fibrillation of the cartilage of the medial intercondylar eminence of the tibia is also seen. If the tissue that has extruded cranially has mineralized, it restricts arthroscopic access to the abaxial part of the joint. Meniscal injuries can be associated with injuries to other structures in the joint, and this can be assessed at arthros-

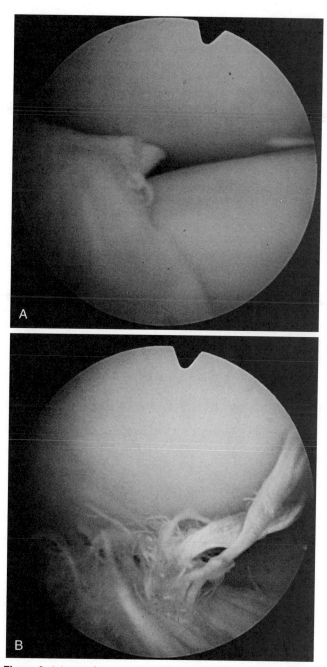

Figure 3. *(A)* An arthroscopic view of a normal right cranial ligament of the lateral meniscus. The cranial pole of the meniscus can just be seen between the lateral femoral condyle and the articular surface of the tibia. *(B)* An arthroscopic view of a torn right cranial ligament of the lateral meniscus.

lameness. Lesions in the cranial meniscal ligaments often involve the meniscus. Tearing of the meniscofemoral and caudal ligaments of the lateral meniscus has not been reported.

Therapy

Acute gonitis, in which no definitive diagnosis can be made on clinical examination, can potentially involve meniscal injury. Normal first aid as for joint sprains is appropriate. Stall rest and nonsteroidal anti-inflammatory treatment, such as phenylbutazone (2 mg/kg p.o. b.i.d. for 1 week then 1 mg/kg for the second week), should be followed by careful evaluation of progress if the lameness subsides. Arthroscopy is indicated if there is no response to initial treatment; it is indicated also in more severe cases and in cases when a provisional diagnosis of meniscal tearing can be made. Loose meniscal and ligamentous tissue should be removed with instruments designed for cutting soft tissue such as an O'Connor punch or motorized synovial resector. The major limitation in this treatment, compared with equivalent endoscopic partial meniscectomies in humans, is the poor access to most of the meniscus. Improved access to the meniscal body has been reported to be obtained by pulling the stifle against a post to open the femorotibial joint opposite the direction of pull. This author has had poor success with this technique. Good access has been obtained experimentally using a distractor device attached to Steinmann pins implanted in the femur and tibia. In some horses a reasonably clean edge to the damaged tissue can be achieved, but frequently the lesion can be seen to extend out of reach between the femur and tibia. Postoperatively complete stall rest for 3 weeks, followed by a controlled exercise program without turn out over the next 6 months, is probably the most suitable regimen.

Prognosis

Generally any injury of the menisci or their ligaments that causes lameness carries a guarded prognosis. Best results are obtained in acute cases in which a satisfactory partial meniscectomy is possible. A degree of meniscal regeneration has been reported in the dog, and this author has seen evidence of some regeneration in two horses. If inaccessible diseased tissue has to be left, although there may be a temporary improvement, mild lameness usually recurs. In some cases this appears to be due to cartilage defects that develop in association with the loose meniscal tissue. Nevertheless, some horses are able to be used for light work.

Supplemental Readings

Butler JA, Colles CM, Dyson SJ, Kold SE, Poulos PW: Clinical Radiology of the Horse. Oxford, Blackwell Scientific Publications, 1993, p 272.
Jeffcott LB, Kold SE: Stifle lameness in the horse: A survey of 86 referred cases. Equine Vet J 14:31–39, 1982.
Lewis RL: A retrospective study of diagnostic and surgical arthroscopy of the equine femorotibial joint. Proc Am Assoc Equine Pract 23:887–893, 1987.
McIlwraith CW: Diagnostic and surgical arthroscopy of the femoropatellar and femorotibial joints. In Diagnostic and Surgical Arthroscopy in the Horse, ed 2. Philadelphia, Lea & Febiger, 1993, pp 113–159.
Mueller POE, Allen D, Watson E, Hay C: Arthroscopic removal of a fragment from an intercondylar eminence fracture of the tibia in a two-year-old horse. J Am Vet Med Assoc 204:1793–1795, 1994.
Prades M, Grant BD, Turner TA, Nixon AJ, Brown MP: Injuries of the cranial cruciate ligament and associated structures: Summary of clinical, radiographic arthroscopic and pathological findings from 10 horses. Equine Vet J 21:354–357, 1989.
Sanders-Shamis M, Bukowiecki CF, Biller DS: Cruciate and collateral ligament failure in the equine stifle: Seven cases (1975–1985). J Am Vet Med Assoc 193:573–576, 1988.
Walmsley JP: Vertical tears of the cranial horn of the meniscus and its cranial ligament in the equine femorotibial joint: 7 cases and their treatment by arthroscopic surgery. Equine Vet J 27:20–25, 1995.
Wright IN: Ligaments associated with joints. Vet Clin North Am Equine Pract 11(2):249–291, 1995.

Pain Associated With the Distal Tarsal Joints of the Hock

THOMAS C. BOHANON
Littleton, Colorado

The proximal intertarsal (talocalcaneal-centroquatral), distal intertarsal (centrodistal), and tarsometatarsal joints constitute the distal tarsal joints of the horse. They are diarthrodial joints, but because of the relatively flat shape of the cuboidal bones of the distal tarsus and the dense connective tissue that surrounds them, these joints contribute little to the range of motion in the hock, which comes mainly from the tarsocrural joint. Bone spavin, or osteoarthrosis of the distal tarsal joints, is the most common cause of hindlimb lameness in the horse, and can manifest itself in a variety of forms from acute and severe lameness to subtle performance-limiting problems. The tarsometatarsal and distal intertarsal joints are most frequently involved, but the proximal intertarsal joint may also be affected.

The etiology of bone spavin is uncertain. Degenerative joint disease of the distal tarsal joints most commonly occurs in performance horses during the active parts of their careers, and is commonly associated with sickle-hocked or cow-hocked conformation. Bone spavin is likely caused by compression and rotation of the distal tarsal bones, which occurs most forcefully at the gallop. Bone spavin can also occur in young horses before they have begun training or had any heavy exercise. In these cases, osteochondrosis affecting the cuboidal bones of the tarsus is probably involved, or degenerative changes may result from crushing of the central and/or third tarsal bones because of excessive exercise as a neonate. This is most common in premature or dysmature foals that are allowed to run free before sufficient skeletal maturation has occurred. In addition to lesions associated with the articular cartilage and periarticular soft tissues, bone spavin may be a result of increased intramedullary pressure in the cuboidal bones of the hock. Bone spavin differs from distal tarsitis syndrome identified in Standardbred race horses, in which lameness originates exclusively from the soft tissues of the distal hock and does not involve degenerative changes at the articular surface of the distal tarsal bones.

DIAGNOSIS

Clinical Signs

Diagnosis of bone spavin can be made with routine techniques available to the equine practitioner. Affected horses usually present with a lameness of gradual onset that is most obvious during the initial part of an exercise period and gradually improves. Advanced cases may have palpable bony enlargement on the medial aspect of the distal hock. Effusion of the tarsocrural joint, or bog spavin, may be present if there are degenerative changes in the proximal intertarsal joint. Cunean bursitis and effusion in the cunean bursa are uncommon. Lameness is best detected at the trot on a hard asphalt surface, and is most obvious when the affected leg is on the inside of a 10- to 15-meter circle. Horses with bone spavin frequently demonstrate a reduced foot flight arc at the trot and have a shortened cranial phase of the stride. When observed from behind while trotting straight away from the observer, affected horses exhibit a gradual axial deviation in the flight path of the foot during the cranial phase of the stride, followed by a rapid abaxial deviation at the conclusion of the stride. The hoof or shoe may show excessive wear in the toe region and on the lateral aspect because of these gait abnormalities. Affected horses frequently show pain to palpation of the lumbar and gluteal muscles in addition to lameness, and many owners present their horse for veterinary attention with a primary complaint of back pain.

Some horses present with a history of performance limitations in their discipline and have minimal or no discernable lameness. Hunter-jumpers may refuse fences or lead changes; change leads at inappropriate times or become disunited; and wring their tails, buck, or lay back their ears while on course. Barrel-racing horses may lose time while racing, because they turn too wide around the barrel. Reining horses may spin or stop poorly because of spavin pain. A history that includes a deterioration in the horse's attitude or willingness to perform may suggest subtle hock pain that does not produce overt lameness.

Hyperflexion of the hock for 90 seconds usually exacerbates lameness but should be performed and interpreted with caution. Because of the reciprocal apparatus, hock flexion is always accompanied by flexion of the stifle and hip, and a positive response may indicate pain in these areas as well. The leg should be held by the hoof to avoid digital pressure and a potentially painful response originating from the proximal sesamoid bones, fetlock joint, flexor tendons, suspensory ligament, or pastern area (Fig. 1).

Diagnostic Anesthesia

Diagnostic intra-articular anesthesia is very useful to document the source of lameness. Because the incidence of communication between the tarsometatarsal and distal tarsal joints is low, each joint should be anesthetized and the results interpreted individually. Significant improvement in lameness 10 minutes after intra-articular injection of 2 to 4 ml mepivacaine hydrochloride° is diagnostic, but complete resolution of lameness may not occur due to intramedullary pain in the tarsal bones that is unaffected by intra-articular anesthesia. Larger volumes of anesthetic should not be used, because of potential for periarticular extravasation that can contact many tissues, including the sensory nerve supply from the distal limb as it passes through the tarsus. Diagnostic anesthesia is of limited value in horses with extremely subtle lameness, or in those that have only a history of performance limitation. In these cases, intra-articular injection of corticosteroids may be helpful, and both the distal intertarsal and tarsometatarsal joints of both hindlimbs are routinely treated. In horses with obvious radiologic changes in the distal tarsal joints, a long-acting corticosteroid such as methylprednisolone acetate can be used, but in horses with subtle or no radiographic changes, triamcinolone acetonide is preferable to

---

°Carbocaine-V, The Upjohn Company, Kalamazoo, MI

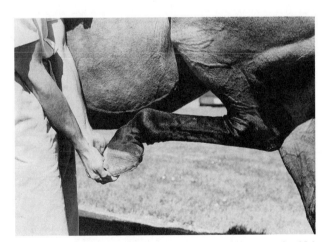

Figure 1. The upper hindlimb flexion test, or spavin test, should be performed without abduction or adduction, which may exacerbate lameness associated with the upper part of the limb. The leg should be held by the toe to avoid digital pressure and a potentially painful response originating from the proximal sesamoid bones, fetlock joint, flexor tendons, suspensory ligament, or pastern area. Holding the limb by the toe also allows the clinician to position the joints of the lower limb in the maximum degree of extension allowed by the reciprocal apparatus.

minimize risk of cartilage damage if the distal tarsal joints are not involved. Improvement in the horse's attitude or way of going, shortly after intra-articular corticosteroid injection, is suggestive that the problem originates from the distal tarsus. This technique requires the rider to interpret results 2 to 7 days after treatment. It is vital to emphasize to the rider the importance of maintaining the horse at a level of exercise consistent with its preinjection training regimen, and to stress objectivity in the interpretation of results.

Intra-articular injection may be difficult in horses with advanced radiographic abnormalities and in those that have received multiple corticosteroid injections, although it is sometimes possible using high injection pressures. If injection cannot be achieved, a diagnosis may be confirmed by exclusion or using nuclear scintigraphy. A negative response to both subtarsal analgesia and intra-articular analgesia of the tarsocrural joint, combined with a positive response to peroneal and tibial nerve blocks, is highly supportive. Nuclear scintigraphy may also be helpful in cases with very subtle lameness or in horses with apparent fusion of the distal intertarsal or tarsometatarsal joint.

Radiography

Lameness associated with the distal tarsal joints may exist with few or no radiographic abnormalities. Conversely, extensive radiographic changes may be present that are not associated with pain or lameness. Four views are recommended and include dorsoplantar, lateromedial, and two oblique projections. Typical radiographic changes are periarticular new bone growth, lysis, sclerosis, narrowing of the joint space, irregular widening of the joint space, subchondral cyst formation, and ankylosis. Dorsal bulging of the central or third tarsal bone observed in the lateromedial projection suggests tarsal bone crushing as a neonate, or osteochondrosis. Bone spavin is commonly a bilateral condition, and radiographs of both hocks are recommended. Often, the most dramatic radiographic changes are associated with the least clinically affected limb. Special attention should be given to direct the x-ray beam parallel to the articular surfaces of the distal tarsal joints, because proximal-to-distal obliquity obscures the joint margins and makes interpretation difficult. Often, the earliest radiographic changes are seen on the dorsoplantar projection as a small osteophyte extending distally from the lateral aspect of the central tarsal bone. This view is also the most reliable for interpretation of joint space narrowing and ankylosis. Radiography may underestimate the degree of ankylosis because fusion may occur in a spot-weld type pattern with apparent persistence of a joint space radiographically.

TREATMENT

The goal of treatment for bone spavin is to eliminate pain and lameness, return the horse to full exercise, and encourage joint fusion, because in most cases fusion results in the elimination of clinical signs. However, horses that respond favorably to intra-articular anesthesia but do not exhibit degenerative radiographic changes may have synovitis and capsulitis without cartilage damage, and treatment regimens for these horses that may hasten articular cartilage damage and promote fusion are discouraged. This situation is most commonly encountered in young horses at the onset of training. A conservative approach to treatment is warranted, including rest, nonsteroidal anti-inflammatory medications, and careful clinical and radiographic follow-up.

The most commonly used treatments include systemic nonsteroidal anti-inflammatory drugs, intra-articular or intravenous hyaluronan (sodium hyaluronate), intra-articular or intramuscular polysulfated glycosaminoglycan, oral chondroitin sulfate, intra-articular corticosteroids, cunean tenectomy, chemical fusion with sodium monoiodoacetate (MIA), and surgical arthrodesis. Clients should be advised to investigate medication regulations for their particular discipline before pursuing a treatment plan.

Nonsteroidal anti-inflammatory medications can be effective and economical in the management of bone spavin for horses with mild lameness that are ridden intermittently or perform at relatively low levels of competition, or are used for pleasure riding. Although all nonsteroidal anti-inflammatory drugs have the potential to produce gastrointestinal ulceration and renal lesions, aspirin* (30 mg/kg p.o. q24h) is relatively safe for long-term administration. Alternatively, phenylbutazone† (4.4 mg/kg intravenously [IV] or p.o. q24h) or flunixin meglumine‡ (1.1 mg/kg IV or p.o. q24h) can be given the day before and the day of exercise with minimal risk of toxicity, provided that the horse is withdrawn from medication for at least 3 days each week.

Hyaluronan is available as an intra-articular or intravenous§ treatment, and is indicated in horses in which there are no radiographic changes, synovitis and capsulitis are not suspected, and long-term treatment is not anticipated. This concept also applies to intra-articular or intramuscular administration of polysulfated glycosaminoglycan‖ and to the various oral chondroitin sulfate products.¶ However, these medications are expensive for long-term therapy, and may delay the ongoing degenerative process that is necessary to achieve ankylosis in horses already exhibiting obvious radiographic changes.

Intra-articular Therapy

Intra-articular corticosteroids are commonly used to treat bone spavin. Methylprednisolone acetate is the most widely used and has the advantage of being relatively inexpensive and long-lasting. Typically, the distal intertarsal and tarsometatarsal joints of both hindlimbs are injected simultaneously, unless the results of intra-articular anesthesia indicate otherwise. The hair is clipped on the medial aspect of the hock in the area of the cunean tendon for the distal intertarsal joint injection, and on the lateral aspect of the hock in the area of the proximal fourth metatarsal bone for the tarsometatarsal joint injection. Both sites are then prepared for aseptic injection of 60–100 mg methylprednisolone acetate# with a 22-gauge 2.5-cm

*Acetylsalicylic acid 10%, Rhone-Poulenc, Inc., Cranbury, NJ
†Vedco, St. Joseph, MO
‡Banamine, Schering-Plough Animal Health, Kenilworth, NJ
§Legend, Miles, Inc., Shawnee Mission, KS
‖Adequan, Luitpold Pharmaceuticals, Inc., Shirley, NY
¶Flex-Free, VitaFlex Nutritional Co., Inc., Staten Island, NY
#Depo-Medrol, The Upjohn Company, Kalamazoo, MI

needle, and the tarsometatarsal joint is injected first. Injection of the distal tarsal joints is difficult, but with practice both the tarsometatarsal and distal intertarsal joints can be reliably entered in most horses. Positive contrast arthrography may aid injection for inexperienced clinicians, or in horses with advanced degenerative changes.

The tarsometatarsal joint is the easiest of the distal tarsal joints to inject. It is entered laterally, 0.5 cm proximal to the head of the fourth metatarsal bone. The needle is inserted in a craniomediodistal direction at a 45° angle to both the sagittal plane and the ground until it contacts bone, usually at a depth of approximately 2 cm. This technique results in the needle tip passing deep, medial, and slightly distal to the palpable lateral edge of the head of the fourth metatarsal bone, positioning it near the articulation between the fourth metatarsal bone and the fourth tarsal bone. The steep angle is critical to position the needle tip sufficiently distal to avoid penetration of the proximal intertarsal joint, which is located only slightly proximal to the head of the fourth metatarsal bone. Penetration of the tarsometatarsal joint usually produces a small volume of synovial fluid in the hub of the needle, but is less likely to do so in horses with severe degenerative changes or those that have had multiple corticosteroid injections. When synovial fluid is not visualized, testing the injection pressure with a small volume of sterile saline solution is a helpful technique in all joint injections, to confirm that the needle tip is in the proper location.

The distal intertarsal joint is injected medially, in the space that exists between the central tarsal bone, third tarsal bone, and fused first and second tarsal bone. This space can often be felt with deep palpation, and is found at the dorsodistal border of the cunean tendon, approximately 2 cm caudal to a vertical line extending distally from the medial malleolus. Ideally, the needle is inserted to the hub in a caudolateral direction, at a 45° angle to the sagittal plane and parallel to the ground. Synovial fluid can be visualized in the hub of the needle approximately half the time. Often, the needle is inserted to a depth of 1.5 to 2 cm and bone is contacted, but presence of synovial fluid in the hub of the needle and ease of injection help confirm the intra-articular position of the needle tip. It is possible to position the needle tip in the cunean bursa if penetration is too superficial. Although synovial fluid may be obtained and injection pressure is slight, this error can easily be detected by visual distension of the bursa, which does not occur with intra-articular injection. In small horses, full penetration of a 2.5-cm needle can result in it passing completely through the distal intertarsal joint space and into loose connective tissue deep to the joint capsule. Confirmation of this positioning error is difficult without positive contrast arthrography, but slight withdrawal of the needle may result in visualization of synovial fluid or easier injection. Occasionally, the tarsometatarsal joint may be entered on the medial aspect of the hock while the clinician attempts to enter the distal intertarsal joint. This occurs because the tarsometatarsal joint capsule also occupies the space that exists between the central tarsal bone, third tarsal bone, and fused first and second tarsal bone, and is only slightly distal to the distal intertarsal joint capsule (Fig. 2). If the tarsometatarsal joint has been previously

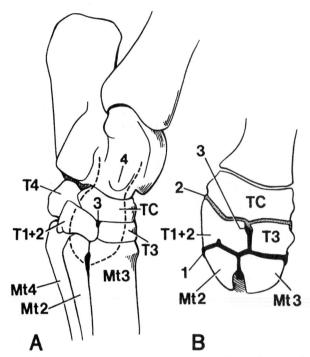

Figure 2. (*A*) Left hock, medial aspect. The broken line indicates a slice removed by sagittal saw cut. (*B*) Appearance of cut surface after removal of slice, slightly enlarged. The cut surface is about 8 mm lateral to the most medial point on the head of Mt2. Heavy black lines represent the tarsometatarsal joint space, and stippled areas represent the distal intertarsal joint space, both of which occupy the space between the third, central, and fused first and second tarsal bones on the medial aspect of the hock. T1 + 2 is the fused first and second tarsal bone; T3 the third tarsal bone; T4 the fourth tarsal bone; TC the central tarsal bone; Mt2 the second metatarsal bone; Mt3 the third metatarsal bone; Mt4 the fourth metatarsal bone; 1 the tarsometatarsal joint; 2 the distal intertarsal joint; 3 the gap between T1 + 2, T3, and TC; 4 the distal tubercle of the talus. (From Sack WO, Orsini PG: Distal intertarsal and tarsometatarsal joints in the horse: Communication and injection sites. J Am Vet Med Assoc 179:355, 1981, with permission.)

injected laterally with methylprednisolone acetate, retrieval of white fluid medially indicates the positioning error. Many clinicians have interpreted this phenomenon as evidence of communication between the tarsometatarsal and distal intertarsal joint. However, the low incidence of communication between the distal tarsal joints documented in multiple refereed publications makes this explanation unlikely, and repositioning of the needle slightly proximal often results in visualization of clear synovial fluid from the distal intertarsal joint.

Treatment with multiple injections of long-acting corticosteroids like methylprednisolone acetate may have the additional benefit of hastening fusion of the affected joints by increasing the rate of cartilage destruction. Triamcinolone acetonide* may be used as a short-acting intra-articular corticosteroid in cases lacking radiographic evidence of degenerative joint disease. Triamcinolone acetonide has potent anti-inflammatory effects but is detectable in synovial fluid for only a few days, and therefore may cause less depression of chondrocyte metabolism compared with methylprednisolone acetate. Triamcinolone acetonide is

*Vetalog, Solvay Animal Health, Medota Heights, MN

used at a dose of up to 12 mg per joint, not exceeding 18 mg as a total body dose.

Cunean Tenectomy

Cunean tenectomy is a relatively simple surgical procedure, which is performed in the sedated standing horse with the aid of local anesthesia. The efficacy of this technique is debated, and there are no controlled studies to either support or refute the validity of the procedure. Many clinicians feel that they see significant and long-lasting improvement in lameness associated with bone spavin following cunean tenectomy. Proposed mechanisms for improvement following this procedure include alleviation of cunean bursitis and elimination of pressure on the medial aspect of the hock where periarticular new bone growth commonly occurs. However, cunean bursitis is rarely part of the lameness, and many horses that have minimal proliferative changes respond favorably to cunean tenectomy. Cunean tenectomy is more likely to improve lameness by decreasing rotational forces on the tarsus that occur when the cunean tendon tightens, because of its oblique anatomic orientation across the dorsomedial aspect of the tarsus. The surgical site is bandaged for 14 days, and the horse is hand walked 10 minutes daily over ground poles, beginning the day after surgery, for 2 weeks. Light riding starts 2 weeks after surgery, and the horse is returned to full work 3 weeks after surgery. This postoperative exercise regimen is important to prevent formation of restrictive scar tissue between the severed tendon ends and the cunean bursa.

Joint Fusion

Intra-articular injection of sodium monoiodoacetate° fuses the distal tarsal joints by causing chondrocyte death, cartilage necrosis, and joint collapse. Sodium monoiodoacetate is not currently licensed in the United States for clinical use in the horse, and can only be legally obtained by a lengthy application process through the federal government. Horses receiving MIA should be treated with phenylbutazone (4.4 mg/kg IV q12h) for 24 hours, beginning 12 hours before treatment. Injection with MIA should be preceded by contrast arthrography of each joint, because communication between the distal intertarsal and proximal intertarsal joint and communication between the tarsometatarsal and proximal intertarsal joint have been documented. The incidence of these communications is low but would exclude the use of MIA as a form of treatment because of the consistent communication that exists between the proximal intertarsal and tarsocrural joints. Injection procedures for contrast arthrography and treatment are identical to those for diagnostic anesthesia described previously. Joints are aseptically injected individually with 2 ml of diatrizoate meglumine,† the needle is capped, and dorsoplantar and lateromedial radiographic views are obtained immediately. In limbs in which contrast arthrography is done on both the distal intertarsal and tarsometatarsal joints, the distal intertarsal arthrogram is performed first. If contrast arthrography reveals no evidence of communication between the distal tarsal joints

and the proximal intertarsal joint, 100 mg of MIA in 2 ml of 0.9% saline solution and sterilized with a 0.2-μm filter° is aseptically injected into each joint. Horses treated with MIA are likely to experience severe post-injection pain from 4 to 18 hours following treatment. Because of this, they should be hospitalized following treatment and medicated with butorphanol tartrate† and detomidine hydrochloride‡ as needed. Treated horses are exercised lightly the day following injection and returned to full work 2 days following injection. Phenylbutazone is typically administered for 3 to 5 days following treatment (4.4 mg/kg p.o. q24h), after which anti-inflammatory medications are usually unnecessary.

Surgical arthrodesis of the distal tarsal joints is also a treatment for bone spavin and may be indicated in cases in which intra-articular injection is not possible. The original technique used a 4.5-mm drill bit to remove 60% of the articular cartilage in the affected joint. However, instability after surgery resulted in frequent complications including severe postoperative pain, infection, weight loss, long recovery times, and persistent lameness. Most surgeons currently recommend a less aggressive drilling technique, and the results are considered favorable. Surgical arthrodesis, like chemical fusion, can be performed bilaterally on both the distal intertarsal and tarsometatarsal joints as a single procedure. Perioperative nonsteroidal anti-inflammatory medication is indicated for 5 to 7 days. Horses can be hand walked after suture removal, and light riding can begin 4 weeks after surgery.

PROGNOSIS

In general, the prognosis for bone spavin is favorable, because most horses return to full function when the affected distal tarsal joints fuse. However, spontaneous ankylosis without treatment is a lengthy, inconsistent, and often painful process, and usually some form of therapy is necessary to keep the horse useful for athletic purposes. Unfortunately, little objective data are available that evaluates specific treatments for bone spavin. Involvement of the proximal intertarsal joint carries a guarded to unfavorable prognosis because of its consistent communication with and concurrent involvement of the tarsocrural joint. Because horses with crushed central and third tarsal bones frequently have involvement of the proximal intertarsal joint, their prognosis is poor.

Injection of the distal intertarsal and tarsometatarsal joints with methylprednisolone acetate can relieve clinical signs for up to a year, but the duration of benefit for most horses with bone spavin is 3 to 4 months. However, the extent and duration of clinical effect often wanes with multiple treatments, and after four to five treatments many horses show minimal improvement following intra-articular corticosteroids. In addition, arthrocentesis and injection becomes increasingly difficult after multiple injections.

In our experience, cunean tenectomy is helpful in alleviating lameness in the majority of bone spavin cases. The

°Iodoacetic acid, sodium salt, Sigma Chemical Co., St. Louis, MO
†Renografin, Squibb Diagnostics, New Brunswick, NJ

°Nalgene syringe filters, Nalge Co., Rochester, NY
†Torbugesic, Fort Dodge Laboratories, Inc., Fort Dodge, IA
‡Dormosedan, SmithKline Beecham Animal Health, West Chester, PA

procedure is safe and relatively inexpensive, and horses return to full exercise with minimal convalescence. Close adherence to aftercare instructions is considered critical to the success of this procedure. However, some horses receiving cunean tenectomy show only temporary improvement or no improvement, necessitating additional treatment.

The prognosis following chemical fusion of the distal tarsal joints with MIA is favorable, and most horses show improvement in the original level of lameness within 2 weeks of treatment. In a recent study of 39 horses with bone spavin, 73% were free of lameness within a month. Joint fusion occurred in 15%, 63%, 85%, and 93% of horses within 1, 3, 6, and 12 months of treatment, respectively. Treatment was considered successful in 8%, 56%, 81%, and 93% of animals at the same time periods. In long-term follow-up (13–51 months) 80% of horses were free of lameness, 94% had fusion of the treated joints, and in 75% treatment was considered successful. Horses that have radiographic evidence of joint fusion but are not sound may respond favorably to drilling obliquely, in a distal to proximal direction, across the proximal aspect of the third metatarsal bone, third tarsal bone, and central tarsal bone. Complications of MIA injection, other than transient pain and swelling, occur in about 16% of horses and include skin and periarticular soft tissue necrosis, septic arthritis, and osteoarthrosis of the tarsocrural joint.

Surgical arthrodesis of the distal tarsal joints has a success rate similar to that of chemical fusion with MIA. Eighty to 85% of horses undergoing arthrodesis of the distal intertarsal and tarsometatarsal joints return to soundness over the subsequent 3 to 12 months.

Supplemental Readings

Bell BTL, Baker GH, Foreman JH, Abbott LC: *In vivo* investigation of communication between the distal intertarsal and tarsometatarsal joints in horses and ponies. Vet Surg 22:289–292, 1993.

Bohanon TC: Contrast arthrography of the distal intertarsal and tarsometatarsal joints in horses clinically affected with osteoarthrosis. Proc 40th Annu Conv Am Assoc Equine Pract, 1994, pp 193–194.

Bohanon TC, Schneider RK, Weisbrode SE: Fusion of the distal intertarsal and tarsometatarsal joints in the horse using intra-articular sodium monoiodoacetate. Equine Vet J 23:289–295, 1991.

Kraus-Hansen AE, Jann HW, Kerr DV, Fackelmann GE: Arthrographic analysis of communication between the tarsometatarsal and distal intertarsal joints of the horse. Vet Surg 21:139–144, 1992.

McIlwraith CW, Turner AS: Orthopedic surgery. In Equine Surgery: Advanced Techniques. Philadelphia, Lea & Febiger, 1987, pp 185–190.

Sack WO, Orsini PG: Distal intertarsal and tarsometatarsal joints in the horse: Communication and injection sites. J Am Vet Med Assoc 179:355–359, 1981.

Wyn-Jones G, May SA: Surgical arthrodesis for the treatment of osteoarthrosis of the proximal intertarsal, distal intertarsal, and tarsometatarsal joints in 30 horses: A comparison of four different techniques. Equine Vet J 18:59–64, 1986.

Soft Tissue Injuries of the Hock

KAREN M. BLUMENSHINE
Santa Barbara, California

SUE J. DYSON
Newmarket, England

PROXIMAL SUPERFICIAL DIGITAL FLEXOR TENDINITIS

The superficial digital flexor tendon descends from the caudal gaskin toward the plantar metatarsus and fans out over the tuber calcis, to which it is attached medially and laterally by strong fibrous bands. Proximal superficial digital flexor (SDF) tendinitis is often confused with plantar ligament desmitis, but may present with greater swelling, and is often associated with a more severe lameness, which persists longer. This uncommon condition may be caused by direct trauma or by a sudden marked increase in load as in slipping, but more often is caused by repetitive overloading of the tendon. It occurs most commonly in horses working at speed.

Clinical Signs and Diagnosis

Acute SDF tendinitis generally occurs unilaterally and results in heat and swelling on the distal plantar aspect of the hock. The tendon is palpably painful. Lameness is moderate and may be exacerbated by proximal limb flexion.

Diagnostic ultrasonography is the most reliable way to confirm the diagnosis and to determine the extent and severity of the injury. Abnormalities include areas of decreased echogenicity, interruption of fiber pattern, loss of definition of the tendon margins, and increase in the cross-sectional area of the tendon.

Treatment

Treatments of tendinitis and desmitis depend on the phase of healing. In general, the healing process can be divided into four phases after injury: the first 2 to 3 days, 3 to 21 days, 21 days to 60 days, and from 60 days to between 6 months and 1 year. The process may be retarded at any time because of reinjury or interruption of normal healing. Therefore, frequent examinations are crucial so that therapy can be adjusted accordingly.

The goal during the acute phase (the first 2 to 3 days) is

to reduce secondary cell death. Perilesional hemorrhage and edema compress local vasculature, thereby reducing nutrient and oxygen supply to tissue already metabolically stimulated by the heat of inflammation. Aggressive therapy is prudent to save viable perilesional cells by inhibiting hemorrhage, edema, and the byproducts of inflammation. Cold therapy, by application of ice, should be used in 30- to 60-minute intervals, three to six times daily. A constant, firm, uniform counterpressure wrap reduces the amount of extravasation and edema within the tendon. The action of the hock always poses a challenge to this, but a strong foundation wrap beginning at the coronet acts to reduce slippage. Rest is indicated.

Nonsteroidal anti-inflammatory drugs are an essential part of therapy. Flunixin meglumine (1.1 mg/kg s.i.d.) provides a rapid onset of activity. Phenylbutazone (1.1–4.4 mg/kg b.i.d.) is more appropriate for long-term maintenance because of its longer half life. Corticosteroids are more potent but may delay healing and reduce repair strength for up to 1 year after administration. Their use may give the clinician an unreliable sense of rapid progression of healing by the reduction of edema, pain, and warmth. Local injection may predispose to soft tissue calcification. In severe cases, systemic ultra-short-acting corticosteroids may be indicated to reduce secondary cell death in normal tendon tissue, which is compressed and compromised by the adjacent lesion. Dimethyl sulfoxide (DMSO) (2.2 mg/kg IV diluted) may be used as a free-radical scavenger to reduce the detrimental effects of the acute inflammatory products.

In the ensuing phase (3 to 21 days after injury), anti-inflammatory therapy is still indicated to minimize subsequent fibrosis and scar formation. Cold therapy may be alternated with a warm therapy interval, which should be three times as long (90–180 minutes) as the cold interval. Fibroproliferation occurs after about 6 days; therefore, it is more difficult to remove the intralesional fluid after that time. However, the cold therapy seems to have merit as long as the tendon is warmer than the surrounding tissues. Rubrifactants or a "sweat" such as a DMSO and nitrofurazone ointment mixture are useful to achieve warmth. DMSO use should be limited once fibroproliferation begins, because it is thought to have a detrimental effect on the quality of collagen formation in healing. Massage by hand, or with water from a pressurized hose, can stimulate circulation. If swelling has been controlled, walking exercise may begin. Tendon splitting or puncture to drain inflammatory products and to promote neovascularization within the lesion may be considered.

During the following phase (3 weeks to 2 months), if healing has occurred normally, collagen is remodelled or replaced in the newly vascularized lesion. To encourage linear alignment of the collagen fibrils, daily walking exercise is indicated, beginning with 10 minutes daily and adding 5 minutes per day each week. The walking exercise may be in hand, on a horse walker, or by riding. Routine monitoring of the tendon for an increase in heat or swelling is important, and exercise should be adjusted accordingly. Too much exercise may disrupt the healing collagen, delay healing, and lead to excessive fibrosis, which predisposes to reinjury. Therefore, uncontrolled turn out is inadvisable. Insufficient exercise results in fibers that are less well aligned, which may predispose to reinjury. By 2 months, there is usually an increase in echogenicity of the lesion, and in longitudinal images some linear echoes are apparent, but they are generally neither dense nor well aligned. If repair has not advanced to this level, or if it is apparent that reinjury has occurred, the time schedule for exercise (i.e., for tendon loading) must be set back to match the stage of healing. If a core lesion persists, a tendon splitting procedure may be warranted.

If the ultrasonographic findings are normal for phase 3, the tendon loading may be gradually increased by jogging the horse on an underwater treadmill, or by controlled jogging on even ground. A phase 4 exercise regimen may consist of 5 minutes of jogging daily for the first week, followed by an additional 5 minutes per day each consecutive week. Careful monitoring of the tendon is prudent.

Shoeing with an extended egg bar or other extended heel support helps prevent the heel from sinking in soft ground and minimizes sudden "overstretching" of the lesion in any stage of healing. If the disposition of the horse prohibits controlled exercise at any level, a mild tranquilizer such as acepromazine maleate (0.044–0.088 mg/kg intramuscularly [IM] or IV) or promazine hydrochloride granules (1.3 mg/kg p.o.) may be administered about one-half hour before exercise.

Inflammation is a natural result of destruction of adhesions that occurs mainly when an increased level of exercise extends the range of motion of the limb. If inflammation occurs, it is prudent to reduce exercise to a walk and re-evaluate the lesion ultrasonographically. The decision of when to allow cantering or galloping to begin depends largely upon the extent and severity of the original lesion, progression of healing, temperament of the horse, and level of compliance of the owner.

Prognosis

The prognosis for a strain-related SDF tendon injury in a hindlimb is better than in a forelimb. Those lesions restricted to the proximal metatarsus have a good prognosis for return to full athletic function, provided an adequate convalescent period is allowed, based upon ultrasonographic monitoring.

DISPLACEMENT OF THE SUPERFICIAL DIGITAL FLEXOR TENDON

At the point where the SDF fans out over the tuber calcis, strong ligamentous bands attach it medially and laterally to the tuber calcis. Displacement of the superficial digital flexor tendon from the tuber calcaneus usually results in an acute onset of severe lameness, although occasionally it is preceded by a low-grade subtle lameness. The latter is presumably due to pain associated with progressive breakdown of the ligamentous attachments of the SDF tendon. The dislocation occurs after rupture of the ligamentous attachments, allowing either medial or, more commonly, lateral displacement. The condition is usually unilateral, although occasionally it occurs bilaterally. Displacement has been seen as a result of degenerative failure of the suspensory apparatus seen in the Peruvian Paso and several other breeds.

Diagnosis

Extensive soft tissue swelling rapidly develops around the tuber calcaneus, and the horse has moderate to severe lameness at the walk. The horse may look anxious, especially if the tendon persistently moves on and off the calcaneus. In some cases, the tendon dislocates only when the limb is in motion and adjusts back to proper alignment at rest. The degree of soft tissue swelling may prohibit accurate assessment of the position of the SDF tendon, and ultrasonographic examination may be useful. After swelling diminishes, the position of the displaced tendon can be readily appreciated.

Treatment

Conservative treatment consists of immobilization in the form of a Robert Jones bandage for 60 days and stall rest for 6 months. Hand walking may begin at 2 to 4 months, if the SDF tendon appears to be stabilized and if exercise does not promote slipping. The use of nonsteroidal anti-inflammatory drugs is controversial. They may be contraindicated because the resultant reduction in soft tissue swelling allows more motion of the SDF tendon on and off the tuber calcaneus. By allowing the swelling to immobilize the SDF tendon in the "off" position, the tendon tends to heal in that position, which gives a better prognosis.

Surgical repair, using mesh or intermedullary pins to reattach the SDF to the tuber calcaneus, or implantation of cortical screws that protrude above the bone surface to serve as a guide for the replaced SDF tendon, have had variable results. If the tendon persistently slips on and off the tuber calcaneus, sectioning the intact ligamentous band of attachment may be considered.

Prognosis

Conservative treatment of cases in which the tendon continues to move on and off the tuber calcaneus is usually unrewarding. Conservative treatment is successful in some cases in which the tendon is permanently displaced, although the likely outcome cannot be predicted accurately. Some horses have returned to full athletic function, including Grand Prix showjumping and 3-day eventing, although a mild gait abnormality has persisted.

GASTROCNEMIUS TENDINITIS

The gastrocnemius muscle arises from the caudal aspect of the femur by two heads that converge into a common tendon by the midtibial region. Proximally the gastrocnemius tendon lies caudal to the SDF tendon and then lateral and finally cranial, inserting on the plantar aspect of the tuber calcaneus. The gastrocnemius bursa lies between the gastrocnemius tendon and the SDF tendon and extends to the midtarsal level. A smaller calcaneal bursa lies beneath the gastrocnemius tendon, just proximal to its insertion. These two bursae may communicate. Gastrocnemius tendinitis may be associated with trauma, but usually no predisposing cause is identified. It occurs in horses involved in a broad variety of disciplines.

Diagnosis

Lameness is usually unilateral and may be from mild to severe; it is generally proportional to the extent of the injury. It may be characterized by shortened duration of weightbearing in the caudal phase of the stride and a lowered arc of foot flight. The lameness is variably accentuated by flexion of either the proximal or distal limb joints. There is usually associated enlargement of the gastrocnemius and calcaneal bursae, resulting in a capped hock appearance, but distension of the gastrocnemius bursa may occur without tendinitis or lameness. Palpable enlargement of the gastrocnemius tendon is rarely appreciated, and it is difficult to elicit pain on pressure, but there is often localized heat, especially after exercise. A tibial nerve block usually improves lameness, but improvement may result from local diffusion of anesthetic solution rather than perineural analgesia itself.

An ultrasonographic examination should be done using a 7.5 MHz probe and a stand-off. Proximally the normal gastrocnemius tendon contains a core of muscular tissue within it, which appears hypoechoic. This core diminishes in cross-sectional size as the gastrocnemius tendon winds laterally around the SDF tendon and disappears distally. Comparison of normal versus injured gastrocnemius tendons, at equal distances proximal to the tuber calcaneus, aids the examiner in assessing the extent of the injury. Abnormalities include enlargement of the tendon, loss of distinct margins, and variably sized hypoechoic areas. Most lesions are restricted to the distal aspect of the gastrocnemius tendon. In injuries that are the result of direct trauma, there may be concurrent damage to the SDF tendon. Occasionally, proliferative new bone is seen on the tuber calcaneus, which is best appreciated in a flexed dorsoplantar (skyline) projection.

Treatment

Treatment to date has been purely symptomatic (see Current Therapy in Equine Medicine 3, page 146). Horses are restricted to stall rest and hand walking for the first 3 months and then re-evaluated ultrasonographically. Usually there is progressive increase in echogenicity, which continues for up to 9 to 12 months after injury. Large lesions usually have persistent hypoechoic defects that persist over a long period, whereas small lesions are shown to have resolved ultrasonographically. Increases in exercise intensity and duration should be based on the ultrasonographic appearance of the tendon.

Prognosis

The prognosis for return to full athletic function is guarded. A recent study followed 15 horses for at least 1 year and up to 3 years after resuming work. All horses had been rested for at least 9 months. Four horses resumed full work (flat racing, polo, and pleasure riding [2]) without further problems. One horse returned to showjumping despite mild persistent lameness. Eight horses resumed hunting, showjumping, horse trials, steeplechasing, and polo but experienced recurrent lameness because of gastrocnemius tendonitis 3 to 18 months after resuming work. Two horses were retired due to lameness associated with an unrelated cause. It is possible that in the future the use of β-aproprionitrile fumarate intralesionally may improve the prognosis.

DISTENSION OF THE TARSAL SHEATH (TRUE THOROUGHPIN)

Distension of the tarsal sheath, "true thoroughpin," is common and results in distinct fluctuant swellings on either side of and approximately 5 cm cranial to the common calcaneal tendon. Rarely, there may also be swelling medially at the level of the tarsometatarsal joint. Beginning about 5 to 7.5 cm proximal to the level of the medial malleolus, the tarsal sheath is 20 to 30 cm long and ends distally in the proximal third of the metatarsus. It encompasses the deep digital flexor (DDF) tendon. The tarsal canal surrounds the tarsal sheath on the plantar aspect of the tarsus.

Idiopathic tenosynovitis of the tarsal sheath usually occurs bilaterally, especially in young horses, even before work begins. Generally there is no associated lameness and often the swellings resolve spontaneously.

Acute tenosynovitis of the tarsal sheath is associated with a sudden effusion in the tarsal sheath, accompanied by pain, inflammation, and usually mild to severe lameness. Occasionally there is no associated lameness. Direct trauma and overstretching, or strain, of the sheath and the associated deep digital flexor tendon are the most frequent causes. Proximal to the protection of the tarsal canal, the tarsal sheath shifts medially during extension of the hock, allowing susceptibility to direct trauma. Acute sheath distension of traumatic origin may be accompanied by DDF tendonitis, periostitis, or a chip or horizontal fracture of the sustentaculum tali. Desmitis, rupture, or avulsion fracture of the insertions of the middle, short, medial collateral ligament, or tarsometatarsal ligament on the distomedial surface of the sustentaculum tali, may also occur.

Chronic tenosynovitis of the tarsal sheath has a persistent synovial effusion in, and fibrous thickening of, the tarsal sheath. It may be accompanied by adhesions to the DDF tendon or stenosis of the sheath. A common sequela to acute tenosynovitis, it can be associated with any of the same associated tendon, ligament, or bone conditions. In cases associated with bone trauma, adhesion formation, and tendon pathology, lameness is usually chronic.

Septic tenosynovitis of the tarsal sheath characteristically has a marked suppurative synovial effusion accompanied by severe lameness, generalized soft tissue edema, heat, and swelling. It most often results from a penetrating wound but may be the iatrogenic result of an injection.

Other rare causes of tenosynovitis of the tarsal sheath include chondrosarcoma extending from the cartilage of the tarsocrural joint and systemic lupus-like synovitis.

Diagnosis

Analysis of synovial fluid aspirated from the distended tarsal sheath can help differentiate the idiopathic, acutely or chronically inflamed, septic, autoimmune, or neoplastic processes.°

A radiographic study is indicated in chronic cases in which lameness is present, even if the distension is cool and nonpainful. This should include a dorsomedial-plantarolateral oblique view of the hock, so that any new bone on the sustentaculum tali may be highlighted. A dorsoplantar (flexed) view may aid in identification of abnormalities restricted to the axial aspect of the sustentaculum tali. Sustentaculum fracture or, rarely, mineralization and/or ossicles in the tarsal sheath may be detected. Exostoses on the sustentaculum tali are usually associated with tendon fibrillation and chronic pain. The prognosis is guarded to poor.

A positive result on a radiographic contrast study of the tarsal sheath may differentiate synovial distension of the sheath from other swelling, such as "false" thoroughpin, and may help identify adhesions of the synovial lining to itself, or to the deep digital flexor tendon, folding or pocketing of inflamed synovium, and tendovaginal masses.

Ultrasonographic examination from the plantaromedial aspect of the hock is also useful in differentiating tarsal sheath synovitis and other swelling in the hock region because the deep digital flexor tendon can be imaged within. Primary DDF tendon damage can be diagnosed and evaluated. Early tendon mineralization is detected more easily by ultrasonographic than radiographic examination. However, accurate assessment of the entire length of the DDF tendon is difficult, and lesions, especially those in a longitudinal plane, may be missed. Acute traumatic injuries may result in blood and fibrin clots that can be seen within the sheath. A septic sheath has a cellular echogenicity and may contain small gas shadows produced by an anaerobic infection or larger gas shadows resulting from a penetrating wound. Other findings may include synovial proliferation, invagination, mineralization, and intrathecal adhesions or masses.

Treatment

Treatment of idiopathic tenosynovitis by applying sweat wraps or by draining synovial fluid and injecting corticosteroids are only of temporary value. In mild cases of tenosynovitis unaccompanied by bone abnormalities, stall rest accompanied by hand walking and systemic anti-inflammatory drugs such as phenylbutazone (2.2 mg/kg b.i.d.) or flunixin meglumine (1.1 mg/kg s.i.d.) often resolve the signs. The more chronic cases, in which bony complications have been ruled out, also lend themselves to this therapy. Intrathecal treatment with corticosteroids is controversial. Methylprednisolone acetate (80 to 120 mg) or triamcinolone acetonide (10 mg) injected into the tarsal sheath, followed by application of a pressure bandage, often relieves the symptoms. Long-term repeated injection of the tarsal sheath with corticosteroids, with or without prior drainage, has been associated with spontaneous rupture of the DDF tendon. This may reflect failure to identify preexisting damage of the DDF tendon. Reports exist of large ossicles forming in adhesions that had attached to the DDF tendon following repeated corticosteroid injection into the tarsal sheath.

Markedly enlarged chronic distensions of the tarsal sheath have responded favorably to arthroscopic or surgical debridement of fibrin tags adhering to the DDF tendon and tarsal sheath, and subsequent imbrication of the sheath in the area of herniation, where indicated, to restore the sheath to the original shape. Postoperative injection of hyaluronate sodium° 5 ml (10 mg/ml) may facilitate lubri-

---

°See *Current Therapy in Equine Medicine, ed 3, page 134.*

°*Synacid (hyaluronate sodium sterile injection), Schering-Plough Animal Health, Union, NJ*

cation and possibly inhibit entheseous formation. In the absence of damage to the DDF tendon, prognosis for return to full athletic function is fair, although a satisfactory cosmetic outcome cannot be guaranteed. Horses with lesions in the DDF tendon within the tarsal sheath have a more guarded outcome. One of the authors (SJD) has seen several cases of acute tenosynovitis unassociated with lameness; the horses have been successfully maintained in work without therapy. The swelling ultimately decreased considerably.

Septic tenosynovitis requires surgical drainage and copious lavage. Five to ten L of sterile lactated Ringer's solution or sterile saline solution per flush is usually adequate. High-velocity flushing and suction is optimum for gentle mechanical debridement. A sterile disposable motorized instrument (Surigilav Plus*) is excellent for this purpose. Hand-powered devices, such as a syringe or a bulb, may be used, but high-velocity fluid debridement is more difficult to achieve. Daily flushing with maintained open drainage is the most recently accepted treatment for optimal healing. Sterile wraps over open drainage should be applied between flushings. Broad-spectrum bactericidal systemic antibiotics should be administered (crystalline penicillin 20,000 IU/kg t.i.d. and gentamicin 2.2 mg/kg t.i.d. or 6.6 mg/kg s.i.d. IV or IM). Administration of nonsteroidal anti-inflammatory drugs such as phenylbutazone (2.2 mg/kg b.i.d.) or flunixin meglumine (1.1 mg/kg s.i.d.) is helpful. Acute-onset aggressively treated septic tenosynovitis has a fair prognosis for return of the horse to previous athletic function, but chronic cases and cases with infection of the DDF tendon have an extremely guarded prognosis.

"FALSE" THOROUGHPIN

Either a cystic or a solid extra-tendovaginal mass in the region of the tarsal sheath may be termed "false" thoroughpin. Abnormalities that may form a mass in the region of the tarsal sheath are: (1) a swelling of the common calcaneal (Achilles) tendon; (2) swelling of the intertendinous calcaneal bursa; (3) hematoma; (4) granulation tissue; (5) organized scar tissue, (6) ganglion; (7) fibrous synovial-lined cavity; or (8) dissected synovial cyst resulting from chronic distension of the tarsal sheath or tarsal sheath herniation. Lameness may or may not be associated.

Diagnosis

Positive contrast radiography helps to differentiate true from false thoroughpin and to identify communication. In a true thoroughpin the DDF tendon is outlined. Diagnostic ultrasonography is also useful to determine if the swelling is solid or cystic and whether it communicates with the tarsal sheath. Identification of a synovial swelling emerging from between the gastrocnemius and superficial digital flexor tendon as it passes over the tuber calcis indicates calcaneal bursitis.

Treatment

In the absence of lameness, therapy is not required, although swelling may persist. In cases with lameness, this

*Surigilav Plus, Stryker Instruments, Kalamazoo, MI

frequently resolves with rest, although there is often a cosmetic blemish. Persistent lameness associated with multiloculated cyst-like lesions has improved following surgical removal, but with disappointing cosmetic results.

PLANTAR LIGAMENT DESMITIS OR "CURB"

The plantar ligament originates proximally on the plantar border of the tuber calcaneus and extends distally, to attach on the proximal ends of the third and fourth metatarsal bones. The distal continuation of this ligament becomes the accessory ligament of the deep digital flexor tendon. The partially cartilaginous, smooth plantar surface of the ligament forms the dorsal wall of the tarsal canal. Desmitis of the plantar ligament, commonly called a curb, is the result of direct trauma or strain and results in a localized soft tissue swelling on the plantar aspect of the calcaneus or proximal metatarsus.

Several other conditions cause curb-like swelling and mimic plantar ligament desmitis. The most common of these is proximal superficial digital flexor tendinitis. Subcutaneous edema, hematoma or fibrosis, or deep digital flexor tendinitis are also associated with similar swellings but may be differentiated ultrasonographically. The head of the fourth metatarsal bone may interrupt the normally vertical plantar outline of the hindlimb and also may be mistaken for a curb. Axial enlargement of the proximal fourth metatarsal bone also results in a plantar dislocation of the superficial digital flexor tendon in the weightbearing position. This is seen most commonly in Warmbloods and can be confirmed radiographically. A curb-like appearance in a neonatal foal or older horse may be the result of defective endochondral ossification of the central and third tarsal bones, resulting in their partial or complete collapse. This has been observed in association with hypothyroidism in young foals. Radiographic examination is indicated for this diagnosis.

Acute plantar ligament desmitis is less common than previously thought. Swelling and pain are present upon digital palpation over the ligament. The degree of lameness is variable and may be increased by exercise. The horse may stand with the heel in an elevated position at rest.

Treatment

Treatment during the first 2 to 3 days of acute desmitis consists of rest and application of ice packs for 30 minutes' duration, repeated every 2 hours, antiphlogistic poultices, and systemic nonsteroidal anti-inflammatory drugs such as flunixin meglumine (1.1 mg/kg s.i.d.), or phenylbutazone (2.2 mg/kg b.i.d.). This intensive treatment not only aids healing but also increases the chances of a better cosmetic end result.

In horses that are not exhibiting lameness, light exercise may begin soon after inflammation subsides. In the more severe cases exhibiting lameness, hand walking for up to 4 to 6 weeks may be indicated before light work begins. The earlier mentioned therapy for reduction of inflammation should continue as long as local inflammation is apparent. Severe traumatic injury in this region may result in periostitis on the plantar aspect of the calcaneus, causing permanent bony enlargement.

SUBCUTANEOUS SWELLING ON THE PLANTAROPROXIMAL ASPECT OF THE METATARSUS

Subcutaneous swelling on the plantar proximal aspect of the metatarsus may be due to edema, hemorrhage, or fibrosis. Although swellings in this location may be due to direct trauma, some cases associated with moderate to severe lameness of acute onset occur with no apparent inciting cause. The pathogenesis is unknown. In these cases, lameness may persist for many weeks to months, although no underlying tendon or bone pathology can be identified. Ultrasonographically there is usually a subcutaneous anechoic area in the acute stage. Systemic anti-inflammatory therapy and local treatment as discussed previously are indicated, together with stall rest. Lameness generally resolves ultimately. Sequential ultrasonographic examinations usually reveal a progressive increase in echogenicity of the area plantar to the SDF tendon and plantar ligament. Some degree of soft tissue swelling usually persists over the long term.

CONDITIONS OF THE DEEP DIGITAL FLEXOR TENDON IN THE TARSAL AND PROXIMAL METATARSAL REGIONS

There are three muscular heads of the deep digital flexor, which merge as a common tendon in the distal third of the crus. The DDF tendon descends in the tarsal sheath, over the groove in the sustentaculum of the fibular tarsal bone.

Tendinitis

Deep digital flexor tendinitis in the region of the distal tarsus or proximal metatarsus is an uncommon condition that may mimic the presentation of a curb. Heat and swelling occur in the proximal plantar metatarsus coinciding with a mild lameness, which may be exacerbated by hock flexion. The lameness may improve following intra-articular anesthesia of the tarsometatarsal joint, or subtarsal analgesia of the plantar and plantar metatarsal nerves.

Diagnosis is confirmed by ultrasonographic imaging of the DDF tendon through a window on the caudomedial aspect of the hock over the sustentaculum tali, or farther distally, from the plantar aspect of the limb. The normal DDF tendon is of uniform echogenicity. Lesions include hypoechoic regions within the DDF tendon, an increase in cross-sectional area of the tendon, and poor definition of the tendon margins.

Because only a few clinical cases of DDF tendinitis have been reported, prognosis is not defined. In the reported cases in young Thoroughbred racehorses, lameness resolved rapidly but enlargement of the DDF tendon remained. Horses were treated conservatively by box rest, followed by a controlled exercise program of increasing intensity. Work was successfully resumed approximately 4 to 6 months after injury.

Slipped Deep Digital Flexor Tendon

The rare condition of a slipped deep digital flexor tendon is the result of a congenital malformation of the sustentaculum of the fibular tarsal bone. The absence of the medial prominence of the groove that guides the DDF tendon and tarsal sheath allows the DDF tendon to slip medially. Instead of a groove, the surface slopes from lateral to medial, so that the flexor tendon displaces medially. The presenting complaint may be a varus deformity of the fetlock of the affected limb. This appears to be caused by the abnormal pull of the displaced DDF tendon. Characteristically, the plantar aspect of the tarsus appears wider than normal. The displaced DDF tendon can be palpated medially until it gradually returns to its normal position, approximately one-third of the distance down the metatarsus. Radiographically, the sky-line view of the hock allows the best visualization of the loss of the normal groove.

In one reported case, surgical repair of a slipped DDF tendon was attempted by transferring an autogenous splint bone to the location of the medial ridge. The horse became usable for pleasure but not for show performance. Generally, soft tissue enlargement may remain in the region after healing. If the surgery is performed during the first 3 to 6 months of age, the varus deformity tends to correct itself.

DESMITIS OF THE COLLATERAL LIGAMENTS OF THE TARSUS

The medial and lateral collateral ligaments of the tarsocrural joint each have two parts: the long and superficial and the short and deep. The long medial collateral ligament arises on the caudal aspect of the medial malleolus of the tibia, widens distally, and inserts on the distal tuberosity of the talus, the medial aspect of the third tarsal, and second and third metatarsal bones. The long lateral collateral ligament arises from the caudal aspect of the lateral malleolus and extends distally, almost straight downward, to insert on the fibular and fourth tarsal bones and the third and fourth metatarsal bones. The short medial collateral ligament arises from the cranial aspect of the medial malleolus, runs caudodistally and inserts via two branches on the proximal tuberosity of the talus and the sustentaculum tali. The short lateral collateral ligament arises from the cranial aspect of the lateral malleolus and extends caudally to insert on a rough area on the lateral aspect of the talus and the adjacent surface of the fibular tarsal bone.

Injuries to the collateral ligaments may be seen in any horse, but the incidence is highest in horses that race, especially over fences, and particularly in horses that have fallen.

Diagnosis

Collateral ligament injury is manifested by mild to severe lameness that is exacerbated by proximal limb flexion. Often there is a history of periodic lameness that has responded to 1 to 2 weeks of rest. In mild cases there is little or no swelling, although in more severe cases there is often distension of the tarsocrural joint capsule. Lameness may be improved, although not alleviated, by intra-articular analgesia of the tarsocrural joint, especially if there is desmitis of the deeper short collateral ligaments. In the acute stage, usually there are no radiographic changes; however, lateral malleolar fractures of the distal tibia may be associated with localized desmitis. Six to 8 weeks after injury entheseophytes at the sites of attachment of the collateral ligaments are often identifiable. Ultrasonography may reveal hypoechoic defects in the damaged collateral ligaments.

Nuclear scintigraphy may be the most sensitive method of determining tears of the attachments of the collateral ligaments in the acute phase. Arthroscopy of the tarsocrural joint may reveal tearing and herniation of fibrils.

Treatment

In the acute phase, phenylbutazone (2.2 mg/kg p.o. b.i.d.) is indicated until the signs of inflammation and positive proximal limb flexion have disappeared. The horse should be restricted to stall rest and controlled walking exercise. Avulsion fractures of the lateral malleolus of the tibia should be removed surgically, although horses treated conservatively do have a fair to good prognosis for return to full athletic function. Ideally horses should be allowed 6 months of box rest, followed by a gradual return to normal work.

SUBLUXATION OR LUXATION OF THE TARSOCRURAL JOINT

Tarsal luxation or subluxation can be produced by complete disruption of the collateral ligaments. Complete luxation of the tarsocrural joint is a catastrophic injury for athletic performance, although horses may be salvaged for breeding purposes. Other structures are generally damaged as well. Luxation or subluxation of the proximal intertarsal or tarsometatarsal joints may be treated by reduction and application of a full limb cast. Surgical arthrodesis, combined with casting, results in a more favorable prognosis for return to work. Minor subluxations of these joints in immature animals may be managed successfully by stall confinement only.

Supplemental Readings

Bramlage LR: Medical treatment of tendinitis. In Robinson NE (ed): Current Therapy in Equine Medicine, ed 3. Philadelphia, WB Saunders, 1992, p 146.
Dik KJ, Leitch M: Soft tissue injuries of the tarsus. Vet Clin North Am Equine Pract 11:235–247, 1995.
Dyson SJ: The value of diagnostic ultrasonography in the hock region: Uses and limitations. Proc 7th Annu Symp Advanc Clin Vet Med, 1994.
McIlwraeth CW: Diseases of joints, tendons, ligaments and related structures. In Stashak TS: Adams' Lameness in Horses, ed 4. Philadelphia, Lea & Febiger, 1987.
Wright IM: Ligaments associated with joints. Vet Clin North Am Equine Pract 11:249–291, 1995.

Implications of Bone Adaptation in the Thoroughbred Racehorse

CHRISTOPHER M. RIGGS
Neston, England

Injuries to bones of the appendicular skeleton are the cause of considerable loss among Thoroughbred racehorses. Approximately 60% of all race course fatalities are related to fractures, and a high proportion of young Thoroughbreds lose time in training as a consequence of less severe bone pathology. Some of these injuries are caused by direct trauma, but a high proportion occur in the absence of a particular incident and can only be associated with high-speed exercise.

The spontaneous nature of some fractures and common occurrence of conditions such as bucked shins suggest that the mechanical properties of the bones affected are insufficient to withstand the loads to which they are subjected during routine training and racing. It is well recognized that the physical characteristics of bones vary in response to changes in the loads placed upon them. It is thought that this adaptive mechanism has evolved in part to minimize the risk of bone injury during routine activity.

Knowledge of the mechanisms of functional adaptation of the skeleton paves the way to an understanding of spontaneous-type bone injury in the racehorse and may provide a basis for the prevention and treatment of such injuries.

FUNCTIONAL ADAPTATION OF BONE

Basic Biomechanics

When a load is applied to a structure, whether it is a bridge or a bone, it deforms. Within certain limits this deformation or strain is elastic and the structure returns to its normal shape, unaltered, once the load has been removed. If the degree of deformation rises beyond a threshold limit, irreversible change or damage to the structure may be caused. A single extreme load may deform the structure beyond an ultimate limit, resulting in its complete and sudden failure (i.e., fracture). Alternatively, although the extent of damage from a single load cycle may be insufficient to cause failure, repetition of such loads results in cumulative damage, which may lead ultimately to complete failure of the structure.

The extent to which a structure is deformed depends on the magnitude and direction of the load applied to it and the mechanical properties of the structure. These properties are determined by two major factors:

1. The geometry of the structure, encompassing mass, and spatial distribution of that mass about the axis of loading
2. The mechanical properties of the material from which the structure is constructed.

In a manmade structure, such as a bridge, these parameters are determined at the time of construction and remain fixed thereafter. The initial design therefore requires accurate predictions of the magnitude and frequencies of the loads to which the structure will be subjected during its expected lifespan. Significant increases in loads from those predicted may result in excessive deformation of the structure, leading to its untimely collapse. Creating a structure with safety margins that are far in excess of those ever expected to be required may circumvent this problem, but will add considerable and possibly unnecessary cost to the project.

The skeleton would be a highly inefficient biologic system if its formation was constrained by such static limitations. Considering the wide variation in physical activity between individuals of the same species, or even within the same individual at different times of its life, mechanical requirements of the skeleton fluctuate, and bones would oscillate between being excessively large and dangerously small. Bone is, however, a living, dynamic tissue. Although the overall shape and construction of most bones is genetically predetermined, their mass, three-dimensional structure, and microstructural characteristics are all capable of change in response to variation in their mechanical environment. As a consequence, the skeleton can adapt to changes in the level or type of exercise to maintain mechanical competence with the minimal appropriate amount of bone tissue.

The Mechanism of Adaptation

The mechanisms by which the change in mechanical environment of a bone is transduced into a biologic response and the precise physiologic aims of the response remain matters for speculation and subjects of active research. One of the more convincing hypotheses in this field has been developed over the years by Lanyon and coworkers. They suggest that a population of cells is able to detect changes in the mechanical environment of the bone and activate cells responsible for bone architecture accordingly. Because stress cannot be measured directly, it is likely that strain is the influencing factor. Indeed, experiments based on avian and mammalian models suggest that changes in the distribution, rate of change, and magnitude of strain within the matrix are capable of stimulating a remodeling response by the bone. The even distribution of osteocytes throughout the bone matrix, together with their extensive network of cytoplasmic interconnections, places this cell population in a good position to sense changes in these mechanical variables. Work documenting rapid increases in metabolic activity of osteocytes in response to mechanical loading further suggests that these cells are responsible for initiating the biologic response. It is proposed by Lanyon that following the appreciation of the strain situation, osteocytes influence the behavior of cell populations at the bone surfaces, which are responsible for modeling and remodeling. The bone's architecture is then adjusted until functional strains match those genetically determined to be appropriate for that particular location. In this way, functional strains are both the objective and the stimulus for the process of adaptive modeling and remodeling.

Physical expression of bone adaptation is performed by two cell populations responsible for formation (osteoblasts) and resorption (osteoclasts) of matrix. Mechanical influences during early life are likely to influence the rate, type, and location of formation of matrix around the bone's circumference. This process, involving addition of new bone to a developing surface, may be referred to as modeling. Subsequent alterations in the mechanical environment of the bone may stimulate changes in this architecture, whereby existing bone is removed and replaced in the same location, replaced in a different location, or not replaced at all. This process may be referred to as remodeling and can occur at periosteal and endosteal surfaces, or within the cortex itself in the form of osteonal remodeling.

IMPLICATIONS OF BONE ADAPTATION IN THE RACEHORSE

Bone Mass

One of the simplest ways in which the mechanical properties of a structure may be enhanced is by increasing the bulk of material from which it is formed. Many examples can be given of functional associations between increased loading of a bone and its hypertrophy. For instance, the cortical thickness of the humerus of the playing arm of professional tennis players is significantly greater in comparison with that of the nonplaying arm. Conversely, reduced loading of bone, for example following application of a rigid external cast, has been shown to lead to bone resorption.

However, there are limitations to the size of bones, and increasing their mass may also have disadvantages, especially in the more distal regions of the limb. The contribution of the mass of a bone to the moment of inertia of the limb is proportional to the square of its distance from the center of rotation. It has been calculated that approximately 50% of the power required by a horse galloping at 15 m/sec is used to accelerate and decelerate bones of the distal limb. A 10% reduction in the mass of bones of the distal limb may produce a 5% saving in the total power required by the horse. Although this may be of little consequence to slower breeds, in horses selected and bred purely for speed, this factor may become significant.

Three-dimensional Shape

The deformations that occur in bones of the appendicular skeleton during locomotion reflect the effects of a combination of:

1. Longitudinal compression due to gravity
2. Bending due to eccentric distribution of axial loads and the pull of attached musculature.

The mechanical competence of a structure loaded in bending is optimized when its mass is distributed as far as possible from the neutral axis (the axis about which the structure bends). The use of I-beams in the construction industry is an example of exploitation of this fact. The hollow structure of all long bones provides a mechanism whereby the bulk of tissue mass may be situated farther from the axis of bending (Fig. 1). The roughly cylindrical nature of some long bones, such as the humerus and femur, provides a structure that is equally stiff in all planes of bending. Close inspection of the more distal bones reveals eccentric distribution of mass about the bone's central axis. This arrangement provides greater bending stiffness in one particular direction. Although the cylindrical form offers greater "protection" from loads in all directions, the eccentric structure reflects an adaptive mechanism, whereby concentration of bone mass in specific locations about its circumference ensures increased stiffness in a particular plane and hence reduced deformation of the bone as a consequence of routine loads during normal locomotion. The loss of safety margins in other planes of bending may be the price for reduction in total bone mass.

Variation in the geometric properties of the equine third metacarpal bone have been well documented by Nunamaker and his group in Pennsylvania. Analysis of cross-sections of bones obtained from Thoroughbred racehorses

revealed significant age-dependent changes in the second moments of area that relate to bending stiffness in a particular direction. The most dramatic changes were noted in horses between the ages of 1 and 2 years. Lesser changes were recorded in horses up to 4 years of age, after which geometric properties remained similar. The correlation between the period of intense bone modeling, bringing about the change in cross-sectional area, and commencement of race training was wholly consistent with the hypothesis of bone adaptation.

The functional significance of this observation was further emphasised following direct observation of deformation of the third metacarpal bone using strain gauges bonded to its dorsal surface in experimental racehorses. Changes in geometry of the bone correlated well with, and presumably accounted for, a decrease in peak strain in older animals. However, the relationships between exercise, modeling, and incidence of bone injury were more subtle than may first appear. Significant changes in the direction of peak strain in the third metacarpal bone were recorded when the speed was increased from a trot (5.5 m/sec) to a fast gallop (16.6 m/sec). Training for prolonged intervals at slower speeds induced a modeling response that was inappropriate for racing speeds. Therefore, peak strains associated with high-speed exercise remained elevated. Considering that the number of loading cycles to failure (the fatigue life of a structure) is related logarithmically to the deformation associated with each cycle, persistence of high peak strains greatly increase the risk of fatigue damage. On the basis of these observations, together with studies by Lanyon, which demonstrated that only a few cycles of load are required daily to activate an osteogenic response, Nunamaker designed a training schedule aimed at reducing the incidence of fatigue damage to the third metacarpal bone. By reducing the extent of the low-speed work and increasing the frequency of short-interval high-speed work, an appropriate modeling response can be stimulated with minimal risk of fatigue damage.

Material Properties

Just as the modeling of a bone can have profound influence on its mechanical competence through changes in its geometric properties, so remodeling can affect it by altering the mechanical properties of the tissue from which it is composed—bone. Characteristics of the material properties of bone may be determined using established engineering techniques on standardized test specimens, from which geometric variation has been eliminated. Studies using these principles have gathered a substantial body of information on the material properties of bone and factors that affect it. The reader is referred to other texts for detailed descriptions of this subject.

Significant differences in the material properties of bone in different animals, samples from different bones in the same animal, and even specimens from different regions of the same bone (Table 1) may reflect adaptive mechanisms that confer some mechanical advantage. For example, bone from the equine third metacarpus is significantly stiffer than that from the proximal phalanx but has a lower energy-absorbing capacity. Bearing in mind the relative lengths of the bones and hence the increased moment of

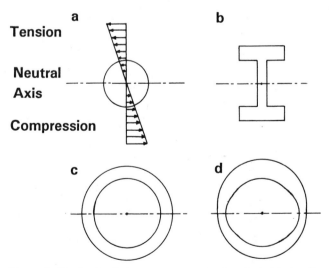

Figure 1. The longitudinal stress across a structure loaded in bending will increase with distance on either side of its neutral axis (a). Consequently, by distributing the bulk of material as far as possible from the neutral axis, stress and strain within the material is reduced (b). When the load may come from any direction, a hollow tube provides the optimal structure (c). If load comes from one predominant direction, but some protection is required in all directions, eccentric distribution of mass around the circumference of the tube may provide the most efficient compromise (d).

TABLE 1. VARIATION IN THE MECHANICAL PROPERTIES OF CORTICAL BONE BETWEEN DIFFERENT SPECIES, BETWEEN DIFFERENT BONES OF THE SAME SPECIES, AND BETWEEN DIFFERENT REGIONS OF THE SAME BONE

	Young's Modulus GPa	Ultimate Stress MPa
Species		
Polar Bear	17–22	107–129
Human	14–28	107–162
Bovine	12–40	54–271
Equine	15–22	121–129
Bone		
Equine		
Third metacarpus	19	124
Proximal phalanx	15	74
Cortex		
Equine Radius		
Cranial	22	161
Caudal	15	105

bending acting on the third metacarpal bone, increase in stiffness of the tissue from which it is composed seems a sensible adaptation. Conversely, the relative proximity of the proximal phalanx to the point of contact of the limb is likely to increase the impact loading of this bone, and hence an increase in its ability to absorb energy is likely to be functionally advantageous.

Variation in the mechanical properties of bone may be explained by differences in the composition and structure of its matrix. For instance, an increase in the degree of mineralization of the organic phase of the matrix results in a concomitant rise in its strength and stiffness. It takes several months for recently formed osteoid to achieve an optimal mineral content (approximately 66% by weight). Consequently, new bone is weaker and less stiff than older bone. The rapid rise in strength and stiffness in bone from the equine third metacarpus over the first year of life, associated with a sharp increase in its mineral content over the same period, is consistent with this fact. However, the material properties of this bone have been found to plateau or even fall slightly thereafter. This observation can be explained by changes in the bone's microstructure. The mechanical properties of remodeled secondary osteonal bone are inferior to those of primary bone in most ways. A number of physical explanations exist for the apparent weakening effects of secondary osteons, and these can be summarized as follows:

1. Secondary osteons frequently have a lower mineral density because of their relative immaturity
2. The active remodeling process results in increased bone porosity owing to the formation of resorption canals
3. Secondary osteons are joined to surrounding bone by a cement line that represents a line of relative weakness.

Long bones in the fetal horse consist of a woven fiber template, upon which fibrolamellar bone is rapidly forming at the time of birth. Circumferential growth is maximal over the first year of life, during which time little remodeling occurs. Between 2 and 3 years of age, a high level of remodeling activity occurs in bones of Thoroughbreds, and

up to 50% of the primary structure may be replaced by 3 years.

The apparent detrimental effects of remodeling on the mechanical properties of bone may be compensated for by other beneficial features of this process, which include:

1. Mineral homeostasis
2. A potential mechanism for repair of the matrix
3. A mechanism by which a bone's microstructure may be modified in response to changes in its mechanical environment.

Some evidence for the latter is provided by the observation that the caudal cortex of the equine radius is extensively remodeled during the first 2 years of life. During this process the orientation of collagen fibers within the matrix is replaced from predominantly longitudinal to transverse. The change in this one microstructural feature has a significant effect on the mechanical properties of the bone, which may be expected to have a beneficial influence on the mechanical competence of the bone as a whole.

To date there has been little direct evidence for an effect of physical activity on the material properties of bone. Longitudinal studies of Thoroughbreds subjected to different training regimens revealed differences in the rate of

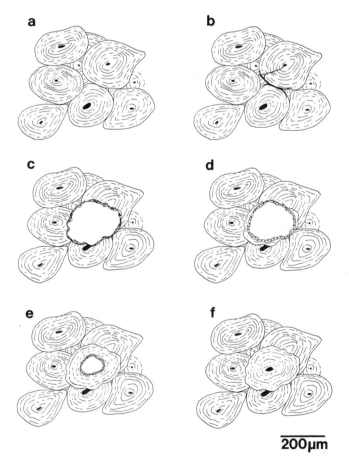

200μm

Figure 2. Repair of fatigue-damaged bone. (a) Intact osteonal bone; (b) microdamage; (c) osteoclastic resorption; (d and e) new bone formation; (f) repaired bone with a new secondary osteon. This process takes 4 to 6 months. (From Riggs CM, Evans GP: The microstructural basis of the mechanical properties of equine bone. Equine Vet Educ 2:197–205, 1990.)

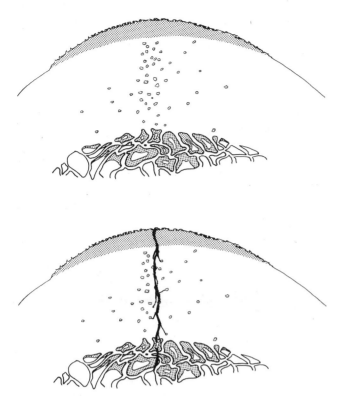

Figure 3. Pathologic processes involved in some fatigue fractures. Accumulation of microdamage in a region of the cortex results in activation of a large number of resorption units. The resultant increase in porosity has a stress-concentrating effect and may predispose the bone to fracture. The periosteal and endosteal callus (stippled), recognizable radiographically, provides minimal mechanical support. (From Riggs CM, Evans GP: The microstructural basis of the mechanical properties of equine bone. Equine Vet Educ 2:197–205, 1990.)

change of ultrasound conduction velocity through the third metacarpus. This parameter, which is related to the stiffness of bone, increased with exercise. Subsequent histomorphometric analysis revealed bones from horses exercised intensively to have undergone relatively less internal remodeling than those from control animals. As a consequence, the bones had lower porosity and higher mineral content (both of which are related to ultrasound conduction velocity). These findings suggest an inhibitory effect of intense cyclical loading on internal remodeling and may have important implications for horses temporarily removed from training.

Fatigue

Fatigue fractures are relatively common in racehorses. The pathologic processes that underlie them illustrate the importance of understanding the dynamic nature of bone and potential hazards of the remodeling process. The elastic modulus (stiffness) of bone decreases as it undergoes fatigue. As in manmade composites, this effect has been related to the appearance of microcracks within the tissue.

These cracks tend to run along lamellar interfaces, such as osteonal cement lines, and extend fatigue life by diverting energy from the propagation of transverse cracks that would cause immediate failure. In an inert structure, continued cyclical loading results in accumulation of microdamage, leading to its eventual failure. Internal remodeling provides a mechanism whereby fatigue-damaged bone may be replaced with healthy tissue, potentially extending its fatigue life indefinitely (Fig. 2). However, the very process of repair may contribute significantly to a bone's failure. Where a region of the cortex has suffered fatigue damage, resorption (the initial phase of remodeling) may be so intense as to increase significantly the local porosity of the bone. This effect results in a temporary increase in the local stress intensity, predisposing the bone to failure at loads within the usual limit (Fig. 3). Continued training during this phase of repair carries a greater risk of catastrophic fracture occurring. In consideration of the fact that it takes a secondary osteon 2 to 3 months to form and a further 4 to 5 months to reach a mineral density approaching that of surrounding bone, the need for extended convalescence periods is appreciated.

The clinical signs associated with fatigue damage and its repair are not specific, making clinical diagnosis difficult. The advent of gamma scintigraphy in racehorse practice has greatly improved recognition of early fatigue fractures before they progress to complete fractures of the bone.

CONCLUSIONS

The advantages of strategic training in preparation of the cardiovascular, respiratory, and muscular systems for intense physical activity have been acknowledged for centuries. More recently, recognition of the adaptive nature of bone has revealed the potential to prepare the skeleton by training. The high incidence of spontaneous-type fractures and other less severe injuries to the skeleton of Thoroughbred racehorses suggests that current training regimens have deficiencies. The work of Nunamaker has made significant advances in our understanding of this field, but lack of basic knowledge of many aspects of bone physiology in the racehorse means that the picture is still far from complete.

Supplemental Readings

Currey JD: The Mechanical Adaptations of Bone. Princeton, NJ, Princeton University Press, 1984.
Gordon JE: Structures: Or Why Things Don't Fall Down. Oxford, Plenum Press, 1978.
Lanyon LE: Functional strain in bone tissue as an objective, and controlling stimulus for adaptive bone remodelling. J Biomechanics 20:1083–1093, 1987.
Martin RB, Burr DB: Structural Function and Adaptation of Bone. New York, Raven Press, 1989.
Nunamaker DM, Butterweck DM, Provost MT: Fatigue fractures in Thoroughbred racehorses: Relationships with age, peak bone strain and training. J Orthop Res 8:604, 1990.

Stress Fractures

ROB PILSWORTH

MIKE SHEPHERD
Newmarket, England

Stress fractures occur in performance horses and rarely in mature general-purpose riding horses. Equine bone evolved in wild horses, which use a short burst of speed to escape from a predator. With the addition of a rider, performance horses sustain these speeds at maximal effort over a much longer distance. These factors subject bone to mechanical force and a number of maximal strain cycles that bone is not evolved to withstand. Because the equine skeleton is pushed to its limit in the athletic performance horse, stress fractures become a clinical problem, but one which, with care and early diagnostic intervention, can be minimized.

Equine bone can break in a variety of ways. A single supra-physiologic load can shatter a previously normal bone, for example, the explosive, multiple, comminuted fracture of the first phalanx. However, evidence from necropsy and imaging surveys indicates that many fractures occur through areas of previously diseased bone. Stress fractures occur after days or weeks of bone weakening at sites of accumulated microdamage. The response to this microdamage is invasion by osteoclasts to clear up debris, and osteoblasts to remodel the bone and lay down new haversian systems. This process, if coupled with continuing super-physiologic loading, leads to eventual collapse of the cortex, because the bone never "catches up."

Understanding the pathogenesis of a stress fracture is important in interpretation of radiographs. The clinician does not encounter signs of acute injury but rather those of a chronic healing fracture, that is, one with sclerosis; periosteal new bone formation; endosteal callus formation; and ragged, ill-defined radiolucent fracture lines. Careful examination of radiographs is necessary to see the subtle periosteal new bone, which is often the only feature of these fractures, and therefore knowledge of the common sites for these fractures can aid in this respect. Because stress fractures occur in areas of repeated microdamage, they have predilection sites that are governed by the mechanical forces operating throughout the long bones during locomotion. These forces are predetermined by the design of the bone, the weight of the horse, and the manner in which the bone is cyclically loaded during rapid gaits.

Because of their etiology, stress fractures are common in young or naive horses. Bone is an exquisitely adapting, constantly changing biologic material, which not only changes in direct response to loading but also changes in the reverse direction during periods of rest. During training of young horses, bone receives repeated and increased loading that leads to modeling and remodeling. Stress fractures therefore commonly occur in young horses being submitted to training for the first time, but they also occur in older horses being submitted to retraining following a prolonged lay-off through ill health or injury. Similarly they can occur in any age class of horse that is stepping up in workload, primarily that involving increasing speed.

STRESS FRACTURES OF THE HUMERUS

Diagnosis

The gait abnormality observed in horses with stress fractures of the humerus is very characteristic. An extremely shortened protraction of the affected limb occurs, coupled with dragging of the toe that often catches the bedding when the horse walks around the box. The head nod is very obvious when the horse bears weight on the affected limb. Severe cases of proximal humeral head stress fracture may even mimic radial paralysis for the first few days. Lameness is usually mild to moderate over several days but becomes increasingly severe with continued daily exercise. A few days of rest often render the horse completely sound, only for the lameness to recur as soon as exercise recommences. Pain can be elicited in many cases by forced protraction of the limb, although manipulation of the humerus itself often produces no signs of pain. During the weightbearing phase of the stride, lameness is pronounced (grade 1 to grade 3 out of 5) and there is an obvious head nod.

Radiographic examination normally confirms the diagnosis by the presence of periosteal new bone formation and callus on the caudal humeral head (Fig. 1A). A second predilection site is the craniodistal aspect of the humerus. Both of these sites are best visualized on a mediolateral projection. Sclerosis of the cortical bone is often also present in these sites, but this may be difficult to appreciate unless extremely good radiographic facilities are available. It is extremely rare to see fracture lines within the area of diseased bone.

Scintigraphic examination reveals an obvious focally increased uptake of isotope, either in the proximocaudal or craniodistal aspect of the humerus, or both (Fig. 1B). Probe point–counting techniques often reveal a focally increased uptake starting at the shoulder and increasing through the humerus, or increases centered around the elbow (Fig. 2). Gamma camera scans show focal isotope accumulation in the caudal humeral head. A normal physeal area is seen in the proximal humerus, and this should not be confused with a stress fracture. This physeal plate curves from caudoproximal to craniodistal on the lateral view obtained with a gamma camera and is clearly differentiated from the common stress fracture site in the caudal humeral head.

Treatment

Treatment options are limited because any attempt at general anaesthesia and surgical repair is accompanied by an extremely high risk of complete fracture as the horse tries to stand during recovery. The fracture is therefore almost invariably treated by rest alone. The required period of rest varies from horse to horse but should be guided by radiographic and, if possible, scintigraphic findings. A minimum of 6 weeks of stall rest is usually advised followed by radiographic examination to monitor the remodeling of the periosteal callus. When the callus is smooth and appears to be inactive, walking exercise can be instituted for a further 6 weeks. Lameness often recurs if racing begins in less than 3 months and necessitates starting the treatment clock again. In our experience, humeral stress fractures take a long time to heal, and attempts to hurry them along are seldom justified.

Prognosis

If sufficient time is allowed for complete bone healing to occur, the prognosis in young horses is excellent and recurrence is extremely rare. If the horse is returned to training prematurely, further lameness or complete fracture of the humerus often occurs.

STRESS FRACTURES OF THE RADIUS

Diagnosis

Diagnosis of radial stress fractures is difficult. The horse has a nonspecific weightbearing lameness which, as with most stress fractures, resolves after only a few days of rest. The lameness is not altered by nerve blocks to the distal forelimb, but a median and ulnar block usually renders these horses sound. Radiographic findings often are limited to endosteal new bone formation, most commonly in the midradial diaphysis, particularly on the caudal cortex. Good-quality films are necessary to visualize this endosteal new bone, the appearance of which alters significantly with time. In any horse suspected of a radial stress fracture, follow-up radiographs are probably justified 2 weeks after the initial onset of lameness when radiographic signs are at their peak.

Scintigraphically, focal accumulations of isotope are seen in the same site as the radiographic lesion and can be detected with the probe or gamma camera. However, these fractures are often bilateral so that there may not be an obvious difference between limbs in the results of scintigraphy evaluation.

Treatment

Rest alone has been used to treat this condition. Confinement to the stall for 1 month is usually mandatory and

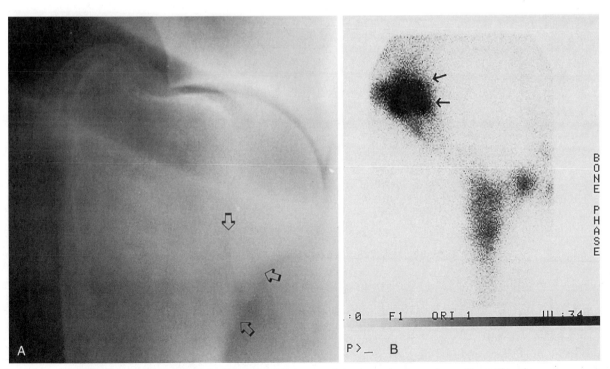

Figure 1. (*A*) A mediolateral radiograph of the proximal humerus showing a lucent line within the proximocaudal aspect of this bone, surrounded by an obvious periosteal callus. These are typical radiographic findings of a proximal humeral stress fracture. (*B*) A lateral scintigram of the right proximal humerus showing an obvious increase in technetium uptake centered on the caudal aspect of the proximal humerus. Note that the presence of the proximal physes in this region typically gives rise to a moderate increase in uptake, although this normal uptake will not be as intense, or situated caudal to the humeral head.

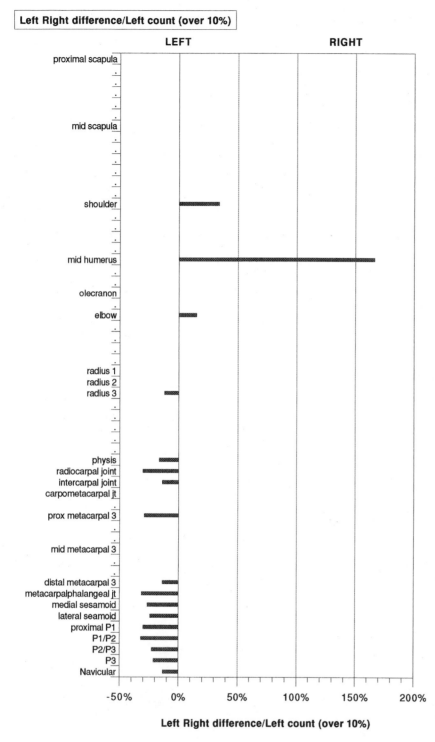

Figure 2. A difference plot, obtained by the probe point–counting technique of bone scanning, showing the difference in technetium uptake between matched anatomic points of both the left and right legs. This example also demonstrates a proximal humeral stress fracture, with a 150% increase in uptake at the mid-humeral sampling point. (See Pilsworth RC, Holmes MA: Proc 37th Annu Conf Am Assoc Equine Pract, 1991, pp 327–350, for a description of the technique.)

is followed by further radiographic assessment. Smoothly remodeled callus and resorbed endosteal callus are indications for resumption of light exercise. Bone healing seems to be unaffected by walking and trotting exercise, after the initial period of stall rest, and these activities save time in bringing horses back to full use.

Prognosis

The prognosis for future athletic function is excellent following bone healing, and recurrence is rare.

STRESS FRACTURES OF THE TIBIA

Diagnosis

Stress fractures to the tibia are one of the commonest causes of acute onset hindlimb lameness in the young racing Thoroughbred and can be one of the most difficult to diagnose. They are not affected by regional or intra-articular nerve blocks.

Horses are often affected by a relatively severe hindlimb lameness, which is observed soon after a bout of exercise. The horse may be non-weightbearing an hour or two following exercise only to walk normally the next day and be sound at the trot after a further 2 or 3 days. Lameness recurs immediately when the horse returns to a canter. The lameness is usually of a weightbearing type, accompanied by dragging of the toe and a reduced arc of foot flight during protraction at the trot, but these signs are seen in hindlimb lamenesses of many etiologies. Lameness is normally grade 2/5 to 4/5 in intensity on the day of first occurrence, but rapidly resolves with rest in cases of simple cortical stress fracture. Cases of incomplete linear or spiral fracture often initially exhibit more severe lameness that is present for several days with little improvement.

Strain-gauge studies have shown that the tibia is subjected to torsional forces during weightbearing. It is almost certainly these forces that produce the microdamage necessary for stress fracture to occur. Replication of these forces by use of the tibial torsion test is therefore often the best way to elicit a pain response in horses affected with these lesions. To test the left hind leg, the clinician faces the rear of the horse and picks up the leg. The leg is held in flexion using the left hand cupped loosely around the inside of the distal metacarpus, holding the proximal sesamoids. The clinician's shoulder is placed firmly against the horse's stifle. The point of the hock is grasped in the right hand, and in one movement the point of the hock is moved laterally; pressure is applied to the stifle using the shoulder as the fetlock and distal metacarpus are moved medially. Not all horses show a positive response to this test, but in horses that do, a good control is to try the same torsion test on the contralateral limb. In most cases there is much less pain in response to the test. Firm digital palpation of the caudal aspect of the tibia, approached medially, is also a useful test to elicit pain, particularly in cases in which the fracture is situated in the distocaudal cortex.

Radiographic signs tend to occur in certain predilection sites. In 2- and 3-year-old horses racing on the flat, the commonest predilection site is the proximolateral aspect of the tibia approximately 8 cm from the stifle joint surface (Fig. 3). In this site periosteal new bone formation and indistinct lucent lines are often visualized on both lateromedial and caudocranial projections. The second most common site is the distocaudal aspect of the tibia approximately 10 cm above the distal tibial physis. In this site an irregular semilunar callus is often visualized on the lateromedial projection, but a sufficiently penetrated caudocranial projection of the same site often shows the presence of incomplete fracture lines. These appear to be surrounded by a hazy zone of sclerosis. The third most common location often seen in older horses, or in young horses returning to training after a lay-off, is the midshaft endosteum (Fig. 4). In these horses the periosteal new bone formation is minimal, but large areas of "swirling" endosteal new bone are visualized in the medial and lateral cortices. On the lateromedial radiographic projection, these areas of endosteal callus can summate to give dense, white, chalk-like opacities. These have been described as bone infarcts, but this diagnosis has not been confirmed histopathologically. Less common predilection sites are on the

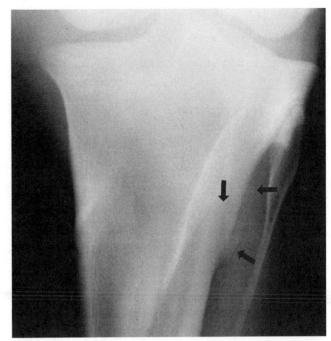

Figure 3. A caudocranial projection of the proximal tibia. There is periosteal callus on the proximolateral cortex, and a short lucent line extending proximally from the site of the callus into the cortex. These features are typical of a proximal tibial stress fracture.

proximomedial and proximocranial cortex immediately below the tibial crest.

Some horses show a combination of radiographic signs in various sites. Similar periosteal new bone formation can often be visualized in radiographs of the contralateral limb, but this does not mean that these changes are normal. Radiographic signs and the presence of pain are not the same thing. It is expected that a stress fracture that has occurred because of accumulated microdamage, during loading-adaptation mismatch, might be present in both legs. However, pain is usually not present until either the cortex begins to collapse or subperiosteal hemorrhage occurs. This may occur in one leg well in advance of the other. In rare cases, full cortical stress fracture occurs in both legs simultaneously. These horses present with a bilateral severe lameness, which is often thought by the trainer to be "muscular" in origin or the result of pelvic bone damage. In these cases, scintigraphic examination is extremely helpful.

Tibial stress fractures were among the first to be described using probe point–counting techniques, and this is still an extremely effective way to make the diagnosis. The tibia is the ideal bone for examination using the probe, because it is easily divisible into discrete sampling points and has a very distinctive anatomy with several bone prominences to ensure that sampling in both limbs is identical. The bone is near the skin surface on the medial aspect over its entire length. Probe point–counting data usually localizes the fracture to proximal, mid-, or distal tibia, but further information about which cortex is affected has to be obtained from subsequent radiographs.

Gamma camera imaging of the tibia easily confirms the diagnosis. The tibia in young horses has an active physis both proximally and distally. The proximal physis is one of

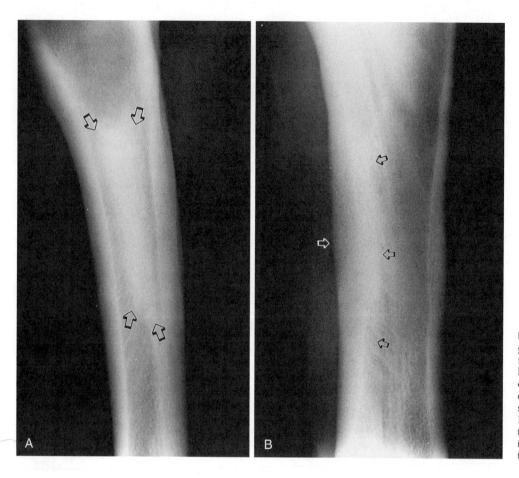

Figure 4. (*A*) A lateromedial radiograph of a midshaft tibial stress fracture, showing an abundant proliferation of endosteal callus. (*B*) A caudocranial radiograph of the same case confirming the callus to be associated with the endosteal surface. Note also the loss in definition to the periosteal surface (*white arrow*), indicative of some periosteal reaction.

the slowest to close and is often still extremely active in 3- and 4-year-old horses. This should not be confused with a stress fracture, and images of both hindlimbs and a familiarity with the normal range encountered in horses unaffected by stress fractures is essential. It is not uncommon for the proximal physes to "close" asynchronously in the two hindlimbs, and this can also lead to confusion in interpretation.

Treatment

Because of the risks of anesthesia in cases of incomplete fracture, only conservative treatment has been used. Usually a period of stall rest is advised, to allow the damaged bone to heal, before starting a controlled exercise program involving walking and trotting. The length of stall rest varies from 1 month in horses that show only periosteal callus in the proximolateral aspect of the tibia, to 3 months for horses in which obvious short segments of fracture line are visible in the distal cortex. In cases of long linear incomplete fracture, the use of a head-tie to prevent recumbency for at least 3 weeks should be considered if the horse's temperament allows. If recumbency is prevented, regular auscultation of the lungs and monitoring of complete blood count and plasma fibrinogen levels and plasma viscosity are essential because there is a real risk of the development of pleuropneumonia. Older horses affected with midshaft endosteal stress fractures are often given between 2 and 3 months of rest. Healing is monitored by radiographing the tibia monthly during the rest period.

Even in cases in which complete healing has not occurred it is often satisfactory to allow these horses to return to walking and jogging exercise at the end of 4 to 8 weeks.

Lameness resulting from incomplete linear fractures in the distal tibia in older horses tends to recur no matter how long the horse is rested. It is therefore probably beneficial for these horses to undergo controlled loading exercise during the early stages of healing; 1 month stall rest is probably adequate to avoid the risk of complete fracture. Extremely long periods of confinement are contraindicated because not only does the tibial fracture become dormant but also the rest of the skeleton "detrains," so that when exercise is finally resumed the horse often sustains a catalogue of orthopedic mishaps such as sore shins, suspensory desmitis, and stress fractures in other sites.

Prognosis

In cases of uncomplicated stress fracture in the younger horse, in which the prominent radiologic sign is periosteal new bone formation, the prognosis is excellent and recurrence is rare. Midshaft endosteal stress fractures carry a slightly poorer prognosis and seem to require longer intervals to allow full bone healing. One problem seems to be that these cases are often left with a residual sclerotic appearance to the midtibia; presumably this affects the flexibility and biologic properties of this bone. Incomplete linear fractures of the tibia carry the poorest prognosis. In some of these, the fracture becomes complete and displaced during box rest, even if the horse is prevented from lying down by a head-tie. Prolonged periods of being tied up can lead to complications such as pleuropneumonia. If the fracture does not become complete and displaced during the initial convalescent period, the horse should be gradually brought back into walking and trotting exercise after 2 to 3 months, depending on radiologic signs.

We have observed several cases in our clinic in which recurrence of incomplete fracture has occurred up to three times following periods of ever-increasing withdrawal from training, stall rest, and an exercise program of slowly increasing intensity. This seems to be particularly true in the older horse, and these cases present a real risk of complete displaced fracture. For these reasons, in cases of recurrence of linear incomplete fracture, retirement should be considered after full healing is achieved on the second occasion.

STRESS FRACTURES OF THE THIRD METACARPUS

Stress fractures of the third metacarpus (MCIII) involve the dorsal cortex of young racing Thoroughbreds. They have also been described on the proximopalmar aspect of this bone close to the origin of the suspensory ligament. The complex of bone damage, lameness, and fracture to the palmar aspect of the condyles has been described as a stress fracture, as have fractures to the dorsomedial aspect of proximal MCIII. The latter affects pacing Standardbreds and has a similar presentation as a stress fracture of the third metatarsus, which is covered in a later section.

Dorsal Cortical Stress Fractures

The dorsal cortical stress fracture most commonly occurs in young racehorses and has a typical presentation. It is distinct from the bucked shin complex, although it may represent an end stage of this condition.

Diagnosis

Obvious unilateral lameness is generally seen, although bilateral stress fracture can occur. A firm and painful palpable swelling over the dorsal or dorsolateral aspect of the MCIII is usually detectable. Radiography is required to confirm the diagnosis and rule out other possible causes. The fractures involve the midportion of the dorsal or dorsolateral cortex of the bone. They curve in a proximopalmar direction from the periosteal surface, seldom reaching the endosteal surface, although endosteal callus is often noticed. They may re-exit through the periosteal surface more proximally, producing the classic saucer-type fracture. These fractures are most easily seen on a lateromedial or dorsomedial-palmarolateral oblique view. Some are extremely difficult to visualize radiographically, and the only obvious radiographic indicators are intracortical lucencies associated with both endosteal and periosteal callus. Scintigraphy can be helpful in assessing whether the callus is currently active.

Treatment

Although surgical procedures are advocated to reduce the period of time off, or as treatment for a nonunion fracture, the majority of stress fractures heal with stall rest alone. During the initial stages, hydrotherapy and systemic anti-inflammatory drugs (phenylbutazone 1–2 g p.o. b.i.d.) reduce pain. A minimum of 8 weeks of stall rest should be followed by radiographic re-examination. If adequate bone healing is evident and the horse is sound, hand-walking exercise should be started followed by a gradual and graded return to full exercise.

If there is little radiographic evidence of healing, further rest or surgery can be considered. In some instances, a period of carefully controlled exercise may stimulate healing. Surgical options include interfragmentary drilling or lag screw fixation. The prognosis for this condition is generally good.

Proximal Palmar Stress Fractures of the Third Metacarpus

These fractures tend to occur in a broad age group of horses, with older horses commonly affected. It is postulated that cyclic compressive forces, immediately after foot contact with the ground, result in cortical disruption and possible intracortical microfractures. If damage exceeds osteogenic repair, a stress fracture results.

Diagnosis

Horses usually present with a unilateral lameness, no worse than grade 1/5 to 2/5, that often follows a chronic history of low-grade lameness. A low foot flight and shortened cranial phase to the stride may be exhibited. The lameness is often abolished by blocking the lateral palmar nerve just deep to the accessoriometacarpal ligament. In some cases the ulnar nerve may have to be blocked to improve the lameness. This discrepancy in blocking response is thought to be due to different afferent innervation of the periosteal and endosteal surfaces in this region. Innervation of the endosteal surface originates from a dorsal branch of the ulnar nerve. Obviously this response to nerve block is not specific because a number of other structures are desensitized.

Because of the nonspecific nerve block effect, a thorough high-quality radiographic evaluation is essential, preferably in association with scintigraphy and ultrasonography. On a dorsopalmar radiograph these fractures appear as multiple or single faint lucent lines surrounded by an area of sclerotic bone. The normal trabecular pattern may be lost in the proximopalmar aspect of this bone because of the encroaching sclerosis from the palmar cortex. On the lateromedial radiograph, a "halo" of endosteal callus may be seen in the same area. Scintigraphy reveals an intense increase in tracer uptake in the proximopalmar aspect of MCIII.

Ultrasonography should be performed to make an assessment of the proximal suspensory ligament and to gain an appreciation of the contour of the surface of the palmar cortex, which is often roughened and irregular.

Treatment

A period of 8 weeks' strict stall rest should be followed by a controlled period of exercise of increasing intensity. This regimen generally results in resolution of lameness and radiographic lesions. One horse reported to be nonresponsive to conservative management was successfully treated by surgical forage of the proximopalmar cortex. The prognosis for full return to normal function is good.

Palmar Condylar Stress Fractures of the Third Metacarpal Bone

The term "palmar condylar stress fracture" has been adopted to describe the condition that often precedes a complete condylar fracture. These fractures, which typically affect young racing Thoroughbreds, result from an osteosclerotic reaction, with secondary sites of microfractures in the palmar aspect of either the medial or lateral condyle, abaxially to the sagittal ridge.

Diagnosis

Horses present with unilateral lameness ranging from 1/5 to 4/5 in severity. Joint distension is absent or slight. The lameness may improve dramatically in a 24- to 48-hour period; therefore, the history may be one of an intermittent lameness of increasing severity. Flexion of the fetlock joint invariably accentuates the lameness. Anesthesia of the medial and lateral palmar and palmar metacarpal nerves at the level of the distal cannon bone renders the horse sound; however, intra-articular anesthesia of the fetlock joint gives variable results.

Scintigraphically these fractures result in a moderate to marked increase in tracer uptake, which is centered on the palmar aspect of the distal MCIII. This fracture can only be demonstrated radiographically using a special projection to give a skyline view of the palmar aspect of this bone. The toe is placed on a block with the fetlock joint flexed and the cannon bone perpendicular to the ground. The x-ray beam is directed upward toward the palmar condyle, with the cassette angled to be perpendicular to the x-ray beam. This positioning should remove the sesamoid bones from the joint space on the radiograph, hence minimizing the possibility of artifactual lesions. The fracture appears as a sagittal lytic line, of variable length, traversing an area of sclerotic bone, abaxial to the sagittal ridge.

Treatment

Treatment consists of stall rest for a minimum of 8 weeks, followed by a radiographic re-evaluation. If satisfactory resolution is apparent, or only a small defect persists, exercise may be reintroduced gradually.

Prognosis

Because these short incomplete stress fractures are probably a precursor to a complete condylar fracture, an early diagnosis is advantageous. In horses that do not develop a complete fracture, this injury carries a good prognosis, and the horse should be capable of regaining a level of performance equal to that before the fracture.

STRESS FRACTURES OF THE THIRD METATARSUS

The third metatarsus (MTIII) can also suffer stress fractures to the dorsal cortex that are similar to but less common than those of MCIII. Pathologic changes similar to those of the palmar aspect of the distal metacarpus occur in the plantar aspect of the distal metatarsus. The clinical signs, diagnosis, and treatment of dorsal cortical stress fractures and plantar condyle stress fractures are as for those of MCIII. A stress fracture of the proximodorsal aspect of this bone has been described in young Thoroughbred racehorses. The following section refers to this proximodorsal stress fracture.

Diagnosis

Lameness is acute in onset, grade 2/5 to 3/5, and usually unilateral. Pressure applied to the proximal dorsal cannon may elicit an obvious pain response. Lameness is abolished by tibial and fibular nerve blocks. Some improvement occurs after intra-articular anesthesia of the tarsometatarsal joint. Scintigraphy reveals an obvious increase, up to 600%, in technetium methylene diphosphate (MDP) uptake in the dorsal aspect of the proximal MTIII. Radiographically these lesions are best visualized with projections either just dorsal or plantar to a true lateromedial approach. Often multiple radiographic views are required to demonstrate the fracture line running through the diseased bone. Other characteristic radiographic abnormalities include osteophyte formation on the proximodorsal MTIII, sclerosis, and thickening of the proximodorsal cortex with periosteal reaction. It is common to observe similar but less marked radiographic changes in the contralateral limb.

Treatment

Successful treatment of these fractures has been reported with 2 months of stall rest, followed by a gradual reintroduction to full exercise. Intra-articular medication with sodium hyaluronate should be considered if follow-up radiography indicates active lesions within the tarsometatarsal joint. The prognosis is generally good; however, because of the joint involvement, residual tarsometatarsal joint disease may be associated with a chronic low-grade lameness.

STRESS FRACTURES OF THE ILIUM

Stress fractures of the ilium are a relatively common cause of hindlimb lameness in the young Thoroughbred racehorse. They develop gradually so that acute lameness generally follows a period of poor hindlimb action. The tuber sacrale on the affected side is lower than on the unaffected side and is very painful when palpated. The horse usually has a plaiting action of the hindlimbs in which each foot is placed cranial or craniomedial to the contralateral foot during trotting. The lameness varies from bad movement to grade 4/5 level. Both sides may be affected, resulting in a bilateral lameness.

The predilection site is approximately 10 cm from midline, across the ilial wing, in a sagittal direction. This area of the ilial wing is directly dorsal to the sacroiliac joint, which is therefore often involved. Damage is almost invariably more severe toward the caudal margin of the ilial wing. A degree of overriding of the fracture margins may be present, which results in the asymmetry of the tuber sacrale.

Diagnosis

The diagnosis is based on the typical clinical presentation, which is confirmed by either ultrasonography or scin-

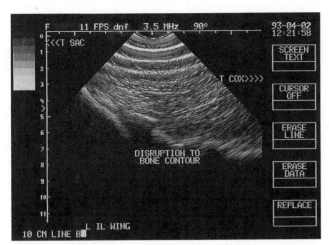

Figure 5. A transverse ultrasonogram of the midsection of the ilial wing approximately 10 cm from the midline. Note the irregularity and roughening to the dorsal surface of this bone created by periosteal new bone formation.

tigraphy. To assess this area ultrasonographically, a 2.5- or 3.5-MHz transducer is required. The skin should be prepared as with other ultrasound examinations, although in thin-coated horses clipping is often not necessary. The tuber coxae and tuber sacrale are easily identified as bony prominences close to the skin surface. The normally smooth and continuous surface of the ilial wing can be assessed running between these two landmarks. A fracture of the ilial wing forms an obvious discontinuity and roughening of the bone surface (Fig. 5). The width of the bone echo is often greater than that of normal bone, indicating active new bone formation.

Treatment

Treatment is stall rest for 10 to 16 weeks. The time required can best be judged by serial ultrasonography. Exercise can resume when the bone surface has a smooth and continuous contour. This result is generally achieved by 12 weeks, but healing depends on the initial degree of damage and the age of the horse.

Prognosis

In a series of 20 horses with ilial stress fractures, 11 successfully returned to racing. The remainder did not race for reasons other than nonhealing of the fracture. Ilial stress fractures have a relatively good prognosis when horses are given an early diagnosis and correct treatment; however, involvement of the sacroiliac joint may adversely affect the horse's action for a prolonged period of time.

PREVENTION OF STRESS FRACTURES

Measures to avoid stress fractures apply equally to all of the fractures described earlier. Bone must be conditioned by a progressive increase in loading, over a period of time that allows adaptation in form and function to these increased demands. Definite differences are apparent between horses in their ability to cope with this process,

either because of an inherent weakness in the bone of some horses or, more likely, the presence of a slower adaptive response. It is therefore very difficult to give dogmatic instructions on how stress fractures can be avoided in all horses. However, bone suffering from the stress fracture syndrome is almost always making a plea for a slower progression of training speeds, or even a long delay before reinitiating training of the 2-year-old. These messsages should be taken seriously if catastrophic fractures are to be avoided.

A horse that has been removed from training for a period of more than 2 months because of illness or injury should be regarded as an unbroken yearling in terms of bone strength. These horses require a prolonged adaptive period once retraining begins, regardless of the chronologic age of the horse. It is relatively common to observe sore shins, and even stress fractures of the tibia, in mature jumpers brought back into work after a summer at pasture.

Bone should always be given time to adapt to each gait before progressing to the next speed or gait. Although strict rules cannot be defined, experience with fractures indicates that bone takes approximately 1 month to react to a significant degree. For this reason, our potential athletes should receive at least 1 month's training in any one gait before progressing to the next speed. It may be of advantage to introduce the next intended speed in short, infrequent bursts of only a dozen or so strides during this 1-month adaptive period.

It is extremely important that signs of lameness in the young athletic horse be taken seriously and investigated fully, if progression of incomplete stress fractures to a complete, displaced fracture is to be avoided. The full range of diagnostic tools, including scintigraphy, is vital for accurate diagnosis. The high cost of these techniques has to be weighed against the potential loss subsequent to a catastrophic fracture. These factors need to be explained to, and understood by, owners and trainers. Continuing to train horses that exhibit gait deficits, training these horses while they receive nonsteroidal anti-inflammatory drugs, or injecting inflamed and painful joints with agents to suppress these signs in the face of continued training cannot be recommended if the progression from loading/adaptation mismatch to stress fractures is to be avoided.

Supplemental Readings

Blevins WE, Widner WR: Radiology in racetrack practice. Vet Clin North Am Equine Pract 6(1):31–61, 1990.

Ferraro GL: Lameness diagnosis and treatment in the Thoroughbred racehorse. Vet Clin North Am Equine Pract 6(1):63–84, 1990.

Goodman NL, Baker BK: Lameness diagnosis and treatment in the Quarter Horse racehorse. Vet Clin North Am Equine Pract 6(1):85–108, 1990.

Mackey VS, Trout DR, Meagher DM, Hornof WJ: Stress fractures of the humerus radius and tibia in horses. Vet Radiol Ultrasound 28:26–31, 1987.

O'Callaghan MW: The integration of radiography and alternative imaging methods in the diagnosis of equine orthopedic disease. Vet Clin North Am Equine Pract 7(2):339–364, 1991.

O'Callaghan MW: Future diagnostic methods: A brief look at new technologies and their potential application to equine diagnosis. Vet Clin North Am Equine Pract 7(2):467–479, 1991.

Palmer SE: Lameness diagnosis and treatment in the Standardbred racehorse. Vet Clin North Am Equine Pract 6(1):109–128, 1990.

Pilsworth RC, Holmes MA: A low-cost, computer-based scintigraphy system for use in lameness investigation in general practice. Proc 37th Annu Conf Am Assoc Equine Pract, 1991, pp 327–350.

Pool RR, Meagher DM: Pathologic findings and pathogenesis of racetrack injuries. Vet Clin North Am Equine Pract 6(1):1–30, 1990.

Riggs CM, Evans GP: The microstructural basis of the mechanical properties of equine bone. Equine Vet Ed 2:197–205, 1990.

Steckel RR: The role of scintigraphy in the lameness evaluation. Vet Clin North Am Equine Pract 7(2):207–239, 1991.

Stover SM, Johnson BJ, Daft BM, Read DH, Anderson M, Barr BC, Kinde H, Moore J, Stoltz J, Ardans AA, Pool RR: An association between complete and incomplete stress fractures of the humerus in racehorses. Equine Vet J 24:260–263, 1992.

Biochemical Bone Markers

PAT HARRIS
Waltham-on-the-Wolds, England

J. A. GRAY
Newmarket, England

Bone is constantly being modeled and remodeled, and its structure, quality, and strength represent a balance between formation and resorption. Disturbances to the mechanisms that maintain the optimal balance, particularly if long-term or repetitive, affect bone quality and structure.

One aim of noninvasive monitoring of bone metabolism is to detect animals at risk of developing bone problems before clinical signs are apparent. Early detection may allow prevention of the problem or decrease its severity. The ultimate aims are to minimize pain and suffering associated with skeletal problems and reduce the resultant wastage of horses.

Interest has recently focused on the use of biochemical bone markers that can be monitored repeatedly in blood and urine samples. It is too early to judge which bone markers will prove clinically useful, or under what circumstances they will do so, but current studies are providing useful data on bone metabolism in the horse and the changes that occur with age and training. A number of these biochemical bone markers are described.

HYDROXYPROLINE

Bone resorption can be indirectly evaluated by measuring urinary hydroxyproline excretion. Urinary hydroxyproline is, however, a relatively insensitive marker. It is also nonspecific because hydroxyproline is present in all connective tissue collagen as well as in some other proteins, and therefore it does not provide information on the rate of collagen breakdown in specific tissues such as skin, cartilage, or bone. In addition, hydroxyproline can be derived from sources other than the degradation of mature collagen. Hydroxyproline is also present in the cell walls of plants, which may be a complication with respect to the herbivorous horse.

HYDROXYLYSINE GLYCOSIDES

These compounds have some advantages over hydroxyproline. They are, for example, unaffected by dietary intake. In humans, the urinary ratio of the two isomers, galactosyl-hydroxylysine (HG or GHYL) and glucosyl-galactosyl-hydroxylysine (HGG or GGHYL), may indicate in which tissue extensive collagen breakdown is occurring. However, in some species other than humans, enzymes within the kidney convert HGG to HG and thereby affect the urinary ratios, and it is unknown whether this occurs in the horse. In addition, these markers give no indication of the stage of collagen metabolism from which they are derived (i.e., mature or newly synthesized collagen degradation).

PROCOLLAGEN PROPEPTIDES

Collagen is synthesized intracellularly as a precursor molecule or procollagen that contains both amino- and carboxydisulfide bonds. It appears that cleavage of these extension proteins is needed to ensure correct fibril and fiber formation. Carboxy terminal propeptide of type I procollagen (PICP) is the trimeric globular protein that is cleaved off as the carboxyl terminal from the type I procollagen molecule before the collagen molecules form collagen fibers. The amount of PICP released is believed to be directly related to the number of collagen fibers formed. Because most type I collagen is found in bone, serum PICP concentration is affected by the metabolic rate of bone and tends to reflect the rate of bone formation during skeletal growth and in metabolic bone disease. Although type I collagen is found in tissues other than bone, under most conditions increases in PICP tend to reflect changes in bone turnover, and blood PICP levels have been shown to correlate with histomorphometric and calcium-47 measurements of bone formation.

The amino terminal extension peptide of the type III procollagen (PIIINP) is similarly cleaved off during conversion of type III procollagen to type III collagen. High serum concentrations of PIIINP in other species have been suggested to reflect enhanced synthesis and deposition of fibrillar type III collagen or an alteration in the degradation and elimination of circulating PIIINP. Type III collagen is mainly found in fibrous tissues and as such is commonly used more as a connective tissue marker, but it can be found in small amounts in normal bone.

The amino acid sequencing for PICP and PIIINP differs little between species, which has resulted in kits designed for use in humans sometimes being applicable to other species. In one study, in dogs, although synovial fluid PIIINP levels were not found to be diagnostic for hip dysplasia, the concentrations were significantly higher in certain dogs with clinical and radiographic evidence of hip dysplasia than for a normal control group. In horses, one study showed that serum PIIINP levels did not increase following surgical incision, but could be used to monitor fibrosis associated with intestinal ischemia. PICP levels are affected by changes in the metabolic rate of bone, and studies have shown that PICP levels are affected by age in the horse, with younger animals having higher values than the older animals and values stabilizing after about 5 years of age. Within each age bracket, "normal" expected values may vary depending on the growth curves for the individual animals. Studies are currently ongoing to evaluate the relationship between age, growth curves, diet, certain clinical abnormalities, and PICP/PIIINP levels (Table 1). Initial results have suggested that increased levels of PIIINP may be found in horses before the clinical development of certain skeletal disorders, although much more work is needed to confirm this.

PYRIDINIUM CROSSLINKS OF COLLAGEN

Within the formed collagen fibers, collagen molecules slowly undergo chemical modification. Intermolecular crosslinks are formed, which start as bivalent structures but with time mature to become multivalent. Crosslinks help to provide the tensile strength that is integral to the function of collagen. In the type I collagen of bone, some of the mature crosslinks are formed from two original hydroxylysine residues and one lysine residue; such crosslinks are known as deoxypyridinoline or Dpd. Mature crosslinks are also formed from three hydroxylysine residues, referred to as pyridinoline or Pyd. Similar structures also occur within the other collagen types. These crosslinks, therefore, are not specific for a particular type of collagen. Pyridinoline (a 3-hydroxy pyridinium derivative) is, however, absent in skin collagen but is a major crosslink within

TABLE 2. COMPARISON OF OSTEOCALCIN, PYRIDINOLINE, AND DEOXYPYRIDINOLINE*

Animal Number	Problem (and Date Diagnosed)	Month of Sample	TPyd nmol/L Urine	TDpd nmol/L Urine	OC ng/m Serum
1	Stress fracture (Jan)	March	943	235	38
		April	940	169	35
2	Chip fracture plus bony exostosis (Nov)	March	1156	260	97
		April	1524	309	105
		May	2136	292	115
3	Wobbler (Apr)	March	1660	281	364
		April	1602	230	364
4	Control	April	955	113	58
5	Control	April	921	149	34
6	Control	April	462	84	62

*In six 2-year-old Thoroughbreds in the same training yard, under the same management regimen, three of which did not show any clinically apparent skeletal problems throughout the year and three of which showed clinically apparent skeletal problems associated with radiologic abnormalities.

OC = osteocalcin; TPyd = total pyridinoline; TDpd = total deoxypyridinoline.

cartilage collagen (type II) and to a lesser extent within bone collagen (type I). Deoxypyridinoline appears to be present in appreciable amounts only in bone collagen, although it is found, at least in humans, in certain ligaments, in the aorta, and in dentine. These crosslinks are present only in extracellular collagen fibers and are not present in immature or newly synthesized collagen. They are only released, therefore, with mature collagen degradation. Urinary levels of these pyridinium crosslinks of collagen have been used in other species as markers of mature collagen degradation and joint deterioration, bone turnover, and bone resorption.

These pyridinium crosslinks of collagen are not found in the diet of a horse, and they are more specific than hydroxylysine, in that neither is found in skin or basement membrane collagen. Although the highest concentration of pyridinoline is found in cartilage, the actual amounts of pyridinoline in human bone are around four times higher than deoxypyridinoline concentrations, and only in rheumatoid arthritis has there been any evidence for urinary pyridinoline originating from nonbony sources in humans. In the horse, the ratio between Dpd and Pyd in bone has been shown by the authors to be lower than the human 4:1 ratio and seems to vary with the skeletal site and between cortical and trabecular bone. The clinical relevance of these differences needs to be determined.

A diurnal variation in the urinary excretion of these compounds in humans has been suggested, which may differ between men and women. Age has an effect in the horse, and there appears to be greater urinary crosslink excretion during the night. In another study in the horse, deoxypyridinoline levels were shown to reflect the increased bone resorption that accompanies acute inflammation of the superficial digital flexor tendon. Table 2 shows the Pyd and Dpd levels in a number of horses with a variety of clinical problems. However, much more work is needed before any confirmed association can be made between the levels of these markers and the subsequent development of such conditions.

At present, in other species, urinary concentrations of Dpd and Pyd are used clinically. However, although urine

TABLE 1. THE RELATIONSHIP BETWEEN FRACTURE INCIDENCE AND MEAN LEVELS OF PICP AND PIIINP IN HORSES FROM TWO THOROUGHBRED TRAINING YARDS*

Yard	Number	PICP	PIIINP	Fracture Incidence
A	13	916 +/− 302	15.8 +/− 3.3	60%
B	30	457 +/− 155	8.9 +/− 2	10%

*A number of randomly chosen horses were sampled throughout the racing season on a monthly basis. A similar percentage of the total number of horses within each yard was sampled. The sample groups were mainly 2- and 3-year-old horses of both sexes.

can be obtained relatively easily from the horse, blood samples are far more acceptable for regular monitoring; therefore, techniques for measuring these crosslinks in both blood and urine have been developed by the authors together with Dr. S. Robins of Rowett Institute.

TELOPEPTIDES

The degradation of type I collagen involves the cleavage of the carboxy terminal pyridinoline crosslinked telopeptide (ICTP). Some controversy has arisen over its potential use as a marker of bone resorption in humans owing to difficulties with assay sensitivity and a failure, with certain therapies, for levels to parallel the fall in other markers of bone resorption. In the horse, ICTP levels have been measured in one study using a human kit, and have been shown to decrease with age. Whether these will be a useful marker of bone resorption in the horse remains to be seen.

BONE-SPECIFIC ALKALINE PHOSPHATASE

Total alkaline phosphatase (AP) measurement lacks specificity, because the enzyme originates from multiple sources including liver, bone, kidney, and the gastrointestinal tract. Numerous iso-forms exist, differing according to their post-translational glycosylation. Bone alkaline phosphatase (BSAP) is an enzyme located on the cell surface of osteoblasts and is known to be associated with bone mineralization. A number of methods to quantify the various iso-forms have been reported including electrophoresis, radioimmunoassay, and heat inactivation.

In the horse, although a number of studies have measured total AP as a marker of bone metabolism, few have investigated the use of the bone-specific iso-enzyme. Total AP and BSAP decrease with age because of the rapid bone formation that accompanies skeletal development in the actively growing animal, decreasing with approaching maturity. The proportion of total AP that is BSAP also tends to decrease with age. BSAP, ICTP, and PICP have been shown to increase with exercise in 2-year-old Thoroughbreds.

OSTEOCALCIN

Osteocalcin (OC) is synthesized by osteoblasts and odontoblasts. Most of the OC produced is incorporated into the bone matrix and the rest is released into circulation. The amount incorporated appears to vary with age, being higher in the young. It is a noncollagenous calcium-binding protein, which forms about 1 to 2% of adult human bone. It is also referred to as *bone gamma-carboxyglutamic acid*, or *bone gla protein* or BGP. Its precise function is not very well understood, but levels appear to correlate with the activity of osteoblasts and thereby with bone formation. Levels in humans rise not only when bone formation levels are increased but also when predominantly bone-resorbing conditions occur, provided that the two processes of formation and resorption are coupled. Levels are decreased with glucocorticoid excess but increased with renal failure due

to impaired clearance and as a consequence of renal osteodystrophy.

Ovine and bovine osteocalcin differ from human osteocalcin by only a few amino acids, and therefore heterologous assays have been used for humans, although problems with the interpretation of the different results that can be obtained with different kits have not been fully resolved. Species-specific assays have, however, been recommended for rat, mouse, chick, and other species. Work by the authors has suggested that equine osteocalcin may differ from that of the bovine and ovine forms; therefore, equine-specific assays may be preferable. Sample handling and storage have been found by the authors to be important, as well. Treatment with certain glucocorticoids may result in a decrease in osteocalcin concentrations within 12 hours of administration.

A number of studies on osteocalcin in the horse have been carried out. These suggest that, as may have been expected, levels are affected by age, but there is no effect of gender. The presence, or absence, of a circadian rhythm may depend on whether the animal is kept under natural or artificial light. Under natural lighting, levels seems to remain fairly constant throughout the day, starting to decrease around 5 to 7 PM, reaching a low around 7 to 8 PM, and then increasing to a peak at 5 AM, followed by a decline to the daytime levels. In rats it has been suggested that collagen synthesis and new bone formation may be diurnally regulated. Ranges of 47 ± 10.1 ng/ml OC for horses younger than 12 months of age and 36 ± 14 ng/ml for older horses have been reported. One study investigated the changes in osteocalcin, parathyroid hormone, 25-hydroxy-vitamin D, calcium, and phosphorus concentrations when 10 unbroken Quarterhorses approximately 18 months old were put into training. Results showed significant activity in bone mineral metabolism during the early stages of training, with a continuing drop in osteocalcin levels as well as radiographic bone aluminum equivalence (RBAE) values for the dorsal, palmar, and medial metacarpal cortices to a low point, around 40 to 60 days after training started. The RBAE values then increased significantly over the next 2 months, as did the osteocalcin levels.

THE FUTURE

A panel of selected biochemical bone markers may be capable of indicating total body bone metabolism and may be of value in the monitoring of certain therapies. However, the effects of exercise, enforced rest, diet, pregnancy, growth spurts, and other such factors on the various bone markers must be explored in large numbers of horses, together with the effects of different bone pathologies. Larger numbers of animals are needed to determine the expected normal ranges for animals that do not go on to develop subsequent skeletal problems. In addition, the half lives of the various markers for the horse need to be determined. Studies are ongoing in a number of institutes in these areas.

In humans, a report concluded that biochemical markers are useful in studying the pathogenesis of osteoporosis, identifying those at risk of developing osteoporosis and related fractures, choosing the appropriate treatment, and monitoring the efficacy of treatment. The potential usefulness of these biochemical bone markers in the horse is therefore great, and readers are advised to keep watching for reports on this area, in particular on the use of osteocalcin, the procollagen propeptides, and the pyridinium crosslinks of collagen.

Supplemental Readings

Bettica P, Moro L: Biochemical markers of bone metabolism in the assessment of osteoporosis. J Int Fed Clin Chem 7(1):16–22, 1995.

Price JS, Jackson B, Eastell R, Goodship AE, Blumsohn A, Wright I, Stoneham S, Lanyon LE, Russell RG: Age related changes in biochemical markers of bone metabolism in horses. Equine Vet J 27(3):201–207, 1995.

Price JS, Jackson B, Eastell R, Wilson AM, Russell RGG, Lanyon LE, Goodship AE: The response of the skeleton to physical training: A biochemical study in horses. Bone 17(3):221–227, 1995.

Robins SP, Black D, Paterson CR, Reid DM, Duncan A, Seibel MJ: Evaluation of urinary hydroxypyridinium crosslinks measurements as resorption markers in metabolic bone disease. Eur J Clin Invest 21:310–315, 1991.

Equine Rhabdomyolysis Syndrome

PAT HARRIS
Waltham-on-the-Wolds, England

The term *equine rhabdomyolysis syndrome* (ERS) has been used to encompass a number of conditions including tying up, azoturia, set fast, Monday morning disease, exertional rhabdomyolysis, and others. The word *exertion* has deliberately been omitted from this general term because exertion per se is not always involved, although some form of exercise is usually the final triggering factor. In the future it may be more beneficial to subdivide this syndrome according to the pathophysiologic processes involved. At present this information is not available.

PATHOPHYSIOLOGY

ERS is a pathologic condition that primarily affects the type II muscle fibers. The condition tends to be recurrent in nature, with variable intervals between episodes, which in themselves may be of variable clinical severity, even within one individual. A theory as to the cause of this syndrome must be able to explain these characteristics. In addition, the theory must be able to explain why only one animal in a group, all on the same management, feeding, and exercise regimen, may be intermittently affected. Exercise is a common triggering factor, but the type and nature of the exercise that precedes an episode varies between individuals and within an individual. The author's current belief is that animals suffering from this condition have an underlying predisposing abnormality. A set of circumstances, or triggering factors, may then be required to initiate the perhaps common process that results in the clinical signs. The triggering factors and predisposing factors are likely to vary from one group of individuals to another. This means that the pathophysiologic processes involved are also likely to differ. In addition, the optimal treatment and preventative regimens that appear to work for one individual may not be ideal for another. It is unlikely that a single theory can explain all manifestations of this syndrome.

A number of predisposing and triggering factors have been proposed, including carbohydrate overload, local hypoxia, vitamin E and selenium deficiency, metabolic pathway abnormalities, hormonal disturbances including reproductive and thyroid hormone imbalances, a malignant hyperthermia-like condition, viral etiology, electrolyte imbalances, as well as temperament. It is a common opinion that appropriate nutrition and management procedures may help to prevent or decrease the incidence of ERS in some cases, which suggests that nutritional and management factors may be important.

EPIDEMIOLOGY

This syndrome appears to occur in most, if not all, breeds of horse, at any time of the year and at any age, although it seems to be more prevalent in 2- to 15-year-olds, perhaps because these tend to be the more active animals. It is more common in females, especially the young filly in training. A familial predisposition has been suggested but not conclusively proven. Traditionally this syndrome was seen in animals that had been exercised following a period of rest without a reduction in feed intake. This type of history is less commonly reported today, and many episodes seem to occur in animals being regularly exercised.

PROGNOSIS

In animals that never have suffered an episode of ERS previously, and in which the potential triggering factor (such as exercising after a period of rest on full feed) can be identified, further episodes may not occur, provided that appropriate management safeguards are instigated and the animal's return to work does not itself initiate another episode. An animal that has suffered a number of episodes is more likely, however, to suffer another at some point in the future. In the author's opinion, one of the more vulnerable periods for a potential sufferer is during the return to work, because many animals tend to suffer repeated episodes during this time.

CLINICAL SIGNS

In its mildest form, ERS may be difficult to distinguish from a number of other conditions, in particular overexertion and certain lamenesses, which can all produce similar signs of a very slight stiffness or a shortened stride. In the more classic cases, the animal may be very reluctant or unable to move (i.e., "set fast") and take obviously shortened strides when forced to walk. Affected animals can become totally unable to move and in extreme cases may become recumbent and unable to rise. Death from ERS is not common.

The condition tends to affect the hindlimbs, usually bilaterally; however, apparently unilateral cases have been seen. The forelimbs are occasionally involved. In mild cases no clinical signs other than stiffness may be apparent, but in more severe cases the affected muscles may be swollen and the animal may resent palpation. Affected animals tend to show signs of pain and distress, including flank watching, profuse sweating, and elevated pulse and respiratory rates. Abdominal disturbances can occur simultaneously, or following an episode of ERS, and need to be considered in the differential diagnosis.

The apparent clinical severity of an episode of the ERS cannot always be related to the intensity or duration of exercise. It may be preferable, therefore, to divide the condition according to the severity of the stiffness and the clinical signs, as shown in Table 1. This division is arbitrary but helpful when discussing likely treatments. Tempera-

ment is an important factor in determining the apparent severity of the clinical signs and can make it difficult to evaluate the severity of the underlying muscle damage.

Little information is available on the prevalence of cardiac muscle involvement in ERS. In one study, functional disturbances of the heart were said to be found clinically and confirmed by histopathologic lesions in a high proportion of the cases.

DIAGNOSIS

Unless a horse is clinically affected, there is no test or series of tests that can confirm that an individual has suffered from or will suffer again from ERS. Diagnosis of ERS is usually based on the history and clinical picture, often supported by laboratory investigations. The latter may also be useful to monitor the recovery from an episode, as well as the animal's return to work (see under Management).

The differential diagnosis varies according to the nature and severity of the clinical signs. It must be remembered that gastrointestinal complications may occur before, during, or after an episode. The main conditions to exclude include monensin poisoning, the exhausted horse syndrome, laminitis, aortoiliac femoral thrombosis, vitamin E- and selenium-responsive myopathies, as well as overexertion, muscle sprains, and the typically fatal atypical myoglobinuria syndrome.

The plasma enzymes most commonly used to evaluate the muscular system are aspartate aminotransferase (AST) and creatine kinase (CK). AST is not muscle-specific, because it is found in most soft tissues. However, marked elevations tend only to be associated with muscle damage. When AST elevations are accompanied by elevations of the more muscle-specific enzyme CK, the result tends to re-

TABLE 1. EQUINE RHABDOMYOLYSIS SYNDROME GRADED ACCORDING TO CLINICAL SEVERITY

Clinical Signs	Grade 1	Grade 2	Grade 3	Grade 4	Grade 5
Mobility	Slight stiffness, shortened stride	Reluctant to move	Unable to move	Unable to move, may become transiently recumbent	Rapidly becomes recumbent
Muscle	NAD	Often NAD	± Firm and swollen, resents palpation	Firm and swollen, may not resent palpation	Firm ± wasting
Excessive sweating	−	±	+	+ +	+ +
Pulse and respiratory rates elevated above expected levels	−	±	+ +	+ +	+ + +
Signs normally attributed to gastrointestinal disturbance	−	±	+	+ +	+ + +
Discolored urine	−	±	+	+ +	+ + +
Comments	Easily confused with other conditions			? Palpation is actually felt by the horse	Gut stasis can occur, shock may develop, death may occur

From Harris PA: In Practice, 11:1, 1989.
Key: NAD = No abnormality detected; − = absent; ± = sometimes present; + = usually present; + + = prominent; + + + = severe.

TABLE 2. EXAMPLES OF PLASMA CK AND AST ACTIVITIES (U/L)

	A	B	C	D	E	F
CK	60	300	10,000	5000	90	0–50
AST	350	230	2000	7000	1000	0–230

A. Typical pattern that may be seen in an animal several weeks after an equine rhabdomyolysis syndrome (ERS) episode, but such levels of AST could reflect previous injury to soft tissue other than muscle. The slight apparent increase in CK may not be clinically significant.
B. Results that could be found in a young racehorse, with no apparent clinical signs, a few hours after its first gallop. These data most likely reflect some overexertion rather than an episode of subclinical ERS.
C. An acute episode of the ERS if clinical signs appropriate.
D. Initial recovery from ERS.
E. Later stages of recovery from ERS. Provided the animal is moving freely and has been in a small paddock for a few days, it can be returned to work. In recurrent cases it may be advisable to wait until the AST levels are also within acceptable levels.
F. Reference values for laboratory used. Note that these values will differ between laboratories.

flect muscular involvement. After a single insult, AST activities peak after about 24 hours and have a half life of 7 to 8 days. In contrast, CK activities peak within 2 to 6 hours and have a half life of around 2 hours. These differences can be used to help evaluate the stage of muscular involvement, as shown in Table 2.

The use of an exercise test to determine susceptibility to exercise-induced muscular damage has been recommended, but the nature of such a test and its interpretation are controversial. In the healthy horse, a number of factors seem to influence the extent of an increase in CK and AST activities following exercise. These factors include the intensity and duration of exercise, its nature, plus the fitness, gender, age, and possibly diet of the horse. Young females seem to be more likely than males to have elevated AST and CK resting activities. Lunging an unfit animal may result in raised plasma muscle enzymes, regardless of a susceptibility or otherwise to muscular damage. In an ERS-prone animal, lunging may precipitate a further episode. The author therefore recommends the protocol discussed under Management. A guide to the interpretation of enzyme levels that may be found with such exercise

tests is given in Table 3. Some horses are able to race and win despite elevated plasma muscle enzyme activities, but whether they would be able to race in a "better class" if they did not have such elevations is unknown. Activities of CK and AST do not always correlate with the degree of muscular damage or the clinical severity of disease, which often reflects the temperament and pain threshold of the individual. AST and CK activities therefore must be interpreted with caution. It should also be appreciated that they reflect the end result (i.e., the muscular damage) and not the cause.

Recently, the use of bone-seeking radiopharmaceuticals was recommended as a means of detecting and localizing skeletal muscle damage following exercise, especially in the investigation of "poor performance" cases.

TREATMENT

The treatment of ERS depends on the apparent clinical severity, the animal's temperament, and the owner's experience. Mild cases may be managed without veterinary

TABLE 3. EXAMPLES OF PLASMA CK AND AST ACTIVITIES (U/L) BEFORE AND 2–6 HOURS AFTER AN EXERCISE TEST

	A	B	C	D	E
Pre-exercise CK	20	55	200	95	45
Post-exercise CK	25	300	600	1100	60
Pre-exercise AST	90	200	630	250	190
Post-exercise AST	195	230	800	1000	235
Clinical signs	None	None	None	None	Stiff

A. "Normal" exercise test results but a chronic intermittent ERS sufferer may have such values and suffer an episode the next day. *Advice:* If such values are found in an ERS sufferer, it would be acceptable to increase workload.
B. Normal resting CK and AST activities, suggesting that there has been no muscular injury sufficient to raise peripheral muscle enzyme activities in the recent past. Increase in CK after exercise. *Advice:* If horse suffered from recurrent ERS and had not been given excessive exercise, its workload should remain constant for a few more days and exercise test should be repeated.
C. Raised AST and CK resting activities suggesting muscular injury in recent past. The increase with exercise suggests continued muscular involvement. *Advice:* Decrease workload, ideally stop exercise, and turn out. Reassess dietary, management, and therapeutic regimens.
D. Raised AST/CK activities although no apparent clinical signs seen. These may have been missed or very subtle. May reflect more widespread, but slight, muscular involvement, insufficient to cause obvious clinical signs, but there is an increased risk in a recurrent ERS sufferer that the individual will suffer a further episode if exercise is continued. *Advice:* as per C.
E. No marked increase in CK and AST; increases seen cannot be considered diagnostically significant. *Advice:* Most likely it is not ERS that is causing the stiffness.

involvement, but in more severe cases, prompt veterinary treatment is required. Because the specific pathogenesis of this condition is unknown, treatment tends to be symptomatic. Forced walking may make the muscle damage worse and increase the condition's severity. Therefore, unless it is certain that mild overexertion is the cause of stiffness, or the stiffness is due to "muscle cramp" rather than ERS, the affected animal should be rested (see Management).

Treatment is divided into that involving the veterinarian directly and the various management changes that can be instigated by owner and veterinarian. Veterinary assistance is often needed to confirm the diagnosis, limit further muscular damage, reduce pain and anxiety, and restore fluid balance to maintain adequate kidney function. Myoglobin per se is not believed to be nephrotoxic unless combined with inadequate kidney perfusion. Fluids should be considered especially for grades 3, 4, and 5 disease (see Table 1). Diuretics should be avoided because they may potentiate alkalosis and exacerbate electrolyte abnormalities.

TREATMENT

Strict stable rest is advisable. If ERS occurs far from the animal's stable, and the horse must be transported home, then this should occur preferably in a truck or wagon rather than a trailer. It must not walk home. Once returned to the stable, the animal should be kept warm and away from drafts, with plenty of bedding. Initially there should be access to water and hay only, a wet bran mash being fed if required. If the affected animal does not urinate within a reasonable period, the bladder should be palpated rectally to determine if catheterization is needed. The passage of obviously discolored urine often indicates that fluids are required. The horse should be stabled until it moves freely, shows no signs of pain, does not resent muscle palpation, and has urine that is no longer discolored.

A compound manufactured coarse feed mix or cube should be introduced gradually into the diet. This feed should be produced by a reputable manufacturer and should have limited amounts of its energy content provided by soluble carbohydrate sources. The energy level of the particular mix or cube used should initially be one stage below that appropriate for the animal's exercise level, and the amount depends on the individual. Supplementary feeds such as oats, barley, and bran should be avoided. Reducing the intake of oats is of benefit in some cases.

Ideally, there should be a period of turn out into a small paddock or indoor arena before exercise recommences. Pastures with lush grass should be avoided, and animals should not be allowed to become chilled in the field. Very rarely, sedation may be required to prevent excessive activity following initial turn out. Animals that suffer a relatively mild episode may require only a few days of turn out. However, if the episode was quite severe, or if the animal had recurrent episodes, the AST and especially CK activities should be measured before starting exercise. Ideally, AST and CK activities should be within the resting range, but this may not be practical owing to time constraints. It is however advisable to wait until the CK activities are less than double the upper normal limit for the laboratory used. A minimum of 4 days on an appropriate

diet, with the horse 2 or 3 days loose in an indoor school or field, is recommended before exercise starts. Exercise should be introduced gradually; lunging should be avoided and only straight line work carried out initially. The initial work should allow plenty of warm-up time, and hills should be avoided. If the animal misbehaves on its own, or in company, it should be exercised with others or alone, as appropriate.

Laboratory Testing

On the third or fourth day after the animal's return to work, blood samples should be taken for measurements of AST and CK activities before and approximately 2 to 6 hours after exercise. This exercise should provide a fair workout with respect to the animal's current exercise regimen but should not be overly strenuous, and the animal should have undertaken work of similar intensity in the recent past. At the start of the return to work, this may be a short walk, with a brief trot. Activity of CK and AST determines whether there has been additional muscle damage since the previous resting sample was taken, and whether damage occurred during the exercise test. If these initial results are within acceptable limits, exercise can be continued. It must be appreciated that enzyme activities can be normal and the animal can still suffer an episode of ERS the following day.

It is useful to repeat the exercise test a week or so later. At this time, having been on the altered diet for over 2 weeks, a blood and urine sample can be collected to determine urinary fractional electrolyte excretion. Such testing may be of benefit 3 to 4 days after any increase in the activity level of the horse, as part of the ongoing monitoring process.

Preventive Measures

At present, there is no procedure or set of procedures that will eliminate further episodes of ERS in all individuals, but improved management and appropriate nutritional supplementation for animals at risk may reduce the likelihood or frequency of future episodes. Preventive measures can be managemental or therapeutic.

Management Procedures

Hay and grazing should be provided as usual, although lush pastures should be avoided. The diet should be as described under Dietary and Therapeutic Adjustments (later); that is, the diet should provide as low an energy intake as possible, while maintaining sufficient body condition and supporting the type of ride required. The horse may not need the amount of feed recommended by the manufacturer, or the compound feed given may be that designed for an animal working at a lower intensity. In such instances, an appropriate vitamin- and trace mineral-fortified general mix may be required. An additional macromineral mix should not be fed, unless laboratory investigations or nutritional advice suggest that they would be useful. However, if the animal is sweating or working hard, it may be beneficial to feed common table salt (up to 2 oz or 56 g per 500 kg). If this causes the horse to urinate excessively, the intake of salt should be decreased by half an ounce for a few days and the situation reassessed. The quantity and energy density of feed should not be increased in anticipation of an increase in the exercise level, but should occur after the increase in workload and only if essential.

Animals should be turned out into a field or arena as much as possible but should not be allowed to stand for long periods or to get cold. Exercise should be provided daily. If this is not possible, animals should at least be turned out on their days off. If the horse is given a day off, the amount of concentrate fed should be halved, from the evening before the rest day until the evening after the exercise. If a viral infection is active on the premises, animals at risk should have their feed decreased and workload reduced until several days after all signs of infection have passed.

Dietary and Therapeutic Adjustments

It is important to realize that although many regimens have been recommended for treatment and prevention of ERS, virtually none has received critical evaluation.

Sodium Bicarbonate

Controversy still exists over the role of lactic acid in ERS. Most animals' blood lactate levels during an episode reflect the type of exercise undertaken before the attack, as well as the horse's fitness, rather than being related per se to ERS. Most afffected horses have a metabolic alkalosis, but pH changes at the fiber level are unknown. Sodium bicarbonate doses of 2 to 4 oz (28–56 g) per day 3 to 6 hours before exercise have been recommended for the prevention of ERS, but their efficacy is unproven. Some investigators suggest that, depending on the animal's fluid status, high doses of sodium bicarbonate may have a negative effect on performance, whereas others have suggested that any beneficial effect may be due to the sodium rather than the bicarbonate content.

Vitamin E and Selenium

It is unlikely that most horses affected by ERS are deficient in vitamin E and selenium, especially if fed a prepared manufactured diet. Any beneficial effect for prevention or treatment, especially with vitamin E, may be due to a reduction in free radical-induced muscle damage. A potential risk of toxicity occurs when supplementing horses with selenium. Oral administration is usually recommended. In areas of the world where horses may be selenium-deficient, a vitamin E and selenium supplement may be advisable, especially during late winter and spring when serum vitamin E levels are at their lowest in northern latitudes. Supplemental vitamin E as α-tocopherol acetate (1.5–4.4 mg/kg of body weight per day) has been recommended. No evidence exists that vitamin E is toxic, but very high levels may interfere with utilization of other fat-soluble vitamins.

Dimethylglycine

Dimethylglycine (DMG) is reported to prevent lactic acid accumulation by increasing oxygen utilization. Although recent studies have shown no beneficial cardiorespiratory or metabolic effects, 1 to 2 mg/kg of body weight per day has been reported anecdotally to be beneficial in

prevention of ERS. The author has had little success with this substance.

Methysulfonylmethane (MSM)

MSM is said to be the oral natural alternative to steroidal and nonsteroidal anti-inflammatory agents. It may be more useful therapeutically than prophylactically. Daily doses of 5 to 15 g have been suggested after a higher loading dose, but the author has had little personal success with this substance.

Thiamine

Up to 500 mg of thiamine daily or around 28 g/day of Brewer's yeast has been suggested for prevention of ERS, but there is no evidence for its efficacy.

Acepromazine

Acepromazine (ACP), 0.005 to 0.02 mg/kg, given about 30 minutes before exercise, has been used for prevention of ERS, especially in some "nervous fillies." Some recent work reported that although ACP administration did not seem to alter circulating catecholamine levels, it did appear to lower the lactate concentrations recorded following exercise. The author has had little success with ACP.

Phenytoin

Phenytoin has been recommended for prevention of ERS by some workers. Care must be taken with respect to clearance time in racing animals and possible drug interactions, as well as the potential side effects such as tranquilization or seizures. Initial doses of 8 to 12 mg/kg b.i.d. have been suggested, unless side effects occur. Ideally, blood levels should then be checked and the dose adjusted to maintain blood levels at 5 to 10 μg/ml 4 to 6 hours after administration. Some animals seem to require a larger morning than evening dose, but others may just need once-a-day administration. A useful protocol is 8 to 12 mg/kg b.i.d. for 3 days, then 10 mg/kg s.i.d. for 1 week before training recommences.

Diazepam

Diazepam has been used at a dose of around 0.25 mg/kg intravenously. The author has no experience of its use.

Thyroxine

Thyroxine supplementation has been suggested to be of value. Limited investigations have suggested that some ERS sufferers may have a "decreased thyroid reserve." The use of plasma T_4 levels as an indicator of thyroid status has been disputed, and the optimal test on which to base the desirability of thyroid supplementation is unclear. However, supplementation with L-thyroxine (5–10 mg/500 kg) or iodinated casein (6–14 mg/kg) has been suggested. The potential negative feedback effects of suddenly ceasing high-level thyroxine supplementation have not been fully explored.

Dantrolene

The effective dose of dantrolene to prevent or treat ERS is currently unknown. In the horse, as compared to humans, bioavailability of dantrolene is low. Dantrolene is potentially hepatotoxic and the effects appear to be highly variable between individuals. It is therefore advisable to monitor hepatic status before and during treatment with dantrolene. Four alternative treatment schedules have been suggested:

1. For severe cases, 2 to 2.5 mg/kg in physiologic saline is administered by stomach tube and followed by 1 mg/kg q6 to 8 hours. Efficacy is unproven and there is a risk of hepatotoxicity.

2. 2 mg/kg in normal saline p.o. is administered initially daily for 3 to 5 days, then every third day for up to 1 month.

3. In horses in training following their initial return to work after an episode of ERS, up to 1 g is given with a small feed 1.5 to 2 hours before exercise for 3 to 5 days.

4. In animals that are repeated sufferers, 500 mg is administered orally for 3 to 5 days, then 300 mg every third day for a period that varies with the response to treatment and the effect of this dose on the patient's liver function. Treatment for more than 3 months is not recommended. The author has had limited success with this schedule in chronic repeated sufferers that have proved unresponsive to dietary, management, and various other therapeutic regimens, and in which a calcium regulation disturbance was suspected.

Electrolyte Imbalances

Episodes of ERS can sometimes be prevented or decreased in frequency by changes in management coupled with correction of an apparent electrolyte imbalance detected by the urinary fractional electrolyte (FE) excretion test (Fig. 1). The FE test must be carried out appropriately and interpreted with care.

Miscellaneous

A serotonin 5-HT$_2$ antagonist has been reported to be of value, both clinically and histologically, in a group of horses with chronic myopathies of unknown cause in which the clinical signs were variable and vague. Rubella virus immunomodulation has been marketed for the treatment of myositis and myofascial pain, although the author has not seen published studies on its clinical efficacy. Antipsychotic drugs have also been used. Certain antihistamines are also marketed for treatment of myoglobinuria, but there is little evidence as to their efficacy. Other agents used include aspirin, dimethyl sulfoxide (DMSO), adrenocorticotropic hormone (ACTH), dichloroacetate, and various B vitamins.

In some chronic intermittently affected horses, episodes may totally cease or decrease significantly in their fre-

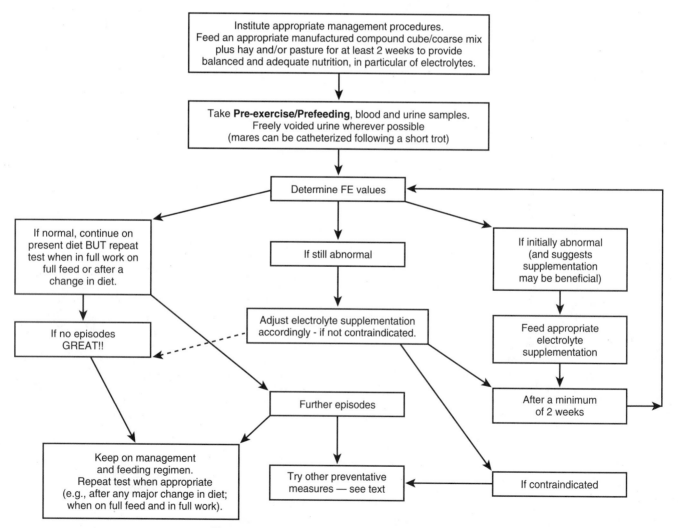

Figure 1. Protocol for fractional urinary electrolyte testing.

quency following a prolonged (6 mo.) period of rest at pasture combined with a controlled return to work. In certain cases, however, episodes may recur after such a break. In some horses episodes may continue during the rest period.

In the future, compounds that help to reduce free radical production or damage may be shown to have a role in preventing ERS. Suggested possibilities include certain branch chain amino acids, carnitine, and creatine.

POLYSACCHARIDE STORAGE MYOPATHY

Recently a distinct subgroup of ERS sufferers has been identified in which up to 40% of the type II fibers contain an acid mucopolysaccharide inclusion. To date, this condition has been identified only in horses with Quarterhorse bloodlines and not in Thoroughbreds or Arabians. The clinical severity appears to be variable, and most have had a history of numerous episodes often within a relatively short period. Affected animals tend to show exercise intolerance to a variable extent. Plasma CK activities may be persistently elevated between episodes. Treadmill exercise

and in vitro studies have suggested that these animals have an abnormal glycolytic metabolism consistent with an impaired activity of the Embden-Meyerhof pathway (glucose-1-P pyruvate) resulting in an insufficient amount of pyruvate for oxidation or anaerobic conversion to lactate. Diagnosis is by examination of biopsy material. Recommended preventative measures include changing to a diet based on good-quality hay with no grain or sweet feed, together with a fat source if required, plus a balanced vitamin and mineral mix, as well as adequate vitamin E and selenium supplementation. Daily exercise and turn out has also been recommended. A similar but apparently more severe condition has been reported in draught horses.

Supplemental Readings

Harris PA, Gray J: The use of the urinary fractional electrolyte excretion test to assess electrolyte status in the horse. Equine Vet Ed 4(4):162–166, 1992.
Valberg S, Jönsson L, Lindhol A, Holmgre N: Muscle histopathology and plasma aspartate aminotransferase, creatine kinase and myoglobin changes with exercise in horses with recurrent exertional rhabdomyolysis. Equine Vet J 25:11–16, 1993.
Valberg S: Exertional rhabdomyolysis and polysaccharide storage myopathy in quarter horses. Proc 41st Annu Meeting Am Assoc Equine Pract 228–230, 1995.

Muscular Disorders

PAT HARRIS
Waltham-on-the-Wolds, England

SUE J. DYSON
Newmarket, England

TRAUMATIC INJURIES

Physical injuries to the muscle can occur in a number of ways, but they are most commonly associated with external trauma or overexertion. The changes that occur within the affected muscle depend upon the extent of the damage to the muscle and the surrounding tissue. Hemorrhage, infection, infarction, and the trauma itself often result in the destruction of the muscle fibers as well as surrounding soft tissue. This tends to cause complete disorientation of the regenerating fibers with marked proliferation of fibroblasts and blood vessels.

Fibrotic Myopathy

Fibrotic myopathy tends to be a chronic, progressive disorder, although clinical signs may apparently be sudden in onset. It commonly affects the semitendinosus muscle, although adhesions to the semimembranosus and biceps femoris may occur, and occasionally only these muscles or the gracilis muscle are affected. The biceps brachii muscle can also be affected. The initiating process usually involves some form of trauma, either external or work-related, followed by inflammation, muscle fiber atrophy, and replace-

ment by fibrous tissue. When mineral deposits form in the affected tissues it is commonly referred to as *ossifying myopathy*. In some cases, no inciting cause can be identified. Cases may occur following excessive exercise over a long period of time, which has resulted in the tearing and stretching of muscle fibers, or as a result of sliding stops in Quarterhorses and Stock horses when the large thigh muscles are contracting while the stifle and hock are extending. Congenital cases, perhaps due to periparturient trauma, have been reported. Cases believed to have occurred as a consequence of intramuscular injections and surgery have also been noted.

Clinical Signs

There is nonpainful mechanical lameness, unilateral or bilateral, associated with a characteristic gait abnormality. The affected limbs are pulled back and down before the end of the protraction phase, so that the foot is slammed down, resulting in a louder sound on impact than that occurring with the unaffected limb. This results in a lengthened weightbearing phase and a shortened cranial or swing phase. The gait has often been referred to as *goose stepping*, and the signs tend to be most obvious at the walk.

The signs may result from mechanical disturbance as a consequence of scar tissue or an altered gamma efferent loop, with an abnormal setting of the muscle spindle, which allows the early unchecked contraction of caudal thigh muscles during the late swing phase of the stride. If the biceps brachii muscle is affected, the horse has a shortened cranial phase of the stride, with a tendency for the foot to land toe first. In both forelimbs and hindlimbs, the area of muscle damage can sometimes be seen as dimpling, or a depression in the skin overlying the muscle. The muscle may be abnormally firm on palpation, although this is not always the situation, especially with congenital cases, which may have only histologic changes.

Diagnosis

Diagnosis is usually based on the clinical signs and history. Diagnostic ultrasound can be useful for confirming the diagnosis and determining whether there is merely fibrosis or if mineralization is also present. Stringhalt is one of the main differential diagnoses. In the latter condition the leg is hyperflexed during the cranial or swing phase, and the stepwise caudal jerking movement does not occur just before the foot reaches the ground.

Treatment and Prognosis

The lameness tends to be unresponsive to routine anti-inflammatory therapy. Some form of surgical treatment is usually recommended, although it is unlikely to be of value if the biceps brachii is involved. A variety of surgical procedures have been recommended including resection of the fibrotic band, a semitendinosus myotenectomy, and a simplified semitendinosus tenotomy. If only the semitendinosus muscle is involved, a tenotomy of the tendon of insertion at the proximal tibia is recommended as the treatment of choice. Although postoperative swelling may be extensive and may persist for several weeks, the long-term functional and cosmetic results have been good.

Gastrocnemius Rupture

Gastrocnemius rupture has been reported in animals attempting to rise after a long period of recumbency; in foals during their initial attempts to rise; in animals that rear and fall over backward; in dystocia cases; and following manual manipulation of a fixed tarsocrural joint. The rupture may occur within the body of the muscle, resulting in a hematoma that may calcify, or, if it occurs in the tendon of insertion, it may be associated with avulsion of a portion of the tuber calcaneus. Initially there is heat, swelling, and signs of pain often associated with elevated plasma muscle enzyme activities. The affected hock is excessively flexed owing to the loss of the gastrocnemius's extensor influence. The animal is recumbent if affected bilaterally. Prognosis is guarded. Immobilization of the affected limb in an extended position combined with support in a sling has been recommended.

Serratus Ventralis Rupture

Rupture of the serratus ventralis muscle is very rare. It usually occurs bilaterally resulting in the dropping of the thorax, so that the thoracic spinous processes are beneath the dorsal borders of the scapulae. It tends to result from dorsal impact trauma over the withers and neck region, or

from jumping a very high fence, or jumping down from a raised platform. It is a very painful condition. The main differential diagnosis is fracture of the dorsal spinous processes at the withers. Prolonged rest in a sling has been suggested, but the prognosis is poor.

"Pulled" and "Sore" Muscles

Muscle strains or tears, often referred to as *pulled muscles*, occur most commonly during exercise. The definitive diagnosis of a pulled muscle can be difficult, especially in more chronic cases. Depending on the muscle involved and the extent of the trauma, obvious external swelling may or may not be apparent. Similarly, there may or may not be apparent pain on muscle palpation. Abnormal muscle tension may be present, especially if the longissimus dorsi muscle is involved. Plasma muscle enzyme activities may or may not be significantly elevated, depending on the extent of damage and the timing, relative to the incident, of the blood sampling (see page 115). A number of techniques including faradic stimulation, thermography, scintigraphy, and diagnostic ultrasound may be used to locate and diagnose a pulled muscle, although it can be difficult in certain cases to pinpoint the area of damage. Treatment is rest together with physiotherapy (e.g., manipulation, ultrasound, faradism; see page 131).

Pulled muscles, in which there has been some disruption of the muscle fiber architecture often with associated hematoma formation, should be distinguished from the over-exerted or sore muscle, in which damage may be at the cellular level and is often only associated with structural damage of the contractile elements. Delayed-onset muscular soreness (DOMS) is a frequently experienced condition in humans, although its etiology is not fully understood, and human biopsy data suggest that the inflammatory changes do not parallel the soreness ratings.

DOMS has been defined as the sensation of discomfort or pain in the skeletal muscles that occurs following unaccustomed muscular exertion, especially when eccentric in nature (i.e., the active muscle lengthens while doing work). The soreness tends to increase in intensity in humans in the first 24 hours after exercise, peaks from 24 to 72 hours, then decreases so that after 5 to 7 days it is gone. In humans there tends to be a sense of reduced mobility or reduced flexibility, and the muscles tend to be sensitive, especially upon palpation or movement. The signs can be very mild, with the slight stiffness disappearing rapidly with routine daily activities, or it can cause severe debilitating pain that interferes with movement. DOMS can adversely affect muscular performance, because of voluntary reduction of effort as well as a reduced ability of the muscles to perform optimally. Specific training involving the activity that produced the DOMS originally decreases the amount of soreness produced by that activity. In humans, exercise-induced muscular soreness can occur without a change in serum enzyme activities or myoglobin concentrations, especially if the condition originates from pathology affecting the connective tissues of the musculotendinous junction, rather than the muscle fiber itself. In such cases increased urinary clearance of hydroxyproline.

Whether DOMS occurs in the horse as a distinct clinical syndrome is not fully known. It has been suggested that a condition similar to DOMS in humans can be seen in horses, particularly those that start training after a period of rest. It causes a stiff gait, palpable soreness, and a reluctance to walk approximately 24 hours after exercise, and raised hydroxyproline concentrations. Free radicals generated during exercise may be involved in both acute and delayed-onset muscular soreness. Whether any relationship exists between acute or delayed-onset muscular soreness and rhabdomyolysis syndrome is unknown.

The best prevention for DOMS is previous appropriate training. The recommended treatment for DOMS varies from rest to light exercise, with or without some form of analgesia. The most effective method of reducing DOMS in humans is believed to involve exercising the sore muscles, although the relief may be temporary. The reduction in muscle soreness with such exercise is not fully understood. A central component may be present, with release of endogenous endorphins, or an effect on the more peripheral neural pathways may be responsible. Heat is often recommended as an aid to recovery, although its importance in the repair process is doubtful. Associated massage as well as the sensation of warmth, however, may help to reduce the apparent perceived level of pain. Continued exercise may be contraindicated in two of the main differentials for muscle soreness (i.e., muscle strains and rhabdomyolysis syndrome).

INFECTIOUS AGENTS

This section describes the more common bacterial infections of muscle. It must be remembered that certain parasites and possibly some viruses may also affect skeletal muscles.

Gas Gangrene and Malignant Edema

Gas gangrene and malignant edema occur most commonly following stake wounds, parturition injuries, castration, and especially intramuscular injections. The most commonly associated pathogens are *Clostridium septicum, perfringens, novyi, sordellii,* and *chauvoei.* Growth occurs under suitable local anaerobic conditions including a low oxidative reduction potential and alkaline pH. The resultant toxin production overwhelms the cellular defense mechanisms, resulting in extensive tissue necrosis. "Gas gangrene" tends to be associated with extensive disintegration of the muscle tissue with bubbles of gas and the presence of a serosanguineous exudate. "Malignant edema" may progress to gangrene, but is more typically a form of cellulitis.

Clinical Signs

Animals are often found recumbent or dead. In less acute cases, lameness is common and may be severe. The affected animal is usually very depressed, with systemic signs of a profound toxemia. Muscular swelling is often present, and crepitation may be felt. The overlying skin often changes from feeling hot and looking discolored to becoming cool to the touch, and the animal appears to be insensitive to palpation.

Diagnosis

Diagnosis is based on the clinical signs and history, although the finding of a nonclotting, malodorous fluid with or without gas on needle aspiration can be helpful. The clinicopathologic changes tend to be nondiagnostic and are similar to those seen in other septic or toxic conditions. Raised plasma muscle enzyme activities are often found, although they do not tend to correlate with the apparent degree of muscle damage. Anaerobic culture or fluorescent antibody identification of the organism in tissue samples is recommended for a definitive diagnosis.

Treatment

Intensive antibiotic therapy in conjunction with surgical debridement or fenestration to remove the necrotic tissue and limit the availability of an appropriate anaerobic environment is usually recommended. Crystalline penicillin (20,000–40,000 IU/kg IV t.i.d. or q.i.d.) is administered either alone or in combination with metronidazole (20–25 mg/kg p.o. t.i.d., or 20 mg/kg IV b.i.d. or t.i.d.). Antibiotic therapy should be continued until infection has resolved; but it should continue for at least 7 days. In the case of, for example, diffuse cellulitis that extends down fascial planes, therapy may be required for several weeks. Supportive treatment such as IV fluids and nonsteroidal anti-inflammatory drugs (NSAIDs) to help combat the "shock" and pain is usually needed. Initial short-term corticosteroid therapy may be beneficial, but corticosteroids should be used with caution in these conditions. Prognosis is poor. Survival is most common when the cause is *C. perfringens.* Extensive skin sloughing may occur in those animals that survive the acute stages of the disease.

Suppurative Myositis: Abscessation

Suppurative myositis can occur from a variety of causes, including intramuscular injections, penetrating wounds, hematogenous spread of infection, or via the extension of an infective focus in an adjacent or distant structure. Initially there is ill-defined cellulitis, which may heal or progress to the more classical organized abscess or, especially in the case of certain staphylococcal infections, may extend, resulting in extensive muscular damage. Abscesses may slowly heal, expand, or fistulate to a body cavity or, most commonly, the skin surface. Once fistulated, they may either collapse and heal (although usually with scar tissue), or they may persist as chronic granulomas that may or may not drain persistently. Chronic granulomas commonly occur with *Staphylococcus aureus* infections in the neck and pectoral region.

Streptococcus equi is a frequent cause of skeletal muscle abscessation in the horse, as is *Corynebacterium pseudotuberculosis,* especially in certain areas of the western United States. The latter organism causes ventral midline, inguinal, and pectoral abscesses. When swollen pectorals are present, infection with this organism is often referred to as *pigeon fever,* owing to the clinical appearance (see page 393 for a complete description of this condition). In general, subcutaneous *C. pseudotuberculosis* infections seem to be less likely than staphylococcal or streptococcal abscesses to result in raised white blood cell counts and fibrinogen levels. Corynebacterial abscesses are often large and are sited deep within the muscle beds. The differential diagnosis includes other bacterial abscesses, seromas, and tumors.

Diagnosis can be confirmed by ultrasound or culture of aspirated fluid. Abscesses in the axillary region, in particular, can be difficult to locate even with ultrasound. The synergistic hemolysin inhibition test is available, which can detect antibodies to *C. pseudotuberculosis*; however, the intensity of the antibody response varies considerably and depends on a number of factors, including the chronicity of the infection. The test can, for example, be very helpful in determining whether internal *C. pseudotuberculosis* abscessation should be included in the differential diagnosis of certain cases.

Treatment for all abscesses includes poulticing to assist maturation, lancing, flushing, and draining. On occasions surgery may be necessary to expose the abscess adequately and to excise it completely. Whether antibiotics should be used is controversial and may depend on the stage of abscessation. Commonly recommended antibiotics include procaine penicillin (20,000 IU/kg IM b.i.d.) or potassium or sodium penicillin (20,000–40,000 IU/kg IV q.i.d.) alone or in combination with rifampin (5 mg/kg p.o. b.i.d.). Sulfamethoprim and erythromycin have also been used on occasion. If antibiotic therapy is used it should be continued for several weeks. It is often recommended for abscesses caused by *Corynebacterium*. Further recommendations are that the contamination of paddocks via a draining lesion be avoided and contaminated bedding be disposed of in a suitable manner. Appropriate fly control may also be of value.

Prognosis is favorable for ultimate recovery, but prolonged resolution, recrudescence, and other undesirable sequelae are possible with corynebacterial abscesses. In a few cases, in addition to the muscular abscesses, internal abscessation occurs, which makes a successful recovery less likely. Affected horses are more likely to have raised white blood cell counts, with neutrophilia and raised fibrinogen levels.

Supplemental Readings

Aleman MA, Spier S, Wilson WD: Retrospective study of *Corynebacterium pseudotuberculosis* infection in horses: 538 cases (1982–1993). Proc 40th Annu Conv Am Assoc Equine Pract, 1994, p 117.
Bramlage LR, Reed SM, Embertson RM: Semitendinosus tenotomy for treatment of fibrotic myopathy in the horse. J Am Vet Med Assoc 186:565–567, 1985.
Clayton HM: Cinematographic analysis of the gait of lame horses V: fibrotic myopathy. J Equine Vet Sci 8:297–301, 1988.
Miers KC, Ley WB: *Corynebacterium pseudotuberculosis* infection in the horse: Study of 117 clinical cases and consideration of etiopathogenesis. J Am Vet Med Assoc 177:250–253, 1980.
Turner AS, Trotter GW: Fibrotic myopathy in the horse. J Am Vet Med Assoc 184:335–338, 1984.
Valberg SJ, McKinnon AO: Clostridial cellulitis in the horse: A report of five cases. Can Vet J 25:67–71, 1984.

Postanesthetic Myopathy

DAVID BARTRAM
Newmarket, England

Postanesthetic myopathy is the most common morbidity associated with general anesthesia and surgery in the horse, occurring in up to 7% of horses anesthetized. The consequences of its development can be devastating. Historically it was thought that postanesthetic lameness was largely the result of a neuropathy. However, it is now generally accepted that muscle damage is the main problem, although it can be accompanied by neural involvement.

Postanesthetic myopathy can occur as a local unilateral problem, such as a masseter or triceps myopathy; a local bilateral problem, such as hindlimb adductor myopathies; or as a generalized myopathy. Muscle groups that can be affected in laterally recumbent horses include the dependent triceps, pectoral, quadriceps, gluteus, chest wall, and masseter. The most common and clinically significant of these myopathies is in the dependent triceps. In dorsally recumbent horses, the gluteal and longissimus dorsi are commonly affected, and myopathy has also been reported in the adductor muscles.

CLINICAL SIGNS AND DIAGNOSIS

Clinical signs usually develop soon after the horse stands, although in some individuals the signs may be delayed for up to 2 hours. Often, the problem is first suspected when recovery from anesthesia is prolonged, with repeated unsuccessful attempts to stand. If the myopathy is either particularly severe or if more than one limb is involved, the horse may be unable to stand unaided. These problems are magnified if there are restrictions to an easy recovery, such as the presence of a full-length leg cast on another limb. Repeated unsuccessful attempts to stand may result in either further injury or exhaustion.

Typically the affected muscle groups are hard, swollen, and painful, and there is usually localized sweating. Severe pain causes sympathetic nervous system stimulation, and so animals are invariably tachycardic, tachypneic, and sweating profusely. The horse often appears agitated. The lameness or abnormal posture that it adopts depends on the muscle groups affected. For example, a horse with triceps myopathy usually has a dropped elbow and is reluctant to bear weight on the affected limb, although extensor function is usually unaffected. This appearance is similar to radial nerve paralysis. Isolated plaques can occur on some muscles such as those in the neck and chest wall without appearing to have any clinical significance. Masseter muscle myopathies can sometimes be associated with clinical signs of facial paralysis, and the signs usually resolve as the myopathy improves. If a horse remains recumbent, one differential diagnosis that must be ruled out is spinal cord malacia. Horses suffering from this are usually able to "dog-sit," and although they may be agitated, they usually do not show signs of pain. They have a complete lack of sensory perception over the hindquarters.

Although diagnosis can usually be made on the evidence of the clinical signs alone, laboratory measurement of serum muscle enzyme activities can be useful to either confirm the diagnosis or to help differentiate it from other causes of lameness or recumbency. Creatine kinase (CK) is the most specific marker of muscle damage, and its serum activities usually peak around 6 to 8 hours after the end of anesthesia. However, after any reasonable period of anesthesia and recumbency, most horses show a significant increase in serum CK activities, perhaps as high as 1500 IU/L, without clinical evidence of lameness. Significant myopathies are usually associated with CK activities of higher than 2000 IU/L, and these may exceed 20,000 IU/L. The CK activity often appears normal immediately after the horse stands, but as blood flow returns to the damaged muscle, and as the horse moves about, the activity rises rapidly over the next couple of hours. Aspartate aminotransferase activities also rise, peaking about 24 to 48 hours after anesthesia, often in excess of 2000 IU/L. It is surprising that in most experimental studies, absolute serum activities of these enzymes correlate poorly with the severity of lameness. This apparent discrepancy may arise from variable contributions from muscle groups not involved in weightbearing, such as the masseter or chest wall muscles. One rare condition that can result in massive CK activity after anesthesia is a generalized myositis resulting from the development of malignant hyperthermia during anesthesia. Clinical signs that develop during anesthesia include hyperthermia, sweating, hyperventilation, tachycardia, and unstable blood pressure.

PATHOGENESIS

Although it seems unlikely that arterial hypoxemia in isolation is a significant cause of postanesthetic myopathy, it is likely to have an additive effect with some of the other predisposing factors. Hypoperfusion of muscle groups seems to be the single most important factor, which is often the result of an increase in intracompartmental pressure. Hypoperfusion is typically produced in dependent muscle groups, especially if the surface on which the horse is placed is particularly unyielding. Another factor opposing blood flow is an increase in venous pressure resulting from venous drainage obstruction. Venous drainage may be reduced if limbs, dependent or otherwise, are flexed or extended in a severe and unnatural manner. These increases in pressure oppose blood flow to the affected muscle groups, and if the mean arterial pressure is insufficient, the tissues are underperfused. Hypotension clearly has a role to play in the development of localized myositis, particularly in dependent or badly positioned limbs, and in severe cases it is also implicated in the development of bilateral and generalized myopathies, by causing a more global hypoperfusion. Generalized myopathies appear to occur independent of positioning.

Time is also a crucial factor, and although most horses tolerate a brief period of hypotension or poor positioning, the longer the animal is anesthetized, the greater the risk of a myopathy developing. Even if the horse is optimally positioned and blood pressure is well maintained, a myopathy is increasingly likely to develop when the horse is anesthetized for more than 2 to 3 hours. However, apparently inexplicable myopathies can develop after uncomplicated anesthesia of a considerably shorter duration.

Compartmental syndrome is a condition that occurs in humans. Pressure within a muscle group bound by fascia increases, causing hypoxic damage, leading to further muscle swelling and increasing pressure even more. Common causes are crush injuries and drug overdose. Although it has been likened to postanesthetic myopathy, it has only once been reported after anesthesia in the horse. It seems likely that its occurrence is limited in the horse because compartmental pressure decreases when the horse stands up.

PREVENTION

Bearing in mind the predisposing factors, it is clear that careful management of the horse under general anesthesia can minimize the risks of development of postanesthetic myopathy. To reduce anesthetic time, surgical sites should be clipped and washed before anesthesia is induced; surgeons should be well prepared and have a surgical plan; and, ideally, inexperienced, unsupervised surgeons should not undertake surgical procedures that are known to take a long time.

To minimize increases in intracompartmental pressure, horses should be carefully positioned on padded operating tables. Obviously, positioning of certain limbs may be dictated by the particular surgical procedure being undertaken. However, it has been recognized that in laterally recumbent horses, the dependent forelimb should be drawn well forward to minimize pressure on the triceps, and the upper limb should be supported at least parallel to the table top to promote venous drainage. Hindlimbs should be supported parallel to, or above parallel to, the table, and they should be sufficiently separated from each other to allow venous drainage. In dorsally recumbent horses, some people suggest that hindlimbs not be allowed to position themselves passively but be supported in slight extension by a hoist. This may prevent hindlimb adductor myopathies, but the author has not seen this particular problem with passive positioning. When the hindlimbs are drawn backward in full extension, for example for dorsal arthroscopic examination of the fetlock joint, time should be kept to a minimum because this position may predispose to quadriceps myopathy.

Arterial blood pressure should be measured directly by cannulation of a peripheral artery. Most anesthesiologists consider that the mean arterial blood pressure should be at least 60 to 70 mm Hg. Keeping the anesthetic depth as light as is compatible with the surgery being performed may minimize the development of hypotension, but frequently this depth is insufficient. Therefore, in horses with a normal circulating volume, hypotension is usually treated by the infusion of an inotropic agent such as the β-adrenoceptor agonist dobutamine (1–5 μ/kg per minute). If hypovolemia is thought to be contributing to the development of hypotension, it should be corrected with intravenous fluid therapy.

Most studies suggest that the two most important predisposing factors are hypotension and prolonged anesthesia. Although there is the clinical impression that both heavily muscled and fitter horses are at an increased risk, most clinical studies have failed to support this relationship. The author has a clinical impression that horses presenting for emergency treatment of their limbs, such as for lacerated tendons, penetrated joints, and fractures, are at particular risk. The horses are not necessarily racing Thoroughbreds, although they frequently have been performing that day. With these cases, the preventative measures mentioned earlier may be particularly important.

Another potential preventative measure is the prophylactic use of the calcium channel blocker dantrolene. This is used to treat malignant hyperthermia in humans, and it is suggested that its use may be appropriate in horses considered to be at risk. The intravenous formulation is prohibitively expensive, and thus the oral formulation is used for prophylaxis. However, there are several reasons that make it difficult to recommend its use at the present time: it has been associated with prolonged recumbency, there is little positive evidence of its effectiveness, the effective dose in the horse is unknown, and it is potentially hepatotoxic.

TREATMENT

Therapy should be symptomatic and supportive. Circulating volume should be maintained to promote perfusion of the damaged muscle, to encourage good renal perfusion and urine production, and to try to prevent myoglobin-induced renal failure. The other main goals are to make the animal comfortable, to prevent it damaging itself further, and to assist it to a standing position with the aid of slings. The horse should be encouraged to drink freely, but if it is showing severe signs of pain and is sweating profusely, it is very unlikely to be able to maintain its own fluid balance in the first few hours. Therefore, a balanced electrolyte solution, such as lactated Ringer's solution, should be administered intravenously. If aggressive fluid therapy is commenced as soon as the condition is recognized, a more rapid and successful outcome may result. Infusion rates may need to be as high as 10 to 20 ml/kg per hour for the first few hours, or at least until the animal is urinating freely. The rate can then usually be reduced to about 4 to 5 ml/kg per hour. Fluid administration should ideally be continued until the horse is able to maintain its own fluid balance.

Analgesia can be provided by the administration of nonsteroidal anti-inflammatory drugs, such as phenylbutazone (4.4 mg/kg), or flunixin meglumine (1 mg/kg). If muscle damage is widespread, the use of a glucocorticosteroid such as dexamethasone (0.1 mg/kg) to reduce inflammation is recommended by some authors. However, in the author's experience, the use of these agents alone rarely makes the animal comfortable enough, and the use of other analgesics and sedatives is often indicated. Opioid analgesics such as morphine (0.1–0.2 mg/kg), methadone (0.1–0.2 mg/kg), or butorphanol (0.1 mg/kg) can be very useful, particularly if combined with acetylpromazine (0.03–0.05 mg/kg), to produce a calming effect. Some authors recommend the use of drugs such as diazepam and glycerol guaiacolate ether to reduce muscle spasm. However, with a horse that is experiencing difficulty standing, it is debatable whether it is appropriate to try to tread the fine line between producing mild muscle relaxation and ataxia, particularly because these drugs have minimal sedative effects when used on their own.

Horses with myositis frequently need sedating, particularly if they are making repeated unsuccessful attempts to stand. These horses become a danger to themselves and the handlers, risk further catastrophic injury and exhaustion, and make effective nursing very difficult. This also applies to particularly agitated horses that are able to stand. The choice of sedative agents lies between the α_2-adrenergic agonists and acetylpromazine. Although the α_2-agonists xylazine, detomidine, and romifidine certainly produce the deepest sedation, particularly if combined with one of the opioids mentioned earlier, they are less than ideal agents to use repeatedly in these animals. Although they produce good analgesia and muscle relaxation, they can produce further ataxia. Other undesirable effects are sweating, hypoinsulinemia and hyperglycemia, and increased urine output, all of which further increase fluid losses. They also produce intense vasoconstriction and reduced cardiac output, which can significantly reduce tissue blood flow, particularly if the drugs need to be used repeatedly. That stated, there is really no alternative for a particularly violent horse; ideally the drugs should be used sparingly and to effect, and the concurrent use of opioids reduces the dose required. Theoretically, a more logical drug to use is acetylpromazine, which, when combined with one of the opioids, can produce good quality sedation with minimal ataxia. It does not produce sweating, and, in theory, the vasodilation that it produces may improve tissue blood flow. It should therefore be considered as a very useful alternative in all but the most violent of horses.

PROGNOSIS

The prognosis for recovery after unilateral myositis is usually good, particularly if therapy is instituted early and aggressively. If muscle damage is severe, there may be some atrophy and fibrosis of the affected areas, which may limit future performance. The prognosis for recovery after bilateral and generalized myopathy, however, is much more guarded; even with the best nursing, such severely affected animals may not recover sufficient muscular function to stand and have to be killed on humane grounds. The nature of these animals is often very important, and if they are mentally unable to tolerate a prolonged period of recumbency, the outlook has to be much more guarded.

Supplemental Readings

Dodman NH, Williams R, Court MH, Norman WM: Postanesthetic hind limb adductor myopathy in five horses. J Am Vet Med Assoc 193:83–86, 1988.
Richey MT, Holland MS, McGrath CJ, Dodman NH, Marshall DB, Court MH, Norman WM, Seeler DC: Equine post-anesthetic lameness: A retrospective study. Vet Surg 19:392–397, 1990.
White NA: Postanesthesia myopathy-neuropathy. In Robinson NE (ed): Current Therapy in Equine Medicine, ed 2. Philadelphia, WB Saunders, 1983, pp 370–374.
White NA, Saurez M: Changes in triceps muscle intracompartmental pressure with repositioning and padding of the lowermost thoracic limb of the horse. Am J Vet Res 47:2257–2260, 1986.

Equine Canker

DAVID G. WILSON
Madison, Wisconsin

Equine canker is a chronic hypertrophic, moist, eczematous pododermatitis that has a characteristic fetid odor. Historically, canker has most commonly been seen in the hind feet of draft breeds; however, in more recent reports, there was no predilection for hind feet and the disease occurred predominantly in light breeds. The cause of the disease is unknown; however, anaerobic gram-negative bacterial rods are consistently observed within the affected epithelium.

CLINICAL SIGNS

Canker is insidious in onset and usually begins in the frog. Given sufficient time, expansion to the sole and even the hoof wall occurs. In its earliest manifestation, there may be an area of moist tissue that is commonly misdiagnosed as thrush. Unlike thrush, in which the predominant feature is destruction of frog tissue, with canker there is proliferation of inadequately keratinized epithelial tissue. As the condition progresses, a distinctly marginated,

punched-out area may develop (Fig. 1). Left untreated, moist, foul-smelling fronds of epithelial tissue proliferate at a remarkable rate, and the condition can affect the entire frog and sole (Fig. 2). Although canker is usually confined to a single foot, multiple feet can be involved to varying degrees. The affected tissue is very vascular and is commonly mistaken for granulation tissue. Lameness is not usually a presenting feature, but it develops as the mechanical protection of the frog and sole is lost. With the onset of lameness, there is always some infection of the deeper tissues of the foot as a consequence of the loss of mechanical protection, not simply an extension of the canker into the deeper tissues.

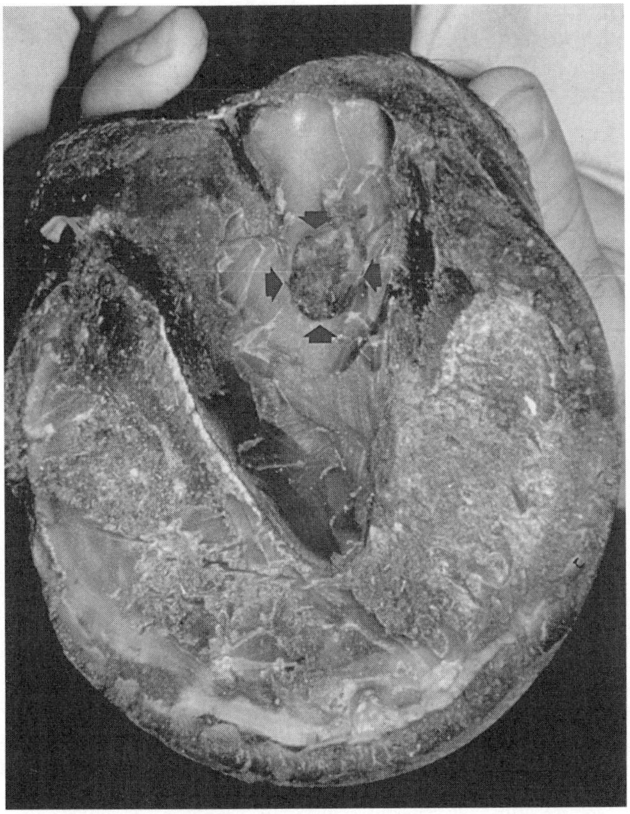

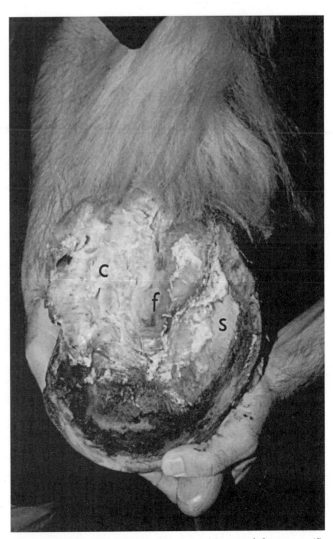

Figure 2. Advanced canker. Canker tissue (c); normal frog tissue (f); normal sole tissue (s).

Figure 1. Early canker *(arrows)*.

DIAGNOSIS

A presumptive clinical diagnosis of canker should be confirmed histologically. Care must be taken to remove the superficial necrotic tissue before a biopsy is sharply collected from the margin of the lesion to include both abnormal and normal tissue. In early stages, there is a focal proliferative papillary hyperplasia limited to the superficial epidermis, with dyskeratosis, keratolysis, and ballooning degeneration of the outer layers. Neutrophils and some mononuclear inflammatory cells sometimes fill the superficial dermal papillae, but deeper dermal inflammation is usually minimal. In long-standing lesions or those in which debridement has been repeated, inflammation can be chronic and deep. A mixed population of bacteria covers the surface of most lesions, and filamentous, beaded, gram-negative rods are frequently seen among ballooned cells.

Bacterial cultures for aerobic and anaerobic bacteria typically yield an assortment of environmental organisms, and *Fusobacterium necrophorum* has been cultured from some horses. From a clinical standpoint, culturing is unnecessary unless there is infection of the deeper tissues of the foot. In that case, the knowledge of bacterial antibiotic sensitivity patterns helps to guide the rational choice of an appropriate antibiotic regimen.

TREATMENT

Historically, canker treatments that involved radical debridement of the foot followed by the application of caustic substances were most often unsuccessful. Current treatment recommendations are founded in the principles of good wound management and the supposition that the anaerobic gram-negative bacteria, which are consistently observed in the affected epithelial tissues, are involved in the pathogenesis. Consistent success is most achievable with a four-component management scheme: early recognition; minor (necessary) debridement; topical application of an appropriate antibiotic; and maintenance of a clean, dry foot environment.

Canker is a disease of the epithelium of the foot, and surgical debridement need not extend beyond the margins of the lesion or into the deeper tissues of the foot unless deep infection is present. Grossly abnormal tissue should be cut away, preserving the germinal layers of the epithelium wherever possible. Debridement is best carried out under general anesthesia with the aid of a tourniquet; however, the procedure can be performed in the standing horse under regional anesthesia. Although complete excision with wide tissue margins is advocated by some, aggressive debridement that results in the loss of germinal epithelium and prolonged healing time is not essential to success. In fact, aggressive debridement may decrease the horse's chance for complete recovery.

Earlier investigators had success with topical penicillin and tetracycline. The author found a combination of parenteral and topical chloramphenicol effective; however, the attendant human health risks associated with the latter forged a move towards topical metronidazole, which is applied daily as a 2% ointment. All of the these antibiotics have activity against anaerobic bacteria, lending some credence to the hypothesis that anaerobic bacteria are involved in the pathogenesis of the condition.

Possibly the most critical element in the successful management of canker is the maintenance of a clean, dry foot environment. This goal is most easily attained by hospitalizing the patient and maintaining a bandage constructed of cotton and held in place with gauze and an adhesive bandage. Short of this ideal, the capable, conscientious handler can be trained to manage the foot. During the first 10 days after surgery, the bandage should be changed daily and the foot should be cleansed with water. This bandage regimen can be continued until the condition is resolved (usually 2 to 4 weeks) or, alternatively, a shoe with a removable treatment plate can be placed. In the author's experience, even the most ingeniously designed treatment plates require some bandage augmentation to maintain a clean, dry foot environment.

PROGNOSIS

Keeping the foot clean, minor debridement, and antibiotic therapy in the form of both systemic and topical chloramphenicol results in close to 100% resolution of the disease in a mean period of 1.4 months compared with 71% resolution in 3.6 months when more aggressive treatment is used. In the previous edition of this book, the prognosis for soundness was listed as guarded. In the author's experience, the prognosis for soundness is excellent, provided that there is minimal involvement of deeper structures in the foot and that the client is in compliance with the treatment. Equine canker is a disease that is underdiagnosed (misdiagnosed as thrush), especially early in the course of the disease. Unfortunately, canker seems to flourish in the face of treatments aimed at resolving thrush, and the condition often becomes severe before a correct diagnosis is made. The evolution away from aggressive debridement and the application of tissue irritants has resulted in dramatic improvement in the prognosis of affected horses. The disasters of the past can readily be the successes of the future with early detection and appropriate treatment of this typically epithelial lesion.

Supplemental Readings

Banic J, Skusek F: Unsere Erfahrungen in der Behandlung des Hufkrebses. Berl Munch Tierarztl Wochenschr 73:186–188, 1960.
Johnson JH: The foot. *In* Mansmann RA, McAllister ES, Pratt PW (eds): Equine Medicine and Surgery, ed 3, vol 2. Santa Barbara, CA, American Veterinary Publications, 1982, pp 1033–1055.
Mason JH: Penicillin treatment of foot canker of the horse. J S Afr Vet Med Assoc 33:223–225, 1962.
Turner TA: Treatment of equine canker. Proc 34th Annu Conv Am Assoc Equine Pract, 1988, pp 307–310.
Wilson DG: Topical metronidazole in the treatment of equine canker. Proc 40th Annu Conv Am Assoc Equine Pract, 1994, pp 49–50.
Wilson DG, Calderwood Mays MB, Colahan PT: Treatment of canker in horses. J Am Vet Med Assoc 194:1721–1723, 1989.

Hypertrophic Osteopathy

T. S. MAIR
Mereworth, England

Hypertrophic osteopathy, also known as hypertrophic pulmonary osteoarthropathy and Marie's disease, is a syndrome characterized by the symmetrical proliferation of connective tissue and subperiosteal bone along the diaphyses of the limb bones. In most cases, the condition is believed to occur as a result of another underlying disease. Hypertrophic osteopathy has been recorded in a number of species, most commonly humans and dogs, in which it is usually associated with intrathoracic disease such as primary or metastatic lung neoplasia. Although hypertrophic osteopathy is uncommon in the horse, it has been recorded in association with various underlying diseases (Table 1). In 42 cases of hypertrophic osteopathy in horses and donkeys, 30 (71%) were associated with identifiable intrathoracic diseases. Extrathoracic diseases, such as ovarian neoplasia, also have been associated with hypertrophic osteoarthropathy. The role of these pathologic processes in the pathogenesis of hypertrophic osteopathy is uncertain. In a small but significant number of cases, no underlying disease process has been identified, even after a full necropsy examination. In one 10-year-old Thoroughbred mare, signs of hypertrophic osteopathy developed during two successive pregnancies; the signs regressed spontaneously after foaling.

The pathophysiology of hypertrophic osteopathy is uncertain. The initial mechanism appears to involve an increase in blood flow to the limbs and fluid retention, followed by proliferation of vascular connective tissue and periosteum, and subsequent bone deposition. However, the precise events leading to increased blood flow are unknown. A number of theories have been proposed, including a hormonal cause, hypoxia, arteriovenous shunts, and neurologic mechanisms. Evidence exists to support each theory, but no single theory appears to offer a completely satisfactory explanation.

CLINICAL SIGNS

Equine hypertrophic osteopathy has been recorded in a wide range of breeds and ages; donkeys are also susceptible. There is no distinct sex predilection. The clinical signs include limb swellings, which involve both soft tissue and bony components. These swellings may be painful or nonpainful on palpation. Involvement is usually bilaterally symmetrical, and both the fore- and hindlimbs are generally involved. The metacarpal and metatarsal bones are most commonly affected, but lesions may also arise in the humerus; radius; carpal bones; proximal, middle, and distal phalanges; femur; tibia; tarsal bones; pelvis; and vertebrae. The limb swellings are frequently associated with stiffness or lameness, and many horses show a reluctance to move. Restricted flexibility of affected joints and resentment to forced flexion may be identified. Other clinical signs vary with the underlying lesion, but may include weight loss, lethargy and dullness, pyrexia, ventral edema, tachypnea or dyspnea, and cough. The bones of the skull including mandible, maxilla, and nasal bones may be affected, resulting in facial swelling.

The clinical course of the condition is quite variable, but most commonly it involves a progressive deterioration over a prolonged period of months to years, with increasing limb swelling and pain. The debilitating nature of hypertrophic osteopathy and the underlying disease often necessitate euthanasia on humanitarian grounds. In a small proportion of cases, resolution of the condition may occur either spontaneously or following treatment of the underlying disease, with a decrease in limb swellings and in associated pain and lameness. Some bony enlargements of the affected areas are likely to remain, but these may have no significant functional effects, and the horse may be able to return to full athletic work.

DIAGNOSTIC PROCEDURES

Diagnosis of hypertrophic osteopathy is based on the clinical features and radiologic findings. Typical radiologic features include periosteal proliferative new bone formation involving the diaphysis and metaphysis of affected bones. The periosteal new bone often has a palisade-like appearance perpendicular to the cortex. The reaction appears active with an irregular outline in most cases, but in

TABLE 1. PRIMARY DISEASES ASSOCIATED WITH HYPERTROPHIC OSTEOPATHY IN THE HORSE

Intrathoracic Diseases

Pulmonary and bronchial tuberculosis
Primary lung tumors
   Example   Granular cell myoblastoma
Bronchogenic squamous cell carcinoma
Metastatic lung tumors
   Example   Squamous cell carcinoma
Pulmonary abscess
Suppurative pneumonia
Granulomatous pneumonia and other granulomatous lesions
Fibrosing pneumonia
Rib fracture and pleural adhesions
Pulmonary infarction

Extrathoracic Diseases

Ovarian neoplasia
   Example   Dysgerminoma
              Granulosa cell tumor
Pituitary adenoma

Miscellaneous

Pregnancy

129

horses that have recovered, the new bone appears smooth and more opaque. Unlike hypertrophic osteopathy in some other species, the articular surfaces of the horse are not usually affected, although the periosteal new bone may approach the joint margins in many cases.

The clinical pathology test results are variable and usually nonspecific. Leukocytosis, neutrophilia, and hyperfibrinogenemia have been recorded in hypertrophic osteopathy cases, but these abnormalities are probably related more to the underlying disease process than to hypertrophic osteopathy itself.

Attempts should be made to identify an underlying disease in all cases of hypertrophic osteopathy; however, diagnosis of an underlying disease is frequently not achieved despite exhaustive examinations. A complete physical examination and hematology and serum biochemistry evaluations should be undertaken, and further examinations performed on the basis of results obtained.

In view of the common association with intrathoracic disease, endoscopic examination of the respiratory tract, bronchoalveolar lavage, thoracic radiography, and thoracic ultrasonography should be performed. It must be remembered that the absence of lesions or abnormalities identified by these techniques cannot be taken as a guarantee that significant intrathoracic disease is not present. Repeated examinations may be necessary. Diffuse pulmonary interstitial infiltrates evident radiographically may indicate the presence of neoplasia or interstitial pneumonia and fibrosis. These findings warrant the collection of a lung biopsy for histopathologic analysis; lung biopsies can be obtained percutaneously using a cutting biopsy needle. Granulomatous pneumonia may be caused by mycobacterial infection, which should be investigated by specific culture techniques, including culture of bronchoalveolar lavage and lung biopsy samples, and by serology testing. Biopsies of peripheral lymph nodes or skin lesions may be helpful in cases of generalized granulomatous disease. Identification of a pleural effusion by radiography or ultrasonography should be followed by thoracocentesis and pleural fluid analysis. Pleuroscopy can be helpful in the investigation of selected cases of pleural disease. Culture of transtracheal aspirates should be performed in cases of suspected bronchopneumonia or pulmonary abscesses.

In the absence of an identifiable thoracic disease, the abdomen should be evaluated by rectal palpation, ultrasonography, and abdominal paracentesis. Laparoscopic examination or exploratory laparotomy may be required on the basis of the results of other examinations.

TREATMENT

The treatment of hypertrophic osteopathy depends on the identification and treatment of an underlying disease. If the underlying condition is successfully resolved, resolution of hypertrophic osteopathy is likely to follow. Recorded equine cases in which regression of the signs and lesions of hypertrophic osteopathy following treatment of the primary disease has occurred include one horse with an intrathoracic abscess, one with chronic bronchopneumonia, one with generalized granulomatous disease, and one with pul-

monary *Mycobacterium avium-intracellulare* infection. Treatment of bronchopneumonia and pulmonary abscesses includes a prolonged course of antibiotics based on the results of bacteriologic cultures and sensitivity tests. An associated parapneumonic pleural effusion may require drainage by repeated thoracocentesis or via an indwelling chest drain. Additional medical treatments that may be helpful in cases of pneumonia and lung abscesses include nonsteroidal anti-inflammatory drug (NSAID) administration and fluid and electrolyte therapy. Generalized granulomatous disease may respond to prolonged systemic prednisolone therapy (2 mg/kg p.o. s.i.d. initially, reducing the daily dose and changing to alternate-day dosing when a response has occurred). Treatment may be required for 8 weeks or longer; the response to treatment appears to be variable between cases. Mycobacterial infections may be treated with prolonged courses of isoniazid (5–20 mg/kg p.o. s.i.d.) and rifampin (5 mg/kg p.o. s.i.d.). Public health risks must be taken into consideration when treating mycobacterial infections.

If no underlying disease can be identified, symptomatic treatment of the affected horse is worthy of consideration. Phenylbutazone (2.2 mg/kg p.o. s.i.d.) or other nonsteroidal anti-inflammatory drugs such as flunixin meglumine (1 mg/kg p.o. s.i.d.) can be helpful in controlling the discomfort associated with hypertrophic osteopathy and may have a beneficial effect on the progression of the disease itself. NSAIDs have been shown to be helpful in controlling hypertrophic osteopathy in other species including humans, but there is only limited information available concerning its use in equine hypertrophic osteopathy.

A small proportion of hypertrophic osteopathy cases in the horse in which there is no obvious underlying primary disease show spontaneous regression of the condition. Treatment may be justified, therefore, in cases in which no primary disease is found, in the hope that regression of hypertrophic osteopathy will take place in time. However, humanitarian and welfare considerations must be taken into account in each case, and these should be regularly reviewed. Repeated examinations at 4- to 6-week intervals, including radiography of affected bones, should be undertaken during treatment to assess progression of the condition. If no improvement is noted within 4 to 6 months, treatment is unlikely to be successful and should be discontinued.

Supplemental Readings

Chaffin MK, Ruoff WW, Schmitz DG, Carter GK, Morris EL, Steyn P: Regression of hypertrophic osteopathy in a filly following successful management of an intrathoracic abscess. Equine Vet J 22:62–65, 1990.
Lavoie JP, Carlson GP, George L: Hypertrophic osteopathy in three horses and a pony. J Am Vet Med Assoc 201:1900–1904, 1992.
Leach MW, Pool RR: Hypertrophic osteopathy in a Shetland pony attributable to pulmonary squamous cell carcinoma metastases. Equine Vet J 24:247–249, 1992.
McClintock SA, Hutchins DR: Case report: Hypertrophic osteopathy in a stallion with minimal thoracic pathology. Aust Vet Pract 11:115–120, 1981.
Mair TS, Dyson SJ, Fraser JA, Edwards GB, Hillyer MH, Love S: Hypertrophic osteopathy (Marie's disease) in the horse and donkey: A review of 24 cases. Equine Vet J 28:256–269, 1996.
Shneerson JM: Hypertrophic osteopathy—an unusual but treatable condition. Equine Vet J 22:1–4, 1990.

Complementary (Alternative) Therapies for Poor Performance, Back Problems, and Lameness

JOYCE C. HARMAN
Washington, Virginia

The poor performance syndrome seen in all sport horses is often the result of musculoskeletal pain and can be successfully treated by use of a combination of acupuncture, chiropractic, and saddle-fitting. Many lamenesses can be treated by use of one or more of the physical therapies such as lasers, ultrasound, electrical stimulation, hydrotherapy, heat, cold, and massage as well as acupuncture and chiropractic. The healing time for injuries is often reduced by use of these modalities; the benefits to the horse industry are great because nobody has time to wait for rest alone to heal injuries. As long as the horse is following a sound rehabilitation program, the return to performance is better than would be expected with conventional treatments of rest, nonsteroidal anti-inflammatory drugs (NSAIDs), or corticosteroids.

Horse owners do not like to have their animals laid off work for long periods of rest after an injury and generally prefer active involvement to help return the horse to work sooner and facilitate the healing. Human sports medicine has made great strides in decreasing recovery time for injuries by taking advantage of various physical therapies and including physical therapists as part of the orthopedic team. Most of these physical therapies can be applied to horses and, when used correctly, can speed up the healing time significantly.

Performance and behavior problems are often the result of soft tissue pain in the neck or back areas. Many causes are responsible for this pain. One of the most frequent is saddle-induced pain, either from a poor fit or improper positioning. Other causes are poor rider balance; lack of rider skill; training techniques that inhibit the natural movement of the back; unbalanced feet; or mouth pain from sharp teeth, rough hands, or a harsh bit. These result in a horse hollowing its back, inverting its neck, and constantly attempting to evade the rider. Conformation and suitability for the sport in mind also play a role, because a horse that has poor conformation has more physical problems than one with suitable conformation. Distal limb lameness may cause chronic back soreness or, more commonly, can be the result of back pain. In many cases, distal limb lameness disappears if the back problem is resolved and does not recur unless the back pain returns.

DIAGNOSIS OF PAIN-INDUCED POOR PERFORMANCE

Performance problems can result in anything from mild protest about being saddled to an unrideable bucking bronco (Table 1). Many, if not most, of the difficulties encountered in training horses can be traced to back pain or neck pain. Although some horses learn to overcome these pain-related performance problems, others do not and are usually sold, thus creating a large economic loss to the industry and the individual horse owner.

The steps to a diagnosis are standard but with a different emphasis. A very complete history needs to be taken, followed by observation of the horse at rest and in motion, with and without tack. The muscles and joints are palpated thoroughly. Standard diagnostic procedures such as nerve blocks and diagnostic imaging can be used.

History

Pertinent history questions include: "What is the primary complaint?" "When is the problem evident?" "What makes the problem better?" "What makes it worse?" Typical responses include: "The problem gets worse toward the end of a ride" and "The horse takes a long time to warm up."

TABLE 1. INDICATIONS OF PAIN-INDUCED POOR PERFORMANCE

Objection to being saddled
Being "cold-backed" during mounting
Slow to warm up or relax
Resistant to work
Resistant to training aids
Difficult to collect or maintain impulsion
Hock, stifle, or obscure hindlimb lameness
Front leg lameness, stumbling, or tripping
Excessive shying
Lack of concentration on rider and aids
Rushing to/from fences and refusing jumps
Twisting over fences
Rushing downhill or pulling uphill with front legs because of reluctance to use hind end
Inability to travel straight
Inability to round back and/or neck
Swishing tail, pinning ears, grinding teeth, tossing head
Hypersensitivity to being brushed or touched
Exhibiting a "bad attitude"
Bucking or rearing regularly
Decreasing speed on the racetrack
Slow out of the starting gate
Avoiding turns
Starts ride doing well, becomes more resistant later
Bucking, rolling excessively in field, or not moving
Difficult to shoe
"Requiring" training aids to perform

131

Because many subtle performance problems show up as behavioral problems (see Table 1), questions about the horse's behavior are important. Some riders are not aware that pain causes training problems.

Observation

The horse should be observed standing at rest without its equipment. The natural stance is examined, because many horses develop a compensatory positioning of the limbs at rest when in pain. Some horses stand stretched out, or "parked out," to rest their back, whereas others stand with their limbs underneath their bodies. The clinician must look at the shoeing, because unbalanced feet lead to alterations in stance and upper body pain. Does the horse always rest one foot, or place one foot in a certain position? Will the horse stand square if asked? Many horses are not able to stand square because of discomfort.

The horse is examined from all angles for symmetry and asymmetry. The horse is observed standing squarely on level ground and viewed for the points of the shoulders, the carpi, and slope of the pasterns, as well as the shape of the feet. With the clinician standing directly behind the horse, asymmetries are noted in the pelvic structure, muscle mass over the hindquarters and in the gaskins, and shapes of the feet.

A stool is placed behind the horse and the examiner stands above the horse's back, looking down. The horse must be standing square, although it may be impossible to have it square in front and behind at the same time owing to discomfort. If the horse cannot stand square on all four legs, the front is observed first, then the rear end, separately. Asymmetrical shoulder positioning can lead to a saddle fitting problem, stiffness, and imbalances in movement. The horse may stand crooked and may be unable to straighten its neck, or there may be a crookedness of the spine that does not correct itself, even when the horse is repositioned.

The horse is observed walking and jogging in hand, while being lunged, with a rider mounted, and after traditional flexion tests. Many horses move freely on the lunge line, but with a rider lose their free movement or change their movement in some adverse way. Significant changes in movement when the rider's weight is added usually indicate back pain, the origin of which may be a poorly fitting saddle, musculoskeletal trauma, poor riding technique, or training aids that put horses into artificial "frames" or head position. The rider may feel that the horse is "off" or just not quite right on a particular limb. To the observer, the main sign is often stiffness or resistance in one direction or another, but the horse is not lame enough for one to see an obvious improvement following diagnostic regional anesthesia. Multiple limbs may be involved, either the ipsilateral or the diagonal limb, with the cumulative picture being one of stiffness. The stiffness is a very important clue, because it usually means the spine is not moving correctly, the muscles are painful or in spasm, or the horse is protecting a painful part, often the back. If the horse moves stiffly and incorrectly, the distal limbs may become affected secondarily, slowly resulting in overt lameness. Correct treatment during the poor performance stage may alleviate the distal limb lameness, and actually allow the horse to perform at a higher level with greater ease.

Palpation

Palpation skills are enhanced by learning acupuncture and chiropractic approaches for treating horses. The information gathered by specific palpation allows the practitioner to make a diagnosis and treatment plan.

The first palpation is a gentle passing of the practitioner's hands over the entire neck, back, and thorax searching for muscle tension, sensitivity, flinching, or discomfort. A well-practiced light touch reveals more than a heavy touch.

The next stage is the acupuncture diagnosis, which involves palpation of the acupuncture meridians for pain or tension. The most common meridian to palpate for back pain is the bladder meridian, which is about 10 cm lateral to the spine in an average-sized horse, beginning in the pocket just behind the shoulder blade and ending near the tail. This meridian is one of the most important and is easily affected by ill-fitting saddles. The meridians along the neck are also palpated. It is beyond the scope of this section to go into further detail about the meridians.

As the practitioner's fingers gain experience palpating acupuncture points, subtle changes can be found. Sensitivity at specific acupuncture points can be used diagnostically not only for back and neck pain but also for distal limb lameness. Because of the nature of the acupuncture meridians and their network of pathways over the body, it is possible to determine which points along the neck and the bladder meridian are sensitive, then relate the findings to locations on the distal limbs. Each point along the back on the bladder meridian is related to one of the other meridians. By knowing the path of the meridian and the internal organ to which that meridian is related, it is possible to locate the spot on the distal limbs where there is a problem. Diagnosing distal limb lameness through use of acupuncture points is an adjunct to other diagnostic techniques. However, sensitivity found along the back also causes the horse to alter its gait when the rider and the saddle are in place, thus accentuating the distal limb soreness. Pain in the back and neck acupuncture points may be the origin of the distal limb problems.

The chiropractic examination is the next stage. All joints in the body including the spine should move smoothly through their entire range of motion. Many horses have lost normal motion throughout their spine, resulting in stiffness and pain. To examine the range of motion, the practitioner gently moves the spine through its normal range, looking and feeling for stiffness. A carrot can be held by the horse's hip, and stifle and down between the front limbs to check neck mobility (the "carrot stretch"), then the back can be raised by pressing on the ventral midline to contract the rectus abdominus ("sit ups" for horses). A normal horse can reach its hip and stifle with its muzzle as well as reach down well between its forelimbs. The back should be able to rise up easily, resulting in the horse extending and lowering its neck. Horses can become upset if this is painful, and if they cannot raise their back while standing still, they cannot raise their back with a rider in place. Loss of normal motion at the junction of the ribs and the sternum, or loss of motion through the

TABLE 2. SADDLE-INDUCED INJURIES

Obvious sores
White hairs under the saddle
Temporary or permanent swellings
Scars deep in the muscle
Atrophy of muscles on sides of withers

withers and midthorax, usually produces pain when raising the back.

The practitioner then performs a palpation for specific motion of the individual joints of the spine and extremities to reveal restrictions. Healthy joints move freely and have spring to them, whereas problem joints often feel stiff. Muscle palpation is also important, starting with a light touch and moving deeper to assess muscle quality. A healthy muscle feels soft and springy; the horse does not object in any way to the palpation. Muscle under tension is tight and hard and has little spring. Muscle spasms and fasciculation can be seen locally and at a distance from the palpation site. Muscle in spasm is more likely to become injured and takes a long time to warm up. Sometimes a horse "splints" its back or holds it rigidly in place while being examined to avoid movement. This reflects pain.

As the palpation is being done, signs of saddle-induced injuries (Table 2) may be found. If a poorly fitted saddle has been used on a horse for any length of time, there is residual back pain and probably loss of normal motion of the thoracic and lumbar vertebrae.

Diagnostic Imaging

When evaluating horses for poor performance, diagnostic imaging of all types can be used to complete the examination. However, it is common to find few radiographic and scintigraphic changes. As scintigraphy becomes more widely available and understanding of the pathologic changes in the spine and upper body is advanced, scintigraphy may become a more useful tool in diagnosing and defining pain in the spinal column. Thermography, although not used widely, has more promise in showing areas of increased and decreased blood flow. Muscles, when contracted or in spasms, have altered blood flow, which shows up well in thermographic images.

TREATING BACK PROBLEMS THAT LEAD TO POOR PERFORMANCE AND SUBTLE LAMENESS

Saddle Fit

In treating the poor performance syndrome and many lamenesses, saddle fit is equal in importance to shoe fit. Treatment of back pain is negated by a poorly fitted saddle. The basics of saddle fit are simple, but the confounding variables are complex, because horses can change shape throughout the season.

No matter what type of saddle is used, it should be placed behind the scapulae; it should fit across the withers, contact the horse evenly along the entire panel, and have a 6- to 8-cm gullet or channel between the panels in which the spine can move. The seat needs to be level and the girth should hang straight down. Each panel should be wide and long enough to spread the rider's weight over a large area, preferably 28 to 31 cm wide under the seat. Most western saddles have too straight a shape to the bottom of the panel and consequently "bridge" the horse's back, making contact at the shoulders and the loins but not in the middle. Most close contact and popular dressage saddles do not have enough panel surface area. The close contact saddles have such a thin panel that they bridge; generally, the saddles have a curve to the point of the tree on each side of the withers that causes a serious pressure point. Many western and English saddles come with so many manufacturing defects and imbalances that it is hard to find an off-the-shelf saddle to correctly fit a horse, but the effort is worthwhile. The riders must also fit in the saddle or they become part of the saddle-fitting problem by being placed in the wrong position in the saddle.

Acupuncture

Acupuncture has proven extremely successful for this author in treating the poor performance syndrome in all sports. When combined with correcting saddle fit, shoeing and riding techniques, the improvement in performance is outstanding, with approximately 85 to 90% of the horses treated returning to the previous level of performance or higher, when one to four treatments are given 2 weeks to 1 month apart. When clients have been unwilling or unable to correct saddle fit problems, have poor quality farriers, or continue with management and training techniques (Table 3) that cause problems, the horse must be maintained with regular treatments. Horses in hard work need more regular treatments than horses in light work. A horse working near its maximal ability, whether training level or Olympic level, requires more frequent therapy. As human athletes have discovered, it is necessary to maintain some regular form of musculoskeletal therapy to maintain maximal performance with minimal injuries, because continued athletic activity puts strain on the musculoskeletal system.

Acupuncture treatment works well in treating many diseases and conditions (Table 4). It is best known for its treatment of back pain and chronic diseases. It is not advisable to treat a horse with acupuncture within 48 hours before a race, because they may be relaxed from the endorphin release that occurs and run poorly. Acupuncture is best performed by a veterinarian with advanced training

TABLE 3. MANAGEMENT AND TRAINING PRACTICES THAT CAUSE DISCOMFORT

Ponying racehorses
Mechanical hotwalkers, horse walkers
Lunging excessively, especially in side reins
Training devices
Paying no attention to the muscles after exercise
Ignoring the importance of warm-up and warm-down
Excessive use of swimming
Blankets that are too tight
Sharp teeth or painful bits
Poor riding, training techniques
Poor shoeing
Conformation incorrect for the sport

TABLE 4.   CONDITIONS TREATED WITH ACUPUNCTURE

Arthritis	Skin conditions	Urinary tract disorders
Bone spavin	Behavior problems	Reproductive problems
Neck stiffness	Allergies	Exertional rhabdomyolysis
Navicular	Diarrhea	Kidney disease
Laminitis	Colic	Liver disease
Wobblers	Respiratory disease	Some neurologic disorders
Back pain	Chronic obstructive pulmonary disease	Radial nerve paralysis

in the technique. Practitioners who just choose a few standard points or follow a single formula find that their results are inconsistent.

Acupuncture points can be stimulated in many ways. This author uses acupuncture with the injection of 3 to 5 ml of vitamin B_{12} into each acupuncture point. The horses are generally receptive to treatment and relax completely. If the horses are tense or needle-shy, a cold laser (Respond Laser 2400, Respond Systems, Madison, CT)* is used as the stimulus. Because acupuncture points are close to the surface of the skin, most brands of lasers work. Many other substances have been injected into acupuncture points, including saline, local anesthetics, anti-inflammatory drugs, and steroids. The internal blistering agents create scar tissue and should never be injected into an acupuncture site.

Other methods to stimulate the acupuncture points include therapeutic ultrasound and electroacupuncture when the practitioner needs to stimulate traditional Chinese needles that lack an injection port. Moxibustion is the burning of the Chinese herb moxa either on a needle placed in an acupuncture point or over the skin at the point. This is especially useful in treating arthritis in the winter. Magnets can be applied with sticky tape or glued onto the hair, using rubber cement or carpet glue. They are useful for long-term (1–2 weeks) stimulation of points, and on foals and needle-shy horses. Implants of gold beads or suture material are useful for long-term stimulation in cases with significant pathology, such as navicular syndrome and degenerative joint disease.

It is important to treat the whole horse with acupuncture, not just the part that appears to have a problem, especially in the case of hock and stifle problems and navicular syndrome. Treating the whole horse involves finding out which meridians are blocked or out of balance, generally through finding sensitive acupuncture points and applying the principles of Chinese medicine to determine which are the best points to treat. If all the acupuncture meridians that need to be treated are balanced, much of the distal limb lameness is improved permanently. If all the meridians are not treated, the resulting pain that shows up along the bladder meridian on the back continues to cause the horse to alter its stride and aggravate the distal limb condition. On the first treatment session, horses frequently have multiple meridians out of balance and have significant pain. With accurate application of acupuncture, fewer needles are required and better results are obtained.

This author uses four to six needles in an average poor-performance case, although many practitioners use more needles and are very successful. A significant improvement with one to three or four treatments is considered a normal response when the whole horse is treated. If a significant positive response, not necessarily a cure but a definite improvement, is not achieved in horses after four treatments, the diagnosis is wrong, the pathology too far advanced, or the treatment incorrect. When the pathology is far advanced, maintenance treatments can often slow the progression of the disease.

Chiropractic

When chiropractic and acupuncture are combined, horses can reach their full potential. When either form of therapy is done alone, the increase in performance is not usually as long-lasting or as good as when both therapies are combined, and repeated treatments are required. If horses are just undergoing chiropractic treatment, this author adjusts them once a week for a month or two, then quarterly, unless they have significant problems, are in heavy competition, or are racing. Horses receiving acupuncture and chiropractic treatments are treated once a month for 2 to 4 months, then quarterly, or less often as needed. The idea is to prevent problems from recurring, rather than to treat them when they recur. Chiropractic work treats most of the behavior problems and stiffness associated with poor performance (Table 5).

Modern chiropractic terminology uses the vertebral subluxation complex (VSC) to describe all the manifestations of the biomechanical and neurologic components of the alteration of normal dynamics and anatomic or physiologic relationships of contiguous articular surfaces in the spine. The physiologic stages of the VSC show that clinical signs of pain do not begin to appear until kinesiopathy, myopathy, neuropathy, vascular abnormalities, connective tissue disorders, and inflammation have all begun. Once signs of pain are present, the next stage is degeneration of the joints. Consequently, the reason for regular chiropractic adjustments is to prevent pain and degeneration. One very well-done study showed, by use of a standardized exercise test, a measurable increase in performance in a group of human athletes treated chiropractically in comparison with a control group. Both groups continued to train normally but the control group did not receive any chiropractic treatment.

TABLE 5.   CONDITIONS TREATED WITH CHIROPRACTIC CARE

Back pain
Neck pain, stiffness
Stiffness in spine or any other joint
Resistance to training
Cold back
Refusing, rushing jumps
Short strided
Unable, unwilling to round back
Subtle lameness
Difficult to "set" head or keep in a "frame"
"Doesn't move like he used to"
Unusual sweating patterns due to nerve damage

*True laser diodes, wavelength 904 nm; penetrates 20 cm, Equine Therapy Catalogue, Lexington, KY

A chiropractic adjustment is a short-lever, high-velocity controlled thrust, by hand or instrument, which is directed at a specific articulation in a single motor unit (i.e., two vertebrae and the associated nerves, tendons, ligaments, and soft tissue). Chiropractic adjustments do not require great strength, just skill in making the short, sharp thrust, and knowledge of how to direct that thrust. This author adjusts all sizes of horses from ponies to draft horses with her hands and has no difficulty. The horses are very receptive and their relaxation makes the job easier, because it is very difficult to adjust even a person when the muscles are tense. A manipulation, as is frequently done in terms of chiropractic, is a forceful passive movement of a joint beyond its active range of motion, generally done with a long lever by jerking a leg or twisting the entire neck. Manipulations can result in damage to the joint capsules and to the joints themselves. Initially improvement in flexibility and performance can be seen, but the long-term joint damage has begun and may not show up for several years.

During the motion palpation of all the joints, the practitioner finds the joints where there is restricted motion and adjusts them chiropractically. Inexperienced practitioners can begin to loosen the spine by inducing the horse to perform some simple exercises such as "carrot stretches" and "sit ups" described earlier, and the owners can continue those exercises. All the other exercises described later begin to make the spine supple and can also be shown to the owners. Owners need to become educated in stretching their athletes (all human exercise books advocate stretching and warm-up). Stretching helps maintain normal joint motion and reduces muscle tension, resulting in a more flexible athlete, less prone to injury. Unfortunately, most of the training devices and techniques used in horse sports maintain the horse's head in a set position and do not allow the spine to move freely. As a result, chiropractic subluxations occur as the muscle and ligaments become tight as a compensation for the artificial restraint of the training device.

Shoeing

Most, but not all of the time, the imbalances in movement and stance can be corrected with acupuncture, chiropractic, and high-quality trimming and shoeing. In some cases, the shoeing must be altered to really correct the problem. Often this is done by placing either a flat pad or a wedge pad in one shoe and not the other. Some horses require a pad in diagonal legs, in ipsilateral legs, and some in only one leg. They may require the pad for 3 to 6 months, or in some cases permanently. Supplemental acupuncture and chiropractic work generally needs to be done to help maintain the changes.

Exercises

"Sit ups" to tone up the rectus abdominus help raise a horse's back to its natural position. They are induced by running a finger or a plastic device like a needle cap along the ventral midline to stimulate contraction of the rectus abdominus. These are done regularly throughout a grooming or handling session, but not constantly because the horse can become irritated. Many horses cannot raise their backs and need chiropractic adjustments to the withers,

sternum, or ribs before they tolerate this exercise. A horse should not be forced to do these lifts, although small gentle movements can be tried on a regular basis to loosen the thoracic girdle. "Carrot stretches" are very beneficial to the entire spine. Audible popping sounds originate from the abnormally moving joints, and may or may not indicate that an adjustment is occurring. "Leg circles" are done by holding the limb in a relaxed position, similar to that used for cleaning out the hoof. Four or five circles are made with the limb, starting small, and getting larger as the limb loosens. Hip joints are particularly responsive to this exercise, and horses become easier to shoe, sounder in their hindlimbs, and more flexible as athletes when their hip joints are loosened with the "leg circles."

TREATING LAMENESS WITH PHYSICAL THERAPY

Physical therapy consists of noninvasive treatment of injuries by use of lasers, ultrasound, electrical stimulation, magnetic therapy, hydrotherapy, heat, cold, stretching, and massage. These can be used in acute injuries, as well as in the rehabilitation of chronic problems (Table 6). Some of the equipment used for horses has been designed for humans and is generally well tested. Muscles, tendons, ligaments, and bone react in similar ways across species; therefore, human equipment can work on horses, although the protocol for the horse may be different. One must be wary of untrained people, including veterinarians, who have learned from a manual or have taken a manufacturer's short course. They may not have a background in the correct use of the equipment or the physiology and proper care of injuries. Heat and cold are simple physical therapies that are powerful tools when used to their fullest. Ice, applied immediately after an injury, and regularly (every 3 hours or so for 20 to 30 minutes maximum) for the first 24 hours, dramatically reduces swelling, especially when pressure is also applied. Bowed tendons and damaged suspensory ligaments heal more rapidly and with less thickening when an owner is dedicated to the application of ice. Ice massage on hematomas for 15 minutes at a time reduces bleeding. Heat can be more difficult to apply in a barn setting, but it is an excellent form of therapy, particularly in chronic injuries in which poor circulation in the distal limbs may inhibit healing. The use of alternating hot and cold in 5 minute cycles for 15 minutes, beginning with

TABLE 6. CONDITIONS TREATED WITH PHYSICAL THERAPY

Pulled muscles
Sore backs
Joint injuries
Bowed tendons, ligament injuries
Nerve injuries
Muscle spasms
Muscle pulls, strains
Scars and adhesions that form after an injury to the muscle
Restriction in the range of motion caused by soft tissue problems
Rehabilitation following fractures and other serious injuries
Wounds

the hot compress, several times a day for a week is excellent for increasing circulation in the case of a tendon or ligament injury. Horses with sore backs often benefit greatly from hot compresses. A large towel is soaked in a bucket filled with very hot water (not too hot for the hands) and the towel is applied to the horse's back or other chronically sore muscle for about 20 minutes, repeating several times a day.

Cold lasers (Equilight Laser, Equilight, Denver, CO)° are perhaps the most useful and versatile of all the physical therapies to improve the healing injuries, especially of the tendons, ligaments, and wounds. Treatment times are 15 to 30 seconds per site; longer treatments can lead to damage rather than healing. Because lasers reduce the swelling and inflammation associated with a tendon or ligament injury, it is easy to think the injury has healed when diagnostic ultrasound indicates it has not. In this author's experience, laser therapy can reduce healing time by as much as one third; however, in the case of a serious bowed tendon, 6 months to 1 year is still necessary for adequate repair.

Therapeutic ultrasound units send sound waves into the deeper tissues and can heat the deep tissue to the point of injury. Ultrasound† increases the circulation, reduces muscle spasms, can increase the elasticity of scar tissue, and reduces edema. Regular use of ultrasound on the back and hip muscles keeps them soft and supple. Caution must be used in the neck area because the vertebrae are close to the surface. Clients who are dedicated to doing a careful job can use ultrasound to keep their horses' muscles in good shape between acupuncture and chiropractic visits. Ultrasound is best used on alternate days so that the tissue has a chance to heal between treatments, and it is best not to use it for extended periods of time because demineralization of bone can occur.

Electrical stimulators‡ apply a gentle electrical current into the muscle. In a damaged muscle the stimulation is an excellent pain reliever and improves blood flow. These stimulators are also excellent in the rehabilitation stage of an injury, because they can exercise a specific muscle or group of muscles and avoid an imbalance between, for example, the flexors and extensors around a particular joint. Electrical stimulators can also be used to activate a weakened group of muscles that are identified by a lack of muscle symmetry. Electrical stimulators are also excellent for pain control, release of muscle spasms, and improved fracture and tendon healing.

Magnetic field therapies are a convenient way to increase circulation and relieve pain. Chronically sore joints respond well, but when magnets are removed the pain often returns because healing has not occurred. Magnets are being successfully used in navicular disease, either by taping the magnet to the bottom of the hoof, over the navicular bone, or placing small magnets at each end of the navicular bone inside a pad or drilled into the hoof wall. Probably all magnets have a similar effect, even those purchased in a craft shop, although these may not be as strong as more specialized magnets. The differences between products do not appear to be great, despite the advertising. Magnets are best applied for short periods of time, less than 2 hours per day, so they provide a stimulus to heal, then allow the body time to heal on its own.

Electromagnetic blankets are very expensive and popular items that increase blood flow, assist in warming up of the muscles, and cause relaxation by release of endorphins. At horse shows, these units are often used in place of a true warm-up. For many show horses relaxation is a good result; however, in a speed class or on the show-jumping phase of a 3-day event, relaxation can be costly. When treatment is stopped the horse generally returns to its pretreatment level of performance or stiffness because the underlying problems are not resolved. Some manufacturers are advocating very long treatment times, but this author recommends no more than 2 hours a day. Many times good results are obtained in less than 1 hour.

Massage and stretching are part of the physical therapy protocols in human medicine. Learning to provide good therapeutic massage takes extensive training (500+ hours), and delivery of such treatment is generally beyond the scope of practitioners because it requires at least 1 hour per treatment. Good massage is a very beneficial adjunct to all of the therapies discussed here, and aids in the recovery of injuries when the horse is laid up and cannot move on its own. Massage of small areas can be done as part of the overall physical therapy treatment.

Along with any form of therapy for muscles, tendons, and ligaments, rehabilitation is critical for maximal strength and fastest return to work. The muscle and tendon fibers need to heal while being stretched and exercised. If not exercised, the scar tissue that forms is stiff and unyielding, and thus when the horse begins to exercise, the areas above and below the injured site are put under a great deal of strain. If the muscle or tendon heals with regular controlled exercise, beginning as soon as the acute painful period is over, about 1 to 2 weeks on average, the scar tissue fibers align with the tendon tissue, resulting in a strong, more flexible scar. If physical therapy modalities such as the laser, ultrasound, electrical stimulation, heat, and massage are applied regularly, the scar tissue is minimized.

CASE HISTORY

An Olympic-caliber advanced event horse was presented with an extremely sore back, atrophied longissimus dorsi, and a history of being weak in the stifle. The rider was unwilling to replace the ill-fitting saddle. The horse was adjusted chiropractically on December 27, 1994 (C2 and C3 from right side; C4 and C5 from left side; T5, T6, and T7 from the right side; L5 and L6 from dorsal, the right sacroiliac joint, and the left hip) and again on January 30, March 16, April 18, and May 22, 1995, during which the horse was competing at the advanced level. Acupuncture was performed at the same time, using slightly different points each time. At the time of the first two treatments the horse was too sore to treat with needles, and thus a laser was used. Subsequently, he was treated very comfortably with needles. The points used included bladder 19, 22, 23, and 24 along the back, gallbladder 29

°*Not true laser light; 4 pads to place on the skin; 10 mw/cm², available from Equine Therapy Catalogue, Lexington, KY*

†*1 MHz pulsed; Chattanooga Corp, Chattanooga, TN; available from Equine Therapy Catalogue, Lexington, KY*

‡*High voltage pulsed unit, Solsen, Garland, TX; available from Equine Therapy Catalogue, Lexington, KY*

and 30 on the hips, and large intestine 17, gallbladder 21 in the neck, as well as triple heater 13 on the right shoulder.

The horse's right shoulder became stiff after his first event of the season and required acupuncture and stretching for two sessions. Both hips became very tight in the latter half of the season and have required extensive stretching, adjusting, and acupuncture. The horse continues to become very sore at events especially at the withers owing to the saddle and is treated just before each major event. The rider, it is hoped, will be willing to change the saddle to prevent this constant soreness. The horse now has a well-developed longissimus dorsi and no sign of stifle problems, and is performing better than ever. However, due to the saddle-fit problem he cannot go more than 6 weeks without a treatment during his competitive season.

Supplemental Readings

Enwemeka CS: The effects of therapeutic ultrasound on tendon healing: A biomechanical study. Am J Phys Med Rehab 68(6):283–287, 1989.

Kendall DE: A scientific model for acupuncture, part I. Am J Acupuncture 17(3):251–268, 1989.

Lauro A, Mouch B: Chiropractic effects on athletic ability. J Chiro Res Clin Invest 6(4):84–87, 1991.

Porter M: Equine Sports Therapy. Wildomar, CA, Veterinary Data, 1990.

Shoen AM (ed): Veterinary Acupuncture: Ancient Art to Modern Medicine. Goleta, CA, American Veterinary Publication, 1994.

Willoughby SL: Equine Chiropractic Care. Port Byron, IL, Options for Animals Foundation, 1991.

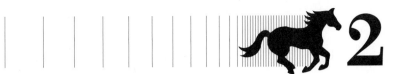
THE MOUTH

Edited by Graham Munroe

Techniques for Examination of the Oral Cavity

GRAHAM MUNROE
EDUOARD CAUVIN
Edinburgh, Scotland

A careful examination of the oral cavity of the horse should form part of the general clinical examination of all equine patients. A detailed evaluation is necessary whenever clinical signs suggest a problem localized to the mouth. If there are problems in other parts of the head, it is wise to thoroughly examine the mouth because of its close anatomic relationship to other systems. Assessment of the conformation and health of the oral cavity, particularly the teeth, also forms an important part of prepurchase and insurance examinations, particularly in the process of ageing by dentition.

HISTORY

As in any clinical examination, the initial step should be to obtain a complete and accurate history. Information should be obtained about the horse's eating habits, quidding, halitosis, biting, riding problems including headshaking, head shyness, vices such as cribbing, loss of condition, and the quality and quantity of the diet. In addition, there may be a history of facial and mandibular swelling, and particularly in the latter case, of draining fistula formation. Apical tooth root infections are a common cause of maxillary paranasal sinus infections and empyema, which lead to a history of chronic unilateral nasal discharge. Oral discomfort may also be manifested in exercising horses by a tendency to mouth breathe or to play with the bit, leading to the possibility of dorsal displacement of the soft palate and choking up.

PHYSICAL EXAMINATION

Even well-trained and well-behaved horses can object to examination of the mouth, and in many cases some form of restraint is necessary. Consideration of the individual animal's temperament and the extent of the examination required determines the appropriate type and amount of restraint. Explanation of the situation to the owner or agent before starting the examination often allays their concerns.

Routine physical methods of restraint, used separately or in combination, include standing the horse in stocks, having an assistant place one or two hands on the horse's nose, holding an ear, and applying a nose twitch. The use of shank chains or bits often obscures the clinician's view of the mouth. In some horses, chemical restraint is required and is best used before making any attempt to examine the horse. Many sedatives and tranquilizers can be used alone or in combination. The authors' preference is a mixture of romifidine° (40 µg/kg) and butorphanol† (20 µg/kg) slowly given intravenously 5 to 10 minutes before the examination is started. Excessive sedation may make the examination more difficult because of ataxia or lowering of the head.

If a horse is very difficult to examine, or when a comprehensive examination is not possible in the standing conscious animal, general anesthesia may be required. The benefits of the improved examination have to be weighed

---

°*Sedivet, Boehringer Ingelheim, Ingelheim, Germany*
†*Torbugesic, Fort Dodge Laboratories, Fort Dodge, IA*

against the risks of anesthesia, but the latter can be minimized with modern anesthetic techniques and monitoring. It may be possible to begin therapy, for example tooth removal, during the same anesthetic period, and suitable preparations should be made to expedite this and minimize time under anesthesia.

Systematic examination of the mouth should begin with evaluation of the external features of the face and jaws both from a distance and also by direct, gentle palpation. The buccal surface of the cheek teeth can be palpated through the cheeks for evidence of sharp edges and pain. Comparison of each side of the head is always useful. Watching the horse eat at some stage during the examination can help clarify an owner's complaints of eating disorders. The lips are next examined, before being separated to allow inspection of the incisors for such factors as conformation, deciduous retention, wear characteristics, and estimation of age. The incisor teeth can also be palpated at this time.

The mouth is then opened by reaching into the interdental space and grasping the tongue, which may be withdrawn, with care, out of the mouth or turned vertically on itself within the mouth and pressure-placed on the hard palate by the clasping hand. Either method allows the mouth to remain open during further inspection. The occlusal surfaces of the incisors and the lower and upper interdental spaces are inspected. If present, the canine and wolf teeth are examined. Examination of the cheek teeth and the caudal oral cavity may be helped by first rinsing the mouth with several large syringes of warm water, particularly if the horse has recently eaten. The caudal oral cavity is first examined visually on the side opposite that on which the tongue is held. This procedure is greatly assisted by the use of a head torch or small flashlight, often held by an assistant. The upper and lower dental arcades with adjacent soft tissue areas are examined. The grasped tongue is moved to the other side to allow examination of the opposite side of the mouth. Following this the dental arcade, especially the lingual and buccal edges, are palpated. This requires considerable care to avoid injury. Traditionally two methods have been suggested, depending on the number of hands that are used. In the two-handed method, the right side of the dental arcade is palpated by grasping the tongue with the right hand and withdrawing it through the left side of the mouth. With the tongue in this position, best achieved through stopping mouth closure, the left hand of the clinician is passed between the right dental arcade and the cheek, with the knuckles toward the latter. The cheek teeth are then palpated with the fingertips. The left dental arcades are palpated in the same way but the clinician's hands are changed around. Other clinicians prefer the one-handed technique, especially when horses resent tongue holding. The horse is approached from the front, and the right side of the mouth is palpated by inserting the right hand into the right interdental space. The palm faces laterally and the hand lies between the lingual aspect of the cheek teeth and the tongue, thereby forcing the latter between the left cheek teeth and stopping the horse from closing its mouth. Either method should be undertaken as quickly as possible to decrease the likelihood of patient resentment. A fetid necrotic smell on the hand after withdrawal from the mouth suggests pocketing of stale ingesta, advanced dental necrosis, or anaerobic bacterial infection.

Complete examination of the standing horse's mouth is difficult and may be only marginally improved by the use of a gag. The use of the Haussman gag in conscious horses is controversial because of the potential danger to attending people. If a detailed examination of the dental arcades, associated soft tissue areas, or caudal oral cavity is required, general anesthesia is recommended. Under these circumstances visualization is enhanced by the use of an endoscope or dental mirrors.

RADIOGRAPHY

Radiography of the horse's head and teeth forms an important part of the examination of the oral cavity. Adequate diagnostic radiographs of the head and teeth, especially lateral views, can be obtained in general practice using portable equipment in the standing sedated horse. The use of rare-earth screens and compatible films improves the quality further. Some views such as 30 to 45° oblique, dorsoventral, or intraoral views give more specific detail but may require the horse to be anesthetized to gain adequate images. The diseased side should be placed next to the cassette. If a draining sinus is present, a radiopaque probe or solution can be inserted into it to help identify the extent and direction of the tract. Externally recognized swellings may also be identified on a radiograph by the use of small radiopaque markers placed on the skin. Radiopaque foreign bodies, such as wire, can be seen clearly on head radiographs, but the more common plant material may be undetectable. The interpretation of radiographs of the head is difficult because of the varying radiographic densities of the tissues present and the complicated anatomy. This is especially so when evaluating the involvement of the teeth and paranasal sinuses. Although the radiologic features of dental disease in horses are well recognized and are described elsewhere in this section (see page 150), even experienced clinicians find definitive interpretation difficult. The use of a number of different radiographic projections can help. The erect lateral view is most useful for assessing the paranasal sinuses, whereas the lateral oblique views, and in the case of incisor teeth the intraoral views, give specific detail on tooth roots.

EXAMINATION OF PARANASAL SINUSES

Up to 50% of cases of chronic paranasal sinus empyema are associated with dental disease, and, therefore, examination of the sinuses is indicated when considering abnormalities of the oral cavity. The nostrils should be examined for the presence of nasal discharge, which is often unilateral, mucopurulent, and increased after exercise or feeding from the floor. A fetid odor is common and indicates turbinate or bone necrosis. Direct external palpation of the maxillary sinuses may reveal heat, swelling, and pain, whereas percussion may detect areas of decreased resonance when compared with the normal side. Erect lateral radiographs of the sinuses using a horizontal beam may demonstrate fluid lines, if liquid material is present, or diffuse opacities, if granulation tissue or inspissated material obscures the normal air spaces.

ENDOSCOPY

Direct visual examination of the upper respiratory tract by endoscopy is useful in detecting secondary effects of oral cavity disease on the respiratory tract. Damage to the nasal septum and turbinates may be detected, but endoscopy is most useful to confirm that the nasomaxillary openings are the source of a nasal discharge and, hence, to confirm sinusitis.

SINUSCOPY AND SINOCENTESIS

Direct endoscopic examination of the rostral and caudal maxillary and frontal paranasal sinuses can be performed routinely in standing sedated animals. A small skin bleb of local anesthetic at the appropriate site allows a skin stab and trephine hole to be made through the facial bones with the aid of a short Steinmann pin and chuck. A sterilized endoscope or arthroscope can then be pushed into the paranasal sinuses and their internal structures, including dental alveoli, may be visualized. Three portal sites are used to allow the major paranasal sinus compartments to be examined. The frontomaxillary portal is made 60% of the distance laterally from the midline of the head to the medial canthus of the eye and immediately caudal to this line. Caudally a view is gained into the conchofrontal sinus, whereas ventrally the caudal maxillary sinus is seen via the frontomaxillary aperture. The caudal maxillary portal is 2 cm rostral and 2 cm ventral to the medial canthus of the eye in the angle formed by the rim of the orbit and facial crest. This approach allows an excellent view of the caudal maxillary sinus. The rostral maxillary portal is made 40 to 50% of the distance from the rostral end of the facial crest to the level of the medial canthus and 1 cm ventral to the line joining the infraorbital foramen and medial canthus, making sure to place the portal in the angle formed by the facial crest and angular vein of the eye. This portal gives a view of the root of the fourth cheek tooth and mucoperiosteal septum separating the rostral and caudal maxillary sinus compartments. Samples can be collected for culture and biopsy via a second trephine hole, under endoscopic guidance, and therapeutic lavage also may be accomplished. The skin is sutured, and healing is usually uncomplicated.

Supplemental Readings

Baker GJ: Oral examination and diagnosis: Management of oral diseases. *In* Harvey CE (ed): Veterinary Dentistry. Philadelphia, WB Saunders, 1985, pp 217–220.

Gibbs C, Lane JG: Radiographic examination of the facial, nasal and paranasal sinus regions of the horse. II. Radiological findings. Equine Vet J 19:474–482, 1987.

Lane JG, Gibbs C, Meynink SE, Steele FC: Radiographic examination of the facial, nasal and paranasal sinus regions of the horse. I. Indications and procedures in 235 cases. Equine Vet J 19:466–473, 1987.

Rose RJ, Hodgson DR: Manual of Equine Practice. Philadelphia, WB Saunders, 1993, pp 4–9.

Differential Diagnosis of Dysphagia

ELSPETH MILNE
Dumfries, Scotland

Dysphagia means difficulty in swallowing (deglutition), although the term is sometimes used generally for difficulty in eating. In this chapter, emphasis is placed on pharyngeal and esophageal conditions that cause true dysphagia. Difficulty in prehension and mastication and nasogastric reflux must always be included in the differential diagnosis of conditions causing dysphagia.

DISORDERS WITH TRUE DYSPHAGIA AS A MAJOR SIGN

Pharyngeal Dysphagia

Swallowing is a complex process with pharyngeal, cricopharyngeal, and esophageal components. The pharyngeal and cricopharyngeal phases are controlled by the nucleus ambiguus with additional input from higher centers, via the glossopharyngeal and vagus nerves. In the pharyngeal phase, the food bolus formed in the oropharynx is moved caudally into the pharynx while the soft palate closes off the nasopharynx and the epiglottic and arytenoid cartilages close the glottis. In the cricopharyngeal phase, the caudal pharyngeal muscles contract and the cricopharyngeal muscles relax, then contract, behind the bolus at the upper esophageal sphincter.

In pharyngeal dysphagia, the major clinical signs are coughing due to aspiration of food and the return of saliva and masticated food from the nares. Congenital causes of pharyngeal dysphagia include cleft palate, congenital neuromuscular pharyngeal dysfunction, pharyngeal and subepiglottic cysts, cricopharyngeal-laryngeal dysplasia (formerly called rostral displacement of the palatopharyngeal arch), and guttural pouch tympany. Pharyngeal cysts and cleft palate are discussed elsewhere in this section. Guttural pouch tympany results from a congenital defect of its pharyngeal ostium and may be unilateral or bilateral. Especially if bilateral, the tympany may cause pressure on the pharynx, which lies ventral to the guttural pouches. Tympany is readily detected by physical examination and radiography. Although a congenital disorder, cricopharyngeal-laryngeal dysplasia may not be evident until several months to years of age. The clinical signs are variable but include dysphagia, regurgitation and, in some cases, abnormal respiratory noise at exercise. Radiographic examination may reveal a shortened larynx and air in the cranial esophagus. Rostral displacement of the palatopharyngeal arch is sometimes present in such cases and can be seen on endoscopy.

Acquired space-occupying lesions that may cause pharyngeal dysphagia include polyps, neoplasia, and foreign bodies. Similar effects may result from external pressure on the pharynx by, for example, infections and snakebite, which cause local edema, guttural pouch distension with pus (empyema) or blood, enlargement or abscessation of the retropharyngeal lymph nodes in *Streptococcus equi* infection (strangles), and peripharyngeal hemorrhage or neoplasia. However, external pressure on the pharynx is likely to cause respiratory stridor before dysphagia is evident, and in clostridial myositis and strangles, systemic signs also are seen. A combination of careful palpation; endoscopy, including examination of the guttural pouches; and radiography are valuable in such cases. Pharyngeal pain associated with pharyngitis, trauma, or fistula formation may also cause dysphagia and can be detected endoscopically.

Neurologic disease associated with pharyngeal dysphagia is most commonly the result of guttural pouch mycosis. The location of the glossopharyngeal, vagus, and accessory nerves across the caudal roof of the guttural pouches renders them subject to damage by mycotic plaques. This may result in unilateral or bilateral pharyngeal paralysis or loss of sensation affecting the pharyngeal mucosa. On endoscopy, a lack of pharyngeal movement may be seen in response to flushing the nasopharynx with water. In mycosis, epistaxis may occur, and secondary empyema may result in a purulent unilateral or bilateral nasal discharge. Other causes of pharyngeal paralysis are lesions such as abscess, trauma, or neoplasia that affect the swallowing center in the medulla. Grass sickness (equine dysautonomia) seen in Europe and mal seco in the southern part of South America can also produce clinical signs suggestive of pharyngeal in addition to esophageal dysphagia. Recent evidence indicates that grass sickness and mal seco are clinically and pathologically identical. Diagnosis of grass sickness relies on histologic examination of the autonomic ganglia (see page 203).

Esophageal Dysphagia

In horses, the proximal two thirds of the esophagus contain striated muscle under neurogenic control of the nucleus ambiguus, whereas the distal third contains smooth muscle and is innervated by the dorsal motor nucleus of the vagus. Both sections of the esophagus contain a myenteric plexus. Esophageal dysphagia results from difficulty in moving a food bolus from the upper to the lower esophageal sphincter or from the esophagus to the stomach and must be distinguished from the gastric reflux that occurs in the presence of gastric or intestinal obstructive lesions. Esophageal dysphagia may be the consequence of congenital anomalies, external compression, intramural lesions, intraluminal lesions and obstructions, and motility disorders.

The clinical signs of esophageal obstruction are regurgitation of saliva mixed with food via the nares and/or mouth at varying times after swallowing coupled with excessive salivation. Esophageal spasm may occur, especially with intraluminal obstructions, and is accompanied by distress, retching, squealing, and episodes of flexion or hyperextension of the neck.

Congenital anomalies are rare, but the major defects are megaesophagus, strictures, duplication cysts, atresia, and persistent right aortic arch. Dysphagia associated with regurgitation of milk may be present from birth, but this depends on the degree of obstruction or interference with motility and may not be evident until solid food is being consumed. Acquired lesions causing external compression on the esophagus are relatively rare as a cause of dysphagia but have been recorded with mediastinal lymphadenopathy and with abscesses or neoplasia in contiguous structures in the neck or thorax. External compression may be detected by palpation if in the cervical region, or by contrast radiography.

Of much greater importance are intraluminal obstructions. Most are the result of accumulation of food material, classically sugar beet pulp, but also cubes, grain, poorly masticated fibrous material, and, rarely, foreign bodies such as stones. Predilection sites are immediately caudal to the upper esophageal sphincter, the thoracic inlet, and sites dorsal to the heart and the distal thoracic esophagus. The condition is not difficult to diagnose based on clinical examination, examination by passage of a nasogastric tube or endoscope, plain radiographs or, if necessary, contrast radiography. Other intraluminal obstructions and intramural lesions may produce similar signs as food obstructions after swallowing. These intraluminal obstructions include intramural abscesses or cysts, esophageal diverticulum, acquired strictures, and neoplasia (especially squamous cell carcinoma). The rapidity of onset can aid in differentiating whether the obstruction is the result of foreign material or soft tissue swellings. Other aids to differential diagnosis are examination after gentle passage of a well-lubricated nasogastric tube (for diagnostic purposes only), endoscopy, and positive or double-contrast radiography. Incomplete obstructions often result in dysphagia after food but not fluid ingestion. Painful lesions such as esophageal laceration, esophagitis due to ingestion of irritants, chronic gastric reflux, repeated nasogastric intubation, or esophageal ulcers associated with gastric ulceration or following food impaction may initially produce more subtle signs than obstruction, but pain on deglutition accompanied by spasm, excessive salivation, and occasionally reflux of ingesta may be seen. The latter may occur progressively because stricture formation may be a sequel to these conditions. Perforation or fistula formation may follow transmural laceration or long-standing obstruction. Emphysema and cellulitis are likely to develop, and saliva and food are visible if perforation is associated with an open neck wound, whereas mediastinal abscessation follows intrathoracic perforation.

Megaesophagus is occasionally seen as a congenital disorder when it may be the consequence of a persistent right aortic arch or a presumed congenital defect of its innervation. Acquired megaesophagus is a major feature of grass sickness, in which contrast radiography reveals barium pooling in the thoracic esophagus and on endoscopy, poor tone in the distal esophagus, together with linear erosions of reflux esophagitis. Megaesophagus has also been associated with "windsucking" behavior despite a report that aerophagia is minimal. When assessing esophageal function by endoscopy or radiography, it is important to remember that sedation with detomidine can cause retrograde peristalsis and pooling of barium in the thoracic esophagus of normal horses and that this effect is exacerbated by prior passage of a nasogastric tube. If equipment is available, fluoroscopy is a valuable aid to the assessment of pharyngeal and esophageal function.

SYSTEMIC DISEASES IN WHICH DYSPHAGIA MAY BE A CLINICAL SIGN

Detailed discussion of these conditions is beyond the scope of this chapter. Most such conditions present as neurologic diseases. Dysphagia may be a component of rabies, the viral encephalitides (eastern, western, and Venezuelan encephalitis), tetanus, botulism, bacterial encephalitis or meningitis, equine protozoal myeloencephalitis, intracranial migration of helminths (*Strongylus vulgaris* and *Micronema deletrix*), leukoencephalomalacia ("moldy corn" poisoning), hepatic encephalopathy, hypocalcemia, hyperlipemia, lead or organophosphorus toxicity, cauda equina neuritis, and neonatal maladjustment syndrome.

DISORDERS THAT MAY BE CONFUSED WITH DYSPHAGIA

Difficulty in prehension may be confused with dysphagia. In the horse, the upper and lower lips are the main prehensile structures with lesser involvement of the incisors and tongue. Clinical manifestations vary with the cause and the type of feed, but they result in difficulty in grasping food or dropping of unmasticated material from the mouth. Causes include lip injuries; incisor malocclusion or pain; tongue lesions; fractures of the mandible, maxilla, or hyoid apparatus; central or peripheral neurologic deficits affecting the facial, trigeminal, and hypoglossal nerves; and nigropalladial encephalomalacia (yellow star thistle poisoning).

Difficulty in mastication may be manifested as inability to open the mouth, or more usually, slow chewing, chewing on one side of the mouth, excessive salivation and dropping of partially chewed boluses from the mouth, or the accumulation of food between the cheek teeth and the cheeks. If dental or oral lesions are present, there is often a fetid smell. Selective eating of feeds that require less mastication may be observed. The most common cause is dental disease affecting the premolars and molars. Difficulty in mastication can also be the result of painful lesions of the oral soft tissues such as stomatitis, glossitis, oral neoplasia, oral foreign bodies, abscesses, and granulomas. Diseases of the temporomandibular joints are rare in horses, but fractures, dislocations, and chronic arthritis have been reported, leading to pain and restriction of jaw movement. Neurologic diseases that affect the facial, trigeminal, or hypoglossal nerves also interfere with mastication.

Reflux of gastric fluid may be confused with regurgitation associated with dysphagia, but clinical examination is likely to reveal other clinical signs of a functional or mechanical obstruction of the gastrointestinal tract, in particular, the presence of colic. The refluxed material, which usually refluxes from the nares rather than the mouth, is generally bile-stained. However, in acute grass sickness, both nasogastric reflux and true dysphagia can occur concurrently.

Supplemental Readings

Cohen ND: Neurologic evaluation of the equine head and neurogenic dysphagia. Vet Clin North Am Equine Pract 9(1):199–212, 1993.
Gibbs C, Lane JG: Radiographic examination of the equine pharynx, larynx and soft tissues of the neck. Vet Annual 31:1–19, 1991.
Hennig GE, Steckel RR: Diseases of the oral cavity and esophagus. *In* Kobluk CN, Ames TR, Geor RJ (eds): The Horse: Diseases and Clinical Management. Philadelphia, WB Saunders, 1995, pp 287–314.

Congenital Abnormalities of the Mouth and Associated Structures

CEDRIC C-H. CHAN
Glasgow, Scotland

GRAHAM MUNROE
Edinburgh, Scotland

The more common and important congenital abnormalities of the mouth are discussed in this chapter; however, most of those involving the teeth are covered elsewhere in this section.

CLEFT PALATE

Cleft palate (or palatoschisis) is an uncommon congenital abnormality in which defects of the primary palate (external nares and lips) and those of the secondary palate (hard and soft palate) can occur. The most common presentation is a defect of the caudal one half to three quarters of the soft palate that occurs as a result of failure of the lateral palatine processes to completely fuse in a rostral to caudal direction during embryogenesis. The heritability of cleft palate in the horse is unknown, but breeding from affected animals is not recommended at present.

Diagnosis

The diagnosis of cleft palate is based upon the history of bilateral nasal discharge containing milk or food after suckling or feeding. Intraoral and nasal endoscopic examination of the oronasal cavity usually reveals an orofacial or oronasal defect. A lack of palatal tissue in contact with the inferior border of the epiglottis and the impression that the epiglottis has "dropped into the oral cavity" are confirmatory features. The extent of the clefting and dehiscence of the soft palatal muscles ("submucosal clefting") should be noted, because these features affect the possibility of treatment. Because concurrent aspiration pneumonia may be present, careful auscultation of the lung fields is necessary and, in some cases, thoracic radiography or ultrasound may be useful. Bacteriologic culture and antibiotic sensitivity testing of transtracheal aspirates should be carried out to direct appropriate antibiotic therapy. The foal's inability to feed properly may lead to a failure of passive transfer of immunoglobulins and chronic malnutrition.

Treatment

The treatment of cleft palate involves surgical repair of the palatal defect and intensive management of concurrent problems, such as aspiration pneumonia. Careful consulta-

tion with the owner is recommended because the surgery has a high failure rate, commonly poor postoperative growth rates, and high associated expense. Surgery should ideally be carried out as early as possible to restore palatal function and decrease the severity of concurrent medical problems. In addition, surgery on younger foals may provide better surgical exposure. The prognosis for repair of the soft palate is slightly better than for correction of the hard palate. However, the prognosis for complete surgical correction is poor in all cases.

Postoperatively, systemic broad-spectrum antibiotics and tetanus antitoxin should be given. Nonsteroidal anti-inflammatory drugs may decrease swelling of the tongue and may minimize discomfort. Foals should be encouraged to suckle as soon as possible after surgery, and older horses should be fed a water-soaked gruel. Feeding by nasogastric tube is to be avoided, if possible, to minimize iatrogenic damage to the surgical repair.

DENTIGEROUS CYSTS

Dentigerous cysts are congenital abnormalities consisting of epithelium-lined cavities containing one or more dental elements, any or all of which may be malformed. Other terms for dentigerous cysts include *heterotopic polyodontia, ear fistula, temporal cyst, ear tooth, temporal odontoma,* and *temporal teratoma.* The latter term is inappropriate because it denotes a true neoplasm. Dentigerous cysts are not thought to be heritable.

These cysts appear to originate from a failure of closure of the first branchial cleft or inclusion of cell nests in this area. Usually the dentigerous cyst is present at the base of the pinna of the external ear, although other locations on the head have been reported. The dental structures may be loosely enclosed in the cyst or may be firmly attached to underlying bone. Teeth within dentigerous cysts often resemble cheek teeth and are usually single.

Diagnosis

Clinically, dentigerous cysts typically present as a firm, nonpainful swelling at the dorsolateral aspect of the cranium, below the ear. This swelling is often associated with a draining tract exuding a sticky, seromucous discharge either around the base of the pinna or directly over the swelling. The cysts are usually present at birth and enlarge during the first few weeks of life. Most are usually diagnosed within the first 2 years of life. Other diagnostic procedures include exploration of the draining tract with a sterile probe and aspiration of cyst contents, which are usually white to honey-colored mucoid exudates. Biopsy is usually unrewarding. A thorough radiographic evaluation can be very useful, and positive contrast fistulography may help delineate the extent of the cyst and its associated fistula.

Treatment

Management of dentigerous cysts involves surgical resection under general anesthesia of all dental and cystic elements. Particular care must be taken during resection owing to the regional neurovascular anatomy and the possibility of calvarium fracture during the removal of bone-attached dental elements. The prognosis following surgery with complete resection is good.

PHARYNGEAL CYSTS

Congenital pharyngeal cysts occur at three possible locations in the pharynx. The most common position is subepiglottic, and these are thought to be a remnant of the thyroglossal duct. Dorsal pharyngeal cysts are less common and may be a remnant of the craniopharyngeal duct or Rathke's pouch. Soft palate cysts may have resulted from aberrant fusion of the embryologic lateral palatine processes.

Pharyngeal cysts can present at any age, although they usually occur in younger animals, and no breed predisposition or hereditability is known. Males have been noted to be twice as likely to be affected as females. Clinically, abnormal respiratory noise is present during both inspiration and expiration, particularly at exercise. Coughing or dysphagia may also be noted. Definitive diagnosis is made by nasal endoscopy of the upper airway. An abnormally raised, circumscribed enlargement directly under the epiglottis, in the aryepiglottic fold, may be present if the cyst is subepiglottic. Dorsal displacement of the soft palate may be seen with cysts in a soft palate or aryepiglottic position. Plain and contrast radiography may be useful in delineating the full extent of the lesion.

Surgical resection of pharyngeal cysts is the treatment of choice. An oral ventral laryngotomy or pharyngotomy approach may be used depending on the nature, size, and location of the cyst. Resection is made easier by not draining the fluid contents before dissection. Transendoscopic Nd:YAG laser removal has also been described. Following complete cyst resection, the prognosis is good.

WRY NOSE

Wry nose (or deviated nasal septum) is a congenital deformity of the nasal and premaxillary bones that results in a laterally deviated rostral face and maxillomandibular malocclusion. Commonly, a concurrent dorsoventral nasal deviation is present, and, occasionally, torticollis may also be observed. The cause of wry nose is speculative. The possibility of hereditability has been cited, but a high incidence of the condition in association with dystocia has been reported, and intrauterine malpositioning was implicated as a primary initiating factor.

Clinical signs associated with wry nose depend on the severity of the deformity. Subtle deviations are insignificant, whereas more severe deviations may lead to respiratory compromise or difficulty in suckling or prehending solid food.

The treatment of wry nose in foals is dependent on the severity of the presenting clinical signs. When respiratory or digestive function is manageable by supportive therapy and not compromised, conservative therapy may be indicated. Indeed, complete return to normal facial conformation is possible with further growth and maturation. If the deformity is greater than 20° off normal, however, the prognosis for a spontaneous recovery is poor, and surgical management may be indicated. The surgery is complex, expensive, and not without significant postoperative complications. A two-stage surgical repair with operations carried out 12 weeks apart has been described. The possibilities for differential bone lengthening and the use of periosteal transection of the concave aspect of the deformity have been suggested.

CHOANAL ATRESIA

Choanal atresia is a rare, possibly hereditary, congenital defect usually present with other concurrent congenital craniofacial and dental malformations. Failure of the bucconasal membrane to rupture during early gestation leads to a loss of communication between the nasal cavity and nasopharynx. The condition has been characterized as unilateral or bilateral, complete or incomplete, and bony or membranous. A bilateral complete choanal atresia is an emergency resulting in severe dyspnea due to the obligate nose breathing of the horse. Unilateral complete or incomplete choanal atresia is generally recognized later in life and is not immediately life-threatening owing to compensation by the unilateral patent choana.

The diagnosis of choanal atresia is based upon physical examination and demonstration of complete or incomplete upper airway obstruction. Nasal endoscopy and positive contrast radiographic study results help confirm obstruction of the choanae. The obstructive tissue can be attached dorsally to the sphenoid, ventrally to the caudal aspect of the hard palate, medially to the nasal septum, and laterally to the palatine bone. Both rostral and caudal aspects are covered with respiratory mucosa. A centrally located "dimple" may be present in the partition, suggesting that the primary deformity may be the result of an inadequate excavation of the nasal cavities.

If bilateral complete choanal atresia is present, emergency tracheostomy is indicated as an immediate lifesaving procedure. Surgical correction of choanal atresia has been reported and may be successful in unilateral cases and bilateral cases that have been stabilized. Redevelopment of obstructive tissue is the most common complication. Facial deformity and dental malocclusion have been noted at follow-up examination. Transendoscopic application of Nd:YAG laser or electrosurgical instrumentation may offer future alternatives.

Supplemental Readings

Bowman KF: Cleft palate. *In* Robinson NE (ed): Current Therapy in Equine Medicine, ed 2. Philadelphia, WB Saunders, 1987, pp 1–3.
Gaughan EM, DeBowes RM: Congenital diseases of the equine head. Vet Clin North Am Equine Pract 9(1):93–110, 1993.

Koch DB, Tate LP Jr: Pharyngeal cysts in horses. J Am Vet Med Assoc 173(7):860–862, 1978.
Valdez H, McMullan WC, Hobson HP, Hanselka DV: Surgical correction of deviated nasal septum and premaxilla in a colt. J Am Vet Med Assoc 173(8):1001–1004, 1978.

Ageing of the Horse by Dentition

JILL D. RICHARDSON
Salisbury, England

Although there is a widely held tradition that the age of a horse can be accurately determined from the examination of the teeth, particularly the incisors, this belief is frequently brought into question by practical experiences. As early as 1912, Galvayne suggested that examination of the incisor teeth provided a reliable method of age estimation even of older horses, but such a close correlation between dental morphology and age does not exist. The increasing frequency of malpractice litigation being brought against veterinarians following false estimation of age emphasizes the importance of a thorough examination of the teeth and of setting realistic goals for the accuracy of the ageing technique.

ANATOMY

The teeth of the horse have a limited period of growth, and the permanent incisors are completely formed by 6 or 7 years old, with the long reserve crowns lying subgingivally in the alveolar bone. The teeth erupt relentlessly throughout the life of the animal to compensate for occlusal wear, and thus the length of the reserve crown decreases with increasing age of the animal.

The deciduous, or temporary, incisors are smaller and whiter and are shell-shaped compared with the permanent teeth, and they have a well-defined neck at the junction of the root and crown. The permanent incisors are, by contrast, broader and thicker in structure, with no marked neck and a yellow or brownish color. The horse has 12 deciduous and then 12 permanent incisors with three pairs in the premaxilla and three pairs in the mandible. Each pair of incisors is described as the centrals, laterals, and corner incisors.

AGEING

The age of young horses can be estimated from the times of eruption of the temporary and permanent incisors, and the times when they come into contact with the equivalent tooth in the opposite jaw. Older horses are aged primarily by an evaluation of the changes in the tables of the lower incisors resulting from the balance between the rates of eruption and attritional wear of the teeth. Eruption times and rates of occlusal wear are, however, not constant features and are influenced by numerous factors including breed, nutrition, familial variation, and the presence of vices such as crib-biting. The later maturing "cold-blooded" breeds may have delayed eruption of the permanent incisors by up to 6 months compared with development in the Thoroughbred. The rate of occlusal wear is influenced by the consistency of the diet, and horses on sandy soils or rough pasture have increased rates of wear compared with horses kept on good soil with better pasture.

The eruption times for the deciduous incisors are commonly stated to be from birth to 7 days for the central teeth, 4 to 6 weeks for the laterals, and 6 to 9 months for the corner incisors. The corresponding ages for eruption of the permanent teeth are 2 years 6 months, 3 years 6 months, and 4 years 6 months for the central, lateral, and corner incisors, respectively, but variations from these general rules do exist. The occlusal surface of the permanent teeth usually comes into wear approximately 6 months after the teeth have erupted.

The table of a newly erupted permanent incisor has an elliptical shape, with its mediolateral length being much greater than its craniocaudal dimension. A deep enamel invagination is present on the table and is called the infundibulum or "cup." When viewed from the side the angle made by the upper and lower central incisors is usually almost vertical, but with increasing wear and age, the occlusal angle becomes gradually more acute. This is because the reserve crown moves nearer to the root, and therefore that exposed in old age has a more horizontal implantation in the jaw.

With increasing wear, the shape of the incisor tables alters from elliptical to round, then to triangular and, finally, oval in old age. As the tooth wears, the infundibulum gradually decreases in size and depth until no physical depression exists, but the enamel ring, or "mark," that previously surrounded the infundibulum is still visible. In addition, as the infundibulum is worn away, its position on the incisor table alters. Initially, it is central, but as the horse ages it becomes smaller and moves to take up a more caudal position on the table nearer to the lingual border of the wearing surface. As attrition continues, not only does the depression of the infundibulum disappear, but also the surrounding enamel ring is ultimately worn away.

The dental star that represents stained secondary dentin, which is laid down within the pulp cavity, is a feature that becomes more apparent with increasing age. As the tooth wears and the infundibulum fades, a transverse line appears on the tables cranial to the disappearing infundibulum. With progressive attrition, the dental star assumes a definite dark coloring and then changes its shape and position. Initially, it is seen as a transverse line, but it then becomes oval and finally rounded, and it changes its location on the table to occupy the center of the incisor table. All of these features are initially seen to occur in the central incisors and later in the lateral and corner teeth. This reflects the state of wear of the teeth at any one time, the centrals being the oldest and the corners the youngest incisor teeth.

Other features that are taken into account in age estimation include the presence or absence of hooks on the upper corner incisors. Hooks arise through disparities of wear along the occlusal surface of the mandibular and maxillary teeth. "Galvayne's groove" is visible on the upper corner incisor on its labial surface. A stained groove appears at the gum margin on the labial surface and extends steadily down the tooth as more of the reserve crown is erupted until it reaches the occlusal surface. At this stage the groove is usually seen along the whole length of the tooth, and with increasing eruption at the gum and wear from the occlusal surface it appears to grow out down the length of the tooth. Thus, in the very old horse the groove may be completely lost from the labial surface of the tooth.

When estimating the age of a horse, the clinician must take into account all of the individual features described earlier and form a balanced opinion of the probable age. However, it is clear from the published literature on ageing by dentition that there is a wide range of guidelines stated for each individual feature; for those characteristics that are altered by attrition, large discrepancies in values exist (Table 1). Recent research has confirmed that some features such as the upper corner incisor hook and Galvayne's groove are of negligible value.

In 1994 a survey was carried out examining the dentition of a large number of Thoroughbreds of known age, and the results have cast serious doubts on the view that the age of a horse can be accurately determined from the dentition. In the study, the age of each horse was estimated by independent experienced clinicians, but discrepancies between estimated and real ages were present in all age groups. The size of the inaccuracies increased as the age of the horse under examination increased. Horses with a real age between 8 and 10 years had their age frequently overestimated by as much as 5 years. Horses aged over 12 years had their ages more often underestimated, and discrepancies of as much as 6 years were not uncommon.

It is this author's opinion that the inaccuracies in the technique are not an excuse for careless examination of the incisors when making age estimation, and when the dental inspection is performed all of the available features should be assessed and a written record made of the findings upon which the estimate of age was founded. Veterinarians

TABLE 1.   PUBLISHED VALUES FOR PERMANENT INCISOR AGEING CRITERIA

Criterion	Central	Lateral	Corner
		Age in Years	
Cups worn out	6–7 (4–8)	7 (7–10)	8 (7–10)
Mark (enamel ring) worn away	12 (10–23)	13 (10–23)	15 (13–23)
Star appears	8 (6–13)	9 (6–14)	10 (8–15)
Tables round	8 (6–12)	9 (6–13)	10 (7–14)
Tables triangular	12 (8–18)	15 (9–19)	17 (9–20)

( ) = age range

should ensure that owners, and in particular purchasers, are aware that age estimation using dental criteria provides only an "informed guess." Clear wording of this on the prepurchase certification should help to discourage litigation.

The reliability of individual dental criteria was also investigated in the same study. The eruption of the incisor teeth and evidence of wear on the corner incisors proved to be the most consistent features, although not infallible. The presence of an upper corner incisor hook and Galvayne's groove were criteria of no value when estimating age. Of the attritional features studied, the dental star showed the highest correlation with age, although it was found to appear at ages younger than those usually stated in previous reports. Other features of use were the occlusal angle of the incisor teeth and the shape of the incisor table. The disappearance of the enamel ring was a feature that did not occur until significantly later than is commonly quoted.

In clinical practice, the ageing of horses is related to individual animals, some of whose dental features will permit an acceptably accurate estimate of age, and some of which will not. It is from this latter group that litigation is most likely to arise. Specific ages cannot be assigned to the dental criteria used in age estimation, and predictions of age for individual horses based on dental criteria must only be given with great reservation. Veterinarians in equine practice who use dentition as a means to age horses are strongly cautioned against making claims of accuracy that defy statistical validation.

Supplemental Readings

American Association of Equine Practitioners: Official Guide for Determining the Age of the Horse, ed 5. Lexington, Kentucky, Am Assoc Equine Pract, 1988.

Richardson JD, Cripps PJ, Hillyer MH, O'Brien JK, Pinsent PJN, Lane JG: An evaluation of the accuracy of ageing horses by their dentition: A matter of experience? Vet Rec 137:88–90, 1995.

Richardson JD, Cripps PJ, Lane JG: An evaluation of the accuracy of ageing of horses by their dentition: A study of the changes of dental morphology with age. Vet Rec 137:117–121, 1995.

Richardson JD, Lane JG, Waldron KR: Is dentition an accurate indication of the age of a horse? Vet Rec 135:31–34, 1994.

Walmsley JP: Some observations on the value of ageing 5–7-year-old horses by examination of their incisor teeth. Equine Vet Ed 5(6):295–298, 1993.

Injuries to the Lips and Mouth

JOHN P. WALMSLEY
Liphook, England

INJURIES TO THE LIPS

Lip injuries are relatively common in horses. They may be caused by sharp projections on feed mangers, doors and walls, or lead rope clips. Because the lips have a good vascular supply, wounds usually heal with or without treatment. The decision to treat these injuries depends on both functional and cosmetic criteria.

Superficial Abrasions

Superficial injuries that have not penetrated the skin or mucous membrane are best treated conservatively. Contaminated wounds should be gently lavaged with saline or dilute povidone-iodine solution. Antiseptic or antibiotic ointments are the most appropriate topical applications for these wounds because they help to prevent desiccation and are better tolerated than sprays. However, because they are easily rubbed off, they should be applied several times daily, particularly after feeding. Wide feed bowls may help to prevent exacerbation of the injury when the horse is eating.

Severe abrasions can be caused by self-mutilation in horses suffering from irritation following, for example, infraorbital neurectomy for head shaking, or head injuries. Apart from treating the cause of the irritation, it may be necessary to muzzle these horses to protect them. Nonsteroidal anti-inflammatory drugs may be useful in alleviating the irritation.

Full-thickness Lacerations

Untreated deep lacerations usually heal with significant scarring that many owners find unacceptable and that may cause a slight functional impairment. In these cases, surgical repair is the best option. Because of the good blood supply, it is not imperative to treat these wounds immediately, and necrotic, severely traumatic wounds may benefit from being left until healthy granulation tissue has developed. The wound should be debrided by saline lavage and sharp dissection until healthy tissue has been prepared for suturing. Oral mucosa and skin are tightly adherent to the underlying muscle, and they should be dissected free for at least 1 cm to reduce the effect of muscle movement on the superficial sutures. The muscle layer can be sutured with vertical mattress sutures of 3.5- or 4-metric nonabsorbable monofilament suture material (e.g., polypropylene) with the ends exiting away from the skin margins. These can be tied as quill sutures if there is wound tension. The oral mucous membrane should then be closed with simple interrupted 3- or 3.5-metric absorbable monofilament material (e.g., polydioxanone) followed by the skin closure with nonabsorbable monofilament material. If the wound is at the commissure of the lips, the repair can be protected by extra tension sutures through both lips rostral to the wound.

Chronic wounds can be reconstructed by dissecting away granulation tissue until the skin, muscle, and mucous membrane layers can be defined. Closure can then be completed as for acute lacerations. Degloving injuries, in which the lower lip separates from the incisor tooth margins, require stabilization of the lower lip with sutures passed from the ventral skin through the mandibular symphysis and back to the skin where they are tied over tubing. The gingival mucous membrane can then be sutured. Following all these procedures, postoperative antibiotics should be necessary for only 2 or 3 days, and nonsteroidal anti-inflammatory drugs are indicated to combat postoperative swelling for about 4 days.

INJURIES TO THE TONGUE

Tongue lacerations are mostly attributable to bits, foreign bodies, and various traumatic causes such as self-inflicted bites during recovery from general anesthesia. Bit injuries, particularly in polo ponies, can be severe. Excessive pulling on the tongue during restraint can tear the frenulum linguae. Following tongue injuries, horses manifest surprisingly little discomfort and rarely stop eating. The abundant blood supply to the tongue ensures that most wounds heal well without treatment, and even quite badly scarred cases function satisfactorily. Untreated deep lacerations near the apex may heal, but the latter becomes uncontrollable since the mucosa heals across the gap left by the severed muscle. Deep wounds that are likely to cause severe scarring or disfigurement are best treated surgically, particularly if the functional integrity of the apex is at risk.

Surgery is best performed under general anesthesia and as soon as possible. A gauze tourniquet caudal to the wound can be used to gain good exposure. Careful sharp debridement and saline lavage are essential to prepare clean healthy tissue for closure. To obliterate dead space, the deep tissues are best closed in multiple layers using synthetic monofilament absorbable material such as polydioxanone. Failure to obliterate dead space results in wound dehiscence. The mucous membrane can then be sutured in an interrupted pattern with absorbable or nonabsorbable monofilament material. Vertical mattress tension sutures placed away from the wound edges are useful. Glossectomy may be indicated in heavily traumatized avascular injuries and can be performed as far caudal as the frenulum without loss of function. Vascular status can be assessed using intravenous administration of 4 to 5 g of sodium fluorescein for a 450-kg horse and testing for homogenous fluorescence under a Wood's lamp 5 minutes later. Reconstructive surgery has been performed on severe deformities but should not be attempted for at least 4 months following the initial injury. Scar tissue should be excised with care because a worse deformity will develop if too much is removed. Closure is completed as in the acute wound.

Following tongue surgery, antibiotics are usually unnecessary, but nonsteroidal anti-inflammatory drugs help control postoperative swelling. The mouth should be lavaged three to four times daily until healing has been achieved. No feeding restrictions are necessary.

SOFT TISSUE ORAL CAVITY INJURIES

Mucosal injuries in the mandibular diastema are often the result of bit trauma and are commonly manifested by obvious discomfort when the rider is using a bridle. Sharp maxillary cheek teeth cause ulceration in the cheek mucosa. This may also show as a bitting problem but is more often seen as a mild dysphagia with food spilled around the manger and material balled up lateral to the cheek teeth. Removal of the inciting cause usually allows the lesions to resolve. A twice-daily mouthwash with potash alum solution made up at the rate of 1 teaspoon to 1 pint of water may encourage healing. This can be administered by sewing a chamois leather around a bit and soaking this in the solution before hanging the bit in the horse's mouth for 15 minutes.

Supplemental Readings

Howard RD, Stashak TS: Reconstructive surgery of selected injuries of the head. Vet Clin North Am Equine Pract 9:185–198, 1993.

Modransky P, Welker B, Pickett JP: Management of facial injuries. Vet Clin North Am Equine Pract 5:665–682, 1989.

Stashak TS: Wound management and reconstructive surgery of the head region. *In* Equine Wound Management. Philadelphia, Lea & Febiger, 1991, pp 89–144.

Dental Disease

PADRAIC M. DIXON
Edinburgh, Scotland

Dental disease is of such major importance in the horse that up to 10% of equine practice time is involved in dental-related work, including prepurchase estimations of age (see page 146), routine dental rasping, and, less commonly, dealing with more serious dental problems such as malocclusions, periapical abscessation, or traumatic injuries. Despite their obvious importance, equine dental studies have been neglected and little is known about the etiopathogenesis of many common equine dental disorders. In addition, many equine dental treatments have not yet been critically evaluated.

CLINICAL ANATOMY

Adult horses have six upper (maxillary) and lower (mandibular) incisors. A vestigial premolar 1 (wolf tooth) is sometimes present in the permanent maxillary dentition. The remaining three premolars (2–4) and three molars (1–3) are of similar size and shape and all are termed *cheek teeth*. Adult male horses, and on occasion females, also have canine teeth in the interdental space (bars of the mouth).

Equine teeth have evolved to become hypsodont (i.e., they possess long crowns, 7 to 10 cm in the cheek teeth). Most of the crown is unerupted and is termed *reserve crown*. These teeth erupt slowly, about 2 to 3 mm/year, for most of the horse's life. Considerable attrition occurs on the occlusal surface of these teeth owing to the constant grinding of large quantities of fibrous food, and this wear is normally compensated for by the prolonged eruption. Equine teeth have complex folding of their peripheral enamel layer. In addition, the upper cheek teeth and all incisors contain infundibula that further increase the amount of exposed enamel folds on the occlusal surface. Because of different rates of wear between the very hard enamel and the softer dentine and cementum, the occlusal surface of equine teeth has an effective self-sharpening mechanism.

The periphery of the erupted crown of equine teeth has a layer of cementum that gives them a chalky, irregular appearance, except for the rostral aspect of the incisors where it is usually worn away. This is in contrast to the brachydont or short-crowned teeth of dogs and humans, in which shiny enamel is always exposed. This equine feature should not be mistaken as evidence of dental calculus.

CLINICAL SIGNS OF DENTAL DISEASE

A common sign of dental disease is oral pain caused by lacerations of the cheeks and the tongue by sharp dental overgrowths that most commonly occur on the lateral edges of the maxillary and medial edges of the mandibular cheek teeth. Pain may cause a partial oral dysphagia that results in particles of masticated food falling from the mouth during chewing and swallowing, a condition termed *quidding*. Because of oral pain, some horses may also chew very slowly, may use just one side of their mouth, or may hold their head in an abnormal position during eating. Affected horses may readily eat grass or mashes but may be reluctant to eat hay. Painful dental lesions may also cause problems with the bit, including headshaking during work.

With advanced dental overgrowths, a mechanical obstruction may additionally prevent the normal vigorous side-to-side chewing movements of the jaws, and mastication is less effective than normal. A reluctance to eat and reduced food utilization may also occur later, leading to weight loss. Ineffective jaw movements may lead to food accumulating in the mouth and can eventually cause periodontal food pocketing. This leads to secondary periodontal inflammation and malodorous breath. Occasionally, "hamster-like" pouches full of food may occur in the cheeks.

In the case of periapical abscessation of the mandibular and rostral maxillary cheek teeth (1–3), the main sign of disease is a localized ventral mandibular or maxillary swelling, respectively, that is usually followed by sinus tract formation. Very rarely the apical abscess of rostral maxillary teeth discharges medially into the nasal cavity, leading to a purulent, malodorous, unilateral nasal discharge. Periapical abscessation of the caudal three or four maxillary cheek teeth usually results in a unilateral purulent nasal discharge as a consequence of the development of secondary maxillary empyema. Maxillary swellings seldom occur with such sinusitis.

EXAMINATION OF EQUINE TEETH

Palpation through the cheeks may reveal gross irregularities of the cheek teeth, particularly of the maxillary teeth, such as a missing tooth or large overgrowth. The presence of pain during this examination usually indicates the presence of sharp enamel overgrowths on the lateral aspect of the maxillary cheek teeth. Painful or mechanical dental disorders prevent the vigorous grinding action of chewing that normally produces loud "crunching" sounds; horses with painful dental disorders instead make quieter "slurping" sounds. Horses may also show restricted mandibular movements that may be confined to one side of the mouth. By fixing the maxilla with one hand, the degree of lateral mandibular movement can be manually assessed.

Because of a combination of factors, including the limited angle of opening of the equine mouth, the rostral positioning of the lip commissures, and the great length of their dental arcade, it is extremely difficult to visually examine the cheek teeth, particularly the caudal teeth, in an unsedated horse. Food retained in the oral cavity, which further reduces visual examination, can be removed by flushing the oral cavity or, failing that, by manual removal. A more detailed oral examination can be performed with the use of a speculum (gag), but for reasons of safety horses should be sedated during this procedure unless they are very docile. The use of a penlight torch or headlight, and a long metal "toothpick" also facilitates visual oral examination. Nevertheless, major lesions, especially of the caudal cheek teeth 2 to 3, and caudal lingual and buccal ulceration, can be missed unless all the teeth and adjacent soft tissues are carefully palpated. It is useful to smell the examiner's hand after oral examination for the presence of foul-smelling odors.

DENTAL RADIOGRAPHY

Many equine cheek teeth disorders are the result of localized periapical abscessation, and little change is usually evident on the erupted crown unless these infections are long-standing, usually more than 12 months, and have spread to other areas of the tooth. Radiography is therefore essential in the investigation of such disorders. Because of the frequent superimposition of radiodense structures of both sides of the head in equine dental radiographs, even skilled clinicians can have difficulty in interpreting some equine dental radiographs. Latero-oblique (at 30–40° to the horizontal plane, higher angles for smaller horses and for mandibular cheek teeth) projections are most useful to outline the dental apices of the cheek teeth. Lateral radiographs (where both dental arcades are superimposed) are useful to outline fluid (pus) lines in cases of secondary maxillary sinusitis. Dorsoventral projections often outline the degree of changes in adjacent tissues, such as distension of the medial maxillary wall or secondary conchal calcification, and they sometimes demonstrate fractured (always sagittal) maxillary cheek teeth that are inapparent on other projections.

The primary radiographic features of periapical abscessation are loss of density and distortion or even loss of the affected apical area. The normal sharp conical shape of a tooth root develops a blunt "clubbed" appearance. This diseased dental tissue usually becomes surrounded by a sclerotic halo of new bone. The adjacent periodontal space is widened, and there may be disruption of the alveolar cortex (lamina dura denta). However, both of these latter features are often seen in recently erupted equine teeth in normal horses and, therefore, these radiographic signs must be interpreted with caution in the young adult. If mandibular or rostral maxillary external sinus tracts are present, it is most useful to insert metallic probes or contrast medium into these tracts during radiography, both to further define the source of the sinus tract and to obtain landmarks for later surgical intervention. Unfortunately, with disease of the caudal cheek teeth (3–6), tracts or swellings do not usually occur because of exudate draining from the alveolus into the maxillary sinus. This renders investigation of apical disorders of these teeth more difficult.

INCISOR TEETH

Significant disorders of the equine incisors are uncommon. Many horses have some degree of brachygnathism (commonly called parrot mouth, overshot jaw, or overbite) that is esthetically undesirable, especially in show horses. However, unless contact between opposing incisors is totally absent, this condition is seldom clinically significant. Prognathism (sow mouth, undershot jaw, overbite) is uncommon in the horse and is clinically insignificant unless severe. Crib-biting causes abnormal wear on the rostral aspect of incisors, and this area should be carefully inspected, especially during prepurchase examinations. Deciduous incisors are occasionally retained and they should be removed under sedation, especially if they are interfering with eruption of the permanent teeth. Supernumerary *permanent* incisors have very long reserve crowns (up to 7.0 cm, 2.5 inches long) that are usually intimately related to the reserve crowns and roots of the normal permanent incisors. Consequently, extraction of these supernumerary teeth is both very difficult and also risks damaging normal teeth. Because supernumerary teeth cause few clinical problems, they are best left alone, with the exception perhaps of show horses.

Fractures of the incisor teeth can occur as a result of trauma, usually kicks, and commonly result in exposure of the pulp cavity. In all of their teeth, young horses have a wide apical foramen and a large amount of vascular pulp that can resist microbial infection. Consequently, pulp exposure in the younger horses does not necessarily lead to tooth loss. Endodontic (root canal) treatment can be performed on such cases to save the tooth. However, in many younger horses, the exposed pulp becomes sealed off at the site of exposure by secondary dentine formation. The tooth remains vital and continues to erupt.

CANINE TEETH

Because the canine teeth do not anatomically oppose each other, calculus, which is often extensive, can accumulate on them. Equine dental calculus does not generally cause secondary periodontal disease, although extensive calculus formation at this site may cause buccal ulceration. This calculus can be readily removed with strong forceps. Occasionally, displaced or grossly enlarged canine teeth interfere with the bit, and such teeth should be extracted. Because of the great length of their reserve crown (up to 7.5 cm, 3 inches), general anesthesia is necessary for this procedure.

WOLF TEETH

With little justification, wolf teeth (PM 1) are blamed for many behavioral problems and for interfering with the bit; therefore, these teeth are frequently extracted. On rare occasions, displaced, enlarged, or partially erupted wolf teeth may cause oral pain or interfere with the bit. These small structures (1–2 cm long) can be readily extracted under local anesthesia, with sedation if necessary, utilizing a variety of specialized elevators.

CHEEK TEETH

Retained Deciduous Teeth

Retention of the remnants of the deciduous cheek teeth, often termed "caps," can occur in horses between 2 and 4 years of age and may cause oral irritation, with quidding, interference with the bit, and, occasionally, transient oral dysphagia. Such signs in this age group warrant an examination of the rostral 3 cheek teeth for evidence of this disorder and, if present, such caps can be removed using a specialized "cap extractor." Retention of caps may also predispose to delayed eruption and the development of "eruption cysts" under the apices of the permanent cheek teeth.

Disorders of Wear

The equine maxillary cheek teeth arcades are normally 30% farther apart than their mandibular counterparts, with both arcades sloping ventrally in the buccal direction (laterally). As previously noted, this absence of complete occlusal

contact between the upper and lower cheek teeth commonly leads to the development of enamel growths laterally on the maxillary and medially on the mandibular cheek teeth. In horses in which the mandibles are even narrower than usual, these dental overgrowths may become large and permanent. This leads to the development of a sharp, sloped occlusal surface, with an excessively long buccal aspect on the upper and lingual aspect on the lower teeth, termed *shear mouth*. This conformation leads to oral and lingual lacerations during eating and to quidding.

The presence of dental overgrowths may cause uneven wear at different teeth and may lead to the occlusal surface of the cheek teeth becoming uneven in a sagittal plane (*wavemouth*). Food impaction and secondary periodontal infection subsequently occur and can lead to teeth loss, especially in older horses with short reserve crowns. The opposing tooth then erupts more rapidly, leading to the dental irregularity termed *stepmouth*. If neglected, these abnormalities of wear are progressive, leading to oral pain and weight loss. Treatment of these disorders includes removal of overgrowths using specialized dental shears, chisels, guillotines, or embryotomy wire followed by vigorous rasping of cut teeth to smooth out sharp edges. Loose teeth can be extracted orally using specialized equine "molar extractors."

The aim of the equine clinician should be, however, to prevent the development of such end-stage conditions by regular twice-yearly dental inspection and rasping of detected overgrowths, thereby encouraging normal chewing activity and allowing the free movement of food and saliva around the oral cavity.

Diastema

Despite their apices and reserve crowns diverging greatly, the occlusal surfaces of the cheek teeth are normally compressed tightly together and the six teeth function as a single unit. This is achieved by the action of the angled first and last cheek teeth compressing together the occlusal aspect of all of the cheek teeth. Even with age, the progressively smaller reserve crowns are usually tightly compressed at the occlusal surface. However, if spaces develop between the teeth, which is termed *diastema*, interdental food impaction occurs and leads to secondary periodontal disease. Some clinicians suggest that mechanically widening the gap between the teeth decreases food trapping in diastema.

Hooks

A common dental abnormality in horses is a rostral positioning of the maxillary arcades relative to their mandibular counterparts, and this is not believed to be related to incisor prognathism. This rostral positioning leads to an obvious overgrowth or hook on the rostral aspect of the first upper cheek tooth that may interfere with the bit. This hook can be readily cut or rasped. However, a similar overgrowth on the caudal aspect of the sixth lower cheek tooth is frequently undetected and lacerates the oral cavity during mastication. Sedation and use of a gag (speculum) is usually necessary to remove the caudal mandibular hooks. Specialized guillotines are available to encircle this caudal hook and allow its removal with little risk of oral damage.

PERIODONTAL DISEASE

Unlike the situation in brachydont animals, primary periodontal disease is not a significant problem in the horse, although, historically, it appears to have been more of a problem than it is at present. During eruption of the permanent dentition, a transient periodontitis occurs in many horses. Because of the prolonged eruption and continuous development of new periodontal fibers in the horse, equine periodontal disease is not necessarily irreversible, as is the case with brachydont dentition. The most severe periodontal disease in horses occurs as a consequence of malocclusions and is caused by food impaction at the periodontal margin, particularly lateral to the mandibular cheek teeth. The causes of this include: chronic enamel overgrowth or shear mouth; supernumerary cheek teeth (usually at the caudal aspect of the maxillary arcade); diastema; displaced and rotated cheek teeth (especially the fifth maxillary), and sagittally fractured cheek teeth. In horses with chronic periapical abscessation of any etiology, infection may eventually track along the periodontal space to the coronal aspect of the tooth.

Because of a combination of diastema and other abnormalities of wear, especially enamel overgrowths, many or most older horses suffer from secondary periodontal disease. The main treatment for this disorder is to promote normal mastication by mechanically leveling the dental arcades and orally extracting very loose or diseased teeth. With dietary management, horses can be satisfactorily maintained after loss of many of their teeth.

PERIAPICAL INFECTIONS

Much disagreement exists on the terminology relating to equine dental infections. Regardless of etiology, these infections are usually most obvious at the apical region and terms such as *apical, periapical, dental,* or, less accurately, *tooth root abscessation* have been used to describe these lesions. Others have proposed that the term *equine dental caries* be used to cover all infections of mineralized dental tissues. The etiology of these infections in many upper cheek teeth is believed to be from food accumulation and fermentation deep in the infundibulum, with destruction of its enamel walls. This process leads to infection of the pulp cavity, and the term *infundibular necrosis* has also been used to describe these lesions. However, localized caries are very common within infundibula and are usually benign. In addition, the lower cheek teeth do not have a true infundibulum.

It is also believed that an imbalance between cheek teeth wear and the formation of secondary dentine that normally prevents the pulp cavity from becoming exposed can occur. This process leads to exposure and, in some cases, to infection of the pulp cavity in both upper and lower cheek teeth. Regardless of etiology, apical infection of upper cheek teeth (most commonly the fourth) appears to arise at the clinical crown, and conservative treatment such as apicectomy (removal of infected apical area) and endodontic therapy are ineffective if concurrent infection of the crown is present. The success of endodontic treatment of maxillary cheek teeth has not yet been fully evaluated, and the usual therapy for maxillary periapical infections is extraction.

In the lower cheek teeth, periapical abscessation most commonly involves the second and third teeth at 3 to 5 years of age. Initially, this infection is totally confined to the periapical region. The radiolucent periapical area, variously known as *dental sacs, pseudocysts,* or *eruption cysts,* surrounding the apices of these erupting teeth normally causes considerable thinning of the underlying mandibular bone. In a minority of cases, the eruption cyst may even burst through the mandible, leading to exposure and infection of the exposed apical region. Impaction or overcrowding of teeth, certain mandibular conformations, or deciduous teeth retention may predispose to this disorder, which is most common in ponies. In the early stages, that is, in cases of less than 3 months' duration, the infection usually remains confined to the apex and adjacent to the sinus tract, and all the pulp cavities remain vital. At this early stage, oral trimethoprim-sulfonamide therapy for 14 days and possibly coupled with local curettage of the eruption cyst may suffice. Later, one or more of the pulp cavities and adjacent dental tissues may become infected. At that stage, removal of the infected pulp and adjacent infected tissues and endodontic therapy or dental extraction are required. Conservative therapy has been more successful with mandibular than with maxillary cheek teeth periapical abscessation, provided that advanced secondary caries is not established. However, most veterinarians currently prefer to extract these infected teeth.

DENTAL EXTRACTION

Extraction of equine teeth is difficult because of the great length of their reserve crown, especially in the younger horse. Difficulty also arises because, in most early cases of periapical infection, the reserve crown has very extensive healthy, strong periodontal ligaments that are difficult to break down. Additional complicating factors are the tight contact between adjacent cheek teeth and the limited oral access to allow accurate identification of affected teeth and placement of extractors. In older horses, however, especially those with periodontal disease, it is easy to extract teeth orally. Oral extraction of teeth does not require general anesthesia, has few postoperative sequelae, and should be considered when feasible.

Tooth repulsion is the most commonly used dental extraction technique in the horse and consists of hammering a metal punch into the apex of the diseased tooth and repulsing the tooth into the oral cavity, which is normally done under general anesthesia. Very extensive force is required to remove teeth in the younger horse, leading to damage to the alveolus and sometimes to the surrounding bones. In addition, the repulsed tooth often shatters during this process. If an external sinus tract from the abscessed apex is absent, creating a surgical access to the infected apex causes additional trauma. Following repulsion, the oral aspect of the alveolus is sealed with wax or bone cement to prevent food from entering the alveolus. Because of many factors, including surgical damage to the alveolus, remnants of dental tissues within the alveolus, and premature loss of the alveolar packing, significant post-operative infection can occur after equine dental repulsion, especially by anaerobic oral bacteria. In many of these cases the chronic local sepsis requires further treatment, including curettage of the alveolus.

An alternative dental extraction technique for the rostral maxillary cheek teeth 2 to 3 is the lateral buccotomy technique, which also requires the use of general anesthesia. A lateral approach is made to the affected tooth; the overlying lateral alveolar wall is removed, and the tooth is longitudinally cut with an electric burr and loosened. The two halves of the teeth are then extracted through the lateral wall, and the alveolus is packed with gauze that is gradually removed over the following days. Minimal postoperative infection appears to occur after this technique, but it is possible to iatrogenically sever the dorsal buccal nerve during this surgery, thereby leading to a partial facial paralysis.

Supplemental Readings

Howarth S: Equine dental surgery. In Practice (Supplement to Vet Rec) 17:178, 1995.

Lane JG: A review of dental disorders of the horse, their treatment and possible fresh approaches to management. Equine Vet Ed 6(1):13–21, 1994.

Pascoe JR: Complications of dental surgery. Proc 37th Annu Conv Am Assoc Equine Pract, 1991, pp 141–146.

Neoplasia of the Mouth and Surrounding Structures

R. SCOTT PIRIE

W. HENRY TREMAINE
Edinburgh, Scotland

Although neoplasia is uncommon in the horse, a significant proportion occurs in the head and neck. Neoplasia should therefore be considered as a possible differential diagnosis with disorders of these regions, particularly those associated with swellings. For the purpose of this chapter, the sites of neoplasia are divided into categories: the oral cavity, including mandible, tongue, lips, gums, and oropharynx; and the nasal cavity and paranasal sinuses. Despite this division, many neoplasms occurring in each of these regions also involve surrounding structures.

ORAL CAVITY NEOPLASIA

Oral cavity neoplasia can originate from dental tissue (odontogenic), bone (osteogenic), or soft tissues of the mouth and oropharynx. Five types of odontogenic neoplasia have been reported in the horse, and their main characteristics are summarized in Table 1. The classification of odontogenic tumors is based on the inductive effect of one dental tissue on another; however, because of the rarity of these tumors and difficulties in their histologic recognition, a degree of inconsistency exists with respect to their nomenclature.

In the horse, in contrast to many other domestic species, osteogenic neoplasms are usually benign and appear to have a predilection for the mandibular symphysis. Benign osteogenic neoplasms include benign osteoma, ossifying fibroma, and fibrous dysplasia. In addition to these neoplasms, a histologically distinct neoplasm of the rostral mandible of young horses has been well described as *equine juvenile mandibular ossifying fibroma*. Malignant bone tumors are extremely rare in the horse, but more than 80% of osteosarcomas in the horse occur in the head region as compared with the high incidence in the metaphyseal region of long bones in dogs, cats, and humans. Chondrosarcomas, fibrosarcomas, and hemangiosar-

TABLE 1. ODONTOGENIC NEOPLASIA OF THE HORSE

Ameloblastoma (adamantinoma)	Mainly affects the mandible in older animals
	Benign but locally invasive
	Often intraosseous and distorts the mandible
	Radiologically appears radiolucent/cystic
	Spheric or multilocular in gross shape
	Rubbery or cystic in gross appearance
Ameloblastic odontoma (odontoameloblastoma)	Mainly affects the maxilla in younger animals
	Benign, slowly expanding, and locally invasive
	Radiologically appears radiolucent/partially mineralized
Complex odontoma	Contains all the elements of a normal tooth but structure is disorganized
	Possibly a self-limiting malformation
	Radiologically appears ossified, possibly cystic mass
Compound odontoma	Contains all the elements of a normal tooth
	Forms tooth-like structures—denticles
	Regarded as a malformation
Cementoma	Dense mineralized structure
	Often associated with teeth apices
	Histologically at least four types

comas, although recorded in the horse, occur with even less frequency than osteosarcomas.

Soft tissue neoplasia of the equine oral cavity and oropharynx is also extremely rare, with melanomas, squamous cell carcinomas, fibrosarcomas, liposarcomas, papillomas, fibromas, and adenomas reported. As is the case in humans, squamous cell carcinoma is by far the most common malignant tumor of the oral cavity and oropharynx, with invasion of surrounding structures a common finding.

Both osteogenic and odontogenic neoplasms usually present as slowly developing, firm, immobile swellings of the mandible or maxilla. A thorough radiographic examination of the affected area is necessary to exclude the possibility of underlying dental disease, especially periapical abscessation, which is the most common cause of mandibular and maxillary swellings. Consideration of the age of the horse may suggest the type of neoplasm because there is a higher incidence of ameloblastic odontomas in young animals, and ameloblastomas usually occur in the older animal. Equine osteogenic neoplasms show no age predilection. Regular dental examinations may allow early detection of neoplasia of the rostral mouth, but the anatomy of the oral cavity allows considerable progression and expansion of a lesion before it causes major clinical signs. The majority of neoplasms in this region are therefore well advanced, with extensive local infiltration, before clinical signs become apparent. The clinical signs of oral cavity and oropharyngeal neoplasia are dependent on the location and size of the neoplasm and may include dysphagia, halitosis, oral discharge, and submandibular lymphadenopathy. Nasal discharge may be evident if the tumor has expanded to involve the nasal cavity or paranasal sinuses.

NASAL CAVITY AND PARANASAL SINUS NEOPLASIA

Neoplasia of the nasal cavity and paranasal sinuses is also rare in the horse. Neoplasms of the paranasal sinuses include adenocarcinoma, unspecified carcinoma, fibrosarcoma, chondrosarcoma, osteosarcoma, angiosarcoma, papilloma, fibroma, adenoma, chondroma, and, by far the most common, squamous cell carcinoma.

Most paranasal sinus neoplasms are malignant and therefore carry a very poor prognosis. The maxillary sinus is the most frequently affected; 68% of tumors of this region are malignant in the horse. Differentiation between neoplasms and other lesions is therefore important. These lesions may include maxillary cysts, nasal polyps, ethmoid hematomas, primary or secondary sinusitis, false nostril atheromata, mycotic rhinitis, and nasal foreign bodies. The clinical findings in horses with nasal cavity and paranasal sinus neoplasia include halitosis, lymphadenopathy, and unilateral or bilateral nasal discharge, which may vary from mucopurulent to serosanguinous in nature and may be constant or intermittent. The presence of nonpainful facial swelling is a common feature. Expansive lesions in the nasal cavity or sinus may result in nasal air flow obstruction and impairment of sinus drainage. Because of the large network of paranasal sinus cavities that provide room for tumor expansion, most neoplasms in these areas are advanced before

the clinical signs are detected. Endoscopy of the nasal cavity and nasopharynx is of value in identifying the presence and nature of a lesion and distortion of nasal conchae. Radiography of the head is of great value in identification of the presence of masses within the sinuses and distortion of the nasal architecture. Direct sinuscopy allows examination of and the collection of biopsies from lesions in the frontal or maxillary sinuses.

TREATMENT

Surgical removal is the treatment of choice for osteogenic and odontogenic neoplasms involving the equine mandible. Surgical excision and curettage are often followed by recurrence, although this may be delayed for many years. Repeated resections may also result in metastasis. Radical tumor resection in conjunction with partial mandibulectomies, and possible stabilization of the resulting defect with internal or external orthopedic devices, has met with greater success. Extraction of maxillary or mandibular cheek teeth may be necessary if dental or periodontal tissues are involved. As previously stated, many neoplasms of the oral cavity and oropharynx are advanced before detection, and therefore surgical removal often leads to poor success rates because of the difficult surgical access and likely incomplete removal of the lesion. Histologic confirmation of malignancy in extensive lesions is an indication for euthanasia.

The use of laser surgery has been advocated for the ablation of certain soft tissue neoplasms of the oropharynx, nasopharynx, and nasal cavity; however, the success of this therapy is largely dependent on early tumor recognition. The neodymium-yttrium-aluminum-garnet (Nd:YAG) laser has advantages over the carbon dioxide laser in that it can be used transendoscopically in the standing horse. Vaporization should begin in the center of the mass, gradually working to the margins. Multiple applications may be required, depending on the size and density of the mass.

Radical surgical resection is indicated for treatment of neoplasia of the paranasal sinuses. Resection can be performed via a nasofrontal or maxillary flap osteotomy under general anesthesia. This approach has the advantage over transendoscopic Nd:YAG laser surgery in that it permits greater exploration of the affected sinus and is indicated for more extensive lesions. Surgery in this area is frequently accompanied by profuse hemorrhage, and the complex anatomy renders complete removal of lesions with an adequate margin impossible in most cases. The incidence of tumor recurrence is therefore high. Radiation therapy is commonly used in other species either as an alternative to, or in association with, excisional surgery for some oronasal neoplasms, and there is currently some interest in the use of chemotherapeutic agents for the treatment of oronasal tumors in the dog and cat. Techniques that have been employed for radiotherapy of skin and mucosal tumors in the head and neck include application of a strontium-90 probe, or implantation of gold-198 grains or iridium-192 wires into the lesion. External sources of radiation such as megavoltage or cobalt-60 have been used in the horse, but to date these techniques have not been regularly used for treatment of oronasal tumors in this species.

Supplemental Readings

Cotchin E: A general survey of tumours in the horse. Equine Vet J 9:16–21, 1977.

Hance SR, Bertone AL: Neoplasia. Vet Clin North Am Equine Pract 9(1):213–235, 1993.
Madewell BR, Priester WA, Gillette EL, Snyder SP: Neoplasms of the nasal passages and paranasal sinuses in domesticated animals as reported by 13 veterinary colleges. Am J Vet Res 27:851–856, 1976.
Sundberg JP, Burnstein T, Page EH, Kirkham WW, Robinson FR: Neoplasms of equidae. J Am Vet Med Assoc 170:150–152, 1977.

Medical Disorders of the Mouth

D E R E K   C .   K N O T T E N B E L T
Liverpool, England

The mouth is subject to primary and secondary diseases and frequently provides a useful aid to the diagnosis of systemic disorders. Primary disorders may also involve other body systems; the exquisite neurologic control of oral function required for prehension, chewing, and swallowing provides opportunities for disorders to arise from relatively minor neurologic dysfunction. Pain with or without oral ulceration usually induces anorexia with or without salivation.

CHANGES IN THE APPEARANCE OF THE ORAL MUCOUS MEMBRANE

The oral mucous membranes provides a "window" on cardiorespiratory function and is an effective indicator of some blood disorders. Changes in the appearance and character of the oral mucous membrane include pallor, cyanosis, icterus, and petechiation.

Oral Petechial Hemorrhages

Oral petechial hemorrhages should alert the clinician to the possibility of underlying disease including vascular and coagulation defects. Idiopathic and autoimmune-mediated thrombocytopenia can cause loss of vascular wall integrity, and mucous membranes that are stressed, such as those of the mouth, are more likely to show petechial or larger (ecchymotic) hemorrhages. Petechiation may reflect a loss of vascular integrity or a failure of clotting mechanisms, particularly with respect to platelet function. Examples of these types of condition include: immune-mediated vasculitis in systemic lupus erythematosus-like syndrome; vascular endothelial damage from endotoxemia or drug reactions; and thrombocytopenia resulting from underlying serious diseases such as lymphosarcoma, internal abscessation, or repeated stimulation of the reticuloendothelial system. Nonthrombocytopenic purpura and petechiation are also features of purpura hemorrhagica in horses with a recent history of viral or bacterial respiratory disease. Clotting defects such as congenital hemophilia and warfarin (coumarin) poisoning result in persistent leakage of red cells into damaged areas, forming hematomas but rarely causing petechiation.

Lampas

Historically, this condition was recognized when the hard palate mucosa of young horses was "swollen" and hung below the occlusal surface of the upper incisor teeth. It was commonly treated by cautery (firing) of the mucosa of the hard palate and, more recently, by injection of corticosteroids into the mucosa. Histologic examination shows that the mucosa is normal, although there is often some submucosal edema. The condition is now regarded as a normal, insignificant consequence of incisor or molar eruption. It appears that there is no justification for treatment. Spontaneous resolution usually occurs, although the mucosa may remain slightly "billowed." Edema of the hard palate of older horses may follow ingestion of sharp grain awns and irritant plant material, in particular those plants with "hairy leaves" or irritant components.

Epulis

This is a benign, nonspecific inflammatory hyperplasia of the gingiva that may present as a tumor-like mass at the tooth-gingival interface, often at the base of the canine teeth. Chronic inflammation of the gum margin from dental tartar or plant irritation is often suggested as the etiology. Many cases are insignificant, especially in the older horse, but some have more severe proliferation. Differential diagnosis includes neoplasia, foreign body reactions, and migrating *Habronema* and *Gasterophilus* species larvae, which induce transient granulomatous reactions (epuloid) at the gum margin. The pathologic character of the tissue should be definitively established. Treatment is rarely warranted but involves removal of the inciting cause and excision of the hyperplastic mass by sharp dissection, laser surgery, or cryosurgery. Recurrences are relatively common.

TONGUE PIGMENTATION

Horses that habitually lick the bark of some trees can develop a black discoloration of the tongue and to a lesser extent other areas of the oral mucosa. Apple and oak trees seem particularly liable to induce this insignificant condition.

ULCERATIVE DISORDERS OF THE TONGUE AND ORAL MUCOSA

Ulceration of Dental Origin

This common problem is discussed elsewhere in this section (see page 147).

Oral Ulceration Induced by Caustics or Irritants

Horses are less inclined than other large animal species to sample irritant chemicals but are still affected occasionally by irritant chemicals such as creosote or caustic disinfectants. The extent of damage depends upon the chemical, its concentration, and the duration and location of contact. Prolonged mastication of foodstuffs containing irritants makes ulceration more common in the mouth than in the esophagus. Most cases have an acute onset of salivation with slowing of eating. The saliva may be blood-stained and halitosis may occur. Weight loss becomes evident later. Horses suffering from phenylbutazone toxicity and the possibly related end-stage renal failure show oral ulceration, particularly on the buccal mucosa. Salivation is increased as a result of the oral discomfort. The blister beetle (*Epicauta* species) toxin cantharidin (see page 666) causes severe oral ulceration, but it may be insignificant compared with the concurrent cardiovascular and intestinal damage.

Treatment of irritant-induced ulceration is symptomatic once the inciting cause is removed. Warm soft foods such as mashes, possibly with added glycerine, are advisable. Attempts to treat oral ulceration topically are difficult and unrewarding.

Pituitary Adenoma, Cushing's Disease, Hyperadrenocorticism

Oral ulceration and diastema formation are common features of this disease complex. Secondary bacterial infections and oral abscessation with periodontal infection is common in these immunosuppressed horses. Interestingly, affected horses show little salivation and are only sometimes reluctant to eat. Affected horses are usually older than 15 years of age and show a variety of other signs including hirsutism, polydipsia, polyuria, laminitis, parasitism, and weight loss. Differentiation from end-stage renal failure, periodontal disease, and phenylbutazone (and more rarely arsenical and mercury) poisoning should be based on clinical evidence and supportive laboratory investigations.

Treatment of the oral lesions independently of the underlying disease is fruitless, and because the oral lesions are a sign of advanced disease, affected animals carry a poor prognosis.

Foreign Body

Foreign bodies such as thorn twigs or wire become lodged in the mouth between the cheek teeth, under the tongue, or between the cheeks and the teeth. They are distressing and induce salivation, fetid breath, and reluc-

tance to eat. Saliva is frequently blood-tinged. Some animals make fruitless attempts to eat, and food may accumulate in the mouth. Loops of nylon baling twine can become looped around the base of the tongue with the free ends in the esophagus, and affected animals present with dysphagia and nasal reflux of food material and saliva. Signs associated with pharyngeal foreign bodies are similar, with obvious distress during swallowing and occasionally bilateral epistaxis. Diagnosis relies on careful visual and endoscopic examination of the mouth with appropriate restraint and equipment protection. Treatment should be directed at removal of the cause and appropriate after-care including antibiosis, tetanus prophylaxis, and analgesia.

PTYALISM

Salivation is an important clinical sign associated with irritation of the oral mucosa. Care should be taken to differentiate overproduction of saliva (ptyalism) from dysphagia. In the former, volumes of saliva are so excessive that they cannot be swallowed, whereas in the latter, there is some obstruction to effective swallowing. Salivation, without nasal reflux of saliva, is seldom the result of esophageal obstruction. Young foals exhibiting salivation and bruxism should be investigated for possible gastric ulceration. Older horses commonly show salivation (ptyalism) when excited or when mouthing on the bit (so-called "bit gnathism"). A stable foam is formed that is difficult for either horse or clinician to clear, making diagnosis difficult.

Profuse salivation of acute onset associated with a fetid breath and blood staining suggests oral ulceration or serious ulceration of alimentary mucosa caudal to the mouth. Oral infestation with migrating *Gasterophilus* species or *Habronema* (or *Draschia*) species larvae may also cause salivation. This may explain why some horses with hypertrophy of the distal third of the esophagus salivate profusely. Organophosphate poisoning causes characteristic neurologic signs accompanied by salivation and diarrhea. Parasympathomimetic drugs and plants with this property necessarily induce salivation. A profuse, peracute-onset of salivation has been reported to be caused by ingestion of the fungus *Rhizoctonia leguminicola* found in preserved fodder. This problem resolves immediately after the source is removed.

Treatment of ptyalism involves the removal of an obvious inciting cause and, provided that swallowing is not abnormal, irrigation of the mouth with copious running water. The administration of parasympatholytic drugs such as atropine should be avoided unless specifically indicated, for example, in organophosphate poisoning.

ORAL HYPERKERATOSIS

Repeated oral irritation can result in oral hyperkeratosis, which can be recognized as a pale, roughened thickening of the oral mucosa, particularly under the tongue. Seldom are there any other clinical signs. The underlying inciting factor may cause salivation and eating difficulties. Most cases are identified incidentally. Differential diagnoses include neoplastic lesions of the mouth. No known viral oral papillomatous condition has been identified such as occurs in cattle and dogs, but equine sarcoid can sometimes affect the buccal wall and invade the mucosa of the mouth. Treatment involves the removal of the cause; treatment achieves spontaneous resolution over some weeks or months.

NEUROLOGIC DISORDERS

Glossal Weakness

A flaccid tongue and reduced tongue-withdrawal reflexes occur in neonatal foals and are probably caused by delayed neurologic development. An affected foal sucks poorly but with normal enthusiasm! Some foals may be patently dysphagic with nasal regurgitation of milk. Differential diagnoses include cleft palate, esophageal obstructions or strictures, and dysphagia arising from neurologic or physical pharyngeal dysfunction. Most cases resolve spontaneously over 2 to 4 weeks, but horses may need supportive therapy.

Tongue Sucking

This vice varies among horses, from those that appear to derive satisfaction from moving the tongue in the mouth, to those that actually suck on the free end of the tongue. Saliva, which may be whipped into a foam, can drool from the mouth. Tongue tone is usually normal but long-term severe habitual sucking may weaken the free end. The vice is irresolvable but can be helped by using a permanent bit in the mouth, particularly when this has some free parts, for example, a mouthing snaffle with keys or an egg-link Pelham bit.

Tongue Flaccidity

Botulism

A flaccid tongue with a weak or absent withdrawal reflex is typically observed in horses with botulism. Muscle weakness and dysphagia as a result of pharyngeal paralysis are prominent signs. Treatment of botulism is difficult requiring intensive nursing to ensure adequate nutritional and fluid intake until the antisera/antitoxin and other supportive measures have an effect. Early diagnosis is essential.

Nigropalidal Encephalomalacia

A history of access to yellow star thistle or Russian knapweed plants is present. Dysphagia with dystonia of masticatory muscles and loss of the ability to grind effectively is characteristic. Fruitless chewing movements cause foaming of saliva at the mouth. The tongue is commonly drawn into a longitudinal trough. Treatment is difficult but the source of the plant has to be removed. Some animals cope adequately if they have only limited deficits, but most die.

Leukoencephalomalacia

Corn contaminated with *Fusarium* species molds causes a dysphagia in which tongue deficits are a relatively minor component and in which horses have a rapid course to death. (See page 668.)

Trigeminal Neuropathy

The masseter muscle mass, together with part of the digastricus and the temporalis muscles, is prone to neurologic dysfunction when the trigeminal nerve is compromised by cranial trauma, idiopathic trigeminal neuritis, polyneuritis equi (cauda equine neuritis syndrome) and, in some geographic areas, equine protozoal myeloencephalitis. When the condition is bilateral, the horse cannot chew effectively. Unilateral cases seldom show significant dysfunction, initially at least. Affected muscles waste progressively. Secondary effects include temporomandibular arthropathy and, after longer periods, dental wear abnormalities including shear mouth. Diagnosis relies upon a detailed clinical cranial nerve assessment. In endemic areas, a diagnosis of equine protozoal myeloencephalitis (see page 329) should be considered in a horse presenting with trigeminal deficits and masseter wasting. Equine protozoal myeloencephalitis can be treated effectively in some cases, but residual deficits are common. Cauda equina neuritis (polyneuritis equi, see page 311) is most often recognized as affecting the cauda equina, but deficits of trigeminal and facial nerve function are a feature of many cases. Treatment of trigeminal deficits depends upon the cause. Most are advanced and long-standing at the time of diagnosis and present limited therapeutic opportunities.

NUTRITIONAL DISORDERS

Masseter Myopathy

This is equivocally caused by selenium/vitamin E deficiency in housed horses under poor management conditions. Acute onset of gross swelling of the masseter muscles is accompanied by severe pain on manipulation of the mandible. Eating is a slow and painful process, and salivation and depression are also noted. Other skeletal muscles may or may not be affected. Serum creatine kinase is usually elevated, and in most but not all affected animals the blood vitamin E and selenium levels are low. Differential diagnosis includes tetanus, circulatory disorders resulting in swelling or edema of the head, and neurologic atrophy of the masseter muscles. Only some cases respond to selenium and vitamin E supplementation, and others may resolve spontaneously. Many fail to respond, and masseter muscle atrophy and mastication problems become increasingly significant. Such cases are untreatable.

ALLERGIC HYPERSENSITIVITY AND IMMUNOLOGIC DISORDERS

Pemphigus Vulgaris, Bullous Pemphigoid

These rare vesicobullous autoimmune diseases are characterized by ulcerative changes in the oral mucosa, mucocutaneous junctions, and skin. The two conditions represent variations in the distribution and severity of the lesions, with bullous pemphigoid showing the most severe oral lesions. Clinical signs are usually advanced on presentation, and thus the early lesions consisting of fragile, pale-colored oral vesicles and bullae are not present. The more common presentation is an accumulation of crusts and collarettes in and around the mouth and mucocutaneous junctions. Cutaneous lesions showing varying degrees of acute and chronic inflammatory changes are commonly present at the coronary bands and around the chestnuts/ergots. Diagnosis can be confirmed from shave and full-thickness biopsy samples taken from fresh lesions and stained by use of immunohistochemical methods. Treatment is frustrating, most horses being only transiently responsive to high doses of oral corticosteroid. The prognosis is always very guarded. Most animals are eventually destroyed.

Oral Amyloidosis

Repeated immune stimulation causes the deposition of amyloid in the oral and nasal cavities, as well as elsewhere. Horses being used for hyperimmune serum production and those with neoplasia or chronic infectious and inflammatory disease are most commonly affected. Within the oral cavity, amyloid deposition produces plaques of varying size and thickness with a delicate overlying mucosa that is easily traumatized. Bleeding, thickened, ulcerated areas with a yellow-orange base in the oral mucosa are a common finding. Less traumatized areas such as the nasal mucosa have a more typical appearance. Serious amyloid deposition in the major internal organs may be life-threatening. Treatment is difficult; some cases resolve following removal of the inciting stimulus, but many cases are the result of a serious underlying disease.

INFECTIOUS DISEASES

Viral Stomatitis

Viral stomatitis is a poorly defined, seldom diagnosed disorder that presents transiently and with signs similar to physical oral irritations caused by plants or chemicals. A herpes-like virus, possibly related to equine Herpesvirus III has been suggested as the most likely cause. Multiple small (1-mm to 1.5-mm diameter) vesicles occur on the mucosa of the lips and gums but the tongue is seldom affected. The vesicles burst, leaving small, rapidly-healing ulcers and erosions. Differential diagnosis includes oral contact with the blister beetle (*Epicauta* species) toxin cantharides, which produces severe vesicle formation and rapid ulceration. However, in the latter condition, the oral signs are relatively minor compared with the other signs of gastrointestinal dysfunction. Horses suspected of having viral stomatitis should be investigated serologically for herpes viruses, although some test results may be negative. No treatment is warranted in cases of true viral stomatitis.

Bacterial Infections

A wide range of bacteria can infect the horse's mouth, but the buccal mucosa seems particularly resistant. Most clinical cases of infections are the consequence of other diseases. Damage to the oral mucosa such as the diastemata, which are a common feature of pituitary adenoma/Cushing's disease, may provide opportunities for pathogenic invasion, particularly because such animals are immunologically compromised.

Candidiasis

Discolored, furry-looking plaques or more extensive diphtheritic pseudomembranous areas over the tongue and the buccal mucosa are characteristic of oral candidiasis, which most often affects immunocompromised foals. The prognosis is usually very poor because of the underlying primary disorder. All cases presented with these signs should be investigated for underlying disease. Conditions that resemble this disease include oral hyperkeratosis. A similar appearance is sometimes seen in adult horses presented with terminal renal failure, hyperlipidemia, or dehydration combined with toxemia. In the latter cases *Candida* may not be involved. Treatment is unrewarding unless the primary problem is addressed.

Gasterophilus and *Habronema* Ulcers

The discrete circular ulcers with characteristically raised margins induced by these parasites are sometimes encountered in the buccal mucosa, and particularly on the mucosa of the lips. The ulcers are usually transient but can sometimes last for some months, occasionally becoming secondarily infected. A specific diagnosis can sometimes be made by use of direct impression smears. The differential diagnosis includes plant awn and irritant ulceration. Treatment with ivermectin or organophosphate anthelmintics is usually effective for both of these conditions.

Supplemental Readings

Knottenbelt DC, Pascoe RR: A Colour Atlas of Diseases and Disorders of the Horse. London, Wolfe, 1994.
Mayhew IG: Large Animal Neurology. Philadelphia, Lea & Febiger, 1989.
Pascoe RR: The T G Hungerford Vade Mecum: Differential Diagnosis of Diseases of Horses, Series B, No 19, University of Sydney Postgraduate Foundation in Veterinary Science, 1994.

Fractures of the Lower and Upper Jaws

TIM R. C. GREET
Newmarket, England

MANDIBULAR FRACTURES

Rostral Mandible

Rostral fractures are the most common of all mandibular fractures and usually involve the incisor arcade. Typically, affected horses have grasped a bucket handle, hinge in the stable door, or a rack chain and then moved without letting go, which results in a compound fracture usually involving several incisor teeth. The fracture fragment tends to hang ventrally and the fracture site frequently becomes contaminated with ingesta. When a small fragment and single tooth are involved, there may only be attachment to the jaw by a small portion of oral mucosa. Such small fragments can be removed safely and easily, and the horses seem to show no complications from such treatment. However, if a larger sized fragment is involved, the most satisfactory way to manage the case is to repair the fracture. The fracture site is lavaged and debrided. The fracture is then reduced and wired in place using one or two cerclage wires secured around the healthy incisor teeth. These can be inserted between adjacent healthy teeth using a drill bit to create a channel. Cutting a groove in the corner incisors using a hacksaw blade minimizes the risk of wire slippage. Twisting the wire readily reduces the fracture but the wire ends should be buried to avoid ulceration of the lips postoperatively. These fractures are treated most satisfactorily under general anesthesia although it is possible to carry out the repair with the patient standing and sedated. If these fractures are not seen immediately, significant contamination with food material occurs, which should be removed and the wound carefully cleansed before repair of the injury.

Although the alveoli of the incisor teeth are usually involved, it is rare for permanent damage to the teeth to occur. Even when temporary teeth are involved and the fracture appears to involve the embryonic permanent tooth, the survival and normal eruption of the affected teeth are common. The wires can be cut for removal approximately 6 weeks postoperatively with the horse sedated. If left untreated, such fractures heal, although there is often some malalignment of the occlusal surfaces of the incisor teeth and some cosmetic disfigurement.

Bilateral Diastemal Fractures

These injuries are less common, are usually the result of a kick or severe traumatic incident, and result in complete rostral mandibular instability. Although it is possible to stabilize the fracture using tension band wiring as described earlier, in such circumstances the use of the canine or premolar teeth may be necessary to afford stability of the injury, although such stabilization is not always satisfactory. The use of a methylmethacrylate thermoplastic brace

to support the rostral mandible in combination with cerclage wiring has been described, although this does not significantly increase stability for bilateral fractures. Two Steinmann pins inserted caudally through either or both mandibles or a dynamic compression plate applied to the ventral surface of the mandibles provides a much better result. Care must be taken when employing such implants to avoid damaging the dental roots. When using compression plates in this manner, it is usually only necessary to stabilize one side of the jaw. A variety of reports describe the use of external fixation devices, although these carry potentially significant risks of postoperative disruption in horses.

Horizontal Ramus

Fractures of the horizontal ramus of the mandible involving the mandibular cheek teeth are not common. In many cases, one or several dental roots may be involved in the injury. These fractures are usually the result of a kick or other traumatic incident and are often compound. Cases occasionally occur as a sequela to extensive periapical tooth abscessation and surrounding bone osteomyelitis, especially where excessive force is used for tooth extraction. In most incidences, no surgical repair is necessary other than to carry out radical debridement of fragments and other contamination. Because the fractures are usually unilateral, the contralateral horizontal ramus acts as a splint support, precluding the need for rigid internal fixation. Such injuries may result in the formation of dental or osseous sequestra, which may need removal at a later stage.

Vertical Ramus

Fractures of the vertical ramus of the mandible are the least common of all fracture types because this area is relatively well protected by the cheek musculature. Fractures most commonly occur in foals following a kick injury, or in adult horses, after a major head trauma. In most cases there is no need to repair the injury because the musculature provides good support and allows satisfactory healing. Occasionally, fractures may involve the temporomandibular joint and these carry a more guarded prognosis than for other types of mandibular fracture. It may be possible to carry out internal fixation of such fractures to allow restoration of articular integrity, although in most cases this is not practicable. In some cases severe disruption to the normal method of mastication is the inevitable result of such an injury. Mandibular condylectomy for such severe cases has been reported, although its value in clinical cases is still unproven.

Chip Fractures and Sequestra

These injuries are relatively common sequelae to other types of mandibular fracture, particularly when kick injuries have occurred to the horizontal ramus of the mandible. In the initial acute stage of the injury, it is often not possible to determine the viability of various fragments. The rich blood supply to the structures tends to minimize the development of areas of devitalized bone. However, persistence of a mandibular wound discharge for several weeks following injury is a strong indication that there may be a sequestrum. Radiologic assessment at this stage is usually the most reliable means of confirming such a problem. Local removal under general anesthesia of osseous or dental fragments results in resolution of the discharge. Rarely there may be secondary major sepsis of a dental root that may require repulsion of the affected tooth at a later date. Other complications such as damage to the parotid salivary duct may also complicate such injuries.

A specific type of sequestrum is recognized in horses when a small fracture develops at the site of contact with a bit. In racing, the use of a narrow metal bit called the Chiffney can produce small fractures that tend to become sequestrated and may need to be removed.

MAXILLARY FRACTURES

Rostral Fractures

Fractures of the maxillary and frontal region are less common than mandibular fractures. They are usually associated with an injury from kicks on the face or running into an object. Fractures involving the rostral portion of the face, in particular the nasal bones, may result in considerable bone displacement and nasal obstruction. Insertion of a temporary tracheostomy tube may be indicated before further evaluation of the lesion by radiographic and endoscopic means. Unstable fractures of the rostral portion of the maxillary or nasal region may require surgical stabilization using wires or compression plates, but in most cases, conservative management with antibiotics and nonsteroidal anti-inflammatory medication results in return to normal function.

Rarely, a severe injury results in complete fracture of both maxillae and the hard palate, which produces considerable facial instability. Such fractures may be open and are probably best treated by conservative means unless the instability is so severe as to compromise respiratory or digestive function.

FRACTURES INVOLVING THE PARANASAL SINUSES

Comminuted fractures of the face overlying the paranasal sinuses are not uncommon. They are often severely depressed, resulting in facial distortion and sometimes respiratory obstruction. These fractures are usually the result of impaction into an object such as a tree or fence, or a severe blow, and are sometimes compound and often contaminated. A flap approach to the sinus may be indicated to remove small bony fragments and other debris, although conservative management is often effective. It may be possible to stabilize the larger fragments using stainless steel wires. It may also be of value to insert a balloon catheter into the sinus for postoperative lavage to minimize the risk of secondary sinusitis.

FRACTURES INVOLVING THE ORBIT AND ZYGOMATIC ARCH

Fractures involving the zygomatic arch may also involve damage to the orbit and the globe. A decision to treat these by medical or surgical means may be made on the basis of the concurrent eye injury. In the majority of cases, such fractures can be managed conservatively, provided that there is no gross displacement. If the fracture is severe and displaced it may impinge upon the coronoid process of the mandible or the temporomandibular joint, resulting in interference with mastication.

FRACTURES OF THE CRANIAL VAULT

Fractures of the parietal bones or of other bones covering the cranial vault may result in significant damage to the brain and consequently may carry a very poor prognosis. Decompression of the underlying cerebral tissue is indicated only if the degree of neurologic dysfunction is not so severe as to preclude recovery. Fractures of the caudal part of the skull, in particular the occipital bone and the base of the cranium, may result from horses falling over backwards. These often produce significant neurologic dysfunction. Surgical treatment is inappropriate, and euthanasia should be carried out if neurologic function is severely disturbed.

In general, most fractures of the facial region can be managed by conservative means. However, reconstruction may be indicated in an attempt to produce a more cosmetic result or to restore impaired respiratory or neurologic function. Superficial bony fragments occurring at any site in the skull may be amenable to surgical removal if sequestration occurs.

Supplemental Readings

Blackford JT, Blackford LAW: Surgical treatment of selected musculoskeletal disorders of the head. *In* Auer JA (ed): Equine Surgery. Philadelphia, WB Saunders, 1992, pp 1075–1092.
Turner AS: Large animal orthopedics. *In* Jennings PB (ed): The Practice of Large Animal Surgery. Philadelphia, WB Saunders, 1984, pp 893–897.
Wheat JD: Fractures of the head and mandible of the horse. Proc 21st Annu Meet Am Assoc Equine Pract, 1975, pp 223–228.

Salivary Gland Disease

ANDREW H. PARKS
S. ANNE BASKETT
Athens, Georgia

Three principal salivary glands are present in horses, the parotid, mandibular, and sublingual, as well as several smaller glands. Fortunately, salivary gland disease is rare and injury to these structures uncommon. The parotid gland is situated superficially, deep to the integument and the auriculopalpebral muscle, between the vertical ramus of the mandible cranially, the wing of the atlas caudally, the ear dorsally, and the linguofacial vein ventrally. The parotid duct originates at the confluence of several smaller ducts near the cranioventral angle of the gland, and passes rostrally medial to the mandible in the intermandibular space. At the rostral margin of the masseter, the duct passes laterally, ventral to the mandible in the facial vessel incisure to terminate in the oral mucosa at the parotid papilla lateral to the fourth premolar.

The mandibular gland is a slender crescent-shaped structure that extends from the atlantal fossa to the basihyoid bone in a sagittal plane lateral to the guttural pouch and larynx, and medial to the parotid gland, and digastricus and pterygoid muscles. The mandibular duct is formed on the dorsal concave surface of the mandibular gland from several ductules. The mandibular duct extends cranially on the dorsal surface of the sublingual gland beneath the oral mucosa of the sublingual fold to terminate at the sublingual caruncle adjacent to the canine tooth.

The stomatic sublingual gland lies between the body of the tongue and the mandible beneath the sublingual fold, extending from the symphysis of the mandible cranially to the second molar caudally.

The parotid gland is a serous gland, and the sublingual and mandibular glands are mixed serous and mucous glands. Saliva is composed principally of electrolytes, mainly sodium, potassium, calcium, bicarbonate, and chloride; glycoproteins; and polysaccharides, amylase, and water. The composition and flow rate vary with diet and physiologic state; a single parotid gland can produce up to 50 ml/minute. The principal function of saliva is to facilitate mastication and deglutition.

The parotid gland is the most susceptible to injury of the three major glands because of its superficial location; for the same reason, signs of disease are more easily observed. A review of the veterinary literature for the last 25 years failed to identify any specific reports of sublingual or mandibular gland disease. In contrast, parotid gland and duct disease were reported several times. Because the sublingual gland and mandibular glands are closer to the oral and pharyngeal mucosa than they are to the superficial integument, abnormalities are more likely to be observed within the oral cavity than superficially. Therefore, diseases involving the sublingual and mandibular glands are more likely to be overlooked and subsequently under-reported. The minor glands appear to be clinically unimportant.

CLINICAL SIGNS

Signs most likely to be associated with abnormalities affecting the salivary gland and ducts include external swelling of either the parotid gland or duct, leakage of saliva from an external wound, and drooling of saliva from the mouth. Closer inspection of the oral cavity may identify swelling of the sublingual gland or mandibular duct, or swelling and erythema around the parotid papilla.

Profuse leakage of saliva from a wound during mastication is pathognomonic for a transected parotid duct. If the salivary gland is damaged, leakage of saliva is closely associated with mastication but may not be as profuse, depending upon the extent of glandular injury. As a consequence, differentiation of saliva from wound exudate may be more difficult.

Swelling of the parotid duct is usually associated with the presence of a sialolith and is unlikely to be confused with anything else. Swelling of the parotid gland may be idiopathic or caused by sialadenitis or neoplasia, or it may be a consequence of duct obstruction. Parotid gland enlargement must be differentiated from swelling of the underlying structures, including the retropharyngeal lymph nodes and the guttural pouch.

Drooling of saliva from the mouth may be caused by either ptyalism or an inability to swallow. Ptyalism is most commonly associated with stomatitis but may also be caused by encephalitis, heavy metal poisoning, and parasympathomimetic poisoning, including poisoning with slaframine. Slaframine is a mycotoxin found on legume hay tainted with *Rhizoctonia leguminicola*. Any source of inflammation from trauma or infection around the pharynx, including the salivary glands, can potentially cause inability or reluctance to swallow, as will neuropathies of the 5th, 7th, 9th, 10th, or 12th cranial nerves. Prolonged loss of saliva, for whatever reason, results in acid-base and electrolyte imbalances. Initially loss of bicarbonate causes acidosis, followed by alkalosis, probably as a result of renal compensation; affected horses become hypochloremic and hyponatremic.

CONGENITAL ABNORMALITIES

Congenital abnormalities of the salivary glands are extremely rare. Two cases of congenital atresia of the parotid duct have been reported. Although transposition of the proximal duct in affected animals is theoretically feasible, ablation of the gland is simpler and less likely to lead to complications. Heterotopic salivary tissue has been reported in a single animal. The presenting sign was a hairlined draining tract caudoventral to the zygomatic process. The tract and associated glandular tissue were removed by surgical excision of the tract, and the animal became asymptomatic.

SIALOLITHIASIS

Sialoliths are concretions of mineral (usually calcium carbonate) and organic material (vegetable matter, bacteria, and cellular debris) that form within the salivary glands or ducts. They are usually single, although up to 26 have been removed from a single duct. Sialoliths vary in weight from a few to several hundred grams. The most common location is in the rostral parotid duct, although they may develop in any of the salivary glands or ducts.

Sialoliths usually cause a firm nonpainful swelling that is freely mobile over the surface of the cheek. Distension of the proximal duct occurs if the obstruction is complete, and occasionally the parotid gland distends. Infrequently, cellulitis, which is caused by septic sialadenitis and sialoangiitis, may obscure the swollen duct and sialolith.

The presence of a discrete, firm, mobile mass in the tissues of the cheek in the proximity of the parotid duct is usually diagnostic for sialolithiasis. Sialoliths are usually evident radiographically as discrete calcified masses, but sialography or computer enhanced radiography may be required to identify small calculi.

Small calculi lodged in the rostral duct may be manipulated through the parotid papilla, or the parotid papilla may be incised. Failing this, an oral sialolithotomy, performed in the heavily sedated standing horse or the horse under general anesthesia, is the procedure of choice to remove calculi lodged in the distal duct. The incision is left to heal by secondary intention.

If the calculus cannot be reached or identified through an oral approach, a transcutaneous sialolithotomy is performed by incising through the skin over the calculus within the duct. The subcutaneous tissues are bluntly dissected to expose the duct, which is incised longitudinally over the calculus. After removal of the calculus, the incision into the duct is closed with a simple continuous pattern with a fine synthetic absorbable suture, followed by routine closure of the subcutaneous tissue and skin. If the duct wall is compromised owing to local trauma or infection, where possible an incision can be made into the oral cavity followed by closure of the lateral surface of the duct, subcutaneous tissues, and skin. The latter procedure is performed to encourage drainage of saliva into the mouth and decrease the risk of cutaneous fistula formation.

TRAUMA

Trauma to the parotid salivary gland and duct is caused by accidental lacerations and as a complication of surgery in the throat latch region. The latter is evidenced by swelling, leakage of saliva through the incision, and incisional dehiscence. Lacerations of the parotid gland and duct are not uncommon because of the location of these structures.

Direct trauma to the parotid gland is usually obvious because of the location and the leakage of saliva; fortunately, the response to debridement and primary closure is good and the incidence of fistula formation is low.

If wounds involving the parotid duct are not observed while the horse is eating, they may often be overlooked until a cutaneous fistula develops. The severed ends of the duct may be difficult to identify. The proximal end can be identified by observing the flow of saliva that occurs during mastication after feeding. However, movement of the jaw makes manipulation of the duct difficult. Administration of small doses of neostigmine (0.004–0.008 mg/kg) subcutaneously stimulates saliva secretion, independent of jaw movement, and may be needed to permit identification of the end of the duct. If it is necessary to identify the distal end of the duct for an anastomosis, a 5- to 8-French polyethylene catheter can be threaded retrograde through the parotid papilla into the distal duct. If further assistance is needed to identify the duct, methylene blue dye can be injected into the duct through the catheter, or the duct can be radiographed after it has been filled with positive contrast material.

Acutely lacerated ducts without loss of duct length may be sutured with fine simple interrupted absorbable suture over a 3- to 5-French polyethylene catheter that has been threaded through both portions of the duct. The distal end of the catheter is sutured to the buccal mucosa; alternatively, the catheter can be retrieved from the oral cavity through a separate incision and anchored externally.

Historically, horses with chronic fistulas of the parotid duct have been treated by simple duct ligation; some veterinarians have encountered difficulty keeping simple ligatures in place. Reports exist in some older textbooks that the isolated proximal duct may be tunneled through the buccal tissues to exit the oral mucosal where the duct is anchored by sutures. No recent reports of this procedure are found. Surgical excision of the parotid duct for treatment of chronic fistulas is tedious and difficult because of the poorly defined gland margins and the intimate relationship of the gland with adjacent delicate structures.

The most reliable treatment is chemical ablation of the gland. The proximal duct is isolated and cannulated. A ligature is placed around the duct and cannula to prevent normograde leakage of the sclerosing agent during injection. Thirty-five milliliters of 10% buffered formalin is infused into the gland where it is retained for 90 seconds before being allowed to drain. Mild swelling and anorexia occur postoperatively. Drainage should cease in 8 to 10 days, and no long-term complications have been reported.

Reconstruction of the parotid duct with interposition of a polytetrafluoroethylene graft has been reported to successfully bridge a deficit in the parotid duct in the treatment of a chronic cutaneous fistula. This technique may also be appropriate for acute injuries in which a portion of the duct was lost.

SIALADENITIS

Bacterial sialadenitis, with or without abscessation, occasionally occurs after ascending infection (a result of obstructed ducts), hematogenous infection, or external trauma. Supportive therapy with analgesics minimizes the discomfort, whereas antibiotics and drainage of abscesses usually resolve the problem. Eosinophilic sialadenitis occurs as part of an eosinophilic epitheliotropic syndrome in horses.

Bilateral swelling of the parotid glands associated with subcutaneous edema is a well-recognized but poorly documented finding. This swelling is most frequently seen after a horse is turned out to pasture. The swelling usually regresses.

MUCOCELE

Mucoceles are an accumulation of salivary secretions in a cavity adjacent to a ruptured salivary duct. Mucoceles are extremely uncommon, and treatment involves creation of an oral salivary fistula or excision of the gland.

NEOPLASIA

Neoplasia of the salivary glands is uncommon, with the exception of melanomas in gray horses. Benign mixed tumors, acinar cell tumors, and adenocarcinomas have also been documented in horses. Because of the rarity of these tumors, generalizations are difficult to make without extrapolating from other species. Horses with slow-growing melanomas probably do not require surgery. Surgical excision is indicated for locally invasive tumors such as acinic cell tumors, benign mixed tumors, and some melanomas. Treatment of horses with tumors that frequently metastasize, such as adenocarcinomas, is usually futile.

Supplemental Readings

Bowman KF: Salivary gland disease. *In* Robinson NE (ed): Current Therapy in Equine Medicine 2. Philadelphia, WB Saunders, 1987, pp 3–6.
Ford TS: Salivary glands. *In* Auer JA (ed): Equine Surgery. Philadelphia, WB Saunders, 1992, pp 306–308.
Morris DD: Salivary gland disease. *In* Robinson NE (ed): Current Therapy in Equine Medicine. Philadelphia, WB Saunders, 1983, pp 183–184.
Stick JA, Robinson NE, Krehbiel JD: Acid-base and electrolyte alterations associated with salivary loss in the pony. Am J Vet Res 42:733–737, 1981.

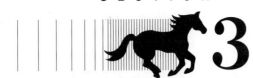

THE GASTROINTESTINAL SYSTEM

Edited by Michael J. Murray

Diagnostic Procedures for Evaluation of the Gastrointestinal Tract

MICHAEL J. MURRAY
Leesburg, Virginia

In addition to a thorough physical examination, rectal examination, and routine laboratory tests, several diagnostic procedures may be selected to enhance the evaluation of a horse with a known or suspected disorder involving the alimentary system. Each procedure is limited in the type and extent of information that can be obtained, and thus the clinician should select the complement of procedures that is most likely to provide the information that is required to make a proper diagnosis and determine the appropriate therapy.

ENDOSCOPY

There are two basic types of endoscopic equipment available: equipment based entirely on a fiberoptic system, and equipment based on a video chip system. Fiberoptic equipment is generally less expensive and more easily transported than video systems. Video systems are well suited for clinical settings; they permit more than one individual to view the procedure and facilitate image documentation. The typical endoscope used in practice consists of an insertion tube that is 100 to 110 cm in length and 9.5 to 14.5 mm in outer diameter. The larger-diameter tube can only be inserted through the nasal passages of older yearlings and adults, whereas a diameter of 10 mm allows passage through the turbinates of young foals. An insertion tube of 100 cm is sufficient for esophagoscopy in foals up to approximately 6 months of age. For older animals, an insertion tube length of 150 to 180 cm is required for esophagoscopy.

An insertion tube length of 110 cm is sufficient to reach the stomach of foals up to 30 to 40 days of age only. A length of 150 to 180 cm is required for weanlings, and 200 cm is usually required for yearlings and adults. An insertion tube length of 200 cm is sufficient to reach the stomach of all adults of warm-blooded breeds, although 280 to 300 cm is required to examine the pylorus in adult horses. A 280- to 300-cm long insertion tube permits duodenoscopy in adult horses.

Gastroscopy can be done using moderate tranquilization (0.5 mg/kg xylazine IV) with the animal standing. In neonates, either no sedation or sedation with xylazine (0.3 mg/kg IV) or diazepam (0.1 mg/kg IV) is adequate. Before gastroscopy in horses, feed should be withheld for 6 to 10 hours. Foals can be allowed to nurse up to 4 hours before gastroscopy. Longer periods of feed deprivation are usually not required, unless the clinician intends to perform gastroscopy with the animal under general anesthesia. This is recommended only in cases in which lateral recumbency is required to examine the entire glandular mucosal surface or to better examine the pylorus, such as with a 200-cm endoscope in a weanling or yearling.

Endoscopy of the rectum and distal small colon can be performed with most flexible endoscopes in use in equine practice and should be preceded, as much as possible, by evacuation and saline lavage of the rectum and distal small colon. The mucosal surface should appear pink to pale red and should have a smooth "velvety" appearance. Mucosal edema or thickening, hyperemia, irregularities, defects, tears, and intraluminal masses are abnormal findings. Because of the concern for trauma to the rectum and small colon, the horse should be adequately sedated and restrained before preparation and examination of the distal alimentary tract.

RADIOGRAPHY

Radiography of the alimentary tract can be a useful diagnostic tool in the evaluation of the oral, esophageal, and abdominal portions of the alimentary system. The size of the patient and the capabilities of radiographic equipment available determine which procedures can be performed. As with all radiographic procedures, safety must be the primary consideration in the development and performance of a radiographic technique. Radiography of the abdomen of weanlings, yearlings, and adult horses requires a high-exposure technique, and is accompanied by significant scatter radiation. Nonetheless, radiography often provides the most valuable information in the evaluation of certain cases.

Many portable units, with settings ranging from 60 kV and 30 mA, to 90 kV and 15 mA, are suitable to take good quality radiographs of the teeth, pharynx, and esophagus in adults, and the entire alimentary tract in young foals. The use of rare earth screens with high-latitude film, in conjunction with a focused grid, enhance the capabilities and quality of films taken with a portable radiography unit. In addition, techniques that take advantage of air/tissue interfaces, such as an oblique view of the teeth, with the paranasal sinuses superimposed on the dorsal arcade of teeth, or the use of positive contrast media, allow the practitioner to produce diagnostic films at lower exposures.

Radiography is particularly useful in the evaluation of disorders of the thoracic esophagus and abdominal viscera in foals. In young foals, radiography can assist in the diagnosis of obstructions caused by meconium impactions, fecal impactions, displacements, volvulus, stricture, and congenital malformations. The use of suspensions of 20 to 40% barium sulfate at 10 to 20 ml/kg can be useful in evaluating the esophagus, stomach, proximal small intestine, intestinal transit, distal large colon, and small colon. Disorders such as megaesophagus, cardia stricture, pyloric stricture, and duodenal stricture can be diagnosed with contrast radiography.

Radiography is indispensable in many cases of colic in young foals in determining whether surgery is indicated (see page 627). In a retrospective report on the use of radiography in abdominal disorders in foals, a positive radiographic diagnosis of abdominal disease was confirmed at surgery or necropsy in 25 of 26 patients. The films were all reviewed by radiologists, emphasizing that the accuracy of the diagnosis is related to the experience and skill of the person interpreting the film.

The average exposure for a 50-kg foal is 30 mA and 80 to 100 kVp. It is normal to see accumulations of gas in the stomach and cecal base. Isolated segments of the small and large intestine also have small amounts of gas. Moderate

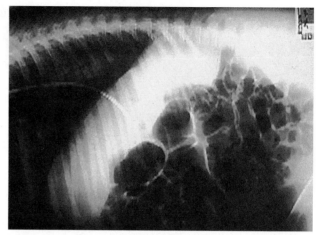

Figure 1. Lateral radiograph of the abdomen of a 6-day-old foal that had signs of abdominal discomfort and mild diarrhea. There is moderate gas distension of several segments of small intestine. The foal had septicemia and enteritis.

gas distension of the small intestine can occur with enteritis (Fig. 1). Marked distension of the small intestine, such as occurs with obstruction or enteritis, can be recognized as multiple hairpin loops with gas/fluid interfaces. Obstructions of the large colon are characterized by long gas/fluid interfaces occurring in the mid- to ventral abdomen.

In young foals with large colon gas distension, retrograde administration of barium sulfate has been used to demonstrate patency of the small colon and the absence of meconium obstructions (see Fischer et al. in Supplemental Readings). Thirty percent barium sulfate (weight per volume [w/v]) solution is administered to sedated foals by gravity administration through a Foley catheter placed per rectum. If the bowel is obstructed, it is difficult to administer more than 100 to 200 ml of contrast material. Adequate filling of the small colon and transverse colon verifies patency of the distal gastrointestinal tract (Fig. 2). For obstructions in the large colon, up to 20 ml/kg barium sulfate suspension should be administered. Both ventrodorsal and

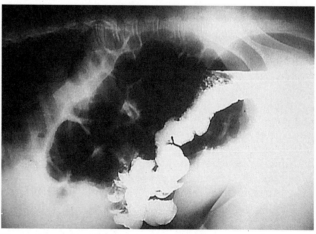

Figure 2. Lateral radiograph of the abdomen of a 1-day-old foal that presented with signs of abdominal discomfort. Retrograde administration of a 20% barium sulfate suspension revealed a patent small colon.

lateral radiographs should be obtained, although in cases of meconium obstruction, the ventrodorsal radiograph may be of greater diagnostic value than a lateral view. Obstructions are noted by an abrupt stop of the dye column. If the dye tapers off, insufficient administration of contrast media has occurred. Meconium retention is readily identified on retrograde contrast radiography.

The adult horse has a large body mass, which makes it difficult to radiograph the abdomen unless high mA settings and high kVp settings are able to be obtained. The cranial abdomen, just caudal to the diaphragm, is often most successfully imaged (Fig. 3). Good quality abdominal radiographs can be obtained on most 500 to 600 mA machines capable of 140 kVp. A high-speed rare earth film screen combination and an 8:1, 80-line/inch grid should be used to minimize exposure times. A 1-mm sheet of lead is placed behind the cassette to reduce scatter. Horses should be fasted for 24 hours before radiography to minimize the volume of digesta in the colons.

Techniques for obtaining abdominal radiographs vary from 300 to 600 mA and 80 to 140 kVp. An average setting for a 500-kg horse is 450 mA and 120 kVp. Less radiation is required for exposures of the diaphragmatic area and the small colon. In some cases, it is helpful to radiograph the animal from both sides. A typical 500-kg horse requires at least three to four radiographs to cover the abdominal cavity. Enteroliths are most commonly seen in the middle of the abdomen, in the area of the right dorsal and transverse colons.

Sand accumulations also can be seen and can be difficult to distinguish from enteroliths if the shape is spherical, such as occurs in the transverse colon. Sand accumulations may obscure enteroliths. If a large accumulation of sand is present, radiographs should be repeated when the sand obstruction has broken up and passed.

ULTRASONOGRAPHY

Ultrasonography can be very useful in evaluating soft tissue structures associated with the alimentary system.

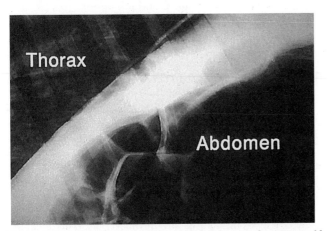

Figure 3. Lateral radiograph of the cranial abdomen of an 8-year-old horse that had enterogastric reflux resulting from entrapment of small intestine in a mesenteric rent. The horse also had moderate gas distension of the large colon that was felt on rectal examination. Gas-distended bowel, which appears to be both small and large intestine, is visible in the cranial abdomen.

Ultrasonography and radiography are often complementary, and in many cases, particularly in adult horses, ultrasonography provides more useful information than radiography. Ultrasonography also is complementary to palpation per rectum, because masses felt per rectum may be better characterized, particularly when using a transrectal probe. Ultrasonography also can assist in making a diagnosis when rectal examination and other examination findings are normal. This is particularly true in the case of abnormalities in the cranial or ventral abdomen of adult horses.

The utility of abdominal ultrasonography is limited by the size of the patient, the quality of the equipment used, and the skill of the examiner. The most limiting features of ultrasonography in its application to the abdominal viscera are the depth of penetration available, 25 to 30 cm, the loss of resolution as depth of penetration increases, and interference by gas within the intestine. Use of transrectal probes can increase the area of the abdominal cavity that can be examined.

When examining abdominal viscera, it is preferable to clip the site to be examined, although in young foals and horses with a short hair coat this may not be necessary. Application of mineral oil to the skin often yields satisfactory results without clipping. When hair is clipped, ultrasound couplant gel should be applied to the site before the examination.

With adults, a 2.5- to 3.0-MHz scanhead is used initially. In foals a 5.0- to 7.5-MHz scanhead can be used. Increasing the scanhead frequency improves the resolution but decreases the depth of penetration. An ultrasonic examination of the abdomen should be performed in a standard manner, so that pertinent structures are examined each time. A protocol for examining the abdomen has been described by Rantanen (see Supplemental Readings).

Gas within the bowel stops the penetration of the sound waves, and often structures deep to the gas/bowel wall interface cannot be examined. This fact can be used to the practitioner's advantage, because clear visualization of proximal and distal bowel walls suggests that fluid, not gas, is present within the bowel lumen (Fig. 4).

Abnormalities that may be detected by ultrasonography include peritoneal effusion, hemoperitoneum, ruptured bladder, adhesions, masses (Fig. 5), small intestinal distension and/or paralytic ileus (see Fig. 4), increased bowel wall thickness, intussusception, and dorsal displacement of the colon over the nephrosplenic ligament. Ultrasonography of the liver may detect areas of heterogeneous echo-reflection in the hepatic parenchyma (neoplasms, abscesses, severe fibrosis), bile duct distension, or choledocolithiasis. In foals with colic, ultrasonography may aid in determining whether there is paralytic ileus, fluid accumulation and distension in the bowel, bowel wall thickening, and bowel wall necrosis (presence of hyperechoic gas within the bowel wall).

PARACENTESIS

Abdominal paracentesis is performed routinely in patients with suspected disorders of the abdominal viscera. Paracentesis typically is performed on ventral midline 5 to 15 cm caudal to the xiphoid. Aseptic preparation of the

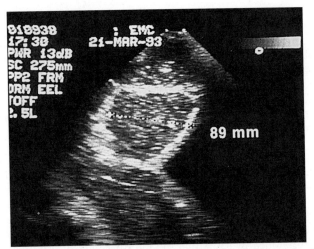

Figure 4. Transabdominal ultrasonographic image (5.0-MHz scanhead) of the right cranial lateral abdomen in a horse that presented with abdominal discomfort. There is distension of small intestinal segments with fluid resulting from incarceration of intestine in the epiploic foramen. Rectal examination did not reveal distended small intestine.

paracentesis site and aseptic collection of abdominal fluid are imperative, otherwise a focal inflammatory response at the paracentesis site will develop. This may be of greatest concern if paracentesis must be repeated; results suggest peritonitis but may be iatrogenic. In foals, a blunt teat cannula is preferred for paracentesis rather than a needle to minimize the chances of inadvertent enterocentesis. Before performing abdominocentesis with a blunt cannula, local anesthetic is infused subcutaneously at the site and a

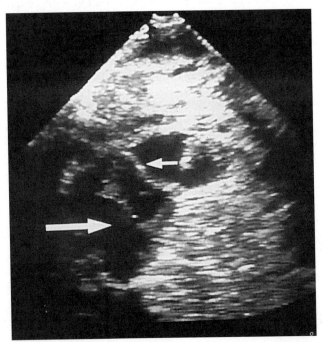

Figure 5. Ultrasonic image (2.5-MHz scanhead) of the cranial ventral abdomen in a horse that presented with weight loss and intermittent abdominal discomfort. A hyperechoic large mass (*small arrow*) is in the ventral abdomen with a marked fibrinous response and pockets of hypoechoic fluid (*large arrow*).

stab incision is made into the skin with a number 15 blade. In adult horses an 18-gauge, 1.5-inch needle may be used, although the chances for inadvertent enterocentesis are greater than with a teat cannula. Enterocentesis in an adult horse usually is benign, other than contaminating the sample. If viscus rupture is suspected, abdominocentesis may have to be performed at several sites.

Many slides should be prepared and air-dried at the time the sample is taken. Cells can degenerate within the collection tube, and bacteria that may have contaminated the sample during collection can be phagocytosed within a few minutes in a collection tube. On cytologic examination this gives the impression of intracellular bacteria being present within the peritoneal fluid. In addition, it is useful to save unstained slides that can be sent to a veterinary pathologist for further evaluation.

BIOPSY

The value of examining biopsies obtained from the alimentary tract depends on the site and method of obtaining the biopsy, amount of tissue obtained, and completeness of the history and request documentation provided to the pathologist who will examine the biopsy. Because small biopsy samples are often submitted, it is essential that a thorough history and an indication of what disorder is suspected be provided. In addition to histologic evaluation, bacteriologic culture, electron microscopy, and direct and indirect fluorescent antibody staining can be performed.

The decision of whether to obtain a biopsy is often based on the ease of obtaining a sample and the relative value of the evaluation that can be made. Very small samples, such as those obtained with an endoscope biopsy instrument, provide limited information, although they are relatively easy to obtain. Full-thickness bowel specimens, obtained via ventral midline or flank laparotomy, provide much more information, yet are more difficult to obtain.

Rectal mucosal biopsies are easily obtained. Many instruments can be used to obtain the biopsy, and a uterine biopsy forceps works well. A fold of mucosa can readily be pinched between two fingers, and a biopsy of this tissue is obtained. The size of the sample is adequate for histologic and bacteriologic examination.

FECAL EXAMINATION

Cytologic, bacteriologic, and electron microscopic evaluations can be performed on fecal samples. In addition, observation of the consistency, color, presence of foreign material such as sand or gravel, and presence of parasites should be included in the examination of the alimentary system. Increased fecal particle size, with loose or watery stool, is suggestive of poor mastication or decreased colonic transit time.

Cytologic examinations are primarily used to evaluate the parasite burden of the animal. Ova of large and small strongyles, tapeworms, round worms, and *Strongyloides westerii* are most common. Coccidia are occasionally observed, but are not considered to be pathogenic. Examination of fecal white blood cells has been advocated in the evaluation of horses and foals with enterocolitis; however, these cells are very labile. Their presence in large numbers indicates that an inflammatory process is present, and that the inflammation is in the distal colon and/or associated with decreased transit time.

Determination of fecal occult blood has been recommended to diagnose gastric ulcers, duodenal ulcers, and other potentially hemorrhagic disorders of the alimentary tract. However, Pearson et al. (see Supplemental Readings) indicated that the test is of limited diagnostic value in the adult horse, because negative results can be obtained when a large amount of blood is present in the proximal portion of the gastrointestinal tract. The sensitivity of most commercially available tests is poor, and negative results can occur in the face of severe gastric bleeding. Even large amounts of hemoglobin are thoroughly degraded by colonic bacteria.

Fecal culture is an essential component in the evaluation of many patients. Bacteriologic culture techniques for fecal samples routinely employ selective media that are designed to isolate *Salmonella*. These media include selenite and tetrathionate broths, brilliant green, xylose-lysine-deoxycholate (XLD), and xylose-lactose-sodium thiosulfate (XLT-4) agars. Less selective media, MacConkey and eosin methylene blue agars, are desirable to culture other potential gram-negative bacterial pathogens, such as *Escherichia coli*. The presence alone of *E. coli* in the feces does not determine its pathogenicity. Enterotoxigenic *E. coli* have been isolated from foals with diarrhea, but special tests, such as polymerase chain reaction (PCR), must be performed to determine whether an isolate produces enterotoxin.

The presence of rotavirus in a fecal sample can be determined by use of an enzyme-linked immunosorbent assay (ELISA),* or an agglutination test.† Both assays test for the presence of viral particles in the feces. The ELISA test is more sensitive than the agglutination test but is less specific. Thus, the agglutination test is likely to give more false-negative results, and the ELISA test is likely to give more false-positive results. The ELISA test is more time-consuming and inconvenient to perform than the agglutination test. When rotavirus is a concern, particularly as a farm problem, a reasonable approach is to screen fecal samples with the agglutination test, and repeat samples that are negative with the ELISA test.

Electron microscopy on feces is not routinely performed but can be useful in determining whether there is a viral component to a herd diarrhea problem. Rotavirus, coronavirus, adenovirus, and parvovirus have been identified by electron microscopy and were determined to be causative agents of diarrhea in foals.

ABSORPTION AND DIGESTION TESTS

Tests that evaluate the ability of the equine intestinal tract to digest and absorb nutrients have a more limited clinical application than in human or small animal medicine but can be useful in the evaluation of horses with chronic weight loss, suspected small intestinal inflammation or neoplasia, gastric and small intestinal partial obstruction, and postoperative malabsorptive disorders. Effective absorption tests that can be routinely performed in a clinical setting are limited to evaluation of the small intestine. For absorption tests to be diagnostic, the intestinal disorder either must be diffuse or must affect the delivery to and transit through the small intestine.

Maldigestion tests are most applicable to foals. Mucosal brush border disaccharidase deficiencies occur in foals as a developmental disorder or as a result of viral and bacterial enteridites. Lactose tolerance can be tested by administering a 20% solution of D-lactose at a dosage of 0.5 to 1 g/kg. This dosage should result in an approximate doubling of the serum glucose within 60 minutes of administration.

Clinically applicable absorption tests include the D-glucose and D-xylose absorption tests. The glucose absorption test has the advantage of being relatively easy and inexpensive to perform. However, cellular uptake and metabolism of glucose, as well as intestinal absorption, influence the results and thus are undesirable variables. The D-xylose absorption test is advantageous because it more directly measures intestinal absorptive capacity. The results of both tests, though, are affected by gastric emptying rate and small intestinal transit time. Absorption and digestion tests should be performed following an 18- to 24-hour fast and should be interpreted as reflecting gastrointestinal transit as well as intestinal digestion and absorption.

The D-glucose and D-xylose tests are performed similarly. Following an 18- to 24-hour fast, a 10% solution of D-glucose or D-xylose, 0.5 to 1 g/kg is administered via nasogastric tube. For the measurement of glucose, blood is collected in sodium fluoride tubes, and for the measurement of D-xylose, blood is collected in heparinized tubes. Samples are taken at 0, 30, 60, 90, 120, 150, 180, 210, and 240 minutes following administration.

Peak levels of D-xylose normally range from 20 to 25 mg/dl and occur 60 to 120 minutes following administration. The normal curve resembles an inverted V. Delay or flattening of this curve may reflect delayed gastric emptying, increased intestinal transit time, and/or impaired intestinal absorption. Accurate interpretation of the results of these tests depends on the results of other diagnostic evaluations. In addition, different types of diet have been shown to significantly affect the height, although not the shape, of the absorption curves. In general, diets that have a higher digestible energy content result in a lower peak in the curve.

Supplemental Readings

Fischer AT, Kerr LY, O'Brien TR: Radiographic diagnosis of gastrointestinal disorders in the foal. Vet Radiol 28:42–48, 1987.

Fischer AT, Yarbrough TY: Retrograde contrast radiography of the distal portions of the intestinal tract in foals. J Am Vet Med Assoc 207:734–737, 1995.

Merritt AM, Kohn CW, Ramberg CF, Cimprich RE, Reid CF, Bolton JR: Plasma clearance of [51Cr] albumin into the intestinal tract of normal and chronically diarrheal horses. Am J Vet Res 38:1769–1774, 1977.

Pearson EG, Smith BB, McKim JM: Fecal blood determinations and interpretations. Proc Am Assoc Equine Pract, 1987, pp 77–81.

Rantanen NW: Diseases of the abdomen. Vet Clin North Am Equine Pract 2(1):67–88, 1986.

Roberts MC, Norman P: A re-evaluation of the D + xylose absorption test in the horse. Equine Vet J 11:239–243, 1979.

*Rotazyme II, Abbott Laboratories, Abbott Park, IL
†Rotalex, Medical Technologies Corp., Somerset, NJ

Rectal Examination of the Colic Patient

NORBERT KOPF
Vienna, Austria

Rectal examination is essential in each case of colic. Findings should always be considered in conjunction with the results of physical examination, nasogastric intubation, abdominocentesis, and laboratory data. Rectal exploration should always be performed before paracentesis in order to recognize extremely enlarged portions of bowel and to prevent accidental penetration of distended loops of intestine. To determine the type of intestinal obstruction, internal palpation is the most useful technique. Palpation findings usually give an indication of the need for surgical intervention or conservative treatment. The value of rectal examination depends on the experience of the examiner and cooperation of the patient. It is impossible to survey the peritoneal cavity completely by internal palpation, because only the pelvic cavity and the caudal portion, or approximately 40%, of the abdominal cavity can be explored.

Frequently, rather subtle signs or hints found during examination yield information pointing to conditions in deeper abdominal regions. In other cases, the location and the type of the obstruction can be identified precisely—for example, incarcerated inguinal hernia and left dorsal displacement of the large colon.

TECHNIQUE

To minimize the risk of damage to the rectum, horses with unrelenting pain should be treated with analgesics or sedatives such as xylazine* (0.1–0.2 mg/kg). Use of a twitch is almost always necessary to prevent straining. An alternative method of restraint is the simple fixation of a hind leg with a rope attached to the pastern and led between the forelegs to the neck. If the veterinarian examines with the right arm the left hind leg is fixed, and vice versa. The anus of the horse and the gloved hand should be lubricated sufficiently to reduce resistance and mucosal irritation when the hand is inserted. First, the mucosa of the ampulla should be examined for any lesions and the withdrawn arm examined for blood or clots. Rectal mucus and the contents of the rectal ampulla are noted and fecal balls are eliminated. The next reinsertion of the arm should be as deep as possible when the rectum is flaccid to facilitate examination of deep regions. The size of the rectal tube in relation to the palpator's hand is assessed from the tension of the rectal wall over the examiner's wrist, hand, and forearm. Limitation by a short mesorectum also will be identified. Often the lumen travels ventrally. The examiner should follow this ventral deviation and then raise the arm dorsally to straighten the rectum. Figure 1 shows the stressed areas,

Rompun, Haver-Lockhart, Shawnee, KS

which are usually predisposed to iatrogenic lesions. Initial manipulation of tissues with a half-inserted arm, and examination of the pelvic cavity first, usually causes tenesmus and propulsive contractions of the rectum. Consequently, thorough investigation of more cranial structures is prevented.

EXAMINATION FINDINGS

Normal Rectal Findings

Rectal findings in the healthy animal (Fig. 2) include well-formed, soft fecal balls in the rectal ampulla that have an aromatic odor. The rectal mucosa is finely folded. The small colon is identified by fecal balls, which can be moved in all directions. At the right side, the cecum often can be recognized as a soft viscus containing some gas. The only portion of the cecum that can always be identified is the ventral taenia. In small horses ventral and medial taeniae can be palpated. If the cecum contains some gas or ingesta, its dorsal adhesion to the abdominal wall can be touched going from the aorta to the right side. At the left flank the caudal edge of the spleen can be found. Usually the caudal pole of the left kidney and the suspensory ligament of the spleen or nephrosplenic ligament can be identified. Two or three fingers can be inserted into the nephrosplenic space

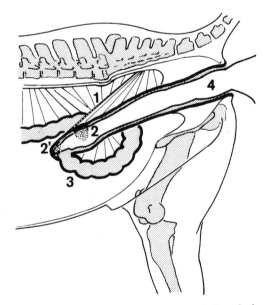

Figure 1. Technique of deep rectal examination. 1, Stretched mesorectum; 2, 2', Areas of increased extension of the rectal wall; 3, Ventral deviation of the small colon; 4, Position of the arm in relation to the abdominal and pelvic cavity.

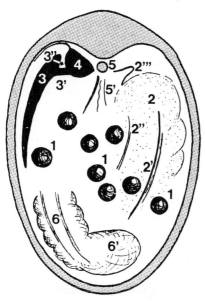

Figure 2. Normal rectal findings. 1, Fecal balls marking the small colon; 2, Cecal base containing some gas; 2′, Its ventral taenia; 2″, Its medial taenia; 2‴, Its adhesion to the dorsal abdominal wall; 3, Spleen; 3′, Its suspensory ligament; 3″, Nephrosplenic space; 4, Kidney; 5, Aorta; 5′, Cranial mesenteric root; 6, Large colon, bands of the ventral portion; 6′, Pelvic flexure.

between the dorsal part of the spleen and the left kidney. In small horses the cranial mesenteric root can be investigated by fingertips as a flaccid folded band running in a ventral direction. Parts of the large colon frequently cannot be identified. By passing the hand along the ventral abdominal wall, it is often possible to feel some bands or the pelvic flexure if it contains ingesta. The caudal part of the abdominal cavity can normally be reached in all directions without any resistance.

Pathologic Findings

The common location of rectal tears is in the dorsal bowel wall at the cranial limitation of the rectal ampulla. Lubricant on the glove with a sanguineous tinge after the first inspection of this area requires careful investigation. Bloody and malodorous brownish fluid is also found in all conditions that compromise the vascular supply of the small colon with or without compromise of its lumen. Injuries of the rectum are best explored by the more sensitive bare hand. The smooth mucosa disappears and the surface is rough.

In cases of intestinal obstruction the rectum frequently contains no fecal material and the rectal mucus is inspissated. Small dry fecal balls coated with pasty mucus signify delayed transport of the feces. By contrast, chronic impaction of the cecum often causes a diarrhea-like stool. To interpret the findings of rectal examination correctly, one must pay particular attention to the consistency, form, position, location, or tenseness of both the intestine and mesentery. The taeniae are important structures for identification of specific segments of the large bowel. Intestinal impactions cause enlargement of the constipated parts of the bowel and have a pasty or doughy consistency. Digital impressions remain for some time.

In dilations of the intestine caused by gas accumulation, impressions disappear at once. By pressing the bowels against the abdominal wall or pelvis, the examiner can identify lesions such as edema and infarction that increase the thickness of the bowel wall. Localized intestinal pain can also be reproduced in this manner. In stallions and geldings, palpation of the vaginal ring should be a routine part of the examination.

Intravaginal inguinal herniation of the small intestine occurs if the peritoneal ring is large. Rectal findings in this condition are an enlarged loop of the small intestine with abnormal fixation at the abdominal wall in the inguinal region, acute pain, and a taut mesentery. External palpation of the scrotum completes this diagnosis.

Obstructions of the small bowel are characterized by distended loops of small intestine that are compressible to varying degrees. The diameter may vary from 5 to 12 cm, depending on the duration of the condition. In cases of high obstruction or in late cases, the dilated second flexure of the duodenum surrounding the dorsal adhesion of the cecum can be recognized. The strangulated part of the small bowel can be identified by the thickening of its wall. In all cases of small bowel obstruction the ingesta inside the large colon become more solid because of dehydration. Dehydration also reduces the size of the large colon, making the constrictions and sacculations of the ventral part of the large colon palpably more distinct (Fig. 3). Touching the strangulated intestinal or mesenteric parts may cause pain. In a high obstruction of the small intestine, distended loops may not be within reach. In this situation, however, gentle traction on the ventral taenia of the cecum in a caudal direction is very painful. *Ileal impaction* can be diagnosed by rectal examination in early cases only. The obstipated ileum feels like a large sausage, the end of which is fixed in the right dorsal region at the base of the

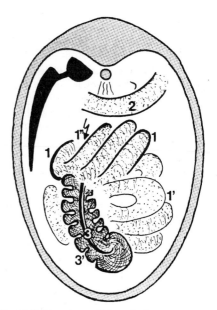

Figure 3. Rectal findings in small bowel obstruction. 1, Strangulated parts of small intestine, distended loops with thickened wall; 1′, Prestenotic loops of small bowel, tympanic without thickening of the wall; 1″ (↯), Painful area; 2, Caudal flexure of the distended duodenum; 3, Large colon containing solid ingesta; 3′, Its contracted sacculations.

cecum; the cecum itself is poststenotic and therefore empty and not palpable. Tension on the taut mesentery of the ileum produces pain. In late cases the constipated ileum cannot be palpated because the distended loops of the caudal portion of the prestenotic jejunum fill the caudal part of the abdominal cavity and the ileum may be dislocated in a cranial direction.

In cases of *ileocecal intussusception* a blunt mass can be felt in the right dorsal region. The mass is fixed at its dorsomedial pole and can be moved like a pendulum in transverse and sagittal directions. Touching the point of fixation often elicits pain. In all cases of small bowel obstruction *gastric dilation* occurs. A dislocation of the spleen in the ventromedial and caudal direction is an indication of tremendous gastric dilation.

Acute dilation of the cecum produces obvious rectal findings as the form of the organ can be recognized very clearly. The ventral taenia, the large-caliber sacculations, and the deep constrictions can be felt. Impactions of the cecum can be diagnosed because of the typical form of this bowel, its dorsal junction to the abdominal wall, and the doughy consistency. Sometimes a relapsing spastic impaction of the overhanging part of the cecal base occurs. It can only be reached in medium-sized horses, is recognized because of its oval form, and can be moved like a pendulum in a transverse direction. In severe cases of recurrent *impaction of the cecum* hypertrophy of the circular layer of the smooth muscles of the base and the body of the cecum can be recognized even if the cecum is not well filled. In all cases of *strangulation of the large colon* there is a large amount of gas distension of the cecum proximal to the obstruction. When the cecum is distended with gas, its apex tends to "float up" and the ventral taenia becomes positioned in an oblique or transverse direction.

One of the most common findings in horses with colic is *impaction of the left ventral portion of the large colon*. The colon is enlarged and the obstipation has a cone-formed end at the pelvic flexure (Fig. 4). The two free taeniae of the ventral large colon can be felt as longitudinal grooves, separated by 90° in relation to the circumference of the intestinal tube. The consistency of the obstipated ingesta depends on the tone of the intestinal wall and can change suddenly during the manual investigation. Because of the enlargement, the sacculations and constrictions are not recognizable. This is a very significant difference from cases of *pseudoimpaction* of the large bowels caused by the dehydration in cases of small bowel obstruction. This difference must be noted to prevent improper interpretation of cases in which the firmness of the contents of the large colon is increased.

Impaction of the ampulla of the right dorsal portion of the large colon has the shape and dimensions of a soccer ball, approximately 30 cm in diameter. Often it will not be within reach. Only in medium-sized horses in which the cranial mesenteric root can be investigated easily can the caudal part of the constipated ampulla coli be reached. The cranial mesenteric root can be pressed against the background of the dome-like protrusion of the constipated dorsal colon and serves as a helpful guide in identifying the location of the obstipated ingesta.

Occlusion of the large colon by enteroliths also occurs at the junction of the right dorsal and transverse colon. If the

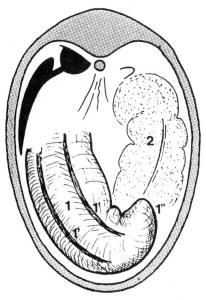

Figure 4. Rectal findings in impaction of the left ventral colon. 1, Enlarged large colon containing doughy ingesta; 1′, Its two free taeniae (Distanced 90° in relation to the circumference of the intestinal tube); 1″, Cone-formed end of the obstipation at the pelvic flexure; 2, Tympanic cecum.

occluding stone can be touched, there is no question about the type of obstruction. The prestenotic parts of the large colon are greatly distended by gas, as in all cases of strangulation and volvulus of the large colon in which the occlusion is total.

Extreme distension of the large colon with gas and tremendous tension on its taeniae are the cornerstones in rectal identification of *torsion or flexion* of this intestinal part. After a few hours, the twisted bowels become edematous, and the thickened intestinal wall, haustra, and longitudinal bands are readily palpated. In some cases the ventral colon can be located dorsal to the dorsal colon. Because of the distension, the large bowel cannot be moved. In some cases it is positioned in a transverse direction, with the curvature of the pelvic flexure dislocated either toward the right flank or in a cranial direction. In dramatic cases of *torsion of the entire large colon* tympany may be so severe that it is impossible to explore the cranial regions of the abdominal cavity (Fig. 5).

A frequently observed condition is the *strangulation of the large colon by the suspensory ligament of the spleen*—the so-called left dorsal displacement of the large colon (Fig. 6). The location of the strangulation can be investigated by rectal palpation. If the dislocated portion of the colon is large, the bands (taeniae) run diagonally to converge at the nephrosplenic space on the left dorsal quadrant of the abdomen. By palpating from the caudal pole of the left kidney toward the left abdominal wall, the examiner can feel the taeniae of the large colon crossing dorsally to the nephrosplenic ligament. The spleen is almost always situated in its normal position but may be hidden by tympanic parts of the dislocated colon. In a few cases of left dorsal displacement of the large colon, only the impacted pelvic flexure is strangulated over the suspensory ligament of the spleen.

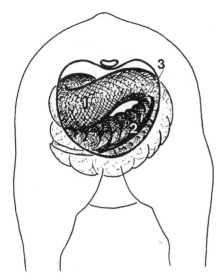

Figure 5. Rectal findings in torsion of the whole large colon. 1, Tympanic dorsal portion; 2, Edematous and gaseous distended ventral part of the large colon in transverse position with clearly contoured sacculations and constrictions; 3, Limitation of pelvic cavity (deeper regions cannot be explored).

In cases of tremendous tympany of the large bowel, enterocentesis of the cecum at the right dorsal flank is indicated to enable rectal diagnosis. After this procedure, evacuation of the cecum can be confirmed. In case of strangulation of the large colon, the stenosed part remains tympanic. However, enterocentesis provides more space for rectal palpation and facilitates determination of the type of dislocation. *Left dorsal dislocation of the large colon over the nephrosplenic ligament* can be corrected

conservatively. The success can be determined rectally step by step. The anesthetized horse is positioned in right lateral recumbency while the clinician is pushing and swinging the relaxed abdominal wall with the palms of the hands. The dislocated tympanic large colon rises to the left flank while the congested spleen sinks down to the middle of the abdominal cavity. With the horse in right lateral recumbency, the liberation of the large colon can be recognized per rectum when the spleen is palpated medial to the tympanic left portion of the large colon (Fig. 7). On turning the horse's body into dorsal recumbency, the conservative reposition is completed, but there is no possibility for rectal confirmation in this position because of the mass of the viscera. Final confirmation should be performed after elevation of the horse.

A similar condition is *right dorsal displacement of the large colon* between the tympanic cecum and the right abdominal wall. The large colon is flexed in a rightward and caudal direction and covers the cecum. The edematous fat of the mesentery containing the large blood vessels between the ventral and the dorsal colon has a jelly-like consistency. In *right dorsal displacement* there is no chance for conservative correction by turning over. Therefore, a very clear distinction of the *left* versus *right dorsal displacement* is essential.

Obstruction of the small colon by foreign bodies or fecal concretions can be diagnosed accurately on rectal examination (Fig. 8). The occluding body is usually situated at the ventral abdominal wall near the pelvic inlet and can be moved in all directions. The broad and prominent antimesenteric band of the small colon can be palpated and helps to identify this bowel section. The tympanic prestenotic loops of the small colon have a diameter of approximately 6 to 10 cm and are curved like wheels.

In cases of impaction or volvulus of the small colon, deep rectal examination often is not possible. Only the forearm can be inserted to touch the distended loops of the small colon. In such cases the caudal mesenteric root can be felt because it is tense. This is not found in any other condition, because the free-floating mesentery of the small colon normally is not noticeable.

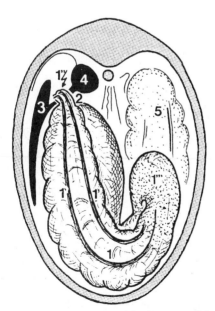

Figure 6. Rectal findings in left dorsal displacement of the large colon. 1, Enlarged large colon with accumulation of gas and ingesta; 1′, Tensed oblique sinistrodorsocranial converging taenia; 1″↯, Location of strangulation with pain on palpation; 1‴, Dislocated tympanic pelvic flexure; 2, Suspensory ligament of the spleen (covered by the large colon); 3, Spleen; 4, Kidney; 5, Prestenotic tympany of the cecum.

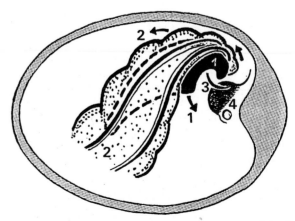

Figure 7. Rectal control of reposition of the dislocation of the large colon over the nephrosplenic ligament in right lateral recumbency of the anesthesized horse. 1, Spleen; 2, tympanic left part of the large colon; 3, nephrosplenic ligament; 4, left kidney; *(arrows)* direction of movement.

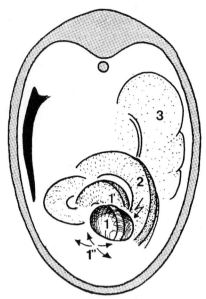

Figure 8. Rectal findings in occlusion of the small colon by an enterolith. 1, Obstructed bowel part with local pain on palpation (⚡); 1′, Prominent free taenia; 1″ Possible directions of manual displacement; 2, Tympany of the prestenotic part of the small colon; 3, Cecum.

Pain elicited on palpation of the visceral surface of the abdominal wall is an indication of acute *diffuse peritonitis*. In cases in which rupture of an abdominal viscus has occurred the dorsal part of the abdominal cavity feels empty and there are floating flaccid intestinal loops in the ventral part. The peritoneum may feel rough because of adherent fecal particles, and in cases of gastric or cecal rupture there is evidence of emphysema in the supraperitoneal space.

To completely assess intestinal or intraperitoneal injury, rectal examination should always be complemented by abdominocentesis. In an analysis of 150 cases at our university, a definitive diagnosis was obtained in 75 patients by rectal palpation alone. In an additional 27% an indication for surgical treatment was obtained by rectal exploration. Only in 6% of these cases was a false diagnosis caused by errors in interpretation of rectal findings. In 9% of the horses rectal examination was not practicable because the horses were too small.

Supplemental Readings

Huskamp B, Daniels H, Kopf N: Magen- und Darmkrankheiten. *In* Dietz O, Wiesner E (eds): Handbuch der Pferdekrankheiten für Wissenschaft und Praxis, vol. 2. Jena, VEB Gustav Fischer Verlag, 1982.

Huskamp B, Kopf N: Die Verlagerung des Colon ascendens in den Milznierenraum beim Pferd (Hernia spatii lienorenalis coli ascendentis). Tierarztl Prax 8:327, 495, 1980.

Huskamp B, Kopf N: Right dorsal displacement of the large colon in the horse. Equine Pract 5:20, 1983.

Huskamp B, Kopf N: Die rektale Untersuchung beim Kolikpferd. In Huskamp B (ed): Opuscula veterinaria. München, wak Verlag- und Kunstberatung, 1995.

Kopf N: Rectal findings in horses with intestinal obstruction. *In* Proceedings of the 1st Colic Research Symposium, University of Georgia, Athens, 1982.

Kopf N, Huskamp B: Die rektale Untersuchung beim Kolikpferd. Prakt Tierarzt 59:259, 1978.

Risk Factors Associated with Colic

NATHANIEL A. WHITE II
Leesburg, Virginia

ETIOLOGY OF COLIC

Most known causes of colic have been established from case reports and case series or from association with easily recognized events. Mild episodes of colic are often described as gas colic, spasmodic colic, or ileus depending on the consistency of feces and the character of bowel sounds heard on auscultation. Most of these mild cases of colic have no known cause, and frequently the clinician cannot establish the segment of intestine involved or the reason for the pain. Other types of colic such as colon impactions and intestinal obstruction due to displacement or strangulation can be diagnosed by palpation per rectum or surgery, but the factors initiating the intestinal disorder are frequently not determined.

Endoparasitism is known to cause colic. Infection with *Strongylus vulgaris* once was reported to cause 90% of all colic in horses. Though this report has never been supported by scientific studies, several reports have shown that *Strongylus vulgaris* larvae cause intestinal motility disturbances, arteritis, thromboembolism, and peritonitis. With the availability of current anthelmintics, colic due to this parasite is now felt to be rare.

Small strongyli are also suspected of causing colic. During a 5-year study of different anthelmintic administration programs, farms had a reduced colic incidence when a bimonthly ivermectin-based control program replaced other non-ivermectin-based programs. Other reports have also linked ascarid, tapeworm, and bot larva infections to episodes of colic.

Several drugs are known to cause bowel injury or dysfunction that can lead to colic. When nonsteroidal antiinflammatory drugs are administered in excessive amounts or for extended periods of time, these compounds are known to cause gastrointestinal ulcers. Horses receiving phenylbutazone (8.8 mg/kg a day for 4–7 days) often develop gastric and intestinal ulcers. Other drugs that cause intestinal stasis and can cause colic include amitraz, an arachnicide, and parasympathetic blocking agents such as atropine or scopolamine. α-Adrenergic agonists and opioid agonists are also reported to cause intestinal stasis or alterations in transit. The duration of action of the most frequently used agents such as xylazine, detomidine, and butorphanol is brief, and there are no reports of these drugs causing colic.

Tumors are relatively rare in horses, and tumors that cause colic a much rarer event. Some tumors reported to cause colic include lymphosarcoma of the spleen and bowel, squamous cell carcinomas of the stomach, intestinal adenocarcinoma, and leiomyoma in the wall of the intestine.

Toxic substances rarely cause colic unless they are inadvertently ingested. Toxic compounds that have caused colic include organophosphates, monensin, and cantharidin from the blister beetle.

Gastric ulcers have been associated with colic in foals and adult horses. Gastric ulcers can cause recurrent colic, and horses with a history of repeated colic episodes should be examined for gastric ulcers. Colic can result directly from the ulcers, or ulcers may be diagnosed concurrent with colon displacements or feed impactions. However, the relationship between ulcers and bowel dysfunction is unknown.

Infectious diseases including salmonellosis, Potomac horse fever, and clostridiosis that are associated with colitis or enteritis can produce signs of colic, though colic is usually not the primary sign seen with these diseases. The pain comes from the inflamed intestine and presumably from endotoxin that is produced or absorbed during infection. An infectious agent is also suspected to cause duodenitis–proximal jejunitis (anterior enteritis), but the agent and the disease mechanism are unknown.

Few epidemiologic studies have evaluated the relationship between environmental or dietary factors and colic. Grain overload normally occurs accidentally or in group feeding situations and can cause colic. Horses with reduced water intake because of frozen water sources are reported to be more susceptible to impaction colic. Sand and foreign body ingestion can cause colic and occur more frequently when horses are fed on the ground, lack proper nutrition, or are bored.

Strangulation of intestine has several known causes including congenital defects like a mesodiverticular band, lipomas, mesenteric rents, and enlargement of the inguinal rings in stallions. Other types of displacements such as the small intestinal volvulus and large colon torsion/volvulus do not have a known cause.

Horses can have colic when they have diseases involving other organ systems. Liver disease causes brain dysfunction and dementia that can give the appearance of colic. Acute pleuritis can cause chest pain, and horses often exhibit similar behavior to that seen with pain from the abdomen. Horses with acute laminitis may stand with a stretched stance and appear to have abdominal discomfort. Horses may exhibit signs similar to those of colic because of muscle pain during acute rhabdomyolysis. Just before foaling some

mares show mild colic apparently related to uterine contractions. Pain from the urogenital system can cause colic, but colic from renal disease is felt to be rare.

COLIC RISK FACTORS

An event, agent, or phenomenon that is associated with a disease risk is called a risk factor (Table 1). A risk factor may be a direct cause of the disease or may be a predictor or indicator of a cause. Some risk factors for colic have been accepted by virtue of common recognition or have been based on numerous anecdotal reports. An example of such a risk factor is in the Standardbred breed, which has an increased risk for inguinal hernia. In this case the Standardbred breed is a marker of the real cause of the problem, the increased size of the inguinal ring. This risk factor is commonly accepted, but a risk ratio, which would give the risk of a Standardbred stallion acquiring an inguinal hernia compared to a stallion of another breed, has not been established.

Geographic location or a particular environment can also be associated with increased risk of certain diseases. As an example, ileal impaction is seen predominantly in the southeastern United States and some other countries. Table 2 includes commonly accepted risk factors derived from clinical experience, descriptive case reports, or hospital case series. Most of these are markers of specific diseases and are accepted as risk factors even though conventional epidemiologic analysis has not been completed to provide risk ratios and other evidence of a direct causal relationship.

Epidemiologic Studies

Several epidemiologic studies on colic have helped to identify certain risk factors for colic. These studies included case control studies reported by Reeves and coworkers (Northeast University study) (Table 3) and Cohen and coworkers (Texas study) (Table 4), and a prospective study

TABLE 1. DEFINITION OF TERMS

When studying risk factors, several terms are used to specifically define the risk of disease or the relationship of a factor to a disease. The following terms are defined to help understand terminology used to describe colic risk factors.

1. **Risk factor**—Factors that are associated with an increased risk of becoming diseased. A risk factor may be a cause or an indicator of a cause of the disease.
2. **Incidence (cumulative incidence)**—Number of new diseases in a known population during a specified period of time.
3. **Incidence density (incidence rate)**—Number of new cases in a population where the time period is defined as the length of time each individual is at risk (usually in years).
4. **Confounder**—An extraneous factor that distorts the effect on another factor being measured. A confounder must be predictive of the disease and may or may not have a causal relationship to the disease.
5. **Marker**—A risk factor that predicts the incidence of disease but is not a cause.
6. **Risk ratio (incidence rate ratio)**—Ratio of the incidence in those exposed to the incidence of those not exposed.
7. **Odds ratio**—Ratio of odds of disease in cases to odds of disease in controls.

TABLE 2. RISK FACTORS COMMONLY CONSIDERED TO BE ASSOCIATED WITH EQUINE COLIC

DISORDER	ASSOCIATED WITH
Meconium impaction	Young age (1–5 days)
Aganglionosis	Paint foal from overo mare
Large colon torsion	Older age, mare, pregnancy
Enteroliths	Highest in California and Florida and on farms with stray wires, nails, other hazards
Gas colic	New grass, new grass and lack of exercise, high-grain diet
Dorsal colon displacement	Large Warmblood breeds
Strangulating lipoma	Horses usually 12 years or older
Epiploic foramen	Older horses (small intestine)
Inguinal hernia	Standardbred, Saddlebred, Tennessee Walking Horse, and Warmblood males
Large colon impaction	Poor dentition, water deprivation, acute stall confinement
Cecal impaction	Older horses
Small colon obstruction	Ponies
Grass sickness	Reported in England, Europe, and South America
Ascarid impaction	Foals after recent worming
Abdominal abscess	More common in mares
Ileal impaction	Southeastern United States

TABLE 4. CASE CONTROL STUDY INVOLVING 821 CASES OF COLIC RECORDED BY VETERINARIANS*

RISK FACTORS	ODDS RATIO
History of previous colic	5.72
History of previous abdominal surgery	5.31
Change in diet in last 2 weeks	2.21

*The next noncolic emergency cases seen by the veterinarians reporting the colic cases were selected to provide similar information for 821 controls.

From Cohen ND, Matejka PL, Honnas CM, Hooper RN, and Texas Equine Colic Study Group: Case control study of the association between various management factors and development of colic in horses. J Am Vet Med Assoc 206:667–673, 1995.

reported by Tinker and coworkers (Virginia-Maryland study) (Table 5). Risk factors were identified in all three studies by selecting factors and determining the odds that exposure to a factor would result in an increased risk of colic. The researchers used logistic regression to statistically analyze and control confounding factors.

History of Colic Episodes

The Northeast University study, Texas study, and Virginia-Maryland study reported that horses having a history of colic were at higher risk for more colic episodes. Other studies have suggested that there is an increased risk after large colon impaction and abdominal surgery for intestinal disease. Several previously identified problems can cause this increased risk, including adhesions or bowel scarring with stricture. In some cases the reason for repeated colic is unclear, and proposed causes, such as increased sensitivity to certain feeds or parasites, have not been documented. It appears that some horses are simply more prone to colic even under optimal management conditions.

Breed and Use

Arabian horses were reported to have a higher risk of colic than other horses in the Northeast University study and the Texas study. This has also been reported in other hospital studies. It has not been determined whether this is related to the breed or to differences in management or use. Horses used for breeding have been reported to be at increased risk in several studies but no specific factor associated with breeding, such as pregnancy, gestation, or lactation, has been directly linked to the increased risk. Nutrition may be a confounder for use because horses used for breeding and strenuous athletic events are more likely to be fed a greater amount of concentrate to maintain weight and performance.

TABLE 3. RISK FACTORS FOR COLIC IN A CASE CONTROL STUDY INVOLVING HORSES PRESENTED TO FIVE UNIVERSITY TEACHING HOSPITALS*

RISK FACTORS	ODDS RATIO
Horse used for breeding (compared with pleasure horses)	1.7
Arabian breed (compared with Thoroughbred breed)	2.0
Day-to-day care by non-owner (compared with owner)	2.2
Pasture access (compared with stabling)	0.8
Number of pastures (compared with 1)	
One pasture	1.0
Two pastures	0.8
Three pastures	0.4
Use of daily anthelmintic (pyrantel pamoate)	0.1
History of previous colic	3.5
Amount of whole grain corn as part of concentrate (compared with control horses that had less corn intake); risk is increased with each additional kilogram consumed	3.4
No water in paddock/pasture (compared with having water)	2.2

*Controls were normal horses from the same farm.

From Reeves MJ, Salmon M, Smith G: Risk factors for equine acute abdominal disease (colic): Results from a multicentered case-control study. Prev Vet Med 26:285–301, 1996.

TABLE 5. COHORT STUDY INVOLVING 1427 HORSES FOR ONE YEAR*

RISK FACTORS	ODDS RATIO
Concentrate intake = 2.5–5 kg/day	4.77
Concentrate intake >5 kg/day	6.33
Change type of concentrate once during year	3.63
Change type of concentrate >once during year	2.17
History of colic during the last 5 years	3.63
Change type of hay >once during year	2.13
Age 2–10 years	2.79
Potomac horse fever vaccine during study	2.04

*A total of 104 case of colic occurred or an incidence of 10.6 cases per 100 horse years. Risk factors listed here were based on the first colic case in each horse affected (total of 86) and all were significant ($P = 0.05$).

From Tinker MK, White NA, Lessard P, Thatcher CD, Pelzer KD, Davis B, Carmel DK: A farm based prospective study for equine colic risk factors and risk-associated events. Doctoral thesis, Virginia Polytechnic Institute and State University, Blacksburg, VA, 1995.

Nutrition

Feeds or feeding activity have long been blamed for colic. Certain types of hay and lush pasture have been anecdotally given as risk factors. Practitioners associate ingestion of rapidly growing lush grass with increased frequency of gas colic. Types of grass and hay such as coastal Bermuda hay or poor-quality roughage are suspected of causing colic in groups of horses. Overfeeding of grain has been reported to cause colic. Both the Virginia-Maryland study and the Texas study found increased colic risk when feed type, grain or hay, was changed. The Virginia-Maryland study documented an increased risk of colic in horses fed mixed grains such as sweet feed and pelleted grains compared with horses fed single grains or no grain. This study also reported that daily feeding of concentrate from 2.5 to 5 kg/day and more than 5 kg/day increased the risk of colic 4.8 and 6.3 times, respectively, compared with horses fed no grain. The amount of grain rather than the type of grain is probably the most important factor, but the increased risk observed for horses fed any type of mixed grains requires further investigation.

Feeding small amounts of grain at frequent intervals has been reported to reduce the fluid shifts in the large colon seen with twice-daily feeding. Although no relationship was found between feeding frequency and colic in the Northeast University study, feeding more than twice daily increased the risk of colic in the Virginia-Maryland study. This was suspected to be due to an increased daily intake of grain rather than the frequency of feeding. The mechanism by which grain excess causes intestinal problems is not known, but is speculated to be the result of feeding high levels of soluble carbohydrate that can alter the microbial population, intraluminal hydration, or pH of the cecum or colon.

Coastal Bermuda grass hay has not been found to be a risk factor for chronic colic in the Texas study and changes in diet, both grain and hay, were related to increased risk of colic in both the Texas and the Virginia-Maryland studies. Gradual change to new types or amounts of feed has long been recommended and is supported by these findings. There is still little information about specific types of feed or the measurement of specific nutrients in the feed, such as minerals or fiber, in relation to colic.

Environment and Management

Housing and confinement on the farms in the Virginia-Maryland study were not risk factors for colic. However, other reports have suggested there is an increased risk of cecal and colon impaction after horses have acute decreases in activity, such as curtailing regular exercise or changing from turn-out activity to strict stall confinement because of an injury or after surgery.

The Northeast University study demonstrated that horses on pasture were significantly more likely to have colic compared with stall-confined horses, although the risk of colic in pastured horses decreased if horses had recent access to two or three different pastures. This study also revealed that turn out in a paddock without water even for a short period increased the risk of colic. It is difficult to prove that decreased water intake is related to colic incidence, but common sense suggests that horses not getting adequate water on a daily basis have increased risk of intestinal or systemic abnormalities.

Studies to this time have not fully appraised the risks associated with exercise or activity level. Although use for racing or eventing was associated with the highest incidence of colic in the Virginia-Maryland study, these activities did not pose an increased risk when compared with other factors (see Table 5). Management factors are difficult to compare between farms and changes in management even more difficult to detect. The increased risk associated with care by trainers and managers compared with owners in the Northeast University study suggests that differences in management are important in the cause of colic. The relationship is probably the result of some other factor commonly associated with horses under the care of trainer or managers.

Management of Health-related Events

Pregnancy. The mare in late pregnancy or lactation has been reported to have a higher risk for colon displacement or volvulus. This was not significant in the Virginia-Maryland study until events were defined within a certain time period before the colic episode and controlled by using random dates for events in horses without colic. When compared with random time for exposure, mares had an increased risk of colic from 60 to 150 days after foaling. Other clinical studies have suggested that the mare is at increased risk just before foaling and during the period of lactation. The physiologic events that predispose to this increased risk are not known, but changes in calcium levels and alterations in diet, including increases in energy in the diet, may be related.

Horse Transport. Horse transport increased colic risk in a study by Uhlinger and in the Virginia-Maryland study. This has been suspected by practitioners, who commonly administer laxatives before shipping to prevent impactions. The mechanism or cause of the increased incidence is unknown.

Fever. It is logical that horses with infection could have alteration of the gastrointestinal tract, predisposing them to colic. Fever within 14 days before a colic episode was frequently associated with increased risk of colic in the Virginia-Maryland study. Because the reported causes of fever in these cases were varied, no specific relationship or cause for each colic episode was established.

Vaccination. When examining all horses for the entire year of the Virginia-Maryland study, there was an increased risk resulting from Potomac horse fever vaccination. If examined using a time frame of 14 days after any vaccination for cases and controls, there was a significant increase in risk of colic after any vaccination. Vaccination has not been previously identified and was not found to increase colic risk in the Texas study. Vaccination as a possible risk factor requires further study, including the possibility that a systemic reaction from a vaccination is sufficient to cause a colic episode. Alternatively, vaccination could be a confounder, and the real cause of colic episodes associated with vaccination has yet to be identified.

Weather. Weather changes are frequently associated with increased frequency of colic, but previous reports have been unable to find statistical proof of any risk. When examined as a direct exposure in the Virginia-Maryland study, weather did not appear to be related to the colic. When events were investigated by looking at a 14-day window preceding colic episodes in both horses with colic and controls, low humidity significantly increased risk. No explanation for this relationship exists unless it is a confounder for management changes, such as altering activity during weather extremes. Further work is needed to review a combination of factors involving weather in a large number of horses.

Miscellaneous. Several events that have been reported or suspected to cause colic but were not found to be significant risks in any of the studies include recent anthelmintic administration and vices such as cribbing. Enough horses received anthelmintics during these studies to confirm that there is no increased risk in horses receiving regularly scheduled medication for parasite control. Cribbing, on the other hand, is considered to predispose to flatulent colic, but the incidence of cribbing was not high enough in the Virginia-Maryland population to make it an increased risk when compared to the other factors. When risk was examined in the Virginia-Maryland study by combining event factors, feeding grain combined with vices and feeding grain combined with transport increased colic risk approximately eight and nine times, respectively, compared with colic in horses that were not exposed to these combinations. Only a few of theses factors were combined and examined by analysis in this study. Other factors may be important and deserve further investigation.

INVESTIGATION OF FARM-BASED COLIC PROBLEMS

Veterinarians are frequently asked what causes individual cases of colic, and typically no specific cause can be determined. Occasionally, a farm or group of horses has an increase in the incidence of colic or a higher rate than is felt to be acceptable by the veterinarian or owner. When groups of cases are available, epidemiologic methods can be employed to help identify risk factors. Although getting help from an epidemiologist is helpful, the practicing veterinarian can initiate the investigation.

To determine a cause of a disease, clinicians must find a factor or factors that significantly increases or decreases risk, and then measure a significant reduction in incidence of disease when the exposure to that factor is reduced. To date, only the first half of this method has been completed for the risk factors reported for equine colic. Even without studying the effect of reduced exposure, it is clear from the factors examined in all these studies that feeding and management factors are related to the frequency of colic. All the event factors point to management changes or factors that can influence physiologic changes and cause colic. Horses that experience a change of activity or diet due to disease, medication administration, or scheduling changes should be considered to be at increased risk for colic. Although individual horses may tolerate change with no problem, some apparently are susceptible to intestinal dysfunction that may be sufficient to cause colic. Although clinicians tend to search for single causes of colic, horses are probably responding to multiple factors, which when combined in the proper sequence, or with a trigger event, result in the disease.

To determine what is causing a high rate of colic on a farm or in a group of horses, identification of risk factors may be necessary. Risk factors can rarely be identified by simple observations, except in the extreme or obvious cases. It is also difficult to identify risk factors for individual horses or for small groups of horses unless other horses managed under similar conditions can serve as controls.

When confronted with a high number of colic cases on a farm, a systematic approach, including careful record keeping and monitoring over an established period, is required to determine risk factors. An initial review with careful monitoring of the management, including on-site observations of the daily routine, can reveal obvious problems, such as excessive phenylbutazone administration or inadequate water intake. However, in most cases these preliminary findings only suggest possibilities and long-term analysis is required to solve the problem. The process can be divided into three stages.

First, the incidence density of colic on the farm should be established. Although not totally reliable, retrospective data can be used to determine if a problem really exists. Uhlinger used veterinary call records to determine incidence density on farms and found this method to be a reliable estimate, although mild colic cases may be missed if the veterinarian is not called. Incidence density is calculated by counting the number of new colic episodes for an extended period, preferably for 1 year, and dividing by the number of horses at risk on the farm during that year. On a small farm this may be difficult because individuals with repeated colic episodes may bias the incidence, making it less reliable as an indicator of the colic problem.

Second, a profile of each horse should be gathered as the basis for future recordkeeping. Factors of interest should include use, specific diet, frequency of feeding, vaccination, medical treatments, and changes in activity, including an exercise schedule, transport, and daily housing schedule. Determination of diet must include analysis of all feedstuffs ingested, including an estimate of intake from pasture and hay. Supplements may add nutrients to the diet and should also be measured.

Third, potential risk factors should be identified by determining the incidence density ratio, which is the incidence density of horses with colic exposed to a factor divided by the incidence density of horses with colic but not exposed to the same factor. An epidemiologist can help in making the appropriate grouping and calculations, including statistical comparisons. The calculated odds ratio becomes the estimate of risk that a horse exposed to that risk factor will have a colic episode, compared to one that is not exposed. If a risk factor is identified, reducing the horse's exposure to the factor provides the best chance of reducing the overall colic incidence.

To make this determination, accurate records of exposure to factors must be made. Although some extra time is required to make daily records, farm owners often are willing to keep daily records, and often the record keeping reveals other discrepancies in management that enlightens owners.

In the Virginia-Maryland study the overall incidence density for colic was 10.6 colic cases per 100 horses. Thirty-four percent of the cases in this study were so mild that they were not initially reported by the farms and in some cases not treated. Even seemingly insignificant cases must be included to ensure that the true incidence is recognized. No doubt colic incidence can vary with different environments and uses, as seen on the different types of farms in the Virginia-Maryland study. However, it seems safe to suggest that incidence density of colic on farms with more than 20 colic cases per 100 horses should be investigated to determine if the colic rate can be reduced by altering diet, monitoring parasite control, or reducing changes in activity, health care, or routine. Much like setting up a preventive health program for infectious disease and parasite control, careful monitoring of nutrition and changes in activity may help owners reduce colic incidence.

Supplemental Readings

Cohen ND, Matejka PL, Honnas CM, Hooper RN: Case-control study of the association between various management factors and development of colic in horses. J Am Vet Med Assoc 206:667–673, 1995.

Cohen ND, Peloso JG: Risk factors for history of previous colic and for chronic intermittent colic in a population of horses. J Am Vet Med Assoc 208:697–703, 1996.

Dabareiner RM, White NA: Large colon impaction in horses: 147 cases (1985–1991). J Am Vet Med Assoc 206:679–685, 1995.

Murray MJ: Gastric ulcers in adult horses. Compend Cont Ed Pract Vet 16:792–794, 1994.

Reeves MJ, Salmon MD, Smith G: Risk factors for equine acute abdominal disease (colic): Results from a multicentered case-control study. Prev Vet Med 26:285–301, 1996.

Tennant B, Wheat JD, Meagher DM: Observations on the causes and incidence of acute intestinal obstruction in the horse. Proc 18th Annu Meet Am Assoc Equine Pract, 1972, pp 251–257.

Tinker MK, White NA, Lessard P, Thatcher CD, Pelzer KD, Davis B, Carmel DK: A farm based prospective study for equine colic risk factors and risk associated events. Doctoral Thesis, Virginia Polytechnic Institute and State University, Blacksburg, VA 1995.

Uhlinger C: Effects of three anthelmintic schedules on the incidence of colic in horses. Equine Vet J 22:251–254, 1990.

Uhlinger C: Investigations into the incidence of field colic. Equine Vet J 13[Suppl]:16–18, 1992.

White NA: Epidemiology and etiology of colic. In White NA (ed): The Equine Acute Abdomen. Philadelphia, Lea & Febiger, 1990, pp 49–64.

Medical vs. Surgical Treatment of Horses with Colic

JAMES N. MOORE
Athens, Georgia

In the past 25 years, significant improvements have been made in the evaluation of horses with colic, the preoperative preparation and anesthetic management of these horses, and the surgical techniques used to correct specific abnormalities. These improvements have made abdominal surgery commonplace in many practices. With the increased availability of exploratory abdominal surgery as a technique to determine the underlying cause of colic, the decision regarding whether to perform surgery or treat the horse medically becomes even more important. Because the horse-owning public requires that their animals receive the best care possible, yet with the minimal recovery time away from their intended function, it is critical that equine clinicians become more adept at identifying horses that should and should not be candidates for abdominal surgery. Because the horse's prognosis for survival depends on its status at the time surgery or intensive medical therapy is initiated, the decision about which form of therapy is indicated must be made before the horse's physiologic condition begins to deteriorate. As part of this decision-making process, the client must be informed about potential problems associated with either form of treatment and the horse's prognosis for survival. The purpose of this discussion is to review the methods used to identify horses requiring abdominal surgery and those that should be treated medically.

There are several classic clinical presentations that have been associated with the need for surgical intervention. These include the following: (1) horses exhibiting signs of severe abdominal pain that fail to respond or respond poorly to analgesics; (2) horses that yield large volumes of gastric reflux upon passage of a stomach tube; (3) horses that have abnormally distended intestine on rectal examination and discolored peritoneal fluid containing an increased number of red blood cells and total protein; and (4) horses with few or no audible intestinal sounds. Unfortunately, these classic indications for surgical intervention may be the exception rather than the rule. Equine practitioners commonly identify some horses with mild or moderate pain that require surgical intervention, thereby underscoring the importance of performing a thorough physical examination on horses exhibiting signs of abdominal pain.

SIGNALMENT AND PREVIOUS HISTORY

The horse's signalment and recent history may provide the veterinarian with data that assist in determining whether surgical intervention is required. As examples, it may be possible to reduce the number of differential diagnoses under consideration by determining the animal's age and gender, whether the onset of clinical signs followed a period of strenuous exercise, the geographic location, whether there have been previous episodes of pain, and the approximate duration of the current colic episode. This information may cause the veterinarian to consider common age-, gender- and breed-related conditions. Ex-

TABLE 1.   COMMON AGE-RELATED CONDITIONS CAUSING COLIC IN HORSES

Aged	Pedunculated lipoma
	Mesocolic rupture
Middle age	Cecal impaction
	Enteroliths
	Epiploic foramen entrapment
	Large colon volvulus
Young	Foreign body obstruction
	Nonstrangulating infarction
	Small intestinal intussusception
Yearlings	Ascarid impaction
Foals	Atresia coli
	Gastroduodenal ulcers
	Meconium retention
	Uroperitoneum

amples of age-related conditions are listed in Table 1. Common gender-related conditions include colonic volvulus, which most commonly occurs in brood mares that have foaled within the previous 90 days, mesocolic rupture in brood mares shortly after parturition, and inguinal hernias in stallions with a recent history of exercise or breeding a mare. Enteroliths commonly cause problems in adult Arabian or Arabian-cross horses; enteroliths may be associated with a history of repeated bouts of abdominal pain, and occur more commonly in the Western United States. Intestinal incarceration and colonic volvulus tend to become painful more quickly than simple obstructions or displacements.

PHYSICAL EXAMINATION

In most instances, the decision regarding the necessity for surgery is based on information obtained from the physical examination. Consequently, a thorough physical examination must be performed, with particular attention paid to the horse's cardiopulmonary and gastrointestinal systems. A strong association exists between the functioning of these two systems and the horse's vital signs, including pulse rate, mucous membrane color, capillary refill time, respiratory rate, and rectal temperature, reflect the adequacy of the intestinal mucosal barrier to bacterial endotoxin. Thus, evaluation of the status of the horse's cardiovascular system in light of the duration of the present colic episode may provide insight into the severity of the intestinal disorder. Because it is equally important to determine when not to do surgery, it is important to recognize that increases in the rectal temperature may be indicative of impending colitis, small intestinal enteritis, pleuritis, or peritonitis, none of which requires surgical intervention.

An important part of the physical examination is the response to passage of the stomach tube. If a large amount of fluid is removed from the stomach, the veterinarian should consider this to be of diagnostic value because fluid tends to accumulate in the stomach from small intestinal disorders rather than from problems involving the large colon. Although the retrieval of large amounts of fluid from the stomach often indicates the need for surgery, a notable exception to this generalization is proximal enteritis-jejunitis.

The results of several clinical studies indicate that information gleaned from the rectal examination provide the veterinarian with the most important data about the horse's underlying disease. Consequently, it is essential that a systematic rectal examination procedure be used to ensure that each accessible area of the abdominal cavity be evaluated (see page 170).

Other historical and physical examination findings should be kept in mind while the rectal examination is being performed. For instance, if a large volume of fluid reflux is removed from the stomach, efforts should be made to feel for distended loops of small intestine. Similarly, if the horse's abdomen is grossly distended, particular attention should be paid to determine if a volvulus, displacement, or enterolith is the cause for the distension. Rectal examination results consistent with the need for surgical intervention include tightly distended loops of small intestine, a grossly distended large colon, a distended loop of small intestine leading to an inguinal ring, an enterolith, an ileocecal intussusception or ileal impaction, and a displacement of the large colon around the cecal base.

One of the most reliable parameters indicating the need for surgery is the persistence of pain despite the administration of potent analgesics, such as xylazine or detomidine, or the recurrence of pain 15 to 30 minutes after administration of these analgesics. This insufficient response to analgesics is often indicative of conditions producing complete intestinal obstruction and requiring surgical intervention. Horses with large colon or small intestinal volvulus most often have extreme pain, reflecting complete obstruction of the intestinal lumen, distension of the intestine proximal to the volvulus, and ischemia. Conversely, other strangulating lesions may cause moderate degrees of pain, which are controlled by analgesics. For instance, the pain associated with entrapment of the small intestine through the epiploic foramen may be controllable with analgesics. Similarly, the results of recent clinical studies indicate that horses with small intestinal strangulating lesions caused by pedunculated lipomas intermittently exhibit signs of pain. This fact complicates the diagnosis of these conditions, especially in stoic horses.

Although no intestinal disorder produces a uniform clinical picture, these generalities may aid the veterinarian in making a rational decision about whether to intervene surgically. Of the aforementioned items, the most important ones to keep in mind when examining a horse with colic are the degree of pain and the rectal examination results (Table 2).

TABLE 2.   COMMON INDICATIONS FOR ABDOMINAL SURGERY

1. Degree of pain	Poor response to analgesics
2. Rectal examination	Distended small intestine
	Displaced colon
	Enterolith or foreign body
3. Fluid reflux from the stomach	More than 4 L
4. Auscultation of abdomen	No borborygmi
5. Peritoneal fluid	Increased protein, erythrocytes, and toxic neutrophils

LABORATORY TESTS

Most laboratory tests provide the clinician with information that is useful in determining the horse's prognosis for survival or which type of supportive therapy may be indicated. No tests make the diagnosis or the decision for surgery. This is true for the determination of acid-base status, blood lactate, blood urea nitrogen, blood glucose, and packed cell volume. Obviously, the veterinarian should neither ignore the results of these laboratory tests nor refuse to use them. In specific instances, laboratory test abnormalities such as neutropenia or a left shift may be useful in identifying diseases with a strong inflammatory component, such as colitis or proximal enteritis.

Excessive reliance should not be placed on visual and microscopic examination of peritoneal fluid. Numerous instances have occurred in which nonviable bowel has been found at surgery when the characteristics of the peritoneal fluid were normal. Consequently, most of the laboratory tests available should be used to evaluate the degree of cardiovascular compromise and determine the animal's response to preoperative medical therapy.

FINANCIAL COMPONENT OF THE DECISION

Based solely on the economics of the situation, it may be difficult to justify performance of emergency abdominal surgery in many horses. It is not uncommon for emotional and sentimental attachment to the animal to exceed the economic value of the horse. Consequently, it is imperative that the veterinarian be sure that the client understands the expected costs of anesthesia, surgery, and postoperative care, and the animal's prognosis for survival. In emergency situations, it is relatively easy for the client to overlook the costs that may be incurred if complications occur; these subjects must be broached and the client should be given time to consider all the information at hand before the final decision is made.

EARLY REFERRAL OF HORSES WITH COLIC

Early referral of horses that require either intensive medical therapy or surgical intervention yields the best chance for a success. Thus, horses that should be referred include those that respond initially to an analgesic but require additional analgesic therapy a few hours later, those that continue to exhibit signs of pain despite administration of analgesics, those that remain in pain but whose peritoneal fluid appears normal, those with distended small intestine on rectal examination but lacking fluid reflux, and those with large quantities of gastric reflux but no distended small intestine palpable on rectal examination. Although some of these horses may not require surgical intervention, this practice probably would result in earlier surgical intervention in other horses. Because the key to success in colic surgery is performing surgery as early as possible, early referrals should improve the outcome for the horse, client, referring veterinarian, and surgeon.

THE TRUE "EXPLORATORY" COLIC SURGERY

One of the most difficult decisions for veterinarians at referral hospitals to make is whether to perform an exploratory celiotomy on a horse that fails to fall into a readily definable disease category. This dilemma arises with certain colonic displacements, intussusceptions, entrapment of small intestine through the epiploic foramen, and proximal enteritis. The veterinarian is often torn between trying to minimize the financial impact of the situation on the client, avoiding surgery on an animal with a condition that is not amenable to surgical intervention, and reducing the deleterious effects of time on a horse with poorly perfused intestine. If, after careful consideration of the physical examination abnormalities and results of laboratory tests, there is sufficient evidence to support the presence of hypoperfused intestine, an exploratory celiotomy should be performed. The benefits of performing surgery earlier on a horse with a condition requiring surgical intervention are obvious. Aside from the costs, potential for incisional problems, and increased lay-up time, there are fewer life-threatening consequences of an exploratory celiotomy in a horse with a condition that must be managed medically.

Supplemental Readings

Ducharme NG, Lowe JE: Decision for surgery. Vet Clin North Am Equine Pract 4(1):51–61, 1988.
Moore BR, Moore RM: Examination of the equine patient with gastrointestinal emergency. Vet Clin North Am Equine Pract 10(3):549–566, 1994.
Schumacher J, Cohen ND, Seahorn TL: Duodenitis/proximal jejunitis in horses. Compend Contin Ed 16:1197–1206, 1994.
Trent AM: Referral of colic cases. In Gordon BJ, Allen D(eds): Field Guide to Colic Management in the Horse: The Practitioner's Reference. Lenexa, KS, Vet Med Publishing Co, 1988, pp 191–200.

Medical Management of Colic

LUCY M. EDENS
Gainesville, Florida

JANA L. CARGILE
Glencoe, Missouri

Acute abdominal pain is the one of the most frequently encountered problems in equine practice. A small percentage of horses with colic will require surgical intervention, whereas the majority can be successfully treated by medical therapy alone. Early and aggressive medical therapy may actually help prevent progression to a lesion that must be resolved surgically. Therefore, it is imperative that the modern-day equine practitioner not only be skilled in recognizing which cases warrant surgical intervention, but also adept at administering, and monitoring the response to, advanced medical treatments.

Gastrointestinal (GI) disorders in horses are accompanied by many alterations to the cardiovascular, musculoskeletal, respiratory, and endocrine systems, all of which can lead to fatal problems if not recognized and addressed. Providing relief of pain, maintaining peripheral as well as organ perfusion, promoting intestinal motility, and treating effects of endotoxemia are all important issues that should be addressed in colic patients. In addition, the list of GI disorders responsive to medical management is expanding, and includes gastric, cecal, and colonic impaction, sand colic, gastric ulceration, duodenitis-proximal jejunitis (DPJ), and right dorsal colitis.

ANALGESICS

The hallmark of gastrointestinal disease in the horse is colic, resulting in clinical signs referable to abdominal pain. The intensity of the visceral pain is frequently comparable to the severity of the accompanying lesion, thus the potency and duration of action of the analgesics used can have a significant impact on the management and outcome of the case. Undoubtedly, most, if not all, horses with acute abdominal disease require analgesics. The success of medical therapy is often dictated by the individual's response to pain relief. Because pain potently induces ileus, pain relief is critical to effective medical management of colic, and to ensure the safety of those handling the animal. Numerous medically treatable gastrointestinal conditions need frequent administration of pain-relieving medications (Table 1). The challenge for the practitioner is to balance the use of analgesics with their potential to mask a more serious condition that needs surgical correction.

Nonsteroidal Anti-Inflammatory Drugs

The most commonly administered and effective analgesics used to manage visceral pain in horses are the nonsteroidal anti-inflammatory drugs (NSAIDs), notably flunixin meglumine, ketoprofen, phenylbutazone, and dipyrone. These drugs exert their effects by reducing the sensitization of nerve endings to pain, and by altering the perception of pain within the central nervous system (CNS). Their mechanism of action is based primarily on inhibition of the enzyme cyclooxygenase. Ketoprofen reportedly also inhibits lipoxygenase activity, although this has not been proven in horses. The benefits of NSAIDs treatment extend beyond merely providing analgesia; by reducing endotoxin-associated mediator production, normal intestinal blood flow can be maintained and intestinal motility restored.

Flunixin meglumine, a cyclooxygenase inhibitor, is one of the most potent (if not the most potent) NSAID for control of colic in horses. This clinical impression, held by most practitioners, is supported by experimental data (refer to the following discussion of endotoxemia). In many cases, a reduced dose of 0.25 to 0.5 mg/kg every 6 to 12 hours provides sufficient analgesia, while minimizing the chances of side effects. The duration of analgesia with flunixin meglumine ranges from 0.5 to 24 hours, depending on the underlying lesion. Repeated dosing is often necessary, which carries minimal risk, provided that intestinal strangulation is not a concern. The symptomatic relief indicated by lowered heart rate and improved mucous membrane color provided by the use of flunixin meglumine may obscure recognition of the presence of a strangulating lesion.

Ketoprofen,* a new NSAID, has had limited experimental and clinical use for the management of equine colic but appears to have comparable efficacy to flunixin meglumine. The suggested dose of ketoprofen is 2.2 mg/kg every 12 hours intravenously (IV) or intramuscularly (IM). The cumulative effect of this drug, as well as other NSAIDs should be kept in mind in regard to their potential to induce gastrointestinal ulceration and renal tubular damage.

Dipyrone and phenylbutazone, also cyclooxygenase inhibitors, provide only minimal analgesia for visceral pain. Dipyrone is a safe analgesic that can be administered intramuscularly (IM), several times within hours, to provide short-term relief for mild abdominal pain. In the authors' opinion, this is the best analgesic to provide to owners and horse trainers because of its wide margin of safety and its potent antipyretic properties. Phenylbutazone provides analgesia comparable to that of dipyrone but has disadvantages of increased risk of NSAIDs toxicity and problems with safe parenteral administration. Therefore, phenylbutazone has minimal use as an analgesic in the treatment of equine colic. Its primary indication for use is treatment of laminitis, which can accompany GI disease. In this instance, phenylbutazone is often administered with flunixin meglumine, using a reduced individual dose for each drug.

*Ketofen, Fort Dodge Laboratory, Fort Dodge, IA

182

TABLE 1.   ANALGESICS USED FOR TREATMENT OF HORSES WITH COLIC

Drug	Method of Action	Suggested Dosage	Comments
Acepromazine	Anti-dopaminergic, α-adrenergic blocker	0.02–0.04 mg/kg IV, IM, s.i.d. to q.i.d.	Do not use in hypovolemic horses
Dipyrone	NSAID°	11 mg/kg IV, IM, s.i.d. to q4h	Weak analgesia
Phenylbutazone	NSAID°	2.2–4.4 mg/kg IV, p.o., s.i.d. to b.i.d.	Weak analgesia
Flunixin meglumine	NSAID°	1.1 mg/kg IV, IM, s.i.d. to t.i.d.	Good analgesia, irritating if given IM
Ketoprofen	NSAID°	2.2 mg/kg IV b.i.d.	Effects comparable to flunixin
Xylazine	α₂-adrenergic agonist	0.2–0.4 mg/kg IV, IM, PRN for severe pain	Potent sedation and analgesia for 10–40 minutes, causes ileus
Detomidine	α₂-adrenergic agonist	10–30 mg/kg IV, IM, PRN for severe pain	Potent sedation and analgesia for 20–90 minutes, causes ileus
Butorphanol tartrate	Opioid receptor agonist-antagonist	0.05–0.10 mg/kg IV, IM, PRN for severe pain	Potent analgesia for 15–90 minutes, often combined with α₂-agonists

°Effects cumulative, use caution to avoid NSAIDs toxicity.

An effective regimen is 0.25 mg/kg t.i.d. for flunixin meglumine, and 2.2 mg/kg b.i.d. for phenylbutazone.

Sedative Analgesics

Initial examination of the horse with acute, severe abdominal pain often requires short-term sedation to minimize the risk of injury to the horse, the horse's handler, and the veterinarian. The onset of action of this category of drugs is more rapid, and the analgesia produced more potent, than that of the NSAIDs. Clinical response to sedative and analgesic effects of short-acting drugs such as xylazine is regularly used to predict whether medical therapy will resolve the problem. The two most commonly used drugs in this category are xylazine and detomidine, which are centrally acting α₂-adrenergic agonists. In addition to inducing sedation and analgesia, α₂-adrenergic agonists induce hypertension-mediated bradycardia, culminating in hypotension and ileus. The ileus and hypotension may persist for up to several hours, exceeding the duration of analgesia and sedation. Although xylazine and detomidine are classified as α₂-adrenergic agonists, they differ significantly in their potency and duration of action. The analgesia provided by xylazine lasts 15 to 30 minutes, and is not typically potent enough to mask the pain induced by a severe strangulating obstruction. Detomidine is 10 times more potent than xylazine, and is capable of masking pain associated with severe intestinal lesions. Recurrence of colic signs within 1 hour of receiving detomidine is an indication for surgery. Because of the prolonged analgesic potency of detomidine, the decision for surgery may be delayed, possibly affecting the ultimate outcome. Therefore, detomidine should be reserved for those cases in which surgery is not an option, or when there is a delay before surgery, for example, during transport.

Butorphanol, an opiate agonist-antagonist, provides analgesia without notable side effects at a dose less than 0.02 mg/kg. By combining butorphanol with an α₂-adrenergic agonist, the amount of α₂-adrenergic agonist can be reduced, yet still can provide a similar degree of analgesia with a slightly longer duration of action. This combination lessens the incidence of side effects. For pain relief in horses with colic due to a condition that requires medical therapy (e.g., large colon impaction), this combination is the authors' preferred analgesic regimen.

Acepromazine must be used cautiously for the management of colic owing to its propensity to induce or exacerbate existing systemic hypotension. In cases of spasmodic colic, it does appear to be effective in enhancing the analgesic effects of NSAIDs when used at a dose of 0.02 to 0.04 mg/kg IV or IM.

INTRAVENOUS FLUID THERAPY

Volume Expansion

Circulating volume must be restored and electrolyte and acid-base imbalances corrected. Effective circulating fluid volume in horses that are moderately to severely dehydrated (7–10%) is best restored by rapid intravenous administration of 30 to 50 L of buffered, polyionic fluids per 500 kg bodyweight. When possible, at least half of the estimated deficit should be given during the first hour. This requires fluid infusion rates of 15 to 30 L/hour for 1 to 2 hours, using 10- to 12-gauge jugular catheters; large-bore, 10- to 12-gauge straight IV fluid delivery systems; and 5 L fluid bags. Further increases in rate of fluid delivery can be accomplished by installing more than one catheter or by use of fluid pumps. Although rates less than 40 L/hour are unlikely to "overload" an adult horse, the relative benefits of rapid fluid administration versus risks of venous thrombosis should be considered, particularly in patients with evidence of coagulopathy. Available large-bore catheters are made of a more thrombogenic material than 14- to 16-gauge catheters, and fluid pumps are associated with an increased incidence of venous thrombosis. One approach is to install a long-term, nonthrombogenic, smaller gauge catheter in one jugular vein and a larger bore catheter in the opposite jugular vein. Using this system, flow rates of 20 L/hour or more can be obtained by gravity. After the initial resuscitation period, the larger catheter can be removed and fluid therapy continued via the smaller catheter.

If enterogastric reflux is not present, fluid deficits are 6% or less, and the horse's disease process will not impair intestinal absorption, oral fluids either by voluntary intake or via nasogastric tube can be given to supply part, or all, of the daily fluid requirements less expensively than IV fluids. This approach to fluid therapy is especially useful to treat large-colon impactions and to maintain hydration of horses with only a low volume of diarrhea. If large volumes of fluid are to be administered enterally, a combination of electrolytes should be added to the solution. This is particularly important in anorectic patients.

Acid-Base and Electrolytes

In moderately to severely dehydrated horses, acid-base and electrolyte status should be evaluated initially and re-evaluated periodically for the duration of fluid therapy. Fluids should provide potassium, 0.04 to 0.08 mEq/kg body weight per hour in horses with normal serum potassium concentration, and up to 0.5 mEq/kg body weight per hour in hypokalemic patients. In horses found to be acidotic on initial evaluation, serum potassium should be monitored closely, because potassium shifts intracellularly during fluid therapy as pH returns to normal. Because potassium is primarily located intracellularly, serum concentrations do not correlate with total potassium deficits.

Volume replacement alone corrects metabolic acidosis in most horses with hypovolemia. Sodium bicarbonate should be used if the initial blood pH is less then 7.2, or the total CO_2 concentration is less then 15 mEq/L. The total deficit can be estimated by using the formula:

$$(27 - CO_2) \times 0.5 \times \text{body weight (kg)}$$

Fifty percent of the calculated deficit can be provided during initial fluid resuscitation by adding 500 ml of 5% sodium bicarbonate to each 5 L bag of calcium-free fluids. The acid-base status should then be re-evaluated and therapy adjusted as needed. Serum calcium concentration, preferably ionized versus total, should be evaluated and supplemented if low. Consideration should be given to the effects of albumin concentration if total calcium measurements are used. Calcium gluconate (23%) can be added to bicarbonate-free fluids (125 to 250 ml per 5 L bag) to provide a total dose of 500 ml. Periodically measuring calcium concentration is the best way to monitor response to therapy.

Magnesium concentrations in horses with GI disease have long been ignored, yet this electrolyte is required for many metabolic functions through its role as a coenzyme for the sodium-potassium adenosinetriphosphatase (AT-Pase) pump. Magnesium absorption occurs in the small intestine; thus, horses with small intestinal diseases (e.g., DPJ) are at greatest risk for deficiency. Hypomagnesemia predisposes patients to neuromuscular weakness, refractory hypocalcemia and hypokalemia, and cardiac arrhythmias (e.g., ventricular tachycardia). Hypomagnesemic patients are also at greater risk for intracellular calcium accumulation within the myocardium, which enhances cardiotoxicity of parenterally administered calcium. Myocardial damage that can accompany endotoxemia may be exacerbated by low magnesium levels. Specific guidelines for magnesium administration in horses do not exist; however, good results have been obtained by supplementing IV fluids with 1 to 5 g/L magnesium sulfate. As with calcium, the best means of monitoring magnesium therapy is to periodically recheck

magnesium concentrations. The authors have observed one horse that became persistently hypomagnesemic after extensive small intestinal resection. This horse responded well to daily oral magnesium chloride supplementation at 25 mg/kg.

Plasma Therapy

Dehydrated horses with a total plasma protein level of 5 g/dl or less may require plasma transfusion to improve intravascular onchotic pressures. Plasma transfusion becomes critical when total plasma protein concentration decreases below 3.5 g/dl, when albumin is less then 1.5 g/dl, or when signs of hypovolemia and hypotension persist, despite volume replacement. Initially, 5 L/450 kg recipient body weight of commercially available plasma° or cross-matched plasma collected from a donor horse should be given. Total protein should be monitored, and multiple transfusions may be necessary.

Hypertonic (7.2%) Saline Resuscitation

In situations in which rapid IV administration of large volumes of fluids is difficult, smaller volumes of hypertonic (7.2%) sodium chloride† solution, given at a dose of 4 to 6 ml/kg body weight, over 10 to 30 minutes, may be beneficial. Hypertonic saline is believed to shift fluid from the intra- to the extracellular space, rapidly expanding circulating volume and improving cardiac output, and may increase myocardial contractility and enhance vascular tone. Although the cardiovascular response of animals given endotoxin improved more after hypertonic saline than an equal volume of isotonic fluids, these results should not be used to conclude that hypertonic saline resuscitation is more advantageous than large-volume isotonic fluid resuscitation. If used, hypertonic saline should always be followed with isotonic fluids given at a rate of two to three times maintenance levels to restore total body water deficits.

ADDITIONAL CARDIOVASCULAR SUPPORT

Following the initial resuscitation period (1–4 hours), obvious clinical improvement should be seen, manifested as improved attitude, decreased heart rate, urination, decreased capillary refill time, moist mucous membranes, strong peripheral pulses, and decreased hematocrit and plasma protein concentration. If an adequate volume of fluids has been administered, and signs of hypovolemia continue, mean arterial pressures should be evaluated by means of a tail cuff manometer or oscillometer. If there is hypotension indicated by a mean arterial pressure less than 60 mm Hg, dopamine (1–3 µg/kg per minute) and dobutamine (2–15 µg/kg per minute) can be given to increase cardiac output (both agents), arterial blood pressure (both agents), and renal and mesenteric blood flow (dopamine). This can be accomplished by adding 200 mg dopamine and 250 mg dobutamine to a 500-ml bag of saline and administering at a rate of 0.5 ml/kg per hour to

---

Polymune, Veterinary Dynamics, San Luis Obispo, CA
†Phoenix Pharmaceutical, St. Joseph, MO

effect, as determined by monitoring blood pressure, heart rate, pulse quality, and urine output.

DECOMPRESSION

Decompression of a distended viscus is an excellent method of relieving pain and providing a proper environment for normal peristalsis. Nasogastric intubation can relieve accumulated gas and enterogastric reflux due to small intestinal obstruction and ileus, or gastric tympany. An indwelling nasogastric tube provides an easy means to frequently decompress the stomach of horses with conditions such as DPJ. However, it is imperative that the tube be checked actively by siphoning on a regular basis for fluid or gas accumulation, because gastric rupture can occur when only passive decompression is applied.

Transcutaneous trocharization of either the cecum or large colon is another method of releasing gas accumulated within the GI tract. Cecal tympany can be relieved easily by inserting a 5- to 6-inch, 14- or 16-gauge needle or cannula in the right paralumbar fossa midway between the last rib and the ventral prominence of the tuber coxae. As the catheter is inserted into the flank it should remain perpendicular to the skin, with insertion continuing until intestinal gases can be smelled escaping from the catheter. External suction combined with transrectal cecal pressure facilitates the procedure. Decompression of the large colon can also be achieved using the same procedure, although greater risk of complications (including leakage of intestinal contents) does exist. Horses should be monitored closely after transcutaneous decompression, and if a fever or other symptoms of peritonitis are seen, antimicrobial therapy should be instituted. Trocharization causes mild to moderate increases in peritoneal fluid protein content and cell count, making interpretation of peritoneal fluid analysis difficult.

REGULATION OF INTESTINAL MOTILITY

Ileus, the absence of propulsive bowel activity, is characterized as either adynamic resulting from short-term alterations of motility, or paralytic, which ensues as a consequence of loss of gastrointestinal motility for longer than 72 hours. Etiologic factors contributing to gastrointestinal stasis include hypovolemia; hypotension; electrolyte derangements; pain; enterocolitis; peritonitis; endotoxemia; ischemia; and distension of the bowel with gaseous, liquid, or solid materials. Gastrointestinal motility is regulated through a series of complex interactions between the autonomic nervous system and hormones; thus, several potential sites for pharmacologic intervention exist. Drugs that modify motility may act by either directly stimulating intestinal contractions or by blocking mechanisms that result in ileus. However, stimulation of intestinal motility and transit is not always successful if severe intestinal damage has occurred. This point cannot be emphasized enough, particularly in disease processes in which chronic or extreme distension may have occurred.

Proper treatment of ileus lies in first identifying and correcting the underlying cause. Routine supportive therapies, including intravenous fluids, NSAIDs, and antimicrobials, provide benefits such as reduced local inflammation and improved blood flow that encourage normal intestinal function. Decompression of the involved intestinal segments should be accomplished, if possible, to aid in the restoration of normal motility. Depending on the site affected, this may be accomplished by nasogastric intubation, transcutaneous cecal or colonic trocharization, or laparotomy (see previous section on Decompression). The use of drugs that impair intestinal motility, most notably the α_2-adrenergic agonists, should be limited. If ileus persists, motility-modifying agents should be considered (Table 2).

Prokinetic drugs available for use in horses include benzamides, cholinomimetics, macrolide antibiotics, α_2-agonists, and lidocaine. Metoclopramide* is a benzamide prokinetic agent that acts via dopamine receptor antagonism, α_2-adrenergic receptor agonist effects, and direct stimulation of acetylcholine (ACh) release from the myenteric plexus. The recently recommended dose of 0.04 mg/kg (bolus, or per hour as a continuous IV infusion) is lower

---

*Reglan, A.H. Robins, Richmond, VA

TABLE 2. DRUGS USED FOR TREATMENT OF ILEUS IN HORSES

Drug	Method of Action	Suggested Dosage	Comments
Metoclopramide	Release of acetylcholine (ACh) from myenteric plexus, dopaminergic antagonist	0.04 mg/kg/hour continuous IV infusion, 0.25 mg/kg IV over 30 minutes	Lower dose may have little prokinetic effect, CNS excitement occurs often at higher doses, premedication with diphenhydramine may minimize CNS effects
Cisapride	Release of ACh from myenteric plexus	0.1–0.2 mg/kg IV, IM	Stimulates ileal, cecal, and colonic contractile activity in normal horses, may also have prokinetic effect on stomach and small intestine
Bethanechol	Cholinomimetic, direct stimulation of smooth muscle	0.025–0.030 mg/kg SQ, q4–6h	Main effect is to increase gastric emptying, may cause urination and increased salivation
Neostigmine	Cholinomimetic, increases ACh by inhibiting cholinesterase	0.022 mg/kg SQ	Duration of effect 10–30 minutes, prokinetic effects in large colon, may inhibit gastrojejunal motility
Erythromycin	Stimulates motilin release	0.1 mg/kg per hour, IV	Induced small intestinal, cecal, and colonic progressive motility in normal horses
Lidocaine	Anti-inflammatory analgesic effects, may directly stimulate smooth muscle	1.3 mg/kg slow IV bolus, then 0.05 mg/kg/min IV infusion	Do not use formulations containing epinephrine If CNS effects (trembling, muscle fasciculations, ataxia) occur, decrease administration rate
Yohimbine	α_2-adrenergic antagonist	75 mg/kg IV	Prevented ileus in horses given a low dose of endotoxin

than that previously recommended (0.25 mg/kg IV), because hyperexcitability may occur at the higher dose. Given as an IV bolus, the low dose of metoclopramide has no effect on intestinal myoelectrical activity in normal horses. However, in colic patients with jejunal resection/anastomosis, those horses given the lower dose of metoclopramide as a continuous intravenous infusion had a significantly shorter duration of postoperative enterogastric reflux than did horses given control treatment or intermittent intravenous boluses of metoclopramide. Cisapride°, another benzamide, directly stimulates ACh release from the myenteric plexus. Experimentally, increased GI motility has been observed after administration of 0.1 to 0.2 mg/kg IV. Clinical efficacy in reducing the incidence of postoperative ileus has been reported using cisapride at a dose of 0.1 mg/kg IM.

Bethanechol† and neostigmine‡ are cholimimetics that exert their prokinetic effect on intestinal smooth muscle directly or indirectly. Gastric emptying is enhanced after the administration of bethanechol (0.025–0.030 mg/kg SQ, q4–6h). Neostigmine appears to be most effective at enhancing ingesta transport in the cecum and the large colon when given at a dose of 0.022 mg/kg SQ. The macrolide antibiotic, erythromycin§ (0.1 mg/kg per hour IV) enhances intestinal motility by stimulating motilin receptors. The disruption of normal colonic motility patterns, cecal hypoperfusion, and ileus caused by endotoxin is reversed by use of yohimbine‖ (75 mg/kg), suggesting that α_2-adrenergic antagonists (yohimbine, tolazoline) may be useful in the treatment of ileus in endotoxemic horses. Lidocaine has been advocated for use as a prokinetic drug in horses, presumably because it has anti-inflammatory and analgesic properties and may directly stimulate intestinal smooth muscle. In horses with ileus, the recommended regimen that appears to have clinical efficacy and minimal side effects is to give a slow (over 5 minutes) IV bolus of lidocaine at a loading dose of 1.3 mg/kg, followed by IV infusion of 0.05 mg/kg per minute, which can safely be continued for up to 24 hours.

DIAGNOSIS AND MANAGEMENT OF ENDOTOXEMIA

When the lipid component of lipopolysaccharide (LPS, also known as endotoxin) binds to host phagocytes, a plethora of hormones and inflammatory factors are released. This complex pattern of mediator release has been termed *systemic inflammatory response syndrome* (SIRS). Much of the SIRS is directed against the vascular endothelium, causing a hypercoagulable state, microvasculature disturbances, tissue ischemia and hypoxia, and, if overwhelming, multiple organ failure and death. Endotoxemia has received much attention in equine literature since the early 1970s, when it was reported that horses given LPS exhibited signs similar to those seen in equine patients with enteric diseases. The extensive equine gut is host to many

gram-negative bacterial flora, and any condition that disrupts the mucosal barrier can cause endotoxemia. Thus, horses with colitis, peritonitis, DPJ, and other forms of colic are likely candidates for endotoxemia. Strenuous exercise, hemorrhagic shock, or burn trauma may also alter intestinal blood flow and mucosal integrity sufficient to cause endotoxemia. Endotoxemia is believed to cause morbidity and mortality in horses by increasing the risk for ileus, disseminated intravascular coagulation (DIC), renal failure, and laminitis.

Diagnosis of endotoxemia in horses is largely based on the presence of a condition associated with endotoxemia, and signs of depression, fever, tachycardia, injected scleral vessels, and hyperemic mucous membranes with a bluish-tinged "toxic" rim to the gums above incisors. Other clinical signs seen commonly during endotoxemia include those associated with hypovolemia such as weak peripheral pulses, cool extremities, prolonged capillary refill time, slow jugular refill, anuria; tachypnea; colic; loose feces; and abdominal distension due to ileus and gas accumulation within the large colon and cecum. Signs associated with coagulopathy such as petechial hemorrhages, prolonged bleeding from venipuncture sites or during nasogastric intubation, immediate thrombosis during venipuncture or catheter placement, and laminitis are also seen in some horses.

Leukopenia, neutropenia, and toxic changes in neutrophils are hallmark hematologic findings during acute endotoxemia. Immature neutrophils are released into circulation, causing a left shift. With chronicity, a mature neutrophilia occurs as a result of bone marrow stimulation. Other common, nonspecific, clinicopathologic findings include increased hematocrit, azotemia, lactic acidosis, increased anion gap, and mild increases of cellular enzymes (lactic dehydrogenase [LDH], aspartate aminotransferase [AST], alkaline phosphatase [ALP], and creatinine kinase). Total plasma protein concentration may be normal, increased, or decreased, depending on the combined effects of dehydration and protein loss through the bowel wall. Low platelet count, prolonged bleeding time, and increased fibrin split products may be seen.

Endotoxin can be measured in plasma by a chromogenic limulus amebocyte lysate (LAL) assay, or in whole blood by a commercially available hemagglutination-inhibition assay.° Because endotoxins are bound quickly to phagocyte cell surface receptors, they are present in circulation only transiently. Because of this, practical applications of endotoxin assays in equine patients are limited. In humans, patients with persistent endotoxemia had a worse prognosis than those without endotoxemia, a positive LAL test (>5 pg/ml) was associated with a higher incidence of organ failure, and use of anti-endotoxin antibodies was most beneficial in patients with a positive LAL test. In horses with abdominal disorders, circulating endotoxin concentration higher than 10 pg/ml was associated with increased risk for mortality. Now that an endotoxin assay kit is readily available, more information on potential uses of endotoxin assays in equine patients may be generated.

The difficulty of treating endotoxemic patients is not surprising considering the array of physiologic disturbances

---

°*Janssen Pharmaceutica, Titusville, NJ*
†*Urecholine injection, Merck & Co., Inc., West Point, PA*
‡*Marsam Pharmaceuticals, Cherry Hill, NJ*
§*Erythromycin lactobionate, Elkins-Sinn, Cherry Hill, NJ*
‖*Yobine, Lloyd Laboratories, Shenandoah, IA*

°*Etox-Dx, KenVet, Ashland, OH*

from which they suffer. Underlying causes of endotoxemia such as strangulated bowel must be removed, if possible, and aggressive supportive care instituted. Treatments specifically directed against endotoxin or host-produced mediators of endotoxic shock are available for use in horses (Table 3), but few controlled clinical studies have been performed to test the safety and efficacy of many of these agents. In equine endotoxemia models, normal horses are first given an agent to be tested or a control treatment, then they are given small amounts of endotoxin. Although these horses experience similar clinical and hematologic signs as horses with enteric diseases, differences exist. For example, normal horses have a decremental response to repeated or continuous endotoxin exposure (endotoxin tolerance), whereas many endotoxemic patients seem to have persistent LPS-induced effects. Extrapolation from the research environment to clinical cases must therefore be made judiciously. Furthermore, these agents should be considered experimental until they have been evaluated in controlled clinical trials or have had extensive clinical use.

Anti-endotoxin Agents

Anti-endotoxin agents are designed to neutralize circulating LPS and prevent subsequent SIRS. These agents prevent ongoing endotoxemia but do not affect the physiologic disturbances already present. Although only small subsets of horses with enteric disease have detectable circulating endotoxins, it is reasonable to assume that continuous or intermittent endotoxemia may occur in horses with enteric disorders. Therapies designed to neutralize circulating endotoxin may be beneficial in these horses, if used early during the course of disease, or if more than 5 pg/ml of circulating endotoxin is detected.

Polymyxin B sulfate* is a cationic antibiotic that binds lipid A and neutralizes endotoxin. In equine endotoxemia models, polymyxin B sulfate treatment (6000 IU/kg IV) reduced circulating cytokine (tumor necrosis factor [TNF] and IL-6) concentrations, rectal temperature, and respiratory rates, versus control treatment. Polymyxin B did not prevent development of laminitis in horses given carbohydrate overload. The recommended dose of polymyxin B

*Polymyxin B sulfate, The Upjohn Company, Kalamazoo, MI

(6000 IU/kg IV daily for ongoing endotoxemia) is much lower than that necessary to produce a systemic antimicrobial effect. Horses given polymyxin B 30,000 IU/kg body weight had transient signs of neurotoxicity including ataxia, head shaking, and hypermetria, suggesting a narrow margin of safety with the 6000 IU/kg dose. Factors associated with enteric disease and endotoxemia may alter the pharmacokinetics of polymyxin B and may predispose to toxicity. Attitude and renal function should be monitored closely if polymyxin B is given. Dextran-conjugated formulations of polymyxin B remain in the intravascular space and neutralize endotoxins at much lower, less toxic doses. In a model of equine endotoxemia, dextran 70-conjugated polymyxin B (5 mg polymyxin B/kg body weight, 165 mg dextran per 70 kg body weight) conferred significant protection against endotoxin effects. Transient tachypnea, sweating, leukopenia, and fever occurred with this protocol, and use of the formulations should be investigated before recommendations for its clinical use can be made.

Equine hyperimmune serum or plasma containing anti-LPS antibodies is available commercially. Donor horses are immunized with bacterial mutants possessing the conserved core glycolipid of either *Escherichia coli** or *Salmonella typhimurium*† to generate anti-LPS antibodies that supposedly cross-react with endotoxins from all gram-negative bacteria. Experimentally, cross-reactivity of anticore antibodies has been difficult to demonstrate. Results from investigations into the efficacy of these products in humans and horses are conflicting, but some studies have demonstrated improved survival with their use. Adverse reactions to these products seem to be rare, and include transient shaking, sweating, and anxiety.

Agents Targeting Eicosanoid Mediators of Endotoxemia

Thromboxane and prostacyclin are produced during endotoxemia in horses and have been associated with pulmonary hypertension and systemic hypotension, respectively. Additional arachidonic acid metabolites (i.e., other prostaglandins and leukotrienes) are also probably produced

*Polymune-J, Veterinary Dynamics, San Luis Obispo, CA
†Endoserum, Immvac, Columbia, MO

TABLE 3. DRUGS USED TO COMBAT THE EFFECTS OF ENDOTOXEMIA

Drug	Method of Action	Suggested Dosage	Comments
Flunixin meglumine	Anti-prostaglandin	0.25 mg/kg IV, IM s.i.d. to q.i.d.	Minimal analgesic effects at this dose, less risk for NSAIDs toxicity
Ketoprofen	Anti-prostaglandin ± anti-leukotriene	2.2 mg/kg IV b.i.d.	Effects comparable to flunixin
Polymyxin B	Binds LPS	6000 IU/kg IV s.i.d.	Human drug, monitor for signs of neuro/renal toxicity
Anti-LPS hyperimmune serum, plasma	Binds LPS	Serum: 1.5 ml/kg diluted 1:2 in IV fluids Plasma: 4–8 ml/kg IV, undiluted	Multiple doses may be required if endotoxemia persists
Pentoxifylline	Immune and rheologic	8.5 mg/kg p.o. b.i.d.	Human drug, concurrent use of NSAIDs may negate benefits
Dimethyl sulfoxide (DMSO)	Reactive oxygen species (ROS) scavenger	1 g/kg IV s.i.d. to q.i.d.	Dilute to 10% in IV fluids
Allopurinol	Xanthine oxidase inhibitor, ROS scavenger	5 mg/kg IV	Human drug

during endotoxemia in horses. Eicosanoids influence vasomotor tone, microvascular permeability, and platelet aggregation, and they activate various inflammatory cells for mediator release.

Corticosteroids and NSAIDs reduce eicosanoid production. Flunixin meglumine (0.25 mg/kg b.i.d. to q.i.d.) is used extensively in clinical cases of equine endotoxemia. Ketoprofen, which may inhibit both lipoxygenase and cyclooxygenase, has had limited experimental and clinical use in equine endotoxemia, but appears to have efficacy comparable to that of flunixin.

Glucocorticoids reduce the production of many inflammatory mediators when given early during experimental endotoxemia, but controlled clinical trials in humans with gram-negative sepsis have failed to show benefits of glucocorticoid use. Because glucocorticoids are associated with increased risk of development of laminitis, their use is not recommended in endotoxemic horses.

Agents Targeting Cytokine Mediators of Endotoxemia

Cytokines are polypeptides that are normally produced in tiny amounts by many cells and exhibit diverse biologic actions via binding to specific cell-surface receptors. During endotoxemia, cellular activation leads to increased production of many cytokines, including tumor necrosis factor-alpha (TNF), interleukin-1, and interleukin-6. Monoclonal antibodies, cell-surface receptors, and pharmacologic agents that neutralize the activity, or modify the production, of cytokines (particularly TNF) are being investigated for use in endotoxemia.

Pentoxifylline* is a methylxanthine derivative that inhibits intracellular phosphodiesterase and reduces TNF production during endotoxemia. It has improved rates of survival in animal models of sepsis. Pentoxifylline also has other immunomodulatory and rheologic properties that may be beneficial during endotoxemia. Because many of these effects are mediated by enhanced prostaglandin activity, concurrent use of NSAIDs during endotoxemia may negate beneficial effects of pentoxifylline. Pentoxifylline (8.5 mg/kg p.o. b.i.d.) has been used experimentally and clinically in a limited number of horses without causing obvious deleterious side effects.

AGENTS TARGETING REACTIVE OXYGEN SPECIES (ROS)

At the cellular level, much of the endotoxin-induced pathology appears to be caused by the effects of free radicals on membranes, enzymes, and structural proteins. Agents that inactivate or block the production of free radicals have reduced mortality in some models of septic shock. Dimethyl sulfoxide (DMSO) is an inexpensive, potent, hydroxyl radical scavenger that is commonly used to treat horses with CNS edema, endotoxemia, laminitis, and other musculoskeletal diseases. Although the effects of DMSO have not been investigated in horses given LPS, DMSO has reduced pathology during experimental endotoxic shock in other species. Dimethyl sulfoxide is commonly given at a dose of 1 g/kg diluted to 10% in IV fluids to prevent hemolysis. Treatments can be given one to four times daily.

Allopurinol* inhibits the activity of xanthine oxidase, thereby causing decreased ROS production, and scavenges ROS. Allopurinol has had limited clinical and experimental use in horses, but did reduce metabolic alterations in horses given LPS. In other studies, allopurinol was not effective at preventing reperfusion injury in ischemic equine bowel.

The cysteine analog N-acetylcysteine has been used to enhance glutathione synthesis and protect against oxidative injury in models of ovine endotoxemia and porcine septic shock. Lazaroids, 21-aminosteroid compounds, scavenge lipid peroxl radicals and inhibit the formation of oxygen radicals by phagocytes. Calves treated with tirilazad mesylate had reduced metabolic, eicosanoid, and TNF responses to LPS infusion, as compared with control-treated calves. The use of these compounds has not been reported in horses.

MANAGEMENT OF COAGULOPATHIES

The likelihood of successful outcome when managing coagulopathies associated with enteric disorders and endotoxemia in horses is increased with early recognition. If signs of hypercoagulability such as venous thrombosis and declining platelet counts are identified, rapid intervention can often prevent or attenuate widespread intravascular coagulation. Prothrombin time (PT), partial thromboplastin time (APTT), fibrin split products (FSP), and platelet counts should be evaluated in horses with signs of coagulopathy. Thrombocytopenia and prolonged PT and/or APTT are suggestive of DIC, which is a dynamic process initiated by promotion of a hypercoagulable state, leading to platelet and clotting factor consumption, and ultimately culminating in a hemorrhagic diathesis. Increased fibrinolytic activity is indicated by elevated FSP, which are byproducts of fibrin degradation and thus are increased by many processes including surgery, hematoma formation, or hypercoagulability. The most widely accepted treatments for DIC are removal of underlying cause, supportive care, and fresh heparinized plasma. Heparin potentiates the anticoagulant and fibrinolytic activities of anti-thrombin III, and may be useful in preventing venous thrombosis and laminitis resulting from hypercoagulable states. However, antithrombin III concentration is not routinely measured in horses and is likely to be low during DIC. Heparin potentiates agglutination of red blood cells, and multiple doses cause a 20 to 35% reduction in hematocrit level, which resolves shortly after therapy is stopped. Intravascular red blood cell (RBC) agglutination can exacerbate microvasculature plugging. For these reasons, heparin use in horses is controversial. Dosing recommendations, which are designed to provide plasma heparin concentrations of 0.05 to 0.20 IU per ml of plasma are: for calcium heparin, an initial dose of 150 IU/kg SQ, followed by 125 IU/kg SQ b.i.d. for six doses, then, if subsequent doses are required,

---

*Trental, Hoechst-Roussel Pharmaceuticals, Somerville, NJ

*Rugby Laboratories, West Hempstead, NY

100 U/kg SQ b.i.d; and for sodium heparin, 40 to 80 IU/kg IV, followed in 2 hours by 40 IU/kg SQ, then 40 IU/kg SQ b.i.d. to t.i.d. for 3 days. If APTT is normal at the beginning of heparin therapy, an appropriate response to treatment is doubling of the APTT.

Safer alternatives to standard heparin therapy in horses may be the use of heparinized plasma, aspirin, or low-molecular-weight heparins. Heparin can be added to fresh room temperature plasma (sodium heparin 125–400 IU/L plasma, up to 200 IU/kg) to provide heparin-potentiated antithrombin III, platelets, and other clotting factors. Low-dose aspirin therapy (10 mg/kg p.o. or rectally, suspended in 60 ml of water, every other day) has been suggested for use in hypercoagulable states in horses. In a recent study in horses, the antithrombotic effect of a low-molecular-weight heparin (2000–8000 daltons) was comparable with that of calcium heparin, without causing erythrocyte agglutination. The dose of low-molecular-weight heparin is 50 IU/kg b.i.d.

ANTIMICROBIALS

In foals younger than 6 months of age, and in adults with gram-negative sepsis, the use of antibiotics is recommended. Adult horses with enteric diseases are usually endotoxemic rather than septic, and antibiotic use in these patients is controversial. Besides adding to the expense of therapy, antibiotics may alter gastrointestinal flora and occasionally exacerbate or cause enteric disease. Some clinicians believe that leukopenia, and possibly depressed immune function, may predispose endotoxemic horses to septicemia. Because clinical signs of sepsis are indistinguishable from those of endotoxemia, these clinicians feel that antibiotic use is warranted in most endotoxemic horses, particularly those with indwelling intravenous catheters. Others prefer to use antibiotics only if specific indications exist such as suspicion of Potomac horse fever, peritonitis, surgical cases, or persistent severe neutropenia.

ADDITIONAL SUPPORTIVE CARE

Once circulating volume has been restored, fluids, bicarbonate, and electrolytes are given as needed to meet maintenance requirements and correct for ongoing losses. Adult horses should be monitored closely for signs of laminitis and treated appropriately if these are seen. Some clinicians apply frog support or sole pads* routinely to all horses with gastrointestinal disease. Adequate nutrition should be provided as soon as possible. Although it is common practice to withhold nutrition for 3 to 10 days in adult colic patients, the adverse effects of inadequate caloric intake on immune function and healing capacity must be considered. If finances allow, most of these patients benefit greatly from providing at least part of their caloric requirements by enteral, if possible, or parenteral routes. Because of the adverse effects of GI disease, anorexia, and antibiotics on GI flora, B vitamins may not be produced or absorbed in adequate amounts. Horses that have been withheld from feed, or are anorectic for 3 days or more, may be given B-complex vitamins to prevent vitamin B deficits and to employ their purported appetite-stimulating effect.

MEDICAL THERAPIES FOR SPECIFIC CONDITIONS

Treatment of Impaction Colic

Impaction of the large or transverse colon is a common cause of colic and often responds to medical treatment directed at controlling pain, maintaining hydration, and administering laxatives via nasogastric tube. Intravenous fluids given at two to five times the maintenance rate may resolve unresponsive impactions. Aggressive medical treatment for 3 to 5 days may be necessary, although softening and movement of the impacted mass should be felt sooner during rectal palpation. Surgical intervention is indicated if systemic deterioration or peritoneal fluid changes occur, or if pain cannot be controlled. The use of prokinetic drugs in these cases is controversial. Some clinicians believe that intestinal contractions induced by neostigmine, which has primary effects in the large colon, may aid in breaking up impacted material. This may also cause increased pain and risk for rupture of compromised gut.

In certain areas, sand impaction is relatively common. This condition is more difficult to treat than feed impaction, thus surgical intervention is required more often. Sand impaction can be difficult to differentiate from feed impaction, and tests for fecal sand do not correlate well with the presence of sand in the colon. History or presence of sand in the feces can indicate exposure to sand. Horses with this condition may have small amounts of diarrhea and clinical signs of endotoxemia. Auscultation of the abdomen on ventral midline, caudal to the xiphoid process, may reveal a characteristic "sand" sound. Abdominal radiographs (if available) can aid in the diagnosis of sand impaction.

Mineral oil, dioctyl sodium sulfosuccinate (DSS), psyllium, and magnesium sulfate are used for laxative effect (Table 4), and may also stimulate colonic motility via a gastrocolic response when instilled into the stomach. The stomach should first be siphoned, and if more than 2 L of fluid is obtained, small-intestinal ileus or delayed gastric emptying is likely. Instillation of additional fluid should be done cautiously, if at all, in these patients. A 500-kg horse with a relatively empty stomach should tolerate a volume of 8 to 10 L over 15 minutes intragastrically. Mineral oil is inexpensive and nontoxic, and acts to lubricate the ingesta to facilitate passage through the intestines. Psyllium is believed to have better ability to penetrate, hydrate, and break up sand impactions than the other laxatives. Psyllium is not toxic and may be used for periods of 1 to 3 weeks, if needed. If used to prevent sand impaction, the length of daily administration should be limited to 3 weeks every 4 to 6 months for best efficacy. The use of both DSS and magnesium sulfate is associated with risk for development of diarrhea, and effective yet safe dosing regimens for these products are debated. Dioctyl sodium sulfate supposedly exerts a laxative effect by reducing surface tension and

---

*3M Animal Care Products, St. Paul, MN

TABLE 4. DRUGS USED FOR LAXATIVE EFFECT IN HORSES WITH COLIC

Drug	Method of Action	Suggested Dose per 500 kg	Comments
Mineral oil	Lubricates ingesta	4 L followed by 2–4 L water	Nontoxic, can give multiple doses
Psyllium	Bulk laxative, believed to penetrate and draw water into impaction	16 oz in 4 to 8 L water	Nontoxic, believed to be the best laxative for treatment of sand impaction, forms a gel in water, mix during administration
Dioctyl sodium sulfosuccinate (DSS, 4% solution)	Reduces surface tension of ingesta, allowing water penetration	4–8 oz in 8 L water	May cause mucosal irritation, systemic toxicity at higher doses
Magnesium sulfate (epsom salts)	Cathartic laxative, osmotic effect to draw water into intestine	0.5–1 g/kg in 8 L water	Higher doses may cause moderate diarrhea, ensure patient is adequately hydrated

allowing water to penetrate impacted material. Experimental evidence suggests that DSS may also increase intestinal secretion and alter mucosal permeability. The recommended dose of DSS is 4 to 8 ounces of a 5% solution per 500-kg horse (10–25 mg/kg), diluted into 4 to 8 L of water. Toxicity indicated by diarrhea and abdominal pain occurs at doses ranging from 0.5 to 1 g/kg, and in one report, suspected toxicity occurred with a 60 mg/kg dose. For these reasons, using DSS only twice (48 hours apart) has been suggested. Magnesium sulfate (1 g/kg) is better at increasing fecal water content and output than is a lower dose (0.5 g/kg), DSS (50 mg/kg), or water alone. Magnesium acts largely via an osmotic effect that, in addition to drawing water into the ingesta, may cause more gastrointestinal distension, and thus stimulate a better gastrocolic response than other laxatives. Drawbacks to the use of higher doses of magnesium sulfate are the risks for development of a mild to moderate diarrhea, and for exacerbating hypovolemia if strict attention is not given to the horse's hydration status during therapy.

Impactions of the stomach, cecum, ileum, and small colon also occur less commonly. If a large amount of feed material is seen via endoscope in the stomach after a 48-hour fast, gastric impaction is diagnosed. Gastric lavage followed by instillation of DSS has been used to resolve this condition. Ileal impaction has been associated with poor-quality roughage, muscular hypertrophy, and tapeworm infection. This condition is usually accompanied by enterogastric reflux, and thus laxative use is contraindicated. Surgical intervention is often required. Cecal impaction is associated with vague clinical signs and a high incidence of cecal rupture, which seems to occur within the first 24 hours of treatment. Because of this, the need for immediate surgical intervention has been debated. In horses surviving longer then 24 hours after diagnosis of cecal impaction, a high percentage (89%) respond to medical therapy. Because of the increased risk of cecal rupture, prokinetics should not be used in horses with this condition. Small-colon impaction is treated in a fashion similar to that for large-colon impaction, but small-colon impaction more often requires surgical intervention. Early aggressive medical therapy is recommended to help avoid the need for surgical intervention. These horses commonly have fever and diarrhea following resolution of the impaction, which may be associated with *Salmonella* infection.

Treatment of Duodenitis-Proximal Jejunitis

Classical signs of DPJ include the presence of colic associated with fever, more than 2 L/hour of enterogastric

reflux (≥50 L/day), mildly distended and compressible loops of small intestine detected during rectal palpation, increased total protein (with normal cell counts) in peritoneal fluid, and clinical improvement in response to medical therapy. Several reviews of DPJ have been written. Treatment of DPJ is largely supportive and involves maintaining hydration and gastric decompression and using anti-inflammatories (flunixin). The use of prokinetic agents is controversial, because beneficial effects of these agents on inflamed bowel have not been demonstrated. The prognosis is generally good for those horses that stop refluxing within 72 hours. The longer ileus persists after this, the more guarded the prognosis becomes. In severely affected horses, DPJ may be extremely difficult to differentiate from strangulating small intestinal lesions. In addition, these horses seem to benefit, at least temporarily, from surgical decompression of their small intestine. For these reasons, early surgical intervention should be considered in horses that have signs compatible with DPJ, but also have any of the following: high cell counts in peritoneal fluid, pain that is not controlled by flunixin meglumine administration and gastric decompression, severely distended small intestine on rectal examination, or continued evidence of systemic deterioration despite adequate fluid and anti-inflammatory therapy.

Treatment of Right Dorsal Colitis

Chronic mild colic, weight loss, diarrhea, low serum total protein and albumin concentration, and a history of receiving inappropriately high doses of NSAIDs support a diagnosis of right dorsal colitis. Glandular lesions near the margo plicatus may also be seen on endoscopic examination of the stomach. The ulcerative lesions are supposedly caused by a decrease in the mucosal production of prostaglandins, which are critical to maintain mucosal blood flow and integrity. Management of this condition can be difficult, and surgical intervention may be necessary to remove affected colon. Use of NSAIDs should be avoided in these horses, and, if gastric ulcers are present, they should be treated appropriately. Plasma transfusions may be necessary. Hay should be withheld, and a complete pelleted ration provided. No medications have been proved to promote healing of colonic ulcers in horses; however, sucralfate, corn oil, and psyllium have all been suggested as relatively inexpensive therapies that may have this effect. Corn oil contains linoleic acid, an arachidonic acid precursor, that may promote prostaglandin production and mucosal repair. Corn oil is palatable to horses, and can be added directly to the ration (total of 2–4 oz daily). Production of short-chain fatty acids, which promote mucosal repair, may be increased with psyllium treatment. Synthetic prostaglandin E_2 analogues promote mucosal healing and prevent gastric and colonic ulceration during administration of toxic dosages of NSAIDs in horses. However, these drugs are relatively expensive, and their efficacy in treating established colonic ulcers in horses has not been evaluated.

Supplemental Readings

Cohen ND, Carter GK, Mealey RH, Taylor TS: Medical management of right dorsal colitis in 5 horses: A retrospective study (1987–1993). J Vet Intern Med 9:272–276, 1995.

Collatos C, Romano S: Cecal impaction in horses: Causes, diagnosis, and medical treatment. Comp Cont Ed Equine Vet 15:976–982, 1993.

Dabareiner RM, White NA: Large colon impaction in horses: 147 cases (1985–1991). J Am Vet Med Assoc 206:679–685, 1995.

Dart AJ, Synder JR, Pascoe JR, Farver TB, Galuppo LD: Abnormal conditions of the equine descending (small) colon: 102 cases (1979–1989). J Am Vet Med Assoc 200:971–978, 1992.

Holbrook TC, Moore JN: Anti-inflammatory and immune support in endotoxemia and septicemia. Vet Clin North Am Equine Pract 10:535–547, 1994.

MacKay RJ: Endotoxemia. *In* Robinson NE (ed): Current Therapy in Equine Medicine, ed 3. Philadelphia, WB Saunders, 1992, pp 225–232.

Martin LG, Wingfield WE, Van Pelt DR, Hackett TB: Magnesium in the 1990's: Implications for veterinary critical care. Vet Emerg Crit Care 3:105–114, 1993.

Moore BR, Hinchliff KW: Heparin: A review of its pharmacology and therapeutic use in horses. J Vet Intern Med 8:26–35, 1994.

Seahorn TL, Cornick JL, Cohen ND: Prognostic indicators for horses with duodenitis-proximal jejunitis: 75 horses (1985–1989). J Vet Intern Med 6:307–311, 1992.

Gastroduodenal Ulceration

MICHAEL J. MURRAY
Leesburg, Virginia

Just as the term *colic* describes a clinical presentation and encompasses a large number of disorders, gastroduodenal ulceration describes a clinical finding, the cause of which is likely to be multifactorial and different from case to case. Within the umbrella term *gastroduodenal ulceration* are included symptomatic and asymptomatic cases, focal or multifocal ulceration involving the squamous and/or glandular mucosal linings of the stomach, gastritis, gastric emptying disorders, duodenitis, duodenal ulceration, and complications resulting from these disorders.

Gastric ulceration affects large numbers of foals, yearlings, and adult horses, and different clinical syndromes and lesion distribution occur in each group. Gastric ulceration may occur as a primary problem, or may occur as the result of another intestinal disorder. Duodenal ulceration occurs primarily in foals, although it has been diagnosed in yearlings. Duodenal ulceration is a rare finding in adult horses.

PATHOGENESIS

In consideration of possible pathogenic mechanisms, the anatomic location of the ulcer must be taken into account. Lesions in the gastric squamous mucosa result primarily from excessive acidity, whereas gastric glandular lesions result primarily from defective mucosal protection. In general, ulceration is considered to result from an imbalance of aggressive and protective factors. The principal relevant aggressive factors are hydrochloric acid and pepsin, whereas relevant protective factors include the mucus/bicarbonate barrier, prostaglandin E_2, mucosal blood flow, cellular restitution, and growth factors that promote angiogenesis and mucosal proliferation. Gastric motility also is important, because delayed gastric emptying and prolonged gastric contractions have been implicated in the pathogenesis of ulcers. Mucosal protection of the duodenum relies on an alkaline or neutral pH, with factors such as PGE_2 and mucosal blood flow of probable relevance.

The squamous mucosa of the equine stomach lacks a mucus/bicarbonate layer, and it has minimal resistance to exposure to hydrochloric acid. Horses secrete acid even when not eating, and gastric pH can fall below 2.0 soon after a horse stops eating. Twenty-four-hour gastric acidity is significantly less in horses with hay available compared with that in horses deprived of feed. Intermittent periods of feed deprivation can induce gastric ulceration in horses, as a result of increased gastric acidity. Bleeding gastric squamous mucosal ulcers can occur in as short a time as 48 hours. Concentrate feeding may contribute to ulcers, by increasing serum gastrin levels and presumably acid secretion, by reducing the horse's roughage intake and, most importantly, the amount of time the horse spends eating. Thus, feeding management may play a pivotal role in the pathophysiology of gastric ulcers in horses. In fact, we have found that horses that are turned out onto pasture full-time typically have no gastric lesions.

Endoscopic studies have revealed a 50% prevalence of gastric lesions in asymptomatic foals. The majority of these lesions were in the gastric squamous epithelial mucosa. The high prevalence of gastric ulceration, particularly in the squamous mucosa, in young foals may be associated with gastric developmental changes that occur in the first days and weeks of life. At birth, the equine gastric squamous epithelium is thin and not highly keratinized. Within days the mucosa becomes hyperplastic and parakeratotic. Desquamation of the squamous epithelium can be observed endoscopically in the first month of life in foals. Histologically, desquamation appears to involve separation of the superficial cornified epithelial layers.

Increasing gastric acidity temporally parallels the proliferation of gastric squamous epithelium, with minimal acidity during the first few days of life and marked acidity present by 7 to 14 days. It is possible that the developing epithelium is less resistant to acid than more mature gastric squamous epithelium, thus predisposing it to peptic injury.

Illness appears to be a risk factor for foals developing glandular mucosal ulcers, because foals that are sick or have a painful musculoskeletal condition have a greater prevalence of glandular lesions compared with normal foals. The lesions presumably are associated with stress, and people in intensive care units are known to be at high risk of developing gastric ulcers. The precise mechanism of stress ulceration is not known, but decreased mucosal blood flow is probably a primary factor. Physiologic stress associated with illness should be differentiated from psychological stress, which is popularly believed to be associated with peptic disease in humans. In fact, such stresses are not correlated with peptic lesions in humans, although psychological stress may be associated with symptoms of dyspepsia.

Much attention has been directed toward *Helicobacter pylori* as a cause of peptic disease in humans. *H. pylori* is now generally accepted as being the principal cause of peptic ulceration and gastritis in humans. The organism is found on the surface of the glandular mucosa, just beneath the mucus layer. Infection with *H. pylori* induces an inflammatory response, particularly in the gastric antrum, and clinical signs are thought to occur usually months to years after infection.

There is no evidence to date of *H. pylori* or related *Helicobacter* species infection in horses. Most gastric lesions in horses occur in the squamous mucosa, and *Helicobacter* species do not colonize alimentary squamous epithelium. Most lesions in the glandular mucosa of foals and adult horses are not associated with a significant inflammatory response, such as that which occurs with *H. pylori* infection in people.

CLINICAL SYNDROMES

Foals

Gastric Ulceration

The clinical signs that typically are associated with gastric ulcers in foals include bruxism, dorsal recumbency, salivation, interrupted nursing, and colic. These signs, though, are observed in the minority of foals with ulcers, and usually are reflective of severe gastric lesions. Signs of salivation or esophageal reflux are indicative of gastric outlet obstruction or pseudo-obstruction, reflecting significant ulceration associated with the pylorus and duodenum.

Most gastric ulcers in foals are located in the squamous mucosa, adjacent to the margo plicatus along the greater curvature and lesser curvatures. The distribution of lesions in the squamous mucosa varies with the age of the foal. In foals younger than 1 month of age, lesions typically originate in the squamous mucosa adjacent to the margo plicatus along the greater curvature. These lesions are frequently associated with desquamation of the squamous epithelium. Desquamation is the shedding of surface epithelial layers, and appears as flakes or sheets of epithelium. Desquamation occurs in the majority of foals up to 35 days of age. In most foals, lesions in the squamous mucosa adjacent to the margo plicatus along the greater curvature resolve without treatment and without causing a clinical problem.

In some young foals, erosive and ulcerative lesions adjacent to the margo plicatus coalesce into larger, or deeper, areas of ulceration. At this point, there may be hemorrhage associated with the lesions. Clinical signs may occur, with diarrhea the most frequently observed sign. In cases with severe or diffuse squamous ulceration, bruxism and colic may be present.

In foals older than 3 months, lesions become more prevalent in the squamous mucosa surrounding the cardia and along the lesser curvature between the cardia and pylorus. Lesions also are found in the squamous mucosa of the fundus and adjacent to the margo plicatus. These lesions can be very severe and are often associated with clinical signs such as diarrhea, poor appetite, poor growth, and poor bodily condition.

Lesions in the gastric glandular mucosa tend to occur less frequently than in the squamous mucosa, but as has been mentioned, glandular lesions can occur in association with illness. These lesions can develop rapidly (within 24 hours), and can cause signs of abdominal discomfort and poor appetite. Lesions at the pylorus can be of particular concern, especially if they become severe and there is secondary submucosal fibrosis. Gastric emptying dysfunction and chronic colic can result.

Duodenal Ulceration

Duodenal ulceration occurs in foals of all ages. Unlike gastric ulceration, subclinical duodenal ulceration probably is uncommon. Lesions occur primarily in the proximal duodenum and range from diffuse inflammation to focal bleeding ulcers. Gastric ulceration frequently occurs as a result of duodenal ulceration, owing to physiologic or anatomic obstruction to gastric emptying, and tends to be severe, often leading to gastroesophageal reflux and esophagitis. The signs of duodenal ulceration include bruxism, colic, and diarrhea, and in many cases the clinical signs may be related to severe gastric and esophageal ulceration that occurs as a result of duodenal ulceration.

Duodenal ulceration can be difficult to confirm ante mortem. Duodenoscopy is the most specific means of diagnosis. Excessive enterogastric reflux of bile through the pylorus suggests duodenal dysfunction. If gastroscopy, but not duodenoscopy, can be performed, gastric lesions, particularly in the squamous mucosa of the lesser curvature dorsal to the pyloric antrum, often are very severe when duodenal ulcers are present. In such cases, histamine type 2 (H_2) antagonist therapy may be less effective in resolving gastric lesions than in cases of primary gastric ulceration.

Other useful diagnostic procedures include radiography, evaluation of peritoneal fluid, measurement of serum liver enzyme activity, particularly biliary-associated enzymes (gamma-glutamyl transferase [GGT], alkaline phosphatase), and serum bile acids. With severe duodenal ulceration, survey radiographs of the cranial abdomen may reveal accumulation of fluid within the stomach and gas ascending

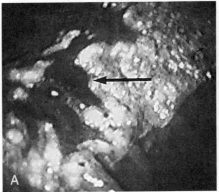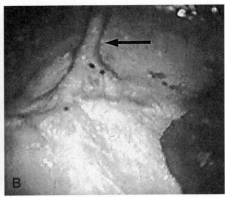

Figure 1. (*A*) Endoscopic photograph from a 5-month-old foal that presented with colic and bruxism and that had been treated with ranitidine (6.6. mg/kg t.i.d.) and sucralfate (2 g, t.i.d.) for 3 days. There is severe ulceration of the gastric squamous epithelial mucosa (*arrow*) that is similar to that seen on admission 3 days earlier. (*B*) Endoscopic photograph of the gastric squamous epithelium 10 days later. Bethanecol (0.35 mg/kg p.o. t.i.d.) was added to the treatment. There is complete healing of the gastric squamous mucosa, although some submucosal scarring is evident by the ridge seen in the squamous mucosa (*arrow*).

the biliary ducts. If barium contrast medium is placed in the stomach, complete emptying is usually delayed (longer than 2 hours), and an irregular mucosal border may be noted in the descending duodenum. If stricture has occurred, this may be noted. If the descending duodenum is to be imaged, the volume of contrast material placed in the stomach should not exceed 0.5 to 1 L in a foal, and 1 to 2 L in a weanling or yearling, or the proximal descending duodenum will be obscured by contrast medium within the stomach.

Complications

Gastric and duodenal ulcers in young foals (younger than 1 month old) may result in significant blood loss, resulting in anemia and hypoproteinemia. Delayed gastric emptying is a common complication to gastroduodenal ulceration, particularly when lesions occur in the duodenum or pylorus. Impaired gastric emptying causes accumulation of acidic gastric secretions, with resultant severe ulceration of the gastric mucosa, particularly the squamous mucosa (Fig. 1). Gastroesophageal reflux and esophagitis may occur.

Perforation is a dramatic, although infrequent, sequel to gastric ulceration. In many cases, perforation is not preceded by signs typical of gastric ulceration, and foals are found acutely depressed, or dead. Most foals presenting with perforation have significant peritonitis, which can have a tremendous fibrinous component. In such cases it is possible for peritoneal fluid cell count and protein levels to be normal, because of sequestration of cells and protein in fibrin clots within the omentum. Careful inspection of a Wright or Gram-stained slide for bacteria may confirm a

perforated viscus. Occasionally, a small perforation along the greater curvature of the stomach or in the duodenal ampulla can be sealed by the greater omentum. Foals with perforated ulcers are febrile and often have signs of shock.

In general, the sequelae to duodenal ulceration are more severe than those to gastric ulceration (Fig. 2). These include severe gastric emptying dysfunction, duodenal perforation with peritonitis and/or adhesions, duodenal stricture with complete or partial obstruction, and ascending cholangitis and hepatitis.

Yearlings

In yearlings, most lesions are confined to the squamous mucosa, particularly adjacent to the margo plicatus. Normal yearlings do not have gastric ulcers, although mild erosions of the squamous mucosa have been noted. Ulcers have been associated with recurrent colic, poor bodily condition, poor appetite, and intermittent diarrhea. Yearlings have been diagnosed with delayed gastric emptying, resulting in severe, often bleeding, gastric ulceration. These patients typically have a history of having had signs of gastroduodenal ulceration as foals, and developed focal duodenal or pyloric fibrosis. One animal was observed to belch. Diagnosis was confirmed by barium-contrast upper gastrointestinal radiography, failure to empty stomach contents following withholding feed for more than 16 hours, or response to prokinetic drugs.

Adult Horses

Gastric ulceration affects a large number of adult horses of all breeds, with clinical signs including poor appetite,

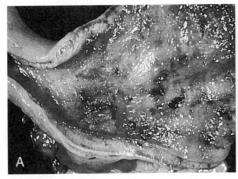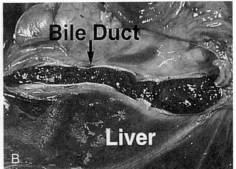

Figure 2. (*A*) Duodenum from a foal that had severe duodenal ulceration with clinical signs of 1 month's duration. The duodenal mucosa was replaced by fibrovascular tissue with a pronounced inflammatory cell infiltrate. (*B*) Liver from a foal that had severe, chronic duodenal ulceration. Feed material had migrated into the common bile duct (*arrow*), as well as into the pancreatic duct.

poor condition, mild to severe colic, attitude changes, and poor racing performance. These signs, some of which are obscure or subjective, have been confirmed as being associated with gastric ulcers based on the results of endoscopic examinations and effective treatment with H_2 antagonists. Gastric lesions are significantly more prevalent and more severe in symptomatic horses than in normal horses.

Horses in race training are at greatest risk of developing gastric lesions, with up to 90% having gastric lesions. In one group of horses, as training progressed, gastric lesion severity increased. Gastric lesion severity was not associated with administration of nonsteroidal anti-inflammatory drugs (NSAIDs) in two studies of Thoroughbred racehorses.

In adult horses, spontaneous gastric lesions occur most frequently in the squamous mucosa and less commonly in the glandular mucosa. Lesions usually occur adjacent to the margo plicatus along the greater and/or lesser curvatures. In several cases, lesions have been associated with hemorrhage, appearing as either active bleeding or darkened coagulated blood. However, bleeding from ulcers in the gastric squamous mucosa is *not* usually associated with anemia or hypoproteinemia, and if these abnormalities are present another cause must be determined. Glandular ulceration is observed with greater frequency subsequent to the administration of excessive NSAIDs.

DIAGNOSIS

Diagnosis of gastric ulceration is based on the presence of age-related characteristic clinical signs, endoscopic findings, and response to treatment. The diagnosis of gastric ulceration in the majority of foals and horses can be definitively determined only by gastroscopic examination. An endoscopic diagnosis of gastric ulceration allows the veterinarian to determine that ulcers are present, the location of the lesions, the severity of the lesions, and the response to therapy. The presence of typical clinical signs, and the results of diagnostic tests such as fecal occult blood and contrast radiography can be unreliable indicators of the presence of gastric ulcers.

Before performing gastroscopy, suckling foals up to 20 days of age are allowed to nurse but not consume solid feed for 6 to 10 hours. Older foals and mature horses should not have solid feed for 6 to 10 hours. This time period is required to ensure adequate emptying of ingesta from the stomach. Young foals may not require sedation for the gastroscopic examination to be performed, although sedation with xylazine (0.3 to 0.5 mg/kg IV) can facilitate the examination. Minimal restraint is usually satisfactory during the procedure, with the most objectionable part of the examination occurring during the initial insertion of the endoscope through the nasal turbinates. Chemical sedation is required if the foal is to be placed in a recumbent position so that the entire glandular mucosa can be examined. Combinations of xylazine (0.5 mg/kg IV) and butorphanol (0.01–0.02 mg/kg IV) or xylazine and diazepam (0.1 mg/kg IV) are useful for this procedure.

Sedation of older foals and horses is necessary. Passage of the endoscope into the esophagus is facilitated by injecting water through the biopsy channel and inducing a swallow. The stomach is distended by insufflation of air through the endoscope and is distended until the nonglandular and glandular regions of the gastric surface can be observed. Distension with air is tolerated by foals and horses and has been associated with signs of abdominal discomfort only rarely in the patients examined by the author.

Viewing along the greater curvature of the stomach, the squamous mucosa of the nonglandular fundus, the margo plicatus, and glandular fundus are observed. The squamous mucosa appears as a pale to white tissue. In foals, the squamous mucosa is very thin in the first several days of life and appears pale pink to pale white. The margo plicatus, the junction between the squamous and glandular gastric mucosal epithelium, is seen from the endoscopist's perspective to proceed dorsally, then ventrally along the greater curvature. The glandular mucosa appears as dark pink to red, with a smooth, glistening texture.

The endoscope is then advanced along the transverse curvature of the stomach, until the lesser curvature and cardia can be observed. At this location the squamous mucosa surrounding the cardia, lesser curvature, and, in foals with an empty stomach, the pyloric antrum and pylorus, can be observed. With a 200-cm-long endoscope, the duodenum can be entered in foals up to 6 months of age. In yearlings and horses, an insertion tube length of 280 to 300 cm is required to perform duodenoscopy.

The pylorus is observed ventral to the cardia. In foals, reflux of bile-tinged fluid from the duodenum into the stomach is occasionally observed and is considered normal. Frequent bile reflux is abnormal, reflective of small intestinal obstruction or adynamic ileus. When observing the cardia and pylorus it is important to recognize that the endoscope is pointing cranially, so that the left side of the animal appears on the left side of the endoscopist's field of view. The endoscope is advanced to the pylorus, and from this point, the normal contractions of the stomach, with some guidance by the endoscopist, are usually sufficient to advance the endoscope into the duodenum. The duodenal mucosa should have a uniform pink "velvety" appearance. The common duodenal papilla may be observed, with bile emptying from the common bile duct.

TREATMENT

The primary objective in the treatment of gastric ulcers in foals and horses is to reduce or neutralize acid secretion so that the gastric mucosal epithelium can heal. Once ulcers form, there are changes in the tissue that promote healing. Suppressing acidity creates an environment within the stomach that is permissive for ulcer healing. Gastric acid secretion can be largely attenuated by use of histamine receptor type 2 (H_2) antagonists. Treatment with H_2 antagonists has been successful in resolving the gastric lesions and in resolving the presenting problem. Cimetidine* and

---

*Tagamet, Smith/Kline Beecham, Philadelphia, PA

TABLE 1. THERAPEUTIC AGENTS FOR USE IN TREATING GASTRIC AND/OR DUODENAL ULCERS IN FOALS AND HORSES

Generic Name (Proprietary Name)

Histamine Type 2 Receptor Antagonists	Dosage
Cimetidine (Tagamet)	18 mg/kg, q8h p.o.
	6.6 mg/kg, q6h IV
Ranitidine (Zantac)	6.6 mg/kg, q8h p.o.
	1.5 mg/kg, q8h IV
Famotidine (Pepcid)*	4.0 mg/kg, q8h p.o.
Nizatidine (Axid)†	6.6 mg/kg, q8h p.o.
Proton Pump Inhibitor	
Omeprazole (Prilosec)	1.5 mg/kg, once daily by nasogastric tube
	0.5 mg/kg, once daily IV
Lansoprazole (Prevacid)	Undetermined as to efficacy or safety in the horse
Antacids	
Maalox TC	240 ml q4h p.o.
Mylanta II	240 ml q4h p.o.
Extra Strength Maalox	240 ml q4h p.o.
Mucosal Protectant	
Sucralfate (Carafate)	2 g (foal) to 6 g (adult), 3 to 4 times daily p.o.

*Dosage based on unpublished data comparing effect of 4.0 mg/kg famotidine with 6.6 mg/kg ranitidine on equine gastric fluid pH.

†Dosage based on equivalent potency with ranitidine in man. Data on effect in horses not available.

ranitidine* are the most frequently used, and both inhibit gastric acid secretion in equids.

Many dosages of H₂ antagonists have been recommended and used in practice (Table 1). Because these drugs are expensive, there is pressure to use as little as possible. When deciding on a dose to use, one must recognize that as the dose of an acid-suppressive agent is lowered the percentage of patients that will respond poorly or not at all increases. Tremendous individual variability exists in the degree and duration of suppression of gastric acidity

*Zantac, Glaxo Inc., Research Triangle Park, NC

by H₂ antagonists between horses (Fig. 3), presumably as a result of differences in drug absorption and first-pass hepatic metabolism. We have found that 6.6 mg ranitidine per kg (p.o. t.i.d.) provides adequate suppression of acidity in the greatest percentage of horses. This dosage schedule resulted in a median 24-hour gastric pH of 4.6 in horses with free access to hay, compared with a pH of 3.1 in horses with free access to hay, but not given ranitidine.

Formulations for intravenous administration of H₂ antagonists are available, but are expensive (approximately three times the cost of oral products). Ranitidine should be given intravenously at 1.5 mg/kg t.i.d. and cimetidine at 6.6 mg/kg q.i.d.

H₂ antagonist therapy should continue for 14 to 21 days to ensure complete healing. In most cases 3 weeks' treatment is required to achieve complete healing. Eighty to ninety percent of adult horses treated with ranitidine p.o. (6.6 mg/kg t.i.d. for 3 weeks) had complete healing of gastric ulcers, whereas at 2 weeks complete healing occurred in only 15 to 40%. It has become apparent from treating horses in training for racing with H₂ antagonists that if the horse is kept in training while being treated, clinical signs may improve but the lesions do not. Thus, for healing of the ulcers to be achieved, treatment with an H₂ antagonist should be accompanied by refraining from training.

Other H₂ antagonists, famotidine* and nizatidine† are on the market for use in humans, but effective dosages in the horse have not been established at this time. From limited experience, it would appear that the effect on gastric acidity from oral administration of 3.3 mg/kg famotidine is similar to that with 6.6 mg/kg ranitidine.

Omeprazole,‡ a drug that completely blocks gastric acid secretion by inhibiting the parietal cell hydrogen ion pump, has been studied in horses, and is a potent inhibitor of gastric acidity. Because of its potency, once-daily treatment is feasible. A dose of 0.7 mg/kg effectively inhibits gastric acidity, although 1.4 mg/kg is superior. Omeprazole (1.5 mg/kg s.i.d.) promoted rapid restoration of normal gastric

*Pepcid, Merck Sharp and Dohme, Rahway, NJ
†Axid, Eli Lilly, Indianapolis, IN
‡Prilosec, Merck Sharp and Dohme, Rahway, NJ

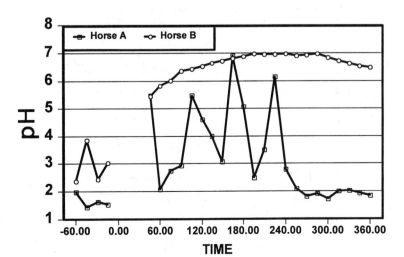

Figure 3. Graph of gastric fluid pH from two horses illustrating the marked interhorse variability in response to oral histamine type 2 (H₂) receptor antagonists. Each horse was administered ranitidine 6.6 mg/kg by nasogastric intubation, and pH measurements were made every 15 min on aspirated gastric fluid 60 minutes before and 45 to 360 minutes after administration of ranitidine. Horse B had complete suppression of gastric acidity for 360 minutes, whereas horse A had intermittent, brief periods of increased gastric fluid pH.

squamous mucosa in a vehicle-controlled study of Thoroughbred racehorses with moderate to severe gastric ulceration. The drug is difficult to administer to horses, because it is manufactured in enteric-coated granules. This is required because the drug is destroyed in an acidic environment. Omeprazole should be administered by nasogastric tube. Because omeprazole is more expensive than H_2 antagonists and is more difficult to administer, we currently reserve its use for patients with severe gastroduodenal ulceration.

The use of antacids in the treatment of gastric ulcers has not been critically examined in the horse. Antacids can effectively reduce gastric acidity, but usually only briefly (30–60 minutes) (Fig. 4) unless large (more than 240 ml) volumes are given. In one report, 240 ml MaaloxTC° decreased gastric acidity for 2 hours. These agents must be given both in large volumes (240 ml or more) and very frequently (four to six times daily) to be effective even in alleviating clinical signs. Antacids may be particularly useful in horses that have evidence of excessive gastric acidity such as moderate to severe hyperkeratosis of the gastric squamous mucosa, but no gastric ulceration.

Sucralfate,† a sulfated polysaccharide, is effective in the treatment of peptic ulcers in people. The mechanism of action likely involves adherence to ulcerated mucosa, stimulation of mucus secretion, binding of salivary epidermal growth factor, and enhanced prostaglandin E synthesis. These are all factors relevant to glandular mucosa, and it is doubtful that sucralfate is effective in treating ulcers in the equine gastric squamous mucosa. We have had horses develop squamous mucosal lesions while being treated with sucralfate for glandular ulcers. Sucralfate appears to be effective in the treatment of ulcers in the gastric glandular mucosa and duodenum in equids. When treatment is initiated without an endoscopic examination, sucralfate should be given as an adjunct to H_2 antagonist therapy, rather than the sole treatment.

Sucralfate has been reported to adhere to gastric mucosa

°Maalox TC, Rhone-Poulenc Rorer Pharmaceuticals, Fort Washington, PA
†Carafate, Marion Laboratories, Kansas City, MO

more readily in an acidic environment. Consequently, some have advocated that administration of sucralfate and an H_2 antagonist be staggered to provide an acidic environment for optimal adherence of sucralfate. However, this is not necessary. A study in rats found similar adherence of sucralfate to gastric mucosa in acidic and neutral pH environments. In addition, the acid-suppressive effect of an H_2 antagonist usually has subsided by the time the next dose is given, and it takes approximately 45 minutes for a dose to affect gastric pH. Therefore, we recommend administering sucralfate and ranitidine concurrently, and results have been entirely satisfactory.

Prokinetic drugs stimulate gastrointestinal motility and enhance gastric emptying. They are used in cases in which delayed gastric emptying is suspected or confirmed. Metoclopramide° has been used in selected cases to prevent gastroesophageal reflux and enhance gastric emptying. An effective dosage is approximately 0.25 mg/kg (IV drip or sq t.i.d. or q.i.d.). Several adverse effects occur with metoclopramide, and it appears to have a very narrow margin of safety.

Consequently, bethanecol,† a cholinergic agonist, is preferred. Recently, bethanecol was reported to enhance gastrointestinal motility while not increasing gastric acid output. In cases of acute gastric atony, 0.025 mg/kg sq q4–6 hours, has been effective in promoting gastric motility and emptying. Oral maintenance dosages (0.35 mg/kg t.i.d. or q.i.d.) are effective. Diarrhea has been observed with the higher dosages, but resolved when the dosage was decreased.

If medical therapy is ineffective or sequelae of duodenal ulceration cause complications, surgical intervention may be required. Gastroenterostomy has been reported to be effective in some cases, through bypassing the affected portion of duodenum and allowing for gastric emptying. However, the reported survival rates in such cases are poor, primarily because of the severity of the disorder when surgery has been attempted. In addition, surgically treated horses require weeks to months of treatment with acid-

---

°Reglan, AH Robins, Richmond, VA
†Urecholine, Merck Sharp and Dohme, Rahway, NJ

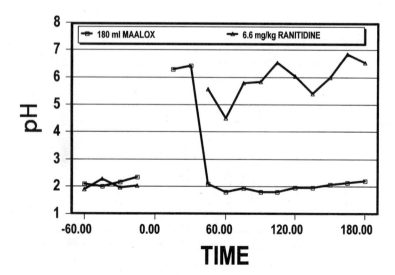

Figure 4. Graph of gastric fluid pH from five horses administered 180 ml Maalox and 6.6 mg/kg ranitidine per nasogastric intubation. The pH measurements were made every 15 min on aspirated gastric fluid 60 minutes before and up to 180 minutes after treatments were given. Administration of Maalox resulted in only a brief increase in gastric fluid pH, whereas ranitidine increased gastric fluid pH for at least 180 minutes.

suppressive and prokinetic drugs until normal gastric emptying is restored.

Supplemental Readings

Baker SJ: Gastric pH in suckling foals: A window of opportunity for ulcer formation? Proc Am Assoc Equine Pract, 1992, p 743.

Feldman EJ, Sabovich KA: Stress and peptic ulcer disease. Gastroenterology 78:1087–1089, 1980.

Furr MO, Murray MJ, Ferguson DC: The effects of stress on gastric ulceration, T3, T4, reverse T3 and cortisol in neonatal foals. Equine Vet J 24:37–40, 1992.

Genta RM, Graham DY: *Helicobacter pylori*: The new bug on the (paraffin) block. Virchows Arch 425:339–347, 1994.

Jenkins CC, Blackford JT, Andrews F, Mattsson H, Olovsson SG, Peterson A, Frazier DL: Duration of antisecretory effects of oral omeprazole in horses with chronic gastric cannulae. Equine Vet J 13[Suppl]:89–92, 1992.

Murray MJ: Gastric ulceration in horses: 91 cases (1987–1990). J Am Vet Med Assoc 201:117–120, 1992.

Murray MJ: Equine model of inducing ulceration in alimentary squamous epithelial mucosa. Dig Dis Sci 39:2530–2535, 1994.

Murray MJ, Grodinsky C: The effects of famotidine, ranitidine and magnesium hydroxide/aluminum hydroxide on gastric fluid pH in adult horses. Equine Vet J 11[Suppl]:52–55, 1992.

Murray MJ, Mahaffey EA: Age-related characteristics of gastric squamous epithelial mucosa in foals. Equine Vet J 25:514–517, 1993.

Murray MJ, Schusser GF: Measurement of 24-h gastric pH using an indwelling pH electrode in horses unfed, fed, and treated with ranitidine. Equine Vet J 25:417–421, 1993.

Acute Colitis

MICHAEL J. MURRAY
Leesburg, Virginia

Colitis refers to inflammation of the large colon, although the cecum frequently is involved (typhlitis). A multitude of inflammatory cells and mediators are activated in horses with colitis, resulting in local colonic inflammation and systemic signs. Severe inflammation can result in loss of the colonic mucosal epithelium (Fig. 1), increased permeability of mucosal and submucosal capillaries, and severe colonic edema. Profuse diarrhea, severe fluid and electrolyte deficits, metabolic acidosis, signs compatible with endotoxemia, and septic shock typically occur in horses with acute colitis. Malabsorption of volatile fatty acids and metabolic alterations that result from excessive production and release of inflammatory mediators lead to an energy deficit and catabolism of body tissues. The severity of illness often demands intensive therapy for several days, and the clinician must consider treatments that modify inflammatory changes and replace losses of fluid, electrolytes, and plasma protein. Because pathophysiologic processes occur simultaneously in horses with colitis, it is important to frequently monitor metabolic parameters so that treatment can be directed to meet the current requirements of the patient, as well as to anticipate medication requirements. Complications, including laminitis, thrombophlebitis, colonic infarction, and dissemination of bacteria from the colon to other organs, frequently occur.

CAUSES

The documented causes of colitis in juvenile and adult horses are limited, and frequently a cause is not determined. The veterinarian has limited diagnostic capabilities in determining the causative agent of colitis, and these include selective fecal culture techniques and serologic tests for *Ehrlichia risticii*. Regardless of cause, aggressive treatment must be begun before the results of tests determining the causative agent are available.

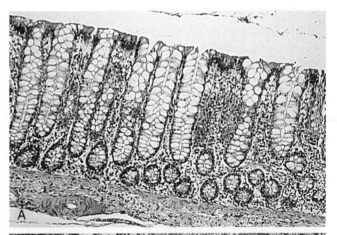
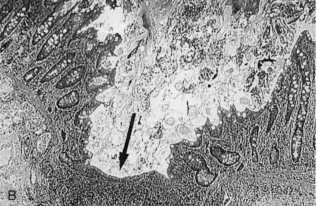

Figure 1. (*A*) Photomicrograph of normal equine large colon mucosal epithelium. The mucosa consists primarily of epithelial cells and clear, mucus-secreting goblet cells. The cells are arranged vertically from lumen to the basement membrane around crypts. (*B*) Photomicrograph of equine large colon 20 hours after inoculation with 10⁹ *Salmonella typhimurium* bacteria. There is loss of mucosal epithelium to the basement membrane (*arrow*); a pronounced inflammatory response; and exudation of inflammatory cells, cellular debris, and serum into the lumen.

Salmonellosis

The most frequently diagnosed infectious cause of diarrhea in horses is infection by *Salmonella* species, which have several virulence factors that contribute to invasiveness, colonic fluid secretory response, and the host's local and systemic inflammatory response. Several serotypes have been associated with equine colitis, and overall more than 3000 serotypes of salmonella have been described. *S. typhimurium, S. agona, S. krefeld,* and *S. St. Paul* are serotypes that have been frequently isolated in horses recently, with dozens of other serotypes isolated sporadically. *Salmonella* organisms are ubiquitous in the environment, and from 1 to 10% of asymptomatic horses tested by fecal culture shed *Salmonella* in the feces. Horses are not considered to be carriers of *Salmonella* because there are apparently no host-adapted *Salmonella* species affecting the horse. Horses can shed *Salmonella* for several weeks to months and may serve as reservoirs of infection.

In acutely affected horses, large numbers of highly infective *Salmonella* bacteria can be shed in the diarrheic feces. Susceptible animals, such as young foals, hospitalized horses, and horses under stress, can be infected by doses of *Salmonella* that are 100 to 1000 times less than those required to infect less susceptible horses. Thus, particular care should be taken in the management of horses and foals with diarrhea in environments such as hospitals, breeding farms, and race tracks in which there are animals at risk. Asymptomatic shedders generally shed a relatively small number of *Salmonella* in the feces and do not appear to pose an important threat to healthy horses, although asymptomatic shedders have been responsible for outbreaks of salmonellosis in hospitals and on breeding farms.

Salmonellosis typically is characterized by an acute, toxemic colitis, resulting in profuse diarrhea. In most cases, with treatment, the severe diarrhea and associated metabolic disorders improve within 7 to 10 days of the onset of illness. Horses that have severe diarrhea and septicemia for 10 days or longer are unlikely to survive, even with intensive therapy, because these horses often have extensive loss of colonic mucosa and chronic colitis. Other clinical syndromes of salmonellosis include fever and leukopenia, colic, and proximal enteritis with gastric reflux.

Equine Ehrlichial Colitis (Potomac Horse Fever)

Potomac horse fever (PHF) is an infectious enterocolonic disorder caused by *E. risticii*. The organism is an obligate intracellular parasite, initially infecting peripheral monocytes and macrophages. It has been observed ultrastructurally in colonic and small intestinal epithelial cells and colonic mast cells. The pathophysiology of the disease is poorly understood, although horses infected with *E. risticii* often have clinical signs and complications similar to those in horses with salmonellosis. The typical clinical scenario of PHF is that 2 to 4 days after infection the horse may have a mild, transient fever that usually is not detected. Ten to 14 days after infection the horse becomes febrile, has a poor appetite, and exhibits mild to severe gastrointestinal signs, ranging from mild colic and soft stool to profuse diarrhea. Clinical signs resembling endotoxemia, including fever, leukopenia, congested mucous membranes,

and hypercoagulability, occur in horses with PHF, as with salmonellosis. Laminitis is a frequent complication, and typically occurs in 25 to 30% of horses with PHF.

Although originally described as a disease of horses living near the Potomac River in Maryland and Virginia, PHF has been confirmed serologically in most states. The association between an affected horse and proximity to a river (within 5 miles) remains strong. At this time, the mode of transmission is still unknown, although in field cases it does not appear to be a horse-to-horse route. Oral transmission with infected cell cultures has been produced experimentally. An insect vector, as well as an intermediate mammalian host, may be involved in the transmission of the disease in field cases.

In areas in which PHF occurs, paired acute and convalescent blood samples should be submitted for indirect fluorescent antibody (IFA) or preferably enzyme-linked immunosorbent assay (ELISA) testing for antibodies to *E. risticii*. Serologic evaluation to confirm the disease is not as straightforward as in many other infectious diseases. A four-fold increase in titer between acute and convalescent sera is considered to confirm infection with *E. risticii*, but failure to "seroconvert" does not rule out infection. Because the onset of clinical signs can be delayed as long as 14 days after infection, horses may seroconvert by the time an "acute" sample is obtained. The magnitude of titer does not always correlate with active infection, because many horses in endemic areas have high titers but no disease. Vaccination also can affect titer, but postvaccination titers can vary greatly.

Once a horse recovers from the disease, the infectious agent appears to be eliminated. Horses do not remain chronic carriers of *E. risticii*. A few horses have had clinical relapses that were responsive to tetracycline 2 to 3 weeks following initial resolution of clinical signs.

Vaccination has appeared to diminish the incidence and severity of disease, but vaccinated animals may still develop PHF. Disease severity has appeared to be less in vaccinated animals, although in the summer of 1994 many vaccinated horses developed severe cases of PHF. All of these horses were located in the area where PHF was originally described. Based on results of polymerase chain reaction testing, a new strain of *E. risticii* appears to have been identified in the horses of that outbreak (personal communication, S.K. Dutta, 1995). Horses in endemic areas probably should be vaccinated in the early spring and early to midsummer on an annual basis.

Clostridial Colitis

Colitis caused by clostridial bacteria is probably common in horses, although there are few reported confirmed cases. Feces must be cultured anaerobically and often in special media. In addition to culturing clostridial organisms, isolation of clostridial toxins from feces of affected animals enhances confirmation of the etiology. *Clostridium perfringens* type A has been described as a cause of peracute toxemic colitis (colitis X), but it is unclear whether this is an important or infrequent etiologic agent in horses. Strains of *C. perfringens* are classified on the basis of the toxins that are produced, with at least a dozen identified to date. *C. perfringens* type A has been cited as an equine pathogen, and this strain produces an enterotoxin as well as up to seven other distinct toxins. A toxin produced by type E (iota toxin) was recently identified in a patient treated by the author. Diarrhea associated with *Clostridium difficile* has been reported in foals, and this organism may be an important agent in some cases of colitis in horses. *C. difficile* produces two toxins, toxin A and B. These toxins have both enterotoxigenic and cytotoxic properties. In addition, toxin A is a potent neutrophilic chemotactic agent and stimulates cytokine release by macrophages. Thus, toxin A can elicit both fluid secretion and a pronounced inflammatory response in the bowel.

An organism that resembles *Clostridium cadaveris* has been reported to have been isolated from experimentally induced colitis in horses and ponies and was implicated as the causative agent in the colitis. This organism does not produce a toxin, and thus its role in inducing diarrhea is not conclusive.

The clinical signs described for clostridial colitis vary from peracute, hemorrhagic, fatal colitis, to signs similar to those of colitis caused by *Salmonella* species. Diagnosis depends upon isolation of pathogenic clostridia and identification of toxin. Suspicion of clostridial diarrhea may be heightened by association with antimicrobial administration. One horse treated in the author's clinic for *Clostridium difficile*-associated colitis had putrid-smelling feces, suggesting involvement of an anaerobic pathogen.

Antimicrobial-Associated Colitis

The onset of acute diarrhea in the horse has been associated with the use of several antibiotics. Lincomycin administered orally and tetracycline administered parenterally have been demonstrated to induce severe diarrhea in horses. Oral administration of trimethoprim/sulfa, erythromycin, metronidazole, penicillin, and parenteral ceftiofur have been temporally associated with onset of colitis in horses. Diarrhea is presumed to result from disruption of normal colonic microflora, which can lead to abnormal volatile fatty acid production and disruption of normal secretory and absorptive patterns in the colon and proliferation of enteropathogens. *Salmonella* species, *C. perfringens*, *C. cadaveris*, and *C. difficile* have been implicated in antimicrobial-induced diarrhea.

Other Causes

The administration of excessive dosages of nonsteroidal anti-inflammatory drugs (NSAIDs) (see p. 724) has been associated with the onset of diarrhea resulting from the development of hypoproteinemia and cecal and colonic mucosal edema. The inhibition of prostaglandin synthesis by NSAIDs disrupts mucosal blood flow and other mucosal-protective mechanisms in the bowel. In addition to hypoproteinemia, these horses often have signs of severe endotoxemia. Many horses with diarrhea and toxemia as a consequence of excessive administration of NSAIDs are slow to respond to therapy and require a long duration of intensive care.

Acute diarrhea in the adult horse has also been associated with conditions such as granulomatous enterocolitis, intestinal lymphosarcoma, peritonitis, heavy metal intoxication, anaphylaxis, and stress.

CLINICAL ASSESSMENT OF HORSES WITH ACUTE COLITIS

Most horses with acute diarrhea have several clinical problems that include fever, dehydration, impaired cardiovascular function, progressive hypoproteinemia, electrolyte and acid-base disturbances, and impaired renal function. Therefore, a thorough examination is required for horses presenting with acute diarrhea.

Clinical Examination

A thorough physical examination should include evaluation of (1) the horse's hydration status by determination of skin turgor, gum moisture, and capillary refill time; (2) signs of toxemia such as injected sclera, conjunctiva, oral mucous membranes, mucous membrane color, and capillary refill time; (3) cardiovascular system by determination of heart rate and rhythm, presence of murmur, character of peripheral pulse, and capillary refill time; (4) respiratory system by evaluating the rate and pattern of breathing, and by thoracic auscultation; and (5) signs of laminitis such as lameness, digital pulse, and palpable heat in the hoof walls. Horses with colitis are often moderately to severely dehydrated, with either purplish or brick-red mucous membrane color. Purple mucous membrane color reflects poor venous return, whereas brick-red color is reflective of venous congestion with partially deoxygenated blood resulting from arteriovenular shunting and poor tissue oxygen exchange. Horses with acute colitis typically are tachycardic, resulting from both hypovolemia and inflammatory mediator release upon exposure to bacterial lipopolysaccharide (i.e., endotoxin). Atrial or ventricular arrhythmias may occur in severely toxemic horses. Heart murmurs may occur as a consequence of flow disturbances in severely dehydrated horses or in toxemic horses with altered cardiac contractility. Rarely, heart murmurs reflect vegetative endocarditis resulting from a septic embolus.

A rectal examination should be done to determine whether there is intestinal distension or possibly displacement. Diarrhea can occur from cecal impaction or large-colon displacement. Palpation of distended small intestine should alert the veterinarian to pass a nasogastric tube for the relief of fluid or gas accumulation. In addition, pronounced edema of the colon can be discerned by rectal palpation.

Laboratory Tests

A complete blood count with plasma protein and total solids and fibrinogen tests should be performed. Packed cell volume (PCV) can be used to assess hydration status, although with endotoxemia splenic contraction increases PCV. Total protein level testing can be used to estimate the degree of protein loss through inflamed intestinal mucosa, as well as loss resulting from protein catabolism in cases of several days' duration. Comparison of clinical hydration, PCV, and total protein level is useful in determining the extent of protein loss, and daily evaluations can be used to determine the rate of protein loss.

Total leukocyte (WBC) count, WBC differential, and WBC morphology are tests used to assess severity of endotoxemia and septicemia; plasma fibrinogen level tests are used to assess the severity of inflammation. Typically, the total WBC and neutrophil counts decrease acutely. This is attributable to bacterial endotoxins and the host's mediators of inflammation. Neutropenia occurs with most cases of acute colitis, not just those caused by *Salmonella*. The morphology of the WBCs reflects the severity of the inflammatory response and degree of sepsis. "Toxic" changes such as basophilia, granulation, vacuolation of the cytoplasm, and scalloped borders of the cell membrane or adherence of neutrophils to RBCs do not reflect injury to the neutrophils by toxins but reflect the cells' responses to stimulation by proinflammatory agents such as tumor necrosis factor and interleukin-1, and the production of inflammatory mediators by the neutrophils that are toxic to bacteria. The degree of these changes in circulating neutrophils can be used to assess the severity of disease and to assess the progress the horse is making. Often, the initial sign that the horse is improving is a decrease in the "toxic" appearance of the neutrophils. A horse that continues to have neutrophils with a scalloped cell membrane adherent to RBCs, together with cytoplasmic vacuolation, granulation, and basophilia for more than 10 days, has a severe colitis that is unlikely to resolve.

Serum chemistry tests that should be performed include electrolytes (sodium, chloride, potassium, and calcium), blood urea nitrogen (BUN), and creatinine and assessment of acid-base status (blood pH and bicarbonate, or total carbon dioxide [CO_2]). Horses with diarrhea typically are hyponatremic, hypochloremic, and hypokalemic. With decreased feed intake, hypocalcemia occurs. The severity of these electrolyte disturbances should be monitored, often daily, to allow for appropriate therapy. Parameters that are measured to assess renal function, BUN, and creatinine levels are frequently increased in horses with diarrhea, for several reasons. Prerenal azotemia resulting from dehydration and decreased filtration across the glomeruli account for some of the increase in these parameters. Hyponatremia and hypochloremia can cause a decrease in glomerular filtration and an increase in BUN and creatinine levels resulting from tubuloglomerular feedback. Horses that are adequately hydrated yet moderately hyponatremic (serum sodium 120–128 mEq/L) often remain azotemic until sodium levels increase above 130 mEq/L. Azotemia also may reflect tubular damage and dysfunction resulting from endotoxemia and septicemia. Urinalysis may reveal glucosuria and an increased gamma-glutamyl transferase (GGT): creatinine ratio owing to proximal tubular cell damage, a specific gravity disproportionately low for the degree of dehydration present, and increased tubular epithelial cells.

The acid-base status can be evaluated by estimating serum bicarbonate on the basis of the total CO_2 or directly from a venous or arterial blood gas analysis. Evaluation of a venous blood gas sample is useful in assessing perfusion and oxygen extraction. An increased venous oxygen partial pressure (>60 mm Hg) is indicative of poor capillary perfusion and oxygen delivery to the tissues. Such horses usually have brick-red mucous membranes.

Multiple fecal cultures for *Salmonella* should be performed on all horses with diarrhea. It is recommended that at least three to five fecal samples be submitted for culture to enhance the chances of isolating *Salmonella*. Samples with little solid matter often yield negative culture results, even when the horse is infected with *Salmonella*. More

formed fecal samples are more likely to result in a positive culture from infected horses. Five to ten grams of feces should be submitted for culture in selective media such as tetrathionate or selenite broth, and brilliant green, XLD, or XLT-4 agars. Culture of a rectal mucosal biopsy can identify some positive salmonellosis cases that are negative on fecal culture.

In areas where equine ehrlichial colitis occurs, paired acute and convalescent blood samples should be submitted for IFA or ELISA testing for antibodies to *E. risticii*. "Acute" serum samples should be taken immediately, because seroconversion may occur early in the course of illness.

TREATMENT

Because the pathophysiology of equine colitis is complex, the treatment of these cases often incorporates several medications. Many of these treatments provide well-documented benefit, whereas with others the efficacy is based on empirical judgment only. In addition, in many cases, the limiting factor to a successful outcome is a complication of colitis, and not a direct effect of colitis.

Fluid Therapy

In cases of acute colitis, fluid administration remains the treatment of primary importance. Severe dehydration can occur rapidly, and most cases require intravenous administration of 40 to 60 L in the first 24 hours of treatment. Large volumes, 40 to 60 L, may be required for several days. An isotonic polyionic fluid such as lactated Ringer's or an equivalent solution is a good initial fluid choice while awaiting laboratory results and assessing the patient's response to treatment.

Fluid requirements are based on the horse's fluid and electrolyte deficits and its anticipated losses. Parameters for estimating degree of dehydration are in Table 1. Horses that have ongoing protein losses may present with "normal" plasma protein levels when severely dehydrated. Hematocrit and physical examination findings are most useful for determining hydration status in such horses. For a 500-kg (1100-lb) horse that is 8% dehydrated, 40 L of fluid are required to correct dehydration, and maintenance fluid

TABLE 1. CLINICAL PARAMETERS FOR ASSESSING HYDRATION STATUS AND ESTIMATES OF DEGREE OF DEHYDRATION

Parameter	Mild (4–6%)	Moderate (7–9%)	Severe (10%+)
Skin turgor	Good to fair	Fair	Poor
Gum moisture	Good to fair	Tacky	Dry
Capillary refill time	1–2 seconds	2–4 seconds	>4 sec
PCV (%)*	40–50	50–65	>65
TP (g/dl)†	6.5–7.5	7.5–8.5	>8.5

*Normal PCV is dependent on breed and level of athletic training. For example, Thoroughbred and Standardbred horses in training can have normal PCV up to 45%, whereas inactive horses have a normal PCV of 32–38%. Normal PCV of draft breeds is 25–30%.

†In horses with significant enteric protein losses, total plasma protein level is similar to "normal" values, even in severely dehydrated horses.

TABLE 2. INTRAVENOUS FLUID DELIVERY, CATHETERS AND CATHETERIZATION SITES

	Advantage	Disadvantage
Catheter		
Polypropylene,° 9 gauge	Large volumes, rapidly	Thrombophlebitis
Teflon,† 12 gauge	Moderate volumes	Thrombophlebitis, kinks
Polyurethane,‡ 14 gauge	Less thrombophlebitis than Teflon	Sometimes difficult to place
Silicon elastomer,§ 16 gauge	Minimum thrombophlebitis, long-term placement	Limited rate of administration
Polyurethane,‖ 16 gauge		
Vein		
Jugular	Ease of catheterization	Sequelae of thrombophlebitis
	Ease of maintenance	
	Ease of access	
Lateral thoracic	Less severe sequelae of thrombophlebitis	Moderately difficult to catheterize
	Relative ease of maintenance, access	
Saphenous	Minimal sequelae of thrombophlebitis	Relative difficulty placing, maintaining catheter

°Cook Critical Care, Bloomington, IN
†Milacath, 12 gauge, Mila International, Covington, KY; and Abbocath-T, Abbott Hospitals, North Chicago, IL
‡Centrasil, Travenol Laboratories, Deerfield, IL; and Milacath-Extended Use, Mila International, Covington, KY
§L-Cath, Animal Health Care, Los Angeles, CA
‖Central Venous Catheter Set, Arrow International, Reading, PA; and Centrasil (Travenol)

requirements may be as great as 120 ml/kg per day, or 60 L in a 500-kg horse.

In a severely dehydrated horse, as indicated by a PCV higher than 65%, dry gums, tachycardia, and poor skin turgor, fluids can be administered at a rate of approximately 1 L/minute IV, using two 5-L bags of fluids administered simultaneously through a two-lead arthroscopic irrigation set, with 12-gauge catheters in place in each jugular vein.

If large volumes of isotonic fluids are unavailable when a horse is first presenting with an acute case of diarrhea accompanied by significant dehydration and cardiovascular compromise, administration of hypertonic saline may help to stabilize the horse's cardiovascular function. Normal saline solution is 0.9% (900 mg/100 ml) sodium chloride, whereas hypertonic solutions are 7 to 8% (7000–8000 mg/100 ml) sodium chloride. Hypertonic saline has been reported to be of benefit in treatment of acute hemorrhagic shock and in a model of equine endotoxemia. Administration of 1 to 2 L hypertonic saline results in improved systemic blood pressure and cardiac output, and buys time until adequate fluid replacement can be administered.

The choice of which catheter system to use and which vein to employ for fluid and medication delivery depends on several factors, including the volume and rate of fluid to be administered, the type of fluid administered, the potential for coagulopathies and venous thrombosis, and the duration of intravenous catheterization required (Table 2). Large-gauge (10- and 12-gauge) catheters permit rapid administration of large volumes of fluid, but they are highly thrombogenic and unsuitable for long-term catheterization in horses. Manufacture of large-gauge polypropylene catheters was recently discontinued. Teflon catheters (14- or 16-gauge) are less thrombogenic but can cause jugular thrombosis in septic patients. These catheters are also prone to forming kinks and cracks with long-term use. Silicone elastomer° and polyurethane catheters† are the least thrombogenic because they are quite flexible and

do not form permanent kinks. These catheters are most appropriate for long-term use in horses with colitis and can be maintained in the jugular veins of septic patients, usually with minimal complications. Catheterization of the lateral thoracic vein is often preferable to the jugular vein, because thrombosis of the jugular veins can lead to severe swelling of the head.

In all cases, intravenous catheters must be placed aseptically (i.e., the operator must wear sterile gloves) and with minimal trauma. Methods of securing catheters to the skin include suturing, stapling, and using super-adhesive glue. It is important that the catheters be well secured, because this minimizes catheter stress and damage to the intima of the vein. The catheter site must be monitored at least daily and kept free of contamination. Signs of swelling, pain, or moisture at the catheter site; venous thrombosis; or fever of unknown origin are grounds for removing the catheter. Catheter complications occur more often than not in severely ill patients, and owners should be forewarned of this likelihood.

As horses begin to recover, they often consume fluids orally, and frequently they select solutions that contain electrolytes in which they are deficient. For example, horses with a mild to moderate bicarbonate deficit often selectively consume water with bicarbonate added. Similar preference may occur for solutions containing potassium with hypokalemic horses. Offering horses a variety of solutions for oral consumption allows animals to specifically select solutions based on their requirements. The author offers buckets containing water, water with baking soda (5 to 10 g baking soda per L), water with potassium chloride (3–6 g Lite Salt per L), and water with a commercial balanced oral electrolyte replacement.

Plasma

Horses with colitis often become hypoproteinemic because of protein leakage through the inflamed colon and catabolism of albumin resulting from negative energy balance. This frequently leads to edema formation in several areas of the body, including the intestinal tract, and can

°Centrasil, Travenol Laboratories, Deerfield, IL
†L-Cath, Animal Health Care, Los Angeles, CA

compromise the clinician's ability to keep the patient properly hydrated through fluid administration. Albumin is the principal plasma protein that regulates plasma oncotic pressure. With colitis, the albumin level typically decreases to less than 2.0 g/dl. Such horses require 5 to 10 L of plasma containing 3.0 g albumin/dl to significantly increase the plasma albumin concentration toward normal. Further plasma transfusions may be required if protein losses continue. Plasma contains other proteins besides albumin, such as fibronectin, elastase and proteinase inhibitors, complement inhibitors, antithrombin III, and other inhibitors of hypercoagulability, and thus may be of benefit beyond improvement of plasma oncotic pressure. With the cost of a 900-ml bag of commercial plasma ranging from $85 to $125, the cost of effective plasma therapy in adult horses is often prohibitive.

Nutritional Supplementation

The nutritional needs of the toxemic patient with colitis must be considered. Affected horses are frequently anorectic, and the disruption of normal physiologic processes in the inflamed cecum and colon limits the effectiveness of these organs in the digestion and absorption of nutrients. In addition, several mediators of inflammation and septicemia alter protein and calorie metabolism, resulting in a catabolic state. Thus, even if the horse will eat, it is likely to be in a severe caloric deficit for some time. Normally, an average horse that is not in work requires 12,000 to 15,000 Kcal/day. A horse with toxemic colitis may require 25,000 Kcal/day! In a catabolic patient, muscle and fat tissue are mobilized and used in lieu of ingested nutrients. The plasma protein pool, including albumin and immunoglobulins, also is catabolized. In many cases of colitis, the decrease in plasma protein may be as much the result of catabolism as leakage through the inflamed colon.

The nutritional requirements of the horse with sepsis and colitis may be supplemented enterally or parenterally. The nutrients in enteral supplements must be digestible and absorbable within the small intestine, because the inflamed colon is diminished in its ability to digest or absorb nutrients. In addition, horses must be introduced to enteral supplements with a high caloric density gradually, over 3 to 4 days; otherwise, excessive fermentable carbohydrate may reach the cecum and colon. Calories, digestible protein, fat, electrolytes, and vitamins should be provided. In most cases, the volume of a feed gruel that can be administered through a nasogastric tube to an anorectic horse is insufficient to supply the horse's nutritional needs. Commercial products are available for enteral nutritional supplementation of horses.°

Parenterally administered solutions containing glucose, balanced amino acid solutions, lipid emulsions, balanced electrolyte and trace minerals, and vitamins have been administered to adult horses with colitis. Parenteral administration bypasses an intestinal tract of questionable absorptive capacity in horses with severe toxemic colitis. Providing for part of the horse's nutritional requirements (10,000–12,000 Kcal/day) is possible with glucose/amino acid solutions that are of moderate cost. Addition of lipid emulsions increases the calories provided to the horse, but also in-

creases the daily cost of treatment by approximately $75. The overall cost of providing nutritional supplementation, enteral or parenteral, to horses with colitis may well be offset by quicker recoveries and diminished requirement for other costly treatments, particularly plasma.

Anti-inflammatory Therapy

The use of nonsteroidal anti-inflammatory drugs (NSAIDs) is a common practice in equine colitis patients. Flunixin meglumine,° in particular, is appropriate in the context of endotoxemia in horses. Several studies have demonstrated that pretreatment with flunixin meglumine prevents several of the pathophysiologic changes associated with the administration of sublethal doses of endotoxin in ponies. Recommended dosages range from 0.25 mg/kg to 0.5 mg/kg q.i.d. The author prefers to give the higher dosage and has not recognized signs of NSAID toxicity associated with this dosage.

A medication with potential anti-inflammatory benefit in colitis cases is dimethyl sulfoxide (DMSO). DMSO scavenges hydroxyl radicals produced by metabolically activated neutrophils. In the acute stages of equine colitis, there is frequently a pronounced neutrophilic invasion of the cecum and colon, and in this context DMSO may be efficacious. A dosage of 100 to 200 mg/kg per day appears appropriate at this time.

Endotoxin Core Antigen Antibody Therapy

Because many of the clinical signs accompanying equine colitis appear attributable to the effects of endotoxin, the development of specific therapy to neutralize endotoxins has been a goal in the past few years. Antibodies to the R-core sugars of lipopolysaccharide (LPS) can provide cross-protection to LPS of a variety of gram-negative organisms, including *Salmonella*. Antibodies are produced by hyperimmunizing horses with a mutant enteric organism that lacks that outer O antigen, such as the J5 *E. coli* strain. Two such products are available for use in horses.† Typically, 2 L containing antibody to *E. coli* J5 core antigen at a titer of 1:20,000 to 1:40,000 are given. The frequency of administration depends on the response to treatment and the clinician's discretion. The efficacy of these products in treating horses with colitis remains undetermined and is probably variable between patients. The author has observed some horses to have a noticeable, although often transient, improvement in attitude, appetite, and heart rate following administration of *E. coli* J5 hyperimmune plasma.

Antimicrobial Therapy

Antimicrobial therapy is indicated in horses with colitis, although the goal of antimicrobial therapy may vary between cases. In cases of colitis caused by *E. risticii*, the efficacy of tetracycline 6.6 to 11 mg/kg IV twice daily has been documented clinically and experimentally. In other cases of colitis, including salmonellosis in which specific antimicrobial sensitivities to the isolated *Salmonella* species have been determined, antimicrobial therapy is unlikely to

---

°*Nutriprime, KenVet, Ashland, OH*

°*Banamine, Schering, Kenilworth, NJ*
†*Polymune J, Veterinary Dynamics, Chino, CA; and Endoserum, Immvac, Columbia, MO*

alter the course of colitis. However, broad-spectrum anti-microbial therapy is indicated to limit spread of enteric organisms to other organ systems. Potentially effective anti-microbials in this context include penicillin/gentamicin (potassium penicillin 10 million IU IV q.i.d., and gentamicin 6.6 mg/kg per day), ampicillin/gentamicin (ampicillin 15–25 mg/kg IV t.i.d.), or ceftiofur (4–5 mg/kg IV t.i.d.). If colitis is thought to be a consequence of antimicrobial administration with potential involvement of clostridial pathogens, metronidazole (15–20 mg/kg p.o. t.i.d.) may be considered.

Anti-secretory Therapy

Medications that minimize or abolish colonic fluid secretion would be of tremendous benefit in the treatment of equine colitis. Medications such as kaolin, bismuth subsalicylate, and activated charcoal are frequently used in cases of colitis in adult horses, but their efficacy as antisecretory agents in this context has not been established. These medications are more effective in foals with diarrhea, probably as a result of an effect on the small intestine rather than on the colon.

PROGNOSIS

The prognosis for horses with acute colitis that receive appropriate fluids, electrolytes, and other supportive treatment is good, with the majority surviving without complications. The most frequent complications that occur include catheter-site infection, thrombophlebitis, and laminitis. Horses that recover usually show signs of improvement within 7 days of the onset of illness, and in the author's experience, invariably by 10 days. Horses that continue to have signs of systemic toxemia and have diarrhea longer than 10 days generally have a poor prognosis for survival.

Supplemental Readings

Burakoff R, Zhao L, Celifarco AJ, Rose KL, Donovan V, Pothoulakis C, Percy W: Effects of purified *Clostridium difficile* toxin A on rabbit distal colon. Gastroenterology 109:348–354, 1995.
Palmer JE, Benson CE, Lotz GW: Serological response of experimental ponies orally infected with *Ehrlichia risticii*. Equine Vet J 7[Suppl]:19–20, 1989.
Palmer JE, Benson CE: Studies on oral transmission of Potomac Horse Fever. J Vet Intern Med 8(2):87–92, 1994.
Shone CC, Hambleton P: Toxigenic clostridia. *In* Minton NP, Clarke DJ (eds): Biotechnology Handbooks: Clostridia. New York, Plenum Press, 1989, pp 265–292.
Spier SJ, Lavoie JP, Cullor JS, Smith BP, Snyder JR, Sischo WM: Protection against clinical endotoxemia in horses by using plasma containing antibody to an Rc mutant *E. coli* (J5). Circ Shock 28:235–248, 1989.
Staempfli HR, Prescott JF, Carman RJ, McCutcheon LJ: Use of bacitracin in the prevention and treatment of experimentally-induced idiopathic colitis in horses. Can J Vet Res 56:233–236, 1992.

Grass Sickness

ELSPETH M. MILNE
Dumfries, Scotland

Grass sickness, also known as equine dysautonomia, is a disease of unknown etiology with a high mortality rate. It was first reported in the east of Scotland in 1907 and is now recognized in many European countries including Norway, Sweden, Denmark, France, Switzerland, and Germany in addition to the United Kingdom. In the southern hemisphere, mal seco (dry sickness), a disease indistinguishable from grass sickness, has been reported in the Patagonia region of Argentina and in Chile and the Falkland Islands. No histologically confirmed cases have occurred in Australia, Asia, Africa, North America, or Ireland. Within the United Kingdom mainland, the eastern side of Scotland and, to a lesser extent, England, has the highest incidence; up to 1% of horses die of grass sickness annually in some areas of Scotland.

EPIDEMIOLOGY

All equidae appear to be equally susceptible, including horses, ponies, donkeys, and captive exotic equidae. A similar disease was reported in brown hares in the United Kingdom, some of which were from premises where equine grass sickness occurred, but no other herbivorous species are known to be susceptible. Clinical and pathologic similarities also occur with feline dysautonomia.

Grass sickness is predominantly a disease of young adult horses, and the peak age range is 2 to 7 years. However, horses of any age from 4 months onward have been affected. The causal agent does not cross the placenta, and foals reared from affected mares appear to be normal, regardless of whether the mare was pregnant or nursing at the onset of clinical signs. There is no gender predisposition.

Grass sickness occurs almost exclusively in grazing horses, although there is controversy regarding whether part-time stabling decreases the risk. Horses housed full-time are very rarely affected. There is a strong association with certain premises and even individual fields, but the type of herbage on the pasture does not appear to affect the risk. Horses that contract grass sickness are significantly more likely to be in good body condition than would be expected from a reference population. Recent movement onto a new pasture or premises predisposes to the occurrence of the disease, and animals on a property for less than 2 months are at greater risk. No evidence suggests that grass sickness is contagious. Although cases usually occur sporadically, however, clusters of cases are not uncommon.

A distinct seasonal distribution characterizes the condition, with the highest incidence in the spring and summer in the northern and southern hemispheres. In the United Kingdom, the peak time is April to July with the greatest number of cases in May, but cases occur in every month of the year. In Argentina, cases of mal seco occur from October to February. At least in Scotland, 10 to 14 days of cool (7–11°C), dry weather tends to precede outbreaks.

ETIOLOGY

The etiology of grass sickness and mal seco is unknown. Factors investigated include toxic plants, chemical or bacterial toxins, viruses, and fungal toxins but none has been proven to be the cause. However, transmission studies have confirmed the presence of a neurotoxin in the plasma of animals with the acute disease. A current hypothesis that grass sickness is associated with a mycotoxin ingested at pasture is still under investigation, but to date, no fungal species is consistently found on pastures where cases have occurred or in gut contents from affected horses. The drier weather conditions that often precede the occurrence of grass sickness may be compatible with a fungal etiology because such conditions can favor toxin elaboration by some fungi. The involvement of *Clostridium botulinum* has also been suggested.

CLINICAL SIGNS

Acute Form

Three forms occur, which overlap in their clinical presentation. In acute cases, with survival less than 2 days, the initial signs are dullness and inappetance, rapidly progressing to varying degrees of colic. Depression is usually present and can be very marked. The abdomen becomes increasingly distended and few gut sounds are audible. The pulse is elevated, often much higher than would be expected from the degree of pain present, and may exceed 100/minute. A normal rectal temperature or a pyrexia of up to 39.5°C may occur. Excessive salivation is usually observed, and spontaneous gastric reflux of green or brown malodorous fluid may occur via the nostrils. Muscle tremor and generalized (or more often patchy) sweating occur. The muscle tremor ranges from slight, particularly over the triceps, shoulders, and flanks, to generalized coarse tremor. Dysphagia is a major presenting sign, although it may not be immediately obvious because of inappetance. Acutely ill horses often "play" with water by flicking the muzzle through water or attacking the water bucket with their feet. Many animals appear to drink, but although laryngeal movements are observed, they may not be followed by esophageal peristalsis. Paralysis of the tongue does not occur. On rectal examination, the rectal mucosa feels dry, and small fecal pellets with varying amounts of mucus may be present. A firm, often very hard, secondary impaction of the large colon is usually present and, in some cases,

distended loops of small intestine are palpable. On nasogastric intubation, the tube may be difficult to pass, but reflux of gastric fluid is generally obtained. If euthanasia is not carried out, acutely ill horses die, often suddenly, sometimes following gastric rupture. The prognosis in acute cases is hopeless.

Subacute Form

In subacute grass sickness, the signs are similar to those of acute cases but are usually less severe. A continuously elevated heart rate is common. Nasogastric reflux is usually absent but colonic impaction is often present and significant weight loss occurs. Most subacutely ill horses die or require euthanasia within 7 days of the onset, but some progress to the chronic stage.

Chronic Form

In the chronic form, the signs may have an insidious onset. Nasogastric reflux is usually absent. The major signs are severe weight loss with a reduction in gut fill leading to a "tucked up" appearance and loss of fat and muscle mass. Affected horses usually have a weak gait with a reduced anterior component to the stride and a tendency to stand with all four feet together, described as an "elephant on a tub" stance. A sleepy expression apparently caused by bilateral ptosis is usually present, and the penis may be pendulous. Varying degrees of muscle tremor, sweating, dysphagia, colic, and reduction in appetite are present, but colonic impaction is rare. Gut sounds are usually reduced, and the pulse may be normal or increased. Animals that are still eating often chew slowly and may drop food from the mouth or accumulate chewed food between the cheeks and the molar teeth. Swallowing is sometimes accompanied by esophageal spasm. If colic occurs, it is usually mild and intermittent. Diarrhea occurs in approximately 30% of chronic cases but often only continues for a few days. Most chronic cases show rhinitis, manifest by a "snuffling" sound from the nasal cavity and accumulation of dry mucoid material on the turbinates or a bilateral mucopurulent nasal discharge. Rectal examination reveals a lack of gut contents and sometimes splenomegaly.

The mortality in chronic cases has been reported to be almost 100%, and it is said that any horses that do survive show permanently poor condition and exercise intolerance. However, better management protocols have improved the prognosis in chronic cases.

CLINICAL PATHOLOGY

No pathognomonic changes in blood chemical or hematologic parameters occur. Blood concentrations of selenium-dependent glutathione peroxidase, vitamin E, vitamin B, and magnesium are within normal limits for grazing horses. Plasma cortisol and catecholamine (epinephrine and norepinephrine) concentrations are significantly higher in acute and subacute grass sickness than in colic cases as well as in "stressed" and normal animals—a finding attributed to increased sympathoadrenal activity. Two acute phase proteins, haptoglobin and orosomucoid, are increased in the serum in acute, subacute, and chronic grass sickness but not in most colic cases. Acute and subacute grass sickness cases tend to have a higher peritoneal fluid protein content than other medical colic cases, although the gross appearance is similar, deep yellow and clear to slightly turbid.

PATHOLOGY

The major gross postmortem findings are predictable from the clinical signs. In acute cases, gastric distension with fluid, erosions associated with reflux esophagitis, excess fluid in the small intestine, and impaction of the colon with hard, dry ingesta occur. A black coating is usually present where the impacted ingesta is in contact with the mucosa. In chronic cases, the main feature is a lack of ingesta and apparent shrinkage of the gastrointestinal tract. However, in mal seco, unlike grass sickness, some chronic cases show colonic impaction at postmortem examination.

Characteristic changes occur in the neurons of the autonomic ganglia, enteric nervous system, and certain brain stem nuclei. These consist of chromatolysis associated with loss of Nissl substance, eccentricity or pyknosis of nuclei, swelling and vacuolation of neurons, and the presence of intracytoplasmic eosinophilic spheroids. The latter are thought to be dystrophic axons. In the central nervous system, the oculomotor, facial, lateral vestibular, hypoglossal, and dorsal motor vagal nuclei, in decreasing order of frequency, and the intermediolateral nucleus of the spinal cord show typical neuronal degeneration. Degeneration and loss of enteric neurons also occur in the submucous and myenteric plexuses. These changes are widespread in the enteric nervous system of acute cases, with the ileum being the most severely affected. In chronic cases, the distal small intestine, especially the ileum, may be the only severely affected area of gut. For this reason, histopathologic examination of ileal biopsies obtained at laparotomy can provide an ante mortem diagnosis of the disease.

The means by which the neurotoxin spreads from the presumed route of entry following ingestion is uncertain, although the widespread degenerative changes suggest hematogenous spread. Experimentally, retrograde axonal transport of the neurotoxin has been demonstrated.

DIAGNOSIS

The diagnosis can only be confirmed by demonstration of the characteristic histopathologic changes in the autonomic or enteric ganglia postmortem, or by ileal biopsy at laparotomy. However, although biopsy can be useful in acute and subacute cases, it is not recommended in chronic cases when subsequent treatment is being considered, because anesthesia and surgery are likely to adversely affect the outcome.

Although no single clinical sign is pathognomonic of the disease, by careful and repeated clinical evaluation, including rectal examination, it is possible to make a confident ante mortem clinical diagnosis in most cases. Diagnosis on clinical grounds is most difficult in acute and subacute cases, which can resemble a variety of other causes of acute and subacute colic. However, dysphagia in a horse with continuous or intermittent colic is strongly suggestive

of grass sickness. Barium pooling in the thoracic esophagus is a suspicious radiographic finding and megaesophagus and linear erosions of the caudal esophagus can also be demonstrated by endoscopy, the latter being most evident in acute cases. In chronic cases, precipitous weight loss accompanied by dysphagia, rhinitis, and abnormal sweating are strongly suggestive of the disease.

Some features of grass sickness are similar to those of equine motor neuron disease (EMND, see page 321), also of unknown etiology, leading to a recent suggestion that these diseases share common etiologic factors. However, there are some notable epidemiologic, clinical, and pathologic differences between grass sickness and EMND, particularly the occurrence of EMND in older horses with no access to pasture, good to voracious appetite and lack of signs of dysphagia, and apparent response to vitamin E supplementation in EMND. The possible association between the two diseases is the subject of further investigations.

TREATMENT

Treatment may be considered in chronic cases only, provided that they are still able to swallow some food, have not become emaciated, and are still reasonably alert. Nursing provides the mainstay of such management, and an improvement in recovery rate for chronic cases from less than 10% to 50% has been associated with the following management regimen.

It is preferable to keep the affected animals housed initially, with short walks in hand several times daily for exercise and access to grass. Rugging seems to decrease sweating and helps to maintain body temperature, which is often subnormal. Ideally, high-energy, high-protein concentrate feeds should be given, but this may be limited by dysphagia and individual preference that may change from day to day. Suitable feeds are sweet feeds, crushed oats, and high-energy cubes, fed wet (soaked in dilute molasses) or dry according to preference, and succulents such as apples or carrots to improve palatability. Up to 500 ml of corn oil can be given daily to increase the dietary fat content. As the appetite and body weight improve, which may not occur for 2 to 5 weeks, increasing access to grazing can be given.

In chronic cases with severe dysphagia, attempts to maintain alimentation by nasogastric feeding for several weeks have been made but are rarely successful, and the indication for such treatment is questionable. A mixture containing 230 g electrolytes, 21 L water, 300 to 900 g dextrose, 300 to 900 g cottage cheese (dry weight), and 2 kg alfalfa meal with or without 150 g corn oil, divided into three meals daily, has been suggested for horses with chronic hypoalimentation. The electrolytes in this mixture consist of 10 g NaCl, 15 g NaHCO$_3$, 75 g KCl, 60 g K$_2$HPO$_4$, 45 g CaCl$_2$.2H$_2$O, and 25 g MgO. The substituted benzamide, cisapride° (0.5-0.8 mg/kg p.o. t.i.d. for 7 days), has been found to increase gut motility in chronic cases. This cholinergic agent facilitates acetylcholine release by acting on the postganglionic cholinergic nerves at the level of

---

°*Prepulsid, Janssen-Cilag Ltd., High Wycombe, Bucks, UK*

the myenteric plexus and lacks central antidopaminergic properties, unlike the related compound, metoclopramide. However, cisapride is expensive and is probably not necessary in cases with normal gut motility. The peak plasma concentration of cisapride occurs approximately 2 hours after oral administration, at least in humans, and mild colic is sometimes observed 2 hours after administration of cisapride to grass sickness cases as increased gut motility is stimulated. Mild to moderate colic also may occur soon after feeding, presumably because of slow gastric emptying. If analgesia is required, nonsteroidal anti-inflammatory drugs such as phenylbutazone (2.2–4.4 mg/kg) or flunixin meglumine (0.5-1.1 mg/kg IV) are suitable because they do not adversely affect gut motility. No reports exist of the successful treatment of mal seco, although, anecdotally, two chronic cases that received oral cisapride are said to have recovered.

In contrast to previous reports, the majority of survivors can resume normal work, in the author's experience. Residual problems in some survivors include mild dysphagia, a change to a more nervous temperament, a tendency to excessive sweating, and seborrhea or multiple small areas of piloerection, all of which tend to improve with time.

PREVENTION

No known means of prevention is available other than permanent stabling with no access to pasture. It is advisable to house horses for the first 2 months after moving them to new premises in a grass sickness-affected area. Clearly, avoidance of the use of fields where the disease has occurred is sensible, especially in the spring and summer. In view of the association with cool, dry weather, it has also been recommended to stable horses in high-risk areas when 7 to 10 consecutive days of such weather has occurred.

Supplemental Readings

Milne E, Wallis N: Nursing the chronic grass sickness patient. Equine Vet Ed 6(2):217–219, 1994.

Milne EM, Woodman MP, Doxey DL: Use of clinical measurements to predict the outcome in chronic cases of grass sickness (equine dysautonomia). Vet Rec 134:438–440, 1994.

Naylor JM, Freeman DE, Kronfeld DS: Alimentation of hypophagic horses. Comp Contin Ed Pract Vet 6:S93–S99, 1984.

Scholes SFE, Vaillant C, Peacock P, Edwards GB, Kelly DF: Diagnosis of grass sickness by ileal biopsy. Vet Rec 133:7–10, 1993.

Uzal FA, Robles CA: *Mal seco*, a grass sickness-like syndrome of horses in Argentina. Vet Res Communication 17:449–457, 1993.

Peritonitis

R O B I N M. D A B A R E I N E R
Leesburg, Virginia

The peritoneum lines the peritoneal cavity and covers the viscera. It forms a closed sac in males but communicates with the external environment in females via the fallopian tubes. The peritoneum consists of a single layer of mesothelial cells resting on a thin basal lamina, which is attached to a loose connective tissue layer containing collagen and elastic fibers, allowing a variable degree of motion. The peritoneum is coated with hydrated microvilli, which serve to minimize friction and thus facilitate free movement between abdominal viscera. Peritoneal fluid is constantly being produced and absorbed.

Cellular defenses are provided by peritoneal macrophages, mast cells, and mesothelial cells. Peritoneal macrophages have antimicrobial activity resulting from their complement receptors, phagocytic ability, and T cell-mediated immune responses. In addition, peritoneal macrophages mediate neutrophil chemotaxis and fibroblast proliferation, which aids in bacteria localization. Peritoneal mesothelial cells are an abundant source of plasminogen activator, which is responsible for normal fibrinolytic activity on peritoneal surfaces.

Peritonitis is defined as inflammation of the mesothelial lining of the peritoneal cavity. Peritoneal inflammation can result from any mechanical, chemical, or infectious insult. The initial reaction to inflammatory stimulus is the release of histamine and serotonin from peritoneal mast cells and macrophages, resulting in vasodilation and increased vascular permeability with transudation of fibrinogen-rich plasma into the peritoneal cavity. The concurrent loss of mesothelial cells and release of tissue thromboplastin reduces the fibrinolytic capabilities of the peritoneal surface and activates the extrinsic coagulation pathway, thereby shifting the fibrinolysis-coagulation equilibrium towards fibrin formation. This response encourages fibrin seals on peritoneal defects and provides the framework for fibroblasts to lay down collagen, which produces fibrous adhesions to localize bacteria. If the inflammatory response is overcome, the mesothelial cell lining is restored and the normal fibrinolytic activity of the peritoneal mesothelial cells returns, initiating removal of the accumulated fibrin clots.

Peritonitis in the horse is usually caused by intestinal leakage or degeneration resulting in the transmural passage of bacteria into the peritoneal cavity. The adverse effects of intraperitoneal bacteria can be enhanced by the presence of excessive peritoneal fluid accumulation, hemorrhage, fibrin, bile, necrotic tissue, ischemia, anaerobes, and fecal matter. Excessive peritoneal fluid enhances the dissemination of localized bacteria and dilutes opsonic proteins such as complement and immunoglobins. In addition, phagocytic cells may float away from bacteria that have been trapped by fibrin. Accumulated red blood cell stromal elements interfere with phagocytosis of numerous bacteria, and hemoglobin is known to increase the pathogenicity of *Escherichia coli* organisms. Fibrin formation can be beneficial in confining bacteria; however, excessive amounts can result in abscess formation and can prevent phagocytes and antimicrobials from reaching the source of contamination. Necrotic tissue, fecal matter, and bile all prolong the debridement phase of peritoneal healing and interfere with peritoneal defense mechanisms.

ETIOLOGY

Inflammation of the peritoneum can result from many causes, which can be classified as primary or secondary, peracute, acute or chronic, and localized or diffuse. Primary peritonitis is uncommon in adult horses but may occur by hematogenous spread of bacteria in the septic or immunocompromised neonate or in young horses exposed to *Streptococcus equi* infection. Peritonitis resulting from another disease process may be caused by perforating abdominal wounds; chemical irritation by bile or urine; neoplasia; breeding and foaling injuries such as uterine or vaginal trauma; intestinal parasitism; hepatitis; nephritis; pancreatitis; ruptured bladder or ureter; urinary infection; ruptured or lacerated abdominal viscera such as spleen, ovary, liver, or diaphragm; castration complications; and factors directly related to gastrointestinal problems, which are divided into preoperative, intraoperative, and postoperative causes.

Uroperitoneum and septicemia-induced peritonitis occur predominately in neonates. Internal abdominal abscesses due to disseminated *S. equi, S. zooepidemicus, or Rhodococcus equi* infection are usually found in weanlings or young horses. Adult horses may develop peritonitis as a result of thromboembolic parasite infestation.

CLINICAL SIGNS

Clinical signs of peritonitis vary and are dependent on the cause and duration of the peritonitis. Localized infections often have limited systemic involvement, whereas diffuse peritonitis can elicit generalized signs of endotoxemia and sepsis. Horses with peracute peritonitis due to intestinal rupture or tearing show signs of acute severe sepsis and shock with tachycardia, tachypnea, sweating, and varying degrees of abdominal discomfort, with death ensuing within hours.

The most common presenting clinical signs for horses with peritonitis include pyrexia (rectal temperature >38.5°C), anorexia, mild abdominal pain, reduced or absent borborygmi, diarrhea, increased heart rate, and clinical evidence of dehydration. Rectal examination often elicits pain, and if adhesions or abscesses are present, distended bowel may be present. In cases of intestinal rupture, either roughened peritoneal surfaces or an abnormally empty abdomen can be palpated because of free gas in the peritoneal cavity. Occasionally abdominal masses or abscesses can be palpated and mesenteric lymph nodes may be enlarged; however, in many cases, no abnormalities can be detected. Parietal pain may be characterized by a "guarded" or splinted abdomen with pain on abdominal ballotment and a reluctance to move or defecate.

Gastrointestinal motility is usually decreased because of sympathetic stimulation from parietal pain, hemoconcentration, or serosal surface trauma. Paralytic ileus frequently results in intestinal stasis with gastric fluid accumulation and intestinal distension, which subsequently intensifies the abdominal pain. The mobilization of fluid into the peritoneal cavity results in an intravascular fluid deficit causing reabsorption of fluid from the large colon and cecum. Findings of intestinal ingesta impactions secondary to these fluid shifts or paralytic ileus are common in horses with peritonitis.

A urogenital examination should be performed in horses with an undiagnosed etiology of peritonitis to rule out vaginal, cervical, or uterine tears in mares, or infected castration sites in males.

DIAGNOSIS

The diagnosis of peritonitis is based on a predisposing factor revealed in the history, clinical signs, and abnormal laboratory findings. Abnormal laboratory values are dependent on the cause and duration of peritonitis. Hematologic abnormalities seen in acute peritonitis include elevated packed cell volume resulting from transudation of fluid into the peritoneal cavity and endotoxemia. Initially, a proportional increase in plasma protein levels occurs, reflecting the degree of dehydration; however, in severe cases, protein eventually is sequestered into the abdomen because of increased capillary permeability resulting in systemic hypoproteinemia. Peripheral blood neutropenia with a degenerative left shift is caused by margination of neutrophils and migration of these cells into the abdomen. Increased plasma fibrinogen levels (up to 1000 mg/dl) can occur after 48 hours. Peritonitis of longer duration or that resulting from internal abscesses is associated with greater variability in laboratory values, but these horses often demonstrate a normal or increased systemic neutrophil count, monocytosis, and increased plasma protein levels as a result of increased immunoglobulin production.

Abdominocentesis

Abdominocentesis and peritoneal fluid analysis confirm the diagnosis of peritonitis, although the cause may remain unknown. The preferred site for obtaining peritoneal fluid is either directly on midline or to the right of midline 2 cm caudal to the xyphoid process. The left side of the abdomen is not used, in order to avoid perforating the spleen. The site should be clipped or shaved and prepared in an aseptic manner and surgical gloves worn to avoid contamination of the abdomen and sample. An 18-gauge disposable needle can be used in most horses and does not require local anesthetic. The needle is placed through the skin quickly and gently rotated until fluid is obtained. Confirmation that the needle is within the peritoneal cavity can be determined by observing the needle move in rhythm with the respiratory rate. In brood mares and overweight horses, a 3-inch 18-gauge spinal needle may be necessary to reach the peritoneal cavity. Abdominocentesis also can be performed using a blunt 4-inch teat cannula or

6-inch female dog urinary catheter. The site is aseptically prepared and 1 to 2 ml of local anesthetic are used to infiltrate the skin and subcutaneous tissue. A number 15 scalpel blade is used to create a small stab incision into the skin and to penetrate the linea alba. Sterile gauze sponges are placed around the hub of the cannula to prevent skin bleeder contamination of the sample, and the cannula is passed into the peritoneal cavity with firm, direct pressure. The cannula is slowly advanced until fluid is obtained. Ultrasonography may be helpful in obtaining abdominal fluid or detecting fibrin tags and ingesta within the ventral abdominal cavity, particularly in foals.

Fluid Analysis

The fluid sample is collected in a sterile tube containing ethylenediaminetetraacetic acid (EDTA) for cytology and total protein concentration tests. Samples for bacterial culture or biochemical assay are collected in a sterile tube with no additives. Bacterial culture can be enhanced by collecting fluid on blood culture media, or using an antimicrobial removal device (ARD)* if the horse has already been treated with antibiotics. Normal peritoneal fluid is clear, light yellow in color, and serous in consistency. A bloody sample may be indicative of skin blood contamination, splenic puncture, or intra-abdominal hemorrhage. Comparison of peritoneal fluid packed cell volume (PCV) and peripheral blood PCV can help differentiate between iatrogenic or abdominal hemorrhage and splenic puncture. The abdominal PCV is higher than peripheral blood PCV if splenic perforation has occurred, and often numerous small lymphocytes are seen on cytology examination. Bloody fluid caused by intra-abdominal hemorrhage usually has a lower PCV but higher total protein content than peripheral blood and erythrocytophagia and few or no platelets are seen (see page 211).

The total nucleated cell count in peritoneal fluid of normal horses is less than 5000 cells per mm³ with a 2:1 ratio of neutrophils to mononuclear cells. The cytologic appearance of the leukocytes and mesothelial cells is normal. A total protein concentration of 0.7 to 1.5 g/dl is considered normal.

Abnormal peritoneal fluid confirms peritonitis, although a normal abdominocentesis does not rule out peritonitis, especially if the disease process is long-standing and localized. Colorless fluid is very dilute and if present in large quantities, the possibility of ascites or uroperitoneum must be considered. Serosanguinous fluid indicates an increase in erythrocytes or free hemoglobin, which can be caused by intestinal degeneration or transmural erythrocyte leakage. Green fluid results from enterocentesis or intestinal rupture, and brown fluid is associated with late-stage tissue necrosis or rupture. Turbid fluid indicates an increased cell count or total protein, and opalescence suggests chylous effusion. Flocculent fluid with fibrin strands is found in cases with an inflammatory exudative process in the abdomen. The quantity of fluid varies between horses and can be increased in acute peritonitis or absent in chronic peritonitis with excessive fibrin production.

Peritoneal fluid parameters consistent with peritonitis

*Antimicrobial Removal Device, Becton Dickinson, Cockeysville, MD

vary widely, depending on the disease process. High nucleated cell counts ranging from 15,000 to 800,000 cells/mm³ with more than 90% neutrophils and toxic or degenerative changes have been reported for horses with peritonitis or internal abscesses. Total protein values are usually higher than 2.5 g/dl because of inflammation of the abdominal viscera or peritoneum resulting in protein exudation, and are usually associated with peritoneal infections, intestinal compromise, or blood contamination of the peritoneal fluid. The presence of fibrin and intracellular bacteria is diagnostic for peritonitis or intestinal strangulation. Cytologic evidence of intra- or extracellular bacteria can result from skin contamination because phagocytosis can occur within the collection tube and should be interpreted in combination with clinical signs.

Peritoneal fluid must be interpreted carefully in horses after abdominal surgery, foaling, castration, or multiple abdominocenteses. Nucleated cell counts between 85,000 and 418,000 cells/mm³ and protein values from 4.7 to 6.5 g/dl were found on postoperative day 5 in six normal horses that had abdominal exploration. Five days after open castration peritoneal fluid can contain 30,000 nucleated white cells/μl with more than 85% being neutrophils. By day 7 after castration, the cell counts became normal with no toxic or degenerative changes. Parturition can cause increased nucleated and red blood cell counts with elevated total protein values in the peritoneal fluid. No significant alterations in peritoneal fluid are seen in normal horses having repeated abdominocentesis when sampled every 24 hours for 5 days. Enterocentesis caused increases in nucleated cell counts up to 113,333 ± 87,532/μl in six of nine horses after 48 hours.

Cytologic examination of the peritoneal fluid should include a Wright's and Gram's stain. Macrophages should be examined closely for evidence of cellular engulfment and erythrophagocytosis. The peritoneal fluid cell morphology is an important diagnostic aid and can be evaluated from the Wright's stain. The Gram's stain demonstrates the presence of bacteria and can guide initial antimicrobial treatments until culture and sensitivity results become available. Microbiologic culture is performed to identify aerobic and anaerobic bacteria, and antibiotic sensitivity testing is done to identify specific antibiotic therapy. The most common organisms isolated from horses with peritonitis include aerobes such as *Escherichia coli*, *Staphylococcus* species, *Streptococcus* species, and *Rhodococcus equi*, and anaerobes including *Bacteroides* species, *Clostridium* species, and *Fusobacterium* species. Bacteria have been cultured or cytologically identified on 48 of 67 horses (71.6%) with peritonitis and *E. coli* the most common bacterium isolated from peritoneal fluid samples. Others have reported only a 16 to 25% isolation rate for infective agents. Anaerobes have been isolated from approximately 20% of equine peritonitis cases, with *Bacteroides fragilis* being most common. Serial cultures of the peritoneal fluid may be necessary to identify emerging or resistant bacterial strains. Optimal bacterial isolation techniques require the use of an enriching broth, blood culture media, and, if appropriate, an ARD device when culturing peritoneal fluid. Failure to identify or culture bacteria from peritoneal fluid does not rule out septic peritonitis.

TREATMENT

Horses with peritonitis require early, aggressive therapy. The treatment of peritonitis is based on (1) stabilization of patient's condition; (2) correction of the inciting cause; and (3) in most cases, administration of antimicrobials and/or anthelmintics. Surgical intervention may be required to identify or correct the cause of the peritonitis.

Stabilization includes treatment of hypovolemia and endotoxic shock. Intensive fluid therapy is usually required to replace fluid losses into the peritoneal cavity and combat perfusion deficits. Imbalances in blood acid base and electrolytes should be corrected and monitored. If intestinal compromise or gram-negative bacterial infections are suspected as the cause of peritonitis, J5 hyperimmune plasma (4.4 ml/kg) may moderate the degree of endotoxemia. J5 is a mutant strain of *E. coli* that lacks the variable oligosaccharide side chains and binds to many gram-negative organisms, providing cross-protection. Minimal benefits would be expected with gram-positive or viral etiologies. If serum hypoproteinemia (total protein <4.0 g/dl) is present, administration of additional plasma should be considered to minimize peripheral and pulmonary edema (see page 291).

Gastrointestinal ileus results from peritoneal trauma, intestinal compromise, or sympathetic stimulation. Gastric or intestinal distension can cause respiratory compromise from increased abdominal pressure and reduced intestinal perfusion, leading to further compromise. Nasogastric intubation is necessary for relief of gastric fluid accumulation and continued intestinal decompression. Parenteral nutritional support should be considered in the compromised anorexic patient or in horses with severe prolonged gastrointestinal dysfunction.

Horses with peritonitis often have clinical signs of endoxemia and tissue trauma eliciting a cascade of inflammatory mediators. Flunixin meglumine,° a nonsteroidal anti-inflammatory drug, inhibits cyclo-oxygenase production of prostaglandins and blocks many detrimental effects of excessive prostaglandin production caused by endotoxemia. Although low doses of flunixin (0.25 mg/kg IV q.i.d.) inhibit prostaglandin production, higher doses (0.50–1.0 mg/kg IV b.i.d.) provide analgesia and may be more beneficial in horses with peritonitis.

Antimicrobials

Antimicrobial therapy should be initiated as soon as the diagnosis of peritonitis is made and peritoneal fluid is obtained for culture and sensitivity. Cytologic examination of the peritoneal fluid can suggest the appropriate antimicrobials until the specific causative organism is identified.

Intravenous administration is preferred, especially in the hypovolemic or shocky patient with compromised tissue perfusion. Broad-spectrum therapy is recommended with a combination of an aminoglycoside such as gentamicin (2.2 mg/kg IV t.i.d.) or amikacin sulfate (6–15 mg/kg IV t.i.d.) and potassium penicillin G (22,000–44,000 U/kg IV q.i.d.) or ceftiofur (2–4 mg/kg IV b.i.d. or t.i.d.). After intravenous administration of aminoglycoside antibiotics, antimicrobial activity in the peritoneal fluid reaches 50 to

80% of serum levels, whereas intestinal tissue concentrations are 10 to 25% of serum concentrations.

Aminoglycosides are bactericidal and effective against the majority of gram-negative intestinal aerobes, but pharmocologic monitoring is important, especially in the hypovolemic septic patient. Important considerations during aminoglycoside use include renal central tubule necrosis and potential neuromuscular blocking effects during general anesthesia. Most gram-positive aerobes and some anaerobes are sensitive to penicillins, but the extended spectrum of antimicrobial activity from sodium ampicillin (11–25 mg/kg IV t.i.d.–q.i.d.) or ceftiofur may be beneficial. Trimethoprim sulfadiazine (30 mg/kg p.o. b.i.d.), chloramphenicol (25–50 mg/kg p.o. q.i.d.), and enrofloxacin (1.5 mg/kg p.o. b.i.d.) are broad-spectrum antimicrobials that have good peritoneal penetration and can be useful if warranted from the culture and sensitivity results. Enrofloxacin has been shown to have adverse effects on cartilage surfaces in young animals and should be reserved for adult horses only.

Anaerobic bacteria, especially penicillin-resistant *Bacteroides* species, are reported in 20 to 40% of equine patients with peritonitis. Percentages of anaerobic involvement may be artificially low because of the difficulty in isolating anaerobic organisms. Metronidazole (15–25 mg/kg p.o. t.i.d.–q.i.d.) is effective against most anaerobic bacteria but should be used in combination with antimicrobials with antibacterial activity against aerobic bacteria. Of 54 horses with positive anaerobic culture results, 95% also had aerobic bacteria isolated from the same specimen. In the face of paralytic ileus, intravenous administration can be used, although financial cost may be prohibitive. Recently, the pharmacokinetics of metronidazole (15 mg/kg t.i.d.–q.i.d.) administered to horses per rectum in a suspension of crushed tablets and water (40 ml) was evaluated, and serum minimal inhibitory concentration (MIC) concentrations were reached after 0.83 hours. Complications attributed to metronidazole administration in horses are rare, with only four of 200 horses (2%) undergoing treatment showing appetite suppression. However, peripheral neurologic deficits and central nervous system dysfunction have been associated with metronidazole treatment in horses and other species.

Anthelmintics are required if verminous arteritis resulting from *Strongylus vulgaris* migration is the suspected etiology of the peritonitis. A history of mild intermittent colic and poor or unknown deworming program may be apparent. A peripheral or peritoneal fluid eosinophilia is suggestive of parasite-induced intestinal damage but is rarely present even in confirmed cases. Fenbendazole (15 mg/kg p.o. for 3 days or 10 mg/kg for 5 days) or ivermectin (0.2 mg/kg p.o.), and aspirin (60 g p.o. s.i.d.) have been recommended.

Abdominal Drainage and Lavage

Controversy exists over the effectiveness of intermittent peritoneal lavage and drainage in horses with peritonitis. The benefits of abdominal drainage and lavage include (1) reduction of bacterial numbers, enzymes, and toxins from the large absorptive peritoneal surface area; (2) removing degenerative neutrophils and cellular debris; (3) elimination of accumulated blood; (4) removal of irritating foreign material such as plant material and urine; and (5) dilution of adhesion-forming substrates such as fibrinogen and fibrin. Some claim that only a small portion of the equine abdomen is effectively lavaged and that lavage may disseminate a localized infectious focus. In the author's opinion, peritoneal lavage and drainage is an important and potentially lifesaving treatment that should be considered in the treatment of horses with peritonitis. The controversial aspect of its use should be "when" and "if" peritoneal lavage is necessary. Peritoneal drainage and lavage should be reserved for acute cases of purulent effusion in the abdomen and in horses not responding to medical therapy as determined by repeated abdominocentesis.

Stabilization, antimicrobial administration, and hydration of the horse should be performed before abdominal drainage or lavage. Placing an ingress catheter in the paralumbar fossa for fluid infusion and an egress catheter on ventral midline for drainage has been described but is probably not effective because the infused fluid usually finds a direct path through the abdomen to the egress catheter, providing inadequate lavage.

Retrograde irrigation and drainage through an ingress-egress catheter placed on ventral midline at the most dependent aspect of the abdomen is most effective for removal of peritoneal exudate in horses. Ultrasonography may be useful in locating a site free of abdominal viscera or uterus if the horse is in late gestation. A variety of drains can be used: Mushroom drains and argyle drains* are most useful, but a large Foley catheter† is also effective. The horse is properly sedated, the drain site is prepared aseptically, and the skin and subcutaneous tissue is infiltrated with 3 to 5 ml of a local anesthetic. A 1-cm stab incision is made through the skin, subcutaneous tissue, and linea alba using a number 11 scalpel blade. Mushroom, argyle, and Foley drains should be stretched over a female canine or Chambers mare catheter to aid insertion. If the bowel is inadvertently punctured, the drain should not be removed until the horse is anesthetized to allow removal of the drain and closure of the puncture site.

With the drain acting as an ingress cannula, 10 to 20 L of a warmed balanced polyionic fluid (Plasmalyte‡ or lactated Ringer's solution) is infused. Abdominal discomfort may be encountered after 10 L of fluid is infused or after rapid infusion. Slowing the infusion rate or further sedation may be required. After fluid infusion, the drain is filled with heparin or heparinized saline and clamped closed and the horse is walked for 20 to 30 minutes to promote distribution of the lavaged fluid. The drain is then opened and allowed to empty into a clean calibrated bucket to record the volume of retrievable fluid. The majority of the infused fluid should be collected; however, some fluid may be resorbed. This process is repeated two to three times daily for 2 to 3 days until the peritoneal fluid white cell count and total protein level show improvement. Between treatments the abdominal drain should be filled with heparin, closed, and protected from the environment by a sterile bandage.

*Argyle Trochar Catheter, Sherwood Medical, St. Louis, MO
†Foley catheter, CR Bard, Murray Hill, NJ
‡Plasmalyte, Baxter Healthcare, Valencia, CA

The addition of povidone-iodine or nitrofurazone to peritoneal lavage solutions has been associated with chemical peritonitis, hypovolemia, hyperosmolarity, and acidosis in normal horses and is not recommended. Adding antimicrobials to the peritoneal lavage solution is probably not necessary; however, plasma concentrations of administered antimicrobials should be measured to ensure proper MIC levels in the face of peritoneal lavage and drainage. Horses treated with peritoneal lavage must also be monitored closely for hydration, protein loss (up to 0.5–1.0 g/dl daily), and electrolyte imbalances. Complications of peritoneal drains include visceral puncture during insertion, ascending infection, subcutaneous leakage and edema, and herniation of intestine or omentum through the drain or drain site.

Intraperitoneal or systemic administration of heparin has been recommended in the treatment of peritonitis in many species. Heparin is thought to inhibit fibrin deposition, thereby minimizing the localization and entrapment of bacteria, which can decrease the effectiveness of antimicrobials. Heparin has decreased the formation of adhesions in ponies after experimentally induced intestinal ischemia. No controlled studies are available in horses describing the outcome of treatment or recommended dosage of heparin therapy in horses with peritonitis.

PROGNOSIS

The prognosis depends on the etiology, severity, duration, and complications of the peritonitis. In a study of 30 horses with peritonitis, 70% were treated successfully with antibiotics and supportive therapy. The mortality rate was 59.7% in a recent retrospective study of 67 horses with peritonitis. The prognosis for mortality in that study was dependent on the inciting cause of peritonitis with postoperative peritonitis having a high mortality rate (56%). Laminitis, diarrhea, paralytic ileus, and coagulopathies can occur subsequent to endotoxemia, and abdominal adhesions or abscess formation can have a negative effect on long-term prognosis. No specific laboratory parameters can predict prognosis in affected horses; however, a rapid response to therapy is considered a favorable prognostic indicator. With early diagnosis and correction of the inciting cause and combining aggressive medical therapy with peritoneal lavage, a fair to good prognosis can be given in acute cases of septic peritonitis in the horse.

Supplemental Readings

Dyson S: Review of 30 cases of peritonitis in the horse. Equine Vet J 15:25–30, 1983.
Hawkins JF, Bowman KF, Roberts MC, Cowe P: Peritonitis in horses: 67 cases (1985–1990). J Am Vet Med Assoc 203:284–288, 1993.
Hosgood G: Peritonitis, part 1: a review of pathophysiology and diagnosis. Aust Vet Pract 16:184–189, 1986.
Markel MD: Prevention and management of peritonitis in horses: Management of colic. Vet Clin North Am Equine Pract 4(1):145–156, 1988.
Rumbaugh GE, Smith BP, Carlson GP: Internal abdominal abscesses in the horse: A study of 25 cases. J Am Vet Med Assoc 172:304–309, 1978.
Semrad SD: Peritonitis in the horse. In Smith B (ed): Large Animal Internal Medicine. St. Louis, C.V. Mosby, 1990, pp 674–679.

Abdominal Hemorrhage

LUCY M. EDENS
Gainesville, Florida

Although uncommon, intracorporeal bleeding and accumulation of blood within the peritoneal cavity, broad ligament, or gastrointestinal organs presents the veterinarian with a diagnostic and therapeutic challenge. The clinical signs can be nonspecific and may mimic other disease conditions that are accompanied by colic and hypovolemic shock. If the results of physical examination and abdominocentesis indicate intra-abdominal hemorrhage, the source of bleeding should be determined, if possible, via rectal palpation and transabdominal or transrectal ultrasonography. Management varies, depending on the etiology and the severity of the accompanying shock. In situations such as bleeding confined to the broad ligament without clinical evidence of hemorrhagic shock, the treatment may be as simple as confinement to a quiet stall. At the other extreme, a horse with acute severe hemorrhage from mesenteric vessels associated with a strangulating lipoma may require a blood transfusion and surgery. Prior awareness of this syndrome is critical to the effective treatment of horses with intra-abdominal hemorrhage, because diagnostic and therapeutic decisions in these cases often must be made rapidly to ensure a successful outcome.

ETIOLOGY

A number of different causes of intra-abdominal hemorrhage have been reported. Probably the most frequently encountered is splenic trauma, usually occurring when the horse receives a kick from another horse to the left caudal abdominal body wall. The bleeding in this situation is generally self-limiting and may go undetected, or may be interpreted as a mild colic. Other causes of splenic hemorrhage include neoplasia, abscessation, and hematoma. Trauma to liver and kidneys has not been reported as an etiologic reason for bleeding, probably because of the protection provided by the overlying ribs. However, post-biopsy bleeding and hemorrhage associated with neoplasia of these organs has been observed. Acute hepatopathies are often accompanied by rapid enlargement of the liver and can infrequently precipitate bleeding from the liver.

Disorders of the reproductive tract, particularly in mares, are another commonly identified cause of hemoperitoneum. Bleeding may arise from a number of different sites within the reproductive tract including the ovaries, uterus, and utero-ovarian blood vessels. Ovarian hemorrhage may occur as a consequence of follicular hematomas or granulosa cell tumors. Uterine bleeding has been attributed to birth-related trauma and neoplasia such as leiomyoma or leiomyosarcoma. Periparturient hemorrhage into the abdominal cavity associated with rupture of the uterine or ovarian arteries is one of the most frequent causes of massive intra-abdominal bleeding in older mares. The proposed etiology of vascular rupture in this situation is that aneurysms form, and subsequently rupture, because of age-related degeneration within the arterial walls. In this situation, unless the bleeding is confined to the broad ligament, fatal hemorrhagic shock rapidly develops.

Intra-abdominal hemorrhage may also arise from the gastrointestinal tract and its associated blood vessels. As with other internal organs, neoplasias, hematomas, and abscesses of the intestinal wall are possible causes of acute or chronic hemorrhage. Rupture of the mesenteric arteries from *Strongylus vulgaris* larval migration was a relatively common cause of intra-abdominal hemorrhage before the advent of ivermectin. Mesenteric bleeding has also been observed to be caused by strangulating lipomas as a result of direct tearing of blood vessels. The most rapidly fatal vascular lesion related to gastrointestinal disease is rupture of the caudal vena cava occurring during incarceration of the small intestine within the epiploic foramen. Because of the deep intra-abdominal location of the vessel, repair is impossible even when diagnosis occurs before death.

Widespread mesenteric hemorrhage may occur with disseminated intravascular coagulation. The amount of blood loss can be significant, particularly in patients that have undergone prior gastrointestinal surgery. Intra-abdominal hemorrhage can also be a complication of postoperative heparin therapy, which is now routinely used in an attempt to preventing intestinal adhesions.

CLINICAL SIGNS

The clinical signs associated with intra-abdominal hemorrhage vary with the severity of the blood loss, whether the blood loss is acute or chronic, and with the accompanying or underlying lesion. The primary sign observed in most horses is colic, which may be attributed to an associated gastrointestinal lesion, increased intraluminal pressure due to bleeding into visceral organs, tissue ischemia resulting from inadequate oxygen delivery to tissues, or possibly from extraluminal pressure on internal organs. In most situations, the signs of colic are mild and intermittent unless accompanied by a more severe gastrointestinal problem. Hemorrhagic shock, arising as a consequence of hypovolemia, is manifested by mucous membrane pallor, tachycardia, tachypnea, and sometimes systolic heart murmur. Often the degree of tachycardia does not correlate with the severity of pain demonstrated by these horses. Thus, moderate to extreme tachycardia in a horse with only mild intermittent signs of abdominal pain should indicate to the veterinarian that this is not a "routine" case of colic. As the quantity of blood loss increases, impaired neurologic function may become apparent, particularly altered behavior. Horses that lose more than 30% of their blood volume frequently appear anxious and agitated. These signs may progress to ataxia and episodes of unconsciousness as the amount of blood lost approaches 40% of total blood volume. In acute hemorrhage, loss of more than 50% of circulating blood volume is incompatible with life.

DIAGNOSIS

Abdominocentesis

Definitive diagnosis is based on demonstrating blood within the peritoneal cavity or within a localized intra-abdominal site. Obtaining blood during abdominocentesis does not always indicate accumulation of free blood within the abdominal cavity. Certainly, subcutaneous blood vessels or the spleen can be sources of significant hemorrhage during the abdominocentesis procedure. However, clinicians should not assume that blood obtained during abdominocentesis is the result of a "splenic tap." It is all too easy for bloody peritoneal fluid to be regarded as merely a contaminated sample, thus delaying the diagnosis of intra-abdominal hemorrhage.

Unfortunately, differentiating between blood contamination of fluid obtained via abdominocentesis and intra-abdominal hemorrhage can be difficult. In both instances, clinicopathologic analysis of the fluid obtained reveals high erythrocyte numbers and an elevated total protein level. Free blood within the peritoneal cavity may settle ventrally and have a packed cell volume, erythrocyte count, and total protein level equal to or exceeding that of peripheral blood; therefore, these parameters cannot be used to indicate the source of blood in peritoneal fluid. With acute hemorrhage resulting either from contamination or true intra-abdominal hemorrhage, platelets often are present. After a few hours of hemorrhage, erythrophagocytosis is frequently observed, and this finding may help rule out contamination during the collection procedure if analysis is performed without undue delay.

A rapid method of determining whether blood has arisen from the peritoneal cavity is to evaluate the color of the plasma after centrifugation. If the sample originated from free blood within the peritoneum, it often has a hemolyzed or pink tinge, especially with chronic hemorrhage.

Because peritoneal fluid analysis may not differentiate blood contamination from true intra-abdominal hemorrhage, further investigation is warranted when bloody peritoneal fluid is obtained. To definitively determine the validity of a hemorrhagic abdominocentesis, either another site should be sampled or an ultrasound examination should be performed.

Hemogram

The classic clinicopathologic changes anticipated with blood loss anemia is a reduction in erythrocyte mass and total plasma or serum protein levels. Because this reduction is due to fluid shifting from the extravascular to intravascular compartment, diluting the remaining blood components, 24 to 48 hours may be required for the full magnitude of these changes to be appreciated in the peripheral blood. Horses have a large reserve of red blood cells within their spleen that are released into circulation upon epinephrine-mediated splenic contraction, enhancing circulating erythrocyte numbers. Because of this, a decline

in total plasma protein is typically observed before the development of the clinicopathologic evidence of anemia.

Rectal Examination

A thorough rectal examination is an important component of the diagnostic work-up in horses with suspected intra-abdominal hemorrhage. In addition to careful palpation of the gastrointestinal tract, the cranial mesenteric artery, left kidney, spleen, and reproductive tract should be examined. When palpating the spleen, pressure should be applied both internally and externally in an attempt to detect areas of soreness that may reflect recent trauma. In mares, both ovaries, the broad ligament, and the uterus should be carefully palpated for abnormalities. If abnormalities can be located on rectal examination, transrectal ultrasonography can be helpful in ascertaining the origin, vascularity, and size of the lesion.

Ultrasonography

High cellularity gives blood a characteristic hyperechoic appearance on ultrasound, which is combined with a rapid "swirling" motion, which is not typical of other exudates. This unique sonographic appearance makes ultrasonography an extremely valuable tool for diagnosing intra-abdominal hemorrhage in horses. In addition to ascertaining the presence of free blood within the abdominal cavity, ultrasound examinations can be used to estimate the volume of blood present and in some situations the source of the bleeding. Abnormalities identified on physical examination or rectal palpation should be investigated ultrasonographically as a possible source of hemorrhage.

Because the spleen is one of the organs more commonly involved in intra-abdominal hemorrhage, it should always be thoroughly evaluated. Hematomas, abscesses, and tumors of the spleen are readily identifiable by ultrasonography; however, the most common cause of splenic hemorrhage, trauma, is typically not readily identified. In mares, the reproductive tract should be examined, and in all horses both kidneys and the liver should be evaluated by ultrasonography.

Coagulogram

Infrequently, coagulopathies are associated with internal bleeding. Therefore, all horses, particularly those with accompanying gastrointestinal disorders, should have a coagulogram performed. Interpretation can sometimes be difficult because any internal accumulation and degradation of blood is accompanied by an increase in fibrin degradation products. Severe acute blood loss results in thrombocytopenia, with levels rarely falling below 40,000 platelets/mm^3. Prothrombin time and activated partial thromboplastin time test results should remain normal unless a coagulopathy exists.

TREATMENT

Formulation of a treatment plan depends on the rate and severity of blood loss, source of the bleeding, and accompanying problems. Some form of fluid replacement usually is required, especially if tachycardia or other evidence of hemorrhagic shock is present. Replacement of

TABLE 1. RECOMMENDED THERAPIES FOR VOLUME RESTORATION AND GUIDELINES
FOR ADMINISTRATION

Treatment	Administration Recommendations	Example of a 500-kg Horse with Hemorrhagic Shock (Estimated Blood Loss 25%)
Isotonic crystalloid solution	Administer at a ratio of 3:1, replacement fluid to estimated volume of blood loss	500 kg × blood volume (8%) × estimated loss (25%) = 10 L whole blood lost 30 L of an isotonic crystalloid solution are needed to restore circulating plasma volume and interstitial fluid deficits
Hypertonic saline solution (7.2%)	4–6 ml/kg administered rapidly over a 10–15 minute period	2–3 L of hypertonic saline solution; should be followed within 2 hours with 15–20 L of an isotonic solution
Equine plasma	Protein deficit (g) = [desired plasma protein concentration (g/L) − measured plasma protein concentration (g/L)] × plasma volume (5% body weight in kg) Liters of plasma required = protein deficit (g) ÷ donor plasma protein concentration (g/L)	[60 g/L−41 g/L (hypothetical)] × 0.05 × 500 kg = 475 g protein deficit 475 g/67 g/L donor plasma = 7 L plasma A crude estimate is that 7 L of plasma (70 g/L) in a 500-kg horse raises the plasma protein concentration by 10 g/L
Whole blood	Total volume of blood transfused = body weight of recipient in kg × 0.08 × ([desired PCV − measured PCV]/donor PCV)	500 kg × 0.08 = 40 L total blood volume 40 × ([20 − 10]/40) = 10 L blood A crude estimate that may be used is that 2.2 ml of whole blood/kg of body weight will increase the PCV of the recipient by 1%, assuming the donor blood has a PCV of 40%

fluid volume may be accomplished with isotonic crystalloid solutions, hypertonic crystalloid solutions, or blood products (Table 1). Synthetic colloidal products such as dextrans or hetastarch are not advocated because of their tendency to inhibit platelet aggregation and alter coagulation protein function. To provide adequate volume, isotonic crystalloids should be administered at an amount three times in excess of the estimated amount of blood lost. This volume of fluid can be difficult to provide in a field situation, and thus an alternative is hypertonic (7.2%) saline, which rapidly ex-

pands plasma volume by promoting fluid to shift from the extravascular to intravascular space and increases blood pressure by enhancing vascular tone. Whenever hypertonic saline is administered, it must be followed by administration of isotonic crystalloid fluids. Some controversy exists regarding the use of hypertonic saline in patients with intra-abdominal hemorrhage, because hypertonic saline has been shown to increase mesenteric bleeding. However, the beneficial effects of hypertonic saline can, in certain situations, be lifesaving, aiding in stabilization of the

TABLE 2. MEDICATIONS FOR TREATMENT OF INTRA-ABDOMINAL HEMORRHAGE

Medication	Dosage Recommendations	Mechanism of Action	Comments
Acepromazine	0.02–0.055 mg/kg IV or IM	Alpha-receptor blockade for venodilation to permit clot formation	Can exacerbate shock and cause acute collapse
Aminocaproic acid	20–80 mg/kg IV, diluted 1:9 in 0.9% saline Administer over 30 to 60 minutes Can be redosed as needed	Stabilizes fibrin clot by inhibiting activity of plasminogen activator	Efficacy in horses has not been proven
Flunixin meglumine	0.5–1.1 mg/kg IV or IM, every 8–12 hours	Cyclooxygenase inhibitor	Used in treatment of hemorrhagic shock to reduce accompanying inflammatory mediator production
10% buffered formalin	0.02–0.06 ml/kg IV, diluted 1:5 in 0.9% saline	Unknown, may be due to activation of coagulation on endothelial cell surface	Monitor closely during administration for adverse reactions
Naloxone	0.01–0.02 mg/kg IV	Opiate antagonist with some dopaminergic activity Reduces cardiac work demands and pulmonary vascular resistance	Clinical efficacy at recommended dose has not been critically evaluated Will increase pain by blocking natural opioids
Prednisone sodium succinate	2–4 mg/kg IV	Glucocorticoid, reduces capillary permeability and increases systemic arterial pressure due to enhanced vasoconstriction	Controversial, may increase tissue oxygen demands

patient's condition pending collection of blood for transfusion, or during transport to a referral center.

Whole blood should be administered in the presence of severe tachycardia (>80 bpm), a packed cell volume (PCV) less than 20% with acute bleeding or PCV less than 10% with chronic blood loss; total plasma protein level less than 4 g/dl; mean arterial pressure less than 70 mm Hg; or neurologic alterations such as agitation. Whole blood can be collected from donor horses and transfused without a crossmatch if the donor and the recipient have not received prior transfusions. It is preferable to use a gelding or a stallion, although a mare that has not been used for breeding is also acceptable. Adult horses can safely donate up to 12 ml of whole blood per kg of body weight without receiving any type of volume replacement (6 L for a 500-kg horse). If additional blood donation is required, it is safe to take up to 24 ml of whole blood per kg of body weight if volume replacement with crystalloid solutions is provided (12 L for a 500-kg horse). It is important to remember that horses with severe anemia requiring replacement of up to 50% of their circulating blood volume, or patients that experience additional blood loss, may require a second blood transfusion 4 to 7 days after the initial transfusion, because the transfused erythrocytes are degraded or removed from circulation. A commercial bovine hemoglobin preparation is available and has been reported to have been successfully used in one horse (see Mason and coworkers in Supplemental Readings). Fresh or frozen equine plasma is another therapy that is useful for treating patients with accompanying coagulation disorders or those in whom whole blood cannot be administered. In addition to replacing coagulation proteins, plasma increases mean arterial pressure in hypotensive horses by enhancing oncotic pressure.

In addition to restoration of normal blood volume, therapy should be directed toward controlling the hemorrhage. If feasible, surgical correction should be a consideration. Medical treatments that have been used to control hemorrhage include venodilatory drugs, antifibrinolytic agents such as aminocaproic acid, opioid antagonists such as naloxone, and buffered formalin solutions (Table 2). Other than surgical correction, the basis for these therapies is largely theoretical, and thus the practitioner must form clinical impressions as to their effectiveness in controlling intraabdominal hemorrhage.

Supplemental Readings

Hooper RN, Carter GK, Varner DD, Taylor TS, Blanchard TL: Postparturient hemorrhage in the mare: Managing lacerations of the birth canal and uterus. Vet Med 89:57–63, 1994.

Maxson AD, Giger U, Sweeney CR, Tomasic M, Saik JE, Donawick WJ, Cothran EG: Use of a bovine hemoglobin preparation in the treatment of cyclic ovarian hemorrhage in a miniature horse. J Am Vet Med Assoc 203:1308–1311, 1993.

Morris DD: Review of anemia in horses, part II: Pathophysiologic mechanisms, specific diseases and treatment. Equine Pract 11(5):34–46, 1989.

Schmall LM, Muir WW, Robertson JT: Haemodynamic effects of small volume hypertonic saline in experimentally induced haemorrhagic shock. Equine Vet J 22:273–277, 1990.

Weld JM, Kamerling SG, Combie JD, Nugent TE, Woods WE, Oeltgen P, Tobin T: The effects of naloxone on endotoxic and hemorrhagic shock in horses. Res Communications Chem Pathol Pharm 44:227–238, 1984.

Hepatic Disorders

THOMAS J. DIVERS
Ithaca, New York

Liver disease occurs commonly in horses, but in the majority of cases, such as those caused by endotoxemia, hypoxia, and other disorders, the disease does not progress to liver failure. Liver disease is diagnosed by observation of elevation of liver enzyme activity in the serum.

DIAGNOSTIC PROCEDURES

Clinicopathologic Evaluation

Enzymes that are released into the blood as a result of hepatocellular disease include sorbitol dehydrogenase (SDH), aspartate aminotransferase (AST), ornithine carbamoxyltransferase (OCT), and isoenzyme 5 of lactate dehydrogenase (LDH-5). Sorbitol dehydrogenase is considered to be the most liver-specific enzyme and has a very short half life of several hours. The enzyme is stable for 12 hours at room temperature and up to 48 hours if the serum is separated and either frozen or refrigerated. Like SDH, LDH-5 also has a short half life but is not liver-specific. The enzyme may also become elevated with muscle disease. Simultaneous measurement of the muscle-specific creatine kinase determines whether the elevation in LDH-5 activity is a result of muscle damage or hepatic disease. AST is not liver-specific but is a sensitive indicator of hepatic disease. It has a much longer half life than SDH or LDH-5 and therefore remains elevated in the serum for several days after the hepatic disease has resolved.

The enzymes gamma glutamyl transaminopeptidase (GGT) and alkaline phosphatase are considered markers of biliary disease, although GGT is probably also released from damaged hepatocytes in the horse. GGT is considered to be liver-specific in the horse, although serum activity may also increase with the rare case of pancreatic disease. In foals younger than 45 days of age, the normal range of GGT activity is greater than in adult horses. Alkaline phosphatase is seldom used in the evaluation of liver disease in the horse because it may be elevated with diseases of many organs and is normally elevated in young foals.

Tests used to determine liver failure include measurement of conjugated bilirubin, prothrombin time (PT), partial thromboplastin time (PTT), and blood ammonia levels. PT and PTT measurements are best used in serial testing over a few days as a prognostic indicator in acute hepatic necrosis. Elevations in blood ammonia are inconsistent in liver failure and are greatest with portosystemic shunts and primary hyperammonemia. A preferred test for liver failure is the measurement of conjugated bilirubin. Although total and unconjugated bilirubin levels are elevated with liver failure, these can also be increased with hemolytic disease or anorexia. Icterus associated with anorexia generally causes bilirubin elevations of 4.0 to 7.0 mg/dl, although in some cases they may be as high as 11 mg/dl.

Several other excretion tests can be used to help determine dysfunction of the equine liver. These include sulfobromophthalein (BSP), aminopyrine, and caffeine clearance tests. These rarely provide clinical information not already gained from the measurement of liver enzyme activity, serum or plasma bilirubins, and serum or plasma total bile acids concentration.

Total bile acids measured in the serum or plasma are highly sensitive for detecting severe hepatic disease in the horse. Although bile acids are used mostly as a function test, they are also frequently elevated in horses with hepatic disease without clinical signs of hepatic failure. Normal horses have plasma or serum concentration of bile acids less than 2 μm/L. Horses that become icteric from anorexia but without liver disease may have elevations in bile acids up to 20 μm/L. A result over 20 μm/L should be considered strong evidence for liver disease. The one limitation to the use of bile acids in the horse is that in young foals bile acid concentrations are normally higher than the normal range for adults.

The finding of bilirubinuria is highly indicative of hepatic failure, although some horses without liver disease may have positive results for bilirubin on commonly used urine dip sticks. Other abnormalities commonly observed in horses with hepatic failure include hypoglycemia, low blood urea nitrogen (BUN), increased aromatic to branch chain amino acid ratio, metabolic acidosis, and polycythemia. None of these is specific for hepatic failure, although an abnormally low BUN is strongly suggestive of such.

Ultrasonography

Ultrasonography of the liver is a valuable diagnostic tool for determining hepatomegaly, hepatic fibrosis, bile duct dilatation, and biliary stones. Ultrasonography is also useful as a guide for determining the site of the liver biopsy. Less common problems that may be detected by ultrasound examination of the liver include portosystemic shunts, hepatic abscesses, tumors, parasitic cysts, or traumatic laceration of the liver. The ultrasound examination is best performed using a 5-MHz sector scanner. The liver can be visualized on the right side just caudal to the lung field in most horses. In some horses the liver normally extends caudally such that it is in apposition with the cranial pole of the right kidney. In older horses with atrophy of the right liver lobe or in horses with acute hepatic necrosis or chronic fibrosis it may not be possible to image the liver from the right side. In almost all horses a small amount of liver can be seen on the left just caudal to the left ventricle and deep to the diaphragm. If the liver can be visualized on the right side, this is usually the preferred site for biopsy. A 14-gauge 11.4-cm biopsy needle is the preferred instrument for performing the liver biopsy.

THEILER'S DISEASE

Theiler's disease is a subacute hepatic necrosis often resulting in hepatic failure and acute encephalopathy in horses. It has been termed *serum hepatitis* because there is often a history of the affected horse receiving tetanus antitoxin 4 to 10 weeks before the onset of clinical signs. In some cases, the affected horse may not have received tetanus antitoxin but may have been in contact with another horse that had received tetanus antitoxin. The disease appears to be more common in late summer or early fall. This apparent seasonal pattern could suggest a vector spread of the disease, or could simply reflect the fact that many foaling mares receive tetanus antitoxin in the spring of the year along with their newborn foals. Most commonly, only one horse on a farm is affected, although outbreaks are reported, and other horses on the farm may have evidence of liver disease, such as elevated enzyme levels, without clinical signs of hepatic failure. A specific tetanus antitoxin product, such as a single company product and/or product with the same lot number, may be responsible for a high number of cases.

Clinical Signs

The most common clinical signs seen with Theiler's disease are central nervous system (CNS) disorder, jaundice, and discolored urine. The CNS signs are variable and may range from acute depression to maniacal behavior. Blindness may be present, and the affected horses may be ataxic. Icteric membranes can be noted in most cases, although in peracute cases, they may not be pronounced. The urine may be abnormally dark, indicating bilirubinuria and, in a few cases, may be red if there is a concurrent microangiopathic hemolytic process.

Diagnosis

The diagnosis is based upon history, clinical findings, and laboratory confirmation of hepatic disease and hepatic failure. Hepatic disease can be detected most easily by measuring serum or plasma activity of GGT, AST, SDH, or LDH-5. GGT levels are elevated in all cases of Theiler's disease and are most often in the range of 100 to 300 IU/L. Aspartate aminotransferase should be measured because horses having values higher than 4000 IU/L have a poor prognosis. The repeated measurement of AST may also be used to assess recovery, because the AST can be expected to decrease within 3 to 5 days if the horse is to improve. GGT, on the other hand, is frequently further elevated during the first 3 days of the illness, despite clinical improvement and eventual recovery in an affected horse. A decrease in SDH in the serum can be expected more rapidly in improving horses than a decrease in AST. Total serum bile acids may also be used to detect liver disease. In horses with Theiler's disease, the measurement of serum or plasma bile acids rarely adds further information than that provided by the measurement of hepatic enzymes. Virtually all horses clinically affected with Theiler's disease have total serum bilirubin values higher than those commonly observed with anorexia. Total bilirubin level in horses showing clinical signs caused by Theiler's disease is generally in the range of 12 to 20 mg/dl. The percentage of bilirubin in the unconjugated form is almost always greater than 70%, although there is some increase in conjugated bilirubin in affected horses. The conjugated bilirubin values are generally 1.5 to 5.0 mg/dl. The PT and PTT times are generally abnormally high in comparison with a control sample, but they rarely offer information not already gathered from the measurement of direct and indirect bilirubin, bile acids, and hepatic enzyme activity in the serum or plasma. Other abnormalities in Theiler's disease are moderate to severe acidosis, hypokalemia, polycythemia, increased aromatic amino acids, and hyperammonemia.

A more definitive diagnosis of Theiler's disease can be made only by liver biopsy. If the history, clinical examination results, and laboratory results are characteristic of Theiler's disease, a biopsy is not imperative, and in many cases may not be easy to perform because the liver is often shrunken and may be difficult to visualize with ultrasound examination. If a biopsy is performed and a sample of liver is successfully retrieved, microscopic examination generally reveals marked hepatocellular necrosis involving the entire lobule, which is most severe in the central and midzonal hepatocytes. There is a very mild to moderate accumulation of lymphocytes and a few neutrophils. The degree of bile duct proliferation is often positively correlated with the duration of the disease.

Treatment

No specific treatment for Theiler's disease has been proposed. Supportive therapy is often successful. Because stressful situations such as moving the animal to another facility or weaning the mare's foal often exacerbate the clinical signs of the hepatoencephalopathy, the affected horse should not be further stressed, if possible. Sedation should be used only when necessary to control fulminant hepatic encephalopathy with injurious behavior. Xylazine can be used to control bizarre behavior to prevent injury of the animal and to allow catheter placement and other therapy.

Intravenous fluids are probably the most important component of treatment for hepatic encephalopathy in horses. Fluids should consist of a balanced electrolyte solution, preferably without lactate, and should be supplemented with potassium 20 to 40 mEq/L, and 5 to 10 g dextrose per 100 ml. Sodium bicarbonate should be given only if blood pH is less than 7.1 and/or bicarbonate is less than 14 mEq/L. Supplemental vitamins can be administered but are not necessary in the treatment.

An effort should be made to decrease ammonia production in the bowel. This can be done by administering neomycin (5.0 mg/kg p.o. t.i.d.) by dose syringe for 2 days. With fulminant hepatic encephalopathy in the horse, the author prefers not to pass a nasogastric tube because nasal bleeding exacerbates the hepatic encephalopathy if the blood is swallowed and because there may be insufficient clotting factors. Lactulose (0.2 ml/kg b.i.d.) may also de-

crease ammonia production in the bowel but is more expensive than neomycin. Both lactulose and neomycin may cause diarrhea if given in excessive dosages or for prolonged periods. Affected animals should be fed high carbohydrate, high branch chain amino acid feeds, with low total protein content. Sorghum and/or cracked corn mixed with molasses are ideal. A grass hay should be fed rather than alfalfa hay. Affected animals should be protected from sunlight to prevent photosensitization.

Prognosis

Affected horses that can be maintained for 3 to 5 days without deterioration of their condition and that continue to eat often recover. A decline in the SDH and PT along with improvement in appetite are the best positive predictive laboratory and clinical indicators of recovery. Horses that have fulminant encephalopathy that cannot be easily controlled with sedatives have a very poor prognosis, although some recover. Those that continue to eat during the first 3 days of the illness generally have a good prognosis. If the affected horse recovers, which many do within 5 to 10 days, its long-term prognosis is excellent. No evidence suggests that severe hepatic fibrosis and/or neoplasia occur following Theiler's disease in the horse.

CHOLANGIOHEPATITIS AND CHOLEDOCHOLITHIASIS

Cholangiohepatitis is a sporadic but common cause of hepatic failure in horses. Adult horses are most commonly affected, and choleliths are rarely seen in horses less than 9 years of age. The disease is thought to be caused by an ascending biliary tract infection usually by a gram-negative rod. Chronically infected horses may develop one or more calculi within the biliary tract, which may produce obstruction, jaundice, and colic. Early in the course of cholangiohepatitis, clinical signs are probably related to the inflammation, which produces fever; hepatic enlargement, which produces colic; and biliary obstruction, which causes severe jaundice and photosensitivity. In chronic cases and those with choledocholithiasis, clinical signs may be a result of biliary obstruction or diffuse hepatic fibrosis.

Clinical Abnormalities

Fever, jaundice, colic, photosensitivity, and anorexia are the most common clinical abnormalities. Weight loss may be apparent in some horses. Fulminant signs of hepatoencephalopathy are rare, although they may be seen in chronic cases with hepatic fibrosis. Colic may be seen in those cases with acute obstruction.

Diagnosis

The diagnosis is based upon history, signalment, and clinical signs. Laboratory findings typical of cholangiohepatitis/choledocholithiasis in horses include marked elevations in serum or plasma GGT, often in the range of 600 to 2500 U/L. Usually increased activity of the hepatocellular enzymes such as AST and SDH is seen in the blood, although the elevation in these enzymes is relatively much less than the increased activity of the biliary enzyme GGT. Bile acids are increased to levels higher than 20 μm/L, even in mildly affected horses. Bilirubin level is increased in those horses that have become jaundiced, and the conjugated or direct bilirubin level typically approaches 35 to 50% or more of the total bilirubin in animals with cholangiohepatitis or choledocholithiasis. Peripheral white blood cell count is increased, predominantly by mature neutrophils. In addition, plasma fibrinogen and total protein levels are frequently elevated. Other laboratory measurements of hepatic function, such as PT, PTT, ammonia, and urea, may be within normal limits despite marked icterus.

Ultrasound examination of the liver is very important in diagnosing cholangiohepatitis and choledocholithiasis. The liver is subjectively enlarged in most cases, although in chronic cases with fibrosis it may be smaller than normal. In many cases, there is obvious bile duct distension (Fig. 1), although this is not seen in all cases. Stones may be seen on ultrasound examination in a few cases. Most commonly they are seen at the eighth to eleventh intercostal space just caudal to the lung border. Stones may be seen as discrete calculi or less discrete sludge deposits within the biliary tract, both of which may cast shadows. In approximately one half of the cases with cholelithiasis, the stones cannot be seen on ultrasound examination because a large portion of the liver cannot be visualized owing to the large lung field in the horse. Most horses with cholangiohepatitis do not appear to have calculi.

If cholangiohepatitis is suspected, a liver biopsy should be performed both to help confirm the diagnosis and, more importantly, in an attempt to culture an offending organism. Either a biopsy or an aspirate of the liver is acceptable. Microscopically, there is bile duct dilatation, bile epithelium proliferation, moderate periportal neutrophilic inflammatory response and, in some cases, periportal fibrosis. Cultures should be submitted to test for both aerobic and anaerobic organisms from the biopsy or the aspirate sample. The success rate of culturing organisms from a biopsy or an aspirate sample is approximately 40% in cases of cholangiohepatitis. Gram-negative organisms are most commonly cultured.

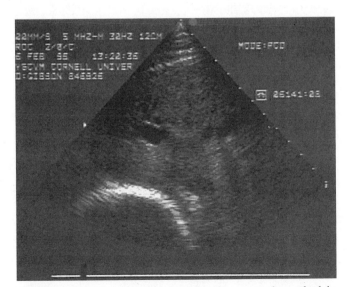

Figure 1. Transabdominal ultrasonography of an equine liver. The bile ducts are distended in a horse with cholangiohepatitis.

Treatment

If there are no visible stones on ultrasound examination and the diagnosis is cholangiohepatitis, antimicrobial therapy based upon culture and sensitivity of the liver biopsy and/or aspirate should be provided for at least 1 month. In many cases, an organism cannot be recovered, in which case initial therapy may be trimethoprim-sulfa (20 mg/kg p.o. b.i.d.). If there is no response, such as decrease in temperature within 3 of 5 days or decrease in GGT, within 14 to 21 days, treatment should be changed. Alternatives include ceftiofur (3.0 mg/kg IV or IM b.i.d.), or enrofloxacin (3.3 mg/kg p.o. b.i.d.). If biliary stones are present, antimicrobial therapy is still indicated. If the calculi are sludge deposits within the biliary tract, antimicrobial and supportive therapy may be effective. If the stones are discrete calculi obviously causing obstruction, antimicrobial therapy is unlikely to work. For obstructing stones, choledocholithotomy is the treatment of choice, although this treatment should not be performed if there is severe hepatic fibrosis, which can be determined by ultrasound examination and liver biopsy.

Prognosis

The prognosis in cases of cholangiohepatitis without stones and without severe hepatic fibrosis is good. Although changing antimicrobials may be necessary to find a drug that is effective, in many cases when an effective drug is found, long-term treatment is curative of the disease. There is no GGT value that indicates a grave prognosis. Some horses with serum or plasma GGT concentrations higher than 2000 U/L have recovered. Those horses with obstructing stones have a poorer prognosis, and horses with severe hepatic fibrosis have the poorest prognosis of all.

HYPERLIPEMIA

Hyperlipemia occurs most commonly in overweight ponies, miniature horses, donkeys, horses with pituitary adenomas, and rarely in horses in late pregnancy. It is characterized by rapid mobilization of lipids from adipose stores, fatty liver, and lipemic serum. Factors that increase lipolysis include late pregnancy, anorexia, and diseases that result in severe stress and catecholamine release, such as laminitis and choke. Horse mares in late pregnancy with lipemia often have diarrhea and are azotemic. Insulin resistance, which is greater in ponies than horses and is increased with obesity and late pregnancy, is thought to be a predominant mechanism in the disease process.

Clinical Signs and Diagnosis

Clinical signs of hyperlipemia in the horse are often acute. Acute anorexia, depression, and nonpainful pitting edema of the ventral abdomen are common clinical signs. Predisposing diseases may have their own set of clinical signs such as diarrhea, choke, laminitis, and chronic obstructive pulmonary disease. The diagnosis is suspected based upon signalment, history, and clinical signs. It is further confirmed by gross observation of plasma, which has a whitish discoloration, and measurement of plasma or serum triglyceride levels, with values being higher than 500 mg/dl. In many cases, there is an increase in hepatocellular enzymes in the serum. Liver function tests generally remain normal, and affected animals rarely become severely jaundiced. Old horses that develop hyperlipemia most often have pituitary adenomas with increases in plasma adrenocorticotropic hormone (ACTH), endorphins, and urine cortisol to creatinine ratio.

Treatment

Specific treatment for hyperlipemia in ponies includes intravenous fluids and nutritional support. Treatment of a primary predisposing disease is of paramount importance. For intravenous fluid therapy, acetated Ringer's solution with 5 g/100 ml dextrose added, and 20 to 40 mEq KCl/ L is indicated for rehydration and maintenance therapy. Lipemic horse mares that commonly have the triad of diarrhea, azotemia, and late pregnancy may require large amounts of intravenous fluids to correct the azotemia.

If the affected animal is eating, it should be fed anything it will eat that is of reasonable nutritional value. Ideally, frequent feedings of small amounts of high-carbohydrate feeds are preferred. If the animal is not eating, it should be given 0.5 g/kg glucose (as a 15% solution) with 10 to 20 g of KCl via nasogastric tube. For valuable horses that are completely off feed, the author recommends the use of parenteral nutrition that can be made by mixing 50% dextrose and an amino acid solution formulated for patients with hepatic failure that are not already hyperglycemic. The final solution should be 20% dextrose with 4 to 5% amino acid. This can be given at a rate of 2 ml/kg per hour if plasma glucose is not greater than 180 mg/dl during treatment. For those cases that cannot be given parenteral nutrition, enteral feeding with a commercially prepared high-calorie product is indicated.

Heparin (100 U/kg q12h IV) may be used in an attempt to decrease the hyperlipemia, although lipoprotein lipase is likely to be at peak values already. Protamine insulin (30 IU/200 kg IM b.i.d.) has been recommended and may be of some benefit, although hyperlipemic animals appear to have increased insulin resistance. Supportive therapy with flunixin meglumine (0.25 mg/kg t.i.d.) may be of value in improving attitude and appetite. Aborting the fetus of the lipemic mare in late pregnancy is fraught with complications and is generally not recommended. If a pituitary adenoma is suspected as the triggering cause of hyperlipemia, affected animals can be treated with either cyproheptadine (0.5 mg/kg p.o. b.i.d.) or pergolide (1–2 mg p.o. s.i.d.) for small ponies or miniature horses, or 5 mg p.o. s.i.d. for larger ponies and adult horses.

Prognosis

The prognosis for animals with hyperlipemia is guarded. Those that continue to eat and have a primary disease that can be quickly reversed have a good prognosis. Hyperlipemic horses totally off feed or with a severe primary disease have a poor prognosis.

TYZZER'S DISEASE

Tyzzer's disease is an acute bacterial infection caused by *Bacillus piliformis*, which causes hepatic necrosis, myocar-

ditis, and colitis in affected foals that are 8 to 42 days of age. It is believed that foals become infected by ingesting soil containing the *Bacillus* organism. The disease is not common but may be endemic on certain farms, affecting a foal every few years. Although rare, more than one case on a farm may be reported in certain years.

Clinical Signs

One of the more common scenarios with Tyzzer's disease is that a young 8- to 42-day-old foal appears healthy before being found dead in the pasture. Some foals are found gravely ill with depression, fever or hypothermia, recumbency, convulsions, and diarrhea. Icterus may occasionally be seen in those foals that live more than 12 hours after onset of clinical disease. On clinical examination, the most pronounced findings are those indicative of cardiovascular collapse, septic shock, and liver failure. These include poor capillary refill, scleral injection, petechiae, pronounced tachycardia, cold extremities, and icterus.

Diagnosis

The diagnosis is based upon age, clinical signs, and evidence of hepatic disease. A moderate to pronounced serum or plasma elevation is present in hepatocellular enzymes (AST, SDH) and in the biliary enzyme GGT, and bilirubinemia. Blood cultures may be performed in affected foals, but they are often negative. Postmortem findings include gross icterus, petechiae, pulmonary hemorrhage, and multifocal small white spots in the liver. These white spots can be confused with or may appear similar to those of *Actinobacillus equuli* hepatitis, which occurs in much younger foals, generally those less than 5 days of age. Microscopic examination of the liver of foals with Tyzzer's disease reveals focal areas of coagulation necrosis with neutrophil infiltration and large bacilli within the cytoplasm of hepatocytes. The *Bacillus* organism is most easily seen with a Warthin-Starry stain (silver).

Treatment

Treatment is generally unsuccessful, although there is a report of successful treatment in a tentatively diagnosed case of Tyzzer's disease. Treatment should include fluid therapy with polyionic fluids with strong ions, along with additional dextrose to make a 5 or 10% dextrose solution. Because of the severe acidosis commonly found in Tyzzer's disease, 5 g sodium bicarbonate should be added to each liter of fluid. Systemic antibiotics should be given at high dosages intravenously. Recommended antimicrobials may be either potassium penicillin (44,000 IU/kg IV q4h) and amikacin (6.6 mg/kg IV t.i.d.), or chloramphenicol (44 mg/ kg p.o. q4h). Other general therapy for septic shock should be provided, such as 1 to 2 L hyperimmune plasma with antibodies against lipopolysaccharide (LPS) and pentoxifylline (8.4 mg/kg p.o. b.i.d.). For those foals that do not respond to fluid therapy and remain severely hypotensive, methylene blue may be administered in hopes of alleviating the hypotensive effects of endogenously released nitric oxide.

Prognosis

The prognosis is extremely grave. There is a single case report of a foal with a tentative diagnosis of Tyzzer's disease that survived. That foal was treated with penicillin and trimethoprim/sulfa.

TOXIC HEPATOPATHY

Toxic hepatopathy may occur in horses for reasons other than pyrrolizidine alkaloid toxicosis (see page 222). Kleingrass (*Panicum coloratum*) is known to produce biliary fibrosis and hyperplasia and to cause icterus and photosensitivity in horses. This is most commonly reported in the southwestern United States from late spring to early fall. In the eastern United States, a similar syndrome is seen sporadically in horses grazing pasture or fed hay containing high concentrations of fall panicum. In the northeast United States and Canada, a similar syndrome is associated with horses grazing alsike clover (*Trifolium hybridum*). Alsike clover grows luxuriantly on heavy clay soil, and an increased incidence is reported during wet seasons. The disease is observed most commonly when the blossom of the plant has been consumed and the predominant forage being fed is the alsike clover. The incidence of hepatopathy associated with any of these three plants varies from year to year, which may indicate a seasonal effect upon the concentration of the toxin within the plant itself. Although all have the potential to have saponin products within the plant, it is also possible that the hepatopathy in some cases is associated with molds that grow on these plants under certain environmental conditions.

Grain that is contaminated with mycotoxins may occasionally produce hepatic failure in the horse. The most common mycotoxin causing liver disease in the horse is *Fusarium*, a mold that is commonly found in corn and is most notorious for causing leukoencephalomalacia in horses. The majority of affected horses with leukoencephalomalacia have hepatic disease, although rarely do they have hepatic failure. Sporadic reports occur of aflatoxicosis causing hepatic failure in horses. These cases are rare and may be associated with contaminated corn or an unusual feed substance for the horse, such as peanuts.

Iron toxicosis has been reported in both adult horses and in foals. In the early 1980s, iron toxicosis was a common cause of hepatic failure in young foals; it was associated with the administration of ferrous fumarate, which was contained in a nutritional supplement intended for newborn foals. The hepatic disease and failure occurred in almost all cases when the ferrous fumarate product was administered before ingestion of colostrum. Some horses may have higher iron contents in the liver and blood than are considered normal for the horse. This may be caused by oversupplementation with oral vitamin and iron supplements. In rare cases, hepatic disease and failure occur from the iron toxicosis. Injectable iron is more likely to cause an acute elevation in body iron concentration than oral supplementation. Other horses have developed severe chronic hepatic fibrosis and liver failure believed to be caused by enhanced absorption (primary hemochromatosis) rather than gross oversupplementation.

Clinical Signs

The clinical signs of plant-induced hepatopathy from Kleingrass, fall panicum, and alsike clover are predominantly depression, photosensitivity, severe jaundice, and weight loss. Fulminant hepatoencephalopathy rarely occurs. Clinical signs of aflatoxicosis and iron toxicosis may be signs of acute hepatic failure, including jaundice and hepatoencephalopathy, and those signs associated with rapid cardiovascular collapse. Horses with liver disease and failure caused by chronic oral administration of iron may be depressed and jaundiced and have weight loss. Petechiae associated with thrombocytopenia were reported in one horse with cholestatic hepatopathy believed to be caused by the oral administration of iron.

Diagnosis

The diagnosis for plant-induced hepatic failure is based upon exposure to those plants, the possibility that multiple animals on a farm may be affected, and multiple horses in a practice area within certain years having similar clinical signs. Severe jaundice in more than one horse on a farm without fever and fulminant signs of hepatoencephalopathy in the affected horses supports the diagnosis of a plant-associated cholestatic disease. Laboratory abnormalities are indicative of cholestatic disease. Serum GGT activities in affected horses are always elevated and are generally in the range of 100 to 800 U/L. Serum AST activity is often mildly elevated in affected horses. Bilirubin concentration is increased, and the direct bilirubin percentage of the total is frequently more than 25%. Ultrasound examination may be within normal limits, or there may be evidence of hepatomegaly and increased echogenicity, indicating hepatic fibrosis. Bile ducts may be readily seen, which suggests biliary fibrosis. A biopsy or aspirate sample of the liver usually reveals large amounts of bilirubin pigment in nucleated hepatocytes, a few neutrophils, degenerative and regenerative changes within hepatocytes, and in some cases pronounced periportal bridging fibrosis with moderate bile duct proliferation.

The diagnosis of aflatoxicosis or *Fusarium* hepatopathy is also based upon history of exposure, most commonly to moldy corn. A variety of neurologic signs may be seen with *Fusarium*-induced leukoencephalomalacia. Fulminant hepatic encephalopathy and jaundice may be present with aflatoxicosis. Biliary and hepatocellular enzyme activity are increased, as are blood ammonia and bile acid concentrations. Biopsy of the liver reveals hepatocellular necrosis, which is most severe in the centrilobular area, and biliary necrosis with some biliary hyperplasia.

In cases of acute iron toxicosis, microscopic examination of the liver reveals hepatic necrosis, which is most severe in the midzonal area. In horses with hepatopathy caused by more chronic accumulation of iron, there is periportal fibrosis, proliferation in bile ducts with cholestasis and marked iron accumulation in hepatocytes with scattered areas of moderately severe hepatocellular necrosis. Hepatic iron is increased to 300 ppm or greater in all affected animals, and serum iron may be increased with acute poisoning. Laboratory findings with hemochromatosis generally reveal elevated levels of PT, PTT, blood ammonia, bile acids, hepatic enzymes in the serum, and, in a few cases, thrombocytopenia.

Treatment

Treatment of plant-induced hepatopathies centers around removal of affected and nonaffected horses from contaminated pastures or removal of the offending hay. Supportive therapy for liver failure and cholestasis is indicated. This includes fluid therapy with polyionic fluids supplemented with additional potassium and dextrose. Although vitamin K may be administered, it is rarely needed. If photodermatitis has occurred, removal from sunlight and treatment with antibacterial creams are indicated. The prognosis in the majority of horses affected with these diseases is good.

For acute aflatoxicosis or acute iron toxicosis, the disease is generally rapidly progressive, causing fulminant encephalopathy and, in the case of iron toxicosis, hemorrhagic tendencies. Treatment is generally supportive with fluids and nutritional sustenance. For iron toxicosis, chelation therapy with deferoxamine can be attempted, but it is unlikely to be successful in either acute iron toxicosis or chronic hemochromatosis. The prognosis in these cases is poor.

OBSTRUCTION OF BILE DUCT IN ASSOCIATION WITH GASTROINTESTINAL DISEASE

Obstruction of the bile duct may occur in young foals that have had duodenal ulcers, and in the healing process, a duodenal stricture is formed at the opening of the bile duct into the intestine. Affected foals have clinical signs of gastric ulcers, are anorexic, have large amounts of gastric reflux, have moderate elevations in serum GGT activity and direct and indirect bilirubin, and become jaundiced. Successful transpositioning of the bile duct has been reported, but the prognosis is guarded to poor. Many foals with duodenal strictures distal to the opening of the bile duct have reflux and ingesta in the biliary tract and cholangitis. This can be seen on abdominal radiographs taken 2 hours after oral barium administration. Surgical repair of the duodenal stricture and antimicrobial therapy may be successful in these foals.

Another cause of obstruction of the bile duct associated with an intestinal disease is biliary obstruction in adult horses associated with certain colonic displacements of 3 days or longer duration. Most commonly this is a 180° torsion of the large colon. Affected horses have mild colic for 3 to 5 days, at which time severe jaundice is noted. Bilirubin levels are higher than those seen with icterus of anorexia, often in the range of 12 to 15 mg/dl with more than 25% of this as conjugated (direct) bilirubin. The activity of GGT in affected horses is generally in the range of 150 to 500 U/L. The exact mechanism as to how the colonic displacement produces the biliary obstruction is not proven and may vary. In some cases it appears to be associated with the large colon displacement causing tension and stretching of the duodenal mesentery at the opening of the biliary duct into the duodenum, resulting in a mechanical narrowing of the duct. If a large colon displacement is suspected in a horse with the laboratory findings outlined, surgery should not be delayed, because liver function returns to normal with correction of the intestinal displacement.

A third and less frequent cause of biliary obstruction associated with intestinal disease is mechanical obstruction of the biliary duct opening associated with granulomatous enteritis and/or eosinophilic or fibrosing pancreatitis. Affected horses generally have severe chronic weight loss, icterus, and frequently laboratory evidence supportive of protein-losing enteropathy and malabsorption, such as decreased plasma protein and abnormally low glucose or xylose absorption test results, along with evidence of hepatic disease (increased GGT).

HEPATIC ABSCESSES AND TUMORS

Hepatic abscesses and primary hepatic neoplasia are both rare in the horse and generally cause signs of ill thrift without hepatic failure. Hepatic abscesses are especially rare in horses, in comparison with cattle, but may be seen sporadically. Abscesses are associated with septic portal vein thrombosis or extension from intestinal disease in close proximity to the intestine, such as an enterolith, causing pressure necrosis and adhesions between the colon and liver. In foals, abscesses may occur in association with ascarid migration, bacterial septicemia, or ascending infection of the umbilical vein.

Primary hepatic neoplasms in horses include cholangiocarcinoma, hepatocellular carcinoma, and rarely lymphoma or other neoplasias. Cholangiocarcinomas generally appear in middle aged or older horses and cause pronounced weight loss before the onset of liver failure. The signs associated with liver failure are predominantly those of severe jaundice associated with obstruction of the biliary tract by the carcinoma. Serum or plasma GGT activity in affected horses is generally very high, ranging from several hundred up to 3000 U/L. Ultrasound examination is very useful in identifying the tumors and facilitating a biopsy of the liver for a definitive diagnosis.

Hepatocellular carcinomas, on the other hand, although infrequent, generally occur in young horses, yearlings to young adults. They are characteristically uniform in their appearance on ultrasound examination, and produce polycythemia as a unique laboratory feature. The predominant clinical findings are depression and weight loss. The presence of carcinoma can be confirmed by liver biopsy and microscopic examination of the liver.

Lymphoma may, on rare occasions, diffusely infiltrate the liver, producing signs associated with hepatic failure. Jaundice, severe depression, and weight loss may be seen. Laboratory findings may include hypoglycemia, mild to moderate elevations in liver enzymes, bilirubinemia, and abnormally low levels of serum IgM.

HYPERAMMONEMIA WITH LITTLE OR NO EVIDENCE OF LIVER DISEASE

Primary Hyperammonemia of Adult Horses

A syndrome of hyperammonemia, blindness, and severe neurologic signs occurs in adult horses, almost always in association with enteric disease, diarrhea, and/or colic.

Blood ammonia values are generally in the range of 200 to 400 μm/L, severe metabolic acidosis is present, plasma bicarbonate concentration is less than 12 mEq/L, and profound hyperglycemia (250–400 mg/dl) is observed. Serum concentrations of liver enzymes, bile acids, and bilirubin are all within normal range. Most commonly, intestinal signs precede the neurologic signs by 24 to 48 hours. With medical treatment, including intravenous fluids with additional potassium chloride and oral neomycin, most horses recover from the neurologic signs within 2 to 3 days. Diarrhea and, in a few cases, protein-losing enteropathy may persist for an additional 3 to 5 days. The cause of this syndrome is unknown, but the uniform appearance of intestinal signs before neurologic signs suggests a primary intestinal problem with overgrowth of urease-producing bacteria within the intestine. No specific etiologic agent has, as of yet, been identified.

Portosystemic Shunts

Portosystemic shunts occur in foals and can be another cause of hyperammonemia and neurologic signs resulting from liver dysfunction without laboratory or microscopic evidence of liver disease. Affected foals are generally 2 months of age when onset of neurologic signs occurs. These signs may include staggering, wandering, blindness, propulsive circling, and seizure. A transient improvement may occur in some cases with minimal clinical therapy, and this improvement is probably associated with decreased protein intake at that time. This diagnosis should be strongly suspected in foals exhibiting repeated episodes of cerebral signs without obvious reasons. Serum hepatic-derived enzyme levels are normal, but blood ammonia and serum bile acid levels are both extremely high and provide strong supporting evidence of the diagnosis of portosystemic shunt. Confirmation and location of the shunt can be obtained by catheterizing the mesenteric vein and performing a portogram. Nuclear scintigraphy can also be used on smaller foals to confirm a portosystemic shunt. The shunt may be seen in some cases on ultrasound examination of the liver.

Clinical signs of affected foals can often be controlled by restricting protein intake and allowing the foal to nurse the dam as the sole source of nutrition, along with orally administered neomycin or lactulose to decrease ammonia production within the bowel, and high-potassium and dextrose intravenous fluid therapy. Successful surgical correction of a congenital portosystemic shunt in a foal has been reported, but the prognosis is guarded.

Hyperammonemia of Morgan Weanlings

A syndrome of ill thrift and hyperammonemia with varying degrees of liver disease also occurs in Morgan foals with clinical signs being noted around weaning time. Liver enzymes are generally increased in affected foals, although bilirubin may be normal and blood ammonia is elevated. Microscopic findings have varied from mild to moderate pathologic disease and include variable degrees of portal and bridging fibrosis with bile duct hypoplasia, karyomegaly and cytomegaly. Copper and iron stains of the liver have been negative. The cause of the liver disease of these foals is uncertain, but affected foals have been related.

CHRONIC ACTIVE HEPATITIS

Chronic active hepatitis is a phrase often used to describe any progressive inflammatory condition of the liver. It most often involves the portal areas most severely, producing bridging necrosis and fibrosis with variable degrees of bile duct proliferation. Often, severe hepatic fibrosis and liver failure eventually occur. Several different causes can produce this disease in the horse, some of which are toxic, some of which are infectious and are reviewed under Cholangiohepatitis (see earlier), and some may be immune-mediated. Immune-mediated disorders may produce a lymphocytic, plasmocytic periportal infiltrate. Any intestinal malabsorption syndrome, such as infiltrative bowel or small intestinal resection, usually results in some degree of periportal disease which, in some cases, is progressive.

Clinical Signs and Diagnosis

The predominant clinical sign of chronic active hepatitis is weight loss. Photosensitivity may be seen in some cases and jaundice may appear in many cases, although there may be considerable time between the weight loss and the onset of icterus. A more generalized scaly skin may be noted in horses with any kind of chronic biliary disease. Affected animals may be depressed, and in those with cholangiohepatitis, fever may be present. An increase in hepatic-derived enzymes is found within the serum; bile acids are elevated, and bilirubin values are variable, although high-normal or increased values are observed in most cases. Serum protein values usually remain within normal range. Horses with suppurative cholangitis and chronic progressive liver disease but no evidence of septic cholangiohepatitis and cholelithiasis or known exposure to a hepatic toxin are often diagnosed as having chronic active hepatitis.

Ultrasound examination generally reveals increased echogenicity of the liver indicative of hepatic fibrosis. The liver may be smaller than normal. Biopsy of the liver reveals bridging necrosis and fibrosis in periportal areas and bile duct proliferation.

Treatment

The treatment of chronic active hepatitis involves general supportive therapy for liver failure, including fluid therapy, if needed, with potassium chloride and glucose supplementation, feeding of low-protein (high branch chain amino acid) high-carbohydrate diets, prevention of sun exposure, and supplementation with vitamins. If the biopsy reveals a lymphocytic plasmocytic infiltrate, prednisolone therapy should be attempted. A dose of 1.5 mg/kg prednisolone should be administered daily by mouth for 5 days, followed by decreasing amounts until the horse can be supported on 0.4 mg/kg of prednisolone every other day. Colchicine has been used in some cases, but efficacy is unproven. Antibiotics should be administered in those cases believed to have septic cholangiohepatitis. The prognosis for chronic active hepatitis is generally guarded to poor. Many animals improve for several weeks or months but seldom survive beyond 2 years.

Supplemental Readings

Bauer JE, Asquith RL, Kivipelto J: Serum biochemical indicators of liver function in neonatal foals. Am J Vet Res 50:2037–2041,1989.

Carlson GP, Vivrette S: Chronic active hepatitis in horses. Proc 7th Annu Meet Am Coll Vet Intern Med, 1989, p 595.

Cornick JL, Carter GK, Bridges CH: Kleingrass-associated hepatotoxicosis in horses. J Am Vet Assoc 193:932–935, 1988.

Fortier LA, Fubini SL, Flanders JA, Divers TJ: Guidelines for the diagnosis and surgical correction of equine and bovine congenital portosystemic shunts [Abstract]. Vet Surg 22:379, 1993.

Humber KA, Sweeney RW, Saik JE, Hansen TO, Morris CF: Clinical and clinicopathologic findings in two foals with *Bacillus piliformis*. J Am Vet Med Assoc 193:1425–1428, 1988.

Johnston JK, Divers TJ, Reef VB, Acland H: Cholelithiasis in horses: Ten cases (1982–1986). J Am Vet Med Assoc 194:405–409, 1989.

Messer NT, Johnson PJ: Idiopathic acute hepatic disease in horses: 12 cases (1982–1992). J Am Vet Med Assoc 204:1934–1937, 1994.

Nation PN: Alsike clover poisoning: A review. Can Vet J 30:410–415, 1989.

Pearson EG, Hedstrom OR, Poppenga RH: Hepatic cirrhosis and hemochromatosis in three horses. J Am Vet Med Assoc 204:1053–1056, 1994.

Watson TDG, Love S: Equine hyperlipidemia. Comp Cont Ed Pract Vet 16:89–97, 1994.

Pyrrolizidine Alkaloid Toxicosis

ERWIN G. PEARSON
Corvallis, Oregon

Pyrrolizidine alkaloid toxicosis, often called *Senecio* or ragwort poisoning, is the most common cause of liver disease in some areas. Poisoning occurs when horses consume sufficient amounts of the alkaloid-containing plants (Table 1). The lethal dose for horses is about 200 mg of pyrrolizidine alkaloid per kilogram of body weight, but the lethal dose varies with the specific alkaloids. Typically, a horse must ingest about 5% of its body weight of dry *Senecio*. The toxicity of other plants varies somewhat, depending on the alkaloid content. Pyrrolizidine alkaloid toxicity is usually delayed and often chronic. Clinical signs may not appear until up to a year after consumption of the alkaloid-containing plant has ceased. The toxin is probably not cumulative, but the toxic effect is thought to persist. The toxic effect is crosslinking and alkylating of double-strand deoxyribonucleic acid (DNA).

CLINICAL SIGNS

The signs of pyrrolizidine alkaloid toxicity are essentially those of liver failure. Weight loss, behavioral change, and icterus are the most commonly seen signs. Hepatic encephalopathy is often part of the clinical picture and includes mental depression, ataxia, yawning, head pressing, continual walking, and stertorous breathing.

DIAGNOSIS

Tests for diagnosing liver disease or failure are described on page 214. History is often not helpful because the horse may not be currently consuming the plant. Serum activity of liver-derived enzymes is usually increased. Gamma glutamyltransaminopeptidase and alkaline phosphatase levels are elevated when the horse shows clinical signs. Sorbitol dehydrogenase (SDH), glutamate dehydrogenase (GDH), and lactate dehydrogenase (LDH) activity may have returned to normal by the time clinical signs are apparent. Serum total bile acid concentration is increased and may be of prognostic value. Sulfobromophthalein (BSP) retention and serum ammonia levels are increased terminally.

A liver biopsy and histopathologic examination of the tissues is needed to help differentiate pyrrolizidine alkaloid toxicity from other liver disease. Megalocytic hepatocytes are the hallmark of pyrrolizidine alkaloid poisoning, but they are not consistently present in all stages of the disease, and they are occasionally seen in aflatoxin poisoning. Most affected horses have biliary hyperplasia, focal hepatocyte necrosis, and portal cirrhosis. Sulphur-bound pyrollic metabolites have been found on the hemoglobin of horses with pyrrolizidine alkaloid exposure.

A poor prognosis is indicated by continual elevation of GGT and alkaline phosphatase levels along with the return

TABLE 1. COMMON PLANTS CONTAINING PYRROLIZIDINE ALKALOID

GENERIC NAME	COMMON NAME	GEOGRAPHIC DISTRIBUTION
Senecio vulgaris	Common groundsel	Western US
Senecio jacobaea	Tansy ragwort	Western Washington, Oregon, California, New England, Eastern Canada, Great Britain, Australia, New Zealand
Senecio douglasii var. *longilobus*	Threadleaf groundsel	Arizona, Colorado, New Mexico, Texas, Utah
Senecio trianularis	Tar weed	Western US
Amsinckia intermedia	Fiddleneck	Western US
Crotalaria sp.	Rattlebox	Southern US (Atlantic to Texas)
Echium plantaquineum	Salvation Jane/Vipers' buglos	Eastern US, California, Australia
Heliotropium europeaum	Common heliotrope	Eastern US, Australia
Symphytum officinale	Comfrey	Cultivated in US
Cynoglossum officinale	Hound's tongue	Western US, Europe

to normal levels of SDH, GDH, or LDH. Horses with serum bile acid concentration of greater than 50 μm/L are less likely to survive. Histologic evidence of bridging fibrosis usually indicates that the animal will not remain alive for more than 6 months. Terminally, the serum albumin level may be reduced and clotting times prolonged.

TREATMENT

Treatment is not likely to be successful in most cases of pyrrolizidine alkaloid toxicosis, especially in those with poor prognostic indicators, as described earlier. The antimitotic effect of the crosslinking of DNA and the bridging fibrosis in the liver makes regeneration of the liver difficult. If treatment is undertaken, removing pyrrolizidine alkaloid-containing plants from the diet is the obvious first step. General dietary or pharmacologic treatment of the liver as described under Theiler's disease may be used (see page 215). Some agents have been proved ineffective in controlled studies. These include butylated hydroxyanisole, cysteine, vitamin B complex, ethoxyquin, magnesium oxide, methionine, and other special vitamin and mineral supplements. Colchicine reduces the progression of fibrosis in some people with hepatic cirrhosis, but there is no scientific evidence that it is helpful in horses with pyrrolizidine alkaloid toxicosis. Branch chain amino acid supplementation may reduce neurologic signs but not prolong life.

Prevention is most important and involves preventing the horses from consuming pyrrolizidine alkaloid-containing plants in pasture, hay, cubes, or pellets. The plants can usually be controlled by using chemical sprays that kill broad-leaf plants, such as 2–4 D. *Senecio* is a biennial, and cultivation eventually reduces its density. Sheep can be grazed on *Senecio* pastures because microorganisms in their rumen make them less susceptible to the toxicity. The plants are eaten by sheep and do not go to seed. Biologic control has been successful in the Pacific Northwest. The cinnabar moth and tansy flea beetle selectively eat tansy ragwort.

Supplemental Readings

Cheeke PR, Schmitz JA, Lassen ED, Pearson EG: Effects of dietary supplementation with ethoxyquin, magnesium oxide, methionine hydroxy analog, and B vitamins on tansy ragwort (*Senecio jacobaea*) toxicosis in beef cattle. Am J Vet Res 46:2179–2183, 1985.

Craig AM, Pearson EG, Meyer C, Schmitz JA: Clinicopathologic studies of tansy ragwort toxicosis in ponies: Sequential serum and histopathological changes. J Equine Vet Sci 11(5):261–271, 1991.

Garrett BJ, Holtan DW, Cheeke PR, Schmitz JA, Rogers QR: Effects of dietary supplementation with butylated hydroxyanisole, cysteine, and B vitamins on tansy ragwort (*Senecio jacobaea*) toxicosis in ponies. Am J Vet Res 45:459–464, 1984.

Johnson AE: Failure of mineral-vitamin supplements to prevent tansy ragwort (*Senecio jacobaea*) toxicosis in cattle. Am J Vet Res 43:718–724, 1982.

Lessard P, Wilson WD, Olander HJ, Rogers QR, Mendel VE: Clinicopathologic study of horses surviving pyrrolizidine alkaloid (*Senecio vulgaris*) toxicosis. Am J Vet Res 47:1776–1780, 1986.

Mendel VE, Witt MR, Gitchell BS, Gribble DN, Rogers QR, Segall HJ, Knight HD: Pyrrolizidine alkaloid-induced liver disease in horses: An early diagnosis. Am J Vet Res 49:572–578, 1988.

Seawright AA, Hrdlicka J, Wright JD, Kerr DR, Mattocks AR, Jukes R: The identification of hepatotoxic pyrrolizidine alkaloid exposure in horses by the demonstration of sulphur-bound pyrrolic metabolites on their hemoglobin. Vet Hum Toxicol 33:286–287, 1991.

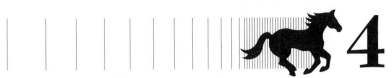

SECTION 4

THE CARDIOVASCULAR
SYSTEM

Edited by Mark W. Patteson

Diagnostic Techniques in Equine Cardiology

PETER W. PHYSICK-SHEARD
Guelph, Ontario

The cardiovascular system displays distinct structural and functional characteristics that are readily accessible to the clinician. They reflect the cyclic behavior of the heart and its associated electrical activity, sound, physical motion, and three-dimensional anatomy, and are exploited during in-depth system examination. Peripheral manifestations of circulatory function (e.g., capillary refill, status of veins) provide further opportunities for assessment of system performance. The ready availability of these dynamic markers makes the cardiovascular system unique among body systems.

Unfortunately, by giving rise to a wide variety of clinical features these characteristics are also a source of confusion. Additional challenges are introduced by the horse's very large cardiovascular functional reserve and by variations that reflect breed, physical conditioning, and a labile response to environmental stimuli. A solid grounding in anatomy and physiology and a systematic approach to examination are necessary if accurate observations and interpretations are to be made. Appropriate application of diagnostic techniques can aid this process greatly.

The following review highlights recent and emerging techniques and draws attention to aspects of more traditional procedures that may not receive sufficient emphasis. Additional emerging techniques are discussed elsewhere in this section.

REVIEW OF PERFORMANCE RECORDS

Most horses are presented for cardiovascular evaluation because they are maintained as athletes, and for this reason the analysis of performance records can be a useful diagnostic aid. Current performance should be compared with normal values for the breed in the same class and to previous individual performance. Seasonal fluctuations in performance and circumstances of individual competitive events should be considered. Currently, performance records are readily available for Standardbred and, to a lesser extent, Thoroughbred racehorses.

Interpretation depends upon the individual horse and competitive event. Typically, racehorses with subacute or chronic cardiovascular disease and insufficiency show a tendency to plateau. Over a season, the affected horse's performance does not necessarily deteriorate and may even improve, but not to the same extent as that of other relatively normal horses with which it competes; affected horses' performances thus seem to be deteriorating. Within a race, affected horses lack stamina and appear to fade. A tendency to unsteadiness may be seen, but only when there has been acute onset of a serious arrhythmia or when cardiovascular reserve is significantly reduced in relation to performance demands. Performance records may reveal the time at which problems first started.

AUSCULTATION

The most valuable diagnostic aid is a thorough physical examination, including careful auscultation of the heart. Specific findings in different disease entities are discussed later in this section. The ease with which sounds are heard is a function of both frequency and amplitude or intensity.

225

Most heart sounds are of low frequency (<600 Hz), well below the optimal range for the human ear (variously described as 1000/2000–4000 Hz), with some very significant sounds below 150 Hz. Low-frequency sounds are often also of low amplitude. This is important, because low-frequency, pansystolic, blowing, band-shaped murmurs that can be difficult to detect are of far greater clinical significance in the horse than easily detected, high-frequency, midsystolic, crescendo-decrescendo sounds.

For effective auscultation of the equine heart a stethoscope must have a frequency response that extends below 50 Hz. Stethoscopes vary greatly in their ability to detect low-frequency sounds, so purchasing an inexpensive model is false economy. A number of newer, and admittedly more expensive, stethoscopes have greatly improved low-frequency response. The best stethoscope for small animal work is not necessarily the best for equine auscultation, and a stethoscope that is optimized for detection of low-frequency cardiac sounds will do an equally impressive job on other body systems, particularly the respiratory system. Use of the bell on a twin-headed stethoscope improves detection of low-frequency sounds, especially if only light pressure is used, but reduces the detection high frequencies. Because heart sounds comprise a mixture of frequencies, the bell should add another dimension to auscultatory skills but should not replace the diaphragm. Use of an electronic stethoscope to amplify sounds is presently rarely effective. These units lack an adequate low-end response and can de-emphasize low-frequency sounds. They also contribute their own interference patterns. Use of electronic filtering to remove this interference usually further distorts or otherwise diminishes the original signal.

During auscultation, background noise from motors and radios should be eliminated. Because a tense, nervous horse is difficult to auscultate, it should be re-examined when it has relaxed but not after administration of agents that alter autonomic balance or blood pressure, because such drugs may modify heart sounds. Overinterpretation of abnormal sounds heard in horses experiencing extreme changes in homeostasis should be avoided. Also, caution should be exercised when examining horses that are agitated or in pain, or those that are only partly warmed up at the start of exercise. Unless there are obvious signs or a history of cardiac disease, unusual findings are noted and reassessed later when the horse's condition is stable.

The cognitive processes used by clinicians during auscultation are likely to vary, but it may be useful when listening for murmurs to "listen for the silence" in systole and diastole. These intervals are essentially silent in the normal horse, and the realization that an interval is not silent is often the first clue that there is a murmur. Clinicians can then use this insight to characterize the extra sounds.

Phonocardiography, in which a graphic representation of heart sounds is recorded on a strip chart alongside an electrocardiogram (ECG), can be very useful in determining the relationship between normal heart sounds (transients) and murmurs, and in characterizing unusual transients such as gallop rhythms caused by unusual emphasis of the third heart sound. However, in the horse the low resting heart rate allows most abnormalities to be adequately characterized by careful auscultation and perhaps simultaneous palpation of the pulse. Limitations in technology and technique rarely allow a phonocardiograph to reveal the subtlety that can be detected by careful auscultation.

HEART RATE VARIABILITY ANALYSIS

The pattern of beat to beat (i.e., instantaneous) variation in heart rate contains information indicative of underlying autonomic nervous system balance. This information could theoretically be used on a real-time basis in clinical medicine or retrospectively when data are gathered during standardized exercise tests to gain insight into contributions made by the autonomic nervous system to various physiologic and pathophysiologic responses. Clinical applications are likely to include monitoring of response to therapy and anticipation of clinical change. Data are derived by the collection of a single-channel ECG signal and its processing, using dedicated hardware and software. The technique has the potential advantage of allowing real-time, stall-side monitoring of autonomic nervous system function. Heart rate variability analysis in the horse requires further validation before it can be applied in clinical medicine, however. The practical utility of the technique may be limited by the horse's labile response to environmental stimuli.

ELECTROCARDIOGRAPHY

Electrocardiography is used for cardiac monitoring; detection and interpretation of cardiac arrhythmias; and detection of changes in myocardial mass, myocardial mass distribution, and chamber size. The first two are valid and important applications in equine cardiology. The last application, vectorcardiography, to detect changes in myocardial mass or mass distribution, has been eclipsed by echocardiography.

A very limited amount of information is available in the equine body surface ECG because the electrical activation of most areas of the myocardium does not proceed according to major wavefronts of depolarization. Alternate vectorcardiographic lead systems have been investigated but the effort and instrumentation necessary to glean the limited information they provide are not justified by the results. ECG leads other than a simple bipolar lead are rarely used, therefore, with perhaps one exception (see later).

In bipolar leads, one electrode (most often an alligator clamp in large animals) is designated the negative electrode, the other the positive electrode. By convention, an electrical signal (wave of myocardial depolarization) passing toward the positive electrode results in a positive deflection on the ECG. Usually a third cable and electrode are employed, the "ground" or "earth" cable, the use of which is necessary to obtain a stable signal. An ECG signal that is large with clearly distinguishable waveforms is easier to interpret and is minimally obscured by noise. Fortunately, in the horse the primary electrical axes of all three waveforms (P, QRS, and T) are oriented approximately along the long axis of the heart (i.e., from base to apex). Wherever the two electrodes are placed, therefore, if a line

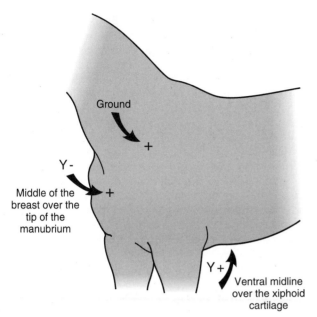

Figure 1. Diagrammatic representation of the equine thorax showing the points of attachment for the Y-lead ECG. The precise position of the ground lead is not critical, as long as it is used.

The ECG machine must be effectively grounded through the electrical outlet. Poor grounding results in electrical interference on the ECG and places the patient at risk of electrocution if the machine malfunctions. As a precaution and an aid to reducing interference, the horse should stand on a dry rubber mat to isolate it from the ground. Metal stocks defeat this precaution. ECG machines should receive regular maintenance. Battery-operated units are fine as long as the battery is charged. The ECG must be run for at least 2 minutes to reduce the chance of missing arrhythmias. The tracing must be labelled with the date and time, horse identifier, lead, sensitivity (gain), paper speed (very important), and location at which the tracing was recorded. It is also important to mount the ECG as a permanent record before it escapes into the bowels of the clinician's truck.

The approach to reading the ECG is as important as collecting it properly. First, the clinician must check the heart rate and be aware of the effect an arrhythmia may have on rate. Instantaneous rate (determined from the interval between adjacent complexes) may be very high or very low. An accurate overall rate may be determined only by counting complexes over a 30- or 60-second interval. Overall rate may be of limited relevance if instantaneous rate is so low or high that cardiac output is significantly compromised, with a danger of syncope. Rhythm is assessed next, with due attention to the wide range of variation normally found in the resting horse. Finally, the clinician must assess the conformation of individual waveforms. Waveform conformations usually encountered in the Y lead in the horse are shown in Figure 2. Although waveform conformation is especially valuable as an aid to the interpretation of arrhythmias, abnormalities may be found even in cases with apparently normal rhythm. Examiners must check carefully to ensure that every QRS has a preceding P wave. The relationships between these three pieces of

joining them is approximately parallel to this axis, a large, easily read signal results. An ECG lead is named according to where on the body the electrodes are attached. With the electrodes attached as shown in Figure 1, the lead is called lead Y. By convention, the negative electrode is attached at the manubrium, which results in a primarily negative-going signal in most horses.

The use of a standardized lead allows efficient comparison between successive tracings and between cases, and for this reason the use of the Y lead is recommended. Limb leads (i.e., leads I, II, and III, where the electrodes are attached to the forelimbs and the left hindlimb) can be used but offer no advantages and several disadvantages, notably susceptibility to movement artifact, and, in some horses, small waveforms. Most standard ECG machines are designed on the assumption that the user will be taking limb leads. To take a Y-lead ECG with a standard machine, the clinician must simply set the lead selector to lead I and attach the left arm cable (the positive electrode for lead I, usually color-coded black or yellow) at the xiphoid cartilage in the midline, and the negative electrode (white or red) at the manubrium. The ground cable (green or black) can go anywhere over the base of the neck where the skin is loose enough to allow its reliable attachment.

An exception to the use of a single lead involves cases in which a waveform appears to be missing from the ECG complex. Occasionally, for example, depolarization of the atria proceeds largely at right angles to the axis of the Y lead, and there will be no obvious P wave. Because the differential diagnosis of this abnormality includes severe electrolyte imbalance and atrial standstill, it is important to look for the P wave. To rule out the possibility of a significantly altered axis of depolarization, the electrodes should be attached sequentially at locations that create two different axes that each run at right angles to the Y lead. If the P wave is still missing it probably is not there at all.

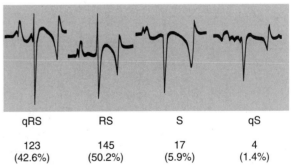

qRS	RS	S	qS
123 (42.6%)	145 (50.2%)	17 (5.9%)	4 (1.4%)

Figure 2. Distribution of Y-lead QRS waveform conformations for 279 horses of various breeds that showed no clinical evidence of cardiovascular disease. The relative size of the R and S waves varies, though the Q wave is invariably small. Overall QRS size and conformation may vary widely in cases of ventricular ectopic origin of excitation. The P and T waves shown are typical for the lead. Frequencies for the P wave are not presented. P waves are most often split (bifid), however, and occasionally biphasic (negative-positive). Little clinical significance can be attached to the conformation of the P wave, other than the observation that variation suggests variation in the origin of the atrial signal or in the path of depolarization. The T wave is highly labile and varies from beat to beat and moment to moment, particularly in response to changes in heart rate and degree of arousal. The clinical significance attached to T-wave changes in humans cannot be extrapolated to the horse.

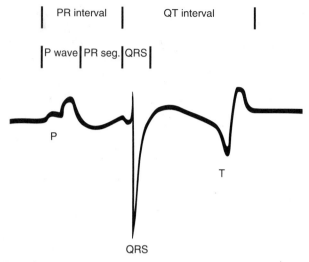

Figure 3. Definition of ECG intervals shown in Table 1. In the equine ECG, definition of the precise beginning and end of waveforms can be difficult. With the exception of progressive changes in QRS duration during drug therapy and electrolyte disorders, no attempt should be made to attach significance to small variation in intervals and durations.

information allow arrhythmias to be detected and, in most cases, interpreted (see page 240).

Scalar measurements of intervals between waveforms and the durations of the waveforms themselves (illustrated in Fig. 3 and presented in Table 1) are of limited practical value. Horses exhibit wide variation in intervals, both within and between subjects (see Table 1) and similarly wide variation in conformation of the P, and particularly the T, wave. What is usually important in reading an equine ECG is not the absolute interval but the pattern and range of variation exhibited. However, careful attention should be paid to ECG intervals in horses receiving certain medications. For example, prolongation of QRS duration can be an indication of toxicity during quinidine sulphate therapy in the treatment of atrial fibrillation. Significant changes in intervals also occur with severe electrolyte imbalances.

ECHOCARDIOGRAPHY

With the exception of electrocardiography, echocardiography has become the most frequently applied and most

useful diagnostic modality in the further evaluation of equine cardiac disease. Errors occur in the application of the modality because of limited awareness both of the physical principles of ultrasound and its use in an animal the size of the horse, and of the most appropriate machine settings to obtain diagnostic and artifact-free images. These errors can lead to misinterpretation or overinterpretation of echo findings and misdiagnoses. The following notes are intended to provide some basic guidance to the application of cardiac ultrasound in the horse, but they are necessarily superficial. The physics of two-dimensional ultrasound are well documented in the veterinary literature and are not discussed here in any detail. However, M-mode and Doppler echocardiography are discussed because a working knowledge of the physics involved in these modalities is essential to their correct use. The reader is strongly advised to read more widely before attempting to apply this technique. Feigenbaum (1994) is an excellent resource.

Ultrasound Machines

Ultrasound machines (echographs) used in veterinary medicine are all basically designed to produce a two-dimensional (2D) scan of the tissues beneath the hand-held transducer. In phased-array transducers, an ultrasound beam is successively redirected, electronically or mechanically, to sweep across an arc, the field of view, which appears on the screen as a sector; hence the term *sector scan* (Fig. 4). Linear array transducers, the type typically used in pregnancy diagnosis, have limited value in cardiac applications because the transducer aperture is large and thus a wide window is required through which to interrogate tissues. Cardiac windows are typically quite small (see later).

There is an important relationship between transducer frequency and depth of penetration and resolution. The smallest object an ultrasound beam can detect is one whose dimension is at least one fourth of the beam's wavelength; the shorter the wavelength (i.e., the higher the frequency), the greater the potential for detection of fine detail. However, a high-frequency ultrasound beam (e.g., 7.5 or 10 MHz) rapidly becomes attenuated as it passes through tissue, because so much of the beam is reflected or scattered by objects in the near-field. Because most adult equine echocardiographic assessments require a penetration depth of 20 cm at the absolute minimum, and ideally

TABLE 1.   SCALAR VALUES FOR THE Y-LEAD ECG

	Heart Rate (bpm)	P Wave Duration (msec)	PR Interval (msec)	PR Segment (msec)	QRS Duration (msec)	QT Interval (msec)
n	279	265	265	265	266	266
Mean	34.85	139.64	312.21	174.61	114.73	510.78
s.e.m.	0.32	1.75	3.35	3.04	1.16	2.59
Range	18–44	45–331	155–530	70–455	60–208	280–620
1st quartile	32	125	280	141.5	100	485
3rd quartile	39	155	340	200	125	540

Data presented are for a group of 279 light horses of various breeds, ages 11 months to 18 years. Animals with clinically significant arrhythmias or other evidence of cardiovascular disease were excluded from this population, but horses exhibiting supraventricular arrhythmias of a type or degree not considered clinically significant were included. For horses with first and second degree partial AV block (1–PAVB and 2–PAVB) the longest PR interval was used. All horses with 1–PAVB (n = 38) were included and all horses with 2–PAVB that did not drop consecutive beats or block more often than every fourth sinus signal (n = 53) were also included. See Figure 3 for definition of intervals. (s.e.m. = standard error of the mean)

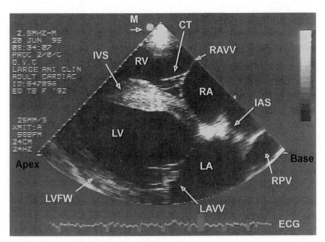

Figure 4. Freeze-frame of a 90° gray-scale sector scan image produced with a 2.5-MHz phased array transducer and 24-cm penetration depth. The image plane is a right parasternal, four-chamber, long-axis view. The ECG at the bottom of the screen scrolls from left to right, with the gray block showing the stage of the cardiac cycle (midsystole in this example) at which the image was taken. This horse has atrial fibrillation. For purposes of orientation, the transducer has a marker (usually a stud) positioned at the "edge" of the 2D beam and maintained by the echocardiographer in a consistent relationship to the horse. The relationship of this marker to the image is indicated by the marker (M) at the apex. In this scan the stud was positioned facing down, so that the apex of the heart is to the left, base to the right. RV—right ventricle; RAVV—right atrioventricular (AV) valve (septal and right anterior cusps); CT—chordae tendineae of the right AV valve; RA—right atrium; IAS—interatrial septum; IVS—interventricular septum; LV—left ventricle; LA—left atrium; LAVV—left AV valve; RPV—a right pulmonary vein; LVFW—left ventricular free wall.

28 to 30 cm, the examiner is limited in adult horses to a 2 to 2.5 MHz transducer. For most practical purposes the detail provided by these transducers is adequate. Higher frequency transducers can be used in foals and in adults for evaluation of structures in the near field.

Transducers both emit ultrasound and receive returning echoes, sound being reflected from interfaces between tissues with significant difference in acoustic impedance (ability to transmit ultrasound). Sound is also refracted and scattered; echocardiographs are designed to maximize detection of reflected sound. The strongest signal arises when ultrasound encounters an interface perpendicularly, and a high proportion of sound waves is reflected directly back to the transducer. Very little sound is reflected by structures and media that are anechoic, such as most fluids, including blood, and these areas appear dark on the screen. A highly echogenic interface close to the transducer may reflect so much sound that little is left to penetrate deeper structures, which are thus hidden. Assessment of deeper tissues may also be complicated by reverberations (an artifact consisting of multiple parallel echo shadows), which may form below such prominent interfaces.

M-mode Echocardiography

If only a single, narrow, stationary beam of ultrasound is used to produce an "ice-pick" view of cardiac structures, a screen image is produced consisting only of a series of bright spots reflecting the location along the path of the beam at which echoic structures were encountered. This is the original B or brightness mode. Because the cardiac structures are moving, the relationship of the dots on the screen changes constantly. If the screen is made to scroll, with time as the x-axis, an M- or motion-mode image is produced (Fig. 5). This was the original mode for assessment of cardiac function, and it continues to be an extremely useful tool for a number of purposes. In particular, it is essential if the timing of cardiac events is to be assessed, and is also ideal for evaluation of high-frequency, low-amplitude axial movement (i.e., movement in the same direction as the ultrasound beam) of valves. Although the image presented on the screen in M-mode has both breadth and depth, it is still a one-dimensional view, the second dimension being time. On most newer machines, M-mode and 2D mode can be combined, an M-mode cursor being selectively positioned on the 2D image to determine precisely where the M-mode, ice-pick view is to be gathered (see Fig. 5).

Spectral and Color-Flow Doppler Ultrasound

Frequent updating of the screen image on an echocardiograph allows movement of cardiac structures to be seen in real time. This movement causes a slight frequency shift in echoes returning from structures with axial movement. This shift, known as the Doppler shift, is proportional to the velocity of the moving structure in the direction of the

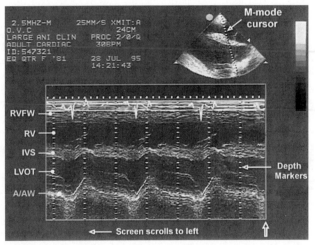

Figure 5. M-mode image produced with a 2.5-MHz phased array transducer. The image plane is a right parasternal, long-axis, four-chamber view with the left ventricular outflow tract brought into the image by angling the transducer beam forward. The resultant sector scan image is shown at the top right. The M-mode cursor has been moved manually on this scan to lie across the right ventricle (RV) and interventricular septum (IVS), and crosses the left side of the heart at the level of the left ventricular outflow tract (LVOT), just below the aortic valve. The M-mode image in the rectangular frame shows how structures intersected by this cursor move with time, and shows three complete cardiac cycles (the ECG can be seen superimposed on the right ventricular free wall, RVFW). The screen scrolls from right to left, with the open arrow (*bottom right*) marking the most recent part of the image. Movement of the interventricular septum and of the base of the aorta and adjacent atrial wall (A/AW) can be clearly seen. Apparent reduction in thickness of the interventricular septum during ventricular systole is paradoxical and reflects downward movement of the heart base during this part of the cardiac cycle; the septum is thinner toward its base. The depth markers show 1-cm increments and appear on the M-mode screen every second.

beam. When sound is reflected from a surface moving toward the transducer, its frequency is increased; when the surface is moving away frequency is decreased. The shift is very small for most slow-moving cardiac structures such as chamber walls or valves.

Blood reflects very little sound and is seen only as a vague swirling cloud, sometimes referred to as "smoke," in heart chambers. Though this smoke is often viewed as significant in humans, it is a frequent observation in horses and is regarded as normal. Whether it is seen is strongly influenced by gain and compensation settings. During most of the cardiac cycle, blood flow generates a minimal Doppler shift in reflected sound. However, during some parts of the cycle blood moves quite rapidly, especially as it passes through the outflow tracts, and produces a Doppler shift, proportional to flow velocity, that can be measured despite the limited amount of reflected sound. The shift is greatest where blood flow disturbances occur, because these are associated with very high local blood flow velocities. Disturbances are found frequently in such clinically significant conditions as valvular insufficiencies and congenital shunts.

Doppler shifts have been exploited in the development of techniques that assess movement of blood within the heart. Two of these techniques, pulsed Doppler and continuous-wave Doppler, are primarily concerned with the detection of normal and abnormal blood flow and measurement of blood flow velocity. Color-flow Doppler additionally allows flow patterns to be monitored visually and supports measurement of velocity in flow disturbances. Analysis of blood flow patterns and flow velocity can be of great diagnostic value and can support assessment of cardiac function. For example, by measuring the diameter of an outflow tract and flow velocity at the level of measurement, and by making some assumptions about flow profile in the vessel, it is possible to estimate cardiac output.

In pulsed Doppler, a "gate," usually represented on the screen as a diamond or similar shape on the M-mode cursor, is positioned on a 2D image in the location at which the examiner anticipates finding flow disturbance (e.g., a regurgitant jet of blood). When pulsed Doppler is then selected the screen switches to a horizontally scrolling display, and pulses of ultrasound at a fixed pulse repetition frequency are generated. Doppler shifts in the frequency of echoes returning from the selected region are measured and translated into blood flow velocity and displayed on the screen as a gray-scale spectral shadow in a mode referred to as *spectral Doppler*. The density of the shadow, sometimes referred to as an *envelope* if it is well formed (Fig. 6), is proportional to the intensity of flow, whereas its height and depth are indicative of blood flow velocity. The direction of the shadow (assuming aliasing to be absent, see later) indicates the direction of blood flow, down usually being away from the transducer, up being toward. With the assistance of the simultaneously collected ECG signal, which should *always* accompany the ultrasound image, the relationship of flow disturbance to the cardiac cycle and to any murmurs heard can be assessed.

In continuous-wave Doppler examination, the system uses a continuous, not a pulsed, ultrasound wave and samples continuously along the entire length of the cursor. Movement anywhere along the cursor is recorded and displayed in a scrolling window, but the precise origin of

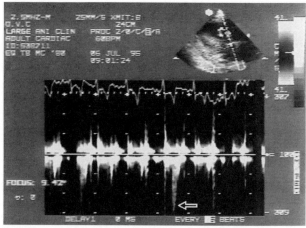

Figure 6. Color-flow and continuous-wave Doppler spectral Doppler display of right AV regurgitation in a 15-year-old horse with atrial fibrillation and left heart failure. The sector scan image at top right shows a right parasternal, two-chamber long-axis view intersecting the right atrium and ventricle and right AV valve and passing through the center of the interventricular septum. A superimposed color-flow display (shown here in gray scale) reveals systolic flow disturbance in the right atrium. The cursor has been positioned to intersect the area of greatest disturbance and the continuous-wave Doppler sampling cursor positioned on top of this area. The rectangular display (scrolling from right to left) shows a gray scale image indicating flow velocity in this region. The open horizontal arrow marks a well-formed envelope, indicating high-velocity flow away from the transducer (i.e., from right ventricle to right atrium). The envelope is not equally clear on all cycles because of difficulty maintaining a constant relationship between the continuous-wave Doppler cursor and the regurgitant stream. After correction for the lack of a coaxial relationship between the beam and the regurgitant stream, maximal flow velocity over six nonconsecutive cycles indicated a mean pressure gradient across the valve of approximately 60 mmHg, consistent (in the absence of pulmonic stenosis) with pulmonary hypertension. The quality of the spectral display in this image could have been improved further by turning off the color display during Doppler interrogation. Brief intense shadows on the spectral display reflect movement of the right AV valve through the sampling beam.

the signal cannot be determined. This is not as great a limitation as one might suspect, however, because it is usually possible to position the cursor so that it intersects only one area of flow disturbance. Availability of simultaneous color-flow Doppler technique (see later) greatly increases confidence that this is indeed the case and assists in positioning the cursor for both continuous-wave and pulsed Doppler methods. Measurement of flow velocity allows estimates to be made of the pressure gradient driving that flow, and can thus be used to detect abnormal pressure gradients, such as pulmonary hypertension in left heart failure (see Fig. 6).

Doppler shift determination of blood flow velocities in general, and use of pulsed Doppler in particular, are subject to some technical constraints. Because of the cardiac windows that must be used in the horse (see later), it is rarely if ever possible to get the ultrasound beam coaxial with (i.e., on top of and parallel with) the direction of blood flow. As a result, measurements usually underestimate true blood flow velocity and can be corrected only with caution. Movement of the heart along its long axis during the cardiac cycle usually results in regurgitant flow constantly moving in relation to the sampling beam. Pulsed Doppler ultrasound technique is also limited in the peak flow velocities it can detect. At high flow velocities, aliasing (a digital sampling error whereby frequencies higher than one half the pulse repetition frequency are measured incorrectly) occurs. Continuous-wave Doppler technique is not subject to this constraint. With pulsed Doppler, maximal detectable velocity falls as the depth of the event of interest increases. This factor can be of great significance in the horse where, for example, aortic regurgitation may be 10 to 15 cm beneath the skin surface.

With pulsed Doppler technique, detection of flow velocity is also a function of transducer frequency, lower frequency transducers being able to detect higher velocities. This consideration contrasts with the relationship between transducer frequency and resolution in other modes of cardiac ultrasonography but works in favor of equine echocardiography. In addition, in contrast to other echocardiographic modes, Doppler signals are best detected if movement is axial (i.e., parallel) with the ultrasound beam, whereas M-mode images are brightest when interfaces are perpendicular to the beam. The best images for M-mode are not usually the best for Doppler flow detection, and vice versa, but in the horse the options for changing views are very limited when compared with small animals and humans.

In color-flow systems, pulsed Doppler-derived Doppler shifts in returning echoes are color-mapped onto the 2D or M-mode screen to provide a real-time visual image of blood flow (Fig. 7). Color and brightness can be selected to display relative velocity and direction of flow, whereas severe blood flow disturbances are represented as a mosaic of colors. This mosaic reflects the presence of multiple different interfaces of high-velocity blood flow of varying direction, typical of severe disturbances of flow, and also aliasing errors because of high velocities. Aliasing results in abrupt transition from one color to another. Variable gain settings allow the threshold at which flow is displayed

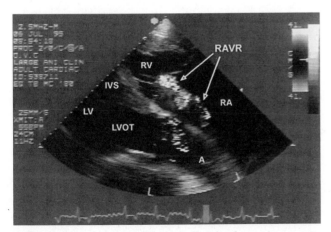

Figure 7. Right parasternal, long-axis, four-chamber sector-scan view with left ventricular outflow tract (LVOT) and superimposed color-flow Doppler (shown here in gray scale). An intense trail originating at the right AV valve and extending approximately 9 cm into the right atrium (RA) reveals right AV regurgitation (RAVR) to be present in this late systolic display. Systolic flow disturbance can also be seen in the aorta (A). The image was acquired with a 2.5-MHz, phased-array transducer with a penetration depth of 24 cm. Note that the color-flow image covers only a 30° sector of this 90° sector scan image. RV—right ventricle, IVS—interventricular septum, LV—left ventricle.

to be determined manually. Color-flow Doppler technique makes identification of flow disturbances in all situations except perhaps regurgitation at the left AV valve relatively simple. Although in the horse the left AV valve is accessible from either side of the thorax, the orientation of the valve is such that regurgitant jets tend to flow almost perpendicular to the direction of the ultrasound beam; such jets can easily be missed.

Despite the information that can be derived from these techniques, clinicians should proceed with caution. Blood flow disturbances are complex, three-dimensional events that change constantly, and echocardiography reveals only a thin slice through the totality of whatever is occurring. Inappropriate use of equipment such as inappropriate color-flow gain settings, overinterpretation, inadequate attention to calibration, failure to allow for the effects of such variables as heart rate, respiratory rate, or psychological state can lead to mistakes. For example, if gain is too high when using color-flow Doppler technique, every chamber of a normal heart can be filled with a pattern suggesting widespread flow disturbance when none is present. Anyone can turn on the color-flow button, but experience and insight are necessary to differentiate between a significant finding, normal variation, and artifact. In addition, when imaging an adult horse, the equipment is usually operating at the extremes of its capacity. Simultaneous display of a wide-sector 2D image and color-flow mapping of even a small sector of blood flow (see Fig. 7) can significantly limit the frequency of screen updating and reduce the quality of the screen image. Events, especially those toward the limits of penetration, may be displayed with limited clarity and an increased probability of artifact. Reducing the angle of the screen image (i.e., reducing the size of the sector) can help greatly but may not be enough to allow a faint signal to be seen clearly. False-negative findings are as likely as false positives.

Color-flow Doppler represents a very significant advance, providing insights into cardiac function. With the information gained, however, some confusion also arises. Of particular significance is the realization that flow disturbances of sufficient magnitude to have obvious clinical significance can be present without there being a detectable murmur.

Standardized Image Planes

The expressions and short forms used to describe intracardiac image planes and measurements in echocardiography can be confusing. The conventions on which these terms are based are easy to understand when the ground rules are clear and the reader appreciates the objective of a measurement. They also provide a necessary lexicon by which examinations can be standardized and findings communicated. The reader is encouraged to refer to the attached bibliography for more detail.

Echocardiographic examination proceeds according to standardized image planes based upon those developed for use in humans by the American Society of Echocardiography. Many of these views, particularly those providing a coaxial view of the outflow tracts (a view from apex to base), are not available to the equine echocardiographer because of equine thoracic anatomy and dimension. The equine heart is examined through the left and right parasternal cardiac windows at the intercostal spaces. Because

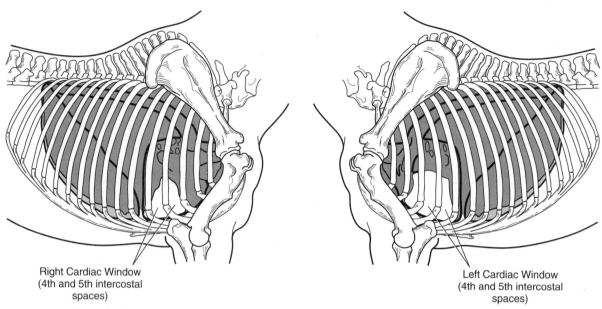

Right Cardiac Window
(4th and 5th intercostal
spaces)

Left Cardiac Window
(4th and 5th intercostal
spaces)

Figure 8. Diagrammatic representation of the equine thorax from the right and left sides showing the position of the heart in the thorax and the relationship between the heart and the overlying lung. The cardiac windows through which the heart can be imaged with ultrasound are small in comparison with the size of the heart, but a great deal of information can still be obtained. In some horses the heart can also be reached through the cranial part of the left sixth intercostal space, and with cooperation and patience, through the left third space. This latter site can be very useful in the evaluation of congenital anomalies in the foal.

all views in the horse are essentially "parasternal" the term is really superfluous. The windows are in fact the sites at which the pericardium is in direct contact with the chest wall (i.e., at which there is no intervening lung) (Fig. 8). The left window is the largest, but most diagnostic information is derived from the right. In addition, no two horses have precisely the same cardiac orientation, relative placement of the ribs, or set of the forelimbs. Clinicians should adapt these planes as necessary to realize diagnostic objectives. This is achieved by interrogating the heart by reference to intracardiac landmarks (see Reef, 1990, and Long and coworkers, 1992).

Cardiac image planes are described as long axis or short axis according to the relationship between the 2D plane of the interrogating beam and the heart. Long-axis views (see Fig. 4) thus show sections through the long axis of the

heart, whereas short-axis views (Fig. 9) show cross sections. Image planes are further defined by which chambers the view intersects. A long-axis view taken toward the caudal margin of the right cardiac window and intersecting both right and left ventricles and atria would be described as a right parasternal, long-axis, four-chamber view (see Fig. 4). The same view could be taken with the transducer beam directed forward, so that the image plane intersects the left ventricular outflow tract, and angled so that the aorta can be clearly seen leaving the left ventricle. This would be described as a right parasternal, long-axis, four-chamber view with left ventricular outflow tract optimized (see Fig. 7). A view taken in short axis from the right and at the level of the right atrioventricular (AV) valve could be described as a right parasternal short-axis view at AV valve level (see Fig. 9). The words *M-mode* would be appended

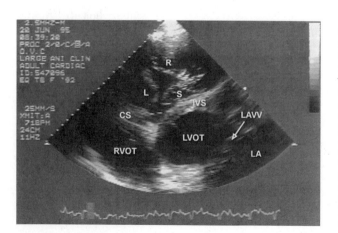

Figure 9. Early systolic, right parasternal, short-axis view of the heart base at right AV valve level. All three of the right AV valve cusps are clearly visible and appear not to meet, but this is an illusion, the plane of the image intersecting the curvature of the valve cusps above their actual point of confluence. The heart valves are not coplanar, and most short-axis heart base images clearly show no more than two valves. In this image the plane optimizes the view of the right AV valve but passes below the pulmonic and aortic valves and above the left AV valve. Note that 24 cm is not sufficient penetration to reach the far side of the heart base in this sector-scan image. Note also the dark shadow down the left side of the scan, a result of rib obstruction (rib "cut-off"). This problem occurs frequently with short-axis views using low-frequency transducers in large animals because the transducer aperture approximates the width of the intercostal space. R, L, S—right and left anterior and septal cusps of the right AV valve; IVS—interventricular septum; CS—crista supraventricularis; RVOT—right ventricular outflow tract; LVOT—left ventricular outflow tract; LAVV—base, septal cusp of left AV valve; LA—left atrium.

if the examiner placed the M-mode cursor across these views and switched to M-mode.

An infinite variety of planes can be used according to the needs of the case. However, when adaptations are employed and especially when intracardiac measurements are taken, the examiner should make careful reference to intracardiac landmarks to standardize the plane and measurements and effectively communicate findings. Measurements can be made of chamber size, wall thickness, and time intervals when using M-mode and should always be referenced to the cardiac cycle (e.g., end-diastole). This is achieved by reference to the obligatory simultaneously recorded ECG. Finally, when gathering intracardiac measurements by cardiac ultrasonography, the examiner should be aware that many measurements are not highly repeatable. The clinician always must take measurements from which clinical inferences are to be drawn such as maximal dimension of the left ventricle in diastole (LVIDD) at least three times from separately collected image planes. The inherent limitations of such measurements as indicators of cardiac status should also be appreciated.

Procedure for Acquiring Echocardiographic Images

Ultrasound does not penetrate air or bone. Bone causes a black shadow on the screen extending from the bone surface (see Fig. 9), whereas air is most likely to produce heavy reverberations on the screen in the area beyond the lung surface. When performing an ultrasound examination it is important to use a coupling gel to exclude all air between the transducer and the patient's chest wall. Clinicians must not use electrode paste; pastes containing salts can damage the transducer and do not work very well. Preparation of the skin should be aimed at avoiding trapped air. Usually the skin is clipped and shaved, which gives the best images. However, soaking the hair at the examination site thoroughly with 70% isopropyl alcohol, then applying coupling gel, taking care not to trap air bubbles, works very effectively on all horses but those with very long coats. When using this technique, the skin should be prepared immediately before imaging. Examination of obese horses, horses with heavy muscling, and those with a very round barrel-shaped chest (e.g., heavy horse breeds) can be difficult, so they must be clipped.

The importance to be attached to the position of the forelimb during examination varies. In general, Standardbreds are the least difficult and heavy horses and Warmbloods more difficult to image, although in all cases examination is easier if the horse can be persuaded to hold the forelimb forward on the side being examined. With the exception, perhaps, of foals being assessed for congenital cardiac disease, examinations should be performed with manual restraint only. Evaluation of foals can be very rewarding because one can use high-frequency transducers and obtain excellent image quality.

Pericardial disease is uncommon in the horse but can be difficult to diagnose in the early stages, when treatment is most likely to be effective. Pericardial effusion can be detected quite effectively with a regular linear array pregnancy diagnosis transducer. Penetration achieved with a 5 to 7.5-MHz transducer is quite sufficient for examination of the pericardial space. Movement of the heart in relation to surrounding tissues helps identify structures. A few practice runs on normal horses will help increase the examiner's confidence when assessing a potential clinical case.

Supplemental Readings

Evans DL: Cardiovascular adaptations to exercise and training. Vet Clin North Am Equine Pract 1(3):513–531, 1985.

Feigenbaum H: Echocardiography. 5th ed. Philadelphia, Lea & Febiger, 1994.

Littlewort MCG: The equine heart in health and disease. *In* Hickman J (ed): Equine Surgery and Medicine, ed 2. London, Academic Press, 1986, pp 1–87.

Long KJ, Bonagura JD, Darke PGG: Standardised imaging technique for guided M-mode and Doppler echocardiography in the horse. Equine Vet J 24:226–235, 1992.

Physick-Sheard PW: Cardiovascular response to exercise and training in the horse. Vet Clin North Am Equine Pract 1(2):383–417, 1985.

Physick-Sheard PW: Diseases of the cardiovascular system. Detailed examination of the cardiovascular system. *In* Colahan TC, Mayhew IG, Merritt AM, Moore JN (eds): Equine Medicine and Surgery, ed 4, vol. 1. Goleta, CA, American Veterinary Publications, 1991, pp 165–187.

Reef VB: Echocardiographic examination in the horse: The basics. Comp Cont Ed Pract Vet 12:1312–1320, 1990.

Reef VB: Evaluation of the equine cardiovascular system. Vet Clin North Am Equine Pract 1:275–288, 1985.

Electrocardiography and Echocardiography in the Exercising Horse

VIRGINIA B. REEF
Kennett Square, Pennsylvania

Electrocardiography has been used for more than 50 years to characterize cardiac arrhythmias in horses, and its usefulness in the characterization of arrhythmias in the resting horse is undisputed. Often, however, the significance of arrhythmias is difficult to determine because the arrhythmia may be intermittent or may change with a change in heart rate or excitement or following exercise.

The ability to monitor cardiac rhythm over a longer monitoring period, such as with continuous 24-hour Holter electrocardiography, can be extremely useful in further characterizing the significance of various arrhythmias. Although both resting and immediate postexercise electrocardiograms (ECGs) can be obtained in horses with performance problems or cardiac arrhythmias, the presence and severity of arrythmias during exercise cannot be determined from pre- and postexercise electrocardiography. For the latter reason, the ability to detect cardiac arrhythmias during exercise by use of radiotelemetry electrocardiography is invaluable for determining their clinical significance. Radiotelemetry electrocardiography is also invaluable for continuously monitoring cardiac rhythm during treatment for a rhythm disturbance.

The usefulness of electrocardiography for determining changes in cardiac chamber size in the horse is limited. Although changes in the configuration of the ECG complexes, particularly the QRS complex, have been reported in horses with cardiac disease, electrocardiography is neither sensitive nor specific for detecting changes in cardiac chamber size or wall thickness. Echocardiography is the technique of choice for evaluating horses with suspected cardiac enlargement. Until recently, echocardiographic examinations were confined to evaluations of horses with suspected cardiac disease. Echocardiographic examinations are performed in horses with murmurs to determine the etiology of the cardiac murmur and its clinical significance. Echocardiograms also are recommended in horses with cardiac arrhythmias, excluding the normal vagally mediated arrhythmias detected in resting horses, and in horses with suspected myocardial dysfunction or pericardial disease. Echocardiograms have also been performed in prospective racehorses to assess cardiac size, looking for an "athletic heart." The evaluation of exercise-induced myocardial dysfunction as a cause of poor performance has only recently been explored in the horse, although it has been used as part of a cardiac stress test in human beings for several years.

TWENTY-FOUR-HOUR HOLTER MONITORING

Continuous ECG recording over a 24-hour period can be successfully performed in horses and has many clinical applications. Contact electrodes, such as are used with heart rate monitoring devices, can be adapted to use with Holter monitors, enabling continuous recording of a horse's ECG during the 24-hour monitoring period. The electrodes are best held in place with a surcingle, and the monitor can be secured to the surcingle at or near the withers for maximal protection of the recording device.

A 24-hour continuous electrocardiographic study of clinically normal horses in which no cardiac disease was detected on routine examination revealed second degree atrioventricular block to be more common than previously reported. One or more periods of second-degree atrioventricular block were detected in 44% of horses during a 24-hour monitoring period, in contrast to the arrhythmia being detected in only 15 to 18% of horses during routine electrocardiography. Sinus arrhythmia was detected in only 10% of horses and sinoatrial block in 3%. Occasional atrial or ventricular extrasystoles were also detected in normal horses during the 24-hour monitoring period but were infrequent, averaging less than one extrasystole per hour. Atrial premature depolarizations were detected more frequently than ventricular premature depolarizations, with a frequency in normal horses of 27% and 15%, respectively. An accelerated idioventricular rhythm was detected occasionally in 4% of horses, and one horse had aberrant ventricular conduction. These observations reveal that occasional premature depolarizations, which are probably clinically insignificant, can occur in clinically normal horses.

Clinically significant arrhythmias may be sustained, easily detected, and characterized with routine electrocardiography, or may be intermittent and, therefore, difficult to diagnose. Often a cardiac arrhythmia was previously detected on auscultation but is absent at the time the horse is presented for an ECG. Performing a 24-hour Holter ECG enables the clinician to evaluate the horse's cardiac rhythm over a longer monitoring period and identify some arrhythmias that are intermittent.

The most common cause of an irregularly irregular rhythm detected immediately following an episode of poor performance is paroxysmal atrial fibrillation. Sinus rhythm usually returns within 24 to 48 hours and, therefore, many horses have a normal resting ECG when examined following this episode. Frequent intermittent supraventricular premature depolarizations may be detected on a continuous 24-hour ECG, supporting a tentative diagnosis of paroxysmal atrial fibrillation. A normal continuous 24-hour ECG would also support a diagnosis of paroxysmal atrial fibrillation, because this rhythm may occur without significant underlying cardiac disease and may resolve without treatment. Occasionally, horses with the history of poor performance have frequent ventricular premature depolarizations detected on a continuous 24-hour Holter ECG, suggesting that ventricular arrhythmias were the cause of the poor performance and irregularly irregular cardiac rhythm detected immediately after exercise (Fig. 1). Underlying ventricular myocardial disease may be present in these horses. A complete cardiac work-up that includes echocardiography, measurement of cardiac isoenzymes, a complete and differential blood count, total protein and fibrinogen concentration, as well as serum electrolyte concentrations should be performed. An ECG obtained during a maximal stress test is not recommended in horses with a history of poor performance and frequent supraventricular or ventricular premature depolarizations detected during a 24-hour continuous Holter ECG, until the arrhythmia disappears or occurs infrequently during follow-up continuous electrocardiographic monitoring (ideally <2–4 premature depolarizations/hour). Continued training of these individuals usually results in repeated episodes of poor performance because these arrhythmias tend to persist if the horse is kept in training. Severe exercise intolerance and collapse may occur if these arrhythmias occur frequently during exercise. Sudden death is also a risk for horses with frequent ventricular premature depolarizations occurring during exercise because these horses are more prone to develop unstable ventricular tachycardia and possibly ventricular fibrillation.

RADIOTELEMETRY

Radiotelemetry enables the clinician to continuously monitor the ECG on an oscilloscope, and a strip chart recorder can be activated to permanently record the ECG as needed. Radiotelemetry is invaluable for obtaining a continuous ECG from a horse during exercise, continuously monitoring a patient with life-threatening cardiac arrhythmias, or continuously monitoring the response of a horse to treatment. The contact electrodes used for the heart rate monitor or 24-hour continuous ECG are adapted to a radio transmitter, which sends the electrocardiographic

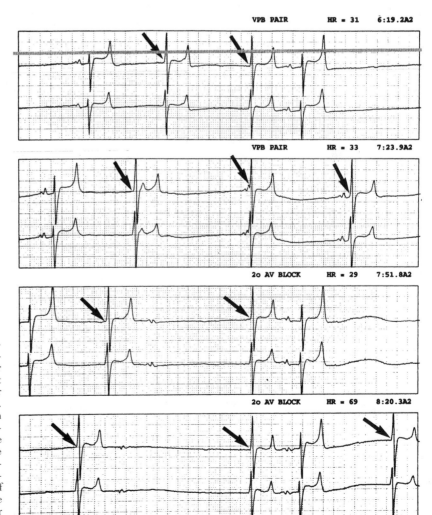

Figure 1. Base-apex ECG obtained during continuous 24-hour Holter electrocardiography from a 3-year-old Standardbred filly with a recent history of poor performance. The filly reportedly stopped in her last race at the half pole, and an irregularly irregular rhythm was detected immediately following the race. Several days later, an ECG and echocardiogram taken in the resting animal were normal, although the cardiac isoenzyme of CK (CK-MB) was elevated. Notice the frequent (>900/24 hours) ventricular premature depolarizations (arrows) detected during this continuous recording. Ventricular arrhythmias, not paroxysmal atrial fibrillation, were the most likely cause of the poor performance and cardiac arrhythmia. The filly was treated with rest and corticosteroids and later returned to racing successfully.

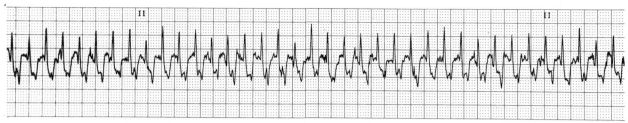

Figure 2. Base-apex ECG obtained via radiotelemetry at peak exercise during a maximal stress test of a 3-year-old Standardbred filly. Notice the rapid sinus tachycardia with a maximal heart rate of 240 beats/minute. The PR interval is very short, there is a small Q wave followed by a large R wave and a deep S wave with ST segment depression, and the T wave is negative. No arrhythmias were detected during or after exercise.

signal back to a receiver. The contact electrodes are held in place with the use of a surcingle or saddle during the monitoring period. Other electrode systems may be used such as alligator clips, adhesive clips, which require clipping off the hair at the site of electrode placement, and needle electrodes. However, contact electrodes carefully placed underneath a surcingle or saddle with the girth tightly cinched provide high-quality tracings in the majority of horses and are usually well tolerated.

The horse's heart rate varies with each level of exercise up to the maximum of 200 to 240 beats/minute that is reached with maximal exercise. The exercising horse should have a sinus tachycardia with a heart rate of 70 to 120 beats/minute during trotting, 120 to 150 beats/minute during cantering, 150 to 180 beats/minute at the hand gallop, and more than 180 beats/minute at the gallop. At peak exercise the normal horse's heart rate should not exceed 240 beats/minute with a rhythm of sinus tachycardia (Fig. 2). The horse's heart rate should recover quickly if the horse is fit, dropping below 100 beats/minute in the first 5 minutes following maximal exercise and returning to baseline within 30 to 45 minutes following exercise. During exercise, the PR and QT intervals shorten significantly with little change in the duration of the QRS complex. Marked changes in the configuration of the T wave occur during exercise in the normal horse with both a change in polarity of the T wave and a marked increase in T wave amplitude detected in normal horses.

The immediate postexercise period is a vulnerable time for the genesis of cardiac arrhythmias. Large fluctuations in autonomic tone occur during this period, which make arrhythmias more likely to occur. Occasional supraventricular or, more likely, ventricular premature depolarizations may be detected during this time, and these are probably clinically insignificant. More frequent ventricular or supraventricular extrasystoles in the immediate postexercise period are probably not normal (Fig. 3). Runs of paroxysmal ventricular tachycardia detected at peak exercise or as the horse is tiring are also not normal (Fig. 4) and may indicate an exercise-induced myocardial problem. Problems with myocardial perfusion, myocardial hypoxia, or pre-existing myocarditis or cardiomyopathy must be considered in these horses. Exercise-induced electrolyte and metabolic disturbances may also be involved in the pathogenesis of some of these arrhythmias. Even short paroxysms of ventricular tachycardia at peak exercise usually result in the horse stopping or slowing significantly during a maximal stress exercise, often within seconds of their occurrence. The detection of frequent ventricular or supraventricular premature depolarizations during peak exercise or in the immediate postexercise period should prompt further cardiac evaluation as to their possible etiology. A continuous 24-hour ECG is recommended to ascertain whether the arrhythmias are occurring frequently at rest during a 24-hour monitoring period. Measurement of levels of the cardiac isoenzymes of creatine kinase (CK) and lactate dehydroge-

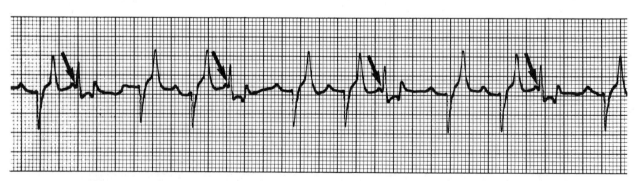

Figure 3. Frequent ventricular premature depolarizations detected during recovery from exercise in a 3-year-old Thoroughbred colt with a history of poor performance. Notice the ventricular premature depolarization *(arrows)*, which occurs after every second normally conducted sinus depolarization. Although these ventricular premature depolarizations are occurring more frequently than normal, their significance is poorly understood because they did not appear during maximal exercise and did not occur until the heart rate had dropped to 100 beats/minute.

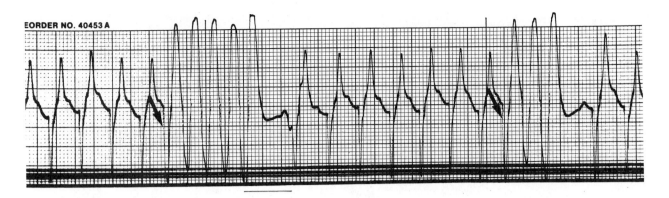

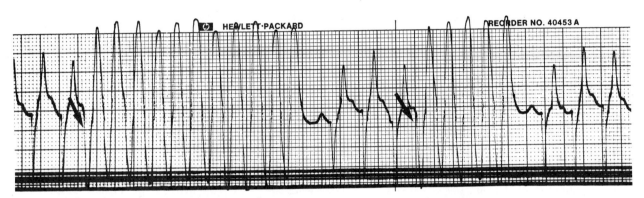

Figure 4. Runs of ventricular tachycardia at near-peak exercise in a 4-year-old Thoroughbred stallion with a history of poor performance. Notice the paroxysms of ventricular tachycardia (*arrows*) with widened QRS and T wave complexes and a nearly sine wave pattern to the wide QRS tachycardia. This rapid wide ventricular tachycardia with a rate of nearly 300 beats/minute could degenerate into a fatal ventricular arrhythmia. The underlying sinus rate is approximately 180 beats/minute.

nase (LDH) pre- and postexercise are indicated to detect an exercise-induced elevation in these isoenzymes, indicating an exercise-induced myocardial injury. The upper airway should be closely evaluated during a maximal stress test, along with the exercising ECG, because horses with significant upper airway dysfunction may also experience ventricular, and, less likely, supraventricular premature depolarizations. The premature depolarizations occur as the

upper airway collapse becomes significant, suggesting that in these horses, the arrhythmias may be the result of arterial hypoxemia and myocardial hypoxia.

Cardiac arrhythmias were detected in nearly 30% of 250 horses with a history of poor performance examined on a maximal treadmill stress test at the author's hospital. All of these horses had no previous history of known cardiac disease or arrhythmias. In approximately 66% of these

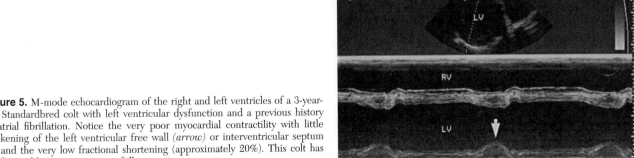

Figure 5. M-mode echocardiogram of the right and left ventricles of a 3-year-old Standardbred colt with left ventricular dysfunction and a previous history of atrial fibrillation. Notice the very poor myocardial contractility with little thickening of the left ventricular free wall (*arrow*) or interventricular septum (S) and the very low fractional shortening (approximately 20%). This colt has not been able to return successfully to racing.

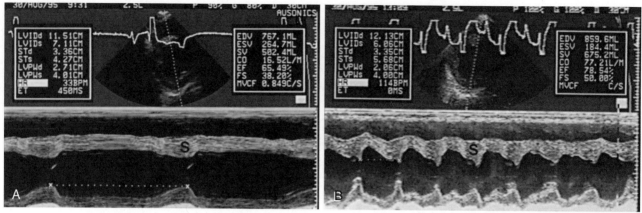

Figure 6. Two-dimensional real time *(top)* and corresponding M-mode echocardiogram *(bottom)* obtained at rest *(A)* and immediately following maximal stress test exercise *(B)* in a 3-year-old Thoroughbred with no evidence of myocardial dysfunction. Notice the increased thickening of the left ventricular free wall and interventricular septum (S) detected in the immediate postexercise echocardiogram resulting in an increase in the fractional shortening (FS) when compared with the resting echocardiogram.

horses, the arrhythmias were infrequent or present only during the recovery period. In the remainder, the cardiac arrhythmias were frequent enough to have accounted for the poor performance and resulted in slowing or termination of the exercise test. Further work needs to be done to characterize the types of exercise-induced arrhythmias that occur in horses and to discern their etiologies and select appropriate patient management and treatment.

POSTEXERCISE ECHOCARDIOGRAPHY

Echocardiographic evaluation of horses presenting for poor performance is useful because significant myocardial dysfunction can be detected in the absence of auscultable abnormalities. Myocardial hypokinesis, dyskinesis, and akinesis in the pre-exercise echocardiogram are indications of left ventricular dysfunction and primary myocardial disease (Fig. 5). However, myocardial dysfunction may be detected in the immediate postexercise echocardiogram in horses that appear normal before the onset of exercise. The normal myocardial response to exercise is an increase in the degree of thickening of the left ventricular free wall and interventricular septum, which persists in the immediate postexercise period (Fig. 6). This increase in left ventricular fractional shortening can be detected in the immediate postexercise period in normal horses with heart rates in excess of 100 beats/minute. As the heart rate returns to normal in the immediate postexercise period, the systolic thickening of the left ventricular free wall and interventricular septum returns to the resting value and an increased shortening fraction is no longer detected. Therefore, it is important that this postexercise evaluation be made immediately following the termination of strenu-

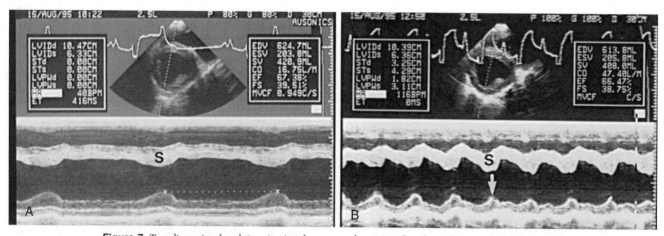

Figure 7. Two-dimensional real time *(top)* and corresponding M-mode echocardiogram *(bottom)* obtained at rest *(A)* and immediately after a maximal exercise test *(B)* in a 3-year-old Thoroughbred colt with evidence of postexercise myocardial dysfunction. Notice the decrease in thickening of the left ventricular free wall *(arrow)* and swinging pattern of motion of the interventricular septum (S) resulting in no change in fractional shortening (FS) when compared with the resting echocardiogram.

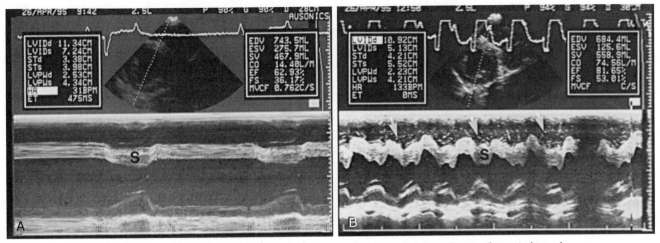

Figure 8. Two-dimensional real time *(top)* and corresponding M-mode echocardiogram *(bottom)* obtained at rest *(A)* and immediately following maximal stress test exercise *(B)* in a 6-year-old Standardbred mare with massive amounts of spontaneous contrast detected in the immediate postexercise echocardiogram. Notice the small bright echoes representing spontaneous contrast in the right ventricle *(arrows)* in the immediate postexercise examination that were absent on the resting examination. S = interventricular septum.

ous exercise when the heart rate still exceeds 100 beats/minute.

A lack of change or a decrease in systolic thickening of the left ventricular free wall and interventricular septum following strenuous exercise is abnormal if observed while the horse's heart rate is higher than 100 beats/minute. This change has been detected in approximately 8% of 250 horses presenting for a maximal stress test at the author's hospital (Fig. 7). The majority of these horses have no other abnormalities detected during the resting or treadmill examination. Ventricular premature depolarizations have been detected occasionally in some of these horses during or immediately after exercise, but they are usually infrequent. Occasionally this echocardiographic change is also detected in horses with significant dysfunction of the upper airway, suggesting that arterial hypoxemia and myocardial hypoxia may play a role in the etiology of this dysfunction. In humans, this exercise-induced myocardial dysfunction is most indicative of coronary artery disease. Although coronary artery disease has rarely been recognized in the horse, exercise-induced myocardial dysfunction does occur and may result in significant elevations of the myocardial fraction of the cardiac isoenzymes after exercise. This elevation of the myocardial fraction of CK and/or LDH after exercise suggests that an exercise-induced myocardial injury is occurring in some of these horses. Investigation of this problem is in the preliminary stages, and additional studies are needed to further evaluate the significance and etiology of these findings so that appropriate treatment recommendations can be made to return the horse to its previous performance level.

Spontaneous contrast is also occasionally detected echocardiographically in the right side of the heart immediately following exercise when it was not detected in the resting echocardiogram (Fig. 8). The etiology of these echoes is still unclear. Platelet aggregations and rouleaux formation are two explanations reported for horses with spontaneous contrast detected at rest. Low flow states also create spontaneous contrast but are not likely to be an etiology in horses in the immediate postexercise period. A high incidence of spontaneous contrast has been detected in resting horses with a history of exercise-induced pulmonary hemorrhage. Further investigation needs to be performed in horses with spontaneous contrast detected in the immediate postexercise period in hopes of determining its cause.

Supplemental Readings

Deegen E, Buntenkotter S: Behaviour of the heart rate of horses with auricular fibrillation during exercise and after treatment. Equine Vet J 8:26–29, 1976.

Fujii Y, Watanabe H, Yamamoto T, Niwa K, Mizuoka S, Anezaki R: Serum creatine kinase and lactate dehydrogenase isoenzymes in skeletal and cardiac muscle damage in the horse. Bull Equine Res Inst 20:87–96, 1983.

Gatti L, Holmes JR: ECG recording at rest and during exercise in the horse. Equine Vet Ed 2:28–30, 1990.

Holmes JR: Cardiac arrhythmias on the racecourse. In Gillespie JR, Robinson NE (eds): Equine Exercise Physiology 2. Davis, CA, ICEEP Publications, 1987, pp 781–785.

Mahoney C, Rantanen NW, DeMichael JA, Kincaid B: Spontaneous echocardiographic contrast in the Thoroughbred: High prevalence in racehorses and a characteristic abnormality in bleeders. Equine Vet J 24:129–133, 1992.

Rantanen NW, Byars TD, Hauser ML, Gaines RD: Spontaneous contrast and mass lesions in the hearts of race horses: Ultrasound diagnosis—preliminary data. J Equine Vet Sci 4:220–223, 1984.

Reef VB: Frequency of cardiac arrhythmias and their significance in normal horses. Proc 7th Am Coll Vet Intern Med, 1989, pp 506–508.

Reef VB, Maxson AD, Lewis M: Echocardiographic and ECG changes in horses following exercise. Proc. 12th Am Coll Vet Intern Med, 1994, pp 256–258.

Ryan T, Vasey CG, Presti CF, O'Donnell JA, Feigenbaum H, Armstrong WF: Exercise echocardiography: Detection of coronary artery disease in patients with normal left ventricular wall motion at rest. J Am Coll Cardiol 11:993–999, 1988.

Senta T, Smetzer DL, Smith CR: Effects of exercise on certain electrocardiographic parameters and cardiac arrhythmias in the horse: A radio-telemetric study. Cornell Vet 60:552–569, 1970.

Diagnosis of Cardiac Arrhythmias

JOHN D. BONAGURA
Columbia, Missouri

Arrhythmias are disturbances in cardiac electrical activity and are manifested in terms of heart rate, impulse formation, and impulse conduction. Rhythm disturbances are classified based on atrial and ventricular rate, anatomic origin of the electrical impulse, mode of impulse formation, and conduction sequence across the heart (Table 1). A wide variety of cardiac arrhythmias are recognized in horses; however, some of these have a physiologic basis and are not clinically significant. Of principal concern to the clinician are those arrhythmias with hemodynamic consequences such as limited cardiac output, reduced blood pressure, and altered organ perfusion, or those with the potential for further electrical instability such as myocardial fibrillation and sudden cardiac death. This chapter reviews the diagnosis of common cardiac rhythm disturbances. Although most serious arrhythmias can be diagnosed using the stethoscope and routine electrocardiogram (ECG), 24-hour, ambulatory, tape-recorded ECG recordings (Holter ECG, see page 234) or exercise ECG recorded with telemetry (see page 235) are needed to identify sporadic or exercise-induced rhythm abnormalities. The therapy of cardiac arrhythmias is detailed later in this section.

Irregularities of the cardiac rhythm are often identified through auscultation. The clinician can use the stethoscope to distinguish normal rhythms from those indicative of structural or functional heart disease. Careful auscultation limits the recording of unneeded ECGs and increases the positive predictive value of the ECG tracing. Key aspects in identifying normal rhythms include noting the heart rate; pulse regularity; atrial (fourth) and first heart sounds; and physiologic state. Sinus arrhythmia, sinus bradycardia, and second-degree atrioventricular (AV) block are common physiologic arrhythmias mediated by vagal activity in standing horses (Figs. 1, 2, and 3). The heart rate is generally less than 40 bpm, atrial sounds precede each first sound, and soft independent atrial sounds may be evident if there is second-degree AV block. These irregularities transiently give way to a regular rhythm, either normal sinus rhythm or sinus tachycardia, if sympathetic nervous system activity increases. Sympathetic activity can be enhanced during the examination process through stimulation such as turning the horse in three or four quick tight circles or other mild exercise. Atrial fibrillation or flutter may be suspected when the pulse strength and rhythm are consistently irregular and distinct atrial sounds do not precede the first sound. The resting heart rate is generally normal unless the horse is in heart failure or has another reason for increased sympathetic tone such as fever or colic. Ectopic beats cause a sudden, premature first heart sound of variable intensity. Paroxysmal or sustained ectopic rhythms lead to periods of rapid, generally regular, rhythm with variable intensity of heart sounds, varying pulse pressure, and absence of the

---

TABLE 1
CLASSIFICATION OF CARDIAC ARRHYTHMIAS

Sinus rhythms	Ventricular rhythms
Normal sinus rhythm	Ventricular escape(s)
Sinus arrhythmia	Ventricular escape rhythm (idioventricular rhythm)
Sinus bradycardia	Ventricular premature complexes
Sinus tachycardia	Idioventricular tachycardia (accelerated ventricular rhythm)
Sinoatrial block	Ventricular tachycardia
Sinus arrest	Nonsustained (paroxysmal)
Atrial arrhythmias	Sustained
Atrial premature complexes	Monomorphic
Atrial tachycardia	Polymorphic
Nonsustained (paroxysmal)	Torsades de pointes (rotating QRS axis)
Sustained	Ventricular flutter
Atrial flutter	Ventricular fibrillation
Atrial fibrillation	Atrioventricular block
Re-entrant supraventricular	First-degree
(reciprocating) tachycardia	Second-degree
Junctional (nodal) rhythms	Third-degree
Junctional escape(s)	Ventricular pre-excitation
Junctional escape rhythm	Hyperkalemia related arrhythmias
Idionodal rhythm	Atrial standstill
Junctional tachycardia	Asystole

Figure 1. Rhythm diagnoses obtained from analyses of 1012 consecutive equine electrocardiograms (representing initial and follow-up examinations in 894 individual horses). (Unpublished observations of Bonagura JD and Miller MS, 1989.) These results are typical of those obtained from routine hospital rhythm strip electrocardiograms, but are unlikely to detect intermittent or exercise-induced rhythm disturbances. The prevalence of second-degree AV block and other vagal arrhythmias is also higher in undisturbed horses examined by telemetry.

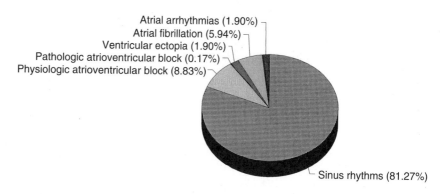

Atrial arrhythmias (1.90%)
Atrial fibrillation (5.94%)
Ventricular ectopia (1.90%)
Pathologic atrioventricular block (0.17%)
Physiologic atrioventricular block (8.83%)

Sinus rhythms (81.27%)

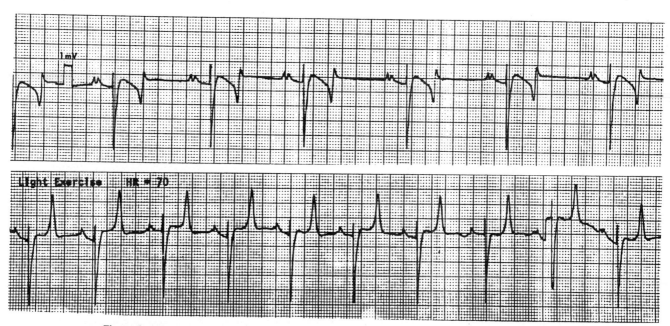

Figure 2. ECG recordings demonstrating sinus rhythms before and after light exercise. Note the physiologic alterations in the heart rate, P wave morphology, PR interval, and ST-T wave (calibration artifact is evident in the second to the last complex).(Base-apex lead, 25 mm/sec.) (ECG courtesy of R. Hilwig.)

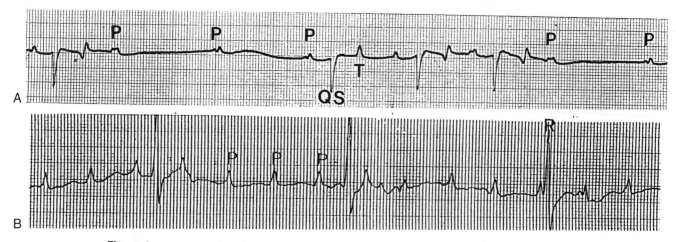

Figure 3. Atrioventricular blocks. *(A)* Sinus arrhythmia, wandering atrial pacemaker (varying P wave morphology), and second-degree AV block. These findings are compatible with varying vagal tone. (Base-apex lead, 25 mm/sec.) *(B)* Third-degree (complete) AV block. All P waves (P) are blocked and a ventricular escape rhythm is evident (lead 2, 25 mm/sec).

S_4 to S_1 sequence. When an abnormal rhythm is suspected from auscultation or the clinical history, an electrocardiogram rhythm strip should be recorded.

SINUS RHYTHM

Sinus node discharge rate is a major determinant of cardiac output and arterial blood pressure. Sinus mechanisms are characterized on the ECG tracing by a consistent relationship between the P waves and the QRS-T complexes (see Fig. 2). In the situation of "wandering atrial pacemaker" the P wave morphology recurrently changes. Sinus rhythms developing at variable heart rates can be explained largely by the impact of autonomic nervous system traffic on the sinoatrial node. Sinus arrhythmias in horses are not consistently linked to phases of ventilation (nonrespiratory sinus arrhythmia). Normal, standing horses may demonstrate vagally mediated sinus bradycardia, sinus arrhythmia, or sinus block with arrest, often with second degree AV block. Excitement or a sudden stimulus may provoke a regular normal sinus rhythm or sympathetically driven sinus tachycardia. Exercise leads to pronounced sinus tachycardia with heart rates often exceeding 200 bpm. Sinus node rate is higher in foals and usually increases slightly in mares during the latter phases of gestation.

Most changes in sinus node rate can be explained by altered autonomic activity, changes in body temperature, influence of a noncardiac disorder, or a drug effect. Disturbances of sinus node function caused by sinus node disease are rare. Persistent sinus tachycardia, typically 60 to 90 bpm, is often observed in horses with congestive heart failure and is related to chronic sympathetic activation. Sedative drugs, anesthetics, and hypoxia can cause sinus bradycardia leading to hypotension in horses undergoing general anesthesia. Anesthetic depression of the sinus node, along with sensitization of latent pacemakers in the coronary sinus or AV junction, can lead to ectopic rhythms in the anesthetized horse. Conversely, an increasing sinus rate during anesthesia may indicate inadequate depth of anesthesia, pain, or hypotension. When the cause of a persistent sinus tachycardia is not obvious, the possibilities of pain, plasma volume depletion, hypokalemia, hypotension, infection, anemia, and sepsis should be investigated and managed. Treatment of most sinus rhythm disorders involves correction of the underlying cause, although an anticholinergic drug (atropine) or sympathomimetic drug (dobutamine) is an appropriate emergency or intraoperative treatment for vagally induced sinus bradycardia or AV block.

ATRIOVENTRICULAR BLOCK

The PR interval of the ECG represents conduction across the atria, the AV node, and the His-Purkinje system. First-degree AV block is characterized by a longer-than-normal PR interval, usually exceeding 0.52 seconds. Second-degree AV block is diagnosed when some P waves are not followed by QRS complexes (see Fig. 3A). Third-degree AV block is present when no P waves are conducted

and the ventricle discharges through a latent, escape pacemaker located in the His-Purkinje system (see Fig. 3B).

Conduction through the normal equine atrioventricular node is highly regulated by autonomic activity, constituting a major mechanism for controlling arterial blood pressure. Atrioventricular conduction generally follows sinus activity: during sinus tachycardia the PR interval shortens, whereas during periods of progressive sinus node depression the PR interval lengthens; however, there are exceptions. For example, Mobitz type I (Wenckebach) second-degree AV block may follow a progressive prolongation of the PR interval; yet, normal horses can also have a block of P waves while having progressive shortening of the PR interval. Arterial blood pressure can be regulated during inappropriate periods of sinus tachycardia by blocking impulses in the AV node even as the sinus rate increases. Examples include a horse that has suddenly stopped submaximal exercise, or an animal that undergoes a brief surge of sinus tachycardia due to anxiety or transient pain. These must be appreciated as variations of normal. The AV node also acts as a filter that modifies ventricular rate response to atrial tachyarrhythmias such as atrial tachycardia and atrial fibrillation. Thus, in situations in which the atrial rate is abnormally increased, the AV node physiologically blocks many of the impulses and prevents 1:1 atrial-to-ventricular conduction. This response is modified by autonomic tone and drugs, such as quinidine, which may enhance AV conduction via a vagolytic effect.

Second-Degree Atrioventricular Block

Second-degree AV block is the most common of the AV conduction delays. This rhythm is characterized by intermittent failure to conduct an atrial impulse to the ventricle. One or more nonconducted P waves is observed before a normal conduction sequence becomes evident. The pattern generally repeats itself. Profound vagally induced second-degree AV block may develop infrequently as a consequence of vagotonia, and must be distinguished from block caused by structural conduction system disease. As indicated previously, physiologic second-degree AV block is characterized by varying PR intervals (usually a Mobitz type I), and the block is abolished following exercise, stress, or vagolytic drugs such as atropine or glycopyrrolate, although a drug trial is rarely if ever needed to establish the diagnosis.

Pathologic second-degree block is an uncommon rhythm indicating a lesion in the AV node, bundle of His, or proximal bilateral bundle branches. Although drug toxicosis or marked surges of vagal tone can cause transient, high-grade, second-degree or even complete AV block, the persistence of this rhythm indicates a congenital, degenerative, inflammatory, or neoplastic condition of the conduction system. The ECG in cases of pathologic second-degree block typically demonstrates two or more blocked P waves until a conducted QRS complex occurs or an escape complex discharges. The PR interval of conducted impulses may be constant (Mobitz type II) or long (concurrent first degree block), and the conduction response to increased sympathetic activity is not appropriate; the block may actually worsen. Widening of the QRS complex, axis deviation in the frontal plane ECG leads, and concurrent second-degree AV block are indicative of diffuse conduction disease and predict future development of complete AV block.

Third-Degree (Complete) Atrioventricular Block

Third-degree (complete) AV block is a rare conduction disorder that may be caused by marked vagotonia, but it is usually irreversible and indicative of structural AV conduction disease. The ECG is characterized by total independence of P waves and QRS complexes (see Fig. 3B). The ventricular rate is controlled by one or more latent pacemakers located below the level of the conduction block. The QRS complexes are either narrow, if the escape rhythm is junctional, or wide, if the escape focus lies within the ventricular Purkinje network. Periods of ventricular asystole, owing to unstable escape activity, may lead to syncope or collapse. Complete AV block appears to be congenital or inherited in miniature (Jerusalem) donkeys and occurs sporadically in mature horses.

ATRIAL ARRHYTHMIAS

Ectopic rhythms originating in the atria are common (see Figure 1). These supraventricular disturbances often develop as "functional" disorders with no overt structural cardiac lesion. Autonomic imbalance (including high sympathetic activity), hypokalemia, beta-adrenergic agonists, infections, anemia, and colic can precipitate atrial premature complexes. Atrial rhythm disturbances are also associated with structural lesions of the valves, myocardium, or pericardium, especially when there is atrial distension or ischemia. Myocarditis, subsequent to a viral or bacterial infection, may precipitate atrial arrhythmias in some horses, although this cause-and-effect relationship is virtually impossible to establish. Atrial premature complexes can precipitate sustained atrial arrhythmias such as atrial tachycardia, atrial flutter, and atrial fibrillation. The large size of the equine atria and the frequent presence of microscopic atrial fibrotic lesions predispose the horse to these sustained arrhythmias. The high level of basal vagal tone present in most horses serves to shorten the action potential duration of atrial myocytes and facilitates the development of sustained atrial tachyarrhythmias that depend on re-entry mechanisms.

Atrial arrhythmias can be manifested as isolated events or sustained abnormal activity. Isolated premature discharges may be an incidental finding, ambiguously related to exercise intolerance, or may coexist with structural disorders such as congenital or valvular heart disease or dilated cardiomyopathy. The sustained atrial arrhythmias (i.e., atrial tachycardia, atrial flutter, and atrial fibrillation) are likely to be clinically significant in most working animals. The overall importance of isolated atrial or other supraventricular premature complexes is often difficult to ascertain. These disturbances are not commonly identified on short rhythm strip ECG tracings (see Fig. 1); however, the frequency of these rhythms markedly increases in horses examined by 24-hour Holter monitor studies (approximately 28%; personal communication, Virginia B. Reef, 1994). Thus, it appears that the incidence of atrial arrhythmias depends not only on the population examined, but on the methods. These rhythm disturbances should be assessed in light of other clinical findings.

Atrial Premature Complexes

Premature atrial impulses are characterized by an abnormal, premature P wave (P') that is often buried in the preceding T wave (Fig. 4A and B). The premature impulse may be nonconducted if it falls within the physiologic refractory period of the AV node, is interpolated (interposed) between normal sinus impulses, or is conducted to the ventricle. The latter is the most common situation, with the impulse conducted with first-degree AV block to be followed by a normal-appearing related QRS complex. Less often, the related QRS complex is abnormal and wide, caused by aberrant (slow, abnormal) conduction across the ventricles. Typically, a brief pause, caused by penetration of the sinus node and resetting of the pacemaker cycle, is observed to follow the premature atrial complex. Care must be taken to distinguish atrial premature complexes from normal variation. Sinus arrhythmia and sinus bradycardia often lead to variations in the P-P intervals, and often a "wandering atrial pacemaker" is present, which gradually alters the P wave morphology.

Atrial premature complexes are more likely to be clinically significant in the following circumstances: frequent at rest; associated with runs of atrial tachycardia; related to poor exercise performance (provided that other causes are excluded); previous diagnosis of paroxysmal or sustained atrial flutter or fibrillation; or in the setting of other signs of cardiac disease such as mitral regurgitation. Documentation of atrial arrhythmias during exercise may be critical for determining if paroxysmal atrial tachycardia or fibrillation is the likely cause of poor performance (see page 235). Clinical judgment must be used, however, because supraventricular premature complexes are common in the immediate post-exercise period, most likely associated with autonomic imbalance. If post-exercise arrhythmias are not related to clinical signs and are not detected during exercise, they are unlikely to be clinically significant. Cardiac rhythm monitoring during exercise may be necessary to be certain (see page 235). In summary, history, auscultation, routine electrocardiography, clinical chemistry and hematology testing, echocardiography, exercise electrocardiography, post-exercise electrocardiography, and continuous 24-hour electrocardiographic monitoring may all be necessary in the evaluation of a horse with intermittent atrial premature complexes.

Atrial Tachycardia

Atrial tachycardia represents a repetitive, ectopic, atrial tachyarrhythmia (see Fig. 4C). Atrial tachycardia may be sustained or nonsustained (paroxysmal). The rhythm is generally precipitated by an atrial premature complex. The ECG demonstrates a rapid and regular atrial rate while the ventricular rate response is normal to increased and usually irregular owing to physiologic AV nodal block of P' waves. Atrial rates of 120 to 300 per minute are typical in horses with sustained atrial tachycardia. At the higher atrial rates, the rhythm may be indistinguishable from atrial flutter. Differentiation of atrial tachycardia from flutter is not critical because both arrhythmias carry the same clinical significance and generally are treated identically. Sustained

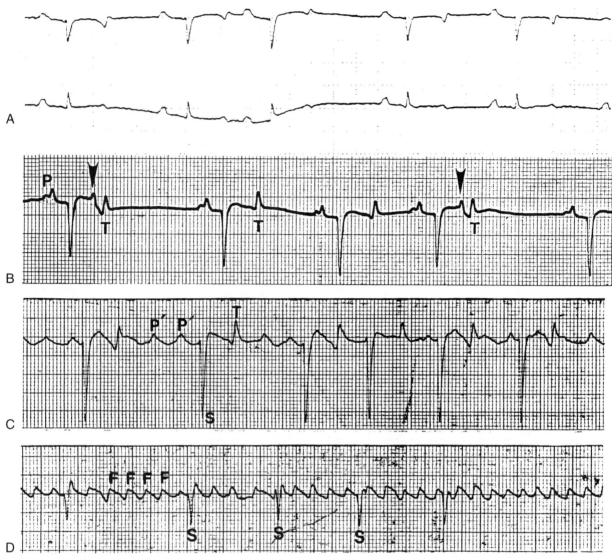

Figure 4. Atrial arrhythmias. (A) Holter ECG recording demonstrating a single atrial premature complex (3rd P-QRS-T complex) with resetting of the sinus node interval (simultaneous thoracic leads at 25 mm/ sec). (B) Nonconducted atrial premature complexes (arrows) deform the ST segment and reset the sinus node, causing a brief pause. Physiologic refractoriness in the AV node to the premature stimulation explains this finding. (Base-apex lead, 25 mm/sec.) (C) Atrial tachycardia with irregular ventricular rate response. Wide, regular abnormal P waves (P′) are evident. (Base-apex lead, 25 mm/sec.) (D) Atrial flutter with rapid and regular, but abnormal, atrial activation evident as saw-toothed F waves with accompanying irregular ventricular response (S waves indicated). (Lead 2, 25 mm/sec.)

atrial tachycardia is most often recognized during treatment of horses with quinidine sulfate (see page 251). Before conversion of atrial fibrillation to sinus rhythm, atrial tachycardia may be observed; thus, in this setting the rhythm indicates a partial therapeutic effect of quinidine on the atrial myocardium. When sustained atrial tachycardia occurs as an isolated finding, structural heart disease or underlying myocardial disease should be suspected and the horse should be considered predisposed to development of atrial fibrillation.

Atrial Flutter

Atrial flutter represents a form of atrial circuit movement or macro-reentry (see Fig. 4D). The clinical circumstances and assessment of this uncommon rhythm disturbance are identical to those of atrial tachycardia. The ECG in atrial flutter is characterized by a very rapid, abnormal, but regular atrial activity, which is usually manifested as a "saw-toothed" ECG baseline. The atrial frequency often exceeds 300 per minute. The R-R intervals are irregular owing to variable AV conduction; therefore, there are fewer QRS and T complexes than flutter waves. The ventricular rate depends on autonomic tone and AV conduction and may be normal or increased.

Atrial Fibrillation

Atrial fibrillation (AF) is probably the most common arrhythmia associated with poor performance and exercise intolerance. Although cardiac output at rest is usually normal in AF, maximal cardiac output during exercise is limited because the atrial contribution to filling is most important at higher heart rates. Exercise intolerance is most obvious in high performance horses. Exercise-induced pulmonary hemorrhage, respiratory distress, congestive heart failure, weakness, and collapse have been reported in association with atrial fibrillation; conversely, the arrhythmia is often an incidental finding.

The electrocardiogram in AF is characterized by an absence of P waves; instead, fibrillation or f waves are seen in the baseline (Fig. 5). These f waves may be coarse (large) or fine (small). Although the number of atrial impulses cannot be counted, the atrial rate usually exceeds 500 per minute. The QRS-T complexes are normal in morphology and duration. Ventricular rate response is quite

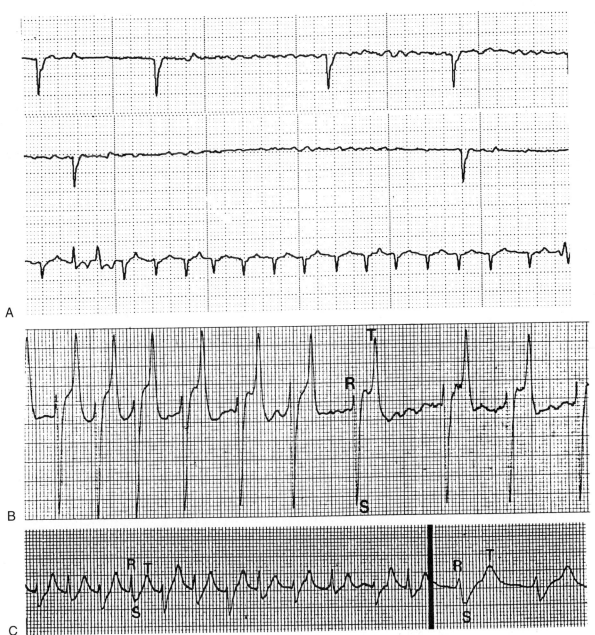

Figure 5. Atrial fibrillation. *(A)* Atrial fibrillation (AF) at variable ventricular rates from a horse as demonstrated by three Holter ECG recordings (thoracic leads, 25 mm/sec). *(Top)* Typical AF with irregular, undulating baseline, irregular ventricular response, and ventricular rate of 39 per minute. *(Middle)* The impact of high vagal tone is evident because there is marked slowing of the ventricular rate response. *(Lower)* Rapid, slightly irregular ventricular rate response following exercise. Two ventricular ectopic complexes are also evident. *(B)* Atrial fibrillation in a horse with congestive heart failure. High sympathetic tone explains the rapid ventricular response. (Base-apex lead, 25 mm/sec.) *(C)* Atrial fibrillation with rapid ventricular rate response resulting from the vagolytic effect of quinidine. The electrical alternans of the QRS complexes is typical of a supraventricular tachyarrhythmia with rapid AV nodal conduction. The ventricular activation process varies with every other beat. The wide QRS complexes are related to quinidine toxicosis (prolonged conduction in the His-Purkinje system). (Lead 3, 25 mm/sec *[left]*; 50 mm/sec *[right]*.)

irregular, although periodicity may be observed infrequently. As for all atrial tachyarrhythmias, the ultimate ventricular rate response depends on the refractory period of the AV node and the strength of the atrial stimuli. In an otherwise healthy horse in atrial fibrillation, vagal tone is high and sympathetic tone low when standing; consequently, the ventricular rate is usually normal (about 30–40 bpm), or even slow (20–28 bpm). If sympathetic activity is increased for any reason, or if vagal activity is reduced, as occurs with quinidine sulfate therapy, the ventricular rate response increases as the AV nodal refractory period shortens. This explains the clinician's simple, but very useful, dependence on measuring pretreatment resting heart rate in horses with AF. Because a horse with structural heart disease is likely to require adrenergic support to maintain cardiac output and arterial blood pressure, persistent resting tachycardia (>60 bpm) is associated with a poorer prognosis.

Atrial fibrillation may be paroxysmal or sustained. The paroxysmal variety may be short-lived, as in the case of exercise-induced atrial fibrillation, or it may convert spontaneously within 24 to 48 hours of onset. Paroxysmal AF may be associated with transient potassium depletion, particularly in horses treated with bicarbonate solutions or furosemide. Sustained AF is probably less common than paroxysmal AF, but it is much easier to diagnose. Most horses with sustained AF have no other evidence of significant underlying cardiac disease, although a thorough evaluation should be done to exclude congenital, pericardial, myocardial, or valvular heart disease.

A number of factors interact in the prognosis of AF. Of these, congestive heart failure represents the most onerous prognostic indicator. Echocardiographic evidence of cardiomegaly, moderate to severe structural heart disease, or a history of recurrent AF are also negative prognostic indicators. Most horses have normal auscultation and echocardiographic signs, although a mild decrease in left ventricular shortening fraction (usually <5% below normal values) may be observed. The management of AF is described elsewhere in this section (see page 253).

JUNCTIONAL ARRHYTHMIAS

Cardiac arrhythmias that originate within the AV conducting tissues or within the most proximal ventricular conducting tissues are likely to be classified as "junctional" or AV "nodal" in origin. Unlike sinus or atrial arrhythmias, the QRS complexes are not preceded by a conducted P or F wave. Junctional tachycardias often lead to dissociation between the sinoatrial (P wave) activity and that of the ventricle (QRS-T), resulting in AV dissociation (Figs. 6 and 7C). Atrioventricular dissociation develops because the premature depolarization interferes with the conduction of normal sinoatrial impulses.

Distinguishing junctional from ventricular ectopic beats, and determining the exact location of the abnormal impulse formation, can be difficult. The distinction between junctional and ventricular ectopic rhythms can sometimes be made by inspection of the QRS complex. Junctional impulses are more likely to result in a QRS complex with a normal width, QRS morphology, and frontal axis. Complexes of ventricular origin, by contrast, are conducted abnormally and more slowly, resulting in a widened QRS, an abnormal QRS orientation, and abnormal T waves. However, junctional tachycardias may be conducted aberrantly, resulting in a similarly bizarre and wide QRS complex.

Junctional rhythms develop at various rates and are typically regular. The clinical significance of these rhythms is probably similar to that described later for ventricular rhythms. If junctional complexes are manifested during periods of AV block or sinus bradycardia, the ectopic rhythms usually arise after a considerable pause. Such complexes are termed *junctional* (or *nodal*) escape complexes, or if linked together, a *junctional escape rhythm*. Escape rhythms are characterized by slow ventricular rates, usually less than 30 per minute. Latent junctional pacemakers may be enhanced by administration of anesthetic drugs or catecholamines. For example, xylazine, detomidine, and gas anesthetic drugs (for example, halothane) depress sinus node function while enhancing the effects of catecholamines on latent junctional and ventricular pacemakers. Such accelerated idionodal rhythms are of little clinical significance, although their presence may prompt reduction of anesthetic dosage. Antiarrhythmic drug suppression of escape rhythms is contraindicated. Junctional complexes that arise early relative to the normal cardiac cycle are designated as premature and may occur as single or repetitive events. Relentless junctional tachycardias can lead to congestive heart failure, although this is uncommon.

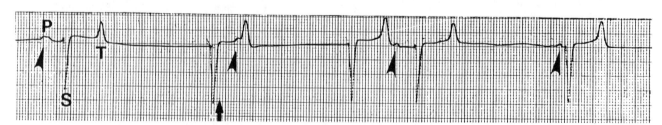

Figure 6. Idionodal (junctional) rhythm in an anesthetized horse. Sinus P waves (*arrowheads*) are indicated. A competing junctional (or high ventricular) pacemaker discharges (*arrow*), causing the second, third, and fifth QRS complexes. The fourth complex is a sinus impulse that is conducted through the AV node (with a prolonged PR interval) and into the ventricle, which is a phenomenon termed *sinus capture*. This rhythm is caused by simultaneous sinus node depression and enhancement of a subsidiary junctional pacemaker.

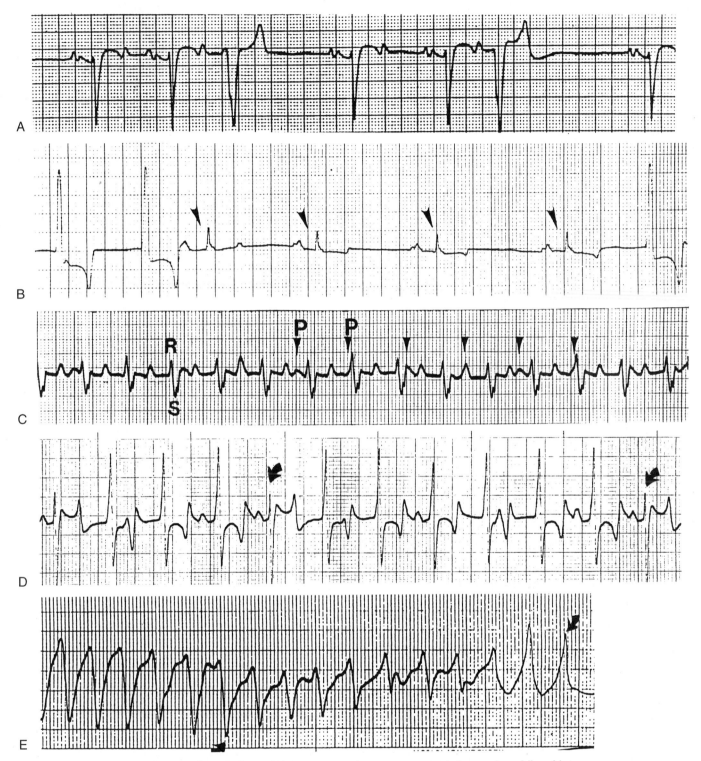

Figure 7. Ventricular arrhythmias. *(A)* Two monomorphic, premature ventricular complexes followed by a compensatory pause. (Base-apex lead, 25 mm/sec.) *(B)* Monomorphic ventricular ectopics (idioventricular tachycardia) alternating with sinus rhythm *(arrows)* (lead 2, 25 mm/sec). *(C)* Sustained ventricular (or junctional) tachycardia with atrioventricular dissociation. Note the independent P waves *(arrowheads;* lead 2, 25 mm/sec). *(D)* Ventricular tachycardia with atrioventricular dissociation. The ventricular rate is about 100 per minute. Occasional sinus capture complexes are evident *(arrows)*. *(E)* Polymorphic ventricular tachycardia. The QRS axis changes (arrows indicate R-waves). (From Bonagura JD, Reef VB: Cardiovascular diseases. *In* Reed S, Bayly W [eds]: Equine Internal Medicine. Philadelphia, WB Saunders, in press.)

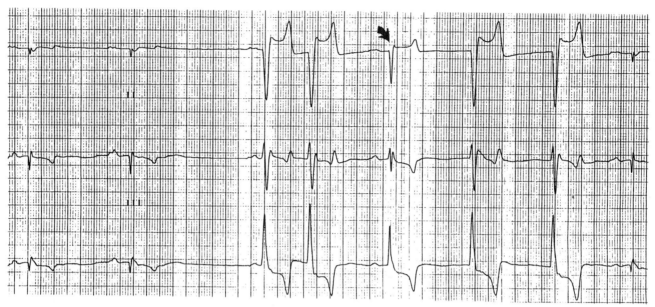

Figure 8. Nonsustained ventricular tachycardia with irregular R-R intervals follows two initial sinus complexes. A fusion complex is also evident *(arrow)*. (Simultaneous leads 1, 2, 3 at 25 mm/sec.)

VENTRICULAR ARRHYTHMIAS

Ventricular arrhythmias are abnormalities of impulse formation arising from abnormal ventricular electrical activity. These ectopic rhythms may be associated with underlying cardiac disease, a prior bout of myocardial ischemia and reperfusion, or a systemic disorder. Ventricular arrhythmias are observed with toxemia or sepsis, primary gastrointestinal disorders including proximal enteritis and large bowel disorders, electrolyte (potassium, magnesium) or metabolic disorders, hypoxia, ischemia, or halothane anesthesia. Catecholamines, anesthetic drugs, myocardial toxins such as the ionophores, viral or bacterial myocarditis, endocarditis, or pericarditis can cause ventricular arrhythmias.

Premature Ventricular Complexes

Premature ventricular complexes (ventricular extrasystoles, PVCs) are characterized by an ectopic premature QRS-T complex, usually followed by a compensatory pause, as the next sinus impulse is blocked by the refractory AV conduction system. If the sinus rate is slow or the ventricular premature depolarization is closely coupled to the preceding normal sinus beat, it may be interpolated (inserted) between two normal beats. Ventricular extrasystoles are characterized by QRS and T waves that are wide and often bizarre in appearance (see Fig. 7). Of course, the premature QRS complex bears no relationship to any preceding P waves, although genesis of the ventricular ectopic beats may be dependent on underlying cardiac cycle length. The morphology of the PVC may be uniform or multiform. The relationship of a PVC to the preceding sinus QRS-T complex is expressed by the "coupling interval" between them. Often the coupling interval is fixed, although it may vary minimally or markedly in cases of ventricular parasystole. A very short coupling interval may place the ectopic QRS on the preceding T wave, a phenomenon called "R on T" and one related to increased

ventricular vulnerability to fibrillation. Ventricular premature complexes occurred in 14% of clinically normal horses during routine 24-hour continuous electrocardiographic monitoring (personal communication, V. B. Reef, 1994).

The distributional pattern of PVCs may include haphaz-

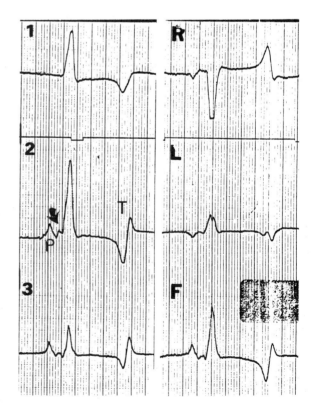

Figure 9. Ventricular pre-excitation. Note the very short PR interval and early ventricular activation or "delta wave" *(arrow)*. (Multiple lead recordings—1, 2, 3, aV$_R$, aV$_L$, aV$_F$—at 50 mm/sec.)

ard distribution, bigeminy, couplets (pairs of ectopic beats), or runs of ventricular extrasystoles. Runs of accelerated ventricular rhythm, usually developing at relatively slow heart rates (<90 bpm), are not uncommon in horses with ventricular ectopic activity (Figs. 7B, 8). These rhythms may be labile, varying in rate with sympathetic activity. Runs of ventricular ectopic beats at a rapid rate, ventricular tachycardia, are more likely to be hemodynamically and electrically unstable, when they develop at rates higher than 100 per minute (see Figs. 7D and E).

Ventricular Tachycardia

Ventricular tachycardia is an ectopic ventricular rhythm characterized by either a regular or irregular ventricular rate (see Figs. 7 and 8). Multiform ventricular tachycardia is characterized by an irregular rhythm and usually is associated with more clinical signs of cardiovascular disease than uniform (unifocal) ventricular tachycardia. Syncope is associated with higher rates of ventricular tachycardia (180/min or higher). Respiratory distress and pulmonary edema may develop from systolic and diastolic dysfunction. Sustained ventricular tachycardia (>120/min) may lead to congestive heart failure.

Ventricular tachycardia should be judged as potentially life-threatening when the rate is rapid (>180–200/min); R on T complexes or multiform ventricular tachycardia are detected; or polymorphic tachycardia with torsades de pointes (varying QRS axis) is observed. Immediate treatment of cardiovascular collapse may be required (see page 254).

The clinical approach to the horse with a ventricular arrhythmia should emphasize ruling out the noncardiac causes and correcting predisposing conditions, particularly when these rhythms attend a serious disorder of another body system or a surgical procedure. When necessary, a thorough cardiovascular examination, including echocardiography, should be performed to exclude overt structural heart disease. Electrolyte levels, including that of magnesium, should be measured. Cardiac isoenzyme concentrations may be measured to identify cardiac injury, although it may be problematic to separate primary (myocarditis) from secondary (ischemic) causes of cardiac isoenzyme elevation. Rest is advisable, and ventricular arrhythmias

often seem to resolve spontaneously following 4 to 8 weeks of rest. It may be judicious to obtain a Holter ECG (see page 234) before beginning training. Once training has begun, an exercise ECG may be useful in determining relative risk. Cases of idioventricular tachycardia generally have a good prognosis if the inciting injury can be traced to a probable bout of myocardial ischemia or an electrolyte disturbance. Ventricular tachycardia and persistent, multiform, ventricular premature complexes are more likely to indicate structural heart disease or "arrhythmogenic cardiomyopathy" and carry a worse prognosis. Affected animals should be carefully followed with serial electrocardiograms, as indicated earlier. Moreover, there is considerable danger in using such an animal, even if follow-up rhythm strips fail to detect a disorder.

OTHER CONDUCTION DISTURBANCES

Once a cardiac electrical impulse is formed, it is conducted rapidly throughout the heart. The sequence of cardiac electric activation is usually dictated by the specialized conducting tissues in the atria, AV node, bundle of His, bundle branches, and Purkinje fiber system. This conduction system permits orderly activation of atrial and ventricular muscle and facilitates effective mechanical activity of the heart. A variety of conduction disorders are recognized, including sinoatrial nodal exit block, atrial standstill (usually due to hyperkalemia), AV block, bundle branch block, and ill-defined ventricular conduction disturbances (see Table 1). The AV blocks have previously been considered.

Accelerated Atrioventricular Conduction

Accelerated AV conduction is an uncommon rhythm that permits conduction around the AV node and results in early excitation of the ventricles. When related to a reciprocating tachycardia (using the accessory pathway as part of a reentrant loop) and sudden weakness, the condition is termed a *pre-excitation syndrome*. The pre-excitation syndromes usually are characterized by short PR intervals and widened QRS complexes (Fig. 9). The prevalence and clinical significance of this electrocardiographic abnormality have yet to be determined in horses. Nevertheless, ECG tracings

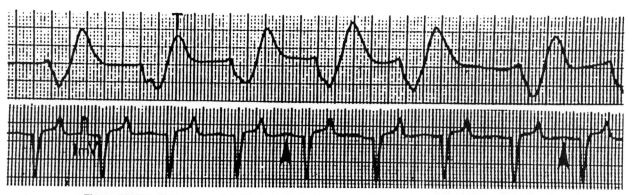

Figure 10. Hyperkalemia in a foal. *(Top)* Atrial standstill and ventricular conduction delay with repolarization abnormalities (T wave indicated). *(Lower)* After therapy with sodium bicarbonate and intravenous saline there is improvement in ventricular conduction and reappearance of low-amplitude P waves *(arrowheads)*. (Base-apex lead, 25 mm/sec.)

occasionally show evidence of ventricular pre-excitation and are characterized by a P-QRS-T relationship but with an extremely short PR interval, early excitation of the ventricle characterized by a slurring of the initial QRS complex (a delta wave), and an overall widening of the QRS complex.

Hyperkalemia

Hyperkalemia can depress atrial, atrioventricular, and ventricular conduction and can shorten ventricular repolarization. Serum potassium is most likely to be markedly elevated following oliguria or rupture of the ureter in foals with a ruptured bladder and uroperitoneum, or after excessive intravenous potassium replacement. Experimentally, changes in the ECG are usually evident when potassium serum concentrations are higher than 6 mEq/L, with severe changes evident when serum concentrations are between 8 and 10 mEq/L. Broadening and flattening of the P wave are the most consistently observed change. Either inversion or enlargement (tenting) of the T waves is also likely. Marked widening of the QRS complex may

be noted as near-lethal concentrations of potassium are approached (Fig. 10A). Ventricular asystole or fibrillation can develop and is related to prolonged ventricular conduction. The Q-T interval is not a reliable indicator of induced hyperkalemia, and other electrolyte/acid-base alterations, including those of serum calcium and sodium, influence the effect of hyperkalemia on the heart.

Supplemental Readings

Bonagura JD, Muir WW: The cardiovascular system. *In* Muir WW, Hubbell JAE (eds): Equine Anesthesia: Monitoring and Emergency Therapy. St. Louis, Mosby-Year Book, 1991, pp 39–104.
Bonagura JD, Miller MS: Electrocardiography. *In* Jones WE (ed): Equine Sports Medicine. Philadelphia, Lea & Febiger, 1989, pp 89–106.
Hilwig RW: Cardiac arrhythmias in the horse. J Am Vet Med Assoc 170:153–163, 1977.
Holmes JR, Henigan M, Williams RB, Witherington D: Paroxysmal atrial fibrillation in racehorses. Equine Vet J 18:37–42, 1986.
Reef VB: Frequency of cardiac arrhythmias and their significance in normal horses. Proc Am Coll Vet Intern Med, 1989, pp 506–508.
Reef VB, Reimer JM, Spencer PA: Treatment of atrial fibrillation in horses: New perspectives. J Vet Intern Med 9(2):57–67, 1995.
Reimer JM, Reef VB, Sweeney RW: Ventricular arrhythmias in horses: 21 cases (1984–1989). J Am Vet Med Assoc 201:1237–1243, 1992.

Treatment of Cardiac Arrhythmias and Cardiac Failure

C E L I A   M .   M A R R
Lambourn, England

In horses, arrhythmias arise as a consequence of primary cardiac disease. Arrhythmias also frequently occur as a result of conditions such as hypoxia, endotoxemia, or electrolyte and metabolic imbalances, or they are associated with the administration of drugs such as anesthetic agents. Before initiating therapy, the clinician should consider the etiology of the arrhythmia and thus determine if it is more appropriate to treat the underlying cause or to attempt to correct the arrhythmia itself using specific antiarrhythmic drugs. In many instances, it is necessary to do both. Specific antiarrhythmic therapy should be considered either when the arrhythmia has reduced cardiac output such that there are clinical signs of low blood flow such as weakness, pallor, weak peripheral pulses, cold extremities, and decreased urine production. Antiarrhythmic therapy also should be considered in the presence of rapid ventricular tachyarrhythmias when there is a danger of ventricular fibrillation.

ANTIARRHYTHMIC DRUGS

In human cardiology, a wide range of antiarrhythmic drugs is approved for use, whereas in horses, the range of

commonly used drugs is less extensive. This arises in part from lack of information on the use of newer antiarrhythmic agents in the horse. In some instances, these products are prohibitively expensive. The majority of antiarrhythmic drugs can be classified according to their electrophysiologic actions. Class I antiarrhythmic agents block the fast inward sodium current of myocardial cells; class II antiarrhythmic drugs block β-adrenoreceptors; class III drugs block the potassium channels and prolong repolarization; and class IV drugs block the slow calcium channel. Class I is further subdivided into IA, drugs that decrease myocardial conduction velocity, increase refractoriness of myocardial cells, and prolong the QRS and QT interval; IB, drugs that shorten the action potential duration; and IC, drugs that decrease conduction velocity.

Drugs that are not included in this classification system are also used in certain equine arrhythmias. Examples are digoxin, which has a variety of negative chronotropic actions, and the vagolytic agents atropine and glycopyrrolate, which are used to abolish vagally mediated arrhythmias.

In selecting treatment for specific equine arrhythmias, it is necessary not only to consider the electrophysiologic effects of particular drugs but also the bioavailability, pharmacokinetics, and adverse effects of these products.

Class I Antiarrhythmic Agents

Quinidine remains one of the most widely used antiarrhythmic agents for the horse. As a class IA drug, its main electrophysiologic effect is to prolong the myocardial refractory period. It is also a vagolytic and an α-adrenergic antagonist. It is used in treatment of atrial fibrillation and of supraventricular and ventricular tachycardia. When administered orally, as quinidine sulfate, peak plasma concentrations are reached within 131 minutes (mean value) and plasma-to-tissue distribution occurs in about 30 minutes. The elimination half life is around 6 hours, although there is considerable individual variation. Quinidine sulfate is administered orally initially every 2 hours until therapeutic concentrations are achieved (usually four or five doses) and thereafter every 6 hours until either the arrhythmia resolves or toxic side effects are seen (Table 1). Quinidine can also be administered intravenously as quinidine gluconate, either as repeated boluses or as an infusion (see Table 1).

The therapeutic plasma concentrations range from 2 to 5 μg/ml but toxic side effects can occur at plasma concentrations only slightly higher than this. Quinidine has both cardiac and extracardiac side effects. It is a proarrhythmic and can induce ventricular tachycardia. It is particularly associated with torsades de pointes, a form of ventricular tachycardia that arises with prolongation of the QT interval. Quinidine's vagolytic action can lead to rapid supraventricular tachycardia (250–300/min) in horses being treated for atrial fibrillation. Because it is an α-adrenoceptor antagonist, quinidine can cause hypotension; at higher doses, it can decrease myocardial contractility. As a result of these effects, sudden death can occur during quinidine treatment. Extracardiac side effects include depression, gastrointestinal ulceration leading to diarrhea and abdominal pain, upper respiratory tract edema and stridor, urticaria, and penile prolapse. Ideally, plasma concentrations of quinidine should be measured in horses receiving quinidine to ensure that they are therapeutic and not toxic concentrations. An increase in the duration of the QRS to more than 25% of its pretreatment value is an early sign of toxicity.

Procainamide is also a class IA antiarrhythmic drug with electrophysiologic and hemodyamic actions and clinical indications similar to those of quinidine. Procainamide is administered orally (see Table 1), and it is metabolized to N-acetylprocainamide (NAPA). NAPA's electrophysiologic actions differ from the parent compound in that it is a class III agent and prolongs the action potential duration. Unfortunately, clinical experience with procainamide is limited. It appears to be less effective than quinidine in treating supraventricular arrhythmias but equally efficacious in ventricular arrhythmias.

Lidocaine is the most widely used class IB antiarrhythmic drug. It increases refractoriness in partially depolarized fibers but has little effect on normally polarized fibers. Lidocaine does not alter atrial myocardial function. It has most effect on Purkinje fibers and ventricular myocardium and, therefore, is most effective in ventricular arrhythmias. It may prevent the onset of ventricular fibrillation by preventing fragmentation of organized wavefronts. It is administered intravenously as boluses or as an infusion (see Table 1). The horse appears to be particularly sensitive to lidocaine's main side effects, which are seizures and excitement. If seizures occur, they should be controlled with diazepam.

Other class I antiarrhythmic drugs include disopyramide (class IA), phenytoin (class IB), and propafenone (class IC). Disopyramide is used in humans for treatment of both supraventricular and ventricular arrhythmias, but its use has not been investigated in the horse. Phenytoin has actions similar to those of lidocaine but appears not to be as efficacious in humans or horses. Propafenone is extremely effective in the treatment of ventricular arrhythmias in humans and is also used in supraventricular arrhythmias. It has been used both orally and intravenously in horses. Intravenously, it has been used successfully in horses with ventricular arrhythmias, but use of the oral preparation in doses extrapolated from experience with humans has been disappointing. Further information on dosage regimens is required before specific recommendations can be made.

Class II Antiarrhythmic Agents

The β-adrenoceptor antagonist (β-blocker) propranolol exerts its electrophysiologic action by competitively inhibiting catecholamine binding at β-adrenergic receptors. Its major hemodynamic effect is to reduce cardiac contractility. It can be used to treat supraventricular and ventricular arrhythmias, but its effects depend on the prevailing sympathetic tone. Unfortunately, its efficacy as an antiarrhythmic drug in the horse is poor. Its negative inotropic and negative chronotropic effects may be disadvantageous, and it should be used with caution in horses with congestive heart failure. Its oral bioavailability is low, and therefore it is administered intravenously (see Table 1). β-Blockers increase the severity of airway obstruction in horses with chronic obstructive pulmonary disease (COPD).

Class III and IV Antiarrhythmic Agents

Drugs belonging to classes III and IV have not been investigated fully in the horse, largely because of their expense. Bretylium, a class III agent, is efficacious in some cases of ventricular fibrillation in humans. The author has used it without success in a small number of foals with ventricular fibrillation. Anecdotal reports exist concerning the use of verapamil, a calcium channel blocker, but specific data relating to its use in the horse are not available. Magnesium sulfate is a physiologic calcium channel blocker. In humans it is used alone, or in combination with other antiarrhythmic agents, for treatment of both supraventricular and ventricular arrhythmias. It has been used successfully in the treatment of ventricular tachycardia in several horses and is also indicated in quinidine-induced ventricular arrhythmias. It is administered intravenously as boluses or an infusion (see Table 1).

Other Antiarrythmic Agents

Both parasympatholytic and sympathomimetic drugs are used in horses with bradyarrhythmias. The vagolytic drugs atropine and glycopyrrolate are administered intravenously to treat vagally mediated arrhythmias. Their main side effect is paralytic ileus. Dopamine is an adrenergic agonist with dose-dependent action. At low doses (1–3 μg/kg per minute), it exerts a dopaminergic effect leading to dilation of the renal vascular bed, improved renal perfusion, and

TABLE 1

DRUGS USED TO TREAT CARDIAC ARRHYTHMIAS IN HORSES—DOSAGE REGIMENS, ANTIARRHYTHMIC ACTIONS, INDICATIONS, SIDE EFFECTS, AND CONTRAINDICATIONS

DRUG	ROUTE	DOSAGE	ANTIARRHYTHMIC ACTION	INDICATIONS	SIDE EFFECTS AND CONTRAINDICATIONS
Atropine	IV, IM	0.01–0.015 mg/kg	Vagolytic	Vagally induced bradyarrhythmias	Ileus, abdominal pain
Bretylium	IV	5–10 mg/kg (from humans, no equine data available)	Class III	Ventricular fibrillation	Not fully investigated
Digoxin	IV	0.0022 mg/kg b.i.d.	Slows conduction through AV node, parasympathomimetic, sympatholytic (also increases myocardial contractility)	Rapid supraventricular arrhythmias, rapid atrial fibrillation	Depression, abdominal pain, ventricular arrhythmias
	p.o.	0.011 mg/kg b.i.d.			
Dopamine	IV	5 μg/kg per min infusion	β-Adrenergic (at these concentrations—also has dopaminergic and α-adrenergic actions that are dose-dependent)	Advanced second degree and third degree atrioventricular block	Vasoconstriction at higher doses
Dobutamine	IV	1–10 μg/kg/min infusion	β-Adrenergic	Advanced second degree and third degree atrioventricular block	Tachycardia and ventricular arrhythmias
Epinephrine	IV, IT	0.1–0.2 ml/kg of a 1:10,000 solution	α- and β-adrenergic	Asystole, cardiopulmonary resuscitation	Vasoconstriction (beneficial in CPR)
Glycopyrrolate	IV	0.005–0.01 mg/kg	Vagolytic	Vagally induced bradyarrhythmias	Ileus, abdominal pain
Lidocaine	IV	0.25–0.5 mg/kg repeated in 5–15 min up to 1.5 mg/kg	Class IB	Ventricular tachycardia	CNS excitement, seizures
Magnesium sulfate	IV	4 mg/kg boluses every 2 min up to 50 mg/kg	Physiologic calcium channel blocker	Ventricular tachycardia	Not fully investigated
Phenytoin	p.o.	10–22 mg/kg	Class IB	Supraventricular premature depolarizations/tachycardia	Sedation
Procainamide	p.o.	35 mg/kg	Class IA	Supraventricular premature depolarizations/tachycardia	Hypotension
Propafenone	IV	0.5–1 mg/kg	Class IC	Supraventricular and ventricular premature depolarizations/tachycardia	Not fully investigated
Propranolol	IV	0.05–0.16 mg/kg	Class II (β-adrenoreceptor blockade)	Ventricular tachycardia	Bradycardia, hypotension, weakness
	p.o.	0.38–0.78 mg/kg t.i.d.			
Quinidine gluconate	IV	2.2 mg/kg bolus every 10 min to 8.8–11 mg/kg total or 0.7–3 mg/kg per hour infusion	Class IA	Atrial fibrillation (recent onset); supraventricular and ventricular tachycardia	Hypotension
Quinidine sulfate	p.o.	22 mg/kg bolus every 2 hours up to five times and then every 6 hours	Class IA	Atrial fibrillation	Gastrointestinal ulceration, abdominal pain, diarrhea, upper airway edema, urticaria, depression; hypotension, penile prolapse; arrhythmias particularly rapid supraventricular tachycardia
Verapamil	IV	0.025–0.05 mg/kg every 30 min	Class IV	Supraventricular premature depolarizations/tachycardia	Not fully investigated

IV = intravenous; IM = intramuscular; p.o. = oral dosage; IT = intratracheal.

increased glomerular filtration rate. At intermediate doses (3–5 μg/kg per minute), it stimulates β-adrenoceptors in the heart, resulting in increased contractility. At higher doses (>5 μg/kg per minute), it leads to increased α-adrenergic tone, which produces vasoconstriction that may be deleterious as blood flow decreases in important vascular beds such as the kidneys. In the horse, dopamine is used as a diuretic, a positive inotrope, and less frequently in the treatment of bradyarrhythmias. Dobutamine is a synthetic sympathomimetic amine that has primarily, but not solely, β-adrenergic effects. The side effects of dopamine and dobutamine include tachycardia and hypertension. Both drugs should be administered as controlled infusions, and arterial blood pressure and the electrocardiograph should be monitored.

Digoxin is a unique compound with a wide range of effects. It is used in congestive cardiac failure for its positive inotropic effect. Digoxin directly prolongs conduction through the atrioventricular node, but its main effect on AV conduction is mediated by an increase in parasympathetic tone and a decrease in sympathetic tone. As an antiarrhythmic agent, it is indicated in supraventricular arrhythmias when the goal is to reduce the ventricular response rate, rather than suppress the arrhythmia itself. Pharmacokinetic studies have demonstrated that there is considerable individual variation in plasma half life of digoxin. Some authors advocate using a loading dose followed by maintenance doses. However, the author prefers to administer 0.011 mg/kg p.o. or 0.0022 mg/kg intravenously b.i.d. Peak concentrations are expected 1 hour after oral administration. Peak and trough plasma digoxin concentrations should be measured and the dosage regimen and intervals adjusted to achieve a plasma concentration of 1 to 2 ng/ml. Concurrent administration of quinidine increases plasma digoxin concentrations. Digoxin has a narrow toxic to therapeutic index, and toxic side effects have been recorded at 2.4 ng/ml. Digoxin is a proarrhythmic and causes anorexia, depression, abdominal pain, and behavioral changes. Digoxin-induced ventricular arrhythmias are treated with phenytoin, lidocaine, and propanolol in humans.

THERAPY AND MANAGEMENT OF SPECIFIC ARRHYTHMIAS

Bradyarrhythmias

The majority of bradyarrhythmias in horses are physiologic rather than pathologic in origin and thus rarely require treatment. Administration of vagolytic agents, such as atropine and glycopyrrolate, is sometimes used as a diagnostic test to confirm that bradyarrhythmias are physiologic rather than pathologic. These drugs are also used to treat horses that develop bradyarrhythmias under anesthesia (see Table 1). Dopamine and dobutamine are also effective in horses that develop bradyarrhythmias under anesthesia.

Advanced second-degree and third-degree atrioventricular block can be caused by inflammatory or fibrotic lesions at the atrioventricular node. In some horses presumed to have inflammatory lesions, high doses of corticosteroids

(dexamethasone 40–100 mg IV) have been effective in reversing the arrhythmia. However, in horses with persistent third degree heart block, a pacemaker may be the only effective treatment. Several workers have used permanent transvenous pacemakers successfully in horses.

Third-degree atrioventricular block can also be associated with hyperkalemia; thus, it is the commonest arrhythmia to arise in foals with uroperitoneum. These foals should be given normal saline and bicarbonate (0.5–2 mEq/kg), insulin (0.5 IU/kg) and dextrose (2–4 g/unit of insulin) to decrease the circulating potassium concentration by increasing cellular uptake.

Atrial Fibrillation

Atrial fibrillation is the most common pathologic arrhythmia in horses. It can occur in the absence of any other cardiac disease. However, atrial fibrillation can also be due to myocardial disease or atrial enlargement in valvular or congenital cardiac disease. In horses with no underlying cardiac disease that are subjected to limited athletic demands, no treatment may be necessary. In racehorses and performance horses, treatment is usually necessary if the horse is to compete successfully. Quinidine sulfate is the drug of choice in horses with atrial fibrillation that have no cardiac murmurs, a normal resting heart rate (40–50 bpm), and no significant cardiac chamber enlargement on echocardiographic examination. Horses with atrial fibrillation of less than 3 months' duration have less risk of recurrence, whereas recurrence rates of 65% have been reported in horses with long-standing atrial fibrillation. The treatment protocol described (see Table 1) should be followed until either the atrial fibrillation resolves or signs of toxicity ensue. Ideally, the electrocardiogram tracing should be monitored continuously throughout treatment to detect quinidine-induced arrhythmias. Rapid supraventricular tachycardia is treated with intravenous digoxin to slow the ventricular response; sodium bicarbonate to reduce the circulating concentrations of quinidine; and polyionic fluids to combat hypotension. Horses receiving quinidine should be confined to a stall to minimize stress. Quinidine administration should be discontinued if the QRS duration exceeds 25% of its value before the onset of treatment. Horses with a condition refractory to treatment with quinidine alone may respond to a combination of digoxin and quinidine. Digoxin increases the effective refractory period in atropinized myocardial cells, increasing the fibrillation threshold; thus, digoxin can complement quinidine's effects. Introduction of oral digoxin (0.011 mg/kg b.i.d.) on day 2 of treatment has been advocated.

Horses with atrial fibrillation of less than 7 days' duration have been treated successfully with intravenous quinidine gluconate. However, the percentage of successful conversions with intravenous quinidine gluconate decreases as the suspected duration of the atrial fibrillation increases. Quinidine is contraindicated in horses with clinical signs of congestive heart failure or rapid resting heart rates. In these horses, palliative treatment with digoxin is appropriate. Potassium depletion has been documented in some horses with paroxysmal atrial fibrillation, and if this is suspected, a potassium chloride supplement (1 oz b.i.d.) should be provided.

Supraventricular Premature Depolarizations and Tachycardia

Isolated supraventricular premature depolarizations rarely require specific antiarrhythmic therapy. In affected horses, it is more rational to investigate and address the underlying causes. Some horses with supraventricular premature depolarizations respond to stall or pasture rest and corticosteroid administration. Similarly, supraventricular tachycardia rarely requires specific antiarrhythmic therapy, unless the ventricular response rate is greater than 100 bpm. Rapid supraventricular tachycardia is treated with digoxin, with the aim of reducing the ventricular response rate. However, occasionally atrial ectopy itself may be suppressed by digoxin.

Ventricular Premature Depolarizations and Tachycardia

The approach to management of isolated ventricular premature depolarizations is similar to treatment of supraventricular premature depolarizations. However, ventricular tachycardia is more likely to require antiarrhythmic therapy. Ventricular tachycardia often occurs as a consequence of other systemic diseases, particularly gastrointestinal disease. Similarly, primary myocardial diseases such as viral or bacterial myocarditis or toxic or immune-mediated cardiomyopathies are most frequently associated with ventricular arrhythmias. Ventricular tachycardia is the most likely cardiac arrhythmia to be life-threatening. Indications for antiarrhythmic therapy include clinical signs of low cardiac output; ventricular rates of greater than 100/minute; multiform ectopic complexes; and the R on T phenomenon, wherein an R wave falls very close to the pre-ceding T wave, indicating that depolarization and repolarization are occurring almost simultaneously.

Lidocaine is one of the most effective drugs for abolition of ventricular arrhythmias, and it is the drug of first choice in ventricular arrhythmias occurring under anesthesia. However, because of the risk of seizures, some clinicians reserve its use in conscious horses to life-threatening ventricular arrhythmias that have failed to respond to other drugs. Quinidine gluconate is also effective, but its hypotensive and negative inotropic effects may be undesirable. Procainamide, magnesium sulfate, propafenone, and propanolol have all been used with variable results.

Ventricular Fibrillation and Asystole

The treatment of these arrhythmias in the horse is rarely successful and is usually undertaken only in horses in which the arrhythmia occurs under anesthesia or in neonatal intensive care units. Electrical defibrillation is the treatment of choice for ventricular fibrillation but is only feasible in horses weighing less than 350 kg. Lidocaine and bretylium are indicated in ventricular fibrillation, whereas epinephrine should be administered to animals with asystole.

TREATMENT AND MANAGEMENT OF CARDIAC FAILURE

The optimal treatment and management of cardiac failure depend on the specific cause. In the horse, congestive cardiac failure can be associated with myocarditis, cardiomyopathy, congenital cardiac defects, and severe left atrioventricular insufficiency alone or in conjunction with other forms of valvular insufficiency (see Acquired Cardiac Disease). Horses with pericarditis usually present with signs of right-sided heart failure. Thus, the first step the clinician must take is to determine the underlying cause of the heart failure. This not only determines treatment options but also provides a realistic prognosis. Horses with pericarditis and some cases of myocarditis can be treated successfully, but in the majority of horses with cardiac failure, the long-term prognosis is poor and treatment is palliative only.

Specific problems should be addressed if possible. For example, pericarditis is treated by drainage and lavage of the pericardial sac and antimicrobial drugs and, if indicated, corticosteroids; bacterial endocarditis requires the use of antimicrobial agents. However, beyond treating the underlying cause, the main goals of therapy in congestive heart failure are to improve tissue perfusion and reduce congestion, thereby improving tissue oxygenation.

Diuretics

Congestive heart failure is characterized by the retention of sodium and water leading to venous congestion and pulmonary and systemic congestion. Diuretics are the first line of therapy to reduce congestion. In many horses with mild chronic heart failure, diuretic therapy can be sufficient to improve the horse's quality of life in the short and medium term. Furosemide is the most effective and popular diuretic used in the horse. It inhibits chloride transport in the distal loop of Henle, increasing the excretion of sodium, chloride, potassium, hydrogen ions, and water. This produces a decrease in plasma volume, extracellular fluid volume, and pulmonary fluid volume; in addition, it decreases congestion and reduces the work of ventilation. Furosemide is administered at 1 to 2 mg/kg IV b.i.d. or t.i.d. or, for longer term dosing, at 0.5 to 1 mg/kg IM or p.o. b.i.d. or t.i.d. Long-term furosemide administration may produce hyponatremia, hypokalemia, hypomagnesemia, and metabolic alkalosis. Electrolyte and metabolic status should be monitored regularly in horses receiving long-term furosemide therapy.

Positive Inotropes

Increasing cardiac output to improve tissue perfusion can sometimes be achieved by use of positive inotropes. In horses, digoxin and the sympathomimetic amines dopamine and dobutamine have been used for this purpose. Dopamine and dobutamine are used for the short-term support of acutely affected horses and are indicated in acute left ventricular or biventricular failure in horses with myocarditis or cardiomyopathy. Digoxin has been used in horses presenting with heart failure resulting from myocarditis and cardiomyopathy, congenital cardiac disease, and valvular insufficiency. The positive inotropic action of digoxin results from its ability to inhibit the enzyme that regulates sodium-potassium exchange in myocardial cells. This leads to an increase in intracellular sodium, activates a sodium-calcium exchange mechanism, and produces a substantial increase in intracellular calcium. The calcium available for contraction is increased, thereby raising contractile force and velocity. In congestive heart failure, digoxin may help to alleviate clinical signs by improving myocardial contractility. However, it also suppresses plasma renin and aldosterone activity, reducing venous pressures. It also inhibits tubular reabsorption of sodium, promotes diuresis, and reduces venous congestion. In horses with congestive heart failure and atrial fibrillation, digoxin slows the ventricular response rate, enabling more efficient ventricular filling. The adverse effects and specific details of therapeutic regimens for digoxin are described earlier (see Table 1).

Vasodilators

Vasodilating agents have had a huge impact on human and small animal cardiovascular therapeutics. However, there is limited information on the use of these agents in the horse. These drugs improve cardiac performance by altering preload and afterload, both of which tend to be increased in congestive heart failure. Reduction of afterload not only improves forward stroke volume and increases cardiac output, but also reduces the regurgitant fraction in dogs and humans with mitral valvular insufficiency. In horses, promazine (1.5 mg/kg p.o.) has been proposed as an economical option for afterload reduction, but the efficacy of this and other afterload reducers such as hydralazine have not been investigated critically.

Supplemental Readings

Baggot JD: The pharmacological basis of cardiac drug selection for use in horses. Equine Vet J 19[Suppl]:97–100, 1995.
Jaillon PJ: Recent antiarrhythmic drugs. Am J Cardiol 64:65J–69J, 1989.
McGuirk SM, Muir WW: Diagnosis and treatment of cardiac arrhythmias. Vet Clin North Am Equine Pract 1(2):353–370, 1985.
Marr CM, Reef VB: Disturbances of blood flow. In Kobluk CN, Ames TR, Geor RJ (eds): The Horse: Diseases and Clinical Managment. Philadelphia, WB Saunders, 1995, pp 157–184.
Muir WW, McGuirk SM: Pharmacology and pharmacokinetics of drugs used to treat cardiac disease in horses. Vet Clin North Am Equine Pract 1(2):335–352, 1985.
Reef VB, Reimer JM, Sweeney RW, Spencer PA: New perspectives in the treatment of equine atrial fibrillation. J Vet Intern Med 9:57–67, 1995.
Reef VB, Levitan CW, Spencer PA: Factors affecting prognosis and conversion in equine atrial fibrillation. J Vet Intern Med 2:1–6, 1988.
Zipes DP: Management of cardiac arrhythmias. In Braunwald E (ed): Heart Disease: A Textbook of Cardiovascular Medicine. Philadelphia, WB Saunders, 1988, pp 628–666.

Congenital Cardiac Disease

A B B Y D. M A X S O N
Kennett Square, Pennsylvania

According to Rooney and Franks, the incidence of congenital cardiac malformation in the horse is low; four cases of congenital cardiac disease were observed in 2500 equine necropsies. The etiology of congenital cardiac disease is likely to be multifactorial, with heredity probably playing a role.

Congenital cardiac malformation should be suspected in a foal with a loud cardiac murmur or a murmur that persists beyond 1 week of age. Cyanosis, persistent tachycardia, tachypnea, exercise intolerance, or stunted growth should prompt a complete examination of the cardiovascular system.

VENTRICULAR SEPTAL DEFECT

Ventricular septal defect (VSD) is the most common congenital cardiac defect in the horse. Most frequently, this malformation is an opening high in the membranous portion of the ventricular septum just ventral to the right or noncoronary cusp of the aortic valve, communicating with the right ventricular inflow tract caudal and ventral to the crista supraventricularis just beneath the septal leaflet of the tricuspid valve (Fig. 1). The defect is caused by a lack of fusion of the atrioventricular endocardial cushion and the muscular ventricular septum. It can occur as a single malformation or as part of a complex of malformations such as tetralogy or pentalogy of Fallot, truncus or pseudotruncus arteriosus, or tricuspid atresia. In uncomplicated VSD, blood is shunted from left to right owing to higher pressures in the left ventricle compared with the right.

Clinical Signs

Clinical signs vary depending on the size and location of the defect and velocity of the shunt flow. Most commonly a loud (grade 3/6 to 6/6) pansystolic band-shaped murmur, with its point of maximal intensity over the tricuspid valve area, is present as a result of the left-to-right shunt. In addition, a slightly softer ejection-type murmur is audible over the pulmonic valve area because of increased blood flow through this valve. If the point of maximal intensity is on the left, a complex malformation should be suspected. A palpable thrill is usually present, and occasionally there is a splitting of the second heart sound (S_2). Small defects have higher resistance to blood flow and may result in louder murmurs than larger defects. Therefore, intensity of the murmur should not be used as a prognostic factor. Large defects may result in lack of support to the right or noncoronary cusp of the aortic valve, and in aortic insufficiency and a diastolic decrescendo murmur in the aortic valve area.

Diagnosis

Diagnosis is most easily made by visualization of the membranous VSD as a discontinuity of echoes between the interventricular septum and aorta on two-dimensional echocardiography (2DE) in the parasternal long axis view

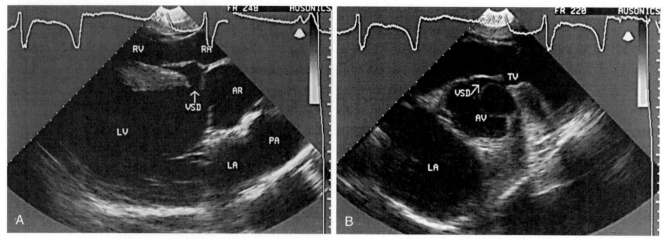

Figure 1. Two-dimensional echocardiogram from a 1-year-old Standardbred colt with a membranous ventricular septal defect. (*A*) Right parasternal long-axis view of the left ventricular outflow tract. (*B*) Right parasternal short-axis view of the aorta. AR = aortic root; AV = aortic valve; LA = left atrium; LV = left ventricle; PA = pulmonary artery; RA = right atrium; RV = right ventricle; TV = tricuspid valve; VSD = ventricular septal defect.

of the left outflow tract. The size of the defect should be measured in two perpendicular planes. Peak shunt velocity through the VSD is measured with continuous-wave Doppler echocardiography. Large VSDs result in volume overload of the left ventricle, pulmonary circulation, and left atrium and may cause chamber dilation that is visible on 2DE. The velocity of the shunt is determined by the size of the defect and the pressures of the right and left ventricles and pulmonary arteries. Aortic insufficiency is semiquantified by Doppler echocardiographic interrogation of the aortic valve. Microbubble contrast material injected into the jugular vein opacifies the right ventricle and produces an area of negative contrast just under the septal valve leaflet of the tricuspid valve in the area of the VSD. In large VSDs, thoracic radiography reveals cardiomegaly, a prominent pulmonary artery, and pulmonary hypervascularization. The electrocardiogram is unremarkable. Cardiac catheterization and oximetry may show a step-up of oxygen saturation or partial pressure of oxygen between the right atrium and pulmonary artery and elevation of pulmonary artery and right ventricular systolic pressures if the defect is moderate to large. Angiographic conformation of the VSD can be made by injection of dye in the left ventricle in young foals.

Prognosis

Echocardiography is extremely useful in guiding the prognosis. If the defect is 2.5 cm or less in diameter, the defect is membranous, peak shunt velocity is greater than 4 m/sec, and there is no aortic insufficiency, the horse may show no clinical signs of the defect. The horse can usually race or compete successfully and has a normal life expectancy. Horses with a membranous defect from 2.5 cm to 3.5 cm in diameter tend to show exercise intolerance at maximal athletic performance, but may be able to perform adequately as pleasure horses. Horses with membranous VSDs larger than 3.5 cm in diameter or muscular VSDs tend to have a decreased life expectancy. They often develop congestive heart failure and show signs of lethargy,

poor growth, dyspnea, and exercise intolerance. These horses have lower peak shunt velocities because the defect is less restrictive and the pressure gradient across the defect is reduced owing to increased right ventricular pressure. Large membranous defects can result in chronic volume overload of the left ventricle, and they lead to congestive heart failure. Aortic insufficiency may contribute to left ventricular volume overload and may result in earlier signs of cardiovascular disease.

PATENT DUCTUS ARTERIOSUS

Patent ductus arteriosus (PDA) is a rare congenital cardiac disorder in the foal. It may occur singly or in conjunction with other cardiac defects. Contracture and functional closure of the ductus arteriosus normally occurs within 96 hours after birth. Although the complete mechanism of closure is unknown, exposure of the smooth muscle in the wall of the ductus arteriosus to oxygenated blood results in contracture. Because of the increase in systemic vascular resistance and decrease in pulmonary vascular resistance after birth, blood shunts from left to right through the PDA.

Clinical Signs

A high-pitched continuous machinery murmur that is loudest over the left heart base is characteristic of a PDA. The murmur has its point of maximal intensity in the left third to fourth intercostal spaces at the level of the shoulder. In some foals, only a bilateral holosystolic murmur is present because pulmonary hypertension may decrease the intensity of the diastolic component. Clinical signs vary depending on the size of the shunt. Some animals may show no clinical signs, except for the characteristic murmur. Foals with a large shunt may have growth retardation or exercise intolerance.

Diagnosis

No clinicopathologic or electrocardiographic abnormalities are associated with PDA. Thoracic radiographs may show nonspecific cardiomegaly and pulmonary hypervascularization. If left-sided congestive heart failure develops as a result of volume overload, then pulmonary venous congestion, interstitial pulmonary edema, and alveolar edema may be present. The PDA is difficult to visualize on 2DE, but dilation of the left atrium and ventricle due to volume overload may be observed. Color-flow Doppler echocardiography can be used to detect flow through the PDA from the aorta to the pulmonary artery. Cardiac catheterization coupled with oximetry reveals a higher oxygen saturation in the pulmonary artery compared with that in the great veins, right atrium, and right ventricle. The increase in oxygen saturation is in proportion to the size of the shunt. If the PDA is large, pulmonary artery and right ventricular pressures are elevated. Definitive diagnosis is made by cardiac angiography or nuclear angiography using a selective aortic angiogram.

Prognosis and Treatment

Prognosis is based in part on the size of the lesion. A horse with a small PDA may show no signs of the defect throughout life. Animals with large defects experience left atrial and ventricular volume overload, pulmonary hypertension, and subsequent left-sided heart failure.

TETRALOGY OF FALLOT

Tetralogy of Fallot is one of the most common complex congenital cardiac malformations in the horse. Four lesions characterize tetralogy of Fallot: (1) biventricular origin of the aorta, which is known as overriding aorta; (2) VSD; (3) hypoplastic pulmonary artery; and (4) secondary right ventricular hypertrophy. If a PDA is also present, the malformation is called pentalogy of Fallot. The condition arises as a result of a developmental abnormality of the bulbus cordis during the fourth week of gestation. The truncus arteriosus is unequally divided by the spiral septum, resulting in abnormal formation of the right ventricular outflow tract and pulmonary valve and incomplete formation of the ventricular septum. Resistance to right ventricular outflow causes secondary hypertrophy of the right ventricle and pulmonary hypoperfusion. Increased flow through the aorta results in aortic dilation. Rarely, cyanosis can result if the deficit is large enough to cause a sufficient amount of unoxygenated blood to enter the aorta from the right ventricle.

Clinical Signs

The severity of clinical signs is dependent on the size of the VSD and the degree of right ventricular outflow obstruction. Foals with tetralogy of Fallot can experience exercise intolerance, difficulty nursing, and dyspnea. A loud (grade 4/6 to 6/6), coarse, band-shaped or crescendo-decrescendo pansystolic murmur with a palpable thrill is audible over the left heart base with its point of maximal intensity in the pulmonic valve area.

Diagnosis and Prognosis

Although not specific for tetralogy of Fallot, thoracic radiographs reveal right ventricular enlargement, hypovascularization of the lungs, and prominence of the ascending aorta. Tetralogy of Fallot is most easily diagnosed with 2DE. The parasternal long axis view of the left ventricular outflow tract and aorta is necessary to demonstrate the VSD and overriding aorta. Aortic root dimension may be increased. Right outflow tract obstruction can be visualized in the parasternal long axis or short axis view of the right ventricular outflow tract. Right ventricular hypertrophy is represented by increased thickness of right ventricular free wall and septum. High velocity turbulent flow is present on Doppler echocardiographic examination of the pulmonary artery. Flow through the VSD is right to left on Doppler echocardiographic examination. Contrast echocardiography and angiography following peripheral venous injection of contrast material results in opacification of the right ventricle followed by simultaneous opacification of the aorta, pulmonary artery, and left ventricle. An increase in right ventricular trabeculation is delineated with angiography as a result of right ventricular hypertrophy. A pressure gradient across the area of pulmonary stenosis, right ventricular systolic hypertension, and equalization of pressures between the right and left ventricle can be demonstrated by cardiac catheterization. Right ventricular systolic pressure exceeds pulmonary artery pressure because of pulmonic stenosis. When oximetry is performed, oxygen content is decreased in the left ventricle and aorta owing to the mixing of unoxygenated with oxygenated blood through the VSD.

Prognosis for long-term survival is poor.

TRICUSPID ATRESIA

Atresia of the tricuspid valve has a grave prognosis, and the defect must occur in conjunction with other congenital cardiac malformations if the foal is to survive. Most commonly, atrial septal defect (ASD) or patent foramen ovale and high VSD are present in conjunction with tricuspid atresia in the horse. Anomalies of the great vessels such as pulmonic stenosis and bicuspid pulmonic valve have also been reported to accompany this defect. Blood in the right atrium shunts across the ASD into the left atrium but, because of the resistance to flow across the ASD, the right atrium becomes dilated. The left atrium, mitral valve, and left ventricle also become dilated because of the volume overload. Some of the mixed arterial and venous blood entering the left ventricle is shunted to the right ventricle and pulmonary artery via the VSD. Rarely, pulmonary hypoperfusion may cause cyanosis.

Clinical Signs

Foals that survive with tricuspid atresia may have cyanotic mucous membranes, dyspnea, weak pulses, and generalized venous distension. Sudden death has been reported. A loud (grade 4/6 to 6/6) harsh, band-shaped or crescendo-decrescendo murmur with a palpable thrill is present over the right heart base.

Diagnosis

Clinical pathologic abnormalities may include polycythemia and arterial hypoxemia. A prolonged P wave resulting from right atrial enlargement may be present on the electrocardiogram. Chest radiographs may demonstrate pulmonary hypoperfusion.

The atretic tricuspid region imaged by 2DE appears as a thick muscular band of echoes that do not open in diastole instead of normal tricuspid valve leaflets. The VSD, enlarged left and right atrium and left ventricle, and hypoplastic right ventricle can also be demonstrated. The path of opacification following peripheral venous injection of contrast material is right atrium to left atrium, through the mitral valve to the left ventricle, followed by simultaneous opacification of the aorta and right ventricle and then the pulmonary artery. The flow from right to left through the ASD and left to right through the VSD can be demonstrated with color-flow Doppler echocardiography. Flow between the right atrium and ventricle is absent.

PERSISTENT TRUNCUS OR PSEUDOTRUNCUS ARTERIOSUS

In persistent truncus arteriosus, only one artery, the common truncus, leaves the heart above a VSD, which allows mixing of blood from both ventricles. The coronary arteries, pulmonary artery, and aorta arise from the one vessel. If a remnant of an atretic pulmonary trunk is present, the malformation is pseudotruncus arteriosus. In pseudotruncus arteriosus, the vascular supply to the lungs comes from bronchial arteries or a PDA. The malformation is caused by failure of development of the spiral septum, which normally equally divides the truncus arteriosus into the aorta and pulmonary arteries. Prognosis for long-term survival is poor.

Clinical Signs

Tachycardia, exercise intolerance, stunted growth, dyspnea, or syncope may be seen. Cyanosis may be present as a result of decreased blood flow through the hypoplastic pulmonary arteries. If pulmonary vascular supply is adequate, cyanosis is minimal. A loud (grade 4/6 to 6/6) crescendo-decrescendo cardiac murmur with a palpable thrill is audible over the left heart base.

Diagnosis

Polycythemia and arterial hypoxemia may be present but are not specific for persistent truncus arteriosus. Two-dimensional echocardiography demonstrates one vessel originating from both the left and right ventricles accompanied by a VSD.

ATRIAL SEPTAL DEFECT

The foramen ovale is formed by openings in adjacent thin membranous sheets, the septum primum and septum secundum, which form the intra-atrial septum. In the foal at birth, the septa primum and secundum become tightly opposed owing to a decrease in right atrial pressure and increase in pressure in the left atrium. Anatomic closure of the foramen ovale occurs within 15 days to 9 weeks after birth. Occasionally the foramen ovale does not completely fuse. Patent foramen ovale is most often an isolated cardiac anomaly and is not usually associated with clinical signs.

True ASD commonly occurs in conjunction with other congenital cardiac malformations and is considered rare in the horse. Persistent foramen primum is a result of failure of closure of the primum portion of the septum and is often accompanied by atrioventricular orifice abnormalities because it is adjacent to the ventricular septum and involved in endocardial cushion formation. Persistent foramen secundum permits blood to shunt from left to right in the area of the foramen ovale. Basilar septal defects occur from defective sinus venosum development.

Blood is shunted from left to right through the ASD because of the higher left atrial pressure. If the defect is of sufficient size, then volume overload, hypertrophy, and dilation of the right atrium, right ventricle, and pulmonary artery can occur.

Clinical Signs

Foals with uncomplicated ASD are often asymptomatic. However, a crescendo-decrescendo holosystolic murmur may be heard over the pulmonic valve as a consequence of volume overload. If the defect is large or complicated by other congenital malformations, additional cardiovascular signs may be present.

Diagnosis

True ASD must be distinguished on 2DE from the normal appearance of the foramen ovale. A gradual discontinuity in echoes of the intra-atrial septum is observed in a normal foramen ovale, whereas an ASD is characterized by a bright echo perpendicular to the site of discontinuity of the atrial septum. During angiography, negative contrast at the site of the left-to-right shunt through the defect is seen on opacification of the right atrium following peripheral venous injection of contrast material. Color-flow Doppler echocardiography can be used to demonstrate shunting through the atrial septum.

OTHER CONGENITAL CARDIAC ABNORMALITIES

In transposition of the great vessels, the aorta originates from the right ventricle and the pulmonary artery originates from the left ventricle. This malformation must be accompanied by shunts for the foal to survive. Interruption of the aortic arch in conjunction with an ASD and VSD has been described in two foals. The ascending aorta originated from the left ventricle and the descending aorta originated from the right ventricle via the pulmonary artery and connecting ductus arteriosus. Differential cyanosis (i.e., cyanosis of the caudal trunk and pelvic limbs only) was present. Persistence of the right aortic arch instead of the left can cause esophageal entrapment by the left ductus arteriosus against the trachea and subsequent dysphagia. Multiple anomalies of the coronary arteries have been described as well as a variety of other congenital cardiac malformations.

Pulmonic valve stenosis is rare as an isolated defect but is more commonly seen in conjunction with a variety of complex malformations. Pulmonic and aortic valve dysplasia such as bicuspid pulmonic valve, aberrant number of aortic valve cusps, and incomplete aortic valve commissure can occur in the foal.

TREATMENT

Successful surgical correction of congenital cardiac malformations has not been documented in the foal. Medical therapy, although not usually warranted based on the final outcome, is directed at the treatment of heart failure until a diagnosis can be obtained. Digoxin and furosemide (see page 252) may be indicated if signs of left or right heart failure are present. Foals with impaired renal clearance should be treated with prolonged dosage intervals of digoxin. Plasma levels should be monitored frequently to avoid digoxin toxicity. Signs of toxicity include anorexia, depression, diarrhea, and cardiac arrhythmia. Plasma potassium should be monitored during treatment with furosemide.

Because of the possible hereditary nature of cardiac defects, owners should be cautioned against breeding affected animals. No information is available on the possible increased risk of a foal having a cardiac defect when parents of affected offspring are rebred.

Supplemental Readings

Cottrill CM, Rossdale PD: A comparison of congenital heart disease in horses and man. Equine Vet J 24:338–340, 1992.
Huston R, Saperstein G, Leipold HW: Congenital defects in foals. J Equine Med Surg 1:146–161, 1977.
McGuirk SM, Shaftoe S, Lunn DP: Diseases of the cardiovascular system. In Smith BP (ed): Large Animal Internal Medicine. St. Louis, C.V. Mosby, 1990, pp 454–465.
Noden DM, De Lahunta A (eds): Cardiovascular system II: Heart. In The Embryology of Domestic Animals. Baltimore, Williams & Wilkins, 1985, pp 231–256.
Reef VB: Echocardiographic findings in horses with congenital cardiac disease. Comp Cont Ed Pract Vet 13:109–117, 1991.
Rooney JR, Franks WC: Congenital cardiac anomalies in horses. Pathol Vet 1:454–464, 1964.

Acquired Cardiac Disease

MARK W. PATTESON
Bristol, England

Heart disease may involve pathology of the valves, myocardium, or pericardium. Pericardial disease is relatively uncommon, although it is important that it be recognized and treated appropriately because it is often life-threatening. Pericardial disease is covered in detail in *Current Therapy in Equine Medicine 3* (pp 402–405). The incidence of myocardial disease is unclear. Severe myocardial disease resulting in cardiac failure is relatively uncommon; however, less widespread myocardial disease may be responsible for the generation of arrhythmias that can affect athletic performance, cause clinical signs of weakness or collapse at rest, or even result in sudden death. Myocardial disease may reduce global ventricular function and limit cardiac output during exercise. The advent of diagnostic techniques such as radiotelemetry, 24-hour electrocardiogram (ECG) monitoring, and post-exercise echocardiography may allow myocardial disease to be detected when previously it would have been unrecognized (see the chapter on exercise ECGs and echocardiography, page 234). Myocardial disease is described in detail in *Current Therapy in Equine Medicine 3* (pp 393–395).

Valvular disease is by far the most important form of acquired cardiac pathology. Valvular disease most commonly results in a reduction in exercise tolerance, or results in a murmur that is an incidental finding and does not cause clinical signs. Although valvular disease is the most common cause of congestive heart failure, its histology is poorly documented; however, it appears that the majority of cases are caused by degenerative myxomatous change.

This results in thickening and irregularity of the endocardial surface of atrioventricular (AV) valves or nodular thickening of the semilunar valves. The left AV (mitral) and left semilunar (aortic) valves are most commonly affected. The myxomatous changes can also affect the chordae tendineae of the AV valves. Endocarditis, with bacterial colonization and erosion of the endocardial surface, adhesion of thrombus, and subsequent formation of vegetative lesions, is uncommon. Endocarditis is discussed in detail in *Current Therapy in Equine Medicine 3* (pp 399–402). Congenital valvular disease is extremely rare in horses.

The cardinal sign of valvular disease is a heart murmur. Identification of valvular disease is complicated in horses by the fact that many horses have functional murmurs caused by normal blood flow in the absence of cardiac abnormalities. It is important that functional murmurs be identified and distinguished from murmurs associated with valvular pathology.

Murmurs are generated by turbulent blood flow. Murmurs may be found in severely anemic animals ("hemic murmurs") because low blood viscosity allows turbulence to develop; however, murmurs related to anemia are uncommon. Abnormally narrow (stenotic) valves or abnormal communications between two chambers (such as an incompetent valve) result in high-velocity blood flow, which may generate turbulent flow. However, valvular stenosis is exceptionally rare in horses. Leakage of blood through the AV or semilunar valves is the most common form of cardiac disease in horses and is described as valvular insufficiency, incompetence, or regurgitation; these terms are synonymous. Occasionally, myocardial disease results in AV valve incompetence if the AV ring dilates.

HISTORY

The incidence of valvular heart disease is not markedly different in horses of different breeds or sex; however, these factors influence the use of the horse, which is a very significant consideration. Degenerative valvular disease is more common in older horses but can also be found in young animals. Cardiac murmurs resulting from congenital heart disease may not be detected in some horses until well into their working lives, and congenital heart disease must be considered as a differential diagnosis in horses of any age (see Congenital Heart Disease, pp 255–259).

The length of ownership and the type and duration of clinical signs should be established. It may be helpful to know when accurate auscultation was last performed. It is particularly important to obtain details of the performance record of the animal. If the horse performs badly, precise details of the way in which poor performance occurs are important and may help to exclude other body system abnormalities. Horses with moderate to severe valvular heart disease usually start a competition well but tire easily and have a prolonged recovery period.

CLINICAL EXAMINATION

General Examination

Identification of a cardiac murmur does not exclude disease of other body systems, and thus the examination should not be confined to the cardiovascular system alone. The horse's demeanor should be assessed; excitement affects heart rate and may affect both cardiac rhythm and the character of murmurs (see later). The animal's bodily condition should be assessed; weight loss is common in horses with congestive heart failure or endocarditis.

Mucous membrane color and capillary refill time should be assessed. Capillary refill time may be delayed if cardiac output is compromised, but a normal capillary refill time does not rule out significant heart disease. Cyanosis is seen only in moribund animals or those with complex congenital disease. In cases of endocarditis the mucous membranes may be injected.

The arterial pulse quality, rate, and rhythm should be assessed. It is important to be familiar with the range of normality in the arterial pulse quality, which can be affected by heart rate and excitement in addition to disease; the facial artery is most easily palpated. It is helpful to palpate the pulse and auscultate heart sounds simultaneously to identify pulse deficits and aid identification of systole and diastole. Palpation of the median artery or an artery in the skin can be useful because the facial artery is usually out of reach.

It is very important to establish a true resting heart rate. Tachycardia can be a mechanism to maintain cardiac output in the face of valvular heart disease; however, there are many other causes of tachycardia. Some minutes may be required to ensure that an elevated heart rate is not due to excitement. If a heart rate in excess of 44 bpm is detected, every effort should be made to establish the cause of tachycardia.

Nasal discharge should be noted; however, respiratory disease is a much more common cause of a nasal discharge than cardiac disease. Frothy white or pinkish fluid can be seen in animals with pulmonary edema. Identification of a discharge may prompt further investigation because poor exercise tolerance caused by respiratory disease may be mistakenly attributed to heart disease. In addition, the laryngeal region should be palpated for muscle atrophy or signs of previous surgery, because laryngeal and other upper airway abnormalities are common causes of poor athletic performance.

Distension of the jugular veins is often the first sign of congestive heart failure and results from raised central venous pressure. The more severe the distension, the more significant the disease. Slight pulsation of the jugular vein at the thoracic inlet is observed in normal horses, because of the change in right atrial pressure associated with the cardiac cycle. The degree of distension of the vein depends on the position of the head. Jugular distension can also result from obstruction of venous drainage, for example, by thoracic tumors as a result of increased intrathoracic pressure or pleural effusions. A distended jugular vein may appear to pulsate because of transmission of the pulse from the underlying carotid artery. True pulsation of the jugular vein is seen if there is moderate or severe right AV valve (tricuspid) regurgitation or electrical AV dissociation. Right-sided congestive heart failure also results in an increase in hydrostatic pressure in systemic veins, and this may lead to the development of dependent edema. However, cardiac disease is only one of a number of conditions that result in dependent edema formation (see Differential Diagnosis of Dependent Edema, pp 269–272).

Auscultation of the lung fields and observation of the respiratory pattern are important features of the examination. Pulmonary disease is the most common cause of abnormal sounds. Most horses with cardiac disease have normal respiratory sounds, but adventitious sounds may be heard in animals with pulmonary edema.

Classically, percussion, palpation, and auscultation are used to identify heart disease. In practice, percussion is a very insensitive technique. Palpation is important to assess the force of contraction and position of the apical impulse. The impulse may be strong in horses with significant valvular disease or excitement-induced tachycardia. However, auscultation is the most important part of the examination.

Auscultation

In addition to assessment of cardiac rhythm, one of the principal aims of auscultation is to classify murmurs according to their timing, duration, character, point of maximal intensity, and radiation so that their source can be identified. Classification is a much better basis on which to evaluate the significance of murmurs than widely-used rules of thumb, such as audibility after exercise. The technique of auscultation is discussed in the section on techniques in equine cardiology (see pp 225–233).

Functional Murmurs

Functional murmurs are generally quiet and short-lasting. They may vary in intensity at different heart rates.

Three types of functional murmurs are well recognized. The most common are early to mid-systolic murmurs with a point of maximal intensity over the left heart base. The most useful distinctive feature of these murmurs is that they end well before the second heart sound is heard. These murmurs can sometimes be identified as being crescendo-decrescendo in character and may be musical. They are usually grade 1/6 or 2/6 in intensity, but occasionally can be up to grade 4/6, especially in foals.

Early diastolic murmurs are most commonly found in young athletic horses but can be heard in any horse. They are high-pitched and have a musical "whoop"-type quality, which is the basis of their description as a "two-year-old squeak." The point of maximal intensity is over the heart base or just ventral to this location. Early diastolic murmurs are usually grade 1/6 or 2/6 in intensity but can be up to grade 3/6. They are often most noticeable at slightly elevated heart rates in the range of 40 to 50 bpm.

Presystolic murmurs are the least commonly identified type of functional murmur. They are most easily detected at slow heart rates, have a low-pitched grating quality, and merge with the fourth and first heart sounds. Although it can be shown using Doppler echocardiography that they are associated with regurgitant blood flow, there is no evidence that these murmurs have any deleterious effects.

Pathologic Murmurs

In the horse, "pathologic" murmurs are associated with regurgitation of blood through incompetent valves or with congenital defects. The pressure gradient across the valves produces characteristic murmurs associated with AV valve and semilunar valve regurgitation. A high pressure gradient is present between the ventricle and the atrium throughout systole, and in AV regurgitation the velocity of the regurgitant jet is usually consistent during this period. Consequently, the intensity of the murmur typically remains constant during systole and is described as "plateau" or "band-shaped" in character. Murmurs associated with incompetence of the semilunar valves are typically decrescendo in quality because the pressure gradient across the valve gradually decreases during diastole. The pressure gradient across the pulmonary valve is relatively low, and a murmur is seldom detected in pulmonary valve insufficiency, even if it is present.

MITRAL REGURGITATION

Mitral regurgitation is usually caused by degenerative disease of the mitral valve. Congenital mitral dysplasia has not been reported in horses, but the valve can be abnormal in some cases of congenital heart disease affecting the endocardial cushion (see Congenital Heart Disease, pp 255–259). Mitral regurgitation may also develop as a result of myocardial disease or congenital heart disease, but this is much less common than primary disease.

Clinical Examination

Presenting Signs

Mitral regurgitation is the most important valvular condition affecting athletic performance. Athletes with mitral

regurgitation may fade toward the end of a race and have a prolonged recovery period. Other animals may cope well with all but uphill work. However, in other cases, clinical signs of mitral regurgitation are subtle and may not be appreciated by the owner, particularly in horses that do not perform arduous athletic work. Congestive heart failure may develop insidiously in the nonathlete without the signs of moderate jugular distension and dependent edema being noticed. Much more commonly, mitral regurgitation is detected as an incidental finding at a routine examination, and the principal problem in these cases is determining the likely effect on the future athletic performance of the animal. In only a few cases is congestive heart failure the first presenting sign. If mitral regurgitation is acute in onset, there is a sudden increase in left atrial pressure that may result in pulmonary edema. This may be sufficiently severe to result in a white or pink-tinged frothy fluid appearing at the nostrils. Tachypnea and hyperpnea may also be noted. Sudden death from left-sided congestive heart failure is uncommon. More commonly, acute left-sided congestive heart failure is not seen, but signs of right-sided failure are observed. This is because the left atrium can dilate if the regurgitation is insidious in onset, and changes in pulmonary vasculature result in pulmonary hypertension and then right-sided congestive heart failure.

General Examination

The arterial pulse quality in mitral regurgitation is usually normal, but in severe cases it may be weak. Arrhythmias are a significant finding; in particular, dilation of the left atrium may lead to the development of atrial fibrillation. Tachycardia is a very important finding and is almost invariably present in cases of congestive heart failure.

Auscultation. The characteristic feature of mitral regurgitation is the auscultation of a grade 1/6 to 6/6 pan- or holosystolic murmur with a point of maximal intensity over the left apical area. A plateau-type or band-shaped murmur is typically identified. The murmur may radiate dorsally and caudally or cranially. In some cases in which the murmur radiates cranially it may be very loud over the left basal area. Occasionally, the character of the murmur is crescendo, often with a musical element. It is thought that these cases may be associated with mitral valve prolapse.

Diagnostic Aids

Echocardiography

Two-dimensional echocardiography (2DE) and M-mode echocardiography are useful techniques for identifying thickening and abnormal movement of the mitral valve. However, the most important feature of echocardiography is that it enables the clinician to assess the significance of the condition. The larger the regurgitant fraction and the more severe the mitral regurgitation, the more volume overload will be present. Volume overload due to mitral regurgitation results in an increase in left atrial diameter and left ventricular internal diameter (particularly left ventricular internal diameter at end diastole). This can be detected echocardiographically. In some cases, dilation of the ventricle or atrium is so marked that a purely subjective assessment identifies severe volume overload (Fig. 1). However, echocardiography is most useful in cases in which

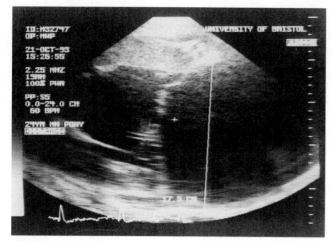

Figure 1. The left atrium is markedly dilated as a result of mitral regurgitation in this 24-year-old pony with atrial fibrillation.

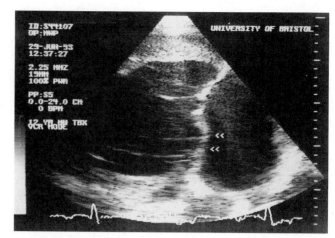

Figure 3. Prolapse of the mitral valve (arrows), with the valve bowing back into the left atrium.

clinical signs are less dramatic and there is mild or moderate volume overload that cannot be identified by any other means. In these cases, accurate measurement of left ventricular diameter and left atrial diameter is essential. Measurements should be made with reference to established methods and a range of values for normal animals (see Supplemental Readings).

The mitral valve is best assessed from the left parasternal long-axis view, although left and right short-axis views and the right parasternal long-axis views can provide useful additional information. Diffuse or nodular thickening of the valve may be seen (Fig. 2). Appreciation of the thickening depends on experience of the normal appearance of the valve and consistent use of the gain settings of the machine. The absence of obvious thickening of the valve or volume overload does not rule out the presence of mitral regurgitation. Abnormal motion of the valve occurs in some cases and may be obvious or subtle. In some cases, prolapse of the valve is seen. Prolapse has the appearance of the valve

bowing back into the left atrium (Fig. 3); however, it should be identified when the beam transects the valve through its widest point because it can be produced artifactually if the beam cuts a small portion of the valve. Flail leaflet can be seen in horses in which a ruptured chordae tendineae allows the tip of the valve to flip back into the atrium during systole. The right commissural cusp is most frequently affected and can be identified most easily in the far-field from the left parasternal long-axis view (Fig. 4).

Although endocarditis is uncommon, the mitral valve is the second most common site for this condition. The presence of a large nodular thickening of the valve along with the relevant clinical and pathology signs supports a diagnosis of endocarditis.

Motion of the interventricular septum and left ventricular free wall can be exaggerated in cases in which there is significant valvular incompetence. The resistance to contraction is reduced because blood can flow retrogradely through the mitral valve, and in addition the chambers are

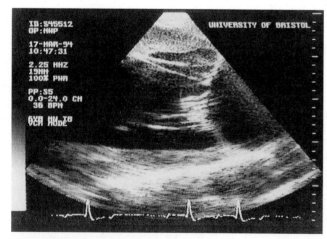

Figure 2. Diffuse thickening of the mitral valve and chordae tendineae.

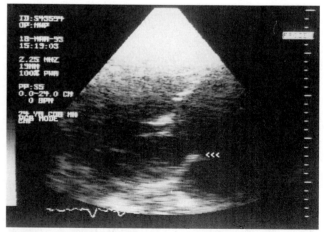

Figure 4. A ruptured right commissural cusp chorda tendinea has resulted in a flail leaflet curling into the left atrium in the far-field in this left parasternal long-axis view (arrows).

dilated as a result of volume overload. Fractional shortening is therefore increased, provided that myocardial function remains normal.

In horses with severe mitral regurgitation, the rapid expansion of the ventricle during early diastole, with exaggerated motion of the septum seen best on M-mode, is particularly striking (Fig. 5).

Doppler echocardiography is a useful tool in the evaluation of horses with mitral regurgitation. The presence of mitral regurgitation can be confirmed by the detection of a jet flowing into the atrium during systole; however, with experience, auscultation is probably as accurate as Doppler echocardiography in identifying the presence of mitral regurgitation. Using pulsed-wave Doppler or color-flow technique, the extent of the regurgitant jet can be mapped as a semiquantitative guide to severity. As a guide, if the jet is detected over a limited amount of the atrium it can be quantified as mild; if it covers up to approximately one half of the atrium it can be described as moderate; if it is more extensive, the mitral regurgitation is severe.

Electrocardiography

Electrocardiography is of value for identifying arrhythmias in cases of mitral regurgitation, but ECGs provide very limited information about chamber size in horses. However, arrhythmias can be significant and may alter the prognosis and subsequent management or treatment of the horse. Atrial premature complexes may indicate atrial myocardial disease caused by stretching, resulting from mitral regurgitation. Ventricular premature complexes may on occasion result from poor myocardial oxygenation in severe mitral regurgitation. The most important arrhythmia complicating mitral regurgitation is atrial fibrillation. Many cases of atrial fibrillation are uncomplicated by underlying pathology; however, significant mitral regurgitation does predispose to the condition. If atrial fibrillation is identified, in most cases it is likely to indicate that the mitral regurgitation is moderate or severe. In addition, the presence of mitral regurgitation may preclude successful treatment of the arrhythmia (see Diagnosis of Arrhythmias and Therapy of Cardiac Conditions, pp 240 and 250).

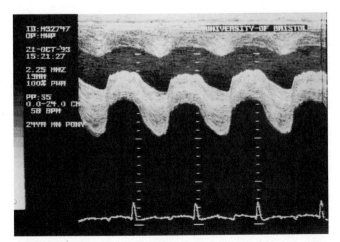

Figure 5. M-mode echocardiogram showing exaggerated septal motion and dilation of the left ventricle with the left ventricular free wall beyond the range of depth display (24 cm).

Clinical Pathology

Measurement of plasma fibrinogen may be helpful if endocarditis is suspected or if a secondary pneumonia is thought to have occurred in a horse with pulmonary edema. However, clinical pathology testing is of little direct value in the assessment of mitral regurgitation. No evidence exists to support the use of cardiac muscle isoenzymes as a diagnostic aid in these cases.

Prognosis and Treatment

Treatment of mitral regurgitation is confined to management of congestive heart failure and pathologic arrhythmias (see Therapy of Cardiac Conditions, p 250). The most important consideration in horses with mitral regurgitation is to decide whether the condition has any effect on exercise tolerance. This decision determines whether mitral regurgitation can be identified as the cause of poor athletic performance in some animals, and what level of athletic activity the horse can be expected to perform safely. Often, the clinician is asked to speculate on the effect on athletic performance in future years.

Clinical guides to prognosis are crude. If congestive heart failure is present, the prognosis for future athletic use is hopeless. In a few cases the horse's condition can be stabilized (see Therapy of Cardiac Conditions, p 250) so that it has a satisfactory quality of life as a breeding animal or pet. If the resting heart rate is elevated, the pulse quality is abnormal, the murmur is very widespread, or pathologic arrhythmias are detected, it is likely that mitral regurgitation is sufficiently severe to restrict the use of the horse. If poor athletic performance has been reported, it is wise to restrict the use of the animal to less arduous events.

Prognostication can be much more accurate following echocardiographic assessment of the condition. In some cases, there is no sign of volume overload, with left ventricular diameter and left atrial diameter within the normal range and no evidence of exaggerated septal motion. In these cases, it is unlikely that the valvular incompetence is affecting athletic performance. In other cases, the left ventricular diameter and left atrial diameter are at the top end or just greater than the normal range and it is possible that exercise tolerance will be reduced. As a rough guide, in an adult Thoroughbred, once left ventricular diameter exceeds 14.5 cm or left atrial diameter exceeds 15.5 cm, the horse is unlikely to be suitable for arduous activities.

Another factor to consider is pulmonary hypertension leading to dilation of the pulmonary artery. This can occur as a result of mitral regurgitation and is a poor prognostic sign. It is usually seen in horses with overt right-sided congestive heart failure but is found occasionally in animals without severe clinical signs. Rupture of the pulmonary artery is a potential sequela that is responsible for sudden death in some horses with mitral regurgitation; if dilation is suspected from echocardiographic examination, the horse should not be ridden.

Serial examinations are very useful for monitoring the progression of the disease and for assisting with prognosis on the likely effects of the condition in the future. Because mitral regurgitation is usually caused by a degenerative valvular disease, one must assume that mitral valve integrity will deteriorate in time. In most cases, this progression takes months or years. Occasionally, sudden deterioration is seen when an arrhythmia such as atrial fibrillation develops or chordae tendineae rupture. Echocardiography should be repeated ideally at 6- to 12-month intervals to allow a quantitative assessment of the progression of the disease and detection of potentially life-threatening developments such as pulmonary artery dilation. Repeated echocardiograms are particularly useful because measurements can be compared with a known starting point rather than comparing single measurements with a normal range.

TRICUSPID REGURGITATION

The etiology of tricuspid regurgitation is uncertain. In a few cases, thickening of the tricuspid valve is seen, but changes have been shown to be uncommon in a postmortem survey. It is therefore difficult to explain the relatively high prevalence of the murmur of tricuspid regurgitation in athletic horses. The condition has been reported in as many as 16% of mature Thoroughbred racehorses. It is possible that the murmur is in some way a consequence of athletic training and is therefore physiologic rather than pathologic in some cases.

Clinical Examination

Presenting Signs

Tricuspid regurgitation is most frequently detected as an incidental finding. It may also be found as a complicating factor in animals with more significant primary heart disease, such as mitral regurgitation that has become sufficiently severe to result in pulmonary hypertension. Many horses appear to cope well with mild or moderate tricuspid regurgitation; however, severe tricuspid regurgitation can result in reduced exercise tolerance or even right-sided congestive heart failure. A useful identifying feature in severe cases is the presence of a jugular pulse, which results from blood flowing retrogradely into the right atrium during systole.

Auscultation

Tricuspid regurgitation is characterized by the auscultation of a grade 1/6 to 6/6 pan- or holosystolic plateau-type murmur with a point of maximal intensity over the right apical area. The apical area is located further forward on the right than the left and may be well under the triceps muscle unless the limb is protracted. In many cases the murmur is localized and is quite soft in quality. The murmur caused by a ventricular septal defect is an important differential consideration when this murmur is detected, but it is usually loud and harsh (see Congenital Heart Disease, p 255). In severe tricuspid regurgitation, the murmur resulting from tricuspid regurgitation can be auscultated over the left hemithorax approximately the second intercostal space, substantially further cranially than the left apical area.

Diagnostic Aids

Echocardiography

Gross valvular abnormalities of the tricuspid valve are rarely seen on 2DE. However, prolapse of the valve is a relatively common finding and can be present in horses in which a murmur typical of tricuspid regurgitation has not been detected. Spontaneous echo contrast is often seen in horses with tricuspid regurgitation. This consists of echogenic "particles" which can be a gray haze ("smoke") or more discrete echogenic dots that fill the right atrium and pass into the right ventricle. These may even be seen to pass in a retrograde direction through the incompetent valve. Just as with mitral regurgitation, significant valvular insufficiency results in volume overload and dilation of the ventricle and atrium. Owing to the trabeculation of the right ventricular wall and absence of reliable landmarks, measurement of right ventricular and right atrial dimensions is difficult. A subjective assessment of their size should be made from a variety of views. If right-sided overload is severe, the interventricular septum may be bowed towards the left ventricle, and may even move toward the left ventricular free-wall during diastole (paradoxical septal motion).

Doppler echocardiography is a very useful method of assessing the severity of tricuspid regurgitation. Good alignment with the jet and the limited depth display required ensure that accurate mapping of the jet can be achieved. Color-flow technique can demonstrate the jet very clearly (see Diagnostic Techniques in Equine Cardiology, p 225). Usually the regurgitant jet runs along the atrial wall bordering the aorta and is most easily detected in a tilted right parasternal long-axis view. It should also be mapped in the right ventricular inflow-outflow view. As a rough guide, the more widespread the jet of tricuspid regurgitation, the more severe the condition.

Electrocardiography

An ECG should be recorded in cases in which arrhythmias are detected on clinical examination; however, in the author's view, the ECG is not helpful in directly assessing right ventricular or right atrial enlargement. In a few cases, atrial premature complexes and atrial fibrillation result from right atrial dilation caused by severe tricuspid regurgitation; however, this is uncommon. More frequently, pathologic arrhythmias are coincidental, but they may be important. For example, detection of multiple atrial premature complexes in a horse with exercise intolerance may be a more significant finding than tricuspid regurgitation (see Diagnosis of Arrhythmias, p 240).

Clinical Pathology

Clinical pathology testing is seldom of any direct relevance to investigation of tricuspid regurgitation, but it can be helpful in ruling out the presence of other conditions that might cause exercise intolerance or dependent edema. A raised fibrinogen level in association with large vegetations on the tricuspid valve is supportive evidence for endocarditis; however, this valve is rarely affected.

Prognosis and Treatment

The prognosis for most horses with tricuspid regurgitation is excellent. When gross valvular abnormalities are absent, it is likely that the condition will not progress. In cases in which valve thickening is seen, the long-term prognosis must be more guarded. It is very difficult to give an accurate prognosis without the aid of echocardiography, unless congestive heart failure has already developed. It is the author's impression that tricuspid regurgitation is more likely to be clinically significant if the murmur is widespread and harsh than if the murmur has a soft quality. Tricuspid regurgitation is much less common in ponies than in Thoroughbred athletes and is more likely to be caused by valvular disease in nonathletes. If there is no echocardiographic evidence of right ventricular or right atrial enlargement, the condition is likely to have limited clinical significance. If volume overload is seen, exercise intolerance may develop. No treatment is possible other than medical stabilization of congestive signs (see Treatment of Cardiac Disease, p 250).

AORTIC REGURGITATION

Aortic regurgitation is usually caused by degenerative disease of the valve, which results in band-shaped lesions on the valve cusps. Nodules are also a common postmortem finding; however, they appear to be less commonly associated with aortic regurgitation. Fenestrations in the leading edge of the cusps are common findings in normal horses. Occasionally, aortic regurgitation develops as a result of a ventricular septal defect. The root of the aortic valve can move into the defect, resulting in prolapse of a cusp during diastole.

Clinical Examination

Presenting Signs

Aortic regurgitation is quite common in older horses, but it may also be found in young animals. It often causes no clinical signs, but in some cases it can result in severe volume overload and can progress to cause congestive heart failure. The effects of aortic regurgitation are much more severe if mitral regurgitation is also present. Poor athletic performance may be associated with aortic regurgitation, but more frequently the murmur is an incidental finding.

General Examination

One feature of particular relevance in horses with aortic regurgitation is the arterial pulse quality. If there is significant volume overload, the stroke volume will be large, but the diastolic pressure decreases more rapidly than normal because of leakage of blood back into the left ventricle. The systolic pressure in the main arteries is high and the diastolic pressure low (i.e., there is a large pulse pressure difference). Consequently, the arterial pulse feels strong but short in quality. This is termed a *water-hammer pulse*.

Despite the fact that endocarditis is uncommon, horses in which aortic regurgitation is detected for the first time should be closely examined for signs of ill thrift, weight loss, and pyrexia because endocarditis most often affects the aortic valve.

Auscultation

Aortic regurgitation is characterized by the auscultation of a grade 1/6 to 6/6 holodiastolic murmur with a point of maximal intensity over the left heart base. The murmur usually radiates ventrally but can radiate cranially and ventrally or to the right hemithorax in some cases. The charac-

ter of the murmur is decrescendo, and it can be very variable in pitch, from a low-pitched rumble to a high-pitched sigh. Often it has a "cooing" quality. The quality is frequently musical, which is associated with pure notes of sound caused by vibrating intracardiac structures. Occasionally the murmur has a late diastolic accentuation associated with the opening of the mitral valve at the time of atrial contraction. During periods of second degree atrioventricular block, the murmur can be heard throughout the long diastolic interval. The intensity of the murmur is a particularly poor guide to the severity of aortic regurgitation. In some cases, it is as loud as grade 6/6, without being associated with severe volume overload.

Diagnostic Aids

Echocardiography

Echocardiography is a very useful tool in evaluating horses with aortic regurgitation because the intensity of the murmur is such a poor guide to severity, and because it helps to identify horses with endocarditis that require intensive treatment. Many horses have been retired prematurely because the murmur is so striking, but quite often exercise tolerance is satisfactory until severe volume overload develops.

Echogenic nodules can be identified in most cases of aortic regurgitation, particularly on the left and right coronary cusps (Fig. 6). However, these nodules can be identified in some horses without aortic regurgitation. Although Doppler echocardiography can be useful to confirm the presence of a regurgitant jet, 2DE and M-mode echocardiography can be used to confirm the diagnosis and give the best guide to severity. High-frequency vibration of the aortic valve and/or the anterior mitral leaflet can be seen in most cases (Figs. 7, 8). In a few cases, a small portion of cusp can be seen to flail into the left ventricle in diastole (Fig. 9). Rarely, the aortic root can rupture and a whole cusp is seen prolapsing into the left ventricle. In severe cases of aortic regurgitation, the mitral valve may close early in mid-diastole owing to raised left ventricular diastolic pressure, or the valve may open little during atrial contraction.

Measurement of left ventricular diameter is the best

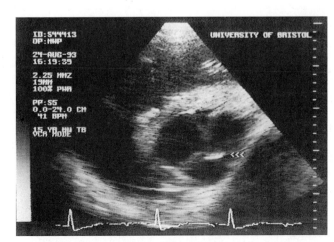

Figure 6. An echogenic nodule on the aortic valve (*arrows*).

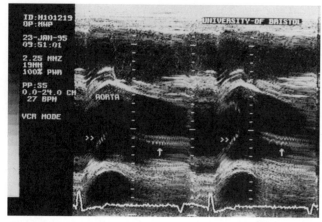

Figure 7. High-frequency vibration of the aortic valve during diastole (*single arrow*).

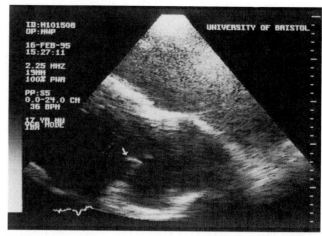

Figure 9. A small portion of the left coronary cusp is seen flailing into the left ventricle during diastole (*arrow*).

overall guide to severity. In many cases there is little evidence of volume overload. In other cases with few apparent clinical signs, volume overload can be substantial. Fractional shortening is increased in many cases because the stroke volume is substantially increased. Septal motion may give the impression of continuous ventricular filling throughout diastole (Fig. 10).

Electrocardiography

As with other valvular conditions, an ECG should be recorded in those cases in which an arrhythmia is detected during clinical examination. Radiotelemetric recording during exercise may help to reveal arrhythmias that may be relevant to exercise intolerance.

Clinical Pathology

It is worthwhile submitting blood samples for a fibrinogen assay and a white cell count in those horses that have a period of malaise or weight loss immediately before the detection of the murmur of aortic regurgitation in order to identify horses with endocarditis.

Prognosis and Treatment

In most horses, aortic regurgitation develops in later life and progresses over a period of months or years. The majority are therefore retired for some unrelated reason, and aortic regurgitation never becomes a clinical problem. In some cases, volume overload develops to the point at which the level of exercise that the horse can perform has to be reduced, or the animal has to be retired. In a few cases, particularly if mitral regurgitation is also present, congestive heart failure develops. In the rare instance of valve rupture, congestive heart failure may develop acutely or sudden death may occur. Many horses appear to be able to cope with volume overload caused by aortic regurgitation better than with similar left ventricular dilation caused by mitral regurgitation. However, occasionally horses with aortic regurgitation do suffer severe exercise intolerance despite only moderate volume overload. It is possible that myocardial disease plays a role in these cases. As with any case, measurements of left ventricular dimensions should not be the only guide used in prognostication.

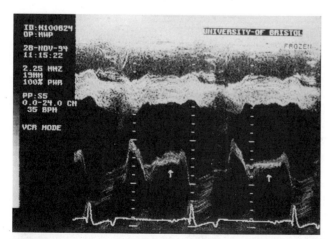

Figure 8. High-frequency diastolic vibration of the anterior mitral leaflet (*single arrow*).

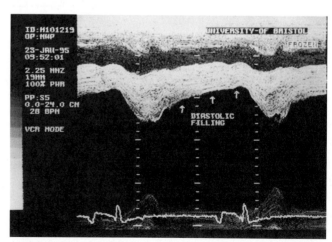

Figure 10. M-mode echocardiogram showing movement of the septum towards the right ventricle throughout diastole in a horse with aortic regurgitation (*arrows*).

Supplemental Readings

Glendenning SA: A distinctive diastolic murmur observed in healthy young horses. Vet Rec 76:341–342, 1964.

Littlewort MCG: The clinical auscultation of the equine heart. Vet Rec 74:1247–1260, 1962.

Long KJ, Bonagura JD, Darke PGG: Standardised imaging technique for guided M-mode and Doppler echocardiography in the horse. Equine Vet J 24:226–235, 1992.

Paterson, DF, Detweiler DK, Glendenning SA: Part II. Comparative aspects of normal and abnormal heart sounds and murmurs. Ann NY Acad Sci 127:242–305, 1965.

Patteson MW: Echocardiographic evaluation of horses with aortic regurgitation. Equine Vet Ed 6(3):159–166, 1994.

Patteson MW, Cripps PJ: A survey of cardiac auscultatory findings in horses. Equine Vet J 25(5):409–415, 1993.

Patteson MW, Gibbs C, Wotton PR, Cripps PJ: Echocardiographic measurement of cardiac dimensions and indices of cardiac function in normal adult Thoroughbred horses. Equine Vet J 19 [Suppl]:18–27, 1995.

Reef VB: Evaluation of the equine cardiovascular system. Vet Clin North Am Equine Pract 1(2):275–288, 1985.

Reef VB: Color flow Doppler mapping of horses with valvular insufficiency. Proc 8th Am Coll Vet Intern Med, 1990, pp 483–485.

Reef VB: Echocardiographic examination in the horse: The basics. Comp Cont Ed Pract Vet 12:1312–1319, 1990.

Reef VB: Heart murmurs in horses: Determining their significance with echocardiography. Equine Vet J 19[Suppl]:71–80, 1995.

Reef VB, Spencer P: Echocardiographic evaluation of equine aortic insufficiency. Am J Vet Res 48:904–909, 1987.

Aortoiliacofemoral Thrombosis

S U E   J .   D Y S O N
Newmarket, England

L E I L A   W O R T H
Kennett Square, Pennsylvania

Aortoiliacofemoral thrombosis, also called aortoiliacofemoral arteriosclerosis, is a poorly understood condition. Authors have suggested that (1) arteriosclerosis is the primary degenerative condition, occurring in widespread locations throughout the body with secondary thrombus formation; and (2) the anatomic configuration of the clinically affected vessels predisposes to turbulent blood flow and stress to the vessel walls, resulting in more severe lesions. If this is true, it is curious that cases were suggested to occur predominantly in young horses of 3 years of age or less, whereas it might be expected to affect older horses if a degenerative lesion was primary. These authors differentiated the progressive condition due to aortoiliacofemoral arteriosclerosis that results in poor performance and ultimately lameness from a rarer, acute-onset condition due to true thromboembolism.

In a survey of 28 equine veterinarians in Europe, South Africa, Australia, and the United States, eight who had been in practice for a minimum of 15 years had not recognized a case of aortoiliacofemoral thrombosis. From the remaining 20 veterinarians, 44 cases were confirmed ultrasonographically. A profound domination of male horses (20 stallions, 16 geldings) was observed but no particular breed predilection (15 Thoroughbreds, 17 Standardbreds, 12 others). However, at one clinic in the United States, 15 of 16 cases were Standardbreds, whereas the overall hospital population consisted of approximately 50% Thoroughbreds. Racehorses (17) and other competition or pleasure horses (18) were similarly affected. Nine were breeding stallions. Nine horses were younger than 5 years of age, 19 between 5 and 10 years of age, 10 between 10 and 15 years of age, and 6 of 15 years of age or older. These figures are similar to the distribution of the equine population, suggesting no age predisposition.

CLINICAL SIGNS

Clinical signs are exercise-induced and generally moderate to severe when first recognized but are frequently preceded by a history of loss of performance. In performance horses the initial clinical signs include hindlimb stiffness during work and suboptimal performance, which is variable in occurrence and degree. The condition generally progresses to an exercise-induced mild to severe unilateral or bilateral hindlimb lameness, which is initially very transient and rapidly resolves following cessation of exercise. As clinical signs become more severe, their duration after stopping of exercise lengthens. Lameness is characterized by hindlimb stiffness, stumbling and repeated knuckling at the fetlock, and an increasing reluctance to move. The horse may ultimately become very distressed and sweat profusely except over the affected limb or limbs, which remain relatively cool. If the horse is allowed to stand still it may repeatedly flex the affected limb in an exaggerated manner, stamp the limb to the ground, and show reluctance to bear weight on the limb. Severely affected cases may become recumbent. Before the horse exercises it may be possible to appreciate a decreased pulse amplitude in the affected limb. Immediately after exercise the saphenous vein may remain collapsed for up to 1 minute. Atrophy of the hindlimb musculature is a variable feature. In breeding stallions, clinical signs are usually first recognized after covering, although frequently there is a history of slowness to cover, pain after covering, pain during thrusting, failure to ejaculate, and/or many mounts before ejaculation. Although several authors have suggested that affected stallions are usually infertile because of decreased testicular blood flow, this was not documented in the recent survey except through failure to ejaculate. Several stallions showed very severe hindlimb pain immediately after covering, and in some this progressed to recumbency.

In the recent survey seven horses had exhibited clinical signs for less than 7 days, several for only a few hours prior to diagnosis. Ten horses had shown signs for more than one week and up to 1 month, while the remaining 27 horses had a longer history of compromised performance.

DIAGNOSIS

In mild cases the clinical signs may be difficult to differentiate from other causes of hindlimb lameness, tying up syndrome, and in some instances, colic. Diagnosis is based on exclusion of other causes of hindlimb lameness; history and clinical signs; muscle enzyme determinations before and after exercise; rectal examination; and ultrasonographic evaluation of the terminal aorta, the internal and external iliac arteries, and, if possible, the femoral arteries. Moderate increases of creatine kinase and aspartate aminotransferase may be seen after exercise in performance horses, but these are of much lesser magnitude than levels seen typically in tying up. Rectal examination may reveal enlargement of the terminal aorta or the internal or external iliac arteries, abnormal vessel firmness, decreased pulse amplitude, or fremitus. A negative finding does not preclude the presence of a thrombus. In the recent survey, 13 of 44 horses had no palpable abnormality, but partial vessel occlusion·was seen ultrasonographically.

Ultrasonographic evaluation of the terminal aorta and internal and external iliac arteries usually reveals a thrombus originating on the dorsal wall of the terminal aorta (Fig. 1). Thrombi in the aorta or iliac arteries frequently occupy more than 50% of the vessel diameter. The thrombi are heterogeneous, with chronic organized areas appearing hyperechoic and newer portions appearing hypoechoic.

TREATMENT

Treatment rationale has been based on pain relief and the use of anti-inflammatory drugs, platelet inhibitors, anthelmintics, fibrinolytic agents, and vasoactive and anticoagulant drugs. Multiple treatments have been proposed including one or more of the following, phenylbutazone (2.2 mg/kg b.i.d. for 2 months), aspirin (5 mg/kg s.i.d. for several months), ivermectin (200 mg/kg weekly for 4 weeks, or monthly for 3 months), fenbendazole (15 mg/kg s.i.d. for 1 to 7 days), dextran 70 (6% in 5% dextrose solution s.i.d. for 4 days, weekly for 4 weeks), sodium gluconate (450 mg/kg IV) preceded by prednisolone sodium succinate (100 mg IV), isoxsuprine (1 mg/kg b.i.d. for 12 weeks), heparin, dimethyl sulfoxide (DMSO), and a combination of streptokinase (100,000 IU), streptodornase (25,000 IU), and plasminogen (500 IU).

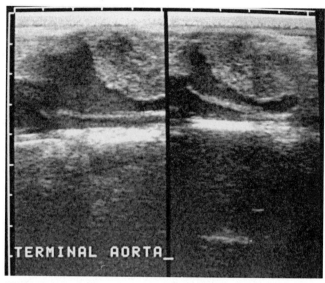

Figure 1. Longitudinal ultrasonographic images of the terminal aorta of an 8-year-old pleasure riding horse with relatively severe clinical signs of aortoiliac thrombosis. A large, well-organized thrombus of heterogeneous echogenicity occupies more than 50% of the lumen diameter.

CONCLUSIONS

In the recent survey, 29 of the 44 horses underwent treatment, and a further three were allowed to live, untreated. Two horses returned to their former athletic function with apparent resolution of clinical signs. Eleven horses improved but clinical signs persisted. Twelve horses showed no response to treatment or deteriorated, and an additional four were humanely destroyed. The three untreated horses remained symptomatic if exercised.

The results of treatment documented in the literature and accumulated from the survey suggest that there is no treatment that reliably influences the outcome. A successful outcome is presumed to be reliant on the development of an effective collateral circulation and reducing the risk of further thrombus formation. Platelets play a central role in the pathogenesis of arterial thrombosis, and platelet activating factor antagonists may provide antithrombotic therapy for the future. Treatment of a preformed thrombus is virtually impossible; fibrinolytic agents such as streptokinase are ineffective after approximately 12 hours of development of a thrombus. Nonetheless, a small proportion of horses improve and occasionally a horse may be able to resume athletic function, but the vast majority have persistent or deteriorating clinical signs, although these may be ameliorated if the horse is retired.

Supplemental Readings

Physick-Sheard, PW, Maxie MG: Peripheral vascular disease. *In* Robinson NE (ed): Current Therapy in Equine Medicine, ed 2. Philadelphia, WB Saunders, 1987, pp 173–176.

Poole AW: Thrombosis in the horse: The role of platelets in its pathogenesis and therapy. Equine Vet Ed 5:99–102, 1993.

Reef VB, Roby KAW, Richardson DW, Vaala WE, Johnston JK: Use of ultrasonography for the detection of aortic-iliac thrombosis in horses. J Am Vet Med Assoc 190:286–288, 1987.

Differential Diagnosis of Dependent Edema

FRANK G. R. TAYLOR
Bristol, England

Dependent edema is common in horses and accompanies a variety of disease processes. The purpose of this chapter is to consider the potential causes of edema in the horse and indicate their differential diagnosis. Details of the diagnosis and treatment of these diseases are contained elsewhere in this volume under appropriate headings.

Within arteriolar capillaries, the high hydrostatic pressure and the relatively low osmotic pressure promote the net movement of water and crystalloid solutes into the interstitial space. Fluid is then removed from the interstitial space by lymphatic drainage, aided by muscular movement, and a net absorption process that operates at the venous end of capillaries. There, the hydrostatic pressure is lower than at the arteriolar end, while the osmotic pressure has increased as a result of water loss. A disturbance in any of these forces, or in the functional integrity of the semipermeable endothelial and basement membranes, can cause the rate of water entering the interstitial space to exceed its rate of removal, thus leading to edema formation. In horses this is most frequently seen in the lowermost parts of the body, the ventral thorax, abdomen, and limbs, and is termed *dependent edema*. Dependent edema is often a clinical manifestation of generalized edema, whereas local edema occurs when local conditions favor its development, as in the head or a single limb.

DIFFERENTIAL DIAGNOSIS OF GENERALIZED EDEMA

Confinement

Rest in confinement is the most common cause of swelling and edema in the limbs of horses. "Filling" of the legs, particularly the hind legs, is a characteristic of some individuals when rested in a box stall overnight. It seems likely that the reduction in movement-assisted lymph flow (the "muscle pumping" of lymph) predisposes to edema. Its rapid resolution during exercise seems to support this view.

Hypoalbuminemia

Hypoalbuminemia results in a lowered intravascular osmotic pressure, which leads to water retention in the interstitium and the development of dependent edema. However, a state of hypoalbuminemia is not invariably associated with dependent edema formation. The most common cause of hypoalbuminemia in horses is a protein-losing enteropathy. Much rarer causes are loss to effusion (e.g., peritonitis and pleuritis), liver failure, and glomerulonephropathy.

Acute protein-losing enteropathy is associated with acute-onset enterocolitides such as salmonellosis, clostrid-iosis, and ehrlichial colitis (Potomac fever). Clinical signs are indistinguishable between these diseases and encompass fever, depression, anorexia, profuse diarrhea, dehydration and, in survivors, a somewhat intractable dependent edema. An additional spur to edema formation in these acute cases is the associated toxemia, which can damage endothelial surfaces, allowing leakage of protein and water into the interstitium.

Salmonellosis is a common cause of acute enterocolitis in horses and is diagnosed on isolation of the organism from the feces. Unfortunately, it is shed intermittently, and at least five fresh samples should be submitted over as many days during the acute phase to increase the chances of culturing the organism.

Clostridial diarrhea in horses is usually associated with *Clostridium perfringens* type A. This organism is ubiquitous in the soil and normally inhabits the equine gut in small numbers only. In poorly defined circumstances it can flourish in the intestine and cause acute disease by production of alpha toxin. Diagnosis is based on the isolation of high counts from fecal material ($>10^4$/g feces).

Ehrlichial colitis is caused by the rickettsia *Ehrlichia risticii* and is probably transmitted by ticks. It is recorded in the United States and Europe and occurs during the summer months. In endemic areas, clinical signs consistent with acute toxic enterocolitis suggest a diagnosis, but paired sera taken over a 7- to 10-day interval are required to confirm infection.

Chronic protein-losing enteropathy could reflect heavy parasitism, but it is usually associated with a progressive lesion of the intestinal mucosa that leads to a state of malabsorption. Such patients lose weight and their appetite may vary, but they show few clinical signs otherwise. Alternative differential diagnoses are liver failure and glomerulonephropathy. In all instances, the results of hematologic examination are nonspecific, although there may be evidence of chronic inflammation.

As well as revealing a state of hypoalbuminemia, serum biochemistry test results quickly indicate renal failure (serum urea and creatinine concentrations elevated), or liver failure (serum liver enzymes and total serum bile acids elevated). If both problems are eliminated, the clinician should rule out the possibility of endoparasites by appropriate anthelmintic treatment. If this treatment has no effect, small intestinal absorption should be evaluated by oral glucose or xylose tests. Confirmation of a state of malabsorption indicates that hypoalbuminemia is the result of protein-losing enteropathy. The cause is usually one of a number of chronic infiltrations by inflammatory cellular elements or a diffuse lymphosarcoma. Definitive diagnosis requires histopathologic examination of an intestinal biopsy.

269

If the hindgut is infiltrated, these patients also develop chronic diarrhea.

Intrathoracic Disease

Intrathoracic space-occupying lesions cause dependent edema by obstructing venous return to the heart and, depending upon the site, the central flow of lymph into the venous system at the vena cava. Mediastinal masses, often lymphosarcomas, obstruct the cranial vena cava and can cause a relatively localized edema of the forelimbs, head, and neck. In addition, the trachea and esophagus may be compressed, leading to dyspnea and dysphagia. The jugular veins are distended but not pulsatile. Thoracic radiography or ultrasonography indicates the position and extent of the lesion. More generalized intrathoracic lesions such as pleuritis, pleural abscessation, and diffuse thoracic neoplasia are often associated with generalized edema, although weight loss and dyspnea are likely to be the predominant clinical signs. In these cases, there is an associated pleural effusion, and analysis of the fluid obtained by thoracocentesis is usually diagnostic.

Vasculitis

Generalized vasculitis is associated with protein and water leakage from small vessels, which causes a drop in the intravascular osmotic pressure, leading to secondary edema. Clinical characteristics of vasculitis include petechiation of the mucous membranes, dependent edema, lethargy, and occasionally fever. The usual causes are infectious agents, although the vasculitis may be immune-mediated. Potential causes are purpura hemorrhagica, equine viral arteritis, equine infectious anemia, and equine ehrlichiosis (*Ehrlichia equi*).

Purpura Hemorrhagica

Purpura hemorrhagica is believed to be a hypersensitivity reaction within blood capillaries to antigenic remnants from a previous bacterial or viral infection. It is often associated with streptococcal infections, particularly *Streptococcus equi* (strangles). When implicated, infection precedes the clinical signs of purpura by 2 to 3 weeks.

The presentation and severity of clinical signs vary greatly between cases, but consistent features are some form of edematous swelling with petechiation of the mucous membranes. The edematous swellings can vary from diffuse urticarial plaques to marked edema of each limb, which terminates as an abrupt ridge in the upper leg ("bottle neck leg"). In some cases there is edema of the muzzle and face. Diagnosis is largely based on the clinical signs of edema with petechiation. If there is no obvious petechiation of the oral mucous membranes, the clinician should carefully check the membranes of the intranasal septum and, in mares, the vulva. Clinical pathology examination shows hyperfibrinogenemia but is otherwise nonspecific.

Equine Viral Arteritis

Equine viral arteritis is a highly contagious disease that is spread by respiratory and venereal routes. The virus replicates in the tunica media of small arteries throughout the body and the resultant vascular damage can lead to lung edema, pleural effusion, dependent edema, conjunctivitis, and placental separation. The result is respiratory disease with widespread tissue inflammation and the potential for abortion in mares. The causal virus has a worldwide distribution and in many countries is subject to control by legislation or codes of practice.

Clinical diagnosis can be difficult because the presenting signs vary greatly in their severity; infection is more common than clinical disease. The petechiation can be confused with that of purpura hemorrhagica (see earlier). However, most clinical cases of equine viral arteritis feature a marked keratoconjunctivitis and photophobia, with swelling of the eyelids that is not usual in cases of purpura. In acute disease, viral isolation is possible from nasopharyngeal swabs; heparinized blood; the stallion's urine or semen; and splenic and lung tissues of the aborted fetus. Viral antibody can be detected in serum, but a fourfold increase in titer over 10 days is needed to confirm recent exposure.

Equine Infectious Anemia

Equine infectious anemia is a viral disease transmitted by biting flies or contaminated needles. The disease has a worldwide distribution, but most outbreaks occur in warm, wet areas where the blood-sucking vectors are abundant. This gives rise to its synonym *swamp fever*. It is a notifiable disease in many countries. In acute disease there is fever, depression, and petechiation of the mucous membranes. At a later stage, there is jaundice, anemia, and dependent edema. A horse showing these clinical signs should be viewed with suspicion and tested for equine infectious anemia. A characteristic of the disease is persistence of infection; recovered cases can relapse after several days or weeks.

The petechiation and edema are thought to be the result of a hypersensitivity vasculitis. The anemia is the result of immune-mediated hemolysis associated with the attachment of viral particles to erythrocytes. In terms of the petechiation and edema, the clinical expression can be similar to purpura hemorrhagica, equine viral arteritis, and ehrlichiosis. The diagnosis is confirmed by an agar-gel immunodiffusion test (the Coggins test), which identifies equine infectious anemia virus-neutralizing antibodies in serum.

Equine ehrlichiosis is caused by a rickettsial organism, *E. equi*, which parasitizes the white cells of the blood and is believed to be transmitted by ticks. It usually occurs in northern California, but individual cases have been reported in other states and elsewhere in the world. The agent is antigenically distinct from *E. risticii*, the cause of Potomac fever. The clinical signs are of fever, depression, jaundice, mucosal petechiation, and dependent edema. Definitive diagnosis is based on demonstrating *E. equi* morulae in the cytoplasm of neutrophils and eosinophils in a peripheral blood smear. Routine Giemsa or Wright's stains reveal blue-gray inclusions, which have a mulberry-like appearance. Serologic confirmation is possible using an indirect fluorescent antibody test, but this is not widely available.

Heart Disease

Acute heart failure is an uncommon cause of dependent edema in horses. The resultant venous congestion raises intravascular hydrostatic pressure and obstructs the central flow of lymph into the venous system at the vena cava. Possible causes include acute myocardial failure associated with ionophore toxicity, and acute left-sided failure associated with rupture of one of the mitral chordae tendineae.

Ionophore antibiotics such as monensin are used as feed inclusions to improve weight gain and to control coccidiosis in cattle, sheep, and poultry. Horses are extremely susceptible to ionophore toxicity, and intermittent reports of accidental poisoning are widespread. The predominant lesion is cardiac myodegeneration, but there are also muscular, hepatic, and renal disturbances. The clinical presentation varies but always includes tachycardia and may include arrhythmias. Serum levels of muscle enzymes are elevated.

Rupture of a chorda tendinea leads to pulmonary edema and hypertension, and subsequently to right-sided heart failure. However, the cardinal clinical sign in these cases is acute dyspnea rather than the development of dependent edema. Echocardiography is of particular diagnostic value in these cases.

Chronic heart failure is also uncommon in horses, but diseases affecting the pericardium, myocardium, and valves lead to venous congestion and dependent edema for the same reasons described under acute failure. Horses with severe valvular incompetence, especially of the mitral valve, may develop atrial fibrillation, and the condition can progress to heart failure with tachycardia and a pulsatile distension of the jugular veins. On auscultation, arrhythmia and obvious murmurs are heard. Chronic myocardial disease is rare in horses but can be associated with chronic ionophore toxicity. Pericarditis is also rare and presents with muffled heart sounds, distended nonpulsatile veins, tachycardia, and dependent edema. Echocardiography is of particular diagnostic value.

Urticarial Lesions

Urticarial reactions are very common in horses. They are localized areas of edema on the body surface but may occur in very large numbers with a widespread distribution. The pathogenesis of urticarial reactions is ill defined; they are often idiopathic and may not be worth investigating unless they persist for several weeks or recur regularly. Biopsies are usually not helpful, except to rule out other skin diseases, and diagnosis leans heavily on the associated history. Causes include systemic drug reactions, most commonly antibiotics and nonsteroidal anti-inflammatory drugs, food allergy or reaction, contact urticaria in response to topical drugs or other applied substances, and seasonal recurrent urticaria associated with ectoparasites or, much more rarely, inhaled allergens such as pollens or molds. Diagnosis is by elimination of the implicated agent.

DIFFERENTIAL DIAGNOSIS OF LOCAL EDEMA

Trauma

Trauma is the most common cause of tissue swelling and local edema in horses, and it usually involves the legs. The local inflammatory response causes an increase in vascular permeability, which favors edema formation. The localized swelling can expand to obstruct local venous and lymphatic

drainage, so that the entire limb distal to the injury becomes swollen. Diagnosis is usually evident on the basis of the history and clinical examination.

Infections

Infections are usually the result of trauma and often take the form of diffuse cellulitis. Examination reveals swelling, pain, heat, and occasionally exudation. Puncture wounds with localized bruising, such as stake wounds or injection sites, may be sufficiently anaerobic to allow vegetation of clostridial spore contaminants, resulting in toxin elaboration and profound systemic illness. In these cases there is localized edema followed by necrosis, gas production evident as crepitus in tissues, a thin serosanguineous exudate, and generalized toxemia. All these signs appear within 24 to 48 hours of injury. The toxemia causes severe depression, tachycardia, and a progressively weak pulse culminating in fatal shock. Tissue culture is diagnostic, but the provisional diagnosis is based on the clinical findings, and immediate aggressive treatment is indicated.

Lymphatic Obstruction

Inflammation of lymphatic vessels and regional lymph nodes in association with local infection is common. Examples are infection with *S. equi* (strangles), and the various infections associated with lymphangitis of the limbs (see later). Lymph nodes can also be distended by neoplastic invasion or metastasis. Distension of local nodes can obstruct lymph flow and render lymphatic valves incompetent, thus allowing a retrograde flow of lymph. Concurrent obstruction of the local vein increases venous pressure and augments the effect of lymphatic obstruction, leading to chronic edema of the dependent area.

Sporadic lymphangitis is a common lymphatic obstruction of uncertain etiology that usually affects one or another of the hindlimbs and is traditionally blamed on a protein-rich diet. Inflammation of the lymphatic tracts and associated regional lymph nodes leads to lymph stasis and, at the extreme, a thickening of the whole limb. The earliest change is acute lameness, but swelling of the limb quickly follows, and it may be sufficiently severe to cause serum to ooze out of taut skin surfaces. Secondary infection and development of cellulitis are possible. Early treatment of the acute case to resolve edema is extremely important. If edema persists for more than 7 days, severe fibrosis can develop in the interstitial spaces, resulting in permanent swelling and reduced function. This chronic disfigurement is usually refractory to all treatments.

Infectious Causes of Lymphangitis

Infections causing lymphangitis usually involve the limbs and produce local swelling and edema. In contrast to sporadic lymphangitis, these conditions are contagious and involve bacterial or fungal agents.

Ulcerative lymphangitis is the most common of these conditions and may be associated with wound infection in conditions of poor hygiene. Transmission by direct contact (e.g., via the grooming kit) and by biting flies is also possible. The result is multiple foci of nodular abscessation along lymphatic tracts, which erupt to discharge a greenish pus. A number of bacterial causes are implicated, including *Corynebacterium pseudotuberculosis, Pseudomonas aerugi-*

nosa, and staphylococcal and streptococcal species. Diagnosis is based on culture results.

Cutaneous glanders or *farcy* is a rare disease caused by *Pseudomonas mallei*. It is the cutaneous form of a debilitating pneumonia that has been eradicated from most of Western Europe and is now confined to parts of Asia. Lymphatic infection is associated with the development of nodules that discharge a honey-like pus. Diagnosis is based on results of culture and serum antibody tests, and an intradermal hypersensitivity test using an antigen extract of the bacterium (Mallein test).

Epizootic lymphangitis is caused by a yeast-like fungus, *Histoplasma farciminosus*, which gains access to superficial wounds to produce skin nodules from which a thick creamy pus erupts. The disease is now of limited occurrence worldwide, being found in parts of the African and Asian continents. The clinical presentation is similar to the cutaneous form of glanders, from which it can be distinguished by smear cytology or Mallein test.

Sporotrichosis is caused by the fungal agent *Sporothrix schenckii*, which invades superficial wounds. The condition is widespread and occurs in Europe, India, and the United States. The organism spreads through the lymphatics, causing cording and minor nodular eruptions, which may discharge a small amount of pus. Diagnosis is confirmed by smear cytology, culture, and biopsy results.

Pythiosis is an infection associated with edema and progressive necrosis of subcutaneous tissues. It is caused by the Protista organism *Pythium insidiosum*, a plant parasite found in stagnant water. The condition is found in swampy, tropical, and subtropical locations. The rapid and malignant development of the lesion gives rise to the synonym *swamp cancer*. Diagnosis is by results of culture at a specialized laboratory and by biopsy examination.

Photosensitization

In horses exposed to sunlight, photosensitization is recognized as erythema, edema, serum ooze, crusting, and, at worst, skin necrosis. Only white nonpigmented areas of the muzzle, forehead, and limbs are affected. Primary photosensitization occurs in conditions of high ultraviolet exposure and is associated with the grazing of plants that contain photodynamic agents, such as St. John's wort or perennial rye grass. Several horses in a group may be affected. Alternatively, secondary photosensitization is associated with liver failure that leads to a decrease in the excretion of phylloerythrin, a product of bacterial activity on chlorophyll. This substance is photodynamic and provokes erythematous reactions in susceptible areas of skin. In all cases of suspected photosensitization, serum liver enzyme levels should be checked for evidence of liver-associated disease. Otherwise, diagnosis is by transferring the animal to shade and checking the pasture for implicated plants.

Snake and Insect Bites

The toxic components of snake venoms vary with the species, and the effects on their victims vary accordingly. Bites usually occur in the summer months and are often about the head, indicating the inquisitive nature of the victim. A marked local edema frequently follows the bite, but in most cases there is insufficient toxin to cause the death of a large horse. Nevertheless, the swelling may be sufficiently severe to cause dyspnea, and secondary infection at the site can lead to bacterial toxemia and death.

Bees and wasps may attack as swarms, producing multiple, painful papules and plaques. Rare fatalities are recorded in horses. Multiple stings about the head can cause a severe local swelling with dyspnea.

Supplemental Readings

Brown CM (ed): Limb and ventral edema. *In* Problems in Equine Medicine. Philadelphia, Lea & Febiger, 1989, pp 138–149.

Dixon P: Swellings of the head region in the horse. In Practice (supplement to the Veterinary Record) 13:257–263, 1991.

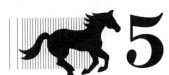

SECTION 5

THE HEMATOPOIETIC SYSTEM

Edited by Chrysann Collatos

Diagnostic Approach to Anemia

JEANNE LÖFSTEDT
Charlottetown, Prince Edward Island

Anemia is a decrease in the absolute red blood cell (RBC) mass and is characterized by a decreased RBC count, decreased packed cell volume (PCV), and except in cases of hemolysis, decreased hemoglobin concentration. Anemia frequently accompanies underlying systemic disease in the horse. Failure to recognize and treat the underlying disease process results in frustrating therapeutic failures. Pathophysiologic classification of anemia as regenerative (i.e., due to hemorrhage or hemolysis) or non-regenerative (i.e., due to systemic disease or intrinsic bone marrow abnormalities) helps to narrow the list of differential diagnoses. Unfortunately, several features of the equine erythron make this classification less straightforward than in other species. This chapter focuses on the clinical signs of anemia, evaluation of the equine erythron, and the approach used to classify anemia as either regenerative or non-regenerative.

CLINICAL SIGNS OF ANEMIA

Anemic horses generally have pale mucous membranes. Physiologic adjustments to inadequate tissue oxygen transport are responsible for many of the other clinical signs. The PCV at which signs become noticeable depends on the rate at which anemia develops and the physiologic demands placed on the animal. Clinical signs of anemia of an acute onset are tachycardia, tachypnea, decreased exercise tolerance, and a systolic murmur associated with decreased blood viscosity and increased turbulence as blood flows through the heart and great vessels. Hypovolemic

shock, characterized by a weak, thready pulse, marked tachycardia, poor jugular filling, and blanched mucous membranes, is seen in horses with acute severe loss of more than 30% of blood volume. Because of physiologic adaptation, anemia that develops slowly is usually advanced before clinical signs such as weight loss and lethargy are recognized. Vital signs often are normal at rest, but they increase dramatically if the horse is stressed. Other clinical findings in anemic patients depend on pathogenesis and may include one or more of the following: fever; icterus; hemoglobinuria; bilirubinuria; signs of external blood loss such as epistaxis, melena, hematuria, bleeding from wounds; or evidence of coagulation abnormalities such as hematomas, petechiae, or ecchymoses.

EVALUATION OF THE ERYTHRON

Peripheral Blood Evaluation

Careful gross inspection of the blood sample may reveal pink plasma (i.e., hemoglobinemia) suggestive of intravascular hemolysis, brown blood (i.e., methemoglobinemia) consistent with exposure to an erythrocyte oxidant, or spontaneous erythrocyte agglutination indicating immune-mediated anemia.

Automated cell counters provide information on PCV, RBC count, hemoglobin concentration, and several erythrocyte indices. PCV and hemoglobin concentration are used to evaluate RBC mass. These parameters vary considerably among breeds of horses and also are affected by age. Generally athletic or "hot blooded" horses such as Thoroughbreds and Standardbreds have considerably higher values (PCV 32–50%; hemoglobin 12–17 mg/dl) than "cold blooded" draft breeds (PCV 24–44%; hemoglobin 12–14 mg/dl). The reported reference ranges for Miniature horses (PCV 24–32%; hemoglobin 9–16 mg/dl) and donkeys (PCV 28–47%; hemoglobin 9.5–16.5 mg/dl) approximate those of draft breeds. The PCV of neonatal foals in the first 14 days of life is similar to that of adult horses, but then decreases dramatically and remains below adult values until 18 months of age. In normal horses, the ratio PCV (%)/hemoglobin (g/dl) is greater than three. This ratio is usually less than three in patients with intravascular hemolysis and hemoglobinemia.

The labile PCV of equids complicates interpretation. Horses have a highly innervated muscular spleen capable of storing up to one third of the potentially circulating red cell mass. In excited or recently exercised individuals, adrenergic stimulation causes splenic contraction and release of stored erythrocytes into the circulation. Under these conditions, the PCV may increase by as much as 50%. Splenic contraction in response to massive hemorrhage also masks the magnitude of blood loss in the horse for at least 24 hours. Serial PCV evaluations are therefore indicated when assessing the hematologic status of the equine patient. Equine erythrocytes exhibit marked rouleaux formation (coin-like stacking), which causes them to sediment rapidly. If blood samples are not thoroughly mixed before the PCV is determined, false decreases in PCV may be recorded, leading to an incorrect diagnosis of anemia.

Erythrocyte indices are usually reported by automated cell counters, but can be calculated if PCV, RBC count, and hemoglobin concentration are known (Table 1). They are helpful in the pathophysiologic classification of anemia (see Table 1).

Descriptions of normal and abnormal equine erythrocyte morphology can be found in a variety of textbooks. RBC morphology is of limited value in the pathophysiologic classification of anemia in the horse, but it provides valuable clues for etiologic diagnosis. Anisocytosis (i.e., variability in RBC size) is caused by presence of macrocytes or microcytes among normal RBCs. Macrocytes may be seen at the peak of the regenerative response in horses; however, in many cases regeneration occurs without appreciable macrocytosis. Polychromasia, which is variation in color of erythrocytes, is caused by presence of reticulocytes that stain bluish because of residual deoxyribonucleic acid (DNA). Polychromasia and reticulocytosis exemplify regenerative anemia in ruminants but are rare findings even in horses with intense erythropoiesis, because equine erythrocytes remain in the bone marrow until fully mature. Howell-Jolly bodies, which are basophilic nuclear remnants in immature RBCs, are sometimes observed in regenerative anemias of ruminants. Howell-Jolly bodies occur in up to 0.1% of erythrocytes of healthy horses and do not represent immature erythrocytes in peripheral blood. Spherocytes, which are small round RBCs lacking central pallor, are observed in some horses with immune-mediated hemolysis. Heinz bodies, which are precipitates of denatured hemoglobin that appear as round aggregates attached to the RBC membrane, are readily demonstrated using new methylene blue stain and are indicative of oxidative stress to erythrocytes. Autoagglutination of erythrocytes, which is observed grossly or microscopically in some cases of immune-mediated anemia, should be differentiated from rouleaux formation by diluting the blood sample 1:4 with 0.9% saline. Rouleaux formation disperses, but autoagglutination persists following suspension in isotonic saline. *Babesia equi* and *Babesia caballi* are intra-erythrocytic parasites of horses raised in subtropical regions. They are rarely encountered in peripheral blood because they develop in the vascular endothelium, and parasitemia commonly precedes clinical disease. Because *Babesia* species may be overlooked on routinely stained blood smears, Giemsa or methylene blue stains should be employed in cases when equine piroplasmosis is suspected.

Osmotic Fragility Tests

Osmotic fragility tests measure resistance of RBCs to in vitro hemolysis when they are suspended in increasingly hypotonic saline solutions. In normal horses, hemolysis commences with exposure to 0.45% saline and is complete with suspension in 0.34% saline. Susceptibility to hemolysis increases as erythrocyte size decreases. Erythrocyte fragility is often abnormal in equine patients with immune-mediated anemia because antibody attachment to RBCs results in membrane loss in the mononuclear phagocyte system (MPS) with a subsequent decrease in RBC size and deformability.

Direct Antiglobulin (Coombs') Test

A positive direct antiglobulin (Coombs') test indicates presence of antibody or complement on the surface of RBCs and is diagnostic of immune-mediated anemia. This test may be positive in idiopathic immune-mediated anemia, neonatal isoerythrolysis, and equine infectious anemia. The Coombs' reagent should contain antisera to IgG, IgM, and C3. The end-point of this test is agglutination, and thus it should not be performed on a blood sample already exhibiting autoagglutination.

RBC Volume Distribution Width (RDW)

A coefficient of variation of RBC volume, RDW is sometimes reported by automatic cell counters. It is increased in horses exhibiting anisocytosis after hemorrhage or hemolysis. Other erythrocyte parameters that have been investi-

TABLE 1.   CALCULATION OF ERYTHROCYTE INDICES AND THEIR INTERPRETATION

Indices	Formulas	Units	Interpretation
Mean corpuscular volume (MCV)	$\dfrac{PCV \times 10}{RBC\ count}$	Femtoliters (fl)	> with regenerative anemia (occasionally) < with iron deficiency
Mean corpuscular hemoglobin (MCH)	$\dfrac{Hb \times 10}{RBC\ count}$	Picograms (pg)	> with intravascular hemolysis < with iron deficiency anemia
Mean corpuscular hemoglobin concentration (MCHC)	$\dfrac{Hb \times 100}{PCV}$	Grams/ deciliter (g/dl)	> with intravascular hemolysis < with iron deficiency anemia

Units for above calculations are % for PCV, 10^6/L for RBC count, and g/L for hemoglobin concentration.

gated as markers of the equine regenerative response are glucose-6-phosphate dehydrogenase (G6PD), creatine, and adenosine-5-triphosphate. Although their concentrations in equine erythrocytes are increased during the regenerative response, these tests are not widely available, which limits their clinical usefulness.

Bone Marrow Evaluation

Bone marrow evaluation is indicated to separate responsive from nonresponsive anemias in horses and for the definitive diagnosis of myeloproliferative disorders. Blood loss and hemolytic anemias, however, are usually diagnosed without bone marrow evaluation. Marrow aspirates or biopsies can be collected from the sternum, ileum, or proximal ribs; the technique is described in detail in the third edition of *Current Therapy in Equine Medicine* (pp 491–492).

Marrow samples are first examined at lower magnification for cellularity, heterogeneity, and individual progenitor series. The myeloid:erythroid ratio (M:E ratio) is estimated by counting 500 cells. The normal M:E ratio ranges from 0.5 to 3.76. A ratio of less than 0.5 is indicative of erythroid regeneration, but it may be the result of myeloid suppression. Reticulocyte counts (i.e., the number of reticulocytes/1000 RBCs) in the marrow can also be used to assess the regenerative response in the horse. Normal equine marrow contains approximately 3% reticulocytes; in cases of regenerative anemia this percentage increases to greater than 50%. Special histochemical stains such as Prussian blue can be used to stain marrow iron and assist in the evaluation of marrow iron stores. In horses with hemolytic anemia, marrow macrophages frequently contain phagocytosed RBCs.

Serum Iron Evaluation

Evaluation of serum iron status is indicated in equine patients with microcytic hypochromic anemia. Serum ferritin concentration reflects storage iron; the reference range reported for normal horses is 152 ± 54.6 ng/ml. As mentioned earlier, special iron stains can be applied to assess the storage pool of iron in the bone marrow. Serum iron concentration measures iron bound to transferrin (i.e., the total amount of transport iron in serum). Reported normal ranges for horses are 120 ± 5.0 µg/dl. Total iron binding capacity (TIBC) measures the amount of iron that transferrin is capable of binding when totally saturated. The reference range for normal horses is 388 ± 8.1 µg/dl. The percentage of transferrin saturation is calculated from the TIBC and serum iron concentration and is approximately 30% in normal horses.

PATHOPHYSIOLOGIC CLASSIFICATION OF ANEMIA

Regenerative Anemia

A regenerative anemia is one in which the bone marrow responds appropriately with increased RBC production to accelerated erythrocyte loss from the circulation. Marked anisocytosis and mean corpuscular volume (MCV) greater than 60 femtoliters (fl), a rare observation, suggests a regenerative anemia, as does a M:E ratio less than 0.5. Acute blood loss and hemolysis are examples of responsive anemias. Acute blood loss and hemolytic anemia are often accompanied by pyrexia and mature neutrophilia. Pigment-induced nephropathy associated with intravascular hemolysis commonly precipitates renal azotemia. Hepatic hypoxia resulting from anemia may cause moderate increases in hepatocellular enzyme activities.

Non-regenerative Anemia

Non-regenerative anemias, or anemias associated with inadequate erythrocyte production, are common in horses. These anemias are mild and slowly progressive. Plasma protein concentration is variable, but is frequently increased in horses with chronic inflammation or neoplasia. Evaluation of bone marrow cytology samples confirms an inadequate marrow response for the degree of anemia. Non-regenerative anemias in horses have been attributed to the following disorders: iron deficiency; chronic inflammatory, endocrine, or neoplastic diseases; and generalized bone marrow failure.

Supplemental Readings

Jain NC: Schalm's Veterinary Hematology, 4th ed. Philadelphia, Lea & Febiger, 1986.
Smith JE, Cipriano JE, DeBowes R, Moore K: Iron deficiency and pseudo-iron deficiency in hospitalized horses. J Am Vet Med Assoc 188:285–287, 1986.
Tablin F, Weiss L: Equine bone marrow: A quantitative analysis of erythroid maturation. Anat Rec 213:202–206, 1985.
Tyler RD, Cowell RL, Clinkenbeard KD, MacAllister CG: Hematologic values in horses and interpretation of hematologic data. Vet Clin North Am Equine Pract 3(3):461–484, 1987.

Blood Loss Anemia

CHRYSANN COLLATOS
Reno, Nevada

ACUTE BLOOD LOSS

The pathophysiologic effects of acute blood loss are the result of decreased circulating blood volume and associated hypovolemic shock. Clinically significant hemorrhage occurs when more than 30% of the body's blood is lost rapidly. Because blood volume comprises approximately 8% of body weight, this implies a 10.8-L loss in a 450-kg horse. Unfortunately, accurate quantitation of blood loss rarely is possible, thus assessment of the presence and severity of hemorrhage is based on clinical signs and sequential measurement of packed cell volume (PCV) and plasma protein.

Severe hemorrhage usually is due to loss of vascular integrity, which may result from iatrogenic (e.g., surgical) or accidental trauma, or from erosion of vessel walls by neoplastic, infectious, or parasitic lesions. Rarely, coagulopathies such as an inherited or acquired factor deficiency, thrombocytopenia, or disseminated intravascular coagulopathy cause clinically significant acute blood loss. Common causes of external hemorrhage due to large vessel rupture include castration complication or accidental trauma. Epistaxis associated with nasal surgery or guttural pouch mycosis also can result in severe blood loss. Rarely, exercise-induced pulmonary hemorrhage, ethmoid hematoma, or nasal neoplasia cause serious epistaxis. Internal hemorrhage occurs most often into large muscle masses, the abdominal cavity, or the thorax. In muscle, jagged fracture fragments or severe soft tissue trauma can lacerate large vessels. Traumatic splenic rupture or spontaneous middle uterine artery hemorrhage in postpartum mares can cause hemoperitoneum. Less often, mesenteric vessels may be damaged by large strongylus migration, mesenteric abscessation, or neoplasia. Similar erosive processes, such as a pulmonary abscess or neoplasia, as well as trauma, can cause hemothorax.

Clinical Signs and Diagnosis

Consistent signs of acute blood loss include tachycardia, tachypnea, pale mucous membranes, and prolonged jugular filling. With continued bleeding, progressive exercise intolerance, muscular weakness, and collapse ensue. Decreased organ perfusion can cause oliguria and ileus. With internal hemorrhage, signs associated with the site of blood accumulation may be present. These include dyspnea and pleurodynia in the case of hemothorax, low-grade colic in the case of hemoperitoneum, or lameness in the case of hemarthrosis or muscle hemorrhage.

The source of massive extracorporeal bleeding usually is obvious. However, with internal or multifocal bleeding, a careful physical examination may be required to discern clinical signs of hemorrhage and to differentiate them from other signs of abdominal, thoracic, or musculoskeletal disease. When a nonhemorrhagic emergency is suspected, such as colic, pleuritis, or acute musculoskeletal trauma, internal bleeding should always be considered if tachycardia, tachypnea, and mucous membrane blanching persist after the patient's condition is stabilized. Auscultation, percussion, centesis, and percutaneous ultrasonography are useful ancillary diagnostic aids. If no source of vascular damage to account for the hemorrhage can be identified, the diagnostic work-up should include a platelet count and clotting profile. The latter should include measurements of prothrombin time, activated partial thromboplastin time, and the concentration of fibrin degradation products.

In the first 12 to 24 hours following acute hemorrhage, the severity of blood loss must be estimated on the basis of clinical signs, unless the actual volume of hemorrhage has been measured. This is because physiologic alterations render PCV and plasma protein levels unreliable indicators of bleeding. Initially, increased sympathetic nervous system activity triggers splenic contraction, releasing stored red blood cells that temporarily support the PCV. Concurrently, decreased hydrostatic pressure within capillaries causes interstitial fluid to move into the vascular space. This begins within 30 minutes of acute hemorrhage and can restore 20 to 50% of blood volume within 6 hours. Subsequently, further translocation of interstitial fluid, absorption of fluid from the gastrointestinal tract, and renal water resorption all act to support intravascular volume but dilute the PCV. Thus, the PCV continues to decrease until the true severity of blood loss can be assessed 24 to 36 hours after hemorrhage ceases. Plasma protein is reclaimed from lymph during fluid shifts after bleeding. As a result, plasma protein, which is a more useful indicator of severity of hemorrhage in the first hours after bleeding, increases more rapidly than PCV thereafter. With internal hemorrhage, the interpretation of PCV and plasma protein values is further complicated by the recycling of up to two thirds of the erythrocytes and most of the protein lost into extravascular spaces within the body. The bone marrow response to hemorrhage is not reflected by an increase in PCV level until 3 to 5 days after hemorrhage has occurred, and normal red blood cell mass may not be restored for 4 to 6 weeks. In general, the clinicopathologic indicators of response to hemorrhage seen in other species are not present in horses. Leukocytosis and thrombocytosis are rare. Occasionally, the mean corpuscular volume increases above 60 femtoliters by 4 to 7 days after hemorrhage.

Treatment

The two immediate goals of treatment for acute blood loss are: (1) stop the bleeding, and (2) reverse hypovolemic shock. External hemorrhage is best controlled with direct pressure or large vessel ligation. With internal hemorrhage, physical and environmental stress must be minimized. Surgical intervention to identify and control sites of internal hemorrhage often is not practical. Although the reports are anecdotal, the antifibrinolytic agents epsilon-aminocaproic acid° (5 g intravenously [IV]) and tranexamic acid† (1 g IV) as well as the narcotic antagonist naloxone hydrochloride‡ (8 mg IV) have been used without deleterious effects to treat postpartum uterine artery hemorrhage. Aminocaproic and tranexamic acid directly inhibit the fibrinolytic action of plasminogen. In humans, these drugs decrease intracranial hemorrhage, bleeding after cardiopulmonary bypass, and dysfunctional uterine bleeding. Naloxone apparently combats the effects of endogenous opioids on cardiovascular dynamics. Equivocal results have been reported in experimental studies investigating the efficacy of naloxone in the treatment of hypovolemic shock. The efficacy of the antifibrinolytic agents and naloxone have not been evaluated objectively in horses.

If clinical signs of hypovolemic shock are present, an intravenous crytalloid solution should be administered rapidly at 40 to 60 ml/kg to provide cardiovascular support. Colloid solutions such as dextran, hydroxyethyl starch, or plasma typically are not immediately available or are cost-prohibitive in large animals. The use of hypertonic saline in the face of uncontrolled hemorrhage is controversial, because some experimental evidence has demonstrated increased blood loss and mortality resulting from the increased blood pressure and cardiac output that follow hypertonic saline administration. If bleeding has been controlled, 7% saline at 4 ml/kg IV (2 L to a 450-kg horse) may be beneficial, particularly if high-volume crystalloid solution administration is not practical.

Following stabilization, the necessity for whole blood transfusion must be assessed. With acute blood loss, if blood pressure and circulatory volume are adequate, myocardial oxygenation is maintained until the hematocrit falls below 15%. The decision for transfusion is based on the overall clinical assessment of the patient. Signs indicating the need for transfusion include: PCV level below 15% and falling; uncontrolled bleeding; quantitated loss of 30% of blood volume; and poor clinical response to shock therapy manifested as persistent tachycardia, tachypnea, weakness, and mucous membrane pallor. (See page 290 for specific recommendations regarding transfusion administration.)

CHRONIC BLOOD LOSS

Chronic blood loss is uncommon in the horse, but when present is most often the result of gastrointestinal parasite

°*Amicar, Wyeth-Ayerst, Pearl River, NY*
†*Cyklokapron, Pharmacia, Mississauga, Ontario*
‡*Narcan, DuPont Pharmaceuticals, Manati, Puerto Rico*

infestation. Other sources of gastrointestinal blood loss include infiltrative diseases such as gastric squamous cell carcinoma, or ulcers resulting from nonsteroidal anti-inflammatory drug toxicity. Urogenital bleeding from neoplasia or infection is possible, and idiopathic urethral hemorrhage in male horses has been reported. Thrombocytopenia or coagulopathy should always be considered when chronic blood loss is suspected.

Clinical Signs and Diagnosis

Gradual loss of red cell mass does not result in overt signs of anemia such as tachycardia, tachypnea, or weakness until the PCV level is below 12%. Pale mucous membranes are noted earlier, as well as clinical signs related to the underlying disease, such as weight loss in the case of parasitism or neoplasia. The primary differential diagnoses for anemia due to chronic blood loss are anemia of chronic disease (see page 283) and low-grade hemolysis (see page 278). Diagnostic procedures should be aimed at characterizing the anemia, identifying a source of blood loss, and ruling out other causes of anemia. Therefore, results of complete blood count, bone marrow evaluation, fecal occult blood, fecal examination for parasite ova, urinalysis, total and indirect serum bilirubin, and Coggins test for equine infectious anemia are indicated. Although iron deficiency anemia is rare in horses because dietary iron usually is abundant, chronic blood loss may result in decreased iron stores, reflected by hypoferremia, increased total iron binding capacity, decreased marrow iron, and a poor regenerative marrow response. The anemia typically is microcytic and hypochromic.

Treatment

Treatment of chronic blood loss is based on identification and elimination of the source of blood loss. As mentioned earlier, dietary iron rarely is inadequate, therefore iron supplementation is not necessary. Administration of parenteral iron is not recommended because of the possibility of serious adverse reactions. If desired, ferrous sulfate can be given (2 mg/kg p.o., s.i.d.).

Supplemental Readings

Easley JR: Erythrogram and red cell distribution width of equidae with experimentally induced anemia. Am J Vet Res 46:2378–2384, 1985.
Jain NC: Blood loss or hemorrhagic anemias. *In* Schalm's Veterinary Hematology, ed 4. Philadelphia, Lea & Febiger, 1986, pp 577–588.
McCarthy PF, Hooper RN, Carter GK, Varner DD, Taylor TS, Blanchard TL: Postparturient hemorrhage in the mare: Managing ruptured arteries of the broad ligament. Vet Med 89:147–152, 1994.
Muir WW: Small volume resuscitation using hypertonic saline. Cornell Vet 80:7–11, 1990.

Hemolytic Anemia

DEBRA C. SELLON
Raleigh, North Carolina

Various pathophysiologic events can result in intravascular or extravascular destruction of erythrocytes. Hemolysis is most often the result of oxidative injury, immune-mediated processes, or infectious diseases. Less common causes of hemolysis include intravenous administration of hypotonic solutions or concentrated dimethyl sulfoxide (DMSO), severe hepatic disease, microangiopathic hemolysis, or snake venom. During intravascular hemolysis the destruction of erythrocytes results in increased free hemoglobin in the blood. This is rapidly bound by haptoglobin and removed from circulation by mononuclear phagocytes. Free hemoglobin exceeding the haptoglobin binding capacity causes the hallmark clinical pathologic features of intravascular hemolysis, hemoglobinemia, and hemoglobinuria. In contrast, extravascular hemolysis is the result of accelerated removal of damaged erythrocytes from circulation by mononuclear phagocytes. The hemoglobin is retained in the phagocyte and ultimately metabolized to bilirubin. Thus, both intravascular and extravascular hemolysis can result in increased serum total and unconjugated (indirect) bilirubin concentrations.

OXIDATIVE INJURY TO ERYTHROCYTES

The normal functional hemoglobin molecule contains iron in the ferrous (Fe^{++}) form. Oxidative stress in the erythrocyte causes conversion of ferrous iron to the ferric (Fe^{+++}) form, resulting in methemoglobin, a molecule incapable of carrying oxygen to tissues. Cellular reducing mechanisms normally maintain methemoglobin concentrations at less than 1% of total cellular hemoglobin concentration. The principal cellular reducing enzyme is methemoglobin reductase; glutathione reductase, catalase, and ascorbic acid (vitamin C) play lesser roles in maintaining low intracellular methemoglobin concentrations. If the reducing capacity of methemoglobin reductase is exceeded, methemoglobin accumulates in erythrocytes, giving blood a dark brown color and reducing tissue oxygenation.

Oxidant stress of erythrocytes can also result in disulfide formation in the globin molecule with denaturation and precipitation of the protein. Precipitated hemoglobin results in formation of spherical, refractile Heinz bodies attached to the erythrocyte cell membrane. Heinz bodies increase osmotic fragility and may enhance cell clearance from circulation by mononuclear phagocytes. Methemoglobinemia and/or Heinz body hemolytic anemia occur when the normal reducing abilities of the erythrocyte are overwhelmed by an extreme oxidant stress or when these reducing abilities are diminished and there is a reduced rate of reduction of physiologically produced methemoglobin. Overwhelming oxidative events with subsequent methemoglobinemia and/or Heinz body formation occur in associa-

tion with ingestion of phenothiazine, wild onion (*Allium canadense*), and wilted red maple leaves (*Acer rubrum*) in the horse. Familial methemoglobinemia associated with decreased erythrocytic glutathione reductase and glutathione has been described in two Trotter mares.

Clinical Signs

Horses with hemolysis resulting from ingestion of an oxidizing toxin usually present with severe depression and lethargy that may progress to ataxia and dementia. Heart and respiratory rates are increased and a holosystolic murmur may be heard on auscultation. Mucous membranes are frequently gray or brown because of methemoglobin accumulation in erythrocytes. Icterus may be apparent. Affected blood has a characteristic chocolate-brown appearance. Intravascular hemolysis results in hemoglobinemia, hemoglobinuria, and bilirubinemia. Packed cell volume may be less than 10%.

Red maple (*Acer rubrum*) trees are common throughout the eastern United States. Leaves have three shallow short-pointed lobes and sometimes two smaller lobes near the base. Leaves have five main veins and wavy saw-toothed edges. Leaves are only toxic when wilted or dried and remain so for up to 30 days. Toxicity is not decreased by freezing temperatures. Horses may die peracutely within 12 to 18 hours of exposure, or clinical signs may be delayed up to 5 days following ingestion of wilted leaves.

Phenothiazine is no longer widely used as an anthelmintic, and reports of Heinz body hemolytic anemia in association with its use are becoming rare. Toxicity depends on individual susceptibility and as yet unidentified environmental factors. Animals in poor physical condition may be more susceptible. Heinz body anemia may also occur in horses with access to unharvested onions or overgrazed pasture containing wild onions. Nitrate poisoning may cause methemoglobin formation in horses but only rarely causes hemolysis.

Diagnosis

Red maple leaf toxicity should be suspected in horses with a sudden onset of moderate to severe anemia with chocolate-brown blood and gray-brown mucous membranes. Clinical pathologic findings of hemoglobinemia, hemoglobinuria, and bilirubinemia are consistent with this diagnosis. Identification of blue-black refractile granules near the cellular margin of erythrocytes stained with new methylene blue (Heinz bodies) confirms oxidant-induced hemolysis. Because erythrocytes containing Heinz bodies are rapidly removed from circulation by tissue mononuclear phagocytes, the absence of Heinz bodies does not rule out the diagnosis. Blood methemoglobin concentrations may be measured spectrophotometrically. Normal concentration is approximately 1.77% of total hemoglobin. Horses that have ingested wilted red maple leaves may have methemoglobin concentrations exceeding 50% of the total blood hemoglobin.

Hemoglobin is toxic to renal tubules, and hemoglobinemia can result in acute renal failure. Renal failure is manifested as increased serum urea nitrogen and creatinine concentrations. Secondary electrolyte imbalances may occur.

Treatment

Treatment of oxidant-induced erythrocyte injury is the same regardless of the source of the toxin. There are four main treatment goals: eliminating further erythrocyte damage, increasing tissue oxygenation, maintaining renal perfusion, and providing general supportive care.

Suspected oxidant-induced erythrocyte injury should prompt the veterinarian to identify the source of the toxin. Search of the pasture for wilted red maple leaves is often successful. Access to toxic leaves should be eliminated. All exposed horses should be treated with activated charcoal via nasogastric tube to decrease toxin absorption, even if several days have elapsed since exposure. Endogenous protective mechanisms of the erythrocyte may be supplemented by administration of intravenous ascorbic acid (vitamin C 30 mg/kg b.i.d. in intravenous [IV] fluids). Dexamethasone may be beneficial in stabilizing cellular membranes and decreasing phagocytosis of damaged erythrocytes. Methylene blue therapy is not helpful in horses and may exacerbate hemolysis. In horses with severe anemia indicated by a PCV level less than 10 to 12%, transfusion with whole blood or packed erythrocytes from a compatible donor should be considered.

Hemoglobin can be extremely toxic to renal tubules. If significant intravascular hemolysis is occurring, diuresis should be induced with intravenous fluid administration. Fluid therapy should be closely monitored to avoid overzealous fluid administration that may potentiate the anemia through a dilutional effect. Potentially nephrotoxic drugs should be avoided if possible.

Cerebral anoxia can result in clinical signs of dementia, and sedation with chloral hydrate or detomidine may be indicated. Blood transfusions have resulted in signs suggestive of acute abdominal pain in some horses, possibly resulting from reperfusion injury following gastrointestinal ischemia. Analgesic or sedative therapy may be helpful in these cases. Horses recovering from the acute oxidant injury may develop severe laminitis.

IMMUNE-MEDIATED HEMOLYTIC ANEMIA

Immune-mediated hemolytic anemia (IMHA) occurs when immunologic mechanisms are directed against circulating erythrocytes. True autoimmune hemolytic anemia (AIHA), with production of antibodies against erythrocyte surface antigens, is uncommon. Secondary IMHA occurs when immune complexes nonspecifically attach to Fc or complement receptors on the surface of erythrocytes. In the horse, IMHA has been reported to result from *Clostridium perfringens* septicemia, respiratory tract infections, purpura hemorrhagica, streptococcal abscesses, lymphosarcoma, and penicillin administration. Three mechanisms can

trigger drug-associated IMHA. (1) The drug combines with erythrocyte membranes and is recognized as foreign by the body. Antibodies against this new antigen are produced, triggering destruction of the drug-coated erythrocytes. (2) The drug forms complexes with a carrier molecule and induces an immune response. When the drug-carrier-antibody complexes attach to erythrocyte membranes, hemolysis results. (3) On rare occasions a drug induces true autoantibody production, leading to erythrocyte destruction. Clinical signs, diagnosis, and treatment of IMHA are similar regardless of the underlying disease process.

Isoimmune hemolytic anemia of foals, neonatal isoerythrolysis, occurs when a mare develops alloantibodies against antigens present on her foal's erythrocytes. These alloantibodies are concentrated in colostrum and ingested by the foal. The resultant hemolysis can be severe and life-threatening. The pathogenesis, clinical signs, diagnosis, and treatment of neonatal isoerythrolysis are described on page 592.

Clinical Signs and Diagnosis

Onset of IMHA can be acute and severe or chronic and insidious. Many horses present for fever, lethargy, and weight loss or with signs referable to a primary underlying disease condition. Mucous membranes may be pale or icteric. Tachycardia with a holosystolic murmur is common. The respiratory rate may be increased. A complete blood count often reveals decreased packed cell volume and erythrocyte count and anisocytosis. If erythrocyte membrane is lost in excess of intracellular contents as immunoglobulin-coated erythrocytes pass through the microcirculation of the spleen, rounded cells with increased osmotic fragility (spherocytes) are formed. In some horses the mean corpuscular volume (MCV) is increased. Serum biochemical analysis reveals increased total and indirect bilirubin. Most hemolysis resulting from immune mechanisms occurs extravascularly. If IgM isotype antibodies are involved, complement may be fixed, with resultant intravascular hemolysis, hemoglobinemia, and hemoglobinuria.

IMHA is confirmed by a positive direct Coombs' test, observation of autoagglutination in ethylenediaminetetraacetic acid (EDTA)-anticoagulated blood, or decreased erythrocyte osmotic fragility. The direct Coombs' test assesses agglutination of patient red blood cells when they are exposed to a reagent containing antiequine immunoglobulin and complement. The Coombs' test may yield a false-negative result if the reagents do not recognize the immunoglobulin class attached to the patient erythrocytes, most antibody-coated erythrocytes have been destroyed in vivo, or corticosteroids have been administered recently to the patient. Because the end-point of this test is erythrocyte agglutination, patient blood that is autoagglutinating when anticoagulated with EDTA is generally not tested. True autoagglutination must be differentiated from rouleaux formation by dilution of the blood with saline. Rouleaux formation disperses in saline, whereas autoagglutinated red cells remain clumped. The Coombs' test is temperature-sensitive and should be performed at room temperature and at 37°C. A negative Coombs' test should be interpreted cautiously, especially if all other clinical signs and diagnostic data support a diagnosis of IMHA.

Treatment

If IMHA is suspected, all drug therapy should be discontinued. If continuing antimicrobial therapy is necessary for a bacterial infection, the class of antibacterial agent administered should be altered. If possible, underlying disease processes should be specifically treated. Identification of an underlying disease process such as neoplasia may dramatically alter the long-term prognosis for the horse.

Specific therapy for IMHA is directed at replacement of erythrocytes and inhibition of the immune response. If the packed cell volume is less than 10 to 12% and the horse is showing signs of severe hypoxia, a blood transfusion may be warranted. Compatible donors can be difficult to find, and administration of new erythrocytes may exacerbate the hemolytic process.

Corticosteroid therapy is indicated to inhibit the horse's immune response. Parenteral corticosteroids are preferred in the acutely affected horse, and dexamethasone° is probably the drug of choice. The amount and frequency of administration should be titrated to the individual horse's response, with the attempt to find the minimal effective dose for each animal. An initial dose of dexamethasone 0.05 to 0.2 mg/kg IV or intramuscularly (IM) may be tried. Ideally, corticosteroids should be administered once daily, preferably in the morning, to minimize interference with the circadian rhythm of endogenous corticosteroid release from the adrenal gland. However, if a horse is experiencing acute, severe immune-mediated hemolysis, twice-daily therapy may be needed until the packed cell volume stops declining. Corticosteroids may potentiate underlying infectious diseases and may predispose to laminitis. Long-term, high-dose corticosteroid administration should be avoided if possible.

INFECTIOUS DISEASES

Equine Infectious Anemia

Equine infectious anemia (EIA) is an infectious viral disease of horses that occurs in all parts of the world. The etiologic agent, equine infectious anemia virus (EIAV), is a member of the *Lentivirus* genus of the family Retroviridae. All members of this viral family cause persistent, life-long infections. In the early 1970s the Coggins test was developed as a serologic test for antibodies against EIAV. This test became the basis for state and federal control regulations that exist today.

Transmission

EIAV is transmitted primarily via mechanical vectors, especially the bites of hematophagous insects such as horseflies and deerflies. These flies have large biting mouthparts that facilitate transmission of relatively large quantities of blood between horses. A painful bite stimulates an infected horse to institute evasive actions such as biting and tail swishing. These flies seek to immediately complete their blood meal. If an uninfected horse is grazing next to the infected horse, the completion of this blood meal is likely to effectively transfer virus between horses. Because of their strong instinct to immediately complete a blood meal, horseflies do not travel long distances before biting again. In addition, the virus only survives 30 minutes

°*Azium, Schering-Plough Animal Health, Kenilworth, NJ*

to 2 hours on the mouthparts of these flies. These considerations have been important for design of control programs, described later.

EIAV also can be transmitted between horses iatrogenically through shared needles, unclean surgical instruments, dental floats, and other contaminated equipment. Virus can be passed transplacentally. Foals are most likely to be born virus-positive if their dam experiences a febrile episode with high-titer viremia during gestation. Only about 10% of foals born to mares with no clinical signs of EIA during gestation are born virus-positive. Venereal transmission appears to be extremely rare.

Clinical Signs

Horses infected with EIAV can present with a wide variety of clinical signs. Acute infection often results in a syndrome of high fever, depression, and thrombocytopenia, with or without accompanying anemia. These horses have a very large quantity of virus in their blood and are considered highly infectious. More chronic infections can cause recrudescent cycles of fever, anemia, and thrombocytopenia with accompanying weight loss and ventral edema. Each febrile cycle is associated with the emergence of a novel antigenic strain of the virus and its replication to a high titer. The frequency and severity of febrile episodes usually decline over time. Most EIAV-seropositive horses appear clinically normal and may have normal platelet and erythrocyte counts. Although these horses have a much lower quantity of virus in their blood than do febrile horses, they remain infectious.

Many of the clinical signs and clinical pathologic abnormalities observed in horses with EIA are the result of a vigorous but ineffective host immune response. Most horses exhibit heterogeneous hypergammaglobulinemia with increases in serum IgG, IgM, and IgG(T) concentrations. During acute disease, anemia is primarily the result of increased clearance of complement-coated erythrocytes from circulation. During febrile episodes intravascular hemolysis may occur. Extravascular hemolysis is more common in chronically infected horses. Depression of bone marrow erythropoiesis is a major contributing factor. Platelets have increased surface IgG and IgM, suggesting that immune processes enhance platelet destruction, but thrombopoiesis is probably also decreased.

Diagnosis

Horses are incapable of clearing EIAV from their body despite mounting a vigorous humoral and cellular immune response. Therefore, serologically positive animals are considered infected for life. The Coggins test is an agar gel immunodiffusion (AGID) test that recognizes antibodies against the highly conserved core protein of the virus. A competitive enzyme-linked immunosorbent assay (C-ELISA) is also approved for diagnosis of EIA in horses. The C-ELISA is slightly more sensitive than the AGID test but is more expensive and labor-intensive. Serologic testing for EIAV can only be done by state and federally recognized laboratories. Foals born to EIAV-infected mares may remain seropositive for up to 6 months after ingestion of colostrum.

Necropsy of an EIAV-infected horse that dies during a febrile episode reveals generalized lymph node enlargement, hepatomegaly, and splenomegaly. Mucosal and visceral ecchymotic hemorrhages are frequently observed. Histopathologically, there is a mononuclear cell infiltrate of liver, lymph nodes, spleen, adrenal gland, and lung. Kupffer cells and splenic and bone marrow macrophages frequently contain hemosiderin deposits. Glomerulonephritis resulting from immune complex deposition in the glomeruli is common. Necropsy of an EIAV-infected horse with no apparent clinical signs is often unremarkable.

Prevention and Control

In the United States, most states require that a horse be seronegative to EIAV within 6 to 12 months of entering that state. Some states also require a negative EIAV test at any change of ownership or for any event involving the congregation of large numbers of horses such as shows, sales, and races. If a horse tests seropositive for EIAV, state regulatory officials are notified before contact of the horse's owners and the testing veterinarian. The farm where the seropositive horse is stabled is quarantined and the seropositive horse is retested. If the result is positive on confirmatory tests, federal law requires that the horse be branded or tattooed to permanently identify it as an EIAV reactor. This identification includes a number assigned to that state, the letter **A**, and a specific number assigned to that reactor. EIAV seropositive horses can only be moved across state lines to return to their farm of origin or be transported to a slaughter sale or research facility. Most states also have specific regulations regarding the disposition of that animal if it remains in the state of origin. In most states, owners have the options of euthanizing the horse, establishing a permanent quarantine, or donating the animal to an approved research facility. Many states vigorously trace back and test all horses known to have had recent contact with the seropositive animal and quarantine and retest all suspect facilities for up to 60 days following the removal of the last seropositive horse from the premises.

A seropositive horse on the premises of any farm can be financially and emotionally devastating. The veterinarian should counsel all horse owners to institute strict control measures. All horses visiting the premises should be required to show proof of seronegative status within the preceding 6 to 12 months. Permanent farm residents should be tested at least yearly. EIAV testing should be included in all prepurchase examinations. Fly control should be encouraged. Any object contacting equine blood should be thoroughly disinfected before use on other horses. Needles should never be used for multiple injections of different horses. Horse owners should be encouraged to pressure organizers of equine events to require proof of negative EIAV status for all participating horses.

Equine Piroplasmosis

Infection with the intraerythrocytic hemoprotozoan parasites *Babesia caballi* or *Babesia equi* results in severe hemolytic anemia. Piroplasmosis is enzootic only in those locales where the tick vector thrives. *B. caballi* has been diagnosed on all continents except Antarctica. In the United States, the tropical horse tick *Dermacentor nitens* transmits the

organism, and infection has been diagnosed in horses in Florida and Texas.

B. equi is only rarely found in the United States; none of the common United States ticks are known to transmit the organism. Although classified in the genus *Babesia*, *B. equi* may be more closely related to *Theileria* species because it undergoes some stages of its life cycle in lymphocytes and lacks the transovarial tick transmission typical of most other *Babesia* species.

Clinical Signs

Previously unexposed adult horses develop signs of acute babesiosis within 1 to 4 weeks of exposure. Fever, depression, pale or icteric mucous membranes, ecchymoses, constipation, colic, and dependent ventral edema may be observed. As their condition worsens, diarrhea may develop. Intravascular destruction of parasitized erythrocytes occasionally results in hemoglobinemia and hemoglobinuria, but extravascular hemolysis is more common. Clinical signs of *B. caballi* infection may last a few days to weeks, but mortality is usually low. In contrast, *B. equi* is frequently fatal and animals may die within 24 to 48 hours of onset of signs.

Horses that survive acute piroplasmosis remain infected asymptomatic carriers of the organism, and stress may precipitate clinical relapse. Horses raised in *Babesia*-endemic areas are often infected with the organism without ever showing recognizable clinical signs. In these animals, initial infection may have occurred when they were foals, which protected them from clinical disease by passive immunity. Horses infected with *B. caballi* are more likely to spontaneously clear the infection than are horses infected with *B. equi*. Once the organism has been eliminated from the body, horses are rapidly susceptible to reinfection and clinical disease.

Diagnosis

Piroplasmosis should be suspected in a horse that has recently arrived in a *Babesia*-endemic area and develops fever, hemolytic anemia, and ventral edema. The diagnosis is confirmed by observation of *Babesia* organisms in blood smears stained with a Giemsa-type stain. The absence of organisms does not exclude a diagnosis of babesiosis. The period of parasitemia may be brief and may occur before the onset of clinical signs. A complement fixation test is available for serologic diagnosis and is usually positive at the time clinical signs become apparent. Differential diagnoses should include purpura hemorrhagica, equine viral arteritis, equine granulocytic ehrlichiosis, equine infectious anemia, and other causes of vasculitis and hemolysis.

Treatment

The location of the horse and the desired goal of treatment often determine the optimal therapy for piroplasmosis. In endemic areas, it may be desirable to suppress clinical signs without eliminating the organism because premunition is dependent on the continued low-level presence of the parasite. Clinical signs of *B. caballi* infection usually resolve following a single injection of imidocarb dipropionate (2.2 mg/kg intramuscularly [IM]). The infection usually can be eliminated by administering imidocarb dipropionate (2 mg/kg s.i.d. IM for 2 days). Side effects of imidocarb administration in horses include salivation, restlessness, colic, and gastrointestinal tract hypermotility. Donkeys may die if treated with imidocarb.

B. equi is more difficult to treat and eliminate than is *B. caballi.* Four doses of imidocarb (4 mg/kg IM q72h) may be tried. There may be strain differences in susceptibility that account for the variable success reported for this treatment regimen. A single dose of the antitheilerial drug buparvaquone (4–6 mg/kg IV or IM) is effective at reducing clinical signs of *B. equi*; however, it will not eliminate infection in carrier horses.

A horse may remain seropositive for up to 8 months following elimination of the organism from its body. All horses entering the United States from *Babesia*-endemic areas are required to have a negative complement fixation test prior to entry.

Equine Granulocytic Ehrlichiosis

Equine granulocytic ehrlichiosis is caused by the rickettsial organism *Ehrlichia equi.* The disease is endemic in the foothills of northern California, but cases have been diagnosed in many other parts of the country, including Colorado, Illinois, Florida, Washington, and New Jersey. A form of granulocytic ehrlichiosis that is antigenically indistinguishable from *E. equi* has been diagnosed in people and dogs. Disease is most common in the fall and winter. The exact mode of transmission has not been determined, but tick vectors are considered likely.

Clinical Signs

Clinical signs of fever, depression, limb edema, icterus, ataxia, and petechiae of the mucous membranes become evident 1 to 9 days after exposure. Horses younger than 1 year of age often exhibit only a slight lethargy and fever. Hematologic abnormalities include mild to moderate anemia, thrombocytopenia, and leukopenia. Without treatment, clinical signs last from 3 to 16 days. Recovered animals are immune to reinfection for at least 2 years.

Diagnosis

Granulocytic ehrlichiosis should be suspected in horses with clinical signs of anemia, thrombocytopenia, fever, and ventral edema. The diagnosis can be confirmed by observation of granular inclusion bodies in the cytoplasm of neutrophils and eosinophils stained with any Giemsa-type stain. Inclusions are most obvious under oil immersion, appearing as pleomorphic, blue-gray to dark blue spokewheel shapes. The appearance of inclusion bodies in neutrophils correlates closely with the onset of fever, with inclusions remaining visible for up to 10 days. Serum may be tested by indirect fluorescence for antibody against *E. equi.*

Treatment

Horses with granulocytic ehrlichiosis usually recover with appropriate supportive care. Elimination of the organism may be hastened by administration of oxytetracycline at 7 mg/kg IV once daily for up to 7 days. Supportive care is recommended, including wrapping edematous legs, giving intravenous fluids, and maintaining stall confinement for severely ataxic horses. In animals that die, necropsy lesions include petechial and ecchymotic hemorrhages, edema, and icterus. Histologically, there is inflammation of small arteries and veins. Mild inflammatory vascular or interstitial lesions may also be observed in heart, brain, kidneys, and lungs.

MISCELLANEOUS CAUSES OF HEMOLYTIC ANEMIA

Hemolytic anemia can occur in horses with microvascular thrombosis resulting from localized or systemic disseminated intravascular coagulation. This microangiopathic hemolytic anemia occurs as red blood cells are damaged while passing through fibrin strands deposited in the lumen of small vessels and may be characterized morphologically by irregularly shaped erythrocytes (schistocytes). Hemolytic uremic syndrome is characterized by acute renal failure, microangiopathic hemolytic anemia, intravascular coagulation, and thrombocytopenia. A similar mechanism may be responsible for the hemolysis observed in areas of turbulent flow caused by hemangiosarcoma or arteriovenous shunts.

Hemolysis may occur iatrogenically following administration of extremely hypotonic or hypertonic fluids. Concentrated (>10%) solutions of DMSO can cause hemolysis if administered intravenously.

A variety of bacterial toxins and snake venoms can cause hemolysis. Lecithinases produced by *Clostridium* species and *Leptospira interrogans* can alter erythrocyte membranes sufficiently to result in hemolysis. Rattlesnake, copperhead, and water moccasin venoms contain phospholipases that may disrupt erythrocyte membranes.

Ingestion of leaves of the northern red oak (*Quercus rubra* L. var. *borealis*) has been reported to cause hemolysis in horses. Associated clinical signs included abdominal pain, constipation, and prolonged coagulation times. Rarely, chronic ingestion of heavy metals such as lead, arsenic, and copper can cause hemolysis in horses.

Severe intravascular hemolytic anemia has been described in some horses with terminal acute or chronic hepatic failure. Prognosis is extremely poor. Hemolysis is associated with increased erythrocyte fragility and morphologic alterations in erythrocytes.

Supplemental Readings

McConnico RS, Brownie CF: The use of ascorbic acid in the treatment of 2 cases of red maple (*Acer rubrum*)-poisoned horses. Cornell Vet 82:293–300, 1992.

Madigan JE, Gribble D: Equine ehrlichiosis in northern California: 49 cases (1968–1981). J Am Vet Med Assoc 190:445–448, 1987.

Robbins RL, Wallace SS, Brunner CJ, Gardner TR, DiFranco BJ, Speirs VC: Immune-mediated haemolytic disease after penicillin therapy in a horse. Equine Vet J 25:462–465, 1993.

Sellon DC: Equine infectious anemia. Vet Clin North Am Equine Pract 9(2):321–336, 1993.

Anemia Resulting From Inadequate Erythropoiesis

CHRYSANN COLLATOS
Reno, Nevada

The average lifespan of the equine erythrocyte is 150 days. Therefore, anemia due to inadequate erythropoeisis is an insidious process associated with scant, nonspecific clinical signs. Causes include anemia of chronic disease, nutritional deficiency, myelopthisic disease, and bone marrow aplasia. Of these, the anemia of chronic disease associated with infectious, inflammatory, or neoplastic disorders is by far the most common. The clinical signs present are those of the primary disease, with anemia detected as a secondary event.

ANEMIA OF CHRONIC DISEASE

This condition is well recognized in mammalian species, and is characterized by a mild to moderate, nonregenerative, normochromic, normocytic anemia. Serum iron and total iron-binding capacity are decreased, but normal to increased iron stores can be demonstrated by serum ferritin or Prussian blue stain for marrow iron. Three mechanisms have been incriminated in the disease process: shortened erythrocyte lifespan, insufficient bone marrow response to demand for red blood cells, and decreased release of iron from the reticuloendothelial system.

Accelerated red cell destruction may be the result of activation of the mononuclear phagocyte system in response to inflammation. In addition, the intravascular response to inflammation may cause increased erythrocyte damage during passage through small vessels, with subsequent removal by the reticuloendothelial system. However, normal bone marrow responds to such increased consumption with an appropriate increase in red blood cell production.

Erythropoietin, the hormone primarily responsible for regulation of erythropoiesis, may be the rate-limiting factor in the marrow's failure to respond to anemia in anemia of chronic disease (ACD). In human and animal models of ACD, although erythropoietin production is increased, there is a deficiency of the hormone relative to the anemia. Administration of pharmacologic doses of recombinant erythropoietin reverses ACD. In addition to the relative erythropoietin deficiency, erythroid progenitor cell activity is inhibited in ACD, as is iron release from the reticuloendothelial system. It appears likely that the abnormal bone marrow and iron metabolism responses in ACD are mediated by cytokines produced in response to inflammatory conditions, including infection and neoplasia. Interleukin-1, tumor necrosis factor, and γ-interferon all have been shown experimentally to play roles in ACD.

Treatment for ACD is solely related to eliminating the underlying disease condition and ensuring that the anemia is not due to blood loss or hemolysis. Diseases associated with ACD in horses include pleuropneumonia, internal abscessation, peritonitis, chronic organ failure, immune-mediated or granulomatous diseases, neoplasia, and chronic viral disease such as equine infectious anemia. Although hypoferremic, horses with ACD have normal iron stores and do not require iron supplementation.

NUTRITIONAL DEFICIENCY

Inadequate erythropoiesis due to dietary inadequacy is exceptionally rare in horses. Vitamin B_{12} and folic acid are important cofactors in erythrocyte maturation. In horses, gastrointestinal bacteria synthesize vitamin B_{12}, eliminating the need for consumption in feed; absorption deficiency, as seen in pernicious anemia in humans, is not recognized. Horses receiving long-term treatment with folic acid inhibitors such as sulfonamides, trimethoprim, or pyrimethamine may benefit from folic acid supplementation. Deficiencies in other micronutrients involved in erythrocyte production such as copper, cobalt, and iron are rare. Iron deficiency anemia in horses is almost invariably the result of chronic blood loss (see page 277). Iron deficiency anemia is diagnosed on the basis of hypoferritemia, hypoferremia, decreased total iron binding capacity (TIBC), and detection of decreased iron stores on examination of bone marrow aspirate. In horses, normal serum ferritin has been reported as 152 ± 54.6 ng/ml, normal iron concentration as 120 ± 5.0 mg/dl, and normal TIBC as 388 ± 8.1 mg/dl.

It should be noted that iron metabolism changes rapidly in foals. Serum iron concentration is very high in the first few days of life; under no circumstances should oral or parenteral iron supplementation be given during this period. Thereafter, there is some controversy regarding the presence of a functionally iron-deficient state in the first 4 to 6 weeks of life because of high iron demands associated with rapid growth and a milk diet that is relatively poor in iron. Whether this physiologic condition exists or not, iron supplementation is not recommended in foals.

ANEMIA DUE TO MYELOPTHISIS OR BONE MARROW APLASIA

Neoplastic infiltration or myelofibrosis can obliterate erythrocyte progenitor cells in bone marrow, resulting in anemia. Such conditions are rare in horses, but pancytopenia resulting from myelofibrosis was reported in one horse. Aplastic anemia results from congenital or acquired developmental failure of hematopoietic progenitor cells. It is rare, but has been reported in a few horses. No definitive cause has been identified, although one horse did have a positive Coombs' test, suggesting an immune-mediated process. In other species, acquired aplastic anemia has been associated with bacterial and viral infections, chronic renal or hepatic failure, irradiation therapy, and drug administration. However, the majority of cases are considered idiopathic. Phenylbutazone has been implicated as a cause of bone marrow aplasia in horses, but this claim has not been substantiated.

Because pancytopenia is usually present, clinical signs are associated with loss of the shorter lived cells—neutrophils and platelets. Therefore, fever, localized infection, and thrombocytopenic hemorrhage can be anticipated. Diagnosis is based on the identification of hypoplastic bone marrow. Bone marrow biopsy is warranted in an animal with persistent pancytopenia, despite the presence of thrombocytopenia. In humans, treatment modalities include drug withdrawal, administration of androgenic hormones and glucocorticoids, and autogenous bone marrow transplantation. One horse with bone marrow aplasia and a positive Coombs' test improved in conjunction with administration of nandrolone decanoate,° an anabolic steroid, and corticosteroids. These drugs enhance erythropoiesis by increasing erythropoietin production and the sensitivity of stem cells to this hormone's action.

Supplemental Readings

Angel KL, Spano JS, Schumacher J, Kwapien RP: Myelophthisic pancytopenia in a pony mare. J Am Vet Med Assoc 198:1039–1042, 1991.

Lavoie J-P, Morris DD, Zinkl JG, Lloyd K, Divers TJ: Pancytopenia caused by bone marrow aplasia in a horse. J Am Vet Med Assoc 191:1462–1464, 1987.

Means RT, Krantz SB: Progress in understanding the pathogenesis of the anemia of chronic disease. Blood 80:1639–1647, 1992.

Sellon DC: Diseases of the hematopoietic system. In Kobluk CN, Ames TR, Geor RJ (eds): The Horse: Diseases & Clinical Management, ed 1, Vol II. Philadelphia, WB Saunders, 1995, pp 1073–1110.

°Deca-Durabolin, Organon Pharmaceuticals, West Orange, NJ

Thrombocytopenia

JENNIFER ADAMS
Corvallis, Oregon

In healthy horses, the platelet count ranges from 1×10^5 to $6 \times 10^5/\mu l$. A platelet count of less than 100,000/μl constitutes thrombocytopenia. Several mechanisms exist: (1) decreased or ineffective production; (2) sequestration of platelets in the reticuloendothelial organs, the spleen, and liver; and (3) increased loss, use, or consumption of platelets.

Decreased or ineffective production of platelets occurs in horses with bone marrow aplasia, neoplastic infiltration of the bone marrow, and myelofibrosis. In addition, bone marrow suppression is associated with phenylbutazone, chloramphenicol, estrogens, and trichlorethylene-extracted soybean meal. In humans, decreased megakaryopoiesis also is associated with congenital stem cell defects, folic acid and vitamin B_{12} deficiency, and bone marrow damage secondary to irradiation therapy.

Sequestration of 30% of circulating platelets in the reticuloendothelial organs, primarily the spleen, is normal in all species. With enlargement of the spleen, the proportion of sequestered platelets also increases. Hyperplasia of the spleen occurs as a nonspecific response to inflammation, and infiltrative splenomegaly is seen with neoplasia. Displacements of the gastrointestinal tract that affect splenic blood flow and diseases that manifest portal hypertension can also cause engorgement of the spleen and can trap large numbers of platelets. Sequestration alone usually decreases the platelet count only moderately. However, when other causes of decreased platelet numbers also are present, sequestration can contribute significantly to the development of thrombocytopenia.

Increased loss, use, or consumption resulting from reduced platelet lifespan are the most frequent causes of thrombocytopenia in the horse. Severe, acute, external hemorrhage may produce excessive loss of platelets transiently. With disorders involving vasculitis, such as purpura hemorrhagica, *Ehrlichia equi* infection, and equine viral arteritis, damage to capillary walls allows extravasation of platelets and red blood cells into surrounding tissues. However, such platelet loss is rarely clinically significant. Horses with tumors of vascular tissues such as hemangioma and hemangiosarcoma, or those with the hemolytic uremic syndrome, may be thrombocytopenic due to excessive coagulation.

Excessive platelet consumption occurs most commonly with disseminated intravascular coagulation (DIC) and acute inflammation associated with infection or endotoxemia. Immune-mediated disease also is often responsible for significant platelet loss. Membrane damage due to attachment of autoantibodies triggers platelet removal by the reticuloendothelial system. In such cases, numerous megakaryocytes usually are seen in bone marrow samples, suggesting ineffective megakaryopoiesis. Release of platelets from the bone marrow is likely to be inhibited by the presence of antibody bound to megakaryocytes. However, the megakaryocytes are not consumed because they are isolated from removal sites in the spleen and from phagocytic macrophages.

Immune-mediated thrombocytopenia (IMT) can be primary or secondary. In primary IMT, antibody production is directed against glycoprotein receptors on the platelet membrane. In secondary IMT, platelet surface glycoproteins either act as haptens or cross-react directly with antibodies aimed against a primary antigen associated with a drug, bacteria, virus, or neoplastic cell marker. Primary IMT is considered idiopathic in horses. Autoantibody to platelets has been identified in humans, dogs, and horses. It usually involves IgG, but IgM and complement activation have been recognized as well. Secondary immune thrombocytopenia (IMT) has been associated or suspected with lymphosarcoma; infectious diseases including equine infectious anemia and Potomac horse fever; inflammatory disease; drug therapy with heparin, aspirin, sulfonamides, phenylbutazone, penicillin, erythromycin; and other immune-mediated diseases including hemolytic anemia, systemic lupus erythematosus, and neonatal isoerythrolysis with thrombocytopenia in mule foals.

CLINICAL SIGNS

Signs specific to thrombocytopenia include petechial and ecchymotic hemorrhages on oral and nasal mucous membranes, sclerae, third eyelid, vulva, and occasionally inside the ear. Epistaxis, melena, hyphema, and hematuria also occur. Life-threatening hemorrhage is extremely rare, but the likelihood of hemorrhage is not correlated with the platelet count. Those cases with underlying disease processes may bleed at higher platelet levels than those with IMT alone. As a general rule, hematomas form at sites of injection or minor trauma, and surgical sites or wounds bleed excessively when the platelet count is less than 30,000 to 40,000/μl. Spontaneous hemorrhage is rare unless the platelet count is less than 10,000 to 20,000/μl. Clinical signs of a primary or concurrent problem that may be present include pale mucous membranes, fever, edema, anorexia, icterus, depression, and colic.

DIAGNOSIS

Clinical pathologic findings in cases of thrombocytopenia include a true platelet count of less than 90,000 to 100,000/μl, prolonged bleeding time, and abnormal clot retraction. When used as an anticoagulant, ethylenediaminetetraacetic acid (EDTA) occasionally produces pseudothrombocytopenia by stimulating in vitro agglutination of platelets. This can be differentiated by the identification of platelet aggregates on a blood smear and repeating the platelet count with a sample in which sodium citrate is the anticoagulant. Heparin can also be used but it too occasionally induces platelet aggregation. Difficult venipuncture and prolonged intervals before measurement may also result in spuriously low platelet counts.

When thrombocytopenia occurs as a result of DIC, fibrinogen and antithrombin III levels may be low, other coagulation tests such as activated partial thromboplastin time (APTT) and prothrombin time (PT) may be prolonged, and fibrin degradation products (FDP) generally are increased. The PT and APTT should be normal with other causes of thrombocytopenia; fibrinogen may be elevated in the presence of primary inflammatory disorders. Bone marrow examination, preferably of a core biopsy, can be diagnostic for aplastic, neoplastic, and infiltrative marrow disorders. Anemia, leukopenia, neutropenia, or pancytopenia frequently accompany bone marrow disorders.

In cases of immune destruction of platelets, normal or increased numbers of megakaryocytes should be present in the bone marrow. Splenomegaly should not be present; however, splenic size is difficult to evaluate in the horse. Demonstration of the presence of an antiplatelet antibody is evidence of immune-mediated destruction of platelets, but the methods to measure the antibody are not yet in clinical use. Increased platelet factor 3 was considered evidence of immune injury to platelets, but results are so inconsistent that the test is no longer considered useful.

The diagnosis of IMT, therefore, is one of exclusion. A thrombocytopenic patient with a normal or hyperactive bone marrow and no signs or history of underlying disease most likely has primary IMT. However, a Coggins test should be submitted to rule out EIA, and an exhaustive search of organ systems for occult neoplasia should be performed to rule out secondary IMT.

TREATMENT

Specific therapy for thrombocytopenia often is not required because platelet counts improve with elimination of a primary cause such as infection or endotoxemia. All medications should be discontinued or substituted with chemically dissimilar agents. A few drugs have very long half lives, and resolution may take considerable time. Otherwise, if platelet counts do not improve within 1 to 2 weeks, IMT is likely and a trial of immunosuppressive therapy with corticosteroids is indicated. Dexamethasone* may be more effective than prednisone,† especially as initial therapy. A dose of 0.05 to 0.2 mg/kg intravenously (IV) or intramuscularly (IM) s.i.d. is given initially. The platelet count should begin to increase within 4 to 7 days. Once the platelet count is higher than 100,000/μl, the dose can be reduced by 0.01 mg/kg each day. Therapy should not stop until the platelet count remains normal for several days to a week. When a dexamethasone dosage of less than 0.04 mg/kg per day is reached, oral treatment with dexamethasone or an equivalent prednisone dosage (0.4 mg/kg) can be substituted. If the duration of treatment has been longer than 14 days, low-dose alternate-day therapy (0.07 mg/kg prednisone) should be used for an additional 10 days to avoid adrenal suppression. Corticosteroids improve platelet numbers by several mechanisms, including reduced expression and affinity of Fc receptors on macrophages, decreased antiplatelet antibody production, increased platelet production, reduced capillary fragility, and impairment of antigen-antibody interactions.

Because most cases of IMT respond to corticosteroid therapy, there are few reports of alternative therapies. Two horses that did not respond to steroids received azathioprine‡ (3 mg/kg p.o. s.i.d.). One horse developed laminitis and was euthanized. The second horse recovered fully and received azathioprine for 24 days, with the dosage gradually reduced after day 7. Azathioprine produces humoral and

*Azium, Schering-Plough Animal Health, Kenilworth, NJ
†Deltasone, The Upjohn Company, Kalamazoo, MI
‡Imuran, Burroughs Wellcome Co., Research Triangle Park, NC

cell-mediated immunosuppression by interference with nucleic acid synthesis, reducing antibody production as well as numbers of lymphocytes. Vincristine* (0.004 mg/kg IV s.i.d.) was used in one horse and in others (0.01 to 0.25 mg/kg IV once or q7days) with concurrent steroid therapy. Vincristine is cytotoxic to rapidly dividing cells via microtubular damage. It is concentrated into young platelets, which then expose lymphoid cells in the reticuloendothelial tissues.

For dangerously low platelet counts ($<$10,000/μl), instances of life-threatening hemorrhage due to thrombocytopenia or neurologic signs associated with hemorrhage into the central nervous system, or for those requiring a pre- or postoperative safeguard, whole blood, fresh platelet-rich plasma, platelet concentrates, and gamma globulin concentrates can be used to increase platelet counts temporarily. Platelet-rich plasma can be produced by centrifugation of citrated whole blood at 1500 to 2000 $\times$ g for 5 minutes. Platelet concentrates are obtained by centrifugation of platelet-rich plasma at 3000 $\times$ g for 6 to 8 minutes. The platelet pellet is allowed to rest undisturbed to allow for disaggregation and then resuspended in a small volume of plasma retained in the bag. Procedures for the production of platelet concentrate and/or platelet-rich plasma using plasmapheresis have been described, with yields of approximately 8 $\times$ 10^{11} platelets in 300-ml volumes. This amount would increase the platelet count by 30,000/μl in a 500-kg horse. Ideally, platelet donors are cross-matched for compatibility to red blood cell antigens to avoid alloimmunization and allergic reactions. Hemapheresis is becoming more common as a means of plasma banking in veterinary medicine. Several veterinary schools use this process, as do companies that market equine plasma products. An equine platelet-rich plasma is commercially available† and has been used successfully in the treatment of one horse with thrombocytopenia. Platelet-rich plasma and platelet concentrate must be handled carefully and used soon after preparation to avoid loss of efficacy. A concentrated equine serum‡ with high levels of IgG is available, but its efficacy

is unknown. To reach the IgG dosage range reported in humans 2.2 to 5.6 L of concentrated equine serum or 7 to 17 L of unconcentrated equine plasma would be required to treat a 500-kg horse.

Splenectomy has been used in dogs and is performed often in human patients that do not respond to medical therapy, with good results in most cases in both species. Removal of the spleen has been reported anecdotally in horses with IMT, but the long-term consequence is unknown. Because the horse's spleen provides a large store of erythrocytes, splenectomy has adverse effects on exercise performance.

PROGNOSIS

If thrombocytopenia is the result of other diseases, the prognosis is dependent on the primary problem and tends to be very good with removal of the offending agent. The prognosis for most cases of primary IMT is also favorable; many resolve without treatment and most of the remainder respond to steroids. Laminitis is a possible complication of dexamethasone therapy.

Supplemental Readings

Carlson GP: Diseases of the hematopoietic and hemolymphatic systems. *In* Smith BP (ed): Large Animal Internal Medicine. St. Louis, C.V. Mosby, 1990, pp 1075–1077.

Duncan JR, Prasse KW, Mahaffey EA: Hemostasis. *In* Veterinary Laboratory Medicine, 3rd ed. Ames, IA, Iowa State University Press, 1994, pp 75–93.

George JN, El-Harake MA, Raskob GE: Chronic idiopathic thrombocytopenic purpura. N Engl J Med 331(18):1207–1211, 1994.

Hinchcliff KW, Kociba GJ, Mitten LA: Diagnosis of EDTA-dependent pseudothrombocytopenia in a horse. J Am Vet Med Assoc 203:1715–1716, 1993.

Humber KA, Beech J, Cudd TA, Palmer JE, Gardner SY, Sommer MM: Azathioprine for treatment of immune-mediated thrombocytopenia in two horses. J Am Vet Med Assoc 199:591–594, 1991.

Morris DD: Alterations in the clotting profile. *In* Smith BP (ed): Large Animal Internal Medicine. St. Louis, C. V. Mosby, 1990, pp 445–446.

Sellon DC: Diseases of the hematopoietic system. *In* Kobluk CN, Ames TR, Geor RJ (eds): The Horse: Diseases and Clinical Management, vol 2. Philadelphia, WB Saunders, 1995, pp 1090–1092.

*Oncovin, Eli Lilly and Co., Indianapolis, IN
†Veterinary Dynamics, San Luis Obispo, CA
‡Seramune, Sera, Inc., Shawnee Mission, KS

Hemostatic Dysfunction

CHRYSANN COLLATOS
Reno, Nevada

Abnormal hemostasis can involve coagulation, fibrinolysis, or both. Hemostatic dysfunction is classified as inherited or acquired in origin. In both cases, clinical signs are related to excessive hemorrhage or thrombosis at sites of vascular endothelial damage. When the defect involves primary hemostasis (i.e., the interaction of platelets with damaged vascular endothelium), clinical signs that may

be seen include mucosal bleeding, petechiae, ecchymoses, epistaxis, hyphema, or melena. With secondary hemostatic disorders (i.e., those involving one or more coagulation factors), clinical signs include unexplained hemorrhage in the form of hematoma, hemarthrosis, hemothorax, hemoperitoneum, or excessive bleeding after surgery or trauma. Hypercoagulable states, or defective fibrinolysis, may be reflected clinically by thrombosis of large vessels such as the jugular vein or by signs related to microvascular thrombosis such as colic or laminitis.

DIAGNOSIS

Diagnosis of hemostatic dysfunction is based on a battery of assays, many of which are not readily available to the practitioner. When hemostatic dysfunction is suspected, initial screening should be performed on blood collected by venipuncture directly into sodium citrate at one part 3.8% citrate to nine parts blood, as well as into a tube containing thrombin and ε-aminocaproic acid (FDP tube). Samples should be evaluated promptly to determine platelet count, prothrombin time, activated partial thromboplastin time, and fibrin degradation products concentration. If possible, companion samples collected from a normal horse should be obtained and analyzed concurrently. Unfortunately, with the notable exception of vitamin K–related coagulopathies, treatment options for most causes of abnormal hemostasis in the horse are limited and often controversial.

HEREDITARY HEMOSTATIC DISORDERS

von Willebrand Disease

von Willebrand disease has been reported in a Quarterhorse filly that experienced several episodes of prolonged bleeding after minor trauma in the first 6 months of life. von Willebrand factor (vWF) forms a bridge between platelets and exposed subendothelium, and therefore is necessary for formation of the primary platelet plug. In plasma, vWF binds to coagulation factor VIII, prolonging its circulating half life. The diagnosis of von Willebrand disease requires specific vWF assays, which measure both the quantity of vWF antigen and its function (i.e., ristocetin and botrocetin cofactor activities). Clotting times are normal in patients with von Willebrand disease, unless a concurrent factor deficiency is present. The clinical importance of von Willebrand disease in horses is unknown, but it should be considered in a horse with normal platelet count and clotting times and a history of unexplained or excessive hemorrhage.

Prekallikrein Deficiency

Prekallikrein circulates bound to high-molecular-weight kininogen. Interaction of this complex with the negatively charged surface of exposed subendothelial matrix and factor XII initiates intrinsic coagulation. Thus, prekallikrein deficiency results in prolongation of the activated partial thromboplastin time, which measures the intrinsic arm of the coagulation cascade. Associated clinical signs usually are absent or minor. Prekallikrein deficiency, a disorder inherited as an autosomal recessive trait in humans, has been reported in a family of Belgian horses and one of Miniature horses. Mild, prolonged bleeding after castration occurred in one of the affected Belgian horses. Definitive diagnosis requires specific factor assays with factor deficient plasmas.

Hemophilia A

Classic hemophilia A, factor VIII deficiency, has been reported in Thoroughbred, Standardbred, Quarterhorse, and Arabian colts. The disease is transmitted as an X-linked recessive trait, and is the most common inherited coagulation defect of horses. Horses with hemophilia A usually experience serious bleeding episodes within the first year of life; however, the bleeding tendency is tempered by the severity of the factor deficiency in each affected individual. The diagnosis is suspected in any young animal with prolonged activated partial thromboplastin time, normal prothrombin time, and unexplained hemorrhage. Specific factor VIII:C assay is necessary for confirmation. Severely affected individuals have factor VIII:C plasma activity that is 10% that of normal pooled equine plasma activity. One horse with 20 to 30% factor VIII:C activity lived to 3 years of age. In horses, hemophilia A is a severe, heritable disease without practical treatment to date. Therefore, most animals die or are euthanized in the first year of life. Carrier mares transmit the defect to approximately 50% of their male foals, and they should not be bred.

Protein C Deficiency

Protein C is a vitamin K–dependent glycoprotein that, when activated by a thrombin-thrombomodulin complex, directly inhibits coagulation factors V and VIII. Protein C deficiency results in a hypercoagulable state characterized clinically by thrombus formation, primarily in large vessels. This condition has been reported in a 2-year-old Thoroughbred colt with clinical signs of venous thrombosis, weight loss, a concurrent diagnosis of nephrolithiasis, and bilateral renal failure. Protein C antigen in this colt was normal, but the activity of the enzyme was markedly decreased, suggesting an inherited disease with production of a functionally abnormal protein.

ACQUIRED HEMOSTATIC DYSFUNCTION

Disseminated Intravascular Coagulation

Disseminated intravascular coagulation (DIC) is a complex pathophysiologic process that can occur as a result of any disease that directly activates the coagulation cascade. Alternatively, severe endothelial damage can cause DIC through exposure of negatively charged subendothelial phospholipid and initiation of platelet aggregation and coagulation. Endotoxemia related to ischemic or inflammatory gastrointestinal diseases is the most common underlying cause of DIC in horses. A cell wall component of all gram-negative bacteria, endotoxin initiates intrinsic coagulation through activation of factor XII, activates extrinsic coagulation through stimulation of mononuclear cell–associated tissue factor expression, directly damages vascular endothelium, and causes thromboxane-mediated platelet activation. In addition, endotoxin inhibits fibrinolysis. Overall, enhanced clot formation and reduced clot resolution occur simultaneously. Other diseases and disease processes that have been associated with fulminant DIC in horses include metritis, pleuropneumonia, hemolytic anemia, viremia, vasculitis, burns, neoplasia, and renal or hepatic failure.

Unregulated hemostasis is the hallmark of DIC. The process begins when systemic hypercoagulation causes microthrombus formation in capillary beds. Tissue ischemia and necrosis ensue; the associated inflammation further stimulates coagulation. The rapidity and severity of thrombus formation is related to the rate of thrombin production, which in turn is determined by the extent to which systemic coagulation has been activated. In addition to cleaving fibrinogen to fibrin, thrombin has several other procoagulant activities, including platelet activation, enhancement of factor V and VIII cofactor activity, and stimulation of fibrin polymerization through factor XIII activation. Thrombin activity normally is kept in balance by the natural anticoagulants, protein C and antithrombin III. However, massively activated coagulation rapidly exhausts available sources of these glycoproteins.

Normally, fibrinolysis begins at the same time as coagulation; thus, fibrin degradation follows fibrin deposition, ensuring maintenance of vascular integrity and tissue perfusion. Fibrin degradation products, which are released as plasmin degrades fibrin, are cleared from circulation by the mononuclear cells of the liver and spleen. During DIC this mononuclear phagocyte system often is compromised by hypoperfusion related to the primary disease and becomes overwhelmed by the combined task of engulfing activated coagulation factors, fibrin, fibrinogen, and fibrin degradation products in addition to pathogens such as endotoxin. Fibrin degradation products begin to accumulate in circulation and contribute to the developing coagulopathy by inhibiting thrombin activity, causing platelet dysfunction, and decreasing fibrin polymerization. Ultimately, coagulation factors become depleted, and the initial thrombotic tendency is replaced by a consumptive coagulopathy, with associated signs of hemorrhagic diathesis. Occasionally, animals develop a chronic, insidious procoagulant state with diseases such as severe gram-negative pleuropneumonia. A compensated form of DIC occurs, with no apparent clinical signs. The patient is at high risk of developing fulminant DIC if additional physiologic stress is experienced.

Clinical Signs

The manifestations of DIC in an individual patient are unpredictable and often are masked by those of the primary disease process. The signs related directly to DIC are determined by the intricate and dynamic balance of hemostatic factors that control the activation and inhibition of both coagulation and fibrinolysis. Horses with acute DIC can show clinical signs related to microthrombosis of any organ system. These include colic, laminitis, oliguria, dyspnea or tachypnea, or even dementia. Of these, laminitis and colic are seen most commonly. The pathogenesis of laminitis is complex, and the precise contribution of digital microthrombosis to this disease is not known. In addition to microvascular occlusion, large vessel thrombosis, particularly at sites of venous catheterization or repeated venipuncture, is commonly associated with DIC in horses. Microangiopathic hemolysis, caused by lysis of erythrocytes as they pass through webs of fibrin strands in capillaries, occasionally occurs as a late manifestation of DIC in horses.

Hemoglobinemia and hemoglobinuria are the associated clinical signs. Uncontrolled bleeding, such as epistaxis, hyphema, and melena, are uncommon in horses with DIC. Signs of microangiopathic hemolysis or frank hemorrhage associated with DIC warrant a grave prognosis.

Diagnosis

The diagnosis of DIC is made on the basis of clinical signs, presence of an underlying disease process, and clinicopathologic abnormalities. The most consistently reported abnormal laboratory findings are thrombocytopenia ($<50,000/\mu l$), increased fibrin degradation products concentration (>40 mg/μl), and decreased ($<60\%$ normal) antithrombin III activity. The latter test is rarely available to the practitioner. As the disease progresses, prothrombin and activated partial thromboplastin times are prolonged; however, these tests are considered crude indicators of DIC. Hypofibrinogenemia, commonly observed in other species, is rare in horses with DIC. Clinicopathologic findings are highly variable and are most useful when interpreted serially. Early in its course, DIC may cause clotting times to be shortened, and fibrin degradation products do not accumulate in circulation until the mononuclear phagocyte system is overwhelmed. In addition, particularly in a field setting, venipuncture and sample handling techniques can greatly affect results of hemostatic testing.

Treatment

Treatment of DIC is highly controversial. Clearly, the underlying disease must be addressed immediately and aggressively, either surgically or medically. Support of tissue perfusion with intravenous fluids is mandatory. Low-dose flunixin meglumine* (0.25 mg/kg IM or IV q8h) has been shown to decrease endotoxin-mediated thromboxane production and generally is administered, although its efficacy in horses with DIC has not been evaluated objectively. If low plasma antithrombin III activity can be documented, or if signs of severe uncontrolled bleeding are present, fresh plasma transfusion may be warranted. Unfortunately, 15 to 30 ml/kg of fresh plasma is recommended, and the cost and availability of such treatment must be weighed against the patient's poor prognosis for survival, regardless of treatment. If hemorrhagic diathesis is not present, fresh plasma may be contraindicated, because administration of additional clotting factors may increase thrombosis. Corticosteroids are contraindicated because they decrease activity of the mononuclear phagocyte system and may enhance the vasoconstrictive effect of circulating catecholamines.

The use of heparin to decrease thrombosis in horses with DIC remains controversial, both because of the potential for detrimental as well as beneficial effects, and because of the difficulty in determining a rational dosage regimen. In healthy horses, plasma concentrations of heparin vary widely between individuals after identical dosages. In addition, the anticoagulant effect of heparin increases unpredictably following repetitive administration of the same dose. Product composition varies widely among commercially available heparin formulations. Heparin exists as a family of molecules with molecular weight varying from 4000 to 40,000 daltons. Low-molecular-weight heparin ex-

---

Banamine, Schering-Plough Animal Health, Kenilworth, NJ

erts an anticoagulant effect by binding to antithrombin III and enhancing its ability to inactivate thrombin. The anticoagulant effect of heparin, therefore, is dependent upon adequate antithrombin III activity. Concurrent administration of 3 L fresh plasma with heparin has been advocated. In one clinical trial in horses with DIC, the survival rate was higher in horses that received heparin than in those that did not; however, only 23 horses were studied and the difference in survival rate was not significant.

Heparin has been associated with thrombocytopenia, hemorrhage, and thrombosis in multiple species. In horses, heparin causes a decrease in hematocrit because of a reversible erythrocyte agglutination phenomenon. Whether such red blood cell agglutination increases the risk of microvascular thrombosis, and specifically of laminitis, is not known. Various dosage regimens for heparin have been recommended. In this author's opinion, if heparin treatment is elected, it should be initiated early in the course of diseases such as strangulating small intestinal lesions, severe colitis, and severe proximal enteritis, which have a high risk for coagulopathy. Heparin should be administered for no more than 3 days, and should be given at a dosage no greater than 40 IU/kg sodium heparin subcutaneously every 12 hours. Packed cell volume should be measured serially and heparin discontinued if a sudden decrease in hematocrit is observed.

Prevention

Clearly, the key to successful treatment of DIC in horses is prevention. Early aggressive intervention for horses with endotoxemia associated with ischemic intestine or severe inflammatory gastrointestinal diseases is crucial. In addition to supportive intravenous fluid and low-dose flunixin meglumine, treatments that have shown anecdotal clinical benefit include dimethyl sulfoxide (100 mg/kg IV q8h as a 10% solution) as a free radical scavenger, acepromazine (0.006–0.01 mg/kg IM or SQ q8–12h) to improve digital and renal perfusion, aspirin (17 mg/kg p.o. every other day) to decrease platelet aggregation, and commercial antisera enriched with antibodies directed against gram-negative bacteria to directly neutralize circulating endotoxin.

Warfarin Toxicity

Exposure of horses to toxic amounts of warfarin or another dicoumarol derivative is uncommon, but can occur following ingestion of rodenticides, ingestion of moldy sweetclover (*Melilotus* species), or in association with the intentional administration of warfarin as a treatment for navicular disease or thrombophlebitis. Most commonly, phenylbutazone, a highly protein-bound drug, is administered in addition to warfarin. Protein-bound warfarin is displaced by phenylbutazone, resulting in the accumulation of a toxic concentration of free warfarin in plasma.

The dicoumarol derivatives all antagonize vitamin K. Hepatic synthesis of the vitamin K–dependent clotting factors II, VII, IX, and X is not impaired, but the factors produced are not functional. The clinical signs associated with dicoumarol derivative intoxication are the same as those with any major clotting factor deficiency, namely unexplained hematomas; hemarthroses; epistaxis; hyphema; melena; hemothorax; hemoperitoneum; or excessive hemorrhage following trauma, venipuncture, or surgery. The diagnosis is made on the basis of a history of exposure, abnormal clotting times, and response to treatment. Prothrombin time and activated partial thromboplastin time usually are prolonged. Factor VII has the shortest circulating half life of the vitamin K–dependent factors, and typically the fall in its activity is first to reach clinical significance; thus, the prothrombin time may be prolonged before the activated partial thromboplastin time. Platelet count, fibrin degradation products concentration, and fibrinogen concentration should be normal unless severe hemorrhage has led to consumptive thrombocytopenia.

Simple withdrawal of warfarin may be effective treatment in horses receiving warfarin therapy that develop low-grade bleeding tendency and mild to moderately prolonged prothrombin time. The clotting time should return to normal within 5 days. In cases of serious dicoumarol derivative toxicity, vitamin K_1 should be given (0.5–1.0 mg/kg SQ, q4–6h). Duration of treatment should be based on clinical response and serial assessment of clotting times, but no more than 3 to 5 days of treatment should be necessary. If life-threatening hemorrhage (>30% blood volume) is suspected, then whole blood transfusion is indicated (see page 290). Under no circumstances should vitamin K_3 (menadione sodium bisulfite) be administered to horses, because it causes acute renal failure.

Supplemental Readings

Brooks M, Leith GS, Allen AK, Woods PR, Benson RE, Dodds WJ: Bleeding disorder (von Willebrand disease) in a Quarter Horse. J Am Vet Med Assoc 198:114–116, 1991.

Edens LM, Morris DD, Prasse KW, Miriam RA: Hypercoagulable state associated with a deficiency of Protein C in a Thoroughbred colt. J Am Vet Intern Med 7:190–193, 1993.

Geor RJ, Jackson ML, Lewis KD, Fretz PB: Prekallikrein deficiency in a family of Belgian horses. J Am Vet Med Assoc 197:741–745, 1990.

Littlewood JD, Bevan SA: Haemophilia A (classic haemophilia, factor VIII deficiency) in a Thoroughbred colt foal. Equine Vet J 23:70–72, 1991.

Moore BR, Hinchcliff KW: Heparin: A review of its pharmacology and therapeutic use in horses. J Vet Intern Med 8:26–35, 1994.

Morris DD: Recognition and management of disseminiated intravascular coagulation in horses. Vet Clin North Am Equine Pract 4:115–143, 1988.

Welch RD, Watkins JP, Taylor TS, Cohen ND, Carter GK: Disseminated intravascular coagulation associated with colic in 23 horses (1984–1989). J Vet Intern Med 6:29–35, 1992.

Blood and Blood Component Therapy

CHRYSANN COLLATOS
Reno, Nevada

WHOLE BLOOD TRANSFUSION

The most common indications for whole blood transfusion in horses are acute hemorrhage associated with trauma or surgery, or hemolysis associated with red maple toxicity or neonatal isoerythrolysis. The decision for transfusion is based on clinical and clinicopathologic assessment of the patient (see page 273). Transfusion is always warranted when acute blood loss or hemolysis results in a packed cell volume (PCV) at or below 12%, or in chronic blood loss when PCV reaches 8%. Transfusion should be avoided unless absolutely necessary, because transfused erythrocytes have a shortened lifespan of 4 to 6 days versus 150 days for nontransfused cells, and they suppress the normal bone marrow response to anemia. Although uncommon, adverse transfusion reactions also are possible, and sensitization of the recipient to heterologous donor red cell antigens is likely.

Volume to Transfuse

An optimal transfusion volume can be calculated using the formula:

$$\frac{(30 - \text{recipient's PCV}) \times (0.8 \times \text{kg body weight of recipient})}{\text{PCV of donor}}$$

However, administration of one third of this calculated volume usually is sufficient to provide adequate oxygen-carrying capacity to supply tissue demands. Generally, if transfusion is warranted, a transfusion volume of 15 ml/kg should be given, or 6 to 8 L, to an adult horse. Volume overload can be a problem in smaller patients, particularly when red cell loss is the result of hemolysis rather than blood loss and the recipient therefore has a normal intravascular volume. The transfusion volume should not exceed 20% of blood volume, calculated at 8% of body weight. Packed red blood cells are easily harvested following gravity sedimentation as described later and resuspended in a small volume of isotonic saline for treatment of hemolytic anemia in patients at risk of volume overload. Alternatively, the use of a bovine hemoglobin preparation as an oxygen transport source has been reported in one Miniature horse for which a compatible red blood cell donor could not be found.

Donor Selection

The ideal equine blood donor weighs at least 450 kg, tests negative for equine infectious anemia virus, has never received a blood or plasma transfusion, if female has never foaled, and has a normal PCV and plasma protein concentration. Equine blood antigens have been grouped into seven blood systems: A, C, D, K, P, Q, and U. Because

horses have more than 400,000 possible blood types, a true universal donor does not exist. However, red cell antigen patterns are fairly uniform within breeds; thus, if no compatibility testing is possible and the donor blood type is unknown, a close relative to the recipient that meets the criteria listed earlier is a good donor candidate. Of the red cell antigens, Aa and Qa are the most immunogenic; thus, if screening is possible, donors should be Aa and Qa alloantigen-negative. In addition, donors should be negative for alloantibodies, particularly those directed against alloantigen Aa. Belgian horses have a low incidence of Aa and Qa antigens. This, combined with their size, makes them good potential donors.

When possible, compatibility testing should precede transfusion. A major crossmatch is an agglutination test in which donor erythrocytes and recipient serum are mixed and observed for agglutination. A minor crossmatch combines donor serum with recipient erythrocytes. Such agglutinin testing does not specifically detect hemolyzing antibodies, which are most likely to cause severe transfusion reaction. Hemolysin testing requires a source of rabbit complement and is not routinely performed in most laboratories. Several laboratories that perform equine blood typing are listed at the end of this chapter. Adverse reaction following an initial transfusion is rare, but antibodies against transfused cells develop within 3 to 10 days in 50% of horses after a single transfusion. Fortunately, if a second transfusion is necessary, it usually is given within 5 days, so the risk of reaction remains low, even if compatibility testing is not possible.

Blood Collection

Container

Blood is best collected into 3-L sterile plastic transfer bags. Larger volume containers are awkward. Evacuated glass bottles are breakable, the vacuum tends to damage erythrocytes and stimulate agglutination, and the glass surface can activate contact coagulation. Many blood product transfer systems are commercially available. In our clinic, we use 3-L bags designed for intravenous fluid administration to calves.° The bags are sturdy, affordable, and reusable.

Anticoagulant

Acid-citrate-dextrose (ACD) and citrate-phosphate-dextrose (CPD) are the recommended anticoagulants for blood collection. Heparin (5–10 IU/ml) and sodium citrate solu-

---

°No. 1953–13, Sanofi Animal Health, Overland Park, KS

tion can be used in an emergency; however, heparin can interfere with endogenous clotting mechanisms, and the lifespan of erythrocytes is markedly shortened by the absence of the dextrose energy source. Stock solution of ACD can be prepared as follows:

11.0 g dextrose (22.0 ml 50% dextrose[*])
9.9 g sodium citrate[†]
3.3 g citric acid[‡]
q.s. distilled water to 300 ml

The anticoagulant is autoclaved and stored at room temperature until needed. Because the desired ACD-to-whole-blood ratio is 1:9, a 300-ml aliquot is added to a 3-L collection bag.

Collection Technique

The donor's PCV and plasma protein should be determined before blood collection. A 500-kg horse with a PCV of 35 to 40% can safely give 8 L blood, 20% of blood volume, every 30 days. The following procedure allows a single person to collect 8.1 L whole blood (three 3-L bags) safely and efficiently. The donor is restrained in crossties or is tied to the wall and lightly sedated with xylazine if necessary. Acepromazine must not be used. Anticoagulant (300 ml ACD) is added to each of three collection bags (3-L volume), and the bags are placed within easy reach of the phlebotomist. Compatible collection tubing[§] is inserted into the first bag. A string is tied around the horse's neck to maintain jugular distension and a 12-gauge, 3.5-inch catheter[||] is placed aseptically, against the flow of blood, in the jugular vein. The collection tubing is attached to the catheter and taped in place, and blood is collected by gravity flow. The bag should be mixed gently several times. As one bag fills, the collection tubing is immediately transferred to the next bag and the full bag is placed aside, with a sterile gauze pad placed over the collection port.

Storage

Typically whole blood is administered immediately. However, whole blood in ACD can be stored refrigerated (4°C) for up to 3 weeks.

Blood Administration

A catheter is placed aseptically in the jugular vein of the recipient. Baseline heart rate, respiratory rate, and temperature are obtained before beginning the transfusion at a rate of 0.1 ml/kg (i.e., a slow drip). A blood administration set with an in-line filter should be used.[¶] If no adverse reaction is seen within 10 minutes, the infusion rate is increased to 20 ml/kg per hour. Blood should be mixed gently and frequently during administration. Signs of an immediate transfusion reaction include tachypnea, trembling, restlessness, tachycardia, urticaria, and sudden collapse. If such signs occur, the transfusion is stopped and flunixin meglumine[#] is administered (1.1 mg/kg IV). In

case of severe reaction, epinephrine (0.01–0.02 ml/kg at 1:1000, IM), high-volume intravenous polyionic fluids, and prednisolone sodium succinate[*] (4.5 mg/kg IV) are considered. For milder reactions, the clinician should wait 15 minutes after administration of flunixin meglumine and then recommence transfusion at a slower rate. If reaction recurs, the blood is discarded, a crossmatch is repeated, and a fresh transfusion source is obtained. If the donor possesses hemolyzing alloantibodies directed against recipient red cell antigens, hemolytic anemia will occur after transfusion.

PLASMA TRANSFUSION

Plasma transfusion is used most commonly to treat partial or complete failure of passive transfer in foals (see page 581). Occasionally, horses with severe hypoalbuminemia, most often that from protein-losing enteropathy, are given plasma to support intravascular oncotic pressure. More recently, plasma collected from horses immunized against specific pathogens, such as *Rhodococcus equi* and *Salmonella typhimurium*, has been marketed as "hyperimmune" products, for use in the prevention of *R. equi* pneumonia in foals, or in the treatment of acute endotoxemia.

Sources

Plasma is best obtained commercially[†] because such products are harvested from horses with excellent immunization status under controlled manufacturing conditions. The immunoglobulin content should be quantitated and clearly indicated on the product description. When necessary, plasma can be collected in a field setting, taking advantage of the rapid sedimentation of equine erythrocytes. Whole blood collected exactly as described earlier can be hung for 2 hours, or left overnight. Plasma then is siphoned or poured off the settled red cells, or a plasma extractor can be used to force plasma from the collection bag against gravity, leaving the red cells behind. Clinicians should expect a plasma yield of 40 to 50% of the total volume of blood collected. Plasma can be stored frozen at 0°C for at least 1 year.

Administration

The volume of plasma needed to achieve a desired increase in IgG or total protein cannot be calculated accurately. Protein is redistributed from the vascular space, and recipients frequently are suffering from disease processes such as septicemia and endotoxemia that are associated with vasculitis and exacerbate circulating protein loss. In general, foals require 1 to 2 L plasma to increase IgG to an acceptable range, and adult horses with clinically significant hypoproteinemia require a minimum of 6 to 8 L plasma to increase the total protein 5 to 10 g/L. The administration technique is identical to that described for whole blood, with the exception that mixing during infusion is not necessary.

The risk of transfusion reaction is low with plasma, but

[*]*Butler, Dublin, OH*
[†]*Sigma Chemical, St. Louis, MO*
[‡]*Sigma Chemical, St. Louis, MO*
[§]*JC5425, Baxter, Toronto, ON*
[||]*Angiocath, Becton Dickinson, Sandy, UT*
[¶]*Fenwal, Baxter, Toronto, ON*
[#]*Banamine, Schering-Plough Animal Health, Kenilworth, NJ*

[*]*Solu-Delta-Cortef, The UpJohn Co., Kalamazoo, MI*
[†]*Veterinary Dynamics, San Luis Obispo, CA, or Lake Immunogenics, Ontario, NY*

recipients may develop immunity to foreign proteins in the plasma, and the risk of reaction increases with repeated transfusion. Particularly with plasma prepared under field conditions, there is also the risk of contamination with trace amounts of endotoxin that can result in an immediate transfusion reaction upon administration. If a reaction occurs, treatment should be as for a whole blood transfusion reaction (see earlier). Unless obtained by plasmapheresis, plasma invariably contains some erythrocyte contamination; therefore, sensitization of the recipient to red blood cell alloantigens of the plasma donor is possible. This may have clinical relevance in fillies that receive plasma transfusions for failure of passive transfer. Owners should be informed of the possibility of neonatal isoerythrolysis in foals born to such fillies if they are used as brood mares. Crossmatching of the mare's blood with that of the intended stallion should be considered before breeding.

ALTERNATIVE BLOOD PRODUCTS

Blood Components

Continuous flow apheresis techniques for blood component separation in horses have been investigated. Many veterinary colleges and commercial companies employ plasmapheresis to harvest equine plasma, returning the erythrocytes to the donor. Techniques for leukapheresis and thrombocytapheresis have been described. Platelet-rich plasma may be a useful product for treatment of immune-mediated thrombocytopenia (see page 284). Although the safety of leukocyte transfusion to equine neonates has been demonstrated, its clinical utility is unknown.

Fresh frozen plasma that is separated from blood and frozen within 6 hours, and cryoprecipitate separated from fresh frozen plasma thawed at 4°C, have been used in human and small animal medicine as a source of clotting factors for animals with inherited or acquired coagulation defects such as DIC, but their use in horses has not been reported.

Growth Factors

Preliminary studies in horses indicate that hemopoietic growth factors may have a role in the treatment of diseases characterized by leukopenia and neutropenia such as ischemic gastrointestinal lesions and neonatal septicemia. In one study, eight healthy foals were given 20 mg of granulocyte colony stimulating factor. The mean total white blood cell count increased over 10-fold by day 7, and no adverse effects were seen. The clinical utility and economic feasibility of such products in equine veterinary medicine remains speculative.

Equine Blood Typing Laboratories

Serology Laboratory
University of California
Davis, CA 95616
Phone: (916)752–2211

Stormont Laboratory, Inc.
1237 East Beamer St., Suite D
Woodland, CA 95695
Phone: (916)661–3078

David Colling
Mann Equitest, Inc.
5550 McAdam Road
Mississauga, ON, L4Z 1P1, Canada
Phone: (416)890–2555

Supplemental Readings

Madigan JE, Zinkl JG, Fridmann DM, Barbis D, Andresen JW: Preliminary studies of recombinant bovine granulcyte-colony stimulating factor on haematological values in normal neonatal foals. Equine Vet J 26:159–161, 1994.
Maxson AD, Giger U, Sweeney CR, Tomasic M, Saik JE, Donawick WJ, Cothran EG: Use of a bovine hemoglobin preparation in the treatment of cyclic ovarian hemorrhage in a miniature horse. J Am Vet Med Assoc 203:1308–1311, 1993.
Morris DD, Bruce J, Gaulin G, Whitlock RH: Evaluation of granulocyte transfusion in healthy neonatal pony foals. Am J Vet Res 48:1187–1193, 1987.
Williamson LW: Highlights of blood transfusion in horses. Comp Cont Ed 15:267–269, 1993.

Vasculitis

S T E E V E   G I G U E R E
Guelph, Ontario

Vasculitis or *angiitis* are general terms that refer to inflammation of blood vessels, regardless of the cause. Vasculitis is uncommon in horses but represents a major diagnostic and therapeutic challenge. Horses of any age, breed, or sex can be affected; however, most are older than 2 years of age. Infectious agents such as equine viral arteritis, toxins, and chemicals all can damage vessel walls directly; however, vasculitis in horses most often results from immune-mediated hypersensitivity reactions resulting from infection, neoplasia, or, occasionally, drug reaction.

In humans, vasculitic syndromes are classified as systemic necrotizing vasculitis (e.g., polyarteritis nodosa), hypersensitivity vasculitis, and several other rarer conditions; each syndrome contains multiple subdivisions. Vasculitic syndromes in horses are not sufficiently defined to allow such categorization. However, most horses with vasculitis have histopathologic and clinical characteristics similar to those of hypersensitivity vasculitis in people. The hallmark of this type of vasculitis is involvement of small skin vessels. Thus, clinical signs related to the skin usually dominate the clinical picture, although other organs can occasionally be involved. Such immune-mediated vasculitis is believed to involve a type III hypersensitivity reaction in which immune complexes are deposited in vessel walls, usually at the endothelial basement membrane. The immune complexes activate complement, with consequent release of C5a and other neutrophil chemoattractants. In the process of phagocytosing immune complexes, neutrophils release lysosomal enzymes and oxygen radicals resulting in vessel wall necrosis with subsequent edema, hemorrhage, and ischemic changes in the tissues supplied by the affected vessels.

CLINICAL SIGNS

Cutaneous lesions occur most frequently on the distal limbs, but the proximal limbs, ventral abdomen, muzzle, pinnae, and periocular area also are commonly affected. Lesions are not necessarily symmetrical; on occasion the lesions follow the vasculature. Early signs of edema and erythema often progress to purpura (i.e., extravasation of red blood cells), crusts, and ulcers. In severe cases, necrosis and sloughing of the affected skin can occur. The edema is warm and pitting; it may be painful, but pruritus usually is absent. Depending on the severity of the lesions, horses may be stiff and reluctant to move. Mucosal hyperemia and petechial hemorrhage are commonly seen. Less often, oral ulcers and/or bullae are present. Severe head edema occasionally causes respiratory stridor. Tachycardia and tachypnea are common. Some horses show signs of systemic illness such as fever, anorexia, depression, and weight loss.

Although skin and mucous membrane involvement usually predominate, vasculitis may also affect kidneys, muscles, joints, gastrointestinal tract, respiratory tract, and nervous system, causing various clinical signs depending on the systems affected. Because vasculitis may be the result of an infection or neoplasia, the clinical signs of the primary disease can complicate the clinical presentation.

DIAGNOSIS

The differential diagnosis of cutaneous vasculitis includes all conditions causing edema of the extremities and ventral midline such as congestive heart failure, hypoproteinemia, peritonitis, pleuritis, and trauma. Appendicular inflammatory disorders such as ulcerative lymphangitis, bacterial furunculosis or cellulitis, sporotrichosis, bullous pemphigoid, pemphigus foliaceus, systemic lupus erythematosus, drug eruption, and certain toxicoses (e.g., stachybotryotoxicosis) should also be considered.

Definitive diagnosis is based on history, clinical signs, and skin biopsy results. Tissue samples collected early in the disease process are most likely to be diagnostic. Multiple formalin-fixed full-thickness punch biopsies (6 mm) should be obtained. Biopsy sites should not be scrubbed or washed. Histopathologic findings include neutrophilic infiltration, leukocytoclasis, endothelial cell damage, and necrosis. Eosinophilic, lymphocytic, or mixed vasculitic syndromes can also be seen.

Direct immunofluorescence testing of biopsies preserved in Michel's fixative may demonstrate immunoglobulin or complement deposition in vessel walls and at the basement membrane. Lesions must be biopsied within 12 hours of their appearance for optimal immunofluorescence testing. However, more chronic lesions are positive on occasion. Although helpful in establishing pathogenesis, immunologic testing is not absolutely necessary for diagnosis, nor does a negative result rule out an immune-mediated process. Weakly positive antinuclear antibody (ANA) test results have been reported in a few cases of vasculitis, but the significance of this finding is unknown. Although very sensitive for diagnosis of lupus erythematosus, a weakly positive result to an ANA test may also be found in many immune-mediated disease processes, as well as in a few normal animals.

Hematologic and biochemical findings are nonspecific and are determined by the underlying disease, multiplicity of organ involvement, and secondary complications. Neutrophilic leukocytosis is present in approximately 50% of cases. Hyperfibrinogenemia, hyperglobulinemia, and mild to moderate anemia also are common. The platelet count and clotting profile usually are normal with cutaneous vasculitis; thus, they are useful diagnostic tools in horses with petechial hemorrhages to rule out consumptive coagulopathy and immune-mediated thrombocytopenia.

ETIOLOGY

The most commonly recognized vasculitic syndrome in the horse is purpura hemorrhagica. Vasculitis can also be associated with equine viral arteritis, equine ehrlichiosis, equine infectious anemia, and photoactivated vasculitis. However, in approximately 50% of cases of vasculitis in horses the etiology is unknown. Some horses have concurrent bronchopneumonia, cholangiohepatitis, granulomatous enteritis, or colitis that could be the source of antigen. Therefore, a primary site of infection or neoplasia should be sought in vasculitides of unknown etiology.

Purpura Hemorrhagica

Purpura hemorrhagica is an acute noncontagious neutrophilic necrotizing vasculitis characterized by subcutaneous edema of the head and limbs and petechial hemorrhages in the mucosae, musculature, and viscera. The disease is typically a sequela to *Streptococcus equi* infection, occurring in approximately 1 to 2% of cases 2 to 4 weeks after an acute infection. Purpura hemorrhagica also occurs as a sequela to strangles vaccination and in horses exposed to *S. equi* that do not develop clinical signs. Rarely, the disease may also follow infection with other *Streptococcus species*, equine influenza virus, or other antigenic stimulation.

The vasculitis is probably immune-mediated; immune complexes consisting of IgA and M protein of *S. equi* have been detected in the serum of affected horses but not in horses that had strangles but did not develop purpura. Affected horses also have higher than normal antibody titers to the M protein and other protein antigens of *S. equi*, and have unusually high plasma C3 concentrations.

In addition to the general signs of vasculitis described

previously, colic associated with hemorrhage, edema, and necrosis of the intestinal wall is possible. Glomerulonephritis and leukocytoclastic vasculitis of the muscles associated with high levels of muscle enzymes (creatine kinase [CK] and aspartate aminotransferase [AST]) also have been reported. The diagnosis of purpura hemorrhagica is usually based on a history of recent respiratory tract infection, clinical signs, and skin biopsies. In the absence of a typical history, the enzyme-linked immunosorbent assay (ELISA) test for detection of antibodies against M protein may support the possibility of a previous occult *S. equi* infection. Nasal swabs for *S. equi* culture may also be positive because nasal shedding usually persists for 3 to 6 weeks following an acute infection. Negative culture results do not rule out previous *S. equi* infection. The clinical distinction of purpura hemorrhagica from other similar idiopathic vasculitic syndromes is problematic but purely academic because the treatment approach is identical.

Equine Viral Arteritis

Equine viral arteritis (EVA) is caused by a ribonucleic acid (RNA) virus of the family Togaviridae. Although serologic surveys indicate that exposure to the virus is common, the clinical disease is uncommon, probably because most cases of acute EVA infection are subclinical or inapparent. Various serologic surveys have shown that 70 to 90% of Standardbred horses are seropositive for antibodies to the virus compared with only 2 to 3% in the corresponding Thoroughbred population. However, neither field nor experimental studies have demonstrated any difference in susceptibility to clinical infection between the different breeds. The incubation period is 3 to 14 days. The primary mode of EVA transmission is believed to be aerosol, but venereal transmission by an acute or chronically infected stallion is also important.

Natural cases of EVA have a wide range of clinical and clinicopathologic manifestations. Pyrexia and leukopenia, especially lymphopenia, are the most consistent findings. Depression, anorexia, ventral and limb edema, nasal and ocular discharge, urticarial-type rash, and abortion in mares are other common clinical features. In contrast to the immune complex component of most other equine vasculitic syndromes, the EVA virus is directly pathogenic to endothelial cells and causes a panvasculitis involving the small arteries and, to a lesser extent, the small veins throughout the body.

A definitive diagnosis of EVA is based on virus isolation and/or results of serologic tests. A fourfold or greater rise in titer on paired serology samples taken 21 to 28 days apart indicates a recent infection. Appropriate specimens for virus isolation from the acutely affected animal include nasopharyngeal or conjunctival swabs placed immediately in a suitable viral transport medium; or ethylenediamine-tetraacetic acid (EDTA), citrate, or heparinized blood samples from which the buffy coat can be isolated.

Equine Infectious Anemia

See page 280.

Equine Ehrlichiosis

See page 282.

Photoactivated Vasculitis

Photoactivated vasculitis is an uncommon form of photosensitization that occurs in summer months in regions with abundant sunlight. Affected horses have no known exposure to recognized photosensitizing compounds and no evidence of liver dysfunction. The disease affects only the nonpigmented portions of the lower limbs. Unlike conventional photosensitization disorders, the nonpigmented skin on other parts of the body is not affected. The most important feature of the condition is painful edema. Associated skin lesions may include erythema and crusting. Histopathology testing reveals vasculitis in the superficial dermis with degeneration of the wall of affected vessels. Although the disease appears to be photoactivated, the exact pathophysiology is unknown.

Diagnosis is based on the history, clinical appearance, and skin biopsy results. Hepatogenous photosensitization is ruled out by results of liver function tests such as measurements of the concentration of bile acids in blood. Exposure to photosensitizing plants is often difficult to rule out. In some horses direct immunofluorescence has shown deposition of IgG or C3 or both in the vessel wall. However, it is not known whether this is evidence of immune-mediated disease or simply nonspecific immune complex deposition, as reported in various forms of porphyria.

TREATMENT

Treatment of purpura hemorrhagica and similar idiopathic vasculitis syndromes consists of: (1) removing the antigenic stimulus; (2) reducing the abnormal immune response; (3) reducing vessel wall inflammation; and (4) providing supportive care. Administration of drugs should be discontinued or, if absolutely necessary, drugs should be replaced with those from a chemically unrelated class. Underlying diseases should be treated aggressively. Whenever possible, bacterial pathogens should be isolated and tested for in vitro antimicrobial sensitivity. Because purpura hemorrhagica is most commonly a sequela to a streptococcal infection, antimicrobial therapy should include penicillin (procaine penicillin G 22,000–44,000 IU/kg IM q12h) or sodium or potassium penicillin (22,000–44,000 IU/kg IV q6h), unless specifically contraindicated. Other antimicrobials should be added if gram-negative organisms are suspected or have been identified. In addition to reducing antigenic stimulus, antimicrobial therapy is indicated to limit potential secondary infections such as cellulitis, pneumonia, or thrombophlebitis.

Because purpura hemorrhagica and other idiopathic vasculitis syndromes probably are immune-mediated, systemic glucocorticoids are usually warranted. Concurrent antimicrobial administration is recommended, and the risk of steroid-induced immunosuppression must be considered when the primary infection is still active or more life-threatening than the vasculitis itself. Dexamethasone* (0.05–0.2 mg/kg IV or IM s.i.d. in the morning) should be administered at the minimal dosage necessary to effect reduction in edema. Alternatively, prednisolone† (0.5–1 mg/kg IM or p.o. q12h) may be used but often is not as effective as dexamethasone in the acute phase of the disease. Once the edema starts to resolve, the dose of gluco-

---

*Azium, Schering-Plough Animal Health, Kenilworth, NJ
†Steris Laboratories, Inc., Phoenix, AZ

corticoids can be reduced gradually (10% per day) over 10 to 21 days. Once the dose of dexamethasone is less than 0.04 mg/kg, the drug can be given orally, or oral prednisone may be substituted, starting with 10 times the dexamethasone dosage. Antimicrobial therapy should be continued throughout the period of glucocorticoid administration and until obvious bacterial infection has resolved. Occasionally, horses respond poorly to therapy or relapse despite continued treatment. Others have their condition stabilize during glucocorticoid treatment but relapse when the dose is decreased.

In human medicine, the addition of the alkylating agent cyclophosphamide to glucocorticoid therapy is more effective than glucocorticoids alone for the treatment of some vasculitis syndromes. To the author's knowledge, there are no reports of the use of cyclophosphamide or other alkalating agents for the treatment of vasculitis in horses, although they have been used for the treatment of immune-mediated anemia and thrombocytopenia. Plasmapheresis has been reported to rapidly decrease the level of circulating immune complexes in humans with acute systemic vasculitis, while awaiting the effect of immunosuppressive therapy. However, plasmapheresis is rarely available to the equine veterinarian.

Supportive care should include aggressive hydrotherapy to reduce or prevent edema, hand walking, and application of pressure bandages to the limbs. Severe respiratory tract edema with stridor or dysphagia may indicate the need for tracheostomy, intravenous fluids, and nutritional support. Nonsteroidal anti-inflammatory drugs are indicated to provide analgesia and reduce inflammation. Phenylbutazone* (2.2–4.4 mg/kg IV or p.o. q12h) or flunixin meglumine† (1 mg/kg IV, IM, or p.o. q12h) are used most commonly.

Horses affected with EVA usually make uneventful clinical recoveries, and therapy is palliative. Prophylactic administration of antimicrobials may be indicated in severe cases. Glucocorticoids are contraindicated because the vasculitis is not immune-mediated. Horses with equine infectious anemia remain infected for life, and treatment also is palliative. Corticosteroids are contraindicated because administration of immunosuppressive drugs can precipitate viral replication and clinical disease. In addition to supportive care, horses with equine ehrlichiosis should be treated with oxytetracycline. Horses with photoactivated vasculitis should be stabled during the day to prevent further exposure to sunlight. Systemic glucocorticoids should be given daily for 10 to 14 days. The dosage can then be reduced gradually. Most horses with photoactivated vasculitis respond adequately to treatment; a few may relapse when reintroduced to sunlight.

PROGNOSIS

The prognosis for vasculitis that is not the result of equine infectious anemia or neoplasia is fair if aggressive therapy is instituted early in the disease process. Most horses recover within 2 to 3 weeks. However, it is difficult to predict the course of the disease in an individual case. There may be a single episode lasting only a few weeks, or the vasculitis may become chronic or recurrent. In some cases, extensive skin necrosis of the distal extremities may lead to severe cellulitis with secondary septic arthritis or tenosynovitis, or it may be followed by excessive granulation tissue formation limiting the usefulness of the horse. The ultimate outcome varies according to the extent of internal organ involvement and the nature of the primary disease process. In some animals, euthanasia may be necessary because of secondary complications such as septic synovial structures, pneumonia, laminitis, thrombophlebitis, myositis, renal failure, or colitis.

Supplemental Readings

Morris DD: Cutaneous vasculitis in horses: 19 cases (1978–1985). J Am Vet Med Assoc 191:460–464, 1987.

Stannard AA: Photoactivated vasculitis. *In* Robinson NE (ed): Current Therapy in Equine Medicine, ed 2. Philadelphia, WB Saunders, 1987, pp 646–647.

Timoney JF: Strangles. Vet Clin North Am Equine Pract 9:365–374, 1993.

Timoney PJ, McCollum WH: Equine viral arteritis. Vet Clin North Am Equine Pract 9:295–309, 1993.

Phoenix Pharmaceutical, Inc., St. Joseph, MO
†*Banamine, Schering-Plough Animal Health, Kenilworth, NJ*

Lymphoproliferative and Myeloproliferative Disorders

DAVID A. SCHNEIDER
Athens, Georgia

Leukemia is the abnormal proliferation of hematopoietic cells and encompasses both lympho- and myeloproliferative disorders. In the horse, neoplasms of the hematopoietic system are rare compared with other species. Leukemia can be classified based on (1) the type of abnormal cell: lymphoid or myeloid; (2) the degree of tumor differentiation: acute or chronic; and (3) the number of abnormal cells circulating in the peripheral blood: aleukemic, subleukemic, leukemic. In addition, tumor cells can be further characterized by histochemical and immunohistologic methods. Lymphoma, plasma cell myeloma, the myeloid leukemias, and erythrocytosis are reviewed.

LYMPHOMA

Lymphoma is a general term for the malignant transformation of solid lymphoid tissue and, in the horse, is synonymous with lymphosarcoma. Although lymphoma is one of the most common internal neoplasms of the horse, the reported prevalence of lymphoma in horse populations, based on United States abattoir surveys, is 0.002 to 0.05%, and based on necropsy surveys is 0.2 to 3.0%. There are no established risk factors for equine lymphoma, and the etiology is unknown. There does not appear to be a breed or sex predilection, and the majority of patients are between 4 and 10 years of age. Individual cases of lymphoma in a fetus, and in horses younger than 1 year or older than 20 years of age also have been reported.

Clinical Signs

A diverse spectrum of clinical signs has been associated with lymphoma. The signs and progression of disease relate to the sites of tumor involvement and are not specific to lymphoma. The most common clinical signs are decreased appetite, depression, weight loss, fever, lymphadenopathy, and dependent edema. In a study of 20 histologically confirmed cases of lymphoma, the clinical findings included, in descending order of frequency, weight loss, fever, peripheral lymphadenopathy, abdominal mass, upper or lower respiratory signs, ocular signs, colic, and diarrhea.

Reported sites of tumor involvement include peripheral and internal lymph nodes, spleen, liver, kidney, intestine, heart, lung, nasopharynx, eye and adnexa, skeletal muscle, skin, reproductive organs, and central and peripheral nervous system. Four anatomic forms of lymphoma and their relative frequencies are well described: multicentric—50%; alimentary—19%; mediastinal—6%; and extranodal—25%. Combinations of these four classic forms of lymphoma occur in approximately 50% of cases.

Multicentric, or generalized, lymphoma is the most commonly reported form and typically involves multiple peripheral and internal lymph nodes and other organs. The most commonly involved peripheral lymph nodes are the mandibular, caudal cervical, retropharyngeal, and superficial inguinal. The most commonly involved abdominal lymph nodes are the mesenteric, colonic, and deep iliac. Splenomegaly occurs in 25% of the cases, and hepatomegaly or perirenal masses are found infrequently. The multiple sites of involvement probably represent metastasis via the blood and lymphatic systems. Notably, this is the most common form to have circulating neoplastic lymphocytes (i.e., "true" leukemia). Clinical signs reflect dysfunction of affected organs, and the course of the disease is rapid once signs become evident.

The alimentary type is the most acute form of lymphoma, causing rapid deterioration; the small intestine and associated mesenteric lymph nodes are most frequently involved. Distant metastasis appears slow to develop. Alimentary lymphoma is commonly detected in horses from 2 to 5 years of age. Signs are nonspecific and include weight loss, decreased appetite, fever, dependent edema, and diarrhea or abdominal pain of varying severity and duration. Affected horses frequently have a blunted oral glucose tolerance response and reduced albumin concentration, suggesting intestinal malabsorption. Immune-medi-

ated hemolytic anemia and hyperglobulinemia may also accompany this condition.

Lymphoma of the mediastinal lymph nodes occurs in adult horses. Common clinical signs are referable to compression of intrathoracic structures and include pleural effusion, tachypnea, dyspnea, and dependent edema. Less common findings include a persistent cough, tachycardia, jugular vein distension, and forelimb lameness. The paraneoplastic syndrome of hypercalcemia has been reported to occur with this form of lymphoma. Neoplastic cells may be observed in the pleural fluid.

The most common extranodal sites of tumor development are, in descending order of frequency, the skin, upper respiratory tract, eyes or adnexa, and central nervous system. Lymphoma of the skin, the cutaneous form, has been reported to be the least and most common form of equine lymphoma. Tumors are readily identified as nonpainful, dermal or subdermal masses that are firm and well-circumscribed and may be haired, nonhaired, or ulcerated. Horses may have a solitary mass or multiple masses ranging in size from a few millimeters up to several centimeters in diameter. The most commonly affected regions include the shoulder, perineum, and axilla. Clinical signs are referable to internal metastasis and are generally not present during the initial examination. Tumors may develop rapidly or slowly and spontaneously regress and reappear.

Extranodal lymphoma of the eye or adnexa is associated with exophthalmus, exposure keratitis, uveitis, chemosis, and conjunctivitis. Occasionally, lymphoma may involve the upper respiratory tract and may cause signs of upper airway obstruction. There may be an associated nasal discharge of variable character. Reports of peripheral nerve sheath and epidural infiltration exist and may be considered rare differentials for lameness and ataxia, respectively.

One case report of primary leukemic lymphoma has been confirmed in the horse. An extensive histologic examination detected neoplastic cells only in the peripheral blood and bone marrow.

Diagnosis

Diagnosis of lymphoma can be difficult, and ante mortem confirmation occurs in less than 60% of cases. The key to ante mortem diagnosis is a persistent diagnostician. Neoplasia must always be considered in an adult horse with recurrent inflammatory and febrile episodes that are not responsive to antimicrobial therapy. The physical examination should include transrectal abdominal palpation and careful thoracic auscultation and percussion. The definitive diagnosis of lymphoma requires the observation of neoplastic cells. The majority of cases are confirmed by aspiration or biopsy results of lymph nodes and other masses. Neoplastic cells may be observed in centesis samples of body cavity fluids and rarely in bone marrow aspirates and peripheral blood.

Cytologic observations consistent with neoplastic transformation of lymphoid cells include mitotic figures, prominent nucleoli, and binucleation. The evaluation of tissue architecture is of great importance in the detection of neoplastic change and can only be obtained with biopsy.

The number of leukocytes and lymphocytes in the peripheral blood is often within normal limits. With leukocytosis, mature neutrophilia and increased serum fibrinogen activity are most commonly observed and indicate the presence of inflammation. Leukopenia or pancytopenia are uncommon findings. The observation of neoplastic lymphocytes in the peripheral blood is uncommon and may be a late manifestation of lymphoma in the horse, indicating dissemination and bone marrow involvement. When neoplastic cells are observed in the peripheral blood, lymphoma is characterized as subleukemic or leukemic if the total white blood cell count is normal or elevated, respectively. Lymphoma is aleukemic when neoplastic cells are absent in peripheral blood.

Anemia is a common finding, occurring in 30 to 50% of horses with lymphoma. Typically, the anemia is mild, normochromic, and normocytic, reflecting bone marrow suppression. Immune-mediated hemolytic anemia may be suspected when based on a positive direct Coomb's test. Thrombocytopenia can be profound and has resulted in bleeding diathesis.

Common alterations of plasma proteins include increased total protein and globulin concentrations, and increased serum fibrinogen activity. Hypoalbuminemia may occur in response to a profound gammopathy or from gastrointestinal loss and rarely from end-stage liver failure as a consequence of hepatic involvement. Miscellaneous biochemical alterations that may be seen include hypercalcemia, elevated liver enzymes, and azotemia.

Prognosis and Treatment

In the majority of patients, rapid deterioration follows the onset of clinical signs. Horses with lymphoma limited to cutaneous involvement, however, have survived for several years. Immunosuppressive glucocorticoid therapy (0.02–0.2 mg/kg dexamethasone° IV, IM, or p.o., s.i.d.) has been reported to be palliative for steroid-responsive malignancies. Cutaneous lesions may regress in 2 to 6 weeks, at which time the dose may be gradually reduced. However, if glucocorticoid administration is reduced too quickly or discontinued, tumors may reappear with a more aggressive behavior.

The use of antineoplastic agents for the treatment of equine lymphoma is not common. The expense and possible toxicity of chemotherapy in the horse are the most common reasons cited for nontreatment.

The following is a recently published multiple-agent induction protocol for horses with lymphoma: cytosine arabinoside† (200–300 mg/m² sc or IM) is given once every 1 or 2 weeks, chlorambucil‡ (20 mg/m² p.o.) is given once every 2 weeks, and prednisone§ (1.1–2.2 mg/kg p.o.) is given every other day throughout the treatment period. Alternatively, cyclophosphamide‖ (200 mg/m² IV given once every 2–3 weeks) can be substituted for chlorambucil. Antineoplastic agents are typically given on alternating weeks but have been given on the same day without apparent consequence. Response to induction therapy should occur within 2 to 4 weeks. If response is not observed,

adding vincristine° (0.5 mg/m² IV once a week) is recommended.

With remission, the induction protocol is used for a total of 2 to 3 months and then is switched to a maintenance protocol. The first cycle of maintenance therapy increases the treatment interval for each antineoplastic agent by one week; prednisone, however, is given for the duration of therapy and is gradually reduced in dose. After 2 to 3 months on the first cycle, if the horse is still in remission, the second cycle is begun, adding one more week to the treatment intervals of each agent. Several cycles of maintenance therapy can be given; however, most horses in remission are treated for a total of 6 to 8 months.

Remission rates and survival times are not yet available for this protocol, although it appears that approximately 50% of multicentric lymphoma patients are brought into remission for several months to a year.† Tumor recurrence has followed the withdrawal of therapy and cutaneous forms seem to respond poorly. Signs of toxicity, including bone marrow suppression and severe gastrointestinal irritation, have been extremely rare using this protocol. Other protocols included single agent L-asparaginase‡ (10,000–40,000 IU/m² IM once every 2–3 weeks), single agent cyclophosphamide (given as described earlier), and combinations of either cytosine arabinoside or cyclophosphamide with prednisone.

Multicentric lymphoma has been successfully managed in a pregnant mare. Administration of the chemotherapeutic agents was discontinued 1 week before foaling to avoid transfer of antineoplastic agents through the colostrum and milk. The mare gave birth to an apparently healthy but small foal. Therapy was not continued and she was euthanized 2 months later because of deterioration in her condition. The use of antineoplastic agents during pregnancy is not without risk to the fetus. Abortion, teratogenesis, carcinogenesis, prematurity, low birth weight, and organ toxicity may occur. However, if given after the first trimester there is no increase in fetal malformations in human patients.

PLASMA CELL MYELOMA

Plasma cells are terminally differentiated B lymphocytes. Malignant transformation can result in three categories of tumors: chronic B cell lymphocytic leukemia, B cell lymphoma, and plasma cell tumors. Plasma cell tumors occur rarely in the horse. No established risk factors exist, and affected animals range from 3 months to 22 years of age. *Solitary plasmacytoma* is the term used when a single extramedullary tumor is involved. However, the most common form involves the bone marrow and is called *multiple myeloma.*

Clinical Signs

Clinical signs are associated with the sites of tumor invasion and include limb edema, ataxia, lameness, epistaxis, lymphadenopathy, weight loss, and anorexia. Second-

---

°*Azium, Schering-Plough Animal Health, Kenilworth, NJ*
†*Cytosar-U, The Upjohn Co., Kalamazoo, MI*
‡*Leukeran, Burroughs Wellcome Co., Research Triangle Park, NC*
§*Deltasone, The Upjohn Co., Kalamazoo, MI*
‖*Cytoxan, Bristol Myers-Squibb, Princeton, NJ*

°*Oncovin, Eli Lilly and Co., Indianapolis, IN*
†*C. Guillermo Couto, personal communication*
‡*Elspar, Merck Sharp and Dohme, West Point, PA*

ary infections commonly involving the lower respiratory or urinary tract may develop. Anemia and hyperglobulinemia are the most common abnormal laboratory findings. With myelophthisic disease, the anemia may be severe and accompanied by leukopenia and thrombocytopenia. Hypoalbuminemia may accompany hyperglobulinemia. A monoclonal gammopathy is detected in nearly all cases by serum electrophoresis and reflects the clonal expansion of a single plasma cell lineage. The monoclonal protein, referred to as a *paraprotein,* may be a complete or partial immunoglobulin, the majority of which are in the IgG class. Urinalysis may reveal proteinuria, and the heat-precipitation method has confirmed the presence of light chains (Bence Jones protein) in the urine of one horse. Occasionally, hypercalcemia may be found as a paraneoplastic condition.

Diagnosis

In human patients, definitive diagnosis is based on the demonstration of bone marrow plasmacytosis (>10% of cells) or an extramedullary plasmacytoma and one of the following: (1) a serum monoclonal gammopathy; (2) detection of a urine monoclonal protein; or (3) osteolytic lesions. The majority of equine cases have a monoclonal gammopathy; however, cases in which the serum globulin content was within normal limits have been described. Further examinations should include skeletal survey radiographs of the long bones and cervical vertebrae and biochemical tests to detect renal or hepatic involvement.

Prognosis and Treatment

Most horses die or are euthanized within 4 months of developing clinical signs, but longer survival times have been reported in a few horses treated with antineoplastic agents. Melphalan,° prednisone, and cyclophosphamide have been used in the treatment of multiple myeloma in an 18-year-old Quarterhorse mare. Diagnosis was confirmed 1 week before foaling. Chemotherapy was started after the foal was weaned at 4 days of age. Dosages were not reported. Plasmapheresis was also performed. The mare was euthanized 7 months after diagnosis because of severe chronic laminitis. A 20-year-old horse with multiple myeloma was treated with melphalan (7 mg/m² p.o. s.i.d. for 5 days every 3 weeks). The horse's condition remained stable for 1 year after diagnosis.

MYELOID LEUKEMIAS

Myeloproliferative disorders are characterized by medullary and extramedullary proliferation of bone marrow constituents including the erythroid, granulocytic, monocytic, and megakaryocytic cell series. Myelodysplastic syndromes are characterized by refractory cytopenia, which generally progresses to acute myeloid leukemia. Classification schemes for myeloid leukemia are based on the degree of differentiation of the transformed cell line. For example, chronic myeloid leukemia involves neutrophils and late precursor cells, whereas acute myeloid leukemia involves myeloblast cells. In general, chronic leukemias are less aggressive than acute leukemias. Reports of myeloprolifera-

°Alkeran, Burroughs Wellcome, Research Triangle Park, NC

tive disorders of horses are rare and are dominated by acute leukemias of the granulocytic cell series.

Clinical Signs

In a review of 11 reported cases of myelogenous leukemia in the horse, the ages ranged from 10 months to 16 years and both genders and various breeds were affected. Common clinical findings included ventral and peripheral edema, petechiation, weight loss, depression, and enlarged lymph nodes. Less common findings were fever, epistaxis, pneumonia, exercise intolerance, and colic. All were found to be anemic, thrombocytopenic, and to have circulating neoplastic cells; the majority had neutropenia and a gammopathy. Secondary infections seem more common in this form of hematopoietic disorders, presumably as a result of immunosuppression. Two horses with myelomonocytic leukemia developed pulmonary aspergillosis.

Diagnosis

Bone marrow examination confirms the diagnosis. Determination of cell lineage may be morphologically obvious. When needed, further characterization is possible histochemically using specific subcellular enzyme content and immunohistologically using cell-surface antigens.

Prognosis and Treatment

Myelogenous leukemias are notoriously resistant to common antineoplastic agents. However, chemotherapy has been attempted in at least two cases of equine acute myelomonocytic leukemia. These horses were given cytosine arabinoside based on a low-dose protocol (10 mg/m² b.i.d. for 3 weeks) adopted from human cancer medicine. The aim of this therapy is to promote terminal differentiation of the neoplastic cell line and diminish clonal expansion. Newer modalities are being tested in human patients including the use of hematopoietic cytokines and bone marrow transplantation.

ERYTHROCYTOSIS

Erythrocytosis, or polycythemia, is the presence of an elevated red blood cell mass and may be further characterized as relative or absolute. Relative erythrocytosis is the result of a normal red blood cell mass in a reduced plasma volume (e.g., in dehydration). The relative volume of red blood cells also can be dramatically, but temporarily, increased following splenic contraction. Absolute erythrocytosis may be primary or secondary. Secondary absolute erythrocytosis develops as a result of increased levels of circulating erythropoietin that may be an appropriate response to chronic tissue hypoxia or may be inappropriate. The latter has been reported in horses with hepatocellular carcinoma. Primary absolute erythrocytosis is an exceedingly rare myeloproliferative disorder characterized by an increase in red blood cell mass without a concurrent increase in erythropoietin production.

Clinical Signs

Clinical signs of absolute erythrocytosis are nonspecific and include lethargy, weight loss, and mucosal hyperemia. Blood hyperviscosity due to the presence of the large numbers of red blood cells significantly alters the hemodynamics of blood flow and may result in bleeding, neurologic signs, and cardiopulmonary signs. In secondary absolute erythrocytosis, clinical signs may also be referable to the primary disease process.

Diagnosis

Diagnosis of absolute erythrocytosis depends on the documentation of an increased red blood cell mass; however, the methodology to do this is not readily employed. Alternatively, the persistence of an increased packed cell volume, total red blood cell count, and hemoglobin concentration in the absence of dehydration or shock can be used to support the diagnosis of absolute erythrocytosis. Cardiopulmonary examination, renal and hepatic evaluation, bone marrow examination, and serum erythropoietin concentration may be used to differentiate primary versus secondary absolute erythrocytosis.

Prognosis and Treatment

The prognosis for horses with absolute erythrocytosis is guarded. The aim of therapy is to reduce the red blood cell mass. Accordingly, it has been suggested that 10 to 20 ml of blood per kilogram of body weight be removed and replaced with an equal volume of balanced polyionic fluid. This therapy is safe and quickly reduces packed cell volume (PCV) and blood viscosity, but needs to be repeated frequently, based on clinical signs and serial PCV monitoring. Chemotherapeutic agents, such as hydroxyurea, have been used in dogs and humans, but no reports are found in horses. A protocol for hydroxyurea treatment was given in *Current Therapy in Equine Medicine*, edition 3, page 516.

Supplemental Readings

Buechner-Maxwell V, Zhang C, Robertson J, Jain NC, Antczak DF, Feldman BF, Murray MJ: Intravascular leukostasis and systemic aspergillosis in a horse with subleukemic acute myelomonocytic leukemia. J Vet Intern Med 8:258–263, 1994.

Byrne BA, Couto CG, Kohn CW: Multiple agent chemotherapy for lymphoma in a pregnant mare. J Am Vet Med Assoc, in press.

Byrne BA, Yvorchuk-St. Jean K, Couto CG, Kohn CW: Successful management of lymphoproliferative disease in two pregnant mares. Proc Annu Conf Vet Canc Soc 1991, pp 8–9.

Couto CG: Lymphoma in the horse. Proc 12th Am Coll Vet Intern Med Forum, 1994, pp 865.

Edwards DF, Parker JW, Wilkinson JE, Helman RG: Plasma cell myeloma in the horse. A case report and literature review. J Vet Intern Med 7:169–176, 1993.

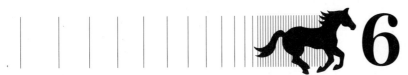
THE NERVOUS SYSTEM
Edited by Robert J. MacKay

Central Nervous System Trauma

B O N N I E   R U S H   M O O R E

Manhattan, Kansas

Injury to the brain and spinal cord occurs in horses during accidental falls, collisions, falling over backward, and direct blows from a kick or handler. Because the calvarium and vertebral canal are solid structures in horses, considerable force is necessary to produce damage to the central nervous system (CNS). Neurologic deficits identified during a thorough systematic examination reflect the neuroanatomic location, severity, and extent of CNS damage. Frequent serial neurologic examination is an essential diagnostic component for evaluation of horses with CNS trauma; the progression of neurologic signs is the most important indicator of prognosis and response to therapy. The therapeutic principles for CNS trauma are to reduce intracranial pressure, mimimize edema formation, and provide supportive care.

PATHOPHYSIOLOGY

Traumatic injuries initially produce destruction of neurologic tissue by contusion, laceration, and hemorrhage. Contusion refers to vascular and nervous tissue damage without loss of cerebral architecture. Laceration of nervous tissues disrupts cerebral architecture and vascular structures, resulting in hemorrhage. Edema within the neural parenchyma develops from direct nervous tissue damage, increased capillary permeability, loss of energy-dependent ion pumps, and release of inflammatory mediators. Expansion of nervous tissue mass as a consequence of hemorrhage and edema within a closed calvarium results in increased intracranial pressure. High intracranial pressure perpetuates a cycle of secondary or delayed nervous tissue destruction owing to pressure-induced necrosis, impaired cerebral blood flow, accumulation of waste products, and membrane lipoperoxidation. Persistently high intracranial pressure may result in herniation of the occipital lobes under the tentorium cerebelli or cerebellum through the foramen magnum.

HEAD TRAUMA

Two basic types of skull fractures occur in horses following characteristic traumatic incidents. Fractures of the frontal and parietal bones of the calvarium result from a direct blow to the frontal region or collision with a solid object, and basilar skull fractures occur when horses fall over backward and strike the poll.

Clinical Signs

Frontal bone fractures, resulting from direct impact, are often open, depressed fractures with direct cerebral laceration by fracture fragments that leads to hemorrhage (Fig. 1). The neurologic signs associated with frontal bone fractures reflect cerebral cortical damage and increased intracranial pressure. Contralateral cortical blindness with a normal pupillary light reflex and decreased facial sensation, depression, compulsive wandering toward the affected cerebral hemisphere, and generalized seizures are common in horses with frontal head injuries. Development of anisocoria or mydriasis with slow pupillary light reflexes indicates increasing intracranial pressure and significant risk of caudal cerebral herniation. Loss of consciousness and development of mydriatic unresponsive pupils indicates that herniation of the occipital lobes under the tentorium cerebelli has occurred.

301

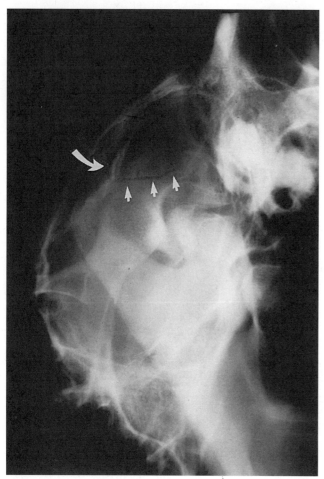

Figure 1. Oblique radiographic view of the calvarium following a frontal impact injury. Note the comminuted depression fracture of the parietal bone (*curved arrow*).

Basilar skull fractures most commonly involve the basisphenoid, basioccipital, and temporal bones, and they result from striking the poll when falling over backward. Basisphenoid fractures occur at the suture between the basisphenoid and basioccipital bones (Fig. 2) and result in compression and hemorrhage of the brainstem. Occipital bone fractures may result from avulsion of the insertion of the rectus capitis ventralis muscle or direct impact. Avulsed occipital bone fragments may be identified superimposed over the guttural pouch on a lateral radiographic view of the skull. Petrous temporal bone fracture may destroy the middle and inner ear, resulting in peripheral vestibular dysfunction and facial nerve paralysis. The basilar artery and venous sinuses are often lacerated by basilar skull fractures, producing massive hemorrhage into the calvarium, guttural pouch, or inner ear.

Neurologic signs associated with basilar skull fractures reflect injury to the brainstem and vestibular system. Following traumatic poll injury, horses usually lose consciousness for a period of minutes to hours, and some never regain consciousness. The most common clinical signs observed in horses that regain consciousness are depression, vestibular dysfunction, facial nerve paralysis, tetraparesis, and hemorrhage from the nostrils and ear. Signs of vestibu-

lar dysfunction result from damage to the inner ear or central vestibular pathways and include circling or falling toward the side of the lesion, head tilt toward the lesion, and pathologic nystagmus. Peripheral vestibular damage produces horizontal nystagmus with the fast phase away from the lesion. Damage to central vestibular pathways may produce horizontal, vertical, or rotary nystagmus with the fast phase usually directed away from the lesion. Damage to vestibular tracts at the cerebellomedullary angle may produce paradoxical vestibular syndrome, whereby the vestibular signs (head tilt, nystagmus, circling) occur contralateral to the lesion. The side of the traumatic lesion is defined by the side of hemiparesis and proprioception deficits. Facial nerve paralysis is characterized by ipsilateral ear droop, ptosis, flaccidity of the lower lip, and muzzle deviation to the contralateral side. Leakage of cerebrospinal fluid or hemorrhage from the external ear is presumptive evidence of petrous temporal bone fracture. Epistaxis may result from fracture of the cribriform plate, fracture of the basisphenoid and basioccipital bones, or hemorrhage into the guttural pouch. Basisphenoid fractures may lacerate the basilar artery and can produce massive life-threatening hemorrhage into the guttural pouch.

Neurologic examination is the most important diagnostic and prognostic tool for evaluation of horses with basilar skull fractures. The examiner should pay particular attention to pupil size, symmetry, and responsiveness to light. Bilateral miosis signifies rostral midbrain swelling, whereas unresponsive bilateral mydriasis is a poor prognostic sign associated with midbrain compression or herniation. The rate and character of respiration should be monitored in patients with abnormal pupil size and symmetry. Changes in the rate of respiration and development of abnormal respiratory patterns indicate increasing intracranial pressure and danger of herniation. The combination of bilateral, unresponsive mydriatic pupil, coma, and erratic respiration is consistent with herniation of the cerebellum through the foramen magnum.

In some instances, a traumatic poll or frontal injury may result in bilateral blindness with mydriatic unresponsive pupils. This injury results from damage or rupture of the optic nerve or the optic chiasm owing to shearing forces

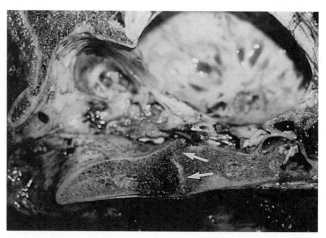

Figure 2. Fracture of the suture between the basisphenoid and basioccipital bones with overriding displacement of fracture fragments (*arrows*).

by the bony optic canals. A basilar skull fracture does not necessarily accompany this lesion, and no other neurologic sign is observed. The prognosis for recovery of vision is poor.

Radiography

Skull radiographs are indicated in horses with head trauma to determine the type, location, and displacement of fractures and fracture fragments. Depressed, comminuted fractures of the frontal and parietal bones are readily identified radiographically (see Fig. 1). Conversely, petrous temporal bone fractures are difficult to see, and multiple oblique views may be necessary to identify a fracture line. In young horses, it is difficult to differentiate a fracture of the basisphenoid/basioccipital suture from the normal physeal growth plate. Absence of an obvious fracture line does not preclude a diagnosis of basilar skull fracture; hemorrhage from the guttural pouch, nose, or external ear following a traumatic poll injury is presumptive evidence of a basilar skull fracture.

Cerebrospinal Fluid Analysis

Cerebrospinal fluid (CSF) analysis is unlikely to provide further diagnostic or prognostic information in horses with closed head injuries. Cytologic analysis and culture of CSF may be indicated in horses with open fractures of the calvarium to diagnose secondary septic meningitis. In addition, CSF analysis may provide supportive evidence of CNS trauma in horses with acute onset of undiagnosed neurologic disease. Alterations in CSF analysis consistent with CNS trauma are xanthochromia, high red blood cell counts, high protein concentration, and increased creatine kinase activity. Sudden decreases in pressure while performing an atlanto-occipital CSF tap may precipitate herniation; therefore, CSF should be obtained at the lumbosacral site in horses with suspected head trauma.

Treatment

The primary therapeutic goals for treatment of CNS trauma are to prevent edema of nervous tissue and to lower intracranial pressure. Because the brain is encased in a rigid calvarium, swelling results in increased intracranial pressure, decreased cerebral blood flow, and pressure-induced necrosis. Medical treatment within 8 hours of injury to prevent edema formation consistently produces a more favorable outcome than does late intervention, which must be directed at resolving existing edema and reducing intracranial pressure.

Glucocorticoid drugs minimize cerebral edema and secondary injury by prevention of membrane lipoperoxidation and inhibition of arachidonic acid metabolites such as thromboxane, prostaglandins, and leukotrienes. These mediators potentiate inflammation, loss of vascular integrity, and vasoconstriction. Dexamethasone (0.1 to 0.2 mg/kg, IV, q8–12h) is the most widely recommended corticosteroid preparation for treatment of CNS trauma in veterinary medicine. In horses, the risk of steroid-induced laminitis associated with dexamethasone must be considered before administration. In humans, massive doses of methylprednisolone sodium succinate* (30 mg/kg IV, followed by 5.4

mg/kg per hour for 23 hours) administered within 8 hours of CNS injury reduce the incidence and severity of residual neurologic deficits. Methylprednisolone administration has not been investigated for treatment of head trauma in horses. Nonsteroidal anti-inflammatory drugs have limited efficacy to reduce CNS edema and inflammation; however, their analgesic properties may relieve malaise and reduce depression associated with the pain of a skull or vertebral fracture.

Dimethyl sulfoxide (DMSO) has several beneficial properties that may prevent formation of cerebral edema in horses with head trauma including membrane stabilization, oxygen free radical scavenging, and inhibition of arachidonic acid metabolites. In addition, DMSO may reduce existing cerebral edema and intracranial pressure via hyperosmolar dehydration. The recommended treatment regimen is twice daily administration (1 g/kg, IV) in 0.9% sodium chloride as a 10% solution; rapid administration of the 10% solution or administration of concentrated DMSO may result in intravascular hemolysis and hemoglobinuria.

Mannitol reduces existing CNS edema via hyperosmolar dehydration, and may reduce intracranial pressure within 30 minutes of administration. Mannitol should not be administered if active intracranial hemorrhage is suspected; leakage of mannitol into the neural parenchyma may draw fluid into the interstitial space and worsen cerebral edema. In cases in which intracranial hemorrhage has stopped, mannitol (0.25–1 g/kg IV over 60 minutes) is administered as a 20% solution, two to three times per day.

Anticonvulsant therapy may be necessary in horses with cerebral edema and hemorrhage. Diazepam* (25–100 mg IV) is effective for controlling focal or intermittent generalized seizures. Although phenobarbital is an effective anticonvulsant in horses, it produces depression and altered consciousness, impairing the clinician's ability to monitor mentation and detect deterioration of neurologic status. Therefore, phenobarbital (5–10 mg/kg IV) administration should be limited to horses with uncontrollable generalized seizures that are unresponsive to diazepam. In addition to antiseizure activity, phenobarbital may protect against ischemic damage by decreasing cerebral metabolism, retarding lipoperoxidation, and decreasing intracranial pressure. Phenobarbitol (10 mg/kg p.o. b.i.d.) may be used effectively for prolonged control of generalized seizure activity. Therapeutic peak and trough blood concentrations of phenobarbital should be maintained between 15 and 40 g/ml.

Broad-spectrum antimicrobial drugs are indicated for basilar skull fractures, petrosal bone fractures, and open frontal bone fractures. Basisphenoid fractures may communicate with the guttural pouch, and petrosal fractures potentially communicate externally via the external auditory canal. Although many antimicrobial agents penetrate the blood-brain barrier during the initial inflammatory process, third-generation cephalosporins readily penetrate the intact blood-brain barrier and maintain high CSF concentrations after inflammation has subsided. In addition, the CNS has poor immunologic competency, necessitating microbicidal activity for successful elimination of infection. Third-gener-

*Solu-Medrol, The Upjohn Company, Kalamazoo, MI

*Valium, Roche Laboratories, Nutley, NJ

ation cephalosporin drugs such as ceftiofur° and cefotaxime sodium† are bactericidal and have broad-spectrum gram-positive and gram-negative activity.

The level of intensive care required to support a head trauma patient depends on the severity of cardiovascular shock, presence of musculoskeletal injuries, and severity of neurologic damage. Recumbent horses require padding at pressure points; a clean, dry environment; and frequent (q4h) positional change to prevent development of decubital ulcers, urine scalding, and pressure-induced neuromyopathy. The head and neck should be elevated from the body to reduce intracranial pressure. Administration of artificial tear ointment is indicated to prevent development of corneal ulceration in horses with facial nerve paralysis. Nutritional support and conservative intravenous fluid therapy are necessary in most recumbent patients.

If horses with head trauma are ambulatory, it is often advantageous to sedate them to prevent further displacement of fracture fragments and self-induced trauma. Xylazine can be safely administered without increasing intracranial pressure if the head is not permitted to hang below the level of the heart. Phenothiazine drugs reduce the seizure threshold; thus, administration is contraindicated in horses with head trauma.

Surgical therapy is indicated for horses with depressed frontal fractures of the calvarium that penetrate nervous tissue, open fractures that communicate with nervous tissue, and deterioration of neurologic status despite medical therapy. Depressed frontal calvarium fractures are reduced by direct traction or elevation of the fracture fragments. Closed head injuries with nondisplaced fractures are not typically managed surgically unless underlying hemorrhage and edema are severe. The most conservative approach to surgical decompression of the calvarium is to place burr holes in the frontal or parietal bones in a triangular pattern. If burr holes are insufficient to relieve intracranial pressure or remove hemorrhage, the holes can be connected to perform a craniotomy. Basilar skull fractures are inaccessible to direct surgical reduction. However, burr holes over the dorsal calvarium may relieve intracranial pressure and prevent secondary pressure-induced necrosis and ischemia in horses with basilar skull fractures that are unresponsive to medical management.

Prognosis

In general, CNS trauma associated with calvarium fracture has a guarded to grave prognosis. Horses that are comatose and fail to respond to therapy within 36 hours are unlikely to recover. Response to medical therapy in 6 to 8 hours indicates a favorable prognosis for life; however, the ultimate usefulness of the horse will not be apparent for many months after injury. During healing, exuberant callus may impinge on nervous tissue and may result in deterioration in neurologic status in horses that had initially responded favorably to therapy.

SPINAL CORD TRAUMA

Foals

The most common sites of spinal cord injury in horses vary with age. Cervical fractures are more common in foals

---

°Naxcel, The Upjohn Company, Kalamazoo, MI
†Claforan, Hoechst-Roussel, Somerville, NJ

and result from hyperextension, hyperflexion, and luxation. Adult horses are more likely than foals to develop fractures of the caudal thoracic and lumbar spine. Regardless of the site of the fracture, the prognosis is dependent on the severity of the initial injury. The most common cervical vertebral fracture in foals is axial dens fracture and atlantoaxial subluxation. Atlantoaxial subluxation may result from resisting head restraint (hyperextension) or somersault (hyperflexion) injuries in young horses.

Clinical Signs

Foals with atlantoaxial subluxation have a stiff splinted neck and, in some instances, audible crepitation when the head is manipulated. Neurologic gait deficits range from none to marked tetraparesis and ataxia. Foals may have a head tilt, without other signs of vestibular dysfunction, owing to mechanical malalignment of the C1 to C2 articulation. Radiographic views of the cervical spine reveal widening of the cranial physis of the axis (Fig. 3). In foals with neurologic gait deficits, cranioventral luxation of axis usually occurs, accompanied by increased distance between the spine of the atlas and axis and between the floor of the atlas and the axial dens.

Treatment

The therapeutic approach for foals with atlantoaxial subluxation is dependent upon the severity of neurologic deficits and the degree of malalignment and instability of the vertebrae. Stall rest and conservative anti-inflammatory therapy (glucocorticoid and nonsteroidal anti-inflammatory drugs) may be successful in foals with relatively stable nondisplaced fractures. Injudicious liberal administration of anti-inflammatory drugs may permit excessive movement by the horse and loss of muscular splinting of the fracture, which may promote displacement of fracture fragments. Exuberant callus formation may impinge on the spinal cord and produce neurologic gait deficits months after the injury. Surgical intervention is recommended for foals with unstable cervical fractures and severe neurologic gait deficits. Surgical approaches for correction of atlantoaxial subluxation in foals include compression plating, Steinmann pin fixation, dorsal laminectomy of the caudal atlas, and ventral cervical fusion.

Adult Horses

In adult horses, compression fractures of the vertebral body and articular facet fractures are the most common fractures of the cervical vertebrae, and they result from head-on collision, falling, and rolling injuries in horses (especially jumping and steeplechasing).

Clinical Signs

Cervical vertebral fractures are always associated with pain, resistance to manipulation, and splinting of the neck. If the exiting nerve roots are damaged by the fracture, focal sweating, loss of cutaneous sensation, and torticollis may be observed. The severity of neurologic gait deficits ranges from none to tetraplegia dependent on the degree of vertebral luxation and spinal cord injury.

Thoracic fractures are more common in adult horses than foals and result from falling over a jump or falling over backward. The first three thoracic vertebrae are most likely to fracture, followed by T12 fractures. Fracture of

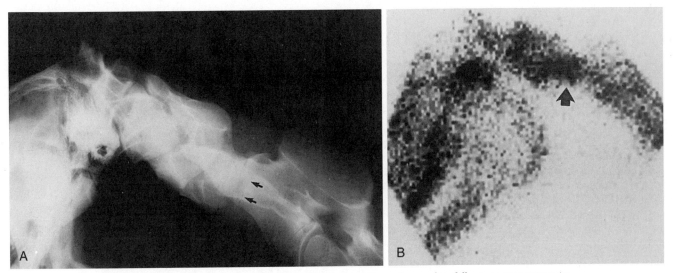

Figure 3. *(A)* Radiographic view of the cranial cervical vertebrae of a weanling following a tying injury. An axial dens fracture is evidenced by widening of the cranial axial physis *(arrows)*. Note the small fracture fragments ventral to the cranial physis. Ventral displacement of the axis, which often accompanies axial dens fractures, is not present. *(B)* Nuclear scintigraphy of the cranial cervical vertebrae. Increased uptake of radionuclide at the cranial physis of the axis *(arrow)* identifies the nondisplaced axial dens fracture.

the thoracolumbar junction is observed in horses that fall and roll down an embankment. Clinical signs in horses with T12 or thoracolumbar fractures include paraparesis and tracking or drifting of the hindlimbs to one side. Dorsal spinous process fractures of T4 to T8 occur in horses that fall over backward. These fractures are not usually associated with fracture of the vertebral bodies, although neurologic gait deficits may result from contusion of spinal cord. Sacral fractures occur with dog-sitting incidents and may result in loss of tail function, urinary incontinence, loss of anal tone, and fecal retention.

Diagnosis of vertebral fracture is often made by history of traumatic incident, clinical signs of tetra- or paraparesis, and neuroanatomic localization by hyperesthesia or loss of cutaneous sensation. Cervical, sacral, and thoracic fractures may be identified by radiographic examination. Fractures of the lumbar vertebrae are not amenable to radiographic examination because of the soft tissue mass surrounding the vertebral bodies in this region. Nuclear scintigraphy may enable the clinician to identify nondisplaced cervical fractures and fractures of the lumbar spine that are inaccessible to radiographic examination.

Treatment

Conservative management, consisting of stall rest and judicious anti-inflammatory therapy, may be rewarding in horses that are ambulatory after vertebral fracture. Surgical stabilization of vertebral fractures is rarely attempted in adult horses, although successful lag screw fixation of vertebral body fracture and dorsal decompression of a transverse, ventrally displaced sacral fracture has been reported. Surgical intervention has not been reported in horses with thoracic or lumbar vertebral fractures in horses. Dorsal spinous process fractures may require surgical removal if sequestration of bone fragments occurs. As with head trauma, the ultimate usefulness of the horse may not be determined until months after spinal cord injury.

Supplemental Readings

Collatos C, Allen D, Chambers J, Henry M: Surgical treatment of sacral fracture in a horse. J Am Vet Med Assoc 198:877–879, 1991.

Mayhew IG: Coma and altered states of consciousness. *In* Mayhew IG (ed): Large Animal Neurology: A Handbook for Veterinary Clinicians. Philadelphia, Lea & Febiger, 1989, pp 133–146.

Reed SM: Management of head trauma in horses. Comp Cont Ed Pract Vet 15:270–273, 1993.

Stick JA, Wilson T, Kunze D: Basilar skull fractures in three horses. J Am Vet Med Assoc 176:228–231, 1980.

Wagner PC: Surgical treatment of traumatic disease of the spinal column. *In* Auer JA (ed): Equine Surgery. Philadelphia, WB Saunders, 1992, pp 1093–1098.

Cervical Stenotic Myelopathy

BONNIE RUSH MOORE
Manhattan, Kansas

Cervical stenotic myelopathy (CSM) is a developmental disease characterized by cervical vertebral malformation, vertebral canal narrowing, and spinal cord compression. Male horses are more frequently affected than females by a ratio of 3:1. The age of onset is typically 1 to 3 years of age, and affected horses are usually rapidly growing and large for their age. The syndrome has been reported in most light and draft horse breeds; however, Thoroughbreds appear to be predisposed. The prevalence of vertebral malformation and spinal cord compression is approximately 2% in the Thoroughbred population, although 10 to 50% of Thoroughbreds have degenerative joint disease of the articular processes without spinal cord compression. Cervical stenotic myelopathy appears to be a manifestation of developmental orthopedic disease, and the pathogenesis is suspected to be similar to that of osteochondrosis.

CLINICAL SIGNS

Horses with CSM exhibit clinical signs consistent with upper motor neuron deficits to all four limbs, characterized by symmetric weakness, ataxia, and spasticity. In most instances, the hindlimbs are more severely affected than the forelimbs; however, forelimb ataxia may be more severe in horses with caudal stenosis (C6-C7) compressing the cervical intumescence. Asymmetrical ataxia and paresis may be observed in horses in which the spinal cord is compressed dorsolaterally by proliferative degenerative articular processes.

A thorough neurologic examination should be performed to assess symmetry and severity of weakness, ataxia, and spasticity. Gait analysis during neurologic examination should be performed at the walk; neurologic deficits can be accentuated by circling, elevation of the head, and manipulation over obstacles and inclines. At rest, CSM-affected horses have a base-wide stance and demonstrate delayed responses to proprioceptive positioning. At a walk, weakness is manifested by stumbling and toe-dragging; horses with prolonged clinical signs of CSM have hooves or shoes that are chipped, worn, or squared at the toe. Ataxia, or proprioceptive loss, is manifested by circumduction of the hindlimbs, posting (pivoting on the inside hindlimb) during circling, and truncal sway at a walk. Moderately to severely affected horses have lacerations on the heel bulbs and medial aspect of their forelimbs from overreaching and interference. Spasticity, which is characterized by stiff-legged gait due to decreased joint flexion, is often observed in moderately affected horses. When urged to move backward, horses with CSM often stand base-wide, lean backward with their body before moving the hindlimbs, and step on their hind foot with a forelimb. The laryngeal adductor response (slap test) is often reduced or absent. The clinical signs of spinal cord compression often progress for a short period of time and then stabilize. Owners often report a traumatic incident that leads to the onset of clinical signs of CSM. This author suspects that, in many cases, the fall is a result of mild neurologic deficits and the traumatic incident exacerbates the clinical signs of spinal cord compression.

Infrequently, there is evidence of nerve root damage such as cervical pain, atrophy of the cervical musculature, cutaneous hypalgesia, and hyporeflexia of cervical reflexes adjacent to the site of spinal cord compression. These signs are more commonly observed in horses older than 4 years of age that have significant arthropathy of the caudal cervical vertebrae (C5 to C7), and the signs result from peripheral nerve compression by proliferative articular processes as the nerve root exits the vertebral canal through the intervertebral foramen. In some instances, arthropathy of the caudal cervical vertebrae may produce cervical pain and forelimb lameness due to peripheral nerve compression, without producing clinical signs of spinal cord compression.

In addition to neurologic deficits, clinical signs of developmental orthopedic disease of the appendicular skeleton, such as physeal enlargement of the long bones, joint effusion resulting from osteochondrosis, and flexural limb deformities, are often present in young horses with CSM.

PATHOGENESIS

The correlation between the incidence of CSM and the incidence and severity of developmental orthopedic disease of the appendicular skeleton is well documented. It is unclear whether there is a causal relationship between osteochondrosis and CSM, or if these syndromes represent separate manifestations of developmental orthopedic disease produced by an underlying inability to form normal cartilage and bone. Nonetheless, the association between the occurrence of osteochondrosis and CSM indicates that the etiology and pathophysiology of these two conditions is similar.

The etiology of osteochondrosis and CSM is likely multifactorial, consisting of genetic and environmental influences. No evidence exists that CSM is directly heritable by simple Mendelian dominant and recessive patterns. The mode of inheritance more likely involves multiple alleles and variable penetrance, which determine genetic predisposition to CSM. A high plane of nutrition, micronutrient imbalance, rapid growth, trauma, and abnormal biomechanical forces most likely contribute to the development of CSM in genetically predisposed individuals.

Dietary factors suspected to play a role in the pathogenesis of osteochondrosis and CSM include copper, zinc, and carbohydrate. Low dietary copper (12 ppm) and high dietary zinc (1000–2000 mg/kg dry weight) concentrations produce osteochondrosis in foals, whereas copper supplementation (55 ppm) significantly reduces the incidence of osteochondrosis of the axial and appendicular skeleton. Copper supplementation does not completely eliminate developmental orthopedic disease, suggesting that other etiologic factors must exist. Excessive carbohydrate in the diet is hypothesized to contribute to the pathogenesis of osteochondrosis through endocrine imbalance. A high carbohydrate meal (130% of Nutritional Research Council [NRC] recommendation) results in postprandial hyperinsulinemia and low serum thyroxine concentration. Insulin stimulates the zone of chondrocyte proliferation, and thyroxine stimulates the zone of chondrocyte maturation at the growth plate. High insulin and low thyroxine concentrations are suspected to promote cartilage proliferation and retention without promoting maturation. Endocrine imbalance associated with a high carbohydrate diet is the basis for the "paced" diet program for prevention and treatment of CSM.

PATHOLOGIC OBSERVATIONS

Spinal cord compression can be dynamic or static in horses with CSM. Dynamic compression occurs owing to vertebral instability and produces intermittent spinal cord compression during ventroflexion of the neck; spinal cord compression is relieved when the neck is in the neutral position. The intervertebral sites most commonly affected by dynamic instability are C3-C4 and C4-C5. Static compression is defined as continuous spinal cord impingement, regardless of cervical position, and occurs predominantly in the caudal cervical region, C5-C6 and C6-C7. In some cases of static compression of the caudal cervical vertebrae, flexion of the neck stretches the thickened ligamentum flavum and relieves spinal cord compression, whereas hyperextension exacerbates compression. Horses with static and dynamic spinal cord compression have narrowing of the vertebral canal from C3 to C6, regardless of the site of spinal cord compression, indicating that generalized vertebral canal stenosis is important in the pathophysiology of CSM.

Pathologic changes of the cervical vertebrae most commonly observed in horses with dynamic compression are instability between adjacent vertebrae, malformation of the caudal vertebral epiphysis (caudal epiphyseal flare), and malformation and malarticulation of the articular processes. Osteochondrosis of the articular processes is not always present at the site of spinal cord compression in horses with dynamic compression. In cases of static spinal cord compression, narrowing of the vertebral canal diameter is exacerbated by thickening of the dorsal lamina, enlargement of the ligamentum flavum, and degenerative articular processes with thickened joint capsules. Osteochondrosis and secondary degenerative joint disease of the articular processes cause excessive force on the ligamentum flavum, joint capsule, and dorsal lamina, producing fibrosis and hypertrophy of these structures. Abnormalities of the dorsal laminae and ligamentum flavum are not observed in young horses with dynamic spinal cord compression and are more common in older horses with degenerative joint disease of the articular processes.

Histopathologic examination of the spinal cord reveals Wallerian degeneration, malacia, focal neuronal loss, and fibrosis at the sites of spinal cord compression. Secondary demyelination occurs in ascending white matter tracts cranial to the affected site, and it occurs in descending tracts distal to the site of spinal cord compression.

DIAGNOSIS

Neurologic disorders capable of producing tetraparesis and ataxia should be considered in the differential diagnoses of CSM. All of the following neurologic disorders are capable of producing clinical signs similar to, or indistinguishable from, CSM on the basis of neurologic examination alone: equine herpesvirus myeloencephalitis, equine protozoal myeloencephalitis, equine degenerative myeloencephalopathy, occipitoatlantoaxial malformation, spinal cord trauma, vertebral fracture, vertebral abscess, and verminous myelitis. Neurologic examination, radiographic procedures, and cerebrospinal fluid analysis are indicated in horses with symmetrical tetraparesis and ataxia to differentiate CSM from these disorders.

RADIOGRAPHY

Accurate assessment of cervical radiographs taken when the horse is standing can determine the likelihood of CSM and may prevent unnecessary myelographic examination. Cervical radiographs should be evaluated for subjective assessment of vertebral malformation and objective determination of vertebral canal diameter. The five characteristic malformations of the cervical vertebrae in horses with CSM include flare of the caudal epiphysis of the vertebral body, abnormal ossification of the articular processes, subluxation between adjacent vertebra, caudal extension of the dorsal laminae, and degenerative joint disease (DJD) of the articular processes. Degenerative joint disease of the articular processes of the caudal cervical vertebrae is the most frequent and severe malformation observed in CSM-affected horses. Nonetheless, degenerative arthropathy occurs in 10 to 50% of nonataxic horses, and is the most frequent and severe vertebral malformation in horses without CSM. Therefore, subjective evaluation of DJD of the articular processes leads to false-positive diagnosis of CSM in the caudal cervical vertebrae. Although the presence of characteristic vertebral malformations supports the diagnosis of cervical stenotic myelopathy, subjective evaluation of cervical vertebral malformation from radiographs does not reliably discriminate between CSM-affected and unaffected horses. Objective assessment of the vertebral canal diameter is more accurate than subjective evaluation of vertebral malformation for identification of CSM-affected horses.

Minimum sagittal diameter (MSD) determination was the first method described to assess stenosis of the vertebral canal from radiographs of the cervical vertebrae. The MSD value is obtained by determining the narrowest diameter measured from the dorsal aspect of the vertebral body to the ventral border of the dorsal laminae (Fig. 1). Reference values for MSD are established for CSM-affected and nonataxic horses weighing more than and less than 320 kg. In the clinical setting, radiographs of the cervical vertebrae are obtained from standing horses. To

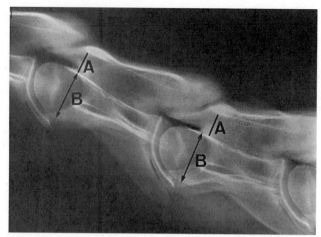

Figure 1. Lateral radiographic view of the third and fourth cervical vertebrae. The sagittal ratio is calculated at each vertebral site by dividing the minimal sagittal diameter (A) by the width of the vertebral body (B). Note flaring of the epiphysis of the caudal vertebral body of C3 and C4.

TABLE 1. LIKELIHOOD RATIOS INDICATING THE PROBABILITY OF CERVICAL STENOTIC MYELOPATHY FOR SAGITTAL RATIO VALUES FOR VERTEBRAE C4 THROUGH C7

Vertebral Sites	Sagittal Ratio	Likelihood Ratio
C4	>0.56	0.04
	0.53–0.56	0.13
	0.50–0.53	1.72
	<0.50	28.6
C5	>0.56	0.04
	0.53–0.56	0.16
	0.50–0.53	2.31
	<0.50	26.1
C6	>0.56	0.03
	0.53–0.56	0.24
	0.50–0.53	1.63
	<0.50	41.5
C7	>0.56	0.04
	0.53–0.56	0.39
	0.50–0.53	1.26
	<0.50	39.0

From Moore BR, Reed SM, Biller DS, Kohn CW, Weisbrode SE: Assessment of vertebral canal diameter and bony malformations of the cervical part of the spine in horses with cervical stenotic myelopathy. Am J Vet Res 55(1):5–13, 1994.

avoid artifacts due to magnification of the radiographic image, the MSD of a vertebral canal is divided by the width of the corresponding vertebral body (see Fig. 1) measured perpendicular to the vertebral canal at the widest point of the cranial aspect of the vertebral body. Determination of this sagittal ratio is more accurate than the MSD for identification of CSM-affected horses over 320 kg body weight. The sensitivity and specificity of the sagittal ratio technique for identification of CSM-affected horses is approximately 89% for vertebral sites C4 through C7. The accuracy of the sagittal ratio technique for identification of CSM-affected horses, without consideration of other bony malformations of the cervical vertebrae, suggests that generalized stenosis of the vertebral canal may be the most important factor in the development of CSM. Accurate measurement of the sagittal ratio value requires a precise, lateral radiograph of the cervical vertebrae. Obliquity of the cervical vertebrae results in indistinct margins of the ventral aspect of the vertebral canal, producing erroneous values for MSD and vertebral body width.

Likelihood ratios have been determined over a range of sagittal ratio values for vertebral sites C4 through C7 in horses larger than 320 kg (Table 1). Likelihood ratios express the odds that a given sagittal ratio value would be expected in a CSM-affected horse. For example, a sagittal ratio value of 0.49 obtained at C5 is 26.1 times as likely to be obtained from a horse with CSM than from a horse that does not have CSM. In this instance, myelographic examination should be performed to confirm the diagnosis and identify the number of affected sites of spinal cord compression. If a sagittal ratio value of 0.55 is obtained, the likelihood ratio is 0.16, indicating that this sagittal ratio value is approximately one tenth as likely to come from a CSM-affected horse as from a horse without spinal cord compression. Therefore, myelographic examination should be postponed until diagnostic tests focused toward alternative etiologies are performed, such as evaluation of cerebrospinal fluid for immunoblot analysis and viral antibody titers.

A semiquantitative scoring system for assessment of

standing cervical radiographs has been developed for identification of CSM in foals up to 1 year of age. The scoring system incorporates objective determination of vertebral canal stenosis and subjective evaluation of vertebral malformation. Stenosis of the vertebral canal is assessed by determination of the inter- and intravertebral MSD, and the maximal score designated for vertebral canal stenosis is 10 points. The inter- and intravertebral MSD are corrected for radiographic magnification by dividing the MSD by the length of the vertebral body (Fig. 2). Malformation of the cervical vertebrae is determined by subjective assessment of five categories: enlargement of the caudal epiphysis of the vertebral body, caudal extension of the dorsal lamina, angulation between adjacent vertebrae, delayed ossification of bone, and DJD of the articular processes. The maximal

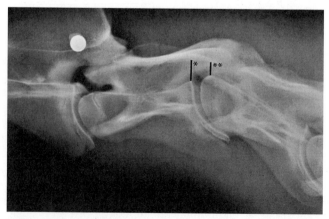

Figure 2. Lateral radiographic view of the third and fourth cervical vertebrae. The single asterisk denotes the intravertebral minimum sagittal diameter for C3, and the double asterisk denotes the intervertebral minimal sagittal diameter for the C3-C4 articulation. Note the marked subluxation of the C3-C4 articulation.

score allotted for each category of vertebral malformation is five points. A total score of 12 or higher (maximal total score 35) constitutes a radiographic diagnosis of CSM. Vertebral canal stenosis and angulation between adjacent vertebrae are the most discriminating parameters in the semiquantitative scoring system to differentiate CSM-affected from unaffected foals. The semiquantitative scoring system is a noninvasive, inexpensive method for predicting and diagnosing the presence of CSM in foals up to 1 year of age.

MYELOGRAPHY

Although the sagittal ratio method is accurate for identification of generalized canal stenosis and determination of the likelihood of CSM, myelographic examination is required for definitive diagnosis of CSM and as a prerequisite to surgical correction. Horses with CSM have generalized stenosis of the vertebral canal, regardless of the site of spinal cord compression. Therefore, use of the sagittal ratio method for determination of specific sites of spinal cord compression results in false-positive diagnosis of the number of sites of spinal cord compression within the CSM-affected population. In addition, the severity of vertebral abnormalities does not always correspond to the site of spinal cord compression, and compression can occur from vertebral canal stenosis at sites that lack bony malformation. Therefore, subjective evaluation of vertebral malformation results in inaccurate diagnosis of the sites of spinal cord compression. Radiographs of the cervical vertebrae cannot replace myelographic examination for identification of the location, number of affected sites, and classification of spinal cord compressive lesions in horses with CSM.

The definitive diagnosis of CSM is defined myelographically by a 50% or greater decrease in the sagittal diameter of the dorsal and ventral contrast columns at diametrically opposed sites. The decrease in the contrast column is quantified by comparing it with the midvertebral site, cranial or caudal to the compressed site. The ventral column is often obliterated at the intervertebral space in normal studies, particularly in the flexed position. Therefore, a decrease of 50% or greater in opposing dorsal and ventral columns must be present for definitive diagnosis of CSM.

In addition to providing the definitive diagnosis of CSM, myelographic examination differentiates between static and dynamic spinal cord compression. Cranial, middle, and caudal cervical radiographs are obtained in neutral and flexed positions, and a hyperextended view is taken of the caudal cervical spine. Horses with dynamic spinal cord compression demonstrate obliteration of the dorsal and ventral contrast columns during ventroflexion of the neck (Fig. 3), whereas spinal cord compression will not be apparent with the neck in the neutral position. Horses with static stenosis have constant spinal cord compression, regardless of cervical position (Fig. 4). In horses with obvious sites of spinal cord compression identified by neutral myelographic views, excessive flexion and extension of the neck should be avoided while obtaining dynamic views, to prevent exacerbation of spinal cord injury.

Myelographic examination is performed under general anesthesia in lateral recumbency. Three non-ionic, water-

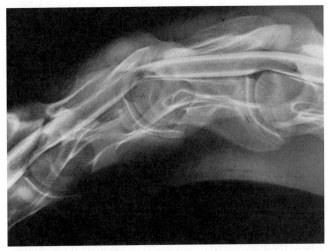

Figure 3. Ventroflexed myelographic view of the third and fourth cervical vertebrae. Dynamic spinal cord compression is identified by obliteration of the dorsal and ventral contrast columns with the neck in the ventroflexed position.

soluble contrast media have been used for equine myelographic studies: iohexol (iodine 350 mg/ml), iopamidol (iodine 370 mg/ml), and metrizamide (iodine 166 mg/ml). Sufficient contrast opacity is obtained using 20 to 40 ml of contrast medium in adult horses. Analytic-grade metrizamide should be dissolved in sterile water (not saline) with 0.005% sodium bicarbonate buffer, and passed through a 0.2 μ millipore filter before use. An equal volume of cerebrospinal fluid is removed before injection of contrast agent into the subarachnoid space at the atlanto-occipital junction. The bevel of the spinal needle (3.5-inch, 18-gauge needle with stylet) is directed caudally, and contrast medium is injected at a constant rate over a 5-minute period. The head and neck are elevated for 5 minutes at 30 to 45° to facilitate caudal flow of contrast medium. Rotation of the head and neck results in obliquity, superimposition, and distortion of the vertebrae, interfering with

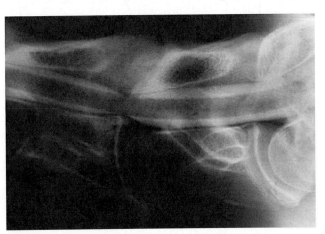

Figure 4. Neutral myelographic view of the sixth and seventh cervical vertebrae. The myelogram was taken with the neck in a neutral position. Static spinal cord compression is identified at the C5-C6 and C6-C7 articulations by obliteration of the dorsal and ventral contrast columns with the neck in the neutral position.

interpretation of the study. Support padding may be necessary under the head, neck, and shoulder to obtain straight lateral projections of the cervical vertebrae.

Although myelographic examination is a relatively safe procedure, it is not without risk. Metrizamide may produce depression, increased ataxia, fever, seizures, meningitis, and muscle fasciculations. The newer non-ionic, water-soluble contrast agents, iopamidol and iohexol, provide superior radiographic contrast with fewer adverse effects than metrizamide. Administration of phenylbutazone (4.4 mg/kg p.o. q24 h) from 1 day before until 1 day after myelographic examination attenuates the clinical signs of depression and fever.

Cytologic analysis and protein concentration of cerebrospinal fluid is usually within reference ranges in horses with CSM. In instances when cerebrospinal fluid analysis is abnormal in horses with CSM, the alterations are consistent with acute spinal cord compression, such as mild xanthochromia or mild increases in protein concentrations. In addition to cytologic evaluation, antibody to equine herpesvirus myeloencephalitis and immunoblot analysis for equine protozoal myeloencephalitis should be determined on cerebrospinal fluid obtained from horses with spinal ataxia.

TREATMENT

Dietary Management

Successful conservative management of CSM has been achieved using the "paced diet" program in foals younger than 1 year of age. The goal of this dietary program is to retard bone growth, enhance bone metabolism, and allow the vertebral canal diameter to enlarge to relieve spinal cord compression. This dietary program is restricted in energy and protein (65–75% NRC recommendations), but maintains balanced vitamin and mineral intake (minimum 100% NRC recommendations). Vitamins A and E are provided at three times NRC recommendations, and selenium is supplemented to 0.3 ppm. Roughage is provided by pasture or low-quality (6–9% crude protein) timothy hay. Dietary regimens are individually formulated according to the age and weight of the foal. Solitary stall confinement is recommended to minimize repetitive spinal cord compression due to dynamic instability. This program of dietary management and restricted exercise has been successful for prevention of neurologic signs in foals with radiographic evidence of CSM and treatment of foals demonstrating clinical signs of CSM. Conservative management consisting of glucocorticoids, dimethyl sulfoxide, and nonsteroidal anti-inflammatory drugs may provide transient improvement in clinical signs; however, spontaneous recovery from CSM without dietary management is not reported. Indiscriminate administration of glucocorticoid preparations to horses with spinal ataxia is not recommended because of the potential of immunosuppressive drugs to exacerbate the clinical progression of equine protozoal myeloencephalitis.

Surgical Treatment

Surgical intervention is the most widely reported treatment for CSM. The goals of surgical intervention for CSM are stabilization of the cervical vertebrae or decompression of the spinal cord. Cervical vertebral interbody fusion provides intervertebral stability for horses with dynamic spinal cord compression. Affected cervical vertebrae are fused in the extended position to provide immediate relief of spinal cord compression and prevent repetitive spinal cord trauma. Seroma formation is common after cervical vertebral interbody fusion; therefore, a pressure bandage is maintained over the surgical site for 2 to 3 weeks to minimize this postoperative complication.

Immediate decompression of static compressive lesions is achieved by subtotal Funkquist type-B dorsal laminectomy in which portions of the dorsal lamina, ligamentum flavum, and joint capsule overlying the compressed site are removed. This procedure effectively decompresses the spinal cord; however, it is associated with significant postoperative complications. Interbody fusion of caudal cervical vertebrae in horses with static compression produces remodeling and atrophy of the articular processes, resulting in delayed decompression of the spinal cord over a period of weeks to months (Fig. 5). Decompression is immediate with subtotal laminectomy; however, because of its relative safety, interbody fusion is selected by some surgeons as the technique of choice for dynamic and static compressive lesions.

Cervical vertebral interbody fusion results in improvement in neurologic status in 44 to 90% of horses with CSM, and 12 to 62% of horses return to athletic function. Subtotal laminectomy results in improvement in neurologic status in 40 to 75% of horses with static compression. Both subtotal laminectomy and cervical vertebral interbody fusion for static compression of the caudal cervical vertebrae are associated with fatal postoperative complications including vertebral body fracture, spinal cord edema, and implant failure. The most important patient factor for determination of postoperative prognosis is duration of clini-

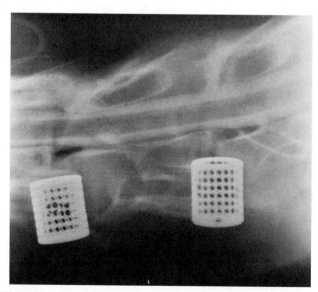

Figure 5. Neutral myelographic view of the fifth, sixth, and seventh cervical vertebrae 5 weeks after ventral stabilization performed for static stenosis (preoperative myelographic examination is shown in Fig. 4). The myelogram was taken with the neck in a neutral position. Spinal cord compression is no longer apparent at the C5-C6 and C6-C7 articulations.

cal signs before surgical intervention; horses with clinical signs less than 1 month prior to surgery are more likely to return to athletic function than are horses with clinical signs of more than 3 months' duration. The number of spinal cord compressive sites and patient age does not appear to affect the long-term outcome of cervical vertebral interbody fusion.

The duration of convalescence and rehabilitation following cervical vertebral interbody fusion is approximately 6 to 12 months. An individual exercise program, which is dependent on capability, projected use, and neurologic status of the horse, should be designed for promotion of muscular strength. Extended exercise at slow speed, including ponying and lunging on inclines, is recommended during rehabilitation. The point at which the horse is competent to return to athletic function following cervical vertebral interbody fusion should be determined by neurologic examination. It is unlikely that significant improvement in neurologic status will occur beyond the 1-year postoperative interval.

Supplemental Readings

Donawick WJ, Mayhew IG, Galligan DT, Green SL, Stanley EK, Osborne J: Recognition and non-surgical management of cervical vertebral malformation in foals. Proc 20th Annu Surgical Forum, 1992, pp 103–105.

Mayhew IG: Tetraparesis, paraparesis and ataxia of the limbs, and episodic weakness. In Mayhew IG (ed.): Large Animal Neurology: A Handbook for Veterinary Clinicians. Philadelphia, Lea & Febiger, 1989, pp 243–333.

Mayhew IG, Donawick WJ, Green SL, Galligan DT, Stanley EK, Osborn J: Diagnosis and prediction of cervical vertebral malformation in Thoroughbred foals based on semi-quantitative radiographic indicators. Equine Vet J 25:435–440, 1993.

Moore BR, Granstom DE, Reed SM: Diagnosis of equine protozoal myeloencephalitis and cervical stenotic myelopathy. Comp Cont Ed Pract Vet 17:419–426, 1995.

Moore BR, Reed SM, Robertson JT: Surgical treatment of cervical stenotic myelopathy in horses: 73 cases (1983–1992). J Am Vet Med Assoc 203:108–112, 1993.

Neuwirth L: Equine myelography. Comp Cont Ed Pract Vet 14:72–79, 1992.

Cauda Equina Syndrome

ROBERT J. MACKAY
Gainesville, Florida

Cauda equina syndrome is a set of abnormal neurologic signs referable to damage of part or all of the cauda equina. There may be urinary and fecal incontinence; analgia of the tail and perianal and perineal skin, rectum, and external genitalia; and paralysis of the tail, anus, and external genitalia. In some cases, involvement of the pelvic limbs is also present. Many possible causes may be responsible for cauda equina syndrome, but most cases are the result of sacrococcygeal vertebral trauma, neuritis of the cauda equina, or equine herpesvirus-1 myeloencephalitis.

For the purposes of this discussion, the cauda equina of horses is that portion of the spinal cord and nerve roots that lies caudal to a transverse plane passing between the third and fourth sacral spinal cord segments. Because of disparate rates of longitudinal growth of the spinal cord and vertebral column, the posterior part of the spinal cord is, in a relative sense, drawn forward within the vertebral canal. As a result, the first three sacral spinal cord segments (S1 to S3) of adult horses lie within the last (L6) lumbar vertebra, and the last two sacral (S4 to S5) and first several coccygeal (caudal) segments are located within the first sacral vertebra. Nerve roots from these caudal segments must course caudally for increasingly long distances within the sacrocaudal vertebral canal before exiting through corresponding intervertebral foramina. Thus, the cauda equina begins at approximately the lumbosacral vertebral junction and includes the terminal segments of the spinal cord (conus medullaris) and the nerve roots of all five sacral and (at least) five coccygeal spinal cord segments.

Sacrococcygeal nerve roots comprising the cauda equina give rise to peripheral nerves and innervate caudal tissues and organs as follows: (1) sciatic and gluteal nerves (S1-S2), which innervate muscles and skin of the pelvic limb not supplied by the femoral or obturator nerves; (2) pudendal and caudal rectal nerves (S2-S4), which supply the external genitalia, are motor to perineal muscles, and sensory to the rectum, anus, perianal and perineal skin to the level of the scrotum or udder; (3) pelvic nerves (S2-S4), which form the pelvic plexus and provide parasympathetic innervation to the bladder, urethra, distal small colon, rectum, anus, and genital erectile tissue; and (4) coccygeal nerves, which innervate skin and muscles of the tail. It should be noted that the sympathetic innervation of the bladder and distal alimentary tract, although intermingled in the pelvic plexus, derives from the first few lumbar spinal cord segments (via the hypogastric nerves) and is therefore not part of the cauda equina.

CLINICAL SIGNS

The initial complaint may be that the horse seems to have a weak tail that is not lifted normally during defecation or urination. Alternatively, the client may first notice frequent dribbling of urine from the penis or vulva of the affected horse, especially during exercise or sudden movement, or signs of constipation and mild abdominal pain. Careful neurologic examination of such horses frequently reveals degrees of the following: (1) weakness of the tail, atrophy of tail muscles, reduced "tail clamp" reflex when the anus or ventral tail area is touched, and reduced sensitivity to painful stimuli over the surface of the tail (resulting from coccygeal nerve root dysfunction); (2) reduced anal tone, evident in some cases as constant dilation of the anus, reduced anal reflex, and insensitivity to painful stimulation of the skin around the anus and perineum, extending up to 20 cm laterally from the anus and down to the udder or scrotum (resulting from pudendal and caudal rectal nerve dysfunction); (3) penile protrusion from the sheath, insensitivity of the penis to painful stimuli, reduced vulvovaginal tone (resulting from pudendal nerve dysfunction); (4) reduced or absent rectal tone and extreme bladder distension noticed during transrectal palpation, and dribbling of urine (resulting from pelvic nerve dysfunction).

Less commonly, there is weakness and ataxia of the pelvic limbs and atrophy of the muscles of the rump and pelvic limbs. These signs are usually mild unless there is involvement of more cranial spinal cord segments. In horses with subtle cauda equina syndrome dysfunction, a reproductive problem may be the presenting sign. For example, breeding stallions may be impotent or occasionally subject to continual penile erections, and affected mares may be prone to retrograde flow and pooling of urine in the uterus. In some horses, there is also a ring of increased or spontaneously painful sensation around the area of reduced cutaneous sensitivity. In these rare cases, the initial complaint may be self-mutilation. In some horses, usually mature males, bladder paralysis occurs without other signs of cauda equina syndrome. It is not known yet whether cauda equina disease is involved in this syndrome.

ETIOLOGY

The cauda equina may be improperly formed during embryonic development (e.g., spina bifida), or may be damaged by injury or compression resulting from fracture, luxation, or malformation of sacrococcygeal vertebrae; abscess; tumor; or hematoma within the caudal part of the vertebral canal; by specific degeneration of cauda equina segments or nerve roots, as with neuritis of the cauda equina or sorghum-Sudan intoxication; by organismal invasion of the caudal spinal cord or nerve roots, as occurs with equine herpesvirus-1 (EHV-1) myeloencephalitis, equine protozoal myeloencephalitis (EPM), meningitis, rabies, or aberrant parasite migration; or by other destruction of the caudal spinal cord, as with tumors of nervous tissue, infarct, or vascular anomaly and malformation.

Trauma

The most common and most important cause of cauda equina syndrome is trauma. Sacral or coccygeal vertebral fracture and luxation may occur as a result of breeding injuries, or when a horse falls over backward or otherwise falls awkwardly, backs violently into a wall, scrapes under an obstruction such as the top part of Dutch doors, or has its tail jerked vigorously or repeatedly. The amount of damage sustained by the cauda equina depends upon the location and severity of fracture or luxation. Fractures of the first two sacral vertebrae may injure all the roots of the cauda equina, including those to the sciatic and gluteal nerves, and thus cauda equina syndrome with pelvic limb signs is possible. Fracture of the third or fourth sacral

vertebrae is more likely to cause cauda equina syndrome without pelvic limb signs, whereas fracture of the fifth sacral or any coccygeal vertebra should cause signs only in the tail. The cauda equina may suffer temporary concussion and neuropraxia; nerve roots may degenerate distal to the site of trauma but may be capable of regrowth, or they may be completely and permanently transected at the fracture site. Signs of neurologic damage should be immediate; however, continued damage at an unstable fracture site, or the formation of epidural hematoma, abscess, strangulating scar tissue, or exuberant callus may cause cauda equina damage at some interval after the original injury.

Neuritis of the Cauda Equina

Neuritis of the cauda equina is a rare condition that appears to be associated with autoimmune response against the sacrococcygeal nerve roots. Affected horses usually are mature or aged; however, the disease was confirmed in a yearling Saddlebred filly. The signs of neuritis of the cauda equina appear insidiously and invariably are progressive over weeks to months. All components of severe cauda equina syndrome, including mild pelvic limb weakness, ultimately are manifested. Signs may be symmetrical or asymmetrical. Despite predilection for sacrococcygeal nerve roots, nerve roots at other locations also may be affected. In addition to cauda equina syndrome, some horses have evidence of cranial nerve involvement, such as masseter atrophy due to trigeminal nerve injury; facial paralysis as a result of facial nerve damage; or head tilt, nystagmus, and staggering gait when the vestibular nerve is involved. These signs of cranial nerve dysfunction may appear suddenly, and then wax and wane. A few horses have been seen in which cranial nerve signs have occurred without cauda equina syndrome. In recognition of the potential for widespread involvement of nerve roots, the disease is also called *polyneuritis equi*.

Sorghum-Sudan Grass Toxicity

Cauda equina syndrome in horses grazing on sorghum species or on sorghum-Sudan grasses has been reported in horses in western and southwestern United States. In addition to classic signs of cauda equina syndrome, weakness and ataxia of pelvic limbs are prominent. The toxic principle in sorghum-Sudan is not known, but causal roles have been suggested for both cyanogenic and lathyrogenic glycosides. Outbreaks of cauda equina syndrome may occur with morbidity of up to 25%.

Epidural Abscess/Neoplasia

Epidural abscessation in the sacrococcygeal vertebral canal usually is a complication of vertebral osteomyelitis or septic discospondylitis. Any of a variety of blood-borne bacteria may seed into the vertebrae, especially into those of young horses. *Rhodococcus equi* may be particularly prone to causing the condition in foals. Cauda equina damage is the result of extradural compression and inflammation of the nerve roots of the cauda equina. Extradural tumors such as lymphosarcoma, malignant melanoma, neurofibroma, and plasma cell myeloma may compress the cauda equina. Accidental injection of caustic substances or bacteria into the coccygeal epidural space likewise could cause cauda equina syndrome. In very rare instances, inflammation of the cauda equina is caused by caudal meningitis. *Listeria monocytogenes* and *Cryptococcus neoformans* have been implicated in this condition in horses.

EHV-1 Myeloencephalitis

Signs of cauda equina syndrome usually accompany EHV-1 myeloencephalitis and occasionally may be seen in horses with equine protozoal myelitis or rabies. In most cases, signs in addition to those attributable to cauda equina dysfunction are seen in horses with any of these diseases (see detailed discussion elsewhere in this section).

DIAGNOSIS

In addition to suggestive aspects of history and signalment, careful clinical and physical examination can at least reduce the number of options that need be considered in a case of cauda equina syndrome. Observation and palpation of the top line of the rump and transrectal palpation of the ventral surface of the sacral and first coccygeal vertebrae may reveal discontinuities or swellings suggestive of sacral or coccygeal fracture and luxation. The examiner must be careful to distinguish fracture displacement from the projection found normally along the ventral aspect of the sacrum. Severe ataxia and weakness of the limbs indicate additional involvement of spinal cord segments cranial to the cauda equina and are more consistent with infectious myelitides (EHV-1, equine protozoal myelitis, rabies) than with neuritis of the cauda equina.

Special imaging techniques can be used to diagnose sacrococcygeal fracture and luxation. Radiography, with or without epidural contrast material, osseous phase nuclear scintigraphy, and transrectal ultrasound examination all may aid diagnosis; however, the equipment and expertise necessary for these techniques often is found only at referral institutions.

Analysis of cerebrospinal fluid (CSF) from the lumbosacral site is useful in many cases of cauda equina syndrome. Horses with neuritis of the cauda equina or equine protozoal myelitis may have mild to moderate increases in protein (>80–150 mg/dl) and nucleated cell (>8–200 cells/μl) concentration. In both cases, the cells are mostly mononuclear, but some granulocytes may be seen. These possibilities can be differentiated by testing CSF for *Sarcocystis neurona* antibody by immunoblot test. Cerebrospinal fluid from horses with EHV-1 myeloencephalitis is usually bright yellow with very high protein concentration (>200 mg/dl) and normal nucleated cell count. In sacrococcygeal trauma, CSF may be normal to bloody in gross appearance, usually without an increase in nucleated cell count. Because the meninges end at the level of the second sacral vertebra, fractures behind this site are less likely to cause changes in CSF than are more cranial fractures. Epidural abscesses are outside the meninges, and thus inflammation at this site is, at most, mildly reflected in the CSF. In contrast, meningitis and parasite migration should cause a dramatic increase in nucleated cell count, particularly of granulocytes.

With the exception of bacterial meningitis and epidural abscess, in which hematologic evidence of inflammation is expected, results of routine blood work in most cases of cauda equina syndrome are unremarkable. Strong supportive evidence for neuritis of the cauda equina is the finding of serum P2 antibody. P2 is a myelin protein of peripheral nerves, and presence of antibody had high sensitivity and specificity for the diagnosis of neuritis of the cauda equina in a small study. Currently, this test is not available commercially.

Epidural lavage, performed by flush and aspiration of 20-ml amounts of sterile saline via an epidural needle, may yield evidence of trauma or inflammation. Coccygeal nerve roots also can be biopsied at this site by use of blind needle biopsy or arthroscope and examined by histopathology sample for changes of neuritis of the cauda equina.

Needle electromyography of horses affected for at least 2 weeks can help define the extent of muscle denervation. Nerve conduction studies within the sacrococcygeal vertebral canal also are possible and provide some prognostic information (see later).

TREATMENT

As an adjunct to treatment of the underlying disease, nursing care is critical in horses with cauda equina syndrome. Horses with paralyzed bladders need to have urine drained at least twice daily by clean urethral catheterization. In some situations, indwelling urethral catheters can be maintained until bladder function is restored. If, after initial catheterization, there still is palpable doughy filling of the bladder because of retained sediment, the bladder should be irrigated with water via a large-bore urethral catheter such as a clean stomach tube to siphon off excessive quantities of crystalline debris, usually calcium carbonate. Antibiotics such as trimethoprim-sulfadiazine may be given to reduce the chance of cystitis, and ammonium chloride powder (1–2 oz p.o. b.i.d.) can be given to adult horses to acidify the urine and reduce sediment formation. If the rectum is impacted by feces, manual evacuations may be necessary and fecal softeners or lubricants such as mineral oil may need to be fed along with a diet of reduced bulk, such as a complete pelleted feed. Careful attention must be given to cleaning and application of barrier cream in areas soiled or scalded by urine and feces. In cases of permanent cauda equina syndrome, the tail can be amputated to simplify this part of nursing care. Administration of a parasympathomimetic drug such as bethanecol (0.05–0.1 mg/kg p.o. b.i.d. or t.i.d.) may stimulate bladder and rectal evacuation in horses with cauda equina syndrome. Effectiveness of this treatment varies greatly among horses; in general, foals appear to respond more efficiently to bethanecol than do adults.

Horses with traumatic cauda equina syndrome usually are treated medically, as is explained under peripheral nerve injuries (see page 318). Anti-inflammatory therapy with combinations of dimethyl sulfoxide, corticosteroids, and nonsteroidal anti-inflammatory drugs can be given for the first 1 to 2 weeks. If the injury was primarily concussive, 2 weeks is sufficient for reversal of neuropraxia or for remyelination. Axons may regrow in intact nerve sheaths at a rate of about 1 inch/month for a maximum of about 6 inches. In practical terms, if no improvement is seen within

2 months, permanent neurologic dysfunction is likely. Measurement of the rate of nerve conduction between a stimulating electrode at the lumbosacral space and an intercoccygeal recording electrode has been described and can help detect cauda equina transection shortly after the injury. Surgical decompression of the cauda equina by dorsal- or hemilaminectomy has been described. In adult horses, the tuber sacrale of the pelvis interferes with the approach to the first and possibly the second sacral vertebra, but decompression of the caudal part of the sacrum is possible. In foals, fractures may be reduced and stabilized with plates and screws. Surgical exploration of the vertebral canal also is indicated in horses, usually foals, with cauda equina syndrome resulting from sacral osteomyelitis and epidural abscess. After laminectomy to decompress the cauda equina, the epidural space may be drained and lavaged and diseased bone removed.

Attempts to treat horses with cauda equina syndrome caused by neuritis of the cauda equina have been universally unsuccessful. Vigorous therapy for autoimmune disease, including corticosteroid therapy and cytotoxic drugs such as cyclophosphamide and azathioprine seems rational, but nerve root degeneration apparently is irreversible by the time of initial clinical presentation. An exception may be the form of polyneuritis equi in which cranial nerve signs predominate. In a few horses of this type, effective control apparently has been achieved with immunosuppressive therapy.

Complete resolution of cauda equina syndrome is likely in horses that survive EHV-1 myeloencephalitis and is possible in horses treated appropriately for equine protozoal myelitis. Some improvement can be expected if horses with sorghum-Sudan-associated cauda equina syndrome are removed to nontoxic pasture. Cauda equina syndrome due to neoplasia or rabies is not treatable.

Supplemental Readings

Chaffin MK, Honnas CM, Crabill MR, Schneiter HL, Brumbaugh GW, Briner RP: Cauda equina syndrome, diskospondylitis, and a paravertebral abscess caused by *Rhodococcus equi* in a foal. J Am Vet Med Assoc 206:215–220, 1995.

Collatos C, Allen D, Chambers J, Henry M: Surgical treatment of sacral fracture in a horse. J Am Vet Med Assoc 198:877–879, 1991.

Fordyce PS, Edington N, Bridges GC, Wright JA, Edwards GB: Use of an ELISA in the differential diagnosis of cauda equina neuritis and other equine neuropathies. Equine Vet J 19:55–59, 1987.

Mayhew IG: Urinary bladder distention, dilated anus, and atonic tail: The cauda equina syndrome. *In* Large Animal Neurology. Philadelphia, Lea & Febiger, 1989, pp 349–357.

Peripheral Neuropathy

LINDA L. BLYTHE
Corvallis, Oregon

Peripheral neuropathy is not uncommon in horses. One or more peripheral nerves arising from spinal nerves and cranial nerves may be affected. The dysfunction of any part of a neuron whose axons innervate a skeletal muscle fiber is called *lower motor neuron disease*. The cell bodies for these neurons are located within the ventral horn throughout the spinal cord and in select motor nuclei in the brainstem, whereas their axons form the motor component of the peripheral nerves. A large number of traumatic, metabolic, toxic, degenerative, congenital, parasitic, infectious, genetic, or neoplastic disorders may affect lower motor neurons within either the central or peripheral nervous system, but these disorders can usually be differentiated and localized by the neurologic examination.

Peripheral neuropathy is often unilateral, affecting one limb. However, peripheral nerve dysfunction due to botulism, tick paralysis, lead poisoning, and idiopathic polyneuritis are exceptions and may involve multiple nerves or neuromuscular junctions. Dysfunction of lower motor neurons within the brachial or pelvic enlargement of the spinal cord is often seen with equine protozoal myeloencephalitis and neuritis of the cauda equina or in the diffuse spinal cord disease called *equine motor neuron disease*. All result in peripheral neuropathy due to axonal die-back.

Stringhalt is a spastic intermittent hyperflexion of one or more hindlimbs that may be a result of peripheral nerve trauma. However, many cases in the United States, Australia, and New Zealand have been associated epidemiologically with ingestion of *Hypochoeris radicata* (false dandelion). The site of the toxic action of this common weed is unknown, but chemical excitation or dysinhibition of lower motor neurons at the spinal cord level may occur. Fungal toxins have been postulated as causative, but no evidence to date for this is in the literature. Shivers, an idiopathic neuromuscular disease seen often in draft breeds of horses, may also be a central nervous system disorder. This chapter focuses primarily on methods of detecting and localizing peripheral neuropathy and on therapy.

CLINICAL EVALUATION

Most of the major peripheral nerves except the olfactory, optic, and vestibulocochlear cranial nerves have mixed function with both sensory and motor components. This fact enables veterinarians to localize lesions to one or more peripheral nerves by (1) evaluating voluntary motor function or its loss by observation of the gait; (2) testing the sensory perceptions of touch and pain; (3) testing reflexes including muscle tone; and (4) detecting neurogenic muscle atrophy. All of these can be evaluated in the field by conducting the standard neurologic examination and, in select cases, by utilization of electronic neurodiagnostic techniques. The latter include electromyography (EMG), nerve conduction velocity, and evoked potentials, which are discussed later. These tools may provide localization and prognostic information and are especially useful in cases of partial denervation or compressive neuropathies. However, the focus of this chapter is on those diagnostic techniques that can be used by the practitioner in the field.

Localization of Peripheral Nerve Lesions by Gait Evaluation and Motor Function

Lameness or obvious motor paresis or paralysis (i.e., frank dragging of a limb) is often the first indication to a horse owner that the horse may have a peripheral nerve dysfunction. Observation of the gait at a walk and trot, on tight turns, and during backing allows a veterinarian to assess the motor function of the major muscle groups that flex and extend the limbs. For the thoracic limb, these include the following: (1) the muscles innervated primarily by the radial nerve, which extend the elbow, carpus, and digit; (2) the muscles that are innervated by the musculocutaneous nerve, which extend the shoulder and flex the elbow; and (3) muscles innervated primarily by two nerves, the axillary and the suprascapular nerves, that serve to stabilize the shoulder joint. Dysfunction of the radial nerve results in a "dropped elbow," which is inability to fix the limb and bear weight and dragging of the toe. With musculocutaneous nerve dysfunction, the most obvious deficit is the inability to flex the elbow, resulting in the horse lifting the limb at the level of the shoulder to flip the carpus and foot forward during a walk. Backing a horse emphasizes the inability to flex the elbow and, as the horse attempts to move the limb caudally, the foot drags on the ground. The muscles innervated primarily by the two nerves that stabilize the shoulder joint are the supraspinatus and the infraspinatus muscles, which are innervated by the suprascapular nerve, and the deltoideus muscle, which is innervated by the axillary nerve. When either of these nerves is dysfunctional, the shoulder joint rotates laterally during the weightbearing phase of the gait. Direct trauma to the point of the shoulder can result in a loss of the suprascapular nerve function, classically called *sweeney*.

In the pelvic limb, the following major muscle groups are essential to the gait: (1) the quadriceps femoris group that serve to flex the hip and extend the stifle, which is innervated by the femoral nerve; (2) the adductor muscles on the inside of the limb, which are innervated by the obturator nerve; and (3) the muscles that extend the hip and flex the stifle (i.e., the biceps femoris, semimembranous, and semitendinous, which are innervated by the ischiatic (sciatic) nerve. Dysfunction of the femoral nerve results in an inability to lock the stifle joint and bear weight either while walking or standing. Obturator nerve dysfunction results in the limb being carried laterally, resulting in a wide-base gait and stance. Dysfunction of the ischiatic nerve involves paresis or paralysis of its innervated muscles and those of its two major branches—the fibular (peroneal) and the tibial nerves. With dysfunction of the fibular nerve, the horse loses the ability to flex the hock and extend the digit, resulting in a dragging of the toe. Tibial nerve dysfunction affects the extenders of the hock and flexors of the digit, resulting in a dropped hock during

the weightbearing phase of the gait. Table 1 lists the innervation of the major muscles of the limbs.

In acute traumatic injuries of the nerves to the limbs, the presence of these gait deficits relative to the major muscle groups is the key to diagnosis of a peripheral nerve injury. Because, classically, peripheral nerve injuries are unilateral, the other three limbs should be functionally normal. In the presence of lameness or paresis of a limb, it is critical to evaluate all four limbs because asymmetrical spinal cord lesions are not uncommon. In addition, although the initial clinical signs can be localized to one limb, progression of a spinal cord problem over the period of days to weeks can result in other limbs becoming clinically affected. This frequently occurs in horses affected with equine protozoal myeloencephalitis. These functional determinations are essential because the treatment of peripheral nerve lesions is different from that for specific spinal cord diseases such as equine protozoal myeloencephalitis.

Dysfunction of cranial nerves can be the result of trauma or the aforementioned multiple etiologies. Facial neuropathy is one of the most common dysfunctions and is characterized by an inability to shut the eye and by lack of tear production, often resulting in a corneal ulcer; a muzzle twisted away from the side of the lesion; a flaccid buccinator muscle resulting in food accumulating in the buccal cavity; and a drooped, paretic, or paralyzed ear. Trauma to the side of the face spares the facial nerve branches that innervate the ear and eye. Petrous temporal bone fractures associated with temporohyoid osteoarthropathy commonly affect the facial nerve as it passes through the petrous part of the temporal bone in the inner and middle ear, as do skull fractures involving basisphenoid bone. In both cases, clinical signs of vestibulocochlear nerve dysfunction are often present.

The muscles that move the eye are innervated by the oculomotor, trochlear, and abducens nerves. When eye muscle paralysis is evident, separation of the responsible cranial nerves can be done by testing as follows. Oculomotor nerve dysfunction causes marked inability to move the eyeball within the orbit, ptosis of the eyelid, and a dilated pupil. The rare trochlear dysfunction leads to a dorsolateral rotation of the eye, resulting in the medial aspect of the horizonal pupil being elevated dorsally. Abducens nerve dysfunction results in a medial deviation of the eye within the orbit and an inability to retract the eye with the retractor bulbi muscle during testing of the corneal reflex.

The mandibular branch of the maxillary nerve innervates the chewing muscles, primarily the masseter and the temporalis. It is rare to see bilateral dysfunction and dropped jaw in horses, as occurs in dogs. The most common indicator of dysfunction of this nerve is a history of difficulty eating and muscle atrophy.

Idiopathic die-back of the left recurrent laryngeal nerve originating from the vagus nerve is common in Thoroughbreds and Quarterhorses and presents as a clinical condition called *roaring*, which is discussed elsewhere in this text. Peripheral branches of the glossopharyngeal, vagus, and hypoglossal nerves may be compressed or inflamed with guttural pouch infections. This results in difficulties in swallowing and dysfunction of the tongue muscles.

Peripheral neuropathies give rise to denervation atrophy

TABLE 1. PRIMARY INNERVATION OF MAJOR MUSCLES OF THE LIMBS IN THE MAJORITY OF HORSES*

	Muscle	Nerve	Spinal Cord Segments
Thoracic limb			
Chest	Pectoral	Pectoral nerves	C7, 8
Shoulder	Supraspinatus	Suprascapular	C6, 7
	Infraspinatus	Suprascapular	C6, 7
	Deltoideus	Axillary	C7, 8
Elbow	Biceps brachii	Musculocutaneous	C7, 8
	Brachialis	Musculocutaneous	C7, 8
	Triceps brachii	Radial	C8, T1
Carpus and digit extenders	Extensor carpi radialis	Radial	C8, T1
	Common digital extensor	Radial	C8, T1
	Lateral digital extensor	Radial	C8, T1
	Ulnaris lateralis	Radial	C8, T1
Carpus and digit flexors	Flexor carpi radialis	Median	C8, T1, 2
	Superficial digital flexor	Ulnar	T1, 2
	Deep digital flexor	Median and ulnar	C8, T1, 2
	Flexor carpi ulnaris	Ulnar	T1, 2
Pelvic limb			
Hip	Gluteals	Gluteal	L5, 6, S1, 2
Limb adductors	Adductor	Obturator	L4, 5
	Gracilis	Obturator	L4, 5
Stifle	Quadriceps	Femoral	L4, 5, ± L3
	Biceps femoris	Ischiatic	L5, 6, S1, ±2
		Caudal gluteal	S1, S2
Hock extenders and digit flexors	Semimembranous	Ischiatic	L5, 6, S1, ±2
	Semitendinous	Ischiatic	L5, 6, S1, ±2
		Caudal gluteal	S1, S2
	Gastrocnemius	Tibial	L5, 6, S1, ±2
	Superficial digital flexor	Tibial	L5, 6, S1, ±2
	Deep digital flexor	Tibial	L5, 6, S1, ±2
Hock flexors and digit extenders	Cranial tibial	Fibular	L5, 6, S1, ±2
	Long digital extensor	Fibular	L5, 6, S1, ±2
	Lateral digital extensor	Fibular	L5, 6, S1, ±2

*Adapted from Ghoshal NC: Spinal nerves. *In* Getty R (ed): Anatomy of the Domestic Animals, ed 5. Philadelphia, WB Saunders, 1975, pp 665–668.

of the innervated muscles, which is an observation that facilitates the diagnosis of peripheral nerve dysfunction. As much as one half of total muscle mass can be lost within 2 weeks of total denervation. Partial denervation can also cause a reduction in muscle mass, but this may be confused after several weeks with disuse atrophy. An EMG evaluation definitively differentiates these two conditions, being abnormal with denervation and normal with muscle atrophy due to disuse.

Localization of Peripheral Nerve Lesions by Sensory Evaluation

Sensory Maps

The sensory innervation of the skin of the horse has been determined by the use of electrophysiologic mapping of the sensory zones of each peripheral nerve. This technique provided an understanding of the cutaneous areas that have multiple innervation (i.e., overlap zones) and those areas of skin that have a single nerve supply (i.e., autonomous zones). These maps of innervation are useful to the practitioner when evaluating the presence and extent of sensory loss, especially in common traumatic brachial plexus injuries. Figure 1 depicts the cutaneous innervation of the thoracic limb and Figure 2 illustrates the five autonomous zones present in the forelimb.

Testing Cutaneous Areas

When peripheral nerves undergo compression due to edema or swelling from trauma, there is an order of axon loss relative to the diameter of the nerve fiber (i.e., the bigger the fiber the more sensitive it is to compression). In a peripheral nerve with both motor and sensory function, the order of loss is first the large motor nerves to the skeletal muscles, followed by the nerves transmitting touch, and, last, the smallest nerves transmitting pain sensation. These facts coupled with knowledge from the sensory maps allow a veterinarian to determine how many nerves are affected and the extent of the damage. If the nerve or nerves are totally transected or have their spinal roots avulsed, all motor and sensory function of the innervated muscles and skin will be absent. If nerves are compressed by post-traumatic edema or a hematoma (e.g., brachial plexus trauma), motor function may be lost, but the presence of perception of touch or pain indicates that the nerves are intact.

When a horse with suspected peripheral nerve damage is examined, initial sensory evaluation is best conducted with light touches of the skin with a very sharp pencil. Starting at the shoulder joint, the clinican should lightly touch the skin from left to right at intervals of 2 cm over the lateral aspects of the brachium and over the skin of the entire limb. If an area of loss of perception to this

in the size of the area desensitized to touch indicates that recovery is occurring and is evident in most cases before the return of motor function.

If perception of both pain and touch is absent, the prognosis is more serious but not hopeless. In these cases, daily retesting for return of the pain sensation is the best monitor of return of nerve function. Persistent loss of pain perception over a week indicates that the nerve has undergone severe damage and that reinnervation may have to coincide with regrowth of the axons. This rate is approximately 1 mm/day or 1 inch/month. The outlining of areas of sensory loss to both touch and pain is also a practical and educational tool for the client to use in monitoring response to therapy.

Localization of Peripheral Nerve Lesions by Reflex Evaluation

Reflex evaluation allows testing of a "hard-wired-in" neural pathway that includes a sensory nerve, a motor nerve, and all interneurons that connect them in the central nervous system. Loss of reflexes is a characteristic of lower

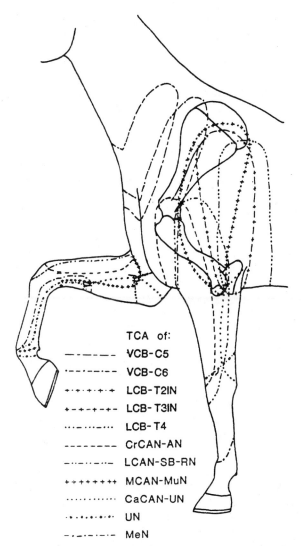

Figure 1. Typical cutaneous areas of the sensory nerves of the thoracic limb as determined by electrophysiologic mapping. Sensory nerves are keyed as follows: VCB-C5 is the ventral cutaneous branch of cervical nerve 5; VCB-C6 is the ventral cutaneous branch of cervical nerve 6; LCB-T2IN is the lateral cutaneous branch of the intercostal nerve from thoracic spinal nerve 2; LCB-T3IN is the lateral cutaneous branch of the intercostal nerve from thoracic spinal nerve 3; LCB-T4 is the lateral cutaneous branch of the thoracic spinal nerve 4; CrCAN-AN is the cranial cutaneous antibrachial nerve of the axillary nerve; LCAN-SB-RN is the lateral cutaneous antibrachial nerve of the superficial branch of the radial nerve; MCAN-MuN is the medial cutaneous antibrachial nerve of the musculocutaneous nerve; CaCAN-UN is the caudal cutaneous antibrachial nerve of the ulnar nerve; UN is the ulnar nerve; and MeN is the median nerve. Note the large areas of nerve overlap where skin is innervated by two or more peripheral nerves.

touch is identified, the clinician may take a felt-tip pen or white poster paint and outline the area with sensory loss (Fig. 3). To do this, a spot is marked wherever there is a difference between the touch being perceived and not perceived. Thereafter, a pair of hemostat forceps can be used to pinch the skin within the area that has a deficit of touch perception. If touch is lost but pain is present, it is a good prognostic sign that the nerve fiber is intact and still transmitting sensation. This area can be subsequently retested each day after treatment is instituted. A decrease

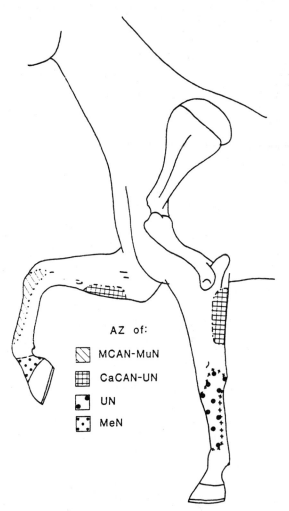

Figure 2. Autonomous zones of the thoracic limb. These are defined as the cutaneous areas supplied by only one sensory nerve. MCAN-MuN is the medial cutaneous antibrachial nerve of the musculocutaneous nerve; CaCAN-UN is the caudal cutaneous antibrachial nerve of the ulnar nerve; UN is the dorsal branch of the ulnar nerve, and MeN is the median nerve.

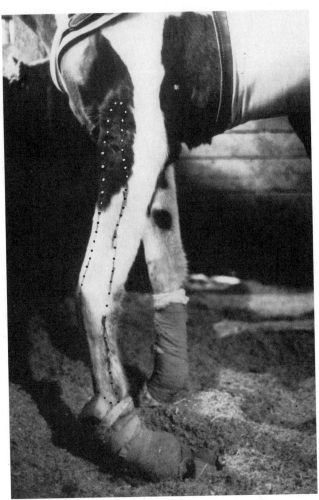

Figure 3. Photograph of a yearling Paint gelding supported by a sling 7 days after a traumatic blow to the shoulder. He is unable to lift the limb or bear weight, and no fractures are radiographically evident. The area of the forelimb contained within the dotted lines had lost both touch and deep pain sensation. No change occurred after 2 weeks of corticosteroid therapy and the horse was euthanized. A large hematoma and tear of the nerves were present in the brachial plexus.

motor neuron disease, peripheral or central. The palpebral and corneal reflexes test the sensory branch of the trigeminal nerve and the motor components of both the facial (closing of eye) and abducens (retraction of the eye) nerves as well as the function of interconnecting neurons in the pons and medulla. The induction of swallowing and coughing tests the glossopharyngeal and vagus nerves and the medulla. A normal slap test results in adduction of the laryngeal arytenoid cartilage following a slap to the contralateral withers and tests the recurrent laryngeal nerve. Focal cervical, cutaneous trunci, and anal sphincter reflexes also test discrete nerve pathways that involve peripheral nerves as well as interconnecting spinal cord or brainstem neurons. Reflex contraction of the anal sphincter when touched tests the caudal sacral spinal cord segments as well as the caudal rectal nerves. Assessment of muscle tone of the limb muscles and tail tests tonic stretch reflex pathways and helps localize a lower motor neuron lesion if flaccid muscle tone is detected. Loss of one or more reflexes allows the veterinarian to localize a problem to and within the nervous system.

NEURODIAGNOSTIC EVALUATION OF THE NERVOUS SYSTEM

With use of EMG, the clinician can detect evidence of either total or partial denervation by observing abnormal electrical potentials, such as fibrillation potentials or positive sharp waves. However, 5 or more days need to have passed since the time of denervation for the abnormal potentials to develop. Other abnormal EMG activity such as "dive bomber" potentials and bizarre high-frequency discharge in resting muscles can indicate presence of either a neuropathy or myopathy such as myotonia. Muscle biopsy and histochemistry tests are useful tools in sorting out and documenting denervation as well as genetic, metabolic, and parasitic diseases of muscles.

Nerve conduction velocities are frequently used in human and small animal hospitals to document total or partial loss of axons in the peripheral nerves or to detect myopathies. Normal nerve conduction velocities have been reported for both sensory and motor nerves in horses, but because of the equipment needed and scarcity of research showing its usefulness in the horse, this diagnostic technique is rarely used. Use of sensory evoked potentials in localizing peripheral or central nervous system lesions is still a research tool.

TREATMENT

Treatment of peripheral neuropathies is dependent on the inciting etiology. Traumatic lesions are the most common, with stretching, tearing, and inflammation of myelinated and unmyelinated nerves. Edema or pressure can cause large-diameter motor and sensory axons to demyelinate. Resolution of the inflammation allows for remyelination to occur, a process that commonly takes 1 to 2 weeks. Cold water therapy, nonsteroidal anti-inflammatory drugs such as phenylbutazone (4 mg/kg b.i.d.) or flunixin meglumine (1.1 mg/kg IM, IV, or p.o. s.i.d. or divided b.i.d.), corticosteroids such as dexamethasone (0.05 mg/kg IV or IM b.i.d.), and dimethyl sulfoxide (DMSO) (1 g/kg IV or via stomach tube s.i.d. or b.i.d.) may be used to reduce inflammation for the initial 2 to 3 days.

Radiographs may be indicated to rule out concurrent fractures. If loss of motor function and sensory perception of touch and pain persist beyond 2 weeks, axonal disruption is probable and optimal nerve regrowth rates can be estimated at 1 mm/day or 1 inch/month. Initial reduction of an area of sensory loss followed in 2 to 3 weeks by a increase in the size of the same area indicates scar tissue obstruction of nerve function during the healing process. In these cases, surgical exploration may be indicated, depending on the anatomic location of the nerves involved.

Surgical exploration may also be indicated if complete transection of a nerve is suspected. In horses affected by sweeney due to traumatic suprascapular nerve paralysis, lack of improvement after 4 to 6 weeks may indicate the need for surgical freeing of the nerve from scar tissue. A surgical notch in the cranial part of the scapula under the nerve reduces tension and facilitates the reparative process. It is important in these cases to test for sensory perception because the suprascapular nerve does not contain sensory fibers. Thus, loss of perception of touch or pain to any part of the affected limb implicates dysfunction of other nerves from the brachial plexus.

Surgical transection of nerves for long-term relief of pain can result in a painful mass of regenerating axons called a neuroma. Most commonly seen following a palmar digital neurectomy, neuromas often need surgical removal. Recurrences are not uncommon.

Suggested Readings

Blythe LL: Neurological examination of the horse. Vet Clin North Am Equine Pract 3(2):255–281, 1987.

Blythe LL, Engel HN, Rowe KE: Comparison of sensory nerve conduction velocities in horses versus ponies. Am J Vet Res 49(12):2138–2142, 1988.

Blythe LL, Kitchell RL: Electrophysiologic studies of the thoracic limb of the horse. Am J Vet Res 43(9):1511–1524, 1982.

Blythe LL, Kitchell RL, Holliday TA, Johnson RD: Sensory nerve conduc-

tion velocities in forelimb of ponies. Am J Vet Res 44(8):1419–1426, 1983.

Cummings JP, de Lahunta, A, Timoney JF: Neuritis of the cauda equina: A chronic polyradiculoneuritis in the horse. Acta Neuropathol Berl 46:17–24, 1979.

Dyson S, Taylor P, Whitwell K: Femoral nerve paralysis after general anaesthesia. Equine Vet J 20:376–379, 1988.

Huntington PJ, Jeffcott LB, Friend SCE, Luff AR, Finkelstein DI, Flynn RJ: Australian stringhalt: (B) epidemiological, clinical and neurological investigations. Equine Vet J 21:266–273, 1989.

Kaneps AJ, Blythe LL: Diagnosis and treatment of brachial plexus trauma resulting from dystocia in a calf. Comp Cont Ed Pract Vet 8(1):64–67, 1986.

Mayhew IG: Tetraparesis, paraparesis and ataxia of the limbs, and episodic weakness. *In* Animal Neurology. Philadelphia, Lea & Febiger, 1989, pp 243–333.

Mohammed HO, Cummings JF, Divers TJ, de la Rua-Domenech R, de Lahunta A: Epidemiology of equine motor neuron disease. Vet Res 25(2–3):275–278, 1994.

Wheeler SJ: Effect of age on sensory nerve conduction velocity in the horse. Res Vet Sci 48:141–144, 1990.

Degenerative Myeloencephalopathy

LINDA L. BLYTHE

A. MORRIE CRAIG

Corvallis, Oregon

Equine degenerative myeloencephalopathy is an idiopathic, diffuse, degenerative disease of the spinal cord and selected parts of the brain in young horses that results in gait deficits. Since equine degenerative myeloencephalopathy was first described in 1977, it has become recognized as one of the major causes of ataxia in young horses in the United States. The reported prevalence of the disease varies throughout the United States. In the initial 1978 survey of 100 "wobblers" in New York State, 24% of horses had this disease. A more recent 1990 histopathologic study of 287 ataxic horses in New York State placed the incidence at 49%. On the West Coast, there appears to be a lesser incidence of disease, with Oregon reporting a 22% incidence of confirmed diagnoses of equine degenerative myeloencephalopathy in 280 wobblers in 1992. Although not proved, development of the disease appears to be associated with an increased dependence on hay or pelleted feed in areas where horses do not have regular access to pasture. In an epidemiologic survey, dirt lot confinement and exposure to either insecticides or wood preservatives were identified as risk factors associated with a higher incidence of equine degenerative myeloencephalopathy. A familial predisposition has been identified in Standardbreds, Appaloosas, Morgans, Arabians, Peruvian Pasos, Thoroughbreds, and Norwegian Fjord horses.

Vitamin E deficiencies during the first year of life have been postulated to be a causative factor in the development of equine degenerative myeloencephalopathy. The accumulating evidence that supports vitamin E as a factor in the pathogenesis of this disease is as follows: (1) the neuropathology is similar to that in induced vitamin E deficiencies in experimental animals and documented clinical cases of human vitamin E deficiency syndromes; (2) low serum vitamin E values in a number of horses is present during the early stages of the disease; (3) supplementation of offspring of families of horses with known equine degenerative myeloencephalopathy has reduced the incidence of the disease or eliminated it; (4) experimental studies have documented an improvement in clinical signs in horses with equine degenerative myeloencephalopathy given massive doses (6000–9000 IU/day) of vitamin E; and (5) plasma α-tocopherol values serially monitored in foals sired by an Appaloosa stallion with equine degenerative myeloencephalopathy from a family of horses with a high incidence of the disease were found to be significantly lower ($P<0.001$) compared with control foals from 6 weeks to 10 months of age. Eight of the nine Appaloosa foals developed clinically detectable ataxia during this period. The mechanism for the low plasma α-tocopherol levels in these horses remains speculative. Oral vitamin E absorption tests have ruled out gastrointestinal malabsorption as a cause.

CLINICAL SIGNS

The onset of this disease is most commonly insidious and progressive, although some owners report an acute onset. Most commonly, horses younger than 2 years old are at risk. The first indication of the disease in horses between 4 and 8 months of age is often a clumsiness that progresses to varying degrees of sensory and motor ataxia. Gait deficits consist of symmetrical ataxia, paresis, and hypometria affecting all four limbs. The degree of involvement can vary from minor deficits in the thoracic limbs with markedly affected pelvic limbs to equal severity in all four limbs. Although the disease is progressive, quadriplegia rarely develops, and clinical signs appear to plateau once the animal matures when it reaches 2 years of age. In some animals, especially in the latter stages of the disease, decreased focal cervical, cervicofacial, cutaneous trunci, and slap test reflexes may be demonstrated. Hyporeflexia of the cutaneous trunci reflex reflects dysfunction primarily of the thoracic segments of the spinal cord. When present, this abnormality can help differentiate this disease from cervical stenotic myelopathy, because equine degenerative myeloencephalopathy is a diffuse disease involving the entire spinal cord, whereas cervical stenotic myelopathy is a focal compressive lesion of the cervical spinal cord. Thus the latter often results in hyperreflexia of the cutaneous trunci reflex.

DIAGNOSIS

No definitive ante mortem method exists for diagnosis of equine degenerative myeloencephalopathy, although the index of suspicion should be high if there has been a familial history of this disease or if signs of hyporeflexia are present. Young horses that present with acute signs of ataxia need radiographic evaluation to rule out traumatic, congenital, or developmental (cervical stenotic myelopathy) bony diseases, and a cerebrospinal fluid (CSF) analysis to rule out equine protozoal myeloencephalitis and the neurologic form of equine herpes virus I myeloencephalitis. In equine degenerative myeloencephalopathy, elevated CSF creatine kinase values may be seen in horses 6 to 18 months of age, reflecting current nervous tissue damage. However, this abnormality is not specific for this disease. In cases with longstanding neurologic deficits, it is more difficult to ascertain cause, beyond ruling it out radiographically or detecting equine protozoal myeloencephalitis with the Western blot antibody test and the PCR test for parasite antigen.

Definitive diagnosis of equine degenerative myeloencephalopathy requires demonstration of the histopathologic lesions of neuroaxonal dystrophy in the cuneate, lateral cuneate, and gracilis nuclei of the medulla oblongata and diffusely throughout the spinal cord. In the latter case, the lesions are often most prominent in the thoracic spinal cord. Histopathologic abnormalities consist of eosinophilic spheroids, astrogliosis, loss of neurons in a number of the sensory relay nuclei, and lipofuscinosis.

Single serum or plasma α-tocopherol values cannot be used as a definitive diagnostic test for equine degenerative myeloencephalopathy. Serum α-tocopherol values vary by 12% (range, 7–17%) over 24 hours. Because of this variation throughout the day, and the narrow difference between normal and deficient α-tocopherol values in horses, an animal can be considered deficient (<1.5 mg/ml) or normal (>2.0 mg/ml) on the same day. In addition, a plasma α-tocopherol value measured at the time of ataxia may not reflect the antioxidant status at the time the horse developed the disease. Measurement of α-tocopherol levels does have value in herd situations when deficiencies of the vitamin are suspected owing to lack of pasture, long-term use of pelleted feed, or increased antioxidant stress resulting from high levels of polyunsaturated fats in the diet.

TREATMENT

Massive vitamin E therapy has resulted in improvement in clinical signs with optimal recovery seen in horses in which the disease was recognized in the early stages, less than 12 months of age. Current recommendations for treatment are D,L-α-tocopherol acetate* at 6000 to 9000 IU/day per 250 to 500 kg body weight, mixed with 30 ml of vegetable oil and 1 quart of mixed grain. Improvement can be seen within 2 to 3 weeks, with continued progress over the next 6 months to 1 year. Prophylactically, oral administration of vitamin E (1500–2000 IU s.i.d.) to foals from equine degenerative myeloencephalopathy-affected lines has been shown to prevent the development of clinical ataxia.

Supplemental Readings

Beech J: Neuroaxonal dystrophy of the accessory cuneate nucleus in horses. Vet Pathol 21:384–393, 1984.

Beech J, Haskins M: Genetic studies of neuroaxonal dystrophy in the Morgan. Am J Vet Res 48:109–113, 1987.

Blythe LL, Craig AM: Equine degenerative myeloencephalopathy. Part I. Clinical signs and pathogenesis. Comp Con Ed Pract Vet 14(9):1215–1221, 1992.

Blythe LL, Craig AM: Equine degenerative myeloencephalopathy. Part II. Diagnosis and treatment. Comp Cont Ed Pract Vet 14(12):1633–1637, 1992.

Blythe LL, Craig AM, Lassen ED, Rowe KE, Appell LH: Serially determined plasma α-tocopherol concentrations and results of the oral vitamin E absorption test in clinically normal horses and in horses with degenerative myeloencephalopathy. Am J Vet Res 52:908–911, 1991.

Blythe LL, Hultgren BD, Craig AM, Appell LH, Lassen ED: Clinical, viral, and genetic evaluation of equine degenerative myeloencephalopathy in a family of Appaloosas. J Am Vet Med Assoc 198(6):1005–1013, 1991.

Craig AM, Blythe LL, Lassen ED, Rowe KE, Barrington R Slizeski M: Variations of serum vitamin E, cholesterol, and total serum lipid concentrations in horses during a 72-hour period. Am J Res 50:1527–1531, 1989.

Craig AM, Blythe LL, Rowe KE, Lassen ED, Barrington R, Walker KC: Variability in α-tocopherol values associated with sample procurement, storage, and freezing of equine serum and plasma samples. Am J Vet Res 53(12):2228–2234, 1992.

Dill SG, Correa MT, Erb HN, de Lahunta A, Kallfelz FA, Waldron C: Factors associated with the development of equine degenerative myeloencephalopathy. Am J Vet Res 51:1300–1305, 1990.

Dill SG, Kallfelz FA, de Lahunta A, Waldron CH: Serum vitamin E and blood glutathione peroxidase values of horses with degenerative myeloencephalopathy. Am J Vet Res 50:166–168, 1989.

Mayhew IG, Brown CM, Stowe HD, Trapp AL, Derksen FJ, Clement SF: Equine degenerative myeloencephalopathy: A vitamin E deficiency that may be familial. J Vet Intern Med 1:45–50, 1987.

*Rovimix 20, Hoffman-LaRoche, Nutley, NJ

Equine Motor Neuron Disease

THOMAS J. DIVERS

HUSSNI O. MOHAMMED

JOHN F. CUMMINGS
Ithaca, New York

Equine motor neuron disease, a neurodegenerative disease causing weakness and muscle atrophy, was first described in 1990, but a later report identified a case that had occurred in 1984. Since the original report in 1990, more than 150 cases have been confirmed in several parts of the world. Although the geographic recognition of the disease is expanding with time, it continues to be most frequently reported in the northeastern region of North America. The attack rate in this region is estimated to be one per 100,000 horses/year and typically the disease is sporadic, affecting only one horse on a farm (most commonly a boarding stable), although small clusters have been documented at two stables. In the more than 100 cases investigated in North America, the greatest risk factors appear to be a lack of pasture and feeding a ration that is (1) rich in grain and (2) contains medium to poor quality grass or cereal grain hay. Many horse breeds and two ponies have been affected, although Quarterhorses and Thoroughbreds are over-represented in the population studies. The Quarterhorse and Thoroughbred over-representation is not a result of genetic predilection but is most likely an epiphenomenon related to the high prevalence of Quarterhorses and Thoroughbreds kept in the boarding stable environments that are apparently conducive to development of the disease. Adult horses of both sexes, 2 to 25 years of age, have been affected with a peak incidence at 16 years.

CLINICAL SIGNS

Horses in the more active phase of the disease have an acute onset of trembling; they lie down more than normal, constantly shift their weight on the rear legs, and hold all four limbs closer together than normal when standing. Less frequent, yet common, additional findings are symmetrical buckling of the forelimbs while standing, abnormally low head carriage, sweating, elevation of the tailhead, and muscle fasciculations. The latter are seen as fine involuntary movement of the muscles even when the horse is lying down. The appetite remains excellent in most cases and transit of ingesta within the intestines is unaffected.

Physical examination reveals pronounced symmetrical muscle atrophy, most severe in the triceps, scapula, quadriceps, lumbar, sacral, and neck muscles. Affected horses may become distressed if made to stand in one location such as stocks for more than a few minutes. Ataxia is not present in horses affected with equine motor neuron disease. Detectable cranial nerve deficits are rare, although abnormal pigment deposition can be frequently observed in the nontapetal area of the retina on ophthalmoscopic examination. A few affected horses rapidly progress to persistent recumbency and respiratory distress requiring euthanasia. The condition in a majority of affected horses stabilizes in 2 to 8 weeks and then they have an "arrested" and/or slowly progressive form of the disease.

In the arrested, no longer rapidly progressive, form of the disease, the most common clinical complaint is failure to gain weight and exercise intolerance, both of which are a result of motor neuron cell death and resulting muscle atrophy. The tailhead may remain abnormally elevated and some horses may continue to be down more than normal. Some improvement in muscle mass may be observed within the first 6 months following the active form of the disease. Horses with the arrested form of the disease may survive for several years but cannot be safely used for riding. A second episode of trembling, and more pronounced recumbency often occurs 1 to 6 years after the initial episode, often necessitating euthanasia. During the chronic phase of the disease, the development of a stringhalt-like gait in one or more limbs is not unusual.

LABORATORY FINDINGS

Routine complete blood count and blood chemistry test results from horses with equine motor neuron disease have been generally unremarkable except for mild to moderate elevations in serum activities of the muscle enzymes, creatinine kinase (CK) and aspartate transaminase (AST), during the active phase of the disease. The muscle enzymes may return to normal in horses with the arrested form of the disease. Cerebrospinal fluid is often normal but may have an increased protein concentration, some of which is caused by intrathecally produced IgG. Glucose absorption tests are abnormal in approximately 30% of affected horses. In a small number of cases, the malabsorption is pronounced and is caused by infiltrative bowel disease. The latter, along with chronic liver disease, are the only abnormalities found in other organ systems, albeit in a low percentage of cases. The most consistently abnormal laboratory finding has been an abnormally low plasma concentration of α-tocopherol (<1.0 μg/ml in >90% of cases). Normal plasma levels of α-tocopherol in the horse are >2.5 μg/ml. The α-tocopherol concentration in muscle, peripheral nerve, and spinal cord of affected horses is also very low. Red blood cell and spinal cord superoxide dismutase (SOD1) activity is also abnormally low. Vitamin A, β-carotene, and ascorbic acid concentrations have been highly variable in affected horses. Serum selenium concentration has been normal in all cases.

PATHOPHYSIOLOGY

The clinical signs are a result of degeneration of somatic motor neurons in the ventral horns of the spinal cord and in selected brainstem nuclei. The nuclei of cranial nerves III, IV, and VI are unaffected. The most severely affected areas in the spinal cord are in the cervicothoracic and lumbosacral intumescences. Motor neurons may appear swollen and chromatolytic or necrotic and undergoing neuronophagia during the active phase of the disease. In the arrested form, focal aggregates of glial cells may be most evident in the ventral horns and indicate sites of previous loss of motor neurons. The death of motor neurons is accompanied by degenerative axonal changes in the ventral roots and peripheral nerves and neurogenic muscle atrophy. There is a preference of type I muscle fiber atrophy with scattered fiber necrosis. Additional findings are extensive deposition of lipopigment in the capillaries of the spinal cord and within the retinal pigment epithelial layer of the eye.

The death of the motor neurons is believed to be a result of oxidative damage. Motor neurons having the highest oxidative activity are therefore at greatest risk for oxidative stress. This would explain the observed predominance of type I muscle fiber atrophy. Horses may be predisposed to equine motor neuron disease by a lack of dietary antioxidants, and during periods of oxidative stress there is increased consumption of intrinsically produced free radical-reducing enzymes such as SOD1. Transient periods of increased oxidative activity may be a result of short-term neurotoxin exposure. With sufficient death and dysfunction of motor neurons, there may be an acute onset of clinical disease. It is believed that clinical signs of equine motor neuron disease only become apparent when approximately 30% of motor neurons are dysfunctional. If this is true, a much larger number of horses may be subclinically affected! The scattered muscle fiber necrosis and lipopigment accumulation in the capillaries of the spinal cord and the retina are characteristic of lipid peroxidation and vitamin E deficiency.

DIAGNOSIS

A tentative diagnosis is made rather easily in patients with active disease, but is often difficult in long-standing cases in which the progression has arrested. In horses with active disease, the acute onset of weakness and associated trembling without ataxia or depression or diminished appetite are nearly diagnostic. The mild to moderate elevation in muscle enzymes supports the diagnosis. A muscle biopsy, preferably of the sacrocaudalis dorsalis medialis, and/or a biopsy of the ventral branch of the spinal accessory nerve

are the preferred ante mortem tests used to help confirm the diagnosis. Electromyography frequently demonstrates denervation, usually in the form of positive sharp waves or fibrillation responses in affected muscles. Abnormalities are not consistent from one muscle area to another. Differential diagnoses include equine protozoal myeloencephalitis, polyneuritis equi, botulism, organophosphate toxicity, myositis/myopathy, and lead poisoning.

TREATMENT

No proven treatment is available for the disease. Vitamin E supplementation (5000 IU p.o. s.i.d.) is recommended because of the frequent finding of low plasma and nervous tissue α-tocopherol concentrations in affected horses and the belief that equine motor neuron disease is an oxidative disease. Prednisolone (0.5–1 mg/kg p.o. s.i.d.) is an additional therapy that has been frequently administered. Many owners have reported some improvement, albeit mild, in the clinical signs following corticosteroid therapy.

PROGNOSIS

The acute and active stage of the disease generally persists in affected horses for 2 to 8 weeks, at which time the signs subside in more than 70% of cases. Many of these horses appear to regain some muscle mass in the following months but remain somewhat disfigured and are not safe for riding. Recurrence of the clinical signs may occur years later and necessitate euthanasia. In approximately 30% of the cases, there is minimal improvement in the clinical signs or progressive deterioration necessitating euthanasia within 1 year from the onset of clinical signs.

Supplemental Readings

Cumming JF, de Lahunta A, George C, Fuhrer L, Valentine BA, Cooper BJ, Summers BA, Huxtable CR, Mohammed HO: Equine motor neuron disease: A preliminary report. Cornell Vet 80:357–379, 1980.

de la Rúa Doménech R, Mohammed HO, Cummings JF, Divers TJ, de Lahunta A, Valentine B, Summers BA, Jackson CA: Incidence and risk factors of equine motor neuron disease: An ambidirectional study. Neuroepidemiology 14:54–64, 1995.

Divers TJ, Mohammed HO, Cummings JF, de Lahunta A, Valentine BA, Summers BA, Cooper BJ: Equine motor neuron disease: A new cause of weakness, trembling, and weight loss. Comp Cont Ed Vet Pract 14(9):1222–1226, 1992.

Divers TJ, Mohammed HO, Cummings JF, Valentine BA, de Lahunta A, Jackson CA, Summers BA: Equine motor neuron disease: Findings in 28 horses and proposal of a pathophysiological mechanism for the disease. Equine Vet J 26(5):409–415, 1994.

Jackson CA, de Lahunta A, Cummings JF, Divers TJ, Mohammed HO, Valentine BA, Hackett RP: Spinal accessory nerve biopsy as an ante mortem diagnostic test for equine motor neuron disease. Equine Vet J 28(3):215–219, 1996.

Mohammed HO, Cummings JF, Divers TJ, Valentine BA, de Lahunta A, Summers B, Farrow BRH, Trembicki-Graves K, Mauskopf A: Risk factors associated with equine motor neuron disease: A possible model for human MND. Neurology 43:966–971,1993.

Valentine BA, de Lahunta A, Diverse TJ, Summers BA, Jackson CA: Is equine motor neuron disease a new neurologic disorder? Prog Vet Neurol 5(4):155–161, 1994.

Temporohyoid Osteoarthropathy (Middle Ear Disease)

LINDA L. BLYTHE

BARBARA J. WATROUS
Corvallis, Oregon

Temporohyoid osteoarthropathy is a progressive disease of the middle ear and the bones comprising the temporohyoid joint. The latter includes the proximal part of the stylohyoid bone and the ventral part of the squamous portion of the temporal bone. Horses from 18 months to older than 20 years of age have been affected, and there is no breed or sex predilection. The pathogenesis of this chronic disease process is believed to originate with a low-grade otitis media that develops into an osteitis of the tympanic bulla and gravitates distally to involve both bones of the temporohyoid joint. Because of lack of evidence of guttural pouch inflammation or otitis externa in the majority of cases, the most probable source of the inflammation is hematogenous. The tympanic membranes of horses with this condition are rarely inflamed, and ruptures are uncommon. As the diseases progresses, the osteitis of the tympanic bulla extends into the temporohyoid joint, which becomes arthritic, enlarged, and subsequently ankylosed owing to bony proliferation. With loss of mobility of the temporohyoid joint, the normal forces generated from movement of the tongue and larynx transmitted through the bones of the hyoid apparatus can cause an acute stress fracture of the skull. Less commonly, midshaft fracture of the stylohyoid bone may occur.

CLINICAL SIGNS

Two sets of clinical signs are associated with the varying stages of progression of this disease process. Early in the syndrome, with otitis media and osteitis of the temporohyoid joint, head shaking, ear rubbing, wild tossing of the head and neck under tack, or reluctance to take a bit may be the only clinical signs. Additional signs may include dropping feed and weight loss. When digital pressure is applied to the cartilages at the base of the ear, the horse may show a painful withdrawal response owing to the arthritic process in the joint. The external ear canal may be narrowed in diameter because of bony proliferation. In some cases, no clinical signs are observed during the early stages of the disease.

The second set of clinical signs present as an acute onset of neurologic deficits of the vestibulocochlear and facial nerve. Clinical signs of vestibulocochlear nerve involvement are consistently present. They include weakness of the extensor muscles on the affected side resulting in asymmetrical ataxia, head tilt with the poll deviated to the affected side, and a spontaneous nystagmus with the slow component to the affected side. The horse may be reluctant or unable to rise, or if standing, may lean on walls for support. These signs may progress over several days.

The facial nerve accompanies the vestibulocochlear nerve from the brain into the internal acoustic meatus of the inner ear and is also affected in the majority of the cases. Paresis or paralysis of the ear, accumulation of food in the buccal cavity, and a muzzle twisted away from the affected side all indicate facial nerve involvement. A corneal ulcer often occurs on the affected side because of inability to close the eyelid and reduction in tear production. A smaller number of horses may have difficulty eating and swallowing because of involvement of the glossopharyngeal and vagus nerves where they exit from the skull behind the temporohyoid joint. Megaesophagus and a clinical syndrome of "roaring" have been seen in one horse with bilateral temporohyoid osteoarthropathy. In one study, 16% of the horses had evidence of bilateral disease, but one side was usually more severely affected than the other. A small number of cases present initially with grand mal seizures resulting from the trauma of the acute fracture of the skull. Bacterial meningoencephalitis may be a sequela and may result in the death of the horse.

DIAGNOSIS

A physical examination with complete neurologic evaluation should be conducted on horses displaying either of the two clinical sets of signs associated with this disease process. Included should be deep but gentle palpation pressure at the base of each ear and examination of the external ear canal for parasites, inflammation, or narrowing. The neurologic examination should include careful testing of all pairs of cranial nerves and blindfolding the horse to detect if the horse has visually compensated for vestibulocochlear dysfunction. Depending on the stage of progression, there are three ways to make a definitive diagnosis of this disease process. Radiographic examination of the skull using ventrodorsal, lateral, and lateral oblique views helps detect those cases in which the bony proliferation has progressed to cause osteitis of the temporohyoid joint.

323

Optimal films are obtained with the horse under general anesthesia and in ventrodorsal recumbency. Symmetrical positioning of the skull is needed for the ventrodorsal view to minimize geometric distortion of the stylohyoid bones, which may otherwise mimic unilateral thickening when oblique skull positioning occurs (Fig. 1). Lateral and oblique views are obtained by rotating the head into the appropriate positions. These views serve to increase the potential for identifying the pathologic fracture and confirming the enlargement of the affected stylohyoid bone.

Endoscopic evaluation of the external contour of the temporohyoid joint from within the guttural pouch can reveal asymmetrical enlargement of the bones composing the joint (Fig. 2) and, in some cases, hyperemia and edema reflected in the guttural pouch lining surrounding the joint.

In early cases in which the bony proliferation is not prominent, tympanocentesis through the external auditory meatus may provide a diagnosis of middle ear inflammation. Under tranquilization, the external ear canal should be gently cleaned with a bactericidal soap and water and alcohol rinses several hours before the procedure. Trying to clean the ear at the time of tympanocentesis with cotton swabs often results in bleeding and interferes with the

collection of a meaningful sample. Under general anesthesia, through otoscopic visualization, a 6-inch needle is inserted through the tympanic membrane and 0.75 ml sterile saline is injected into the middle ear. After 10 seconds, the fluid is aspirated and submitted for cytology and culture and sensitivity testing. Care must be taken when inserting the needle through the tympanic membrane as the sudden change in resistance can result in traumatic hemorrhage in the middle ear. Practicing the technique on a cadaver before performing it on a clinical case is highly recommended.

In horses with neurologic deficits, cerebrospinal fluid (CSF) should be sampled at the atlanto-occipital space to determine if meningoencephalitis is present and for culture and sensitivity testing. Increased protein and white blood cell counts, primarily neutrophilic, indicate inflammation of the central nervous system.

The authors have seen cases in which temporohyoid osteoarthropathy was present but no clinical signs were evident at the time. Once the osteitis progresses to fusion of the temporohyoid joint, the arthritic pain ceases. The horse then only develops clinical signs when a skull fracture occurs or the infectious process involves the vestibulocochlear and/or facial nerves directly.

A sample of CSF should be submitted to the diagnostic laboratory* for *Sarcocystis neurona* titers and a PCR test because equine protozoal myeloencephalitis (EPM) can cause a similar clinical syndrome. Differential diagnosis for cases with neurologic deficits include the aforementioned EPM; traumatic injuries; acute otitis interna due to bacteria, viruses, or fungi; migrating parasitic larvae; tumors; abscesses; and focal or diffuse bacterial or viral encephalitides. For horses presenting with the abnormal behavior of head shaking, the differential diagnoses should include parasitic otitis externa due to mites or ticks, neuritis of the infraorbital nerve, seasonal allergic inflammation of the middle and inner ear, laryngeal hemiplegia resulting in dyspnea under tack, photophobia, and learned behavior problems.

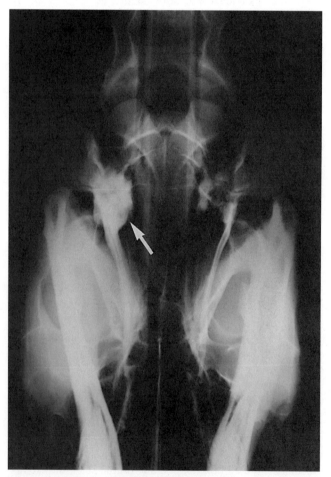

Figure 1. Ventrodorsal radiograph of an 11-year-old Appaloosa mare with a history of 9 days' duration of acute-onset progressive asymmetrical ataxia. Right facial nerve paralysis developed 7 days after onset of ataxia. A bony mass *(arrow)* replaces the right temporohyoid joint, which is indicative of chronic osteitis and ankylosis. The shaft of the right stylohyoid bone is also thickened.

TREATMENT AND PROGNOSIS

Treatment of the early cases with abnormal head-shaking behavior is aimed at eliminating the initiating infectious process and reducing pain and inflammation. Broad-spectrum antibiotics for 30 days are given to eliminate infectious agents in the middle ear and surrounding bony structures. However, once the osteitis and arthritic processes have begun, they often persist after the antibiotic treatment until fusion of the temporohyoid joint occurs. Pain relative to this arthritic condition may remain a problem. Control of pain is with analgesics and/or nonsteroidal anti-inflammatory drugs when the horse is being ridden or trained. In addition, the client must be advised that fusion of the joint, although eliminating the pain from the arthritic condition, predisposes the horse to subsequent skull fracture resulting from continual movement of the hyoid appa-

Equine Biodiagnostics, A165 AST CC Building, University of Kentucky, Lexington, KY 40506-0286.

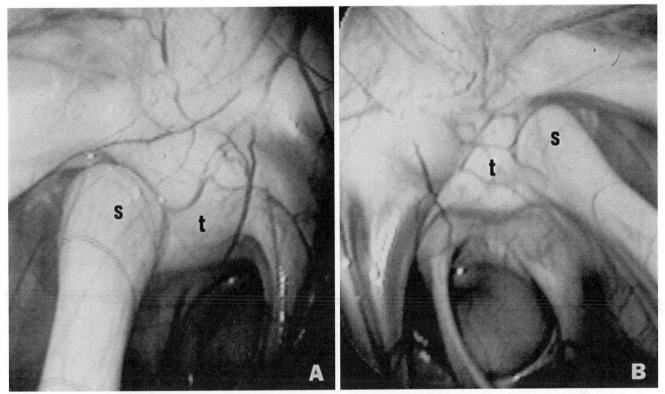

Figure 2. Guttural pouch endoscopic photographs of osteoarthropathy of the right temporohyoid joint (A) compared with the normal left side (B). Note the thickened, smooth contour of the tympanic bulla (t) on the right side that articulates with an enlarged proximal part of the stylohyoid bone (S). The translucency of the tympanic bulla seen on endoscopic examination of a normal horse is often obscured by bony thickening of the affected side. This is not readily apparent in these photographs. The ventrodorsal radiographs of this horse were also diagnostic. (Photographs courtesy of Dr. Hal Schott.)

ratus associated with movement of the tongue and larynx. A surgical procedure has been developed to create a midshaft pseudoarthrosis in the stylohyoid bone to prevent the skull fracture sequela. This surgery has also been successfully used to reduce movement at the fracture site in horses that have neurologic signs resulting from the acute stress skull fracture.

When neurologic deficits are present, systemic use of broad-spectrum antibiotics is indicated. Antibiotics that penetrate the CNS, such as trimethoprim/sulfa (15 mg/kg b.i.d. for 30 days) or chloramphenicol (25 mg/kg t.i.d. or q.i.d.) are preferred. If the blood-brain barrier is suspected to be compromised, other broad-spectrum antibiotics may be selected, especially if results of culture and sensitivity tests on samples from middle ear or CSF indicate their use. Oral or IV dimethyl sulfoxide (DMSO) administration (1 mg/kg s.i.d. for 2–3 days) reduces inflammation and increased intracranial pressure during the initial postfracture inflammatory stages. If seizures are occurring, IV diazepam is given to effect during the acute phase. Most horses do not have to be put on subsequent phenobarbital or antiseizure medications after the initial few days. Nursing care is essential in those horses unable to rise in the initial few days. In cases of facial nerve paralysis, a corneal ulcer is often present and has to be concurrently treated with topical antibiotics and artificial tears. The prognosis for recovery of horses with neurologic signs is very good, provided that the initial infectious and inflammatory damage

to the brain can be arrested and reversed in the initial 2 to 3 days. In 36 cases seen by the authors, only two horses have failed to survive and function normally. Facial nerve paresis may be a permanent sequela in a few horses, and most horses fully compensate visually for unilateral vestibulocochlear nerve loss.

Supplemental Readings

Blythe LL, Watrous BJ, Pearson EG, Walker LL: Otitis media/interna in the horse–A cause of head shaking and skull fractures. Proc Am Assoc Equine Pract 1990, pp 517–528.

Blythe LL, Watrous BJ, Schmitz JA, Kaneps AJ: Vestibular syndrome associated with temporohyoid joint fusion and temporal bone fracture in three horses. J Am Vet Med Assoc 185(7):775–781, 1984.

Blythe LL, Watrous BJ, Shires GMH, Kaneps AJ, von Matthiessen PW, Riebold TW: Prophylactic partial stylohyoidostectomy for horses with osteoarthropathy of the temporohyoid joint. J Equine Vet Sci 14(1):32–37, 1994.

Cook WR: Headshaking in horses: An afterword. Comp Cont Ed Pract Vet 14:1369–1371, 1992.

Lane JG, Mair TS: Observations on headshaking in the horse. Equine Vet J 19(3):331–336, 1987.

Madigan JE: Headshaking in the horse: Shedding new light on an old problem. Proc 12th ACVIM Forum, 1994, pp 565–566.

Mair TS: Case Reports: Headshaking associated with *Trombicula autumnalis* larval infestation in two horses. Equine Vet J 26(3):244–245, 1994.

Power HT, Watrous BJ, de Lahunta A: Facial and vestibulocochlear nerve disease in six horses. J Am Vet Med Assoc 183:1076–1080, 1983.

Watrous BJ: Head tilt in horses. Vet Clin North Am Equine Pract 3(2):353–370, 1987.

Botulism

WILLIAM V. BERNARD
Lexington, Kentucky

Botulism is a flaccid neuromuscular paralysis that can affect all mammals. Horses, however, are one of the most susceptible species. The disease can affect both foals and adult horses. In foals, the disease has been called the *shaker foal syndrome* and, in adults, it is known as *forage poisoning*. The neuromuscular paralysis is a result of interference with acetylcholine release at the motor endplate. The disruption of acetylcholine release is caused by the exotoxin of the gram-positive bacterium *Clostridium botulinum*. This exotoxin is one of the most potent neurotoxins known.

EPIDEMIOLOGY

C. botulinum grows preferentially in neutral or alkaline soils and grows and produces toxin in an anaerobic environment. *C. botulinum* spores are found in 18.5% of the soils sampled in the United States. However, the distribution of spores is variable and is most likely related to the geographic frequency of the disease. Type B toxin is the most common cause of clinical botulism in horses in the United States. It is found in high concentrations in soils of central Kentucky and along the mid-Atlantic seaboard. The shaker foal syndrome is frequently seen in central Kentucky, owing to the large population of susceptible foals and prevalence of the organism. Type C toxin causes disease in European countries but is not a frequent cause of disease in the United States. The type C organism is found in high concentrations in the soils of Florida. Type C was also the offending organism in a California outbreak.

In the horse, the disease generally occurs on an individual case basis; however, outbreaks can occur. Contaminated feed sources are the usual cause of outbreaks. The organism thrives in anaerobic-decaying vegetable or animal matter. Therefore, moist or spoiled feeds and feeds contaminated with animal parts or carcasses can become a source of infection. Stagnant water sources, especially those contaminated by carcasses, have been identified as the cause of outbreaks in cattle.

ETIOLOGY AND PATHOGENESIS

Three routes of botulism infection have generally been accepted to exist: ingestion of preformed toxin, toxicoinfectious, and wound botulism. Ingestion of preformed toxin is thought to be the most common route of infection and gives rise to the syndrome known as *forage poisoning*. Toxicoinfectious botulism is the elaboration of toxin within the gastrointestinal tract. Toxin is produced when spores are ingested and vegetate or when the local gastrointestinal environment is favorable to an overgrowth of *C. botulinum*.

Gastric ulcers in foals have been suggested to be potential sites for the elaboration of toxin. The "wound" route of infection includes abscesses or damage to tissue that results in an anaerobic environment conducive to the growth of *C. botulinum*. Toxin is locally produced and subsequently spreads throughout the body. Infected umbilical remnants have been suggested to be a source of this type of infection in foals. Wound botulism has been reported as a consequence of castration in the horse.

The neuromuscular paralysis of botulism is a result of an interference with the release of acetylcholine. This blockage of acetylcholine release can occur at neuromuscular junctions, peripheral cholinergic nerve terminals in autonomic ganglia, and in postganglionic parasympathetic nerve endings. The central nervous system and sensory nerves are not affected. Two proposed mechanisms of toxin action include: (1) interference with calcium function at the nerve terminal, thereby inhibiting the release of acetylcholine; and (2) blockage of exocytosis of synaptic vesicles.

CLINICAL SIGNS

Clinical signs of botulism are generally related to a flaccid neuromuscular paralysis. Signs may be mild to severe and are dependent upon the amount of toxin ingested or elaborated. The central nervous system is not affected by the botulism neurotoxin; therefore, the horse should be bright and alert. This can help the clinician in differentiating botulism from other diseases that cause similar clinical signs. Botulism also should be on the list of differential diagnoses for a horse that is recumbent and cannot stand or the horse that is found dead.

Foals

The disease in foals has been reported as early as 2 weeks of age. The signs vary from mild to severe. Severe signs of disease may include paralysis, which has progressed to an inability to stand, or foals found dead. If the disease is mild and gradual in progression, some of the first signs noted are varying degrees of muscle weakness, spending large amounts of time lying down, and dribbling milk from the nostrils or mouth. The initial muscle weakness can appear as a stiff-stilted gait that can be difficult to differentiate from mild proprioceptive deficits. The foal may walk slowly and have difficulty keeping up with the mare. If signs progress, muscle tremors may be evident and the foal can have difficulty standing, may stand for only brief periods, or may become recumbent. Muscle weakness is evident when foals lie down because they often collapse to the ground instead of lying down gracefully. The term *shaker foal* was derived from the severe muscle tremors that are frequently seen with the disease. Other signs of neuromuscular paralysis include poor tail, tongue, and eyelid tone or dysphagia. Poor tongue tone results in difficulty nursing and milk dripping from the sides of the mouth. If ingestion or elaboration of toxin has been extensive, foals may be recumbent and in respiratory distress. Respiratory rate and effort increase and chest excursion is reduced, as evidenced by an increase in the abdominal component of breathing. Respiratory difficulties result from paralysis of intercostal and the diaphragmatic musculature. Death due to botulism is a result of respiratory paralysis.

Adult Horses

Botulism can affect a horse of any age. The clinical signs relate to a flaccid neuromuscular paralysis and can vary from a mild motor weakness to near total paralysis. The severity of signs and rapidity of onset or progression of clinical signs is toxin dose-related. The first clinical signs are a loss of tongue, tail, and eyelid tone. These signs are infrequently noted by the owner. Subsequently, signs related to poor tongue tone and paresis or paralysis of pharyngeal musculature are observed. These signs can include dysphagia, dropping of food from the mouth, excess salivation, feed material at the nostrils, or a fetid odor to the mouth. The tongue may be easily pulled from the mouth and may hang from or be difficult to retract back into the mouth. The eyelids and tail may be easily manipulated with very little resistance. The appetite is often normal, but mastication is slow and swallowing is difficult. Affected horses may often stand at and play in water or attempt but be unable to drink. Evidence of weakness may also be evident in the gait. The gait may be stiff, short-strided, or shuffling in appearance. If weakness progresses, muscle tremors may be evident. Exercise can exacerbate tremors. Muscle tremors are most common in the triceps and flank area and are symmetrical. These horses tire easily, spend large amounts of time lying down, and may become recumbent. Bladder paralysis, ileus, and constipation may become a problem in advanced disease and are exacerbated by recumbency. Stridor may result from paresis of pharyngeal musculature or displacement of the soft palate. In advanced stages or in overwhelming toxemia, respiration becomes labored with decreased chest expansion and increased abdominal effort. Death ensues from respiratory failure.

DIAGNOSIS

The diagnosis of botulism is based on historical evidence and clinical signs. Botulism should be on the list of differential diagnoses in a horse exhibiting signs of a flaccid paralysis. Historically, owners may report signs referable to a progressive muscle weakness, as described in the previous section. A failure to vaccinate or an incomplete vaccination schedule in endemic areas is a common historical factor in foals with botulism. Failure of passive transfer is another possible source of vaccine failure in endemic areas.

When considering botulism as a diagnosis, it is helpful to remember that the central nervous system (CNS) is unaffected. Therefore, the patient should be "bright and alert." This can be useful in differentiating botulism from diseases that result in central nervous system signs. When

the disease is slowly progressive in onset, dysphagia is often one of the first signs noted by owners. The differential diagnosis of dysphagia should include obstructive lesions in the pharynx, guttural pouch lesions, and dysphagia resulting from CNS lesions. The most common brainstem lesion resulting in dysphagia is protozoal myelitis, but any encephalitis or encephalopathy such as leukoencephalomalacia, yellow star thistle poisoning, and rabies can result in dysphagia. Other conditions causing neuromuscular paralysis include white snake root toxicity, organophosphate poisoning, tick paralysis, and hypocalcemia.

Clinicopathologic abnormalities can be useful in excluding other diseases but are few and generally nonspecific in horses with botulism. Examination of cerebrospinal fluid (CSF) can be useful in differentiating CNS diseases that cause abnormal CSF from botulism, which does not. In many species but not the horse, mouse inoculation tests can identify toxin in the serum of individuals with botulism. The amount of toxin necessary to kill a horse may be so small that it is not detectable by the mouse inoculation system. In addition, the toxin spends very little time in circulation because it is rapidly bound to the motor endplate. Electromyographic evaluation during repetitive nerve stimulations has been useful in evaluating botulism in humans. However, in horses, it is unreliable as a diagnostic aid and is difficult to perform.

Culturing the feces of horses suspected of having botulism can be useful to confirm a diagnosis. However, the organism is difficult to culture and few laboratories are equipped to do so. In addition, decisions regarding the diagnosis need to be made long before results are available. *C. botulinum* can be cultured from 20% of affected adult horses, and spores can be found in approximately 80% of affected foals. Spores are rarely found in the gastrointestinal contents of a normal horse not at risk for botulism.

TREATMENT AND PROGNOSIS

The development and use of the polyvalent equine-origin botulism antitoxin containing types A, B, C, D, and E has greatly improved the chances for survival of a horse with botulism. Before the advent of the antitoxin, the mortality rate approached 90%. With the use of the antitoxin and appropriate nursing and nutritional therapy, prognosis for survival is greater than 70% in adult horses and is higher in shaker foals. The antitoxin is produced by hyperimmunization of horses with *C. botulinum* toxoid and is expensive. The recommended dose for the adult and foal is 400 and 200 ml, respectively. It must be used early in the course of the disease and its use does not guarantee recovery. The antitoxin is of critical importance in the severely affected animal, but horses with slowly progressive mild disease can survive without it. Clinical signs are not reversed by antitoxin, and owners must be warned that patients may actually worsen after antitoxin administration. The reason for this is that antitoxin binds circulating toxin but does not bind toxin that is already attached to the motor endplate. This bound toxin can result in a deterioration of clinical signs as it proceeds to block acetylcholine release.

Prognosis is related to the rapidity of onset and progression of flaccid paralysis. Patients that present with a gradual onset and slow progression of signs have most likely been exposed to a small dose of toxin as compared with the patient with rapid onset and progression of signs, which has most likely been exposed to a large dose of toxin. The recumbent horse or horses with rapid-onset disease may succumb despite the administration of antitoxin.

Nursing care and nutritional support become the critical factors in case management once antitoxin has been administered. In the recumbent patient or the patient that spends large amounts of time lying down, decubital ulcers can be prevented by use of deep bedding, limb wraps, padding, and frequent turning from side to side. Topical treatment of sores may become necessary.

Respiratory care is important to the outcome of the patient. Turning the recumbent patient from side to side, or maintaining the patient in sternal recumbency, can reduce hypostatic congestion of the lungs, improve ventilation/perfusion matching, and prevent hypoxemia. If the horse is dysphagic but continues its attempts to eat, a muzzle may be useful in preventing aspiration of food into the air passages. This may be particularly important if the horse is coughing while attempting to eat. Broad-spectrum antimicrobials may be beneficial if there is suspicion that aspiration has occurred or in recumbent patients that are more susceptible to infection.

Nutritional support is generally required unless the disease is extremely mild. A nasogastric tube can be sutured in place or passed several times per day. A gruel of alfalfa meal; a slurry of alfalfa meal mixed with cottage cheese, dextrose, and electrolytes; or specialized products produced for enteral use in the horse can be pumped down a nasogastric tube several times per day. The recumbent patient should be fed in sternal position and supported during gastric emptying. Care should be taken not to overfeed and not to administer excessive quantities at one feeding because ileus can be a problem, particularly in the recumbent patient. Mineral oil may be beneficial if constipation occurs or if dry, hard feces are produced. Nutritional support of the suckling foal is simplified by a milk diet. Caution should be taken not to overfeed the foal because some degree of weight loss is more acceptable than the secondary complications of colic, gastric distension, ileus, or diarrhea. The clinician should attempt to reach a feeding level of at least 10% of the foal's body weight divided over several feedings. Frequent small feedings, every 1 to 2 hours, are beneficial. If 10% of the body weight can be fed without difficulties, the amount can be increased toward 20% of the body weight. Intravenous parenteral nutrition or fluid therapy may be necessary if the patient is unable to tolerate oral feeding.

Broad-spectrum antibiotic therapy is advisable if aspiration pneumonia is suspected. Potassium or sodium penicillin (22,000–44,000 IU/kg IV) should eliminate any proliferating *C. botulinum* if wound botulism is suspected. The use of oral antibiotics is controversial because they may either kill the vegetative, gastrointestinal form of the bacterium, resulting in increased toxin release, or they may result in upset of the gastrointestinal flora and allow overgrowth of *C. botulinum*.

The use of drugs such as neostigmine that potentiate neuromuscular transmission are contraindicated. The effect of these drugs is only transient. Patients receiving these drugs often worsen dramatically after a brief period of improvement. Ventilatory support may become necessary if respiratory paralysis develops. The adult horse is very difficult to ventilate, but the foal can be successfully ventilated if equipment and expertise are available.

PREVENTION

Vaccination of horses with *C. botulinum* toxoid has proven to be very successful in prevention of the disease when appropriate schedules are followed. The incidence of the shaker foal in central Kentucky has been dramatically reduced by vaccination programs. The mare should initially be given a three-dose series with 1 month between vaccines and the last vaccine in the last month of gestation. This regimen provides maximal colostral antibody levels. Mares should then subsequently receive a yearly booster vaccination during their last month of gestation. If protection is required in nonbreeding stock, the initial three-dose series should be used with a yearly booster. Vaccination of horses in areas where the disease is not prevalent may not be necessary. However, vaccination of individuals maintained in endemic areas and mares that are shipped to endemic areas is recommended. Vaccine breaks can occur if the initial series is incomplete, the third vaccine does not provide adequate colostral immunity, there is failure of colostral transfer, or if yearly boosters are not provided.

Supplemental Readings

Bernard W, Divers TJ, Whitlock RH, Messick J, Tulleners E: Botulism as a sequel to open castration in a horse. J Am Vet Med Assoc 191:73–74, 1987.

Kinde H, Bettey RL, Ardans A, Galey FD, Daft BM, Walker RL, Eklund MW, Byrd JW: Clostridium botulinum type-C intoxication associated with consumption of processed alfalfa hay cubes in horses. J Am Vet Med Assoc 199:742–746, 1991.

Whitlock RH: Botulism, Type C, experimental and field cases in horses. Proc 13th Annu Meet Am Coll Vet Intern Med, 1995, pp 720–723.

Whitlock RH, Messick JB: Foal botulism (Shaker Foal syndrome), clinical signs, diagnosis, treatment and prevention. Proc 33rd Annu Meet Am Assoc Equine Pract 1987, pp 359–366.

Equine Protozoal Myeloencephalitis

CLARA FENGER
Lexington, Kentucky

Equine protozoal myeloencephalitis (EPM) is a neurologic disease of horses that most commonly results in asymmetric incoordination (ataxia), weakness, and spasticity, although it may mimic almost any neurologic condition. The onset of disease may be peracute, acute, or chronic. Chronic EPM is often insidious in onset and difficult to diagnose until late in disease; it may culminate in death if untreated. In the most mild cases, the only clinical sign may be an ill-defined hindlimb lameness, or a minor respiratory noise. In the most severe cases, horses may be unable to swallow or stand. The causative organism is *Sarcocystis falcatula*, which is a protozoal parasite. The clinical signs are caused by direct neuronal damage by the parasite and damage resulting from inflammation.

ETIOLOGY

Horses are infected by ingesting infective *S. falcatula* sporocysts. *Sarcocystis falcatula* has an obligate two-host-species life cycle, including the natural intermediate host of passerorid, psittacorid, or columborid birds, and the definitive host, opossums (*Didelphis virginiana*). The parasite encysts in the muscle tissue of the bird. When this tissue is eaten by opossums, the organism undergoes sexual reproduction in intestinal epithelium and forms infective sporocysts contained within an oocyst. Oocysts and sporocysts are found in the intestinal contents but the fragile oocyst is commonly disrupted by the time feces are passed. The birds become infected by ingesting sporocysts that contaminate their feed or water. Sporozoites emerge from sporocysts, penetrate the intestines, develop into tachyzoites, and undergo a series of replicative cycles in endothelial cells throughout the body. In birds, the natural intermediate hosts, later generations of tachyzoites emerge from endothelial cells of capillaries and venules in muscle and encyst in myocytes, forming sarcocysts. These later generations of tachyzoites develop into a slowly dividing stage, called bradyzoites. Bradyzoites divide slowly over the course of the host's lifetime. *Sarcocystis falcatula* infection can cause the death of the bird host by hemorrhage resulting from schizogony in the pulmonary vascular endothelium, but the sarcocysts are not usually pathogenic. When the intermediate host is killed or dies and is eaten, these cysts are activated in the gastrointestinal tract of the definitive host, and the cycle starts again. Most *Sarcocystis* species are found encysted in the muscle tissue of the intermediate host, but some *Sarcocystis* species, as well as the closely related protozoa *Toxoplasma gondii*, have been found in cysts in the central nervous system.

Horses are an aberrant intermediate host of *S. falcatula*.

Sporocysts are ingested and excyst, and sporozoites enter the horse, but tissue cysts have not been found. Instead, in some horses, tachyzoites migrate to the central nervous system, where they continue to undergo asexual reproduction intracellularly in neurons and microglial cells, without forming tissue cysts. Therefore, horses cannot transmit *S. falcatula* to other animals.

This disease requires a minimum of 4 weeks from ingestion of sporocysts to the development of clinical signs. Experimental administration of *S. falcatula* sporocysts to foals has resulted in seroconversion within 3 weeks and the presence of antibodies in the cerebrospinal fluid (CSF) within 4 weeks. Clinical signs of neurologic disease have been apparent in experimental trials of horses as early as 4 weeks after infection. However, these horses received high sporocyst doses (2–40 million), and natural infection with these numbers is probably uncommon.

The development of clinical EPM may require as long as 2 years. Horses have been exported from North America as long as 2 years before the development of severe clinical signs. No cases of EPM have been reported outside of the American continents, except in horses that were imported from the American continents. However, no comprehensive studies have been performed to determine if exposure occurs outside the Americas.

Postmortem evaluation of horses with EPM commonly reveals no gross abnormalities. When gross lesions are present, they are evident as malacic regions. On cross section, the edematous tissue may bulge, and areas of hemorrhage may be evident. Most commonly, histopathology reveals infiltration of the region with mononuclear cells and occasional eosinophils, which may be concentrated around blood vessels. Granulocytes may also be observed. Parasites are uncommonly observed, particularly when horses have been treated with either trimethoprim or pyrimethamine in combination with a sulfonamide. Individual tachyzoites may be observed within or between cells, or schizonts may be observed within cells. Schizonts may be difficult to find, unless they are mature, appearing in a classic rosette pattern. Parasites may be found within neuronal cell bodies, microglial cells, or rarely within the endothelial cells of the blood vessels.

EPIDEMIOLOGY

The incidence of EPM is unknown. The clinical signs of this disease can be subtle and can progress slowly or not at all, which means that many horses that are mildly affected may never be diagnosed. The disease is usually sporadic but may occur as an epizootic. Seroprevalence in the eastern and midwestern United States is about 40 to 50% but appears to be much higher among the racing horse population. Seroprevalence studies of other regions have not been completed. Exposure to this organism is widespread throughout the American continents and matches the natural range of the oppossum very closely. The disease appears to be over-represented in Standardbreds and Thoroughbreds, although it has been identified in most breeds of horse. Ponies appear to be resistant.

Exposure rates for different farms or training facilities may vary from zero to 100% of the horses at a given location. Premises with very high seroprevalence appear also to have an above-average prevalence of clinical disease. Most horses that are seropositive probably ingest the sporocysts, mount an immune response, and clear the organism before it can infect the CNS. Alternatively, they may become chronically infected, but are able to combat the organism sufficiently to prevent the development of severe clinical signs.

Foals that have tested seropositive for *S. falcatula* receive their antibodies from the dam, and no foals have been identified that are seropositive before consuming colostrum. Foals that are serially tested for serum antibodies throughout the first few years of life commonly appear to become exposed to this organism before they reach 1 year of age.

CLINICAL SIGNS

Horses with EPM exhibit a wide array of clinical signs that are the result of primary and secondary problems. The "three A" presentation of asymmetric ataxia and atrophy is classic. However, because the parasite reaches the CNS hematogenously, it may proliferate and cause dysfunction at any site. Neurologic signs are referable to the site or sites of infection and are the result of both direct damage to neurons and indirect damage by edema and inflammation in response to the parasites.

Most commonly, clinical signs result from infection of the spinal cord and include ataxia and weakness, which is usually worse in the hindlimbs than in the forelimbs. Placing reactions of affected limbs are abnormal, and the horse may appear weak and may be easily pulled over to one side. Focal muscle atrophy may be evident anywhere, but the gluteal muscles appear to be the common site, probably because muscle atrophy is much easier to detect here than in other muscle groups. Generalized muscle atrophy or loss of condition may also occur without obvious asymmetry. Apparent lameness, particularly atypical lameness or slight gait asymmetry of the rear limbs is commonly caused by EPM. Occasionally, the only evidence of neurologic deficits in a horse with EPM may be a lameness that fails to be alleviated by local anesthesia.

Signs of cranial nerve dysfunction occur in about 10% of EPM cases. Any nucleus of the cranial nerves may be affected by infection of the brainstem. Airway abnormalities, such as laryngeal hemiplegia, can be indicative of vagus nerve damage; dorsal displacement of the soft palate can indicate injury to trigeminal, glossopharyngeal, vagus, accessory, or hypoglossal nerves; and atrophy of the temporalis or masseter muscles can be associated with trigeminal

nerve damage. The latter may or may not be accompanied by dysphagia, which may also be caused by abnormalities of the glossopharyngeal, hypoglossal, or vagus nerves. Difficulty with prehension, mastication, and deglutition of food may be difficult to assess unless the horse is observed eating. The stall, manger, and water bucket should be examined for evidence of quidding (that is, dropping chewed feed), and the horse's nose should be checked for evidence of aspiration or reflux of chewed material. Abnormalities of the facial and vestibulocochlear nerves are often observed together, because of the proximity of the nuclei to each other in the brainstem. Vestibular signs include nystagmus, a head tilt, and base-wide stance (see *Current Therapy in Equine Medicine 3*, p 575). Facial nerve paralysis is associated with muzzle deviation away from the affected side, ptosis, and ear droop, all of which may be subtle early in infection.

Infections of the cerebrum, basal ganglia, or cerebellum are less commonly observed. In the cerebrum, protozoal infection may be focal; it may be associated with seizures and an abnormal electroencephalogram. Rarely is protozoal infection associated with depression. Alternatively, asymmetric amaurosis (central blindness) and facial hypalgesia may be observed. Primary infection of the cerebellum is uncommon and results in cerebellar ataxia, which is usually not associated with conscious proprioceptive deficits or weakness. A narcolepsy-like syndrome without other obvious neurologic signs suggests infection of the reticular activating system.

Injury to muscles, tendons, or ligaments can be a result of nerve damage or ataxia. For example, upward fixation of the patella, which is a common early finding among horses with neurologic disease, probably results from quadriceps weakness and laxity of the medial patellar ligament. Exertional rhabdomyolysis may occur because a limited number of muscle fibers are doing most of the work.

Behavioral problems can result from discomfort. Severe back soreness is a common side effect that commonly results from asymmetric gait. Bad attitudes towards training may be a direct result of protozoal infection in the amygdala, the region of the brain that controls emotions, but is most likely the result of a lack of confidence or pain associated with secondary problems.

Detection of the early signs of EPM is often easiest by observing horses during training. Frequent bucking, constant head tossing, or excessively high head carriage can be signs of discomfort. Weakness of the hindlimbs is manifested as traveling heavy on the forehand, with minimal forward extension during galloping. This gait may result in multiple minor injuries of the forelimbs, including bucked shins, splints, and bowed tendons. Horses may have difficulty maintaining a specific lead while galloping, and may cross-canter or frequently switch leads. Forelimb gait abnormalities include short, choppy strides; dragging one or all of their feet while walking or trotting; and "floating" in the forward phase of the stride at the trot. Other signs may depend on the athletic endeavor. Thoroughbred racehorses may have difficulty breaking from the starting gate or maintaining position around the turns of the race track. Standardbred racehorses commonly lean on one or the other shaft of the sulky, and may have difficulty negotiating turns. Dressage horses may have a history of a gait abnormality, which is evident only when the horse is permitted to travel on a loose rein and is much improved when the horse is "in a frame." A gait abnormality that occurs while training and cannot be attributed to a musculoskeletal abnormality may result from EPM. Horses exhibiting these signs while training should be evaluated more closely for the presence of neurologic abnormalities.

DIAGNOSIS

Diagnosis of EPM is based on (1) clinical signs, (2) response to treatment, (3) analysis of CSF for the presence of anti-*S. falcatula* antibodies, and (4) cytologic analysis of the CSF. Clinical signs provide a level of suspicion for EPM but are not diagnostic. About one third of horses with EPM show some response to treatment within the first 10 to 14 days of treatment. If the horse fails to respond within 2 weeks, additional diagnostic aids should be used.

A CSF analysis is essential to diagnose most cases of EPM. The CSF may be taken from either the atlanto-occipital (A-O) or lumbosacral (LS) space, but the LS space is preferred (see *Current Therapy in Equine Medicine 2*, p 341; and *Current Therapy in Equine Medicine 3*, p 527). Because the CSF flows in a caudal direction and most horses are infected in the spinal cord, sampling from the LS space is most likely to reveal inflammation, high creatinine kinase activities, and anti-*S. falcatula* antibodies. Cytologic analysis of CSF classically reveals increased total protein concentrations (>80–100 mg/dl, depending upon the specific assay used in the reference laboratory), a mononuclear pleocytosis (>8 cells/μl), and elevated creatine kinase (CK) activity (>10 IU/L). CK activity may be increased spuriously as a result of contamination of the CSF sample with a needle plug of epidural fat or ligamentum flavum. No evidence of inflammation may be present, and CK levels may be normal if the infection is localized and small. Intrathecal production of anti-*S. falcatula* antibodies, on the other hand, occurs regardless of the size or location of the focus of infection.

Antibodies reach the CSF either by leakage from the plasma across a damaged blood-brain barrier or by local intrathecal production, but only the latter indicates the presence of *S. falcatula* in the CNS. The high seroprevalence for EPM in normal horses dictates that a CSF sample that tests weakly positive (i.e., is suspected based on immunoblot test) for the presence of anti-*S. falcatula* antibodies should be further evaluated to ensure the intrathecal origin of antibodies. Quantitation of albumin and gamma globulin levels in simultaneously obtained serum and CSF samples and calculation of CSF indices[*] can determine the presence of serum leakage into the CSF. A combination of antibody detection and determination of indices to detect antibody leakage into the CSF provides the most accurate laboratory diagnosis for EPM.

Several tests are available for detection of anti-*Sarcocystis* antibodies in CSF. Immunoblotting or Western blotting[†] uses the *S. falcatula* organism. Another test, a type of

immunofluorescent antibody assay (IFA),[*] uses *Sarcocystis cruzi*, a protozoan that utilizes dogs and cattle for its life cycle, and relies on detection of cross-reactive antibodies. Agreement between the immunoblot and IFA tests is best at higher concentrations of antibodies, but the results are disparate at lower concentrations of antibodies.

An additional laboratory procedure[†] detects the presence of parasite deoxyribonucleic acid (DNA) in horse CSF and does not rely on antibody production. The CSF is harvested into a chelating agent, such as ethylenediaminetetraacetic acid (EDTA). This test appears to be more sensitive than the immunoblot test in very early EPM infections, before the onset of a detectable immune response, and in long-term cases in which the immune response has waned. The immunoblot appears to be a better test in most other cases, because parasite DNA is difficult to detect during an aggressive immune response.

TREATMENT

The basis of therapy for EPM is antibiotics directed against the parasite. Additional treatment may also be necessary to eliminate inflammation of the nervous tissue, treat secondary problems, and offset side effects of the antibiotic treatment. Current maintenance dosage recommendations for antiprotozoal therapy are pyrimethamine[‡] (1.0 mg/kg p.o. s.i.d.; 20 tablets for 450-kg horse) and trimethoprim-sulfamethoxazole or sulfadiazine (15–30 mg/kg in a combined dose p.o. b.i.d.). Alternatively, a different sulfonamide (12–24 mg/kg b.i.d.) can be used in combination with the pyrimethamine, because trimethoprim at achievable concentrations has no effect on the protozoa and is unnecessary in the treatment of EPM. In addition, because trimethoprim has the same mechanism of action as pyrimethamine, it may potentiate the toxicity of the pyrimethamine without adding to the efficacy of treatment. Horses should remain on both drugs for the duration of treatment, because closely related protozoa, including *Falciparium* species and *T. gondii*, become resistant to pyrimethamine in the absence of sulfonamides.

Potentiation of pyrimethamine by sulfonamides may permit treatment of some horses with lower doses of pyrimethamine. However, pyrimethamine (1.0 mg/kg) does not achieve minimum inhibitory concentration for protozoa in the CSF without the presence of a sulfonamide. Use of lower doses of the drug is therefore probably dangerous, because it could encourage selection for a resistant population of protozoa. A lower dose (0.5 mg/kg s.i.d.) should be reserved for mares in foal and horses that exhibit signs of toxicity at the higher dose.

The method of administration of medication is extremely important. Many horses treated by adding the drugs directly to the feed have failed to respond until the medication was administered by dose syringe into the mouth. Horses that do not eat their grain all at one time probably do not achieve drug levels high enough to arrest the parasite. Hay, grain, and folic acid supplements may interfere

---

*Equine Biodiagnostics, Lexington, KY
†Equine Biodiagnostics, Lexington, KY

*Immunoparasitology Laboratory, Oklahoma State University, Stillwater, OK
†Equine Biodiagnostics, Lexington, KY
‡Daraprim, Burroughs-Wellcome, Research Triangle Park, NC

with absorption. In addition, the pyrimethamine should be administered as a single daily dose and not divided into twice-daily doses. Peak drug levels appear to be necessary to achieve minimal inhibitory concentrations.

Sufficient duration of treatment is equally as important as sufficient dose. Horses relapse at a rate of about 40% within the first few months after the medication is discontinued. Most of these horses have been treated for less than 3 months, or with less than 1 mg/kg of pyrimethamine. Some horses that appear to relapse may actually suffer from a new infection. Horses that do not relapse have usually been treated for 4 months or longer. Current recommendations are to treat for a minimum of 4 months, or 4 weeks beyond a plateau of clinical signs, whichever is longer. Horses should be carefully watched for the early recurrence of clinical signs within the first few months after treatment is discontinued. When relapses occur, the protozoa that persist may be resistant to medication, and therefore the duration of the second treatment should be at least twice as long as the first. Some horses that have relapsed when the medication is discontinued ultimately have relapses every time the medication is withdrawn and therefore need to remain on treatment for life. Extreme caution should be taken when recommending that medication be discontinued, because there is currently no alternative medication.

Anti-inflammatory therapy is indicated in the initial treatment of most cases of EPM. The minimal recommendation for treatment is flunixin meglumine (1.1 mg/kg b.i.d. for 3–4 days, then s.i.d. for 3–7 days). This nonsteroidal anti-inflammatory drug has a larger volume of distribution than phenylbutazone, and penetrates into the CNS at higher concentration. Caution should be used when administering nonsteroidal anti-inflammatory drugs to horses with evidence of gastrointestinal ulcers (see page 724), which occasionally accompany EPM. Acute onset of EPM may require the addition of dimethyl sulfoxide (DMSO; 1 g/kg in a 10% solution IV). Administration by nasogastric tube may also be effective. The DMSO can be administered daily for up to 3 days, and then every other day for 3 to 4 treatments, if necessary. Acute onset of severe ataxia or other evidence of brain disease resulting from EPM may warrant the administration of corticosteroids. These potent CNS anti-inflammatory drugs may be administered for several days to combat inflammation, without adversely affecting the prognosis. Long-term administration should be avoided to prevent immunosuppression.

About 10% of horses experience a "treatment crisis," in which the neurologic signs worsen while on medication. This may be the result of an inflammatory response to the dying parasites. This crisis usually responds to the anti-inflammatory treatment described earlier. Supplementation with vitamin E (8000 IU s.i.d.) may be a helpful adjunct to treatment because of its antioxidant properties.

Side Effects of Anti-folate Antibiotics

Several side effects have been identified with the use of the antibiotic doses recommended for treatment of EPM. Diarrhea can be associated with trimethoprim/sulfa combinations. The colitis of unknown mechanism may be severe and may culminate in death. This complication is rare, but

all horses that are placed on this treatment combination should be closely observed for the development of loose stool. Some horses may tolerate lower doses of the pyrimethamine and trimethoprim/sulfa without developing diarrhea.

Anemia has been identified in 10 to 20% of horses by the end of the second month of treatment, unless the horse is also given folic acid and brewer's yeast. Complete blood counts evaluated at this point in treatment reveal a normocytic to macrocytic anemia with packed cell volumes (PCV) as low as 20 vol%. This level is not life-threatening, and the PCV level usually stabilizes and returns to normal within 2 weeks of cessation of treatment. Monitoring of PCV is recommended at least monthly in all horses on treatment for EPM. Pyrimethamine and trimethoprim inhibit the parasite by competitively inhibiting dihydrofolate reductase and interfering with production of the active form of folic acid, tetrahydrofolate. These drugs can also interfere with folic acid metabolism by the horse, resulting in folic acid deficiency and subsequent anemia. Because the protozoa cannot use preformed folic acid, supplementation with folic acid* (40 mg s.i.d.) may prevent the effects of folic acid deficiency without interfering with antiparasitic activity. Once anemia or leukopenia has occurred, folic acid may be effective for treatment but, in many cases, folinic acid† may be necessary to reverse these effects of treatment. No recommended dose exists for folinic acid, but the dose used in humans predicts a dose of 100 to 200 μg/kg (50–100 mg for a 500-kg horse).

Brood mares that are diagnosed with EPM should be placed on treatment with caution. Anecdotal evidence suggests that mares may abort or suffer early embryonic loss if treated during the first trimester of pregnancy, abort during the second trimester, or have abnormal foals in the last trimester. Several foals with a neonatal maladjustment-like syndrome have been born to mares that were treated for EPM for several months in late gestation. These foals are born normal, then lose the suckle reflex. Bone marrow suppression of both erythrocyte and leukocyte lines is observed. Because of these observations, all brood mares in foal should be given supplements of folic acid (80 mg s.i.d.) if treated for EPM. Alternatively, the dosage of medication may be decreased, or treatment may be withheld until after the foal is born, depending upon the requirements of the individual case.

Leukopenia, thrombocytopenia, anorexia, and febrile episodes have been sporadically observed in horses on treatment for EPM. These episodes appear to respond to withdrawal of the medication for several days and do not necessarily recur when the medication is reinitiated. Horses that exhibit these episodes have no respiratory or gastrointestinal signs and appear normal in every other body system. The cause of these episodes is unknown.

PREVENTION

Prevention of EPM is best accomplished by limiting opossum access to horse-raising properties. Opossums are

---

Buckeye Feed Mill, Columbus, OH
†Leucovorin, Immunex, Seattle, WA

nocturnal scavengers. Both feed and garbage cans should have tight-fitting lids to discourage this animal from frequenting barns. Grain should be kept swept away from aisles and shed rows, and swept-up grain should not be fed to horses. Food intended for domestic animals, such as cat and dog food, should not be left in the barn or near pastures overnight. The range of individual opossums is small, usually less than 1 mile in diameter, which suggests that trapping and relocating opossums is likely to decrease morbidity of EPM.

TRAINING AND REHABILITATION

Because an ataxic horse is potentially dangerous, the owner and trainer should be advised that riding is performed at that individual's own risk. Regardless of this recommendation, many owners and trainers continue training the mildly affected horse. This tends to improve the neurologic signs. Horses should usually be kept out of training during the first 10 days of treatment to permit secondary problems to resolve. If significant asymmetry exists, even with mild neurologic deficits, training should include lunging, driving, or working in a round pen without a rider. Jogging or trotting appears to encourage fitness while preventing many secondary problems.

Horses that are likely to fall should not be ridden under any circumstance. Formal training often does not benefit these horses, because the neurologic deficits lead to a lack of confidence and difficulty with training. These horses should be completely rested. Pasture rest is preferable to stall rest, unless the horse is actually falling, because voluntary exercise can improve the effects of neurologic deficits.

PROGNOSIS

Most EPM-affected horses that are treated with the recommended dosages of antibiotics for at least 3 months improve. Recovery to normal may occur in 50 to 75% of cases but depends upon the severity and duration of neurologic signs when the disease is identified. It is impossible to predict which individuals will respond well and which will have permanent residual damage, because clinical signs are the same whether they result from damaged neurons or edema and inflammation surrounding neurons. For the latter reason, the best prognostic indicator is a rapid response to anti-inflammatory medication and some response to antiprotozoal treatment within the first 10 to 14 days. In general, horses that are severely affected do not return to normal, and horses that are mildly affected are more likely to return to normal. However, there are sufficient exceptions in both categories to confound any attempt to predict prognosis based on the initial examination. Horses in which the signs are detected early in the course of disease are likely to respond well, but it is difficult upon first examination to determine how long mild clinical signs may have been present.

Supplemental Readings

Clarke CR, MacAllister CG, Burrows GE, Ewing P, Spillers DK, Burrows SL: Pharmacokinetics, penetration into cerebrospinal fluid, and hematologic effects after multiple oral administrations of pyrimethamine to horses. Am J Vet Res 53:2296–2299, 1992.

Fayer R, Mayhew IG, Baird JD, Dill SG, Foreman JH, Fox JC, Higgins RJ, Reed SM, Ruoff WW, Sweeney RW, Tuttle P: Epidemiology of Equine Protozoal Myelitis in North America based on histologically confirmed cases. A report. J Vet Intern Med 4:54–57, 1990.

Fenger CK, Granstrom DE, Langemeier JL, Stamper S, Donahue JM, Patterson JS, Gajadhar AA, Marteniuk JV, Xiaomin Z, Dubey JP: Identification of opossums as the putative definitive host of *Sarcocystis neurona*. J Parasitol 81(6):916–919, 1995.

Equine Herpesvirus-1 Myeloencephalitis

TIM J. CUTLER

ROBERT J. MACKAY
Gainesville, Florida

Since its first description almost 50 years ago, equine herpesvirus-1 (EHV-1) myeloencephalitis has been encountered with increasing frequency. Occurrence is generally sporadic, but devastating outbreaks with morbidity of up to 40% and mortality of up to 90% can risk the future of an equine operation. Outbreaks are no longer restricted to breeding operations, but also may pose a significant risk to racing establishments. The disease has also been reported in nonhorse equidae and in llamas and alpacas. Distribution is worldwide, although most cases have been reported from North America and Europe.

EPIDEMIOLOGY

The neurologic form of equine herpesvirus-1 infection frequently occurs concurrently with, or subsequent to, signs of respiratory disease. The incubation period is typically 4 to 7 days, but may extend to 2 weeks. EHV-1 myeloencephalitis may affect animals of any age, although cases are seen most often in pregnant or recently foaled mares. Pregnant mares rarely abort during the myeloencephalopathic phase of disease, but other in-contact mares may.

Source of virus may be a newly arrived animal or recrudescence from latency in lymphoid tissue. Immunocompromise from exposure to stressful situations including weaning, castration, parturition, transport, and presumably racing or the use of exogenous corticosteroids likely increases the risk of EHV-1 myeloencephalitis. Subclinical shedders may be an important source of virus. Aborted, stillborn, or clinically affected neonates also are highly infectious. Close contact with donkeys or mules has been implicated in two epizootics. In the environment, the virus generally remains infective for less than 2 weeks but may survive for 5 to 6 weeks on suitable fomites such as horsehair or oily burlap.

CLINICAL SIGNS

The predominant clinical sign is acute onset of symmetrical ataxia and weakness of trunk and limbs, which develop acutely and progress rapidly for up to 48 hours before stabilizing. Recumbency may occur during this period. Although evidence of brain involvement is apparent histopathologically, clinical signs usually are referable to spinal cord disease, particularly of caudal thoracic, lumbar, or sacral segments. Thus, the signs of paresis and ataxia are often limited to, or are much more severe in, the pelvic limbs. Thoracic limb signs indicate involvement of the cervical or cranial thoracic spinal cord; however, this is less commonly seen. Infrequently, there are signs of cranial nerve dysfunction such as nystagmus, head tilt, and staggering gait or tongue weakness. Signs of mental depression are seen rarely. Cauda equina syndrome is a common part of the clinical syndrome. Dribbling of urine may be present from the vulva or prepuce; other signs are bladder distension, tail weakness, fecal retention, penile prolapse or persistent erection, or perineal sensory deficits.

Other signs associated with the disease include lower limb edema, especially in the pelvic limbs, and scrotal edema in stallions. Concurrent signs of respiratory disease such as coughing and nasal discharge in affected or in-contact horses may be seen. (See page 444 for description of EHV-associated respiratory disease.) A moderate to high fever (102°–105°F) may be the only sign preceding the neurologic form of disease.

DIAGNOSIS

Cerebrospinal fluid (CSF) should be aspirated from the lumbosacral or atlanto-occipital spaces for analysis. The techniques are described in *Current Therapy in Equine Medicine 3*, pages 526 to 527. Cerebrospinal fluid from horses affected with EHV-1 myeloencephalitis characteristically is xanthochromic (i.e., yellow due to breakdown of heme pigment), and protein concentration usually is above the normal range (i.e., >80 mg/dl, and can be as high as 300 mg/dl). In contrast, the nucleated cell count is almost invariably normal (<8 cells/μl).

In areas where equine protozoal myeloencephalitis (EPM) is common and CSF and serum routinely are tested for *Sarcocystis neurona* antibody by immunoblot, an element of caution is indicated in interpreting the results. It is predictable that when serum concentration of *S. neurona* antibody is high, an EHV-1-altered blood-CSF barrier may allow passage of antibodies from blood into CSF, leading to an invalid diagnosis of EPM. Such false-positives can generally be detected by IgG index and albumin quotient determinations of blood-CSF barrier permeability.*

Definitive ante mortem diagnosis can be made by isolation of the virus from CSF; however, because of the endothelial location of the virus and the short duration of T lymphocyte–associated viremia and the high concentration of neutralizing antibody, attempts at isolation from CSF seldom are successful. Isolation of virus from other sites such as respiratory tract or blood lends support to the diagnosis. Blood for viral isolation should be collected with sodium citrate as the anticoagulant. Nasopharyngeal swabs for viral isolation should be placed in viral transport media containing antibiotics and sent quickly to the laboratory. Isolation of the virus from close in-contact animals has been successful on some occasions when direct isolation from the affected horse was negative. This may be useful to support the diagnosis in the absence of more definitive test results. Failure to isolate the virus does not exclude the diagnosis of EHV-1 myeloencephalitis. A fourfold or greater increase in serum virus neutralization or complement fixation antibody titer between samples taken during the acute stage of the disease and 2 to 3 weeks later is consistent with the diagnosis, albeit retrospectively. In addition, a higher single serum titer than that encountered in response to vaccination (probably >1:400) may be very indicative of the disease.

Equine herpesvirus-1 myeloencephalitis can be diagnosed definitively by histopathology examination. Small arterioles, particularly those supplying ventral and lateral white matter tracts, are most affected, although venular involvement also occurs. Predominantly, there is mononuclear vasculitis, endothelial necrosis, and thrombosis of small arterioles associated with neuronal swelling and necrosis. Hemorrhage may be extensive. Demonstration by fluorescent antibody or immunohistochemical stain of viral antigen in CNS tissue also is diagnostic. Again, attempts at viral isolation from CNS tissue are warranted, although it is only occasionally successful. Polymerase chain reaction has been employed to detect EHV DNA and differentiate EHV-1 from EHV-4 in nasopharyngeal secretions. The promise of increased sensitivity with this test is encouraging for the future laboratory-based diagnosis of EHV-1 myeloencephalitis.

TREATMENT

The main aim of therapy is supportive care. No specific antiviral therapy has been evaluated. Because EHV-1 mye-

---

**Equine Biodiagnostics Inc, Lexington, KY 40506-0286.*

loencephalitis likely is immune-mediated, corticosteroid administration is an important part of treatment. Most clinicians begin with high doses of dexamethasone,° then gradually reduce the dose over 3 to 5 days. A fair degree of variation is seen in recommended dosages, from 0.05 to 0.1 mg/kg IM b.i.d. for 1 to 3 days (see *Current Therapy in Equine Medicine 3*, page 551) to 0.1 to 0.25 mg/kg IM b.i.d. for 3 days. Clinical judgment is indicated in selecting a dose, based on the severity of disease, confidence in the diagnosis, and the potential hazards of steroid-induced immunosuppression and laminitis. One or two doses of corticosteroids apparently has little adverse clinical effect on other treatable neurologic diseases, most notably EPM. The oxygen free radical scavenger dimethyl sulfoxide (DMSO) is a useful adjunctive therapy, particularly in severe cases. It is administered at 1 g/kg IV, as a 10 to 20% solution, in saline or 5% dextrose b.i.d. for up to 3 days. Concurrent administration of a nonsteroidal anti-inflammatory drug such as flunixin meglumine† (1.1 mg/kg IV b.i.d.) may also be useful.

Rectal examination should be performed to determine bladder size and fecal load in the rectum. A greatly enlarged bladder, indicative of emptying dysfunction, requires catheterization at least twice daily, until normal micturition returns, an event that should not be confused with constant dribbling from an overdistended bladder. As an alternative, particularly when prolonged catheterization or frequent visits to the affected animal are impractical, an indwelling catheter system may be placed. The authors have had success in mares with use of a Foley catheter (24–28 French) attached to 3 to 4 feet of stomach tubing ending in a Heimlich valve that is braided into the tail. This has the advantage of avoiding urine scald without a heavy collection system and also appears to prevent ascending infection by promoting constant orthograde flow of urine. Bag-collection systems have been described that require attachment to a pelvic limb, but these are not suitable for active or fractious horses. Prophylactic administration of antimicrobial drugs, such as trimethoprim/sulfamethoxazole‡ (15–20 mg/kg p.o. b.i.d.) is advisable to prevent urinary tract infection if the bladder is repeatedly catheterized or a continuous urinary catheter system is in place. In males, an indwelling system is more difficult to manage, and it may be necessary to perform a perineal urethrostomy. If there is obstipation, multiple daily manual evacuations of the rectum are required. The use of fecal softeners

such as psyllium, mineral oil, and/or bran mash has been advocated. Highly digestible diets (e.g., Equine Senior°) may also be useful.

PROGNOSIS

The critical factor in determining the prognosis is whether the patient becomes recumbent. In recumbent horses the mortality rate is high, the duration of recovery is usually months to years, the chance of residual impairments is high, and complications of management such as decubital ulcers and difficulties in defecation and micturition are added. If recumbency does not occur during the first several days, the prognosis is good. Some horses improve to normal in 3 to 5 days; however, most take several months during which gradual improvement occurs. Residual gait abnormalities or bladder dysfunction may be present.

PREVENTION

Both modified live and inactivated viral vaccines are available for immunization against EHV-1, with or without EHV-4. The debate about vaccinating against EHV-1 myeloencephalitis centers around its probable immune-mediated pathogenesis. No currently available vaccine appears to be protective against myeloencephalitis, and it has been suggested that vaccines may even predispose the vaccinate to the disease. In particular, first-time vaccination of in-contact animals during an outbreak is not advised because such practice theoretically may precipitate disease. Vaccination of animals known not to have had contact with the diseased animal is more controversial but has been advocated. Management of EHV respiratory disease outbreaks is discussed on page 444 and in *Current Therapy in Equine Medicine 3*, page 322, and, as a minimum, similar preventive efforts should be undertaken in cases of EHV-1-associated neurologic disease.

Supplemental Readings

Kohn CW, Fenner WR: Equine herpes myeloencephalopathy. Vet Clin North Am Equine Pract 3(2):405–419, 1987.
Little PB, Thorsen J: Disseminated necrotizing myeloencephalitis: A herpes-associated neurological disease of horses. Vet Pathol 13:161–171, 1976.
Ostlund, EN: The equine herpesviruses. Vet Clin North Am Equine Pract 9(2):283–294, 1993.

°Dexamethasone injectable, The Butler Company, Columbus, OH
†Banamine, Schering-Plough Animal Health, Kenilworth, NJ
‡SMZ-TMP, United Research Laboratories, Bensalem, PA

°Purina Mills, Lake City, FL

Rabies

SHERRIL L. GREEN
Stanford, California

Rabies in horses is sporadic and outbreaks are infrequent. The equine species, however, is highly susceptible to the disease. With increasing urbanization and the continual resurgence of rabies in the wildlife population, it remains an important threat to livestock. In endemic areas, the frequency of rabies in horses appears to coincide with epizootics in the sylvatic reservoirs (i.e., skunks, raccoons, foxes, and bats). Oral rabies immunization of wildlife has met with some success, but the disease persists in many parts of the world, including Canada, the United States, and Central and South America. Most equine practitioners inevitably encounter a "rabies suspect." Prophylactic antirabies immunization is justifiably recommended for veterinary technicians, veterinarians, and other animal health workers.

CLINICAL SIGNS

It can be difficult to recognize rabies because the disease can present with such a wide range of clinical signs. The diagnosis may be further confounded by the uncertainty of the route and time of exposure and the variable incubation period. The disease is usually transmitted to the horse via a bite wound from an infected wild animal or an infected domestic dog or cat, but the encounter is rarely observed, and wounds are difficult to find. Animals of any age can be infected, including suckling foals, which are generally inquisitive and are inclined to have contact with stray domestic or wild animals. The exact incubation period in the horse is unknown but is generally thought to be 2 weeks to several months. The neurotropic rabies virus, a rhabdovirus, can remain latent at the site of the inoculation before it travels centripetally up the peripheral nerves to the central nervous system (CNS). It then spreads centrifugally to highly innervated body organs. The clinical course of the disease is related to the dose and site of inoculation (i.e., proximity to the brain) and the pathogenicity of the specific rabies virus strain. In horses, natural infection is invariably fatal.

Traditionally, the clinical syndromes associated with rabies virus infection have been described as three forms: dumb or brainstem, paralytic/ataxic or spinal cord, and furious or cortical. However, rabid animals display a broad range of clinical signs. Aggressiveness and indiscriminate attack are alerting, but equine rabies is not invariably manifested as the furious form. The initial clinical signs may include progressive ascending ataxia and paresis, lameness, colic, dysphagia, hyperesthesia and self-mutilation, or fever. A spectrum of other signs has been described, but recumbency, loss of tail and anal sphincter tone, and loss of sensory perception of the hindlimbs often precede death. The disease is generally rapidly progressive. Horses usually die of cardiac or respiratory arrest 4 days or so after onset of the clinical signs. Survival for up to 10 to 15 days after onset has been reported but is uncommon.

DIAGNOSIS

Rabies must be the primary working diagnosis when rapidly progressive unexplained neurologic disease renders a horse recumbent. Other neurologic disorders in the list of differential diagnoses include equine herpesvirus infection; eastern, western, or Venezuelan encephalomyelitis; equine protozoal myelitis; choke; trauma; ingestion of toxins (yellow star thistle plants, lead, or moldy corn); hepatoencephalopathy; or botulism.

Rabies remains a disease in which the ante mortem diagnosis is based on the history and clinical signs. The virus is not highly immunogenic, and there are no hematologic abnormalities specific for rabies virus infection. The cerebral spinal fluid (CSF) analysis may be occasionally helpful, but testing often yields normal results, especially at the onset of the disease. A mild CSF pleocytosis, with a predominance of lymphocytes and macrophages, may be present. However, xanthochromia and an elevated total protein concentration are not consistent findings. It is not always practical to collect CSF from patients in the field, and the risk of exposure to low levels of the virus in CSF should be considered. Results of serology testing, CSF neutralization tests, and positive fluorescent antibody testing (FAT) on skin or tactile hair follicles, corneal scrapings, or salivary gland have limited usefulness because of false positives, false negatives, and difficulties in their interpretation.

The most reliable tests remain those that are performed on brain or spinal cord tissue collected at postmortem examination. Veterinarians should consult with their local laboratories regarding specific guidelines for shipping and handling postmortem specimens. In general, the whole head, shipped in a sealed, refrigerated container, should be submitted to the appropriate state public health laboratory for histopathologic and fluorescent antibody testing. Necropsy on the carcass should be postponed until rabies can be ruled out.

Most laboratories use the fluorescent antibody test for viral antigen in brain tissue as the standard diagnostic test, in conjunction with histopathologic examination. The fluorescent antibody test is highly accurate and can be completed in less than 24 hours. Histologically, the characteristic eosinophilic intracytoplasmic Negri bodies, found in the neurons of the hippocampus and Purkinje cells of the cerebellum, are pathognomonic for rabies. Negri bodies are usually present in animals that have survived the disease for 4 or 5 days. However, the detection of Negri bodies can depend on the thoroughness of the necropsy. Intracerebral inoculation of mice with brain tissue can be used to isolate and identify the specific strain of rabies virus, but these procedures are expensive and time-consuming, and are usually performed only under special circumstances.

MANAGEMENT AND PREVENTION

Management of a suspected rabies virus–infected horse and postexposure procedures for people who have come into close contact with the animal should be undertaken with the advice of local health department authorities. The suspected rabies-infected horse should be quarantined. Contact with human beings should be restricted, preferably to one or two individuals who have been vaccinated against the disease. The virus is susceptible to most disinfectants, and it may be helpful to reassure clients that transmission of the virus from an infected horse to a human being has not been documented. More horses are considered "rabies suspects" than are actually infected with the virus. However, considering the risk associated with this highly fatal zoonotic disease, it seems prudent to be cautious.

The National Association of State Public Health Veterinarians (NASPHV) currently recommends that any vaccinated or unvaccinated horse that has been bitten by a wild animal, regardless of whether the wild animal is available for testing, should be considered exposed to rabies. Exposed vaccinated horses should be revaccinated and observed for 90 days. An unvaccinated horse should be euthanized, or if the owner is unwilling, the horse should be kept quarantined for 6 months. The unvaccinated horse should probably not be vaccinated for rabies during this period.

Annual vaccination of horses against rabies, beginning at 3 months of age, is recommended in areas where the disease is endemic. The currently marketed inactivated rabies vaccines should be given intramuscularly in the thigh. Vaccines appear to be safe and effective. A list of rabies vaccines licensed in the United States for use in horses is regularly published by the NASPHV in the *Compendium on Animal Rabies Control*.

Supplemental Readings

Compendium of Animal Rabies Control, 1995. National Association of State Public Health Veterinarians. J Am Vet Med Assoc 206:14–18, 1995.
Fishbein DB, Robinson LE: Rabies. N Engl J Med 329(22):1632–1638, 1993.
Green SL: Equine rabies. Vet Clin North Am Equine Pract 9(2):337–347, 1993.
Green SL, Beacock SM, Vernau B: Equine rabies: Clinical signs, diagnosis and comments on vaccination. Proc 36th Annu Conv Am Assoc Equine Pract, 1990, pp 357–361.
Hamir AN, Moser G, Rupprecht CE: A five year (1985–1989) retrospective study of equine neurological diseases with special reference to rabies. J Compar Pathol 106:411–421, 1992.

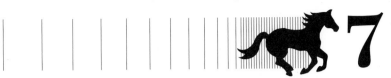

SECTION

7

THE EYE

Edited by Philip Boydell

Ocular Pharmacology and Therapeutics

DAVID L. WILLIAMS
Newmarket, England

The aim of this review is two-fold. It summarizes therapeutic regimens for equine ocular disorders, giving guidelines on ocular drug delivery systems and outlining appropriate drugs for equine ocular disorders. First, however, it seeks to discuss some of the pharmacologic principles upon which equine ocular therapeutics is based. Further details of the therapy of individual diseases are provided in appropriate chapters.

PHARMACOLOGIC BASIS FOR OCULAR THERAPEUTICS

Anatomy and Physiology of the Eye Related to Drug Administration

From a pharmacotherapeutic perspective, the important anatomic and physiologic features of the eye are those that define drug administration, depot storage, distribution within the eye to sites of action, metabolism, and removal from the eye. With regard to topical application, the anatomy of the cornea and adnexa is important. The lipid-dense water-impermeable corneal epithelium may be contrasted with the corneal stroma, a veritable wall of water, stabilized by proteoglycans. Topically applied drugs must cross these two potential barriers before reaching the aqueous. Highly hydrophilic compounds cannot cross the epithelial layer, as demonstrated by the lack of uptake of the highly polar compound fluorescein by the normal cornea. Highly lipophilic compounds are sequestered in the epithelial layer and have poor penetration across the cornea. Compounds in which ionic and nonionic forms exist at physiologic pH have excellent transcorneal penetration;

chloramphenicol is such a drug, ideally suited to providing intraocular antibiosis after topical administration.

The vascular supply to the eye, the distribution of drugs from uveal vasculature to the rest of the anterior segment and the vitreous, together with the influence of the blood-retinal barrier and the avascularity of the majority of the paurangiotic equine fundus are important factors in ocular drug distribution. Systemic administration of nonsteroidal anti-inflammatory drugs is important both as an emergency measure and for long-term prophylaxis in recurrent uveitis, but the systemic route is probably not central to other ocular therapeutics.

Pharmacokinetics of Topically Applied Therapeutic Agents

The bioavailability of topically applied drugs with regard to the cornea and intraocular anterior segment structures depends on several factors. Predominant in surface action of applied drugs is the duration of residence of the drug in the tear film. Considerable work has shown that the volume of an applied drop has a profound influence on tear film residence. In small animals, the volume of an ophthalmic drop overloads the tear volume, and thus much of the applied drug is lost by nasolacrimal overflow. One study demonstrated that 90% of an applied drug is lost in the human eye within the first minute or two after application. The large size of the equine eye reduces these effects, but topical drops are still likely to be lost from the ocular surface through the nasolacrimal duct with the likelihood of systemic absorption after topical application. Such effects may be important with regard to drugs such as atropine (see below). Reflex tearing as well as simple tear overflow contributes to this drug loss. The large topically

339

applied volumes in systems such as transpalpebral lavage systems may give considerably lower bioavailability and drug penetration than would be expected considering the absolute dose of drug given. Smaller volumes increase the percentage of applied drug penetrating the cornea, thus giving advantages for ocular therapeutics as well as reducing possible adverse systemic effects.

Optimizing Topical Drug Delivery

The duration of drug residence at the ocular surface can be increased considerably by the use of gel formulations. Carboxypolymethylene high viscosity gels such as carbomer 940 increase drug residence in the conjunctival sac to up to 8 hours. Although studies of prednisolone acetate in a carbomer formulation have been reported in the rabbit, the only drug licensed for veterinary use in a carbomer formulation is fucidic acid, giving antibacterial effects against gram-positive organisms for up to 24 hours after single topical administration. Such once-daily administration would clearly be invaluable for steroid application to uveitic equine eyes.

Other advances in ocular drug delivery concern the development of systems delivering considerably smaller doses of drugs than is possible in drop formulations. As discussed earlier, such systems can considerably increase the bioavailability of applied drugs. Ophthalmic rods have been discussed (see Miller, 1992 in Supplemental Readings) but have not found significant application in the equine ophthalmic field. A more recent, and potentially more promising, development is that of NODS, the novel ophthalmic delivery system. In this case, a carboxypolymeric tab is placed in the inferior conjunctival fornix where it dissolves, releasing a low concentration of drug locally. The reduced volume in which the drug is delivered gives a considerably increased corneal penetration and thus greater bioavailability. Although the system has not been investigated in the horse to date, NODS atropine could give more rapid mydriasis than do atropine drops or ointment without significant systemic absorption of drug.

Presoaked pig scleral collagen shields and hydrophilic contact lenses can be used, allowing drug retention, although reports have varied considerably in the rate of depletion of drugs from these corneal bandages. These differences are explicable in terms of different shield or lens thickness, presoaking time, and drug concentration. Contact lenses for use in the horse are available from several sources.° The size and curvature of such lenses is critical; lenses should cover the cornea and overlap the limbus slightly. Lenses of the incorrect curvature trap air bubbles in their center, leading to poor fitting and rapid dislodgement. Contact lenses have been used in the treatment of bacterial keratitis, but some workers have reported bacterial colonization of lenses. Thus, care should be exercised in their use. In addition, extended use may lead to corneal edema, presumably because of a reduction in oxygen supply to corneal endothelium. Collagen shields† dissolve over approximately 72 hours, but during that time they can be a useful reservoir for drug solution in which

they are rehydrated before use. Ocular inserts such as hydroxypropyl cellulose pellets° have been produced and can act as drug reservoirs in the conjunctival cul-de-sac, but drugs to be used must be included at the time of manufacture. Currently the only drug available in such a formulation is pilocarpine.†

The practical problems and current solutions with regard to topical delivery in the horse are detailed later. Considerable further research is needed before the use of potentially valuable delivery systems such as rods, shields, NODS, or conjunctival implants can be adequately discussed in the horse.

Subconjunctival Delivery

Drugs injected subconjunctivally might be supposed to enter the eye by trans-scleral penetration. A significant volume of injected solutions, however, has been shown in other species to exit from the injection site and be absorbed by topical transcorneal penetration. Entry by the trans-scleral route can be optimized by a deeper injection at a sub-Tenon's level. Such injections do, however, require considerable sedation. In any case, subconjunctival injections should be attempted only after topical ocular surface anesthesia. The main indication for subconjunctival delivery is the injection of antibiotics for the emergency management of anterior segment infection. Corticosteroid depot injections can also be given in this manner for treatment of corneal inflammation. In either case subconjunctival medication supplements topical therapy rather than replacing it.

Local Deleterious Effects of Topical Drugs

Given the frequent use of topical antibiotics in cases of equine ulcerative keratitis, little consideration is made of the possible effects of such agents on corneal epithelial proliferation or migration. It is widely recognized that topical steroids delay epithelial wound healing and thus should not be used in corneal ulcers. Where corneal inflammation occurs concurrent with ulceration, topical nonsteroidal agents should be used, as detailed in Table 1. The more mildly epitheliotoxic effects of topical antibiotics and ophthalmic preservatives such as benzalkonium chloride are less well noted. Gentamicin has particularly been implicated as increasing epithelial wound healing time, and drug combination ointments are potentially problematic in this respect. Having noted this, the beneficial effects of a topical antibiotic in ulcerative keratitis generally outweigh deleterious effects. When ulcer healing is delayed in a specific animal, however, it is worth considering changing to another antibiotic, specifically one indicated by bacteriologic culture and sensitivity results.

Systemic Effects of Topically Applied Drugs

As discussed earlier, systemic overflow of topically applied drugs may be a problem in some animals. The use of frequent and long-standing topical atropine could, conceivably, have deleterious gastrointestinal effects. Although

°*The Cutting Edge, Diamond Springs, CA, or Veterinary Hydrophobics, Englewood, CO*
†*Opticor, Pitman Moore, Washington Crossing, NJ*

°*Lacrisert, Merck Sharp & Dohme, West Point, PA*
†*Ocusert, Alza Pharmaceuticals, Palo Alto, CA*

TABLE 1. OPTIMAL THERAPEUTIC REGIMENS FOR EQUINE OCULAR DISORDERS

Condition	Suggested Optimal Therapeutic Strategy
Ulcerative keratitis: antibiosis	Topical tobramycin is the preferred antibiotic initially given hourly at 10 mg/ml using a subpalpebral lavage system
Ulcerative keratitis: collagenase inhibition	Autologous serum with 4 mg/ml EDTA and 5% acetyl cysteine again given hourly by lavage
Keratomycosis	Miconazole 10 mg/ml given three times daily
Equine recurrent uveitis: anti-inflammatory therapy	Topical 0.1% prednisolone acetate given four times daily with flubriprofen or suprofen. Systemic anti-inflammatories such as flunixin meglumine in the short term and aspirin 25 mg/kg in the long term should be employed
Equine recurrent uveitis: mydriasis	1–3% atropine given four times daily initially but then reduced to avoid gastrointestinal stasis

there is little documented evidence of such problems, animals under such treatment should be hospitalized and gut motility evaluated regularly while under treatment.

APPROPRIATE THERAPEUTIC REGIMENS IN OCULAR DISEASE

Topical Delivery Systems

The need to provide frequent topical ocular medication to painful eyes is especially important in equine uveitis and ulcerative keratitis. In these conditions, horses often vigorously resent regular instillation of medication and thus placement of a drug delivery system allowing interference with the eye to be minimized is advantageous. Two systems have been reported. The nasolacrimal lavage system involves a length of tubing placed from the nasal punctum of the nasolacrimal duct up the duct. Drug solutions can then be installed topically up the nasolacrimal duct. Although having the advantage of ease of placement, this system has the considerable disadvantage that drug delivery also flushes potentially infectious material from the nasolacrimal duct back to the ocular surface. The technique is therefore not discussed further here.

The preferable technique is one of transpalpebral drug delivery, as illustrated diagrammatically in Figure 1. The technique uses a through-and-through placement with the tube anchored with a knot on the dermal (external) surface of the lid. This is preferable to a technique using a single-lid passage of a flare-ended tube. In this technique, the flared end causes at best ocular irritation and at worst corneal damage; securing the tubing after a second passage through the lid may be more time-consuming to perform but avoids the possibility of corneal damage. Polyethylene tubing (PE 190) or a premature infant naso-gastric feeding tube is used, with holes cut at the appropriate site to allow the drug to bathe the ocular surface. Horses, and especially

those in considerable ocular discomfort, need profound sedation before the placement is attempted. Local anesthesia, with intradermal lignocaine and topical administration of proparacaine or proxymetacaine should also be given. Two key features of tube placement should be noted. First, the guide used to penetrate the lid, either a 14-gauge needle or preferably a 10-gauge flexible angiocatheter, always passes from the conjunctival (internal) to the dermal (external) side of the lid. In this way the cornea is always protected from abrasion or penetration. This does necessitate removal of the hub of the needle or catheter for the second pass through the lid, ensuring that the guide can be passed through the lid over the tubing after placement through the lid. The second feature to note is that the tubing should be placed as deep in the conjunctival fornix as possible, to ensure that corneal abrasion does not occur while the delivery system is in place. When the delivery system is in place, a small quantity of drug is injected into the tubing, followed by a considerable bolus of air to force the solution through the delivery system to the ocular surface. The alternative is to use a constant infusion device to deliver a constant small flow to the ocular surface. Such equipment can readily be fastened to the halter, as can injection ports if frequent bolus deliveries are given.

Habronemiasis

Infective larvae of the flies *Habronema* and *Draschia* may migrate aberrantly in the ocular adnexa, causing severe granulomatous blepharodermal or blepharoconjunctival lesions. Treatment is both larvicidal and anti-inflammatory. Orally administered ivermectin is efficacious systemically for the former, and topical 0.03% ecothiophate has been recommended for conjunctival lesions. Topical corticosteroid or a nonsteroidal anti-inflammatory agent should be used for the latter, although success is not guaranteed because drug penetration into such granulomatous lesions is often suboptimal. Topical preparations containing organophosphates, dimethyl sulphoxide, and petrolatum ointment have been described for this condition, but significant questions remain concerning efficacy and potential local toxicity.

Periocular Neoplasia

Squamous cell carcinoma and sarcoid are the two most frequently occurring periocular neoplasms. Although total excisional biopsy is the ideal treatment, both respond well to double-cycle cryosurgery with rapid freeze to −25°C and slow thaw. Brachytherapy with strontium 90, iodine 125, iridium 192, and radium 222 has also been advocated by some, with strontium 90 giving the best cure rate. Immunotherapy for sarcoid has been reported using intralesional injection of the mycobacterial cell wall extract bacillus Calmette-Guérin (BCG) preparations. Systemic pretreatment with the nonsteroidal anti-inflammatory flunixin meglumine is recommended to avoid anaphylaxis on later injections, in consideration that up to six treatments may be required.

Keratoconjunctivitis Sicca

Keratoconjunctivitis sicca is an infrequently occurring disease in the horse but as in the dog it appears that topical cyclosporine is an effective lacrimogen in this species. The

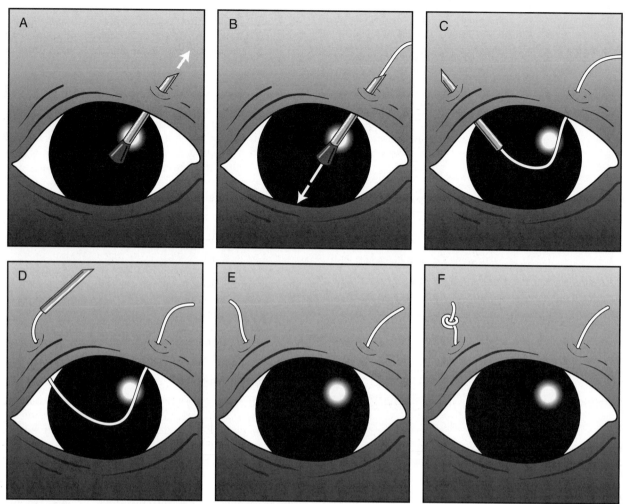

Figure 1. Insertion of a cannula for transpalpebral drug delivery. *A,* Cannula placed through lid from conjunctival to dermal surface. *B,* Tubing drawn through cannula from dermal to conjunctival surface and cannula withdrawn. *C,* Cannula placed through lid from conjunctival to dermal surface, ensuring that the hub has been removed. *D,* Tubing drawn through cannula and then cannula withdrawn over tubing. *E,* Tubing in place well above globe surface, ensuring that no plastic is abrading. *F,* Tubing secured by knotting.

use of 0.2% ointment for the horse has not been reported in the literature, but this product appears as effective in the horse as it is in the dog.

Ulcerative Keratitis

Collagenolytic keratomalacia in ulcerative keratitis, normally caused by gram-negative bacteria such as *Pseudomonas,* is a severe, sight-threatening emergency. Treatment must be aimed both at aggressive topical antibiosis and at the suppression of enzymatic collagenolysis. The choice of relevant antibiosis in an ocular surface infection relies on results of cytologic and bacteriologic investigations. Initially, cytologic investigations show whether gram-negative, gram-positive, or mixed bacterial populations are involved. In stromolytic infections, gram-negative rods such as those of *Pseudomonas* are most commonly seen.

The frequent administration of topical aminoglycosides such as gentamicin is indicated for gram-negative infections. The prevalence of resistant organisms necessitates culture and antibiotic sensitivity investigations of bacteriologic specimens and often calls for aminoglycosides other than gentamicin. Tobramycin is probably the most effica-

cious agent, although problems with resistance to this drug may occur if its use becomes widespread. These problems strongly indicate that gentamicin should not be used as a first-line antibiotic in general ophthalmic use; good clinical practice should restrict its use to *Pseudomonas*-related ulcerative keratitis. Although carbenicillin has good activity against *Pseudomonas,* generally enhanced by gentamicin, the two drugs are incompatible in solution.

Another drug with good activity against gram-negative organisms is polymyxin B. Although polymyxin does not penetrate the intact corneal epithelium, it is readily absorbed by ulcerated corneal stroma. Its sulphate form is several times more potent than the methane sulphonate prodrug sometimes supplied for systemic use. The ophthalmic preparation of polymyxin B and bacitracin has a broad range of activity, because bacitracin acts to inhibit lipid phosphorylation in cell wall synthesis in gram-positive organisms.

The use of fortified topical antibiotics consisting of artificial tear preparations with added crystalline gentamicin made up to a higher concentration than that in commercially available topical drops can be very useful when rapid bactericidal effects are needed. Concentrations of antibiotics diluted in artificial tears are shown in Table 2, together with doses for subconjunctival medication.

Although aggressive antibiosis is important in ulcerative keratitis with stromal melting, inhibition of collagenolysis is critical. The collagenolytic enzymes involved are calcium dependent, and thus the use of calcium chelators such as ethylenediaminetetraacetic acid (EDTA) is valuable. Alpha$_2$-macroglobulins from autologous serum can also be employed to inhibit collagenolysis, as can acetyl cysteine. The optimal treatment regimen in severe stromolytic ulcerative keratitis should therefore include hourly instillation of 5% acetyl cysteine in autologous serum in which is dissolved EDTA (4 mg/ml) and gentamicin (15 mg/ml) or tobramycin (10 mg/ml).

Herpetic Keratitis

In the horse, herpetic keratitis and keratouveitis apparently have been reported, but the significance of these conditions is difficult to assess. Diagnosis has in the past relied on response to antiviral agents. Because they were given together with steroids, it is unclear whether the anti-inflammatory or anti-viral activity was responsible for amelioration of the punctate lesions. Little is known of the efficacy of anti-viral agents against equine herpesvirus type 1—the agent suggested to cause viral keratitis in the horse. Although initial studies suggested that keratitis responsive to idoxuridine and dexamethasone was of viral etiology, recently idoxuridine has not been found to be particularly efficacious on its own. If the virus is similar in response to the feline herpesvirus, idoxuridine or adenine arabinoside are less efficacious than trifluorothymidine. Although in humans acyclovir is an excellent antiherpetic agent, the thymidine kinase of feline herpesvirus does not adequately metabolize the pro-drug 9-(2-hydroxyethyoxymethyl) guanine to its active form, and thus acyclovir is not particularly efficacious in the cat. Its action against equine herpesvirus is, as yet, unclear. In the cat, trifluorothymidine is the optimal antiviral treatment to date, and thus it may be valuable in treatment of potentially viral equine punctate keratitis.

Keratomycosis

The horse has an unusually high incidence of secondary mycotic keratitis after corneal ulceration, this especially occurring after topical corticosteroid use. Although natamycin has been shown to be efficacious in vitro in 97% of isolates from equine mycotic lesions in a large study, two problems are the limited stromal penetration of the

drug and the potentially disastrous toxic induration of subconjuntivally administered agent. The drug is also the most expensive of the antimycotic products available. Although only 67% of fungal species isolated are sensitive to miconazole, the good corneal penetration, safety of subconjunctival administration, and low cost render it worthy of inclusion in the equine ophthalmic pharmacologic armamentarium. Miconazole at 10 mg/ml* for intravenous use may be used topically, or 5 mg may be given subconjunctivally. Natamycin is available as a 5% ophthalmic suspension.†

Intraocular Inflammation

Anterior uveitis in any species requires both intraocular anti-inflammatory medication and mydriatic cycloplegic therapy. The recidivistic nature of equine recurrent uveitis renders the long-term maintenance of vision a difficult task. Aggressive treatment is essential both to halt the inflammatory mechanisms in the disease and to restore and maintain pupillary dilation. Both topical prednisolone acetate and dexamethasone alcohol have good transcorneal penetration. Topical nonsteroidals such as flubiprofen or suprofen may also be useful. Although they have previously been recommended in recalcitrant cases, it is worthwhile combining a topical steroid and a nonsteroidal agent in primary treatment of a severe case of equine anterior uveitis allowing these to have a synergistic effect. The systemic use of steroids is not generally indicated, but a short course of systemic nonsteroidal anti-inflammatory agents such as phenylbutazone or preferably flunixin meglumine may be useful. Long-term oral aspirin at 25 mg/kg s.i.d. apparently reduces the number and severity of recurrent inflammatory episodes, although half-life of the agent in the horse is short and platelet function is inhibited even at low doses given chronically.

Mydriasis requires frequent topical instillation of atropine. A recent review (see Gelatt et al. in Supplemental Readings) has emphasized that 1 and 3% atropine are mydriatics of preference in the normal equine eye, whereas tropicamide, homatropine, cyclopentolate, and scopolamine provided good mydriasis for reduced periods. Phenylephrine (10%) had no mydriatic activity in their study. As discussed earlier, this treatment may have gastrointestinal side effects, and all horses on topical atropine should be monitored for gut motility. The use of atropine ointment reduces systemic absorption of topical drug and may be valuable to use because of this but is more difficult to apply in the horse. Pupillary dilation is significantly more difficult to achieve and maintain in the uveitic than the normal eye; frequent administration of atropine is needed early in the disease to achieve mydriasis. In more chronic disease the synergistic effects of combined atropine, tropicamide, and cyclopentanoate can enable synechiae refractory to single drug treatment to be broken down.

Glaucoma

Clinical trials of drugs acting to reduce aqueous production or facilitate drainage are problematic in the horse, given the low frequency of glaucoma as an ocular problem.

TABLE 2. ANTIBIOTIC DOSES FOR TOPICAL AND SUBCONJUNCTIVAL ADMINISTRATION

Antibiotic	Fortified Eye Drops (Drug Diluted in Artificial Tears)	Subconjunctival Injection
Amikacin	10 mg/ml	25 mg
Bacitracin	10,000 iU/ml	10,000 iU
Carbenicillin	100 mg/ml	250 mg
Chloramphenicol	5 mg/ml	100 mg
Tobramycin	12 mg/ml	40 mg

*Monistat, Janssen Pharmaceutica, Titusville, NJ
†Natacyn, Alcon, Irvine, TX

The greater importance of uveoscleral outflow in the horse as compared with small animal species renders treatment of equine glaucoma potentially different from that in other species. Atropine, for instance, increases uveoscleral outflow and therefore has less of a deleterious effect in a potentially glaucomatous eye than it does in other species. Topical pilocarpine, which is useful in other species, is a poor therapeutic option in the horse because it decreases uveoscleral outflow. In cases of glaucoma associated with uveitis, anti-inflammatory medication combined with topical atropine may, although it is somewhat controversial, be a justifiable therapeutic regimen.

CONCLUSIONS

In several examples given here, it is obvious that the clinical application of ocular pharmacotherapeutics must be undergirded by a thorough understanding of the pharmacology of the drugs, the anatomy and physiology of the eye, and the interaction between therapeutic agents and ocular tissues, which is important in the absorption of drugs, their distribution within the eye, and their action on various tissues within the globe. Given what might be seen as somewhat academic points, the practice of ocular therapeutics relies on practical steps to ensure adequate drug delivery and tried and tested protocols for different commonly seen equine ocular diseases.

Supplemental Readings

Gelatt KN, Gum GG, MacKay EO: Evaluation of mydriatics in horses. Vet Comp Ophthal 5(2):104–108, 1995.

Kern TJ, Brooks DE, White MM: Equine keratomycosis: Current concepts of diagnosis and therapy. Equine Vet J [Suppl]2:33–38, 1983.

Miller TR: Principles of therapeutics. Vet Clin North Am Equine Pract 8(3):479–497, 1992.

Patton TF: Pharmacokinetic evidence for improved ophthalmic drug delivery by reduction of instilled volume. J Pharm Sci 66:1058–1059, 1977.

The Prepurchase Ophthalmic Examination

DENNIS E. BROOKS
Gainesville, Florida

WHAT DOES THE HORSE "SEE"?

The horse has a total visual field of nearly 360°, so that it can just about see its tail with its head pointed forward. The horizontal shape of the pupil allows for tremendous peripheral vision, and a small frontal binocular field of 65° develops postnatally. A horse viewing an object at a distance of 20 feet has approximately the visual acuity of a person viewing the object at 33 feet, or has 20/33 vision. The retina is able to detect the colors yellow, green, and blue. The horse has weak accommodative ability of the lens, and therefore has limited near focus capability, although adaptations of the equine retinal ultrastructure exist that are helpful for near vision. The optic nerve is unique in that it contains a substantial proportion of axons of large diameter. Large ganglion cells possess large-diameter axons and are involved with motion detection, stereopsis, and sensitivity to dim light, suggesting that the horse has strong adaptations for these visual characteristics.

Variations of the normal equine fundus are numerous and are primarily related to coat color. The tapetal fundus is usually yellow to blue-green with the nontapetum various shades of brown. Horses with blue irides may have no tapetum and no pigment in the nontapetal region, and thus display the orange choroidal vascular pattern. The retinal blood vessels are normally small and extend only a short distance from the optic disc. Small dots (stars of Winslow) are distributed in a uniform pattern throughout the tapetal fundus and represent end-on views of choroidal capillaries.

The optic disc is oval to round, pink to orange in color, and located slightly temporal in the inferior quadrant of the nontapetal fundus.

EXAMINATION OF PERFORMANCE HORSES: COMPARING THE TWO EYES

A complete ocular examination of both eyes, using a focal light source such as a transilluminator, and direct ophthalmoscope, should be part of every examination of the performance horse. Examination of the eyes before purchase is carried out by a veterinarian representing the buyer and is designed to detect a disease, such as cataracts or uveitis, that may lead to decreased vision. Minor signs of eye disease overlooked at this examination may be followed by vision loss, rider injury, and lawsuits. The purpose for which the horse is to be used determines the emphasis placed on observed ocular lesions. For example, a horse with a large corneal scar may be unsuitable for young children but may be satisfactory for a more mature rider. Some horses may need to be re-examined before being determined to be suitable (Table 1).

Epiphora, eyelid abnormalities, corneal scarring, conjunctival and adnexal tumors, cataracts, evidence of active or inactive uveitis, and retinal scarring are common problems noted during prepurchase examinations. Some lesions may be acquired or breed-associated (Table 2).

TABLE 1. CLASSIFICATIONS BASED ON PREPURCHASE EXAMINATION OF THE EYE

Suitable: No visible lesion or a nonprogressive lesion is present. No vision loss or vision threatening disease was detected.
Unsuitable: Eye disease is present leading to insufficient vision for safety. Inherited disorder in a breeding animal.
Provisionally suitable: Suspicious disease or lesion present. Suggest ophthalmologist examine the horse.
Re-examine: (1) after therapy; (2) after no therapy
Unsuitable lesions:
 1. Blindness for any reason (one or both eyes)
 2. Mature cataract
 3. Acute or chronic uveitis lesions (anterior or posterior synechiae, and small or large peripapillary chorioretinal scars)
 4. Large corneal scar in the visual axis
 5. Ocular neoplasia
 6. Cornea striae or "band opacities"
 7. Posterior subcapsular cataract (often progressive)
 8. Partial or total retinal detachment in one eye
 9. Large numbers of vitreal floaters
10. Optic nerve atrophy

The source of any epiphora should be determined by placing fluorescein dye in the eye. After several minutes the dye should appear in the nasal passages if the nasolacrimal ducts are patent. The use of fluorescein dye also helps the clinician detect small corneal ulcers that may also be associated with tearing.

Eyelid defects may be associated with exposure keratitis. The nictitans should be carefully examined to see if it is able to protect the cornea in the presence of a lid defect. The most common adnexal tumors in horses are squamous

TABLE 2. BREED-RELATED EYE DISEASE IN HORSES

Appaloosa
 1. Congenital stationary night blindness
 2. Congenital cataracts
 3. Glaucoma
 4. Equine recurrent uveitis
 5. Optic disc colobomas
Arabian
 1. Congenital cataracts
Belgian draft horses
 1. Aniridia and secondary cataracts
Morgan
 1. Cataracts—nuclear, bilateral, symmetrical, and nonprogressive
Quarterhorse
 1. Congenital cataracts
 2. Entropion
Thoroughbred
 1. Congenital cataracts
 2. Microphthalmia associated with multiple ocular defects
 3. Retinal dysplasia associated with retinal detachments in some cases
 4. Entropion
Color-dilute breeds
 1. Iridal hypoplasia—photophobia
Standardbreds
 1. Retinal detachments
 2. Congenital stationary night blindness
Paso Fino
 1. Congenital stationary night blindness
American Saddlebred
 1. Cataracts
Warmbloods
 1. Glaucoma

cell carcinomas. They are always of concern. If small, they should be removed and the tumor site irradiated or frozen. If large, the buyer should be warned, because ocular disfigurement and metastasis may occur.

The cornea should be clear, smooth, and shiny, rather than dull and roughened. Dull-appearing corneas may be edematous or scarred. Corneal scars from previous injuries or ulcerations may pose no problem for the horse's vision if they are small or are located near the limbus. Large scars in the central cornea may be associated with less than satisfactory vision and should be evaluated carefully. The presence of corneal striae or corneal endothelial "band opacities" in nonbuphthalmic horse eyes warrants a high degree of suspicion for equine glaucoma. The intraocular pressure (IOP) should be carefully measured with applanation tonometry, not digitally, to determine if IOP is elevated. Serial IOP measurements over a 12- to 24-hour period may be necessary to detect transient but significant elevations in IOP. Linear corneal opacities also may be found in eyes that are normotensive at the time of examination.

Cataracts are always important because they are generally progressive. They can be staged according to their degree of maturity with incipient (focal), immature (partial lens opacity and the horse still has vision), and mature (complete lens opacity and blindness) types. Veterinarians should be aware that normal aging of the horse lens results in cloudiness of the nucleus beginning at 7 to 8 years of age, but that this is not a true cataract. Cataracts of the posterior lens sutures and cataracts associated with persistence of the hyaloid artery are also reported. Lens opacities are seen best with the pupil dilated and the examination taking place in complete darkness. Many cataracts in horses are the result of previous bouts of uveitis. Nuclear cataracts in Morgan horses do not progress, but are hereditary. Cataract surgery using the phacoemulsification technique in horses has become routine with quite good results, but it is still generally expensive and the postoperative care very labor intensive.

Equine recurrent uveitis (ERU) is the most common cause of blindness in horses (see page 363). In ERU, it is difficult to predict when, or if, clinical signs will recur. Buyers should be made aware of evidence of previous episodes of active ERU. Corneal scarring, iris synechiae and depigmentation, cataracts, aqueous flare, vitreal floaters, and chorioretinal degeneration manifested by "butterfly lesions" are common signs of uveitis. The nontapetal region ventral to the optic disc should be carefully examined with a direct ophthalmoscope because this is the area where focal retinal scars are seen. Large areas of retinal depigmentation and degeneration suggest that the animal has a blind spot of varying size, at least the size of the scar, and therefore vision is reduced.

Retinal detachments may be congenital, traumatic, or the result of ERU and are serious faults because of their association with complete or partial vision loss. Vitreal floaters can develop with age or may be sequelae to ERU. They may rarely cause some head shyness in a few horses, but they are generally benign in nature. Optic nerve atrophy can be related to ERU, glaucoma, or trauma and is associated with blindness. Proliferative lesions of the optic nerve may be noted in older horses, but lesions are generally not sight- or life-threatening.

Vision should be assessed during the examination by ophthalmoscopy and testing of the menace reflex. Appaloosas particularly should be examined in the light and dark to detect evidence of night blindness. Maze testing with blinkers alternatively covering each eye may provide information as to subtle or unilateral visual deficits.

To avoid litigation, the veterinarian must inform the potential buyer what was and what was not done during the examination because of the limitations of the equipment available. In legal thinking, the veterinarian must show that all aspects of the ocular examination were considered, even if sophisticated equipment such as a slit lamp for detailed study of the eye was not available.

In most cases the veterinarian is examining an eye that lacks overt clinical signs of disease. The results of the ocular examination should be related to the intended use of the animal and an assessment made of the possibility that a lesion could subsequently interfere with vision. The intended functions of the horse must be considered in the determination of whether ocular lesions present are unimportant or if it is "safe" for the horse and its rider to satisfactorily perform those functions. Some eye problems may not preclude the use of the horse in a manmade arena where unexpected visual stimuli are unlikely to be present, and when the rider is experienced and aware of a shortcoming in the vision of the horse.

Many examples exist of horses with varying degrees of blindness that are able to perform at a high level in various types of equestrian competitions, and horses with "suspicious" or subtle signs of ocular disease should not necessarily be excluded. The importance of ocular lesions of uncertain significance may be determined if the horse is re-examined over several months. If the horse examined is a brood mare, the genetic nature of an ocular lesion should be considered (see Table 2).

Supplemental Readings

Lavach JD: Large Animal Ophthalmology. St. Louis, C.V. Mosby, 1990.
Roberts SM (ed): Equine Practice: Ophthalmology. Vet Clin North Am 8(3), 1992.

The Cornea

ANDREW G. MATTHEWS
Kilmarnock, Scotland

The cornea occupies the greater area of the open palpebral fissure in the horse, and its exposed location renders it susceptible to exogenous insult. The normal cornea in the adult horse varies from 0.8 mm to 1.5 mm in thickness centrally to peripherally, and is comprised of a highly refractile and intensely hydrophilic collagenous stroma bounded anteriorly by a nonkeratinized stratified squamous epithelium and posteriorly by a modified basement membrane (Descemet's membrane) and an endothelial monolayer. Transparency is maintained by the physical and functional integrity of the epi- and endothelial barriers preventing stromal imbibition of water from the aqueous tear film and aqueous humor. Hydration of the stroma results in the characteristic turgescence and opacity of corneal edema. The cornea's avascular structure and paucity of mesenchymal cells render it highly susceptible to infection following minor penetrating injury. In the horse, most infections involve opportunist pathogens derived from the normal commensal population of the conjunctival fornices and proximal nasolacrimal drainage system. The corneal response to injury and subsequent infection initially involves the sequestration of perilimbal capillary-derived leukocytes at the site of injury, resulting in the local release of host leukocyte- and epithelial cell-derived lysosomal hydrolases and inflammatory cytokines and, following microbial seeding, exogenous toxins and hydrolases. This precipitates the sequence of molecular events that ultimately results in corneal ulceration. The extent and progress of ulceration are determined by the intensity of the host response, the depth and dosage of microbial inoculation, and the keratopathogenicity of the pathogen involved. However, the clinician should be aware that in the horse, particularly in the United Kingdom, corneal ulcers are frequently sterile and appear to derive principally from the host-response mechanisms.

Corneal repair follows the initial destructive response to insult and is accompanied by neovascularization of the affected area at a depth determined by the depth of the insult. Perivascular melanosis may develop concurrently, and in extensive injury, a dense leukomatous opacity associated with stromal fibrosis is a potentially permanent sequela. Judicious use of topical dexamethasone sodium phosphate ointment* (0.1% q.i.d.) during the later phase of restorative repair once re-epithelialization has occurred may limit the extent of permanent opacity.

DEGENERATIVE KERATOPATHIES

Corneal edema may be primary or secondary. Primary edema arises from a functional defect in the endothelium that permits the net ingress of water into the stroma. The condition is rare in the horse, and no specific endothelial abnormalities have been identified. The affected eye is typically painless with a turgid, opaque cornea. Subepithelial bullae may form and cause transient discomfort. There

---

*Decadron, Merck Sharp & Dohme, West Point, PA

is no specific treatment. Temporary clearing may be effected by the use of topical hyperosmotic solutions or ointments, such as 5% sodium chloride or 10% glycerine, although these are too irritant for other than very short-term use. Secondary edema results from epithelial injury or from endothelial disruption caused by anterior chamber pathology, such as anterior uveitis or glaucoma. In these cases, treatment is aimed at eliminating the primary cause.

Both intrastromal deposition of refractile crystalline material and subepithelial calcium deposits may follow recurrent nonulcerative or ulcerative keratitis and keratouveitis of varying etiologies. There is no specific treatment, although application of a topical chelating agent, such as 0.05% potassium or disodium ethylene diaminetetraacetic acid (EDTA), in conjunction with local epithelial debridement, may accelerate clearing in the case of subepithelial calcium deposition.

EXPOSURE KERATITIS AND KERATOCONJUNCTIVITIS

These conditions result from disruption of the precorneal tear film and compromise of the external ocular surface protection mechanisms; they are encountered in cases of exophthalmos, eyelid deformity or neoplasia, ptosis, and rarely in conjunction with keratoconjunctivitis sicca. Keratoconjunctivitis sicca may be caused by toxic, traumatic, parasitic, or immune-mediated injury to the lacrimal gland, but more often results from disruption of the parasympathetic nerves supplying the gland via the facial nerve owing to fractures of the stylohyoid bone or of the vertical ramus of the mandible close to its temporal articulation. The affected cornea is typically dull, vascularized, and slightly edematous with recurring superficial ulceration. In keratoconjunctivitis sicca, chronic or recurrent low-grade conjunctivitis may be the sole presenting sign, and in these cases diagnosis is based upon demonstration of reduced tear production using a Schirmer tear test. Treatment involves the topical instillation of artificial tear preparations or ocular lubricants° as frequently as is required to maintain a healthy corneal appearance. The primary cause of the problem should be identified and, when possible, treated. Topical 0.2% cyclosporin A† b.i.d. may restore some basal tear secretion in cases of keratoconjunctivitis sicca of suspected immune origin.

CHEMICAL KERATITIS

Chemical injuries occur rarely in the horse and are most frequently associated with agricultural sprays. Alkali injuries result in severe and progressive stromal breakdown, whereas acid injuries remain relatively superficial and often appear as areas of shallow punctate ulceration delineated by the palpebral margins. Immediate emergency treatment involves copious and protracted irrigation of the eye with isotonic saline or tap water. Alkali injuries should be treated along the same lines as a "melting ulcer"

°Tears Naturale II, Alcon, Irvine, TX
†Optimmune, Schering-Plough, Kenilworth, NJ

TABLE 1. PRIMARY SELECTION OF ANTIBIOTICS FOR TREATMENT OF BACTERIAL KERATITIS BASED ON GRAM-STAINING CHARACTERISTICS OF ORGANISMS IDENTIFIED IN CORNEAL SMEARS

Organism Identified	Antibiotic
No smear prepared—empirical therapy	Gentamicin
	Chloramphenicol
	Neomycin/bacitracin/gramicidin
Gram-positive cocci	Neomycin/bacitracin/gramicidin
	Gentamicin
	Cephazolin
Gram-negative cocci	Chloramphenicol
	Tetracyclines
	Trimethoprim/sulfonamide
Gram-positive rods	Penicillin G
	Gentamicin
Gram-negative rods	Gentamicin
	Tobramycin
	Amikacin

(see later). Acid injuries may subsequently require only topical broad-spectrum prophylactic antibiotics (Table 1).

INFECTIOUS KERATITIS

Viral Keratitis

Viral keratitis is relatively rare in the United States but is common in the United Kingdom. Affected eyes are acutely painful. Typically the corneal lesions involve the epithelium and subjacent anterior stroma and appear either as multiple punctate opacities with central ulceration or as a discrete lacelike opacity containing minute epithelial fissures. Rarely, dendritic or circumscribed superficial ulcers may form. Treatment is restricted to those preparations available for topical use in human herpetic keratitis (1% trifluorothymidine;° 3% acyclovir†). Solution or ointment preparations should be instilled into the eye every 1 to 2 and 3 to 4 hours, respectively, for 5 to 7 days.

Bacterial Keratitis

Bacterial keratitis is a common sequel to penetrating corneal trauma. Typically the pathogens involved are gram-negative organisms, which are often found in small numbers among the normal periocular commensal microflora. Imbalance of the commensal population toward more keratopathogenic species may result from the inappropriate use of topical antibiotics or from disruption of the corneal surface protection mechanisms. Once established, these potential pathogens appear able to adhere to anterior stromal receptors exposed by external trauma, which triggers their rapid replication and dissemination throughout the cornea and the initiation of the keratolytic host response. The clinical presentation of bacterial keratitis varies depending upon the intensity and duration of the host-pathogen interaction. Commonly, there is either frank circumscribed stromal ulceration or an irregular and ill-defined area of ulceration with under-run epithelial margins en-

°Viroptic, Burroughs Wellcome, Research Triangle Park, NC
†Zovirax, Burroughs Wellcome, Research Triangle Park, NC

TABLE 2. DOSAGES OF ANTIBIOTICS FOR SUBCONJUNCTIVAL INJECTION IN THE TREATMENT OF BACTERIAL KERATITIS

Antibiotic	Subconjunctival Dosage (Injection Volume <1 mL)
Amikacin°	25–75 mg
Cephazolin†	100 mg
Chloramphenicol succinate‡	50–100 mg
Gentamicin§	20–40 mg
Penicillin G	500,000 IU
Tobramycin‖	5–15 mg

°Amikacin sulfate, Elkins Sinn, Cherry Hill, NJ
†Kefzol, Eli Lilly & Co., Indianapolis IN
‡Chloromycetin succinate, Parke-Davis, Morris Plains, NJ
§Gentocin, Schering-Plough, Kenilworth, NJ
‖Nebcin, Eli Lilly & Co., Indianapolis, IN

trapping purulent or organic detritus. Less commonly the pathogen elicits a very intense and rapidly keratolytic host response resulting in the so-called "melting" cornea, seen typically in *Pseudomonas* species infection.

Treatment is initially aimed at elimination of the pathogen and control of keratolysis. Broad-spectrum empirical antibiotic therapy should begin immediately and can subsequently be modified according to the gram-staining characteristics of the presumed pathogen identified in corneal smear preparations (see Table 1) or from the results of culture and antibiotic sensitivity testing. When *Pseudomonas* species infection is suspected on the basis of clinical appearance, tobramycin or amikacin are the antibiotics of choice. Antibiotics should be delivered topically by direct instillation into the lower conjunctival fornix or via a subpalpebral or dedicated nasolacrimal delivery system.° To maintain local therapeutic levels of antibiotics, commercially available ointments must be instilled into the eye every 3 to 4 hours. Solutions should be instilled every 1 to 2 hours, or every 3 to 4 hours if used in conjunction with once-daily subconjunctival injection of the antibiotic. The combination of topical instillation and subconjunctival injection is the optimal regimen for maintaining effective therapeutic levels of most antibiotics in the external eye. The dosages for subconjunctival injection are shown in Table 2. Fortified topical antibiotic solutions can be prepared from parenteral preparations (Table 3) and have the advantage of delivering higher therapeutic levels to the external eye.

Topical enzyme inhibitors, such as 0.05% potassium EDTA or heparin sodium (1000 IU/ml), are well tolerated and can very effectively control the stromolytic host response. These are of primary therapeutic importance in treating sterile ulcers and in melting ulceration, and should be instilled into the eye every hour until healing is underway. Antibiotic and antienzyme solutions should not be instilled simultaneously to avoid dilution of the active principal ingredient.

Ancillary treatment modes include the use of topical mydriatic cycloplegics such as 1% atropine sulphate† to

°Nasolacrimal cannula, Portex, Hythe, England or Sims Canada Ltd., Markham, Ontario
†Atrophate, Schering-Plough, Kenilworth, NJ

relieve pupillary spasm, regular flushing of the ocular surface with sterile isotonic saline to remove inflammatory debris, and systemic administration of nonsteroidal antiinflammatory drugs (NSAIDs) to stabilize the blood-aqueous barrier and alleviate ocular pain. In deep refractory ulceration, particularly if descemetocele threatens or there is subepithelial entrapment of detritus, surgical debridement of the ulcer margins in conjunction with temporary tarsorrhaphy or conjunctival flap grafting is indicated as a means of supporting the damaged cornea and encouraging healing. Collagen shields and therapeutic soft contact lenses are available for use in the horse as corneal dressings. However, difficulties in their placement and retention in the injured eye present drawbacks to their general use. Their value as drug reservoirs capable of maintaining continous high levels of antibiotics in the external eye has not been assessed.

Mycotic Keratitis

Mycotic keratitis is a serious complication of minor corneal trauma, particularly in eyes in which protracted topical corticosteroid use may have compromised protective cell-mediated immune responses. The disease is relatively common in the United States where geographic and climatic factors may influence its prevalence but is rare in the United Kingdom. Mycotic keratitis should be suspected in all nonresponsive deep keratopathies. The fungi involved are usually saprophytes resident in the normal commensal population of the external eye, such as *Aspergillus* species, *Penicillium* species, and *Fusarium* species. Yeasts, such as *Candida* species and *Torulopsis* species, are less commonly involved.

Clinically, affected eyes are typically ulcerated at the time of initial presentation with a distinct raised ulcer margin and dense white or feathery perilesional infiltrates. The depth of the lesion varies, deeper lesions being more difficult to treat. Perforation and endophthalmitis are occasional but disastrous complications. Diagnosis is based upon demonstration of hyphae in methylene blue or Gomori methenamine silver-stained corneal scrapings prepared from the margins and base of the lesion or in corneal sections prepared following keratectomy. Treatment using topical antimycotic preparations (Table 4) must be aggressive and should be continued until hyphae are no longer demonstrable in sequential corneal scrapings. Surgical keratectomy of the affected cornea during treatment increases drug penetration and improves the therapeutic response, particularly in deep infections.

TABLE 3. CONCENTRATIONS OF FORTIFIED ANTIBIOTIC SOLUTIONS FOR TOPICAL USE IN BACTERIAL KERATITIS

Antibiotic	Concentration for Topical Use, Prepared in Balanced Salt Solution or in Artificial Tears
Amikacin	15 mg/ml
Cephazolin	50 mg/ml
Chloromycetin succinate	5–10 mg/ml
Gentamicin	5–15 mg/ml
Penicillin G	$1–2 \times 10^6$ IU/ml
Tobramycin	15 mg/ml

TABLE 4. ANTIMYCOTIC THERAPY FOR FUNGAL KERATITIS

Drug	Treatment Protocol	Comment
Natamycin 5% suspension°	Apply topically 1–2 h	Poorly soluble with consequently limited corneal penetration
Amphotericin B†	0.15% solution in 5% glucose applied topically 2–4 h	Relatively toxic and retards healing
	Can also be injected subconjunctivally 125 μg 3 times weekly	Some activity against yeasts
Miconazole 1% solution‡	Apply topically 1–2 h, along with 10 mg injected subconjunctivally once daily for 5 days	Low toxicity and good corneal penetration
	Reduce frequency of topical application after 7–10 days	
Flucytosine 1% solution§	Apply topically 1–2 h	Active against yeasts only

°Natacyn 5% ophthalmic suspension, Alcon, Irvine, TX
†Fungizone intravenous, Apothecon, Princeton, NJ
‡Monistat 1% solution, Janssen Pharmaceutica, Titusville, NJ
§Alcobon 1% solution, Roche Laboratories, Nutley, NJ

Topical enzyme inhibitors and mydriatic cycloplegics should be used as described under bacterial keratitis, and conjunctival flap grafting may accelerate healing during the later stages of treatment. When perforation or endophthalmitis occurs, the eye should be enucleated. In all cases the prognosis remains guarded until healing is complete.

Stromal Abscesses

Epithelial closure over purulent detritus occasionally follows corneal injury, resulting in stromal abcessation. Abscesses may be sterile, although both bacteria and fungi may be identified in corneal scrapings or, in the case of deeper abscesses, in keratectomy sections of the lesions. Treatment requires debridement or keratectomy of the affected stroma in all but the most superficial lesions, followed by topical antibiotic or antimycotic therapy, as determined by the nature of the specific pathogen identified. Deep abscessation may present a serious threat of perforation and endophthalmitis, and great care is necessary during surgical intervention in these cases. Parenteral ampicillin, gentamicin, or cephalosporins are the antibiotics of choice in cases in which bacterial endophthalmitis threatens.

Parasitic Keratitis

The microfilaria of *Onchocerca cervicalis* are capable of aberrant migration from the palpebral skin to the bulbar conjunctiva and perilimbal cornea. An immunogenic inflammatory response is believed to be initiated by the death of the microfilaria, resulting in a diffuse infiltrative anterior stromal keratitis typically involving the temporal perilimbal cornea. In longer-standing cases, the lesion adopts a vascularized and granular appearance. A presumptive diagnosis is made on the basis of the clinical signs and, in some cases, a history of recent ivermectin administration. The demonstration of microfilaria in conjunctival biopsy preparations supports the diagnosis. Treatment involves suppression of the ocular inflammatory reaction, by use of topical corticosteroids in conjunction with parenteral corticosteroids or NSAIDs. Oral filaricides such as diethylcarbamazine citrate° (4.4.–6.6 mg/kg s.i.d. for 21 days) or ivermectin° (0.2 mg/kg) should be used once the ocular inflammatory response is controlled.

IMMUNOGENIC KERATITIS

A wide range of superficial and deep keratopathies are presumed to have an immunogenic origin. These may derive from derangement of the mechanisms that determine the immune privilege of the normal cornea. Clinically these disorders vary in presentation, but in general they are characterized by stromal edema and focal fluid accumulation, occasional subepithelial bullae formation, superficial and deep neovascularization, subepithelial and stromal pigmentation, and eventual fibrosis. Affected eyes cause only minimal discomfort, and the keratopathy may be recurrent with a varying periodicity. Topical immunosuppressive treatment with 0.1% dexamethasone sodium phosphate or 1% prednisolone acetate,† or by use of 0.2% cyclosporin A twice daily, may be curative in some cases. However, it may be necessary to continue treatment for protracted periods according to the clinical response.

CORNEAL NEOPLASIA

Primary tumors of the cornea are relatively rare, and usually are of epithelial origin. Corneal epithelial keratosis, intraepithelial carcinoma in situ, and squamous cell carcinoma are differentiated by the degree of epithelial and stromal involvement and the expression of cellular malignancy. The two former conditions do not breach the basement membrane. Keratosis presents clinically as a well-defined and superficial papillomatous lesion. Carcinoma in situ appears as well-demarcated irregular whitish-pink superficial corneal infiltrate. Squamous cell carcinoma appears as a progressive dense whitish-pink nodular lesion, commonly with some bulbar conjunctival involvement. Treatment in all cases is excision by lamellar keratectomy under general anesthesia. In the case of squamous cell carcinoma involving the deeper layers of the stroma, com-

°DEC Capsules, R.P. Scherer North America, St. Petersburg, FL

°Eqvalan, Merck Agvet, Iselin, NJ
†Predforte, Allergan, Irvine, TX

plete surgical excision may not be possible and radiotherapy or enucleation is necessary. In these cases the prognosis is always guarded because local intraocular or periocular extension and distant metastasis are possible.

Supplemental Readings

Barnett KC, Crispin SM, Lavach D, Matthews AG: The cornea. *In* Color Atlas and Text of Equine Ophthalmology. London, Mosby-Wolfe, 1995, pp 98–135.

Grahn B, Wolfer J, Keller C, Wilcock B: Equine keratomycosis; clinical and laboratory findings in 23 cases. Prog Vet Compar Ophthalmol 3:2–8, 1993.

Matthews AG: The aetiopathogenesis of infectious keratitis in the horse. Equine Vet J 26:432–433, 1994.

Miller TR: Principles of therapeutics. Vet Clin North Am Equine Pract 8(3):479–497, 1992.

Nasisse MP, Nelms S: Equine ulcerative keratitis. Vet Clin North Am Equine Pract 8(3):537–555, 1992.

Ocular Trauma

R. GARETH JONES
Leicester, England

The eye is well protected by the bony orbital rim and protective mechanisms such as the palpebral reflex in which the eyelids rapidly close and the globe is retracted. However, owing to the prominence of the equine eye and the environment in which horses are kept, ocular injuries are relatively common. The nature of the injurious agent has a major bearing on the degree of ocular damage.

In the case of blunt trauma and contusion, slight compression can be resisted by ocular elasticity but, if the force is great, shearing causes disruption of intraocular structures and violent recoil causes rupture of the ocular tunic or the orbit. Kicks, collisions with gate posts, whip injuries, and road traffic accidents are examples of such injuries. In abrasive injuries, tissue is partially torn, which can be particularly injurious to the eye if associated with foreign material or bacterial contamination. Lacerations or penetrations by sharp objects such as nails, wire fences, or curry combs may cause a complete tear or perforation of ocular tissue.

Foreign bodies such as hay, seeds from bedding, or soil hurled from a racetrack can inoculate bacterial organisms within tissue or act as an inciting focus after the initial incident. Chemical irritants such as shampoos and aerosol sprays also can cause injury. Acidic substances coagulate proteins, which act as a barrier to further penetration, therefore the damage is limited to the ocular surface. Conversely, alkalis cause a breakdown of glycosaminoglycans so that the intraocular penetration and the degree of damage is much greater. Thermal burns can cause necrosis and ulceration of tissue with the risk of secondary bacterial infection.

ASSESSING THE PATIENT

History

The cause of the injury, the duration since the incident, the details of treatment instituted, previous ocular or systemic disease, and the tetanus vaccination status should all be recorded. The presence of pain, swelling, or visual deficit should be noted.

Restraint

Following trauma, examination can be precluded because of extensive eyelid swelling, subconjunctival hemorrhage, and marked blepharospasm. Topical application of drugs may also be difficult. Retraction of wet, swollen eyelids may be aided by application of dry gauze sponges, but this is contraindicated in perforating injuries owing to the risk of violent struggling and expulsion of the intraocular contents. Adequate restraint is essential to perform a complete ophthalmic examination (Table 1).

Examination

The traumatized eye should be examined to assess the degree of damage to determine a prognosis for vision and preservation of the eye. The clinician must approach the animal gently and carefully because injured eyes are often extremely painful. A complete physical examination should be conducted when indicated.

Ocular examination should include an assessment of vision: Can the horse see from both eyes, one, or neither? The degree of pain is assessed by the demeanor of the animal and the presence of blepharospasm or photophobia. Orbital margins are palpated for fractures, crepitus, and cellulitis. Swelling or laceration of the eyelids, the position of the globe within the orbit, and the nature of any discharge—serous, mucoid, or purulent—are noted. Conjunctiva are examined for hemorrhage, chemosis, or laceration. Foreign material in the conjunctival sac is sought by direct inspection or flushing with normal saline. The cornea is examined for laceration, opacities, edema, or

TABLE 1. METHODS OF RESTRAINT FOR EXAMINATION OF OCULAR INJURIES

Twitch
Sedation—intravenous detomidine hydrochloride (0.04 mg/kg)
Auriculopalpebral nerve block (motor function only)
Topical anesthesia—proxymetacaine hydrochloride drops
General anesthesia—occasionally indicated in perforating injuries

TABLE 2. ESSENTIAL OPHTHALMIC EMERGENCY KIT

Focusing pen torch
Fluorescein dye (Fluor-I-Strip-A.T., Ayerst Laboratories, Philadelphia, PA)
Topical anesthetic, proparacaine hydrochloride 0.5% (Alcaine, Alcon, Fort Worth, TX)
Topical mydriatic, tropicamide 1% (Mydriacyl, Alcon, Fort Worth, TX)
Lacrimal irrigating cannulae, 32-mm long, outside diameter 0.91 mm
Suture material, polyglactin, 0.7 and 1.0 metric (Vicryl, Ethicon, Somerville, NJ)

foreign bodies, and fluorescein dye applied to check for ulceration. The anterior chamber is examined for flare, exudate, blood, or anterior lens luxation. While examining the iris, pupil size and shape are recorded, checking the direct and consensual pupillary light responses. Lens position is noted and the eye examined carefully for lens capsule rupture. The posterior segment is examined for vitreous hemorrhage, retinal detachment, and optic nerve damage. Ancillary aids such as ultrasonography may be useful in cases with anterior chamber opacity or orbital abnormalities. Equipment necessary for an ophthalmic emergency kit is listed in Table 2 and drugs used for treatment of ocular trauma are listed in Table 3.

PERIOCULAR AND GLOBE TRAUMA

Orbital Fractures

Pain and marked periocular swelling occur, depending on time since injury. Facial deformity and crepitus may be palpable, and the globe may be displaced. Subcutaneous emphysema or epistaxis may be present if there is a fracture involving the periorbital sinus. Lateral and oblique skull radiographs can demonstrate the extent of a fracture line and may show fluid lines within the periorbital sinus.

The fracture may be left to heal without surgery, provided that there is no gross displacement of the globe. Systemic antibiotics are indicated when the sinuses are involved. Topical antibiotics should be applied if there is corneal ulceration or exposure, and systemic anti-inflammatories reduce pain and eyelid swelling.

If there is major disruption of the orbit, surgery is indicated to reduce the fracture by elevation of large fragments and to allow removal of small avascular pieces of bone. Blood and debris should be flushed away with normal saline. Temporary tarsorrhaphy prevents exposure keratitis if the globe is displaced.

Blunt Ocular Trauma

Severe contusion to the globe can cause hyphema, iridal tears, anterior uveitis, lens luxation, vitreal hemorrhage, and retinal detachment. The rapid elevation of intraocular pressure may be sufficient to rupture the ocular tunic at the limbus where it is thinnest. Ocular examination determines whether the globe is intact and the degree of disruption to the intraocular structures. Large irregular tears in the ocular tunic warrant a poor prognosis.

Mild contusions may result in moderate hyphema, which may clear spontaneously. Stall rest is indicated. Topical steroids and atropine should be used if there is an associated anterior uveitis. Systemic anti-inflammatories provide analgesia.

On occasion, a scleral tear may be hidden under an intact conjunctiva, and thus a surgical exploration is indicated if the globe is hypotonic. Lens removal may be necessary if it is anteriorly luxated. If there is gross disruption of ocular contents or contamination, enucleation is indicated.

TABLE 3. COMMONLY USED OPHTHALMIC DRUGS

Category/Drug	Indication	Dose
Topical		
Antibiotics		
Neomycin/bacitracin/polymyxin	Superficial corneal ulcer	q2–6h
Gentamicin (fortified)	Deep/infected corneal ulcer	q2–6h
Antifungals		
Miconazole 1%	Fungal keratitis	q2–4h
Collagenase inhibitors		
Acetyl cysteine 5%	Infected/melting ulcer	q2–6h
Corticosteroids		
Prednisolone acetate 1%	Anterior uveitis	q2–6h
Mydriatics		
Tropicamide 1%	Short-acting for diagnostics	Once
Atropine 1–4%	Anterior uveitis	To effect
Epibulbar		
Antibiotics		
Gentamicin	Infected ulcer/endophthalmitis	80 mg/2 ml
Corticosteroids		
Triamcinolone acetate	Anterior uveitis	40 mg per eye q12 days
Systemic		
Nonsteroidal anti-inflammatories		
Flunixin meglumine	Inflammation	0.5 mg/kg IV
Phenylbutazone	Inflammation	2–4 mg/kg s.i.d. p.o.

EYELID TRAUMA

The horse is prone to injury to the eyelids; abrasion, contusion, and laceration can occur. Owing to the vascular supply, such injuries can present with profuse hemorrhage and dramatic swelling, obscuring ocular examination.

Eyelid Lacerations

The eye should be examined closely for damage beneath the eyelid and for foreign material, corneal ulceration, and anterior uveitis. Wounds should be gently cleaned with 2% povidone-iodine solution, and systemic antibiotics should be administered if there is a deep laceration or contamination. Cold compresses and systemic anti-inflammatory drugs reduce swelling and effect hemostasis. Topical antibiotics should be used for corneal protection during the healing phase.

Eyelid lacerations should be repaired promptly with minimal debridement to prevent deformity. A two-layer closure is usually employed to prevent tension on the wound, and particular care is taken to accurately appose the lid margin. Old wounds, infected wounds, or ones in which more than 30% of lid length has been lost should be treated with blepharoplastic techniques.

Nasolacrimal Duct Injury

Injuries at the medial canthus may damage the nasolacrimal puncta, canaliculi, or duct. This results in epiphora and excoriation of the skin if the repair is not accurate. Microsurgery incorporating indwelling catheters may be indicated.

Third Eyelid Injury

Careful search is made for foreign material on the bulbar aspect of the third eyelid. Third eyelid lacerations should be carefully repaired using accurately placed absorbable suture to avoid corneal damage. If possible, the margin should be restored and complete resection performed only as a last resort.

Conjunctival Injury

Most conjunctival lacerations heal readily and need not be sutured. Scleral wounds should be sought beneath an extensive laceration.

CORNEAL TRAUMA

Corneal trauma may range from superficial abrasive injuries to full-thickness lacerations. The trigeminal nerve fibers are located in the anterior stroma, and thus paradoxically superficial ulcers cause more ocular pain than deep ulcers.

Ocular examination determines the presence of ulcers, foreign material, or corneal laceration. Other specific injuries include chemical and thermal burns. Fluorescein dye is essential to stain corneal ulcers and demonstrate aqueous leakage. The ulcer should be classified as superficial, deep, or infected. The aim of therapy is to restore the anatomy, prevent infection, and aid healing.

Corneal Ulcers

Therapy for superficial ulcers involves removing the cause and administering routine topical antibiotics to control infection. For deep or infected ulcers, specificity is necessary (see later). Topical steroids are contraindicated if the cornea is ulcerated. Ointments are avoided if there is any risk of the preparation entering the eye, because the base acts as an inflammatory focus. If a secondary uveitis is present, it should be controlled with systemic anti-inflammatory drugs and topical atropine.

Corneal Lacerations

Surgery is necessary to repair full-thickness lacerations and restore the integrity of the globe or, with deep ulceration, to avoid impending perforation. Good illumination, magnification, and the correct instrumentation improve the chance of accurate surgical repair. Uveal prolapse should be replaced as soon as possible, the anterior chamber should be restored with balanced salt solution, and the laceration should be repaired by direct corneal suturing. A conjunctival pedicle graft can be used to support a deep ulcer or a laceration that is extensive and in which the cornea is leaking.

Corneal and Intraocular Foreign Bodies

The extent of damage depends on the type of material, the position within the eye, the size, the number, and the length of time since the injury. For example, lead shot is inert and can generally be left alone, whereas iron compounds should be removed as soon as possible, before they oxidize.

Vegetable matter is a common vector for contamination of the eye with bacterial or mycotic organisms. Cytology and culture testing should be performed to determine the choice of topical antimicrobials and, according to sensitivity, fortified preservative-free preparations used. The drug should be used intensively while healing occurs, and frequent application can be facilitated using subpalpebral lavage systems (see page 339).

Topical steroids must be avoided in the presence of ulceration or if infection is suspected. Secondary anterior uveitis is controlled with a combination of topical atropine and systemic anti-inflammatory drugs.

Removal of a superficial foreign body such as a grass seed may be possible with hydropulsion following sedation and local anesthesia. Deep corneal foreign bodies should be removed by keratectomy following general anesthesia. Intraocular foreign bodies should be removed by a limbal approach so that scarring is away from the central axis.

Chemical Irritants

The degree of damage should be evaluated following nerve block. Most chemical burns warrant a poor prognosis for salvage of the eye.

Copious lavage with more than 2 L tap water or normal saline should be continued until the chemical is eliminated. Urinalysis sticks may confirm that the pH has returned to normal. Topical antibiotics, atropine, and collagenase inhibitors should be used until healing is complete. Systemic antibiotics and analgesics can prove beneficial. Therapeutic soft contact lenses can be used to protect an ulcerated cornea.

Thermal Burns

The eye must be examined closely for eyelid lesions, corneal ulceration, and uveitis. Special efforts are made to treat shock and smoke inhalation and apply moist antibiotic dressings to skin burns.

Immediately, the eye is lavaged with cold running water for 20 minutes. The cornea is protected with topical antibiotics and tear replacements, and collagenase inhibitors are used if there is corneal sloughing. Uveitis is treated with systemic anti-inflammatory drugs and topical atropine. Conjunctival grafts may be necessary to support a weak cornea.

OPTIC NERVE TRAUMA

The animal presents with sudden unilateral or bilateral blindness. The history may be of a blow to the occipital area on rearing up in a confined space or of falling over backward and striking the head on the ground. Posterior movement of the brain results in neuropraxia or an avulsion injury to the intracranial portion of the optic nerve. Subsequently, wallerian degeneration occurs.

Ocular examination reveals an absent menace response on the affected side and absent afferent pupillary light response. No other ophthalmoscopic signs may be evident. The fundus, in particular, may appear normal initially, and only after a delay of several weeks is optic nerve and peripapillary degeneration seen.

Treatment is medical with high doses of systemic steroids or nonsteroidal anti-inflammatory drugs. Prognosis for sight is guarded.

FACIAL NERVE TRAUMA

Facial nerve injuries may follow trauma to the head causing keratoconjunctivitis sicca and lagophthalmos. The exposed, dry cornea is prone to keratitis and ulceration. Absent palpebral reflex and low Schirmer tear test on the affected side suggest facial nerve injury. Other signs of facial nerve paralysis may also be present.

The cornea should be lubricated with topical tear replacement and topical antibiotics used if the cornea is ulcerated. Lid surgery to reduce the size of the palpebral fissure may be indicated in chronic cases.

REFERRAL TO A SPECIALIST

The prognosis for many ocular injuries is the same whether the animal is seen by a general practitioner or an ophthalmologist. However, inappropriate treatment can have a detrimental effect, resulting in synechiae formation, cataract, and phthisis bulbi, which can all cause blindness. If facilities are not available to treat an ocular injury effectively or if microsurgical repair is necessary, referral to a veterinary ophthalmologist should be considered (Table 4).

TABLE 4. CONDITIONS REQUIRING IMMEDIATE REFERRAL TO AN OPHTHALMOLOGIST

Corneal laceration	Intraocular foreign body
Deep corneal foreign body	Nasolacrimal duct laceration
Deep or infected corneal ulcer	Orbital fracture

Supplemental Readings

Blogg JR: The eye in veterinary practice, vol 3, Eye Injuries. Malvern, Australia, Chilcote Publishing, 1987.

Brooks DE, Wolf ED: Ocular trauma in the horse. Equine Vet J 2[Suppl]:141–146, 1983.

Turner LM, Whitley RD, Hager D: Management of ocular trauma in horses, part 2, Orbit, eyelids, uvea, lens, retina and optic nerve. Mod Vet Pract 67:341–347, 1986.

Whitley RD, Turner LM: Management of ocular trauma in horses, part 1, cornea and sclera. Mod Vet Pract 67:233–238, 1986.

Wilkie DA: Ocular injuries. In Robinson NE (ed): Current Therapy in Equine Medicine, ed 3. Philadelphia, WB Saunders, 1992, pp 460–463.

Periocular Disease

SUE PATERSON
Altrincham, England

PHILIP BOYDELL
Manchester, England

The periocular region is a transitional zone to which both the dermatologist and ophthalmologist may lay claim. Ocular disease can extend to involve the periocular skin, or ocular discomfort can lead to traumatization of this area. However, there are some diseases that primarily involve the skin and represent localized dermatologic disease rather than an extension from the eye. The clinician should elicit a thorough history and perform a complete physical examination in every case. This allows detection of systemic disease and provides clues to the possible underlying etiology of the condition. A full ophthalmologic examination is essential.

DIAGNOSIS

Samples of crust and hair should be collected if dermatophytes or *Dermatophilus* is suspected. Similarly, stained impression smears of exudative lesions and fine needle aspirates of nodules and swellings may be useful. Skin biopsy is indicated (1) if neoplasia is suspected; (2) in persistent ulcerative conditions; (3) in a dermatosis that is unresponsive to conventional therapy; (4) in any suspected condition in which therapy is dangerous or expensive; and (5) in the presence of any unusual or potentially serious skin disease. Routine hematology and biochemistry testing can be helpful but is not essential in every case unless there is a suggestion of systemic involvement.

NEOPLASIA

Equine sarcoids can occur anywhere on the body but are commonly found at periocular sites. Four basic gross types of sarcoid are recognized: (1) verrucous, (2) fibroblastic, (3) mixed, and (4) occult. Any of these forms can occur around the eyes. The removal of a periocular sarcoid is a difficult surgical task, and other forms of therapy have been advocated for lesions at this site (see page 372). Immunotherapy with mycobacterial products (percutaneous Bacillus Calmette-Guérin [BCG]), cryosurgery, or radiation brachytherapy, particularly with iridium wire implants, have all been shown to have good effect in clinical trials.

Squamous cell carcinoma is commonly found on the eyelids of older horses with a mean age of 12 years. Lesions are solitary, beginning as nonhealing ulcers, or verrucous proliferative lesions. Horses with white skin and hair are predisposed. Although lesions are locally aggressive they are slow to metastasize. The therapy of choice is wide surgical excision. However, this is not always possible. Debulking surgery or cryosurgery followed by radiation therapy with gold, cobalt, iridium, or strontium has been used. One of the authors (SP) has found fluorouracil cream to be useful in some cases.

Mastocytoma in the horse is recognized as a benign hyperproliferative disease rather than neoplasia. The Arabian is said to be predisposed. Nodules are usually single and may be any size from 2 to 20 cm. The surface of the nodule may be ulcerated, normal, or alopecic. Examination of fine needle aspirates from lesions can prove diagnostic, revealing aggregates of well-differentiated mast cell often accompanied by eosinophils. The lesions appear to be self-limiting and have never been reported to metastasize. Intralesional or sublesional corticosteroid injection is probably the treatment of choice for mastocytosis involving the periocular skin.

Melanoma and neurofibroma have also been reported to occur commonly on the eyelids. Melanomas in this site are generally pigmented and carry a good prognosis after surgical removal. Eyelid papillomas can occur in young horses. These lesions have a viral etiology and regress spontaneously with time.

BLEPHARITIS

Dermatophytosis, dermatophilosis, and staphylococcal folliculitis can all affect the periocular skin. However, there is usually involvement of other areas of the horse.

PARASITES

Demodex caballi, the larger (264–453 μm) of the two demodex mites to affect the horse, can be commonly identified in skin scrapings from the eyelid and muzzle of clinically normal horses. Some individuals will show mild asymptomatic alopecia and scale. The significance of this parasite is unclear. The biting flies such as *Culicoides* species (gnats) and *Simulium* species (black flies) feed around the heads of horses. Their bites produce immediate pain and pruritus, followed by papules and wheals, leading to self-inflicted traumatization. Control is aimed at stabling during high-risk fly-feeding periods, and use of insect repellents. Treatment of severe cutaneous reactions may be accomplished with systemic glucocorticoid therapy. Nuisance flies such as *Musca* and *Hydrotaea* species feed on wound exudate and ocular and nasal discharge. They can be seen feeding at the medial canthus of horse's eyes in the summer, when they can act as vectors for the stomach nematode *Habronema* species. Habronemiasis is commonly seen at the medial canthus. This represents a form of aberrant parasitism when the infectious larvae gain access to traumatized skin in a presumably hypersensitive host. Lesions develop rapidly and appear as areas of ulcerated, exudative granulation tissue. Yellow granules ("leeches") may be seen in diseased tissue. Eyelid granulomas and blepharitis are sequelae in some animals. Diagnosis is based on examination of smears from lesions and on histopathologic findings. Management comprises a combination of surgical excision, glucocorticoids, and antiparasitic therapy.

Pediculosis can affect the face of horses. The small biting louse *Damalinia equi* can induce patchy periocular alopecia due to rubbing. Lice are seen most commonly in the autumn and winter months.

IMMUNOLOGIC DISEASE

Pemphigus foliaceus can present initially as a diffuse crusting and scaling on the face of the horse. Careful examination may reveal evidence of more generalized involvement. Biopsy of primary pustular lesions, if possible, helps to make a definitive diagnosis. Anti-inflammatory therapy with prednisolone or gold is indicated. The prognosis is dependent on the age of onset. Horses less than 2 years of age generally carry a better chance of clinical remission.

Equine cutaneous lupus erythematosus is an uncommon clinical syndrome described by Stannard (see Supplemental Readings). The disease affects adult horses. The dermatologic sign is depigmentation affecting the skin surrounding the eyes, lips, nostril, and genitalia. In addition to leukoderma, there is erythema and scale, which differentiates this disease from vitiligo. Diagnosis is based on compatible histopathologic signs and a positive antinuclear antigen (ANA) titer. Treatment is not indicated in what is thought to be a benign condition without systemic involvement.

PIGMENTARY DISEASE

Juvenile Arabian leukoderma (pinky syndrome) commonly presents with loss of pigmentation involving the eyelid, periocular skin, muzzle, nares, and genitalia (see page 363). The major differential for this disease is cutaneous lupus, although the latter tends to be more inflammatory. The cause of this disease is unknown and it can follow one of three patterns: (1) permanent depigmentation, (2) repigmentation, or (3) intermittent relapsing repigmentation and depigmentation. Successful anecdotal therapy has included castration, as well as vitamin and mineral supplementation. It is possible that such "cures" have coincided with spontaneous repigmentation. The disease can occur in mature horses of other breeds, making diagnosis more difficult.

Photosensitization can be seen on the face and periocularly on unpigmented, hairless skin (eyelids) or haired, lightly pigmented skin. Photosensitization may be primary due to exogenous photodynamic agents, or secondary due to the accumulation of phylloerythrin from liver damage. Routine liver function tests are essential in all cases of photosensitization, as well as a careful search for any possible environmental photosensitizing agents. Treatment should include removal of the animal from sunlight and prevention of exposure to the photodynamic substance. In the acute stages of the disease, anti-inflammatory corticosteroids may be indicated.

ENTROPION

This condition typically involves the lower eyelid. The margin is inverted, causing irritation of the cornea and conjunctiva. In young horses it may be associated with reduced eyelid tone, or small globes, or mild enophthalmos. Treatment may be limited to a lubricating ointment or temporary eversion of the eyelid margin. A more permanent eyelid strip resection may be required at a later date. The condition may be acquired in older horses as a sequel to traumatic damage and distortion of the lid. Several methods of surgical correction have been described.

Suggested Readings

Ackerman LJ: Practical Equine Dermatology. Goleta, CA, American Veterinary Publications, 1989, pp 37–50, 149–153.
Dugan SJ: Ocular neoplasia. Vet Clin North Am Equine Pract 8(3):609–626, 1992.
Lavach JD: Large animal ophthalmology. St. Louis, MO, C.V. Mosby, 1990.
Scott DW: Large Animal Dermatology. Philadelphia, WB Saunders, 1988, pp 207–283, 388–389, 420–452.
Stannard A: Proceedings Equine Dermatology Work Shop, E.S.V.D. Newmarket, 1994, pp 55–56, 86–87, 132–133.

Congenital Ocular Disease

GRAHAM MUNROE
Easter Bush, Scotland

Congenital ocular abnormalities in the horse, although not common, form an interesting and important group of equine eye conditions. Early recognition and diagnosis of these conditions is important to prevent unnecessary suffering and, in some, to expedite treatment. Owners are often concerned with the prognosis for both normal performance and breeding, and, therefore, the possible progression or inheritance of a given problem is of vital importance. This chapter does not attempt to discuss all congenital ocular abnormalities, but rather it highlights those of importance or those that have not been covered in previous editions of this text. Table 1 lists the majority of congenital eye conditions found in the horse.

MICROPHTHALMIA

Microphthalmia refers to an abnormal smallness of the eye, which can be uni- or bilateral, and is one of the more commonly reported congenital ocular abnormalities in foals. The etiology is unknown, and many cases are sporadic and idiopathic. In others, obvious causes such as toxic, mechanical, infectious, or even nutritional insults lead to degeneration or dysplasia of a partially formed optic vesicle, with the severity of the microphthalmia depending on the gestational stage at which the insult occurs. All breeds are affected, but some, such as the Thoroughbred, have a higher incidence. The role of inheritance has not been proven in the horse.

The size of the globe varies considerably from a near-normal structure with normal function to a microscopic structure with only pigmented remnants. Subtle microphthalmia, especially if unilateral, may require a full ophthalmologic examination and corneal measurements before the defect can be confirmed. Even a 10% reduction in globe size results in severe visual deficits. Severe microphthalmia is more easily diagnosed because of the associated enophthalmos, blindness, and passive prolapse of the nictitans. The lid margins and aperture are reduced in size, the cornea and globe either are not visible or are abnormally pigmented, and the orbit is smaller than normal. The poor nasolacrimal drainage and subsequent ocular discharge are associated with the abnormal anatomy of the globe, orbit, and eyelid. Secondary conjunctivitis is common owing to environmental irritation and infection.

No treatment is available and bilaterally severely affected foals are usually euthanized. Animals with a unilateral problem can be worked, will adapt, and may still make effective athletic horses in some cases. Enucleation of the affected globe may be necessary to prevent conjunctivitis, ocular

TABLE 1.   CONGENITAL OCULAR ANOMALIES OF THE HORSE

Anomaly	Description	Comments/Treatment
Orbit and Globe		
Anophthalmia	Absence of any ocular tissue	Rare
Microphthalmia	Abnormal smallness of eye	See text
Multiple abnormalities	Abnormalities of several parts of the eye including corneal/lens abnormalities, colobomata and retinal detachment	Sporadic Blind eye(s) Enucleation
Buphthalmos	Congenital increase in intraocular pressure	Rare
Cyclopia/synophthalmia	Single globe located in middle of forehead	Abnormalities of brain and skull may lead to death
Strabismus	Deviation of globe from proper axis	See text
Eyelids		
Entropion	Inversion of lower eyelid margin and eyelashes	Most common congenital eyelid defect in foals
Ectropion	Eversion of lower eyelid margin	Abnormal exposure leads to conjunctivitis and keratitis Ophthalmic ointments Surgical correction
Coloboma	Full-thickness absence of lid structures, usually margin	Can accompany other multiple abnormalities Surgical correction in large defects
Ankyloblepharon	Adhesion of lid margins	May indicate premature birth Rest of eye normal Digital separation
Dermoids	Choristomas—congenital mislocation normal tissue	Eyelid margin Surgical resection
Color dilution	Part or whole eyelids devoid of pigment, especially in Appaloosa, Paint, Pinto	Increased environmental irritation especially to sunlight Skin protectants/tattooing
Conjunctiva and Third Eyelid		
Dermoids	Palpebral/bulbar conjunctiva and third eyelid	Surgical resection ± keratectomy
Symblepharon	Adhesion between two conjunctival sites or cornea and conjunctiva	Reported in association with microphthalmia
Hypoplasia of nictitans	Part of microphthalmia complex	
Nasolacrimal System		Congenital impatency can be anywhere in the system Uni- or bilateral None is thought to be inherited
Atresia of nasal punctum	Nasal punctum and often a variable length of duct are missing	Most common
Atresia of eyelid punctum	One or both puncta	Uncommon
Misplaced puncta	Single puncta	Uncommon
Cornea		
Dermoids	Most common site See also conjunctiva, eyelids, and nictitans	Superficial keratectomy
Microcornea	Smallness of cornea	Usually part of microphthalmia/multiple defect complexes
Megalocornea	Enlarged cornea	As above
Melanosis	Pigmentation of epithelium and superficial stroma of central cornea ± vessels	Superficial keratectomy Other abnormalities including dermoids & PPM
Persistent pupillary membranes	Attachment to corneal endothelium Focal opacity	Check for other abnormalities
Opacities	Microphthalmia Irregular punctate Thin vertical band and linear	
Sclera		
Subjunctival hemorrhages	Normal and NMS foals	See text
Uvea		
Heterochromia iridis	Combinations of brown, white and blue Part of, one, or both irides	Light-colored breeds Insignificant
Aniridia	Complete absence of iris	See text
Iridal hypoplasia	Partial absence of iris	
Coloboma	Segmental partial or complete absence of iris	See text
Anterior uveal cysts	Stromal Posterior pigment epithelium Granule iridica cysts	Rare in foals
Persistent pupillary membrane	Remnants of anterior vascular sheath of lens	See text

TABLE 1. CONGENITAL OCULAR ANOMALIES OF THE HORSE *Continued*

Anomaly	Description	Comments/Treatment
Lens		
Cataracts	Focal: PPM Persistent hyaloid structures Anterior/posterior sutures Nuclear Diffuse mature cortical	See text
Dislocation/luxation	Anterior/posterior	See text
Coloboma	Notch-like defects in equator	Predisposition to subluxation. Rarely affect vision Associated with iris/ciliary body coloboma
Lenticonus/lentiglobus	Conical or globular lens contour especially posteriorly	Associated with cataracts Other problems such as microphthalmia
Microphakia/aphakia	Small/absent lens	Visual dysfunction related to degree of deformity
Vitreous		
Persistent hyaloid apparatus	Delayed resorption	See text
Fundus		
Colobomata	Typical/atypical	See text
Equine night blindness	Visual disturbance in reduced light	See text
Optic nerve hypoplasia	Disc may be smaller than normal, pale and chalky, with scant or no retinal vessels Not inherited	May be associated with other ocular abnormalities Bilaterally affected are usually blind Unilateral cases may not be noticed until weaning
Optic nerve atrophy	Congenital inflammatory injury to nerves or ganglion cells	Associated with hydrocephalus and possibly viral infections
Retinal detachment	Isolated lesion, or with cataracts, lens luxation, microphthalmia, corneal dystrophy, retinal dysplasia	Usually bilateral and complete with blindness Folded gray veil projecting vitread from the optic disc and hyperreflective tapetum No effective treatment
Retinal dysplasia	Nonprogressive abnormal retinal differentiation often in association with other ocular abnormalities	Bizarre focal or diffuse changes in fundic pigmentation, tapetal reflectivity/color and vascularity Varying degrees of vision defects
Retinal cysts	Within inner/plexiform layers Bulge into vitreous	Associated with multiple ocular abnormalities Individually little effect on vision
Retinal hemorrhage	Single or multiple	See text
Congenital chorioretinitis	Single or multiple small foci depigmentation in non-tapetal fundus	Infections in prepartum mare Affect vision if extensive

PPM = persistent pupillary membrane; NMS = neonatal maladjustment syndrome.

discharge, and irritation caused by flies. Microphthalmia can commonly occur as part of a complex of multiple ocular developmental abnormalities.

STRABISMUS

Strabismus is a deviation of the globe from the proper axis for a given species. The abnormal position is attributable to excessive tension of certain of the extraocular muscles or excessive slackness of their opponents. The primary lesion is thought to be at the level of the cranial nerve nuclei. Strabismus is rare in the horse, although it is more common in the Appaloosa than other breeds, and has been reported in mules at a frequency of one in 200, where it is usually convergent and asymmetrical. Besides a visible abnormality in eye position, affected animals usually have poor vision, assume abnormal postures or head tilting to improve vision, and can be difficult to examine. Surgical correction has been reported in some cases.

CONGENITAL SCLERAL ABNORMALITIES OF THE FOAL

Scleral hemorrhages or splashing have been described in normal neonatal foals and in association with neonatal maladjustment syndrome (NMS). Although these hemorrhages are positioned over the sclera, they are subconjunctival/conjunctival (bulbar). They are thought to result from increased peripheral venous pressure and compressive blunt trauma to the orbit during passage through the birth canal at parturition, leading to rupture of conjunctival and/or episcleral vessels. The hemorrhage can be uni- or bilateral. A complete ophthalmic examination should be performed to reveal other ocular abnormalities such as hyphema, retinal hemorrhage, and retinal detachment. The foal should be carefully examined to exclude the presence of other mucosal or cutaneous hemorrhage that may indicate a coagulopathy. Subconjunctival hemorrhages due to blunt trauma should resolve over 7 to 10 days without treatment. In severe cases, those in which a hematoma or chemosis is present, topical ophthalmic lubrication may be required.

ANIRIDIA

Aniridia is the complete absence of the iris and is rare. Bilateral aniridia, or more correctly iridal hypoplasia, with associated secondary cataracts and dermoids, has been reported as an inherited condition in Belgian draft horses and in the Quarterhorse. Clinical examination reveals an abnormally large, unresponsive, round pupil bilaterally, with the equator of the lens and ciliary processes visible. There may be photophobia, blepharospasm, and lacrimation. Vision may or may not be affected.

COLOBOMA OF THE IRIS

Segmental partial or complete absence of iris tissue may occur as the sole defect, or in association with ciliary body, choroidal, or lens colobomata. They may affect the pupillary margin, or appear as holes within the iris substance. The condition may be hereditary in some species and can be uni- or bilateral. Coloboma causes variations in pupil size and shape. A failure of closure of the embryonic fissure accounts for iris colobomata associated with fundic and optic nerve colobomata in the inferionasal quadrant (typical coloboma). All other segmental defects are atypical and of unknown pathogenesis. They produce clinically insignificant lesions that do not impair vision.

ANTERIOR PERSISTENT PUPILLARY MEMBRANE (PPM)

These remnants of iris embryogenesis are commonly observed in young foals. The membrane is derived from the iris mesenchyme, constituting the anterior vascular sheath for the lens, and forming a delicate membrane stretching across the pupil. The membrane normally atrophies in early life but, when this process is incomplete or delayed, remnants persist as strands attached to the lesser circle or collarette of the iris. The pigmented strands arise from the iris stroma about midway between the pupillary margin and the iris base. When they protrude from the iris surface, or traverse the iris face and insert elsewhere on it, PPMs cause few problems. Strands that traverse the anterior chamber to fuse with the cornea are associated with nonprogressive, deep corneal opacities at their site of attachment, whereas those that attach to the lens capsule are often associated with anterior capsular or cortical cataracts. Remnants can also be associated with other abnormalities such as microcornea, cataract, and iris coloboma. A hereditary pattern has not been identified, and treatment is not usually recommended.

CATARACTS

The opacity of the lens or its capsule is termed a *cataract*. In a report on congenital ocular defects, cataracts comprised 35% of all defects in the horse, and many authors consider them to be the most commonly reported ocular abnormality of the foal.

Congenital cataracts are present at birth, although they may take up to 3 months to manifest themselves. They are often bilateral and the sole defect, but may exist with other problems such as microphthalmia, persistent pupillary membranes and hyaloid structures, and aniridia. The precise etiology of most congenital cataracts in the horse is unknown but possible causes include inheritance, trauma

(prenatal and foaling), poor nutrition, in-utero infections, exposure to toxic substances, and radiation.

A foal with a congenital cataract should have a complete gestational history taken and a thorough ophthalmic examination performed. The foal may present with complaints of visual deficits, clumsiness, or repeated lacerations. The foal should be assessed for vision, other abnormalities, and ocular reflexes; assessment should also be made after mydriasis with 1% tropicamide.

Congenital cataracts may involve the lens diffusely or focally. Focal cataracts may involve any area of the lens but are usually small, with a minimal effect on vision. Anterior capsular or cortical opacities can be associated with persistent pupillary membranes that adhere to the lens capsule. These focal opacities may progress to diffuse cortical involvement if the underlying epithelial proliferation and migration are impaired. Cataracts resulting from persistent hyaloid structures are less likely to progress to diffuse cortical involvement, because the lens epithelium does not extend posteriorly beyond the lens equator. Focal opacities involving the anterior and/or posterior suture lines are often nonprogressive. Under magnification they have a vacuolar appearance.

Focal dense nuclear opacities result from an abnormal influence during fetal or embryonal development. They may occur as a solid opacity, a hollow sphere, or as concentric irregular rings. In all types the periphery of the lens remains transparent, and progression is rare. The location and extent of a focal opacity determine its effect on visual function, but often mydriasis, naturally in dim light or artificially with drugs, improves vision. Vision also improves with age, because new layers of normal cortex increase the total lens size relative to the cataract volume.

Diffuse, mature cortical cataracts usually cause blindness, which may not become apparent until weaning time owing to the close mother-foal relationship. Microphthalmia is present in about 50% of cases. The dense nature of the cataract prevents examination of the fundus, and the diffuse type prevents mydriasis improving vision. Foals with this type of cataract may be candidates for lens extraction surgery.

LENS DISLOCATION OR LUXATION

Congenital dislocation or luxation of the lens is uncommon in the horse, with the primary defect being abnormal zonules in form or number. The problem is often bilateral, associated with other congenital anomalies, and not thought to be inheritable. The lens is often cataractous, and may luxate into the anterior chamber or the vitreous cavity. Anterior luxations may cause marked corneal edema and, occasionally, glaucoma. Iridodonesis, a deepened anterior chamber, and an aphakic crescent accompany posterior luxations. Lens extraction is indicated when luxation into the anterior chamber has occurred, provided that there are no other ocular anomalies.

PERSISTENT HYALOID APPARATUS

The term *persistent hyaloid apparatus* (artery) is a relative one in the equine species, because resorption of the system is quite slow, with remnants remaining well into foal life and even adulthood. It is a comparative term derived from human ophthalmology, where the condition causes serious visual defects. In the horse, persistence of the posterior pupillary membrane and hyaloid artery is usually incidental in otherwise normal foals. In those cases in which ocular problems exist, various conditions have been recorded. Posterior capsular and subcapsular cataracts, often axial, may arise owing to persistence of the hyaloid system and usually appear at the attachment of the hyaloid vessel. They are nonprogressive and have a minimal effect on vision. Uncommonly, a plexus may remain attached to the posterior lens surface, which, if extreme, can cause visual disturbance without the presence of cataracts. If the vessels contain blood, some persistent hyperplastic primary vitreous (PHPV) may cause visual impairment, depending on the extent and density of the fibrovascular membrane on or near the posterior lens surface. None of these conditions is thought to be inherited in the horse.

COLOBOMATA OF THE FUNDUS

In general, colobomata of the equine fundus may be divided into two categories, typical and atypical, according to their anatomic relationship with the embryonic optic fissure. They are usually unilateral and are not thought to be inherited in the horse.

Typical, or true, colobomata are rare and arise as a result of imperfect closure of the optic fissure in the embryonic eye. They are located along a plane extending vertically into the nontapetal fundus from the inferior pole of the optic disc. In severe cases the problem is bilateral, and the foal is blind with a searching nystagmus. The colobomata may involve any of the structures of the posterior segment, either singly or collectively.

Atypical colobomata are more frequently found and are considered to be fundic variants or incidental findings by some authors. They are found within the nontapetal fundus either peripapillary, or near to the tapetal/nontapetal junction. They develop outside the plane of the optic fissure and may involve neurosensory retina, retinal pigment epithelium (RPE), and choroid. They do not affect vision significantly. Considerable variation in appearance occurs, with the most common form being single, or occasionally multiple, sharply demarcated, circular or ovoid, zones of depigmentation overlying normal choroid. In the peripapillary area, these lesions are traversed by normal blood vessels. They usually appear as blue or blue-gray lesions, without evidence of inflammation or hyperpigmentation, and are not progressive.

EQUINE NIGHT BLINDNESS (CONGENITAL STATIONARY NIGHT BLINDNESS)

This is a congenital, nonprogressive disease that produces visual disturbance in conditions of reduced light or at night. A breed predisposition is found in the Appaloosa, in which it is presumed to be hereditary based upon sibling studies. The mode of transmission has not been defined but is thought to be recessive, or sex-linked recessive, with the defect on the X chromosome. A wide variation occurs in the degree of abnormality, with some horses appearing normal during daylight but handicapped at night. Others are impaired even in bright illumination. Foals may cock or raise their heads in a star-gazing manner, and seek light. Some may exhibit bilateral dorsomedial strabismus. No ophthalmoscopic abnormalities are detected and diagnosis is based on history, behavior, and electroretinography (ERG). The problem is thought to result from a defect in neural transmission from photoreceptor cell to the bipolar and Müller cells. No treatment is available.

RETINAL HEMORRHAGES

Small retinal hemorrhages have been observed in foals suffering from the neonatal maladjustment syndrome (NMS). These hemorrhages are seen immediately after birth and resolve, without treatment, within 4 to 10 days. Affected foals may also show pupillary abnormalities, being dilated and nonresponsive, miotic, or asymmetrical. Apparent blindness accompanies a variety of neurologic and odd behavioral signs. More recently, it has been suggested that papilledema and changes in optic disc coloration seemed to be more closely related to the cerebral edema seen in these cases, and that not all cases of NMS had retinal hemorrhages. Retinal hemorrhages are also commonly encountered in neonatal foal examinations in otherwise perfectly normal foals, and they appear to be of no clinical significance. The level of the hemorrhage within the retina of the equine neonate has not been studied histologically. They are not associated with long-term visual or neurologic deficits. Recent work suggests that they are the result of a combination of anoxia and asphyxia and increased intracranial and intravascular pressure occurring at birth.

Supplemental Readings

Barnett KC, Crispin SM, Lavach DJ, Matthews AG: Colour Atlas and Text of Equine Ophthalmology. London, Mosby-Wolfe, 1995.
Kern TJ: Ocular fundus and central nervous system causes of blindness. *In* Robinson NE (ed): Current Therapy in Equine Medicine, ed 2. Philadelphia, WB Saunders, 1983, pp 393–395.
Latimer CA: Diseases of the adnexa and conjunctiva. *In* Robinson NE (ed): Current Therapy in Equine Medicine, ed 2. Philadelphia, WB Saunders, 1987, pp 440–445.
Moore CP: Diseases of the cornea. *In* Robinson NE (ed): Current Therapy in Equine Medicine, ed 2. Philadelphia, WB Saunders, 1987, pp 450–456.
Roberts SM: Congenital ocular anomalies. Vet Clin North Am Equine Pract 8(3):459–478, 1992.
Senk GW: Ocular discharge in young horses. *In* Robinson NE (ed): Current Therapy in Equine Medicine, ed 2. Philadelphia, WB Saunders, 1983, pp 385–388.
Whitley RD: Cataracts. *In* Robinson NE (ed): Current Therapy in Equine Medicine, ed 2. Philadelphia, WB Saunders, 1987, pp 456–458.

Glaucoma

DENNIS E. BROOKS
Gainesville, Florida

The glaucomas are a group of diseases resulting from alterations of aqueous humor dynamics that cause an intraocular pressure (IOP) increase above that which is compatible with normal function of the optic nerve. All glaucomas consist of five stages: (1) an initial event or series of events that affects the aqueous humor outflow system; (2) morphologic alterations of the aqueous outflow system that eventually lead to aqueous outflow obstruction and intraocular pressure (IOP) elevation; (3) elevated IOP or ocular hypertension that is too high for normal ganglion cell and optic nerve axon function; (4) progressive optic nerve axon degeneration; and (5) progressive visual deterioration that eventually leads to blindness.

The glaucomas are frequently categorized into primary, secondary, and congenital types. Although all types of glaucoma have a causative mechanism, primary glaucomas possess no overt ocular abnormality to account for the increase in IOP, whereas secondary glaucomas have an identifiable cause, such as intraocular inflammation, neoplasia, or lens luxation. Primary bilateral glaucoma has not been reported in the horse. Secondary glaucomas due to anterior uveitis and intraocular neoplasia are most commonly recognized. Congenital glaucoma is reported in foals and is associated with developmental anomalies of the iridocorneal angle, goniodysgenesis.

ETIOLOGY

Aqueous humor is produced in the ciliary body by energy-dependent and energy-independent mechanisms. The enzyme carbonic anhydrase plays an important role in aqueous production. Aqueous humor passes into the posterior chamber, through the pupil into the anterior chamber, and then exits through the iridocorneal angle, the conventional outflow pathway, or through the uveovortex and uveosclera, the unconventional outflow pathways. Perfusion and morphologic studies indicate potentially extensive unconventional outflow pathway involvement in the horse. Tonographic studies of the conventional outflow pathways show that the horse has an aqueous outflow facility nearly three times that of the dog. In spite of this high aqueous flow/low-resistance outflow system, obstruction of aqueous humor movement at the pupil, iris face, iridocorneal angle, or any other part of the aqueous outflow system can result in an increase in IOP in the horse.

The sieve-like scleral lamina cribrosa groups the retinal ganglion cell axons into bundles, and supports the axons as they exit the globe at the optic nerve to pass to the optic chiasm. The normal equine scleral lamina cribrosa is complex, with a tendency of the laminar pores in the dorsal-nasal quadrant to have thicker interbundle connective tissue that may protect axons in this region from damage due to increased IOP. The axoplasmic flow of the optic nerve axons is normally subjected to a large pressure gradient between the intraocular and intraorbital spaces at the scleral lamina cribrosa. The elevated intraocular pressure (IOP) found in glaucoma exacerbates this pressure gradient, and is associated with disruption of optic nerve axon axoplasmic flow and posterior displacement of the lamina cribrosa. The optic nerve of the horse is unique in that it contains a large proportion of axons of large diameter, which are more susceptible to elevated IOP than smaller diameter axons. Large retinal ganglion cells possess these large-diameter axons and are involved with motion detection, stereopsis, and sensitivity to dim light. The consequences of the loss of such axons to the visual capabilities of the horse are not known.

Glaucoma in horses is being recognized with increased frequency, although the prevalence of glaucoma in the horse is surprisingly low, 0.07% in the United States, considering the horse's propensity for ocular injury and marked intraocular inflammatory responses. Anterior uveitis often leads to formation of preiridal fibrovascular membranes that may limit aqueous absorption by the iris, and physical and functional obstruction of the iridocorneal angles with inflammatory cells and debris. The extensive low-resistance equine conventional aqueous humor outflow pathway, and the prominent unconventional outflow pathways in the horse, may minimize development of glaucoma in many cases of anterior uveitis because substantial aqueous humor drainage occurs despite considerable damage to the conventional pathways.

RISK FACTORS AND CLINICAL SIGNS

Horses with previous or concurrent equine recurrent uveitis (ERU), horses older than 15 years, and Appaloosas are at increased risk for the development of glaucoma. Although glaucoma is an uncommon complication of ERU, the presence of active or inactive uveitis appears to be a major factor in the development of glaucoma. Elevated IOP is clearly the primary risk factor for rapid progression of optic nerve damage and blindness in the horse, although partial vision may be retained for extended periods despite dramatically high IOP. Large fluctuations in IOP occur in horses with glaucoma and horses with ERU, which may make documentation of elevated IOP difficult.

The presence of corneal striae or corneal endothelial "band opacities" in nonbuphthalmic horse eyes warrants a high degree of suspicion for the finding of elevated IOP, but these signs may also be found in eyes that are normotensive at the time of examination. Corneal striae are linear, often interconnecting, white opacities found deep in the cornea, caused by stretching or rupture of Descemet's membrane, and may be associated with increased IOP.

Commonly seen in buphthalmic eyes, the finding of striae in nonbuphthalmic glaucomatous eyes may suggest that Descemet's membrane in the horse is more sensitive than in other species to tension on the cornea associated with transient elevations of IOP.

The diagnosis of equine glaucoma is made with the documentation of elevated IOP or the presence of clinical signs specific to glaucoma, such as buphthalmia. Equine glaucoma may not be easily recognized in the early stages of the disease owing to the subtle nature of the clinical signs. Generally, there is a low index of suspicion of glaucoma, the pupils are often only slightly dilated, and overt discomfort is uncommon. Afferent pupillary light reflex deficits, corneal striae, decreased vision, lens luxations, mild iridocyclitis, and optic nerve atrophy/cupping may also be found in eyes of horses with glaucoma.

Measurement of IOP in the horse requires applanation tonometry,* which is not routinely available in general practice. For this reason, whenever glaucoma is suspected, early referral should be considered. The mean IOP in the horse ranges from 17 to 28 mm Hg, with the IOP of the two eyes of the same horse being within 5 mm Hg. Failure to utilize auriculopalpebral nerve blocks during tonometry may result in slight overestimates of IOP, but is recommended in fractious horses. Horses that require sedation for ocular examination may show dramatic decreases in IOP, as illustrated by a study in which xylazine† decreased IOP by 23%. The IOP in glaucomatous horses does not remain consistently elevated because large fluctuations in IOP occur. Frequent IOP measurements during the day may be necessary to detect transient IOP spikes. This widely fluctuating IOP not only interferes with the diagnosis of glaucoma, but complicates the monitoring of the response to therapy.

TREATMENT

Therapy for equine glaucoma is difficult to rationalize and apply when the initiating events that result in compromise to aqueous humor outflow, mechanisms by which these events lead to aqueous outflow obstruction, and nature of the obstruction itself are not understood. It follows that at present there are few means of detecting the initiating events, much less treatments to prevent the outflow obstruction and optic nerve atrophy. Treating the cause of the outflow obstruction, if known, and reducing the elevated IOP are the primary goals of therapy. Various combinations of drugs and surgery may be necessary to reduce the IOP to levels that are compatible with preservation of vision. Glaucoma is particularly aggressive and difficult to control in the Appaloosa.

Oral glycerin‡, the systemically administered carbonic anhydrase inhibitors acetazolamide§ and dichlorphenamide,‖ the topical miotics demecarium bromide¶ (0.25% b.i.d.) and pilocarpine# (2% q.i.d.), and the β blocker

timolol maleate* (0.5 % b.i.d.) have been utilized to lower IOP in horses with varying degrees of success. The drugs that appear to be most successful in reducing IOP in horses are those that reduce aqueous humor formation (i.e., β-adrenergic antagonists and carbonic anhydrase inhibitors).

Conventional glaucoma treatment with miotics may provide varying amounts of IOP reduction in horses. A large number of horses have increased IOP when administered topical miotics such as demecarium† or pilocarpine.‡ This may be due to the differences in aqueous humor outflow in horses compared to other species, as well as the high prevalence of anterior uveitis found in equine glaucoma cases. Because miotics can potentiate the clinical signs of uveitis, miotic therapy is generally considered to be contraindicated in glaucoma resulting from uveitis, and should be used cautiously in horses with mild or quiescent anterior uveitis.

Glaucoma in some horses may, paradoxically, respond to topical corticosteroid and atropine therapy, even if active uveitis is not clinically evident. Anti-inflammatory therapy, consisting of topically and systemically administered corticosteroids, and/or topically and systemically administered nonsteroidal anti-inflammatory medications (phenylbutazone§ 1 mg/kg p.o. b.i.d.; flunixin meglumine‖ 250 mg p.o. b.i.d.) also appear to be beneficial in the control of IOP. Because of the prominent role of uveoscleral outflow in the horse, and the variable response to miotics in equine glaucoma, topical atropine,¶ with its effect of enhancement of unconventional outflow and stabilization of subclinical inflammation, may be a better choice of drug to improve aqueous outflow and decrease IOP in horses with glaucoma resulting from anterior uveitis. Atropine therapy for equine glaucoma should only be used in conjunction with careful IOP monitoring because it also is reported to exacerbate high IOP in some cases.

Timolol maleate* (0.5% BID), a nonselective β-adrenergic antagonist, is effective at lowering IOP in horses, and may be used alone or in combination with other drugs. Oral carbonic anhydrase inhibitor therapy, utilizing dichlorphenamide# (1 mg/kg p.o. b.i.d.) or acetazolamide** (1–3 mg/kg daily p.o.) may be beneficial in lowering IOP when combined with β-adrenergic antagonists and miotics. The safety of systemic carbonic anhydrase inhibitors has not been determined in the horse, and the drugs may be cost-prohibitive for extended therapy. Oral glycerin†† (0.75 ml/kg via nasogastric tube) may be expected to decrease IOP by dehydrating the vitreous, but again, the safety of treating glaucoma with oral glycerin in the horse has not been established.

When medical therapy is inadequate, neodymium:yttrium-aluminum-garnet (Nd:YAG) laser cyclophotoablation may be a viable alternative for long-term IOP control because it is very effective at controlling IOP and main-

*Tonopen, Mentor O & O, Santa Barbara, CA
†Rompun, Miles Inc., Shawnee Mission, KS
‡Glycerine, Butler, Columbus, OH
§Acetazolamide, Schein Pharmaceuticals, Port Washington, NY
‖Daranide, Merck, Sharp & Dohme, West Point, PA
¶Humorsol 0.25%, Merck, Sharp & Dohme, West Point, PA
#Piloptic 2%, Optoptics Lab, Fairton, NJ

*Timoptic 0.5%, Merck, Sharp & Dohme, West Point, PA
†Humorsol 0.25%, Merck, Sharp & Dohme, West Point, PA
‡Piloptic 2%, Optoptics Lab, Fairton, NJ
§Phenylbutazone, Butler, Columbus, OH
‖Banamine, Schering-Plough, Kenilworth, NJ
¶Atropine sulfate 1%, Goldline Lab, Ft Lauderdale, FL
#Daranide, Merck, Sharp & Dohme, West Point, PA
**Acetazolamide, Schein Pharmaceuticals, Port Washington, NY
††Glycerine, Butler, Columbus, OH

taining vision in the horse. The author recommends 55 laser sites per eye for contact Nd:YAG laser cyclophotoablation in the horse, 5 to 6 mm posterior to the limbus, at a power setting of 12 watts for 0.3 seconds' duration per site. Preliminary clinical evidence indicates that laser cyclophotoablation is most efficacious at lowering IOP and maintaining vision in horse eyes that are non-atropine-responsive. Filtration gonioimplant surgeries to increase outflow of aqueous humor are experimental in the horse but have been successful. Chronically painful and blind buphthalmic globes should be enucleated or have an intrascleral prosthesis implanted.

Supplemental Readings

DeGeest JP, Lauwers H, Simoens P, De Schaepdrijver L: The morphology of the equine iridocorneal angle: A light and scanning electron microscopic study. Equine Vet J 10[Suppl]:30–35, 1990.

Dziezyc J, Millichamp NJ, Smith WB: Comparison of applanation tonometers in dogs and horses. J Am Vet Med Assoc 201(3):430–433, 1992.

Miller TR, Brooks DE, Gelatt KN, King TC, Smith PJ, Sapenza JS, Pellicane CP: Clinical findings and response to treatment in 14 horses. Vet Comp Ophthalmol 5(3):170–182, 1995.

Pickett JP, Ryan J: Equine glaucoma: A retrospective study of 11 cases from 1988 to 1993. Vet Med 88(8):756–763, 1993.

Samuelson D, Smith P, Brooks D: Morphologic features of the aqueous humor drainage pathways in horses. Am J Vet Res 50(5):720–727, 1989.

Smith PJ, Gum GG, Whitley RD, Samuelson DA, Brooks DE, Garcia-Sanchez GA: Tonometric and tonographic studies in the normal pony eye. Equine Vet J 10[Suppl]:36–38, 1990.

Smith P, Samuelson D, Brooks D: Aqueous drainage paths in the equine eye: Scanning electron microscopy of corrosion cast. J Morphol 198:33–42, 1988.

Smith PJ, Samuelson DA, Brooks DE, Whitley RD: Unconventional aqueous humor outflow of microspheres perfused into the equine eye. Am J Vet Res 47(11):2445–2453, 1986.

Van der Woerdt A, Gilger BC, Wilkie DA, Strauch SM: Effect of auriculo-palpebral nerve block and intravenous administration of xylazine on intraocular pressure and corneal thickness in horses. Am J Vet Res 56(2):155–158, 1995.

Wilcock BP, Brooks DE, Latimer CA: Glaucoma in horses. Vet Pathol 28(1):74–78, 1991.

Cataract

PHILIP BOYDELL
Manchester, England

Cataract refers to any opacity of the lens and results from disturbance of normal lens anatomy, whatever the cause. There are several possible etiologies. Hereditary cataract has been described in Belgians, Morgans, Thoroughbreds, and Quarter horses, but reports are rare. This may be due to the fact that horses are bred mainly for function rather than appearance, unlike the situation in the dog, and affected animals are unlikely to be used in breeding programs. Bilateral cataract is occasionally seen in mature horses; age-related changes may be involved.

Congenital cataract may be accompanied by other ocular defects, notably microphthalmos, or may be the sole abnormality. Where these occupy a large portion of the neonatal lens, the opacity may interfere with normal development of central visual pathways, and early removal is indicated. Some lesions are small and do not progress, becoming less significant as the lens grows around them. The majority of cataract seen in horses may be attributable to eye disease or injuries. These are generally unilateral and accompanied by other signs of ocular disease such as corneal lesions, iris changes, and retinal degeneration.

CLINICAL SIGNS

The assessment of visual function in horses is difficult on anything other than a general basis, and the horse's behavior in specific environments and lighting conditions provides the best clinical guide. The safety of the horse, rider, and other people in the environment must be considered in a case when vision is suspect. This is true after intraocular surgery, and the author advises that such animals be worked only in a controlled environment by an experienced rider.

After assessment of visual function, ocular examination should begin with distant direct ophthalmoscopy. This demonstrates the extent of any opacity as a silhouette against the retinal reflection. It must be remembered that sight can appear to be normal even if there is a large bilateral opacity. The extent and position of the opacity can then be defined more accurately by ophthalmoscopy or preferably slit lamp biomicroscopy. For a full examination, use of a mydriatic such as tropicamide is necessary to allow inspection of the equatorial region of the lens. When the opacity precludes ophthalmoscopic inspection of the posterior segment, ultrasonography should be performed. If there is some doubt about retinal function, electroretinography can confirm the presence or absence of retinal activity.

Cataract may be classified by the position of the opacity within the lens, although, if progressive, the changes may eventually involve the majority of this structure. Some congenital opacities may be restricted to the suture lines or the nucleus. When the cataract forms in response to an inflammatory stimulus, the initial changes may be capsular or subcapsular, and other evidence of ocular inflammation may be detected (see Uveitis).

TREATMENT

When cataract is diagnosed, underlying conditions should be treated appropriately. If the cataract is immature, the administration of mydriatic agents such as tropicamide° or atropine† may allow more light to enter the eye, possibly enhancing vision.

Slit lamp biomicroscopy of the anterior segment and, if possible, the posterior segment, is mandatory. When the opacity precludes ophthalmoscopic inspection of the posterior segment, ultrasonographic examination should be performed to detect anatomic changes. If there is some doubt about retinal function, electroretinography demonstrates the existence or absence of retinal activity.

No medical treatment is available for cataract itself, and a decision to perform expensive and nonguaranteed surgery must be made following a detailed assessment of the eye. Any other signs of severe eye disease may be considered a contraindication for surgery. Evidence of active uveitis adversely affects the prognosis for the restoration of satisfactory vision, although chronic changes may themselves benefit from a surgical approach (see below).

If the lens is to be surgically removed in one piece, its

°*Mydriacyl 1%, Alcon, Fort Worth, TX*
†*Atropine sulphate 1%, Goldline, Fort Lauderdale, FL*

size requires a large incision. Small-incision surgery using aspiration assisted by phacofragmentation techniques is preferable. In young patients the lens material is quite soft, and aspiration alone may be sufficient. In older animals aspiration may require the crystalline lens to be broken up by phacoemulsification, with vitrectomy cutting devices or with manual phacofragmentation. Details of the procedures are not relevant in this volume, and cases should be referred to an experienced surgeon for assessment and treatment.

The control of postoperative uveitis is of paramount importance because the inflammatory response is the major reason for failure of surgery and the temperament of the patient must be such as to allow easy drug administration for some time.

Supplemental Readings

Dziezyc J, Millichamp NJ, Keller CB: Use of phacofragmentation for cataract removal in horses: 12 cases (1985–1989). J Am Vet Med Assoc 198:1774–1778, 1991.
Whitley RD, Meek LA: Cataract surgery in horses. Comp Cont Ed Pract Vet 11:1396–1401, 1989.

Equine Recurrent Uveitis

BERNHARD M. SPIESS
Zurich, Switzerland

Anterior uveitis and chorioretinitis are common in domestic animals. In horses and mules equine recurrent uveitis (ERU) is the most frequently diagnosed inflammatory disease of the uveal tract, affecting up to 12% of the population according to some reports. Synonyms for ERU are *periodic ophthalmia, moonblindness,* and recurrent iridocyclitis. It is the leading cause of blindness in horses worldwide.

Uveitis may also be the result of neonatal septicemia, blunt and penetrating trauma to the globe with or without rupture of the lens capsule, and corneal ulceration. Nonulcerative keratouveitis of unknown etiology has also been described. Although the information given herein specifically relates to ERU, it is applicable to most forms of uveitis.

THE UVEAL TRACT

Anatomy

The uveal tract, or vascular coat of the eye, comprises the iris and pupil, the ciliary body, and the choroid. The pupil is horizontally elliptical and the pupillary margin is lined by a pigmented ruff. It is more rounded in dim light and is only a narrow horizontal slit in bright light. The central margins of the upper margin, and to a lesser extent the lower margin, exhibit corpora nigra of variable size and

shape. The iris is separated by the collarette in a lighter central and a darker peripheral part. It is usually brown, but blue or white irises (wall eye, china eye) occur.

The ciliary body can be separated in two parts: The pars plicata is located immediately posterior to the iris and consists of the ciliary processes, which are covered by pigmented and nonpigmented ciliary epithelium, representing the inner and outer leaves of the embryonic optic cup. The pars plana is the transition zone between the ciliary processes and the peripheral neuroretina.

The choroid is the posterior uvea. It consists—from sclera to retina—of the lamina fusca, the suprachoroidea, a large vessel layer, the fibrous tapetum (in the dorsal part of the fundus), the choriocapillaris and Bruch's membrane.

Physiology

Four principal functions are attributed to the uveal tract: (1) limitation of the entrance of light by the iris and pupil; (2) secretion of aqueous humor by the ciliary epithelium; (3) accommodation as a result of actions of the ciliary body; and (4) nutrition of the retina by the choroid. The pupil constricts in reaction to light. The corpora nigra are believed to act as shades, further limiting the entrance of light. In the horse, the normal pupillary light reflex is somewhat sluggish compared with other species.

Aqueous humor (AH) production is a combination of diffusion, ultrafiltration, and active secretion by the ciliary epithelium. AH is a clear fluid filling the anterior segment of the globe. Its refractive index is similar to that of water. The entrance of large molecules into the AH is limited by the blood-aqueous barrier. The epithelial component of this barrier consists of the tight junctions of the lateral intercellular spaces of the nonpigmented ciliary epithelium. The endothelial component of this barrier consists of the tight junctions of the endothelium of iris vessels.

Contraction of the ciliary body muscles causes relaxation of the zonules of Zinn, which suspend the lens. Because of the elasticity of the lens it becomes more spherical and thereby increases its refractive power for near vision. The accommodative capability of the equine eye is very limited.

The paurangiotic retina of the horse depends on the choroid for nutrition. Bruch's membrane and the retinal pigmented epithelium (RPE) constitute the epithelial part of the blood-retina barrier. The retinal capillaries are nonfenestrated, and the endothelium has tight junctions. Transport mechanisms allow the passage of nutrients from the choriocapillaris to the retina.

Immunology

Following inflammation, the uvea behaves like a lymph node with persistence of memory B cells. Repeated stimulation with the original antigen causes rapid recurrence of uveitis. Even antigen exposure to other parts of the body has this effect. Exposure to a different antigen may cause uveitis through nonspecific lymphokine-mediated stimulation of memory cells. Inflammation of the uvea results in a permanent increase of vascular permeability. Any antigen may then stimulate uveitis by deposition of immune complexes in permeable vessel walls. Autoimmune uveitis may be a late result of microbe-induced injury of the uveal tract.

Inflammatory Reactions

Inflammation of the uvea results in the breakdown of the blood-aqueous and blood-retina barriers. Cells and proteins enter the AH, retina, and vitreous humor. In the acute stage, the iris and ciliary body are initially infiltrated by polymorphonuclear leukocytes (PMNs). At later stages plasmacytes and lymphocytes predominate. In the iris stroma, perivascular lymphoid infiltrates may persist. The anterior chamber is filled with exudate containing lymphocytes and serum proteins. Clotting factors enter the AH, converting the soluble fibrinogen into fibrin. The same exudate may be present in the vitreous. Organizing fibrinous exudates in the anterior chamber and in the vitreous may result in formation of connective tissue with devastating effects on ocular morphology and function. A cellular infiltrate is usually present in the anterior choroid. Perivascular lymphocytic infiltration may be seen in the optic papilla. Peripapillary degenerative retinal lesions may occur after repeated episodes of inflammation.

ETIOLOGY

The etiology of ERU is still an enigma. The currently accepted theory is that of an immune-mediated disease with various causes that manifests itself by recurrent delayed hypersensitivity reactions at variable intervals. Many

microbial organisms have been incriminated as causative agents of ERU, but only *Leptospira* species and *Onchocerca cervicalis* microfilariae have been identified with some consistency. ERU has been experimentally induced by inoculation with *Leptospira,* and naturally occurring infections with rising serum and AH antibody titer have been reported. The importance of *Leptospira* in the pathogenesis of ERU is subject to geographic variations. Nutritional factors and heredity have also been considered at some point; however, they are no longer generally accepted. A study in the United States demonstrated that Appaloosas had a higher risk of developing uveitis than Thoroughbreds, whereas Standardbreds had a lower risk relative to Thoroughbreds. These results suggest a breed predisposition for ERU. In most clinical cases even extensive work-up fails to firmly establish a cause for endogenous uveitis.

CLINICAL SIGNS

Acute anterior uveitis is a very painful condition. Clinical signs are summarized in Table 1. Severe blepharospasm and lacrimation are present. Photophobia is usually evident. The conjunctiva are congested, giving the eyelids a swollen appearance. The episclera is injected, although this is difficult to see owing to the blepharospasm. Corneal edema may be present, and after a few days superficial and deep neovascularization becomes apparent. Breakdown of the blood-aqueous barrier causes cloudy AH with flare and cells. In severe uveitis, anterior chamber hemorrhage may occur. Keratic precipitates, aggregates of inflammatory cells and fibrin on the endothelial surface of the cornea, may be seen in acute and chronic cases. Rubeosis iridis, neovascularization of the iris, is usually present; however, it is difficult to see on the dark iridal surface. Posterior synechiae can be present as firm adherences of the posterior surface of the iris to the anterior lens capsule, or as pigment deposits on the anterior surface of the lens. Repeated inflammatory episodes cause focal cataracts, which can progress to maturity. ERU is the leading cause of cataracts in horses. Inflammatory exudates are seen as cloudy vitreous. In the quiescent stage of the disease, vitreous floaters may be observed. If the fundus can be examined, peripa-

TABLE 1. CLINICAL SIGNS OF UVEITIS

Acute Stage	Quiescent Stage
Pain	Persistent corneal edema
Blepharospasm	
Lacrimation	
Photophobia	
Conjunctival hyperemia	Keratic precipitates
Corneal edema	Focal cataract
Keratic precipitates	Posterior synechiae
Aqueous humor flare	Pigment deposits on lens
Anterior chamber exudate	Vitreous floaters
Miosis	Butterfly lesions
Cloudy vitreous	Phthisis bulbi
Hypotony	Buphthalmos

pillary chorioretinal inflammatory and postinflammatory changes may be seen. They are often referred to as *butterfly lesions.* Occasionally, contraction of organizing vitreous exudates may cause complete rhegmatogenous retinal detachments.

Acute anterior uveitis is accompanied by hypotony of the globe. Intraocular pressure (IOP) can be assessed by digital palpation and can be measured by applanation tonometry. Normal IOP in the horse is approximately 20 mm Hg. In acute anterior uveitis, IOP is markedly reduced. Hypotony may persist in the quiescent stage of the diseases, leading to phthisis bulbi.

Secondary glaucoma and buphthalmos seem to be uncommon sequelae of ERU. Recurrences are at unpredictable intervals that tend to become shorter with time. After an initial acute inflammatory episode most recurrences are within 12 months.

Ophthalmic Examination

Because of the painful nature of anterior uveitis, a complete ophthalmic examination is usually possible only after sedation of the animal and adequate akinesia of the eyelids. For a description of how to complete an ophthalmic examination, see page 344.

TREATMENT

In the majority of cases the etiology of uveitis is unknown and nonspecific anti-inflammatory and cycloplegic therapy is indicated. If an etiology can be established, appropriate antimicrobial therapy must accompany symptomatic treatment of uveitis. Treatment generally aims at stabilization of the blood-ocular barriers and at preventing permanent intraocular damage that interferes with vision.

Topical Anti-Inflammatory Therapy

Topical corticosteroids are the mainstay of uveitis treatment, but if the horse cannot be medicated topically, a subpalpebral lavage system can be installed. Corneal penetration of these drugs is critical if therapeutic anterior chamber concentrations are essential. Prednisolone-acetate 1%° or dexamethasone alcohol† 0.1% are initially instilled 4 to 6 times daily. Both drugs have superior penetration capabilities. In severe uveitis, 20 mg methylprednisolone‡ can be injected subconjunctivally. These injections can be repeated at intervals of 3 to 4 days if necessary.

Nonsteroidal anti-inflammatory drugs (NSAIDs) can be administered topically, alone or in combination with corticosteroids. Diclofenac sodium§ or indomethacin‖ instilled q.i.d. has been used successfully to control uveitis in horses. Topical cyclosporin A 1% or 2% in corn oil is a promising drug to control ERU; however, because of its limited corneal penetration, therapeutic intracameral concentrations cannot be achieved.

°*Pred Forte, Allergan, Irvine, CA*
†*Maxidex ointment or suspension, Alcon Laboratories, Fort Worth, TX*
‡*Depo Medrol, The Upjohn Company, Kalamazoo, MI*
§*Voltaren Ophtha, Ciba Vision, Summit, NJ*
‖*Indophthal, Novopharma, Schaumburg, IL*

Systemic Anti-Inflammatory Therapy

Systemic anti-inflammatory drugs are often necessary to control acute uveitis. Flunixin meglumine° (1.0 mg/kg IV s.i.d.) has been used successfully. At this dose flunixin can be safely given for 5 to 7 days. Prednisolone tablets (1 mg/kg p.o. s.i.d.) initially are well tolerated. Low doses of prednisolone given orally on alternate days in the quiescent stage of the disease may prevent recurrence in horses not used for competition. Alternatively, aspirin (10 to 15 mg/kg p.o.) can be given once or twice daily.

Cycloplegic Therapy

Mydriatic and cycloplegic therapy is very important in the management of uveitis. Atropine sulfate 1% or 2% is given t.i.d. until the pupil is fully dilated and then tapered to effect. More frequent applications of atropine may cause colic in horses and should therefore be avoided. In cases of severe ciliary spasm, 1 to 1.5 ml of the following combination of drugs injected subconjunctivally can prove very useful: epinephrine (0.33 mg/ml), atropine sulfate (3.30 mg/ml), and cocaine chloride (1.0 mg/ml). Alternatively, phenylephrine (5 mg) and injectable atropine sulfate (1–4 mg) may be injected subconjunctivally.

Intraocular Medication

When massive anterior chamber exudates are present, intracameral injection of 25 μg of tissue plasminogen activator† (TPA) reduces clot size and clears the anterior chamber within hours.

Supportive Therapy

During the acute stage of ERU, horses should be kept in a darkened stall and exercise should be limited. Horses suffering from uveitis rarely try to rub their eye. If self-trauma is a problem the animal should be cross-tied. Protective hoods and full eye cups are not recommended.

Surgical Therapy

Based on excellent results in human endophthalmitis, vitrectomy has been advocated in recent years as a possible surgical treatment of ERU. The goal of pars plana vitrectomy is to remove vitreous exudates and inflammatory mediators and products. Of 12 operated horses, 10 have their sight and are free of recurrent episodes of ERU over a follow-up period of up to 3 years. Blind painful eyes should be enucleated or eviscerated. Implantation of a silicone prosthesis may be of cosmetic benefit.

PROGNOSIS

Initially, an accurate prognosis is difficult to render. The time period between acute episodes, the response to therapy in the acute stage, and the damage done by a single inflammatory episode are important prognostic parameters. However, long-term prognosis for control of uveitis and retention of vision is guarded at best. Even in the clinically

---

°*Banamine, Schering-Plough, Kenilworth, NJ*
†*Actilyse, Boehringer Ingelheim, Ridgefield, CT*

quiescent stage of ERU, subclinical low-grade anterior and posterior uveitis causes progressive intraocular damage, such as synechiation, opacification of lens and vitreous, and chorioretinal and optic nerve lesions, resulting in visual impairment or blindness. Diligent daily control by both owner and veterinarian, aggressive treatment of acute inflammatory episodes, and long-term control of uveitis even in the quiescent stage may retard visual disability for many years.

Supplemental Readings

Jones TC: Equine periodic ophthalmia. Am J Vet Res 3:45–71, 1942.
Lavach JD: Periodic ophthalmia. *In* Large Animal Ophthalmology. St. Louis, MO, C.V. Mosby, 1990, pp 162–171.
Werry H, Gerhards H: Surgical treatment of equine recurrent uveitis: A preliminary report: Tierärztl Praxis 20:178–186, 1992.
Whitley RD, Miller TR, Wilson JH: Therapeutic considerations for equine recurrent uveitis. Equine Pract 15:16–23, 1993.

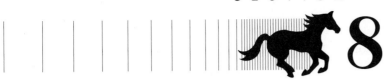
THE SKIN

Edited by M. Amy Williams

Topical Therapy

DAN CARTER

JOHN MACDONALD
Auburn, Alabama

Dermatologic conditions of horses are common and often are of concern to the owner because of the effect on the appearance or comfort of the animal. Treatment of dermatologic conditions poses several limitations, with size of the species being the most important. Systemic therapy is often impractical because of the expense of the medication, whereas topical therapy poses the disadvantages of incomplete response and labor-intensive procedures. Appraisal of the attributes and limitations of both systemic and topical therapy is necessary before starting specific treatment. Topical therapy is often used to augment other forms of treatment and enhance the recovery time, whereas in other circumstances it may be used as the exclusive treatment for the condition. Horse owners have often used topical "home remedies" that can alter the appearance of the lesion and make diagnosis difficult. The attending veterinarian should obtain a minimum data base including skin scrapings, fungal culture, and cytology tests. The results of such tests plus knowledge of the common dermatologic diseases of the region should provide sufficient evidence to develop a list of differential diagnoses and formulate a diagnostic plan.

COMMON DERMATOLOGIC CONDITIONS AMENABLE TO TOPICAL THERAPY

Diseases With Crusting and Scaling

Diseases causing excessive scaling and crusting represent some of the more common dermatologic problems of horses. These diseases may have a similar appearance upon initial presentation. Although the symptomatic topical therapy may be similar, it is best to attain a definitive diagnosis before embarking on a course of therapy. Conditions of crusting and scaling of skin frequently seen in practice include grease heel (scratches, dew poisoning, chronic idiopathic equine pastern dermatitis), dermatophilosis (rain rot, rain scald, streptothricosis), dermatophytosis (ringworm), and pemphigus foliaceus. The distribution of the lesions may provide a clinical impression of etiology such as "scratches" on the palmar pastern or dermatophilosis on the dorsal rump. Although a specific etiology may be suspected but not confirmed, some diseases may be ruled out with simple diagnostic procedures. For example, biopsy may rule out pemphigus foliaceus.

Mild cases of crusting scaling diseases may only require gentle cleansing with a nonmedicated shampoo* to remove scales, crusts, exudates, and debris. Shampoos should be mild and nonirritating and should help remove antigens, which may contribute to pruritus. Shampoos have limited residual effect because of limited contact time and complete rinsing. Time-consuming cleansing can be a deterrent to client cooperation and can result in treatment failure. A medicated antiseborrheic shampoo may be needed in more serious cases to provide the keratolytic and keratoplastic characteristics that aid removal of the stratum corneum to promote better scale formation and epidermal cell keratinization. The active ingredients or combination of ingredients in antiseborrheic shampoos determine the relative potency, with sulfur salicylic acid combinations† the least potent and tars‡ the most potent. Benzoyl peroxide products provide

---

Blue Groom Aid, Evsco Pharmaceuticals, Buene, NJ; or Show Shampoo, The Butler Company, Dublin, OH; or Allergroom, Allerderm, Hurst, TX

†Sebalyt, DVM Pharmaceuticals, Miami, FL; or Sebbafon, The UpJohn Company, Kalamazoo, MI; or Sebolux, Allerderm, Virbac, Hurst, TX

‡Nu-Sal, SmithKline Beecham Animal Health, Exton, PA; or T-Lux, Allerderm/Virbac, Hurst, TX; or Equitar, DVM Pharmaceuticals, Miami, FL; or Adams Pragmatar Shampoo, SmithKline Beecham Animal Health, Exton, PA

antibacterial as well as mild antiseborrheic effects. Cost of some of the medicated products may be prohibitive to some clients, especially when purchased in small quantities such as the 12- to 16-ounce bottles dispensed for small animal patients. Many shampoos are available in gallon sizes and may prove more cost effective.

Many commonly used shampoos contain a detergent base with iodine or chlorhexidine as the active ingredient. Iodine shampoos, polyalkyeneglycol-iodine°, or generic povidone-iodine scrub are effective against a variety of bacterial and fungal infectious conditions, are relatively inexpensive (povidone-iodine scrub $.15/ounce; polyalkyeneglycol [Weladol] $.64/ounce), and are widely available over the counter, but they can be irritating to mucous membranes, eyes, and respiratory tissues, and they dry the hair and skin. Skin irritation and hair loss in the inguinal or axillary region can occur when iodine products are not properly rinsed away. Chlorhexidine shampoos or generic chlorhexidine scrub, are also effective against a variety of fungal, bacterial, and viral agents. Chlorhexidine has often been reported to be less irritating than iodine shampoos but, in the authors' experience, it may also cause irritation of the eyes and vulva. Both products can cause excessive drying of the skin and hair coat after repeated use.

Humectants and emollients are moisturizing agents used primarily to lubricate, rehydrate, and soften dry scaling skin. After the use of agents that may dry the skin, such as benzoyl peroxide, iodine, or tar shampoos, a humectant or emollient rinse may provide a local effect in protecting, softening, and increasing pliability of the skin. Humectants† hydrate the stratum corneum by attracting transepidermal water and work best when applied to the skin while it is moist. Emollients‡ smooth the roughened surfaces of the stratum corneum by filling the spaces between dry flakes with oil droplets. Emulsified oils help hold water in the stratum corneum and prolong hydration by inhibiting evaporation. Lanolin-derived emulsions are used less now because of the high incidence of contact sensitivity.

Infectious Dermatoses

Dermatophilosis ("rain scald") caused by *Dermatophilus congolensis* and dermatophytosis (ringworm) caused by *Trichophyton* species or *Microsporum* species are usually self-limiting diseases often associated with fall or winter weather. Some horses with decreased immune function (for example, those with an adenoma of the pars intermedia of the pituitary) can suffer increased incidence or severity of the diseases. Initial treatment with an antiseborrheic shampoo to remove crusts and debris followed by daily antiseptic shampooing of the affected areas for 7 to 10 days, and then twice-weekly treatment until there is complete resolution of lesions, is advisable. Exposure to sunlight produces significant improvement in normal horses with these diseases. Additional treatment with a disinfecting rinse or topical ointment may be necessary in refractory cases. Available rinses include povidone-iodine solutions,

chlorhexidine (0.5–2%), lime sulfur (2–5%)°, and sodium hypochlorite (0.5%). These may be applied locally to the lesions and allowed to dry. The use of captan† is no longer recommended because of potential human health risks. Lime sulfur rinses are effective, but the product has an objectionable odor and may stain skin and fabrics. The topical antifungal medications, miconazole‡ benzalkonium chloride§ and tolnaftate,‖ may hasten recovery time, reduce severity, and prevent transmission to other animals and humans. The available antibacterial topical preparations rarely contain the commonly used systemic antibiotics, which reduces the usefulness of bacterial culture and sensitivity tests.

The vehicle or base of a topical medication can influence the penetration and biologic activity of the active ingredients. In general, for a given active ingredient, the more occlusive vehicles such as ointments are more potent than creams or gels. Ointments may provide visible evidence of treatment, resulting in greater owner satisfaction during the course of treatment.

Systemic therapy with griseofulvin or ketoconazole is expensive, can be toxic, and has arguable efficacy. Ketoconazole is not well absorbed orally in the horse. Most veterinary dermatologists consider griseofulvin ineffective for treatment of dermatophytosis in the horse.

Grease heel is a multifactorial crusting and scaling condition of the horse pastern. Factors frequently associated with grease heel include contact dermatitis due to moisture, photosensitization, and infectious agents including *Staphylococcus aureus* or *intermedius*, dermatophilosis, and dermatophytosis. Chorioptic acariasis mites may be suspected in refractory cases of grease heel, especially in draft horses. Treatment protocols should address the multifactorial nature of the condition. Initial treatment with a combination antibacterial and keratolytic shampoo aids removal of the thick and often painful crusts that accumulate. Topical application of an astringent (zinc sulfate or lead acetate) may enhance drying if moisture appears to be the inciting cause. Lanolin-based products have been used for many years to repel moisture and soften crusts. Treatment with a combination of topical medications is often used. These include commercially prepared penicillin/neomycin/polymyxin/hydrocortisone,¶ triamcinolone/ nystatin/neomycin/thiostrepton# and home-prepared combinations of dimethyl sulfoxide (DMSO)/thiabendazole and dexamethasone/sulfanilamide in various proportions. These may be applied under a soft bandage to extend contact time. Oral administration of ivermectin has shown efficacy against *Chorioptes* mites in other host species, suggesting that it may be effective in horses. Horses that develop cellulitis of the distal limbs as a consequence of infectious agents such as *Staphylococcus* species or dermatophilosis may benefit from the addition of systemic therapy with trimethoprim/sulfa or penicillin.

°Weladol, Mallinckrodt Veterinary, Mundelein, IL
†Humilac, Allerderm/Virbac, Hurst, TX; or Micro Pearls Humectant Spray, Evsco Pharmaceuticals, Buena, NJ
‡HyLyte, Efa Cream Rinse, DVM Pharmaceuticals, Miami, FL; or Micro Pearls Cream Rinse, Evsco Pharmaceuticals, Buena, NJ

°Lym Dyp, DVM Pharmaceuticals, Miami, FL
†Orthocide, Ortho Products, Division of Chevron Chemical, San Francisco, CA
‡Conofite, Mallinckrodt Veterinary, Mundelein, IL
§Dermacide, The Butler Company, Dublin, OH
‖Tinavet, Schering-Plough Animal Health, Kenilworth, NJ
¶Forte Topical, The Upjohn Company, Kalamazoo, MI
#Panalog, Solvay Animal Health, Mendota Heights, MN

Immune-Mediated Skin Disease

Pemphigus foliaceus is an autoimmune disease associated with circulating and tissue-bound autoantibodies against intercellular epidermal antigen. Clinical signs include crusts, scales, alopecia, and erosions often with a generalized distribution or originating on the ventral half of the body or head. Less frequently blisters, ventral pitting edema, pyrexia, pruritus, and concurrent signs of systemic illness may be seen. Pemphigus foliaceus has been reported to occur most often in Appaloosa horses. Diagnosis is based on clinical signs and skin biopsy. Treatment will likely be lifelong and includes systemic corticosteroids and/or chrysotherapy.° In addition to systemic treatment, gentle cleansing with a sulfur/salicylic acid shampoo helps remove scales and crusts and may also give relief from pruritus or pain and minimize secondary bacterial infection during healing of erosions.

Allergic dermatitis in the horse may cause pruritus, hair loss, wheals, hives, plaques, scales, and crusts. A hypersensitivity to parasites, such as *Onchocerca* and insects such as *Culicoides,* black flies, stable flies, and horn flies may be responsible. The most common insect hypersensitivity is of the genus *Culicoides,* which occurs worldwide. Other causes of allergic dermatitis include contact dermatitis, drug reactions, inhaled allergens, and possibly food hypersensitivity. Treatment for this group of diseases may initially require avoidance of the offending agent through management factors. Food allergies may require withholding a suspected antigen for 30 days to determine an association to dermatitis. Recent evidence indicates that a significant absorption of antigen occurs through the skin. Frequent skin cleansing with a mild shampoo may provide relief by removing exudates, bacteria, and antigens.

The practical value of topical local anesthetics and antihistamines is limited. Systemic therapy with antihistamines is often unrewarding. As hypersensitivity intensifies, effectiveness of corticosteroid therapy may decline. Treatment with a topical corticosteroid spray or ointment† may provide relief for localized lesions such as ventral midline dermatitis due to insect hypersensitivity, but can be expensive. Newer products containing oatmeal and an analgesic‡ have been helpful for focal areas.

Insecticides and insect repellents are frequently used directly on horses as sprays or wipes. The use of organophosphates (coumaphos, dichlorvos) and organochlorines (methoxychlor, lindane), although very effective insecticides, appears to be declining with the changing environmental awareness and concern over health risks to both horses and humans. The use of repellents, pyrethroids, and other botanicals seems more appropriate. Pyrethrins are derived from certain species of chrysanthemum and have the advantage of safety when repeated treatment is needed. Pyrethrins may be safely applied daily as a spray or wipe. Synthetic pyrethroids° have insecticidal and repellent properties and are often incorporated with pyrethrins to obtain a more residual effect.

Topical medications used for treatment of skin diseases can induce contact dermatitis or exacerbate a primary dermatitis, resulting in a confusing clinical picture. Fly sprays have frequently been implicated as significant sources of antigen, and topical application may result in allergic or irritant dermatitis. Treatment should include cleansing with a mild shampoo and avoidance of the offending compound. Environmental control of insects through the use of insecticides, repellents, and stalling of horses in insect-proof stables during periods of insect activity, usually early evening and morning, may prove to be the best solution.

Sarcoids

Equine sarcoid is the most common skin tumor of horses. It is fibroblastic and may be viral in origin. Sarcoids may appear as nodular growths around the eyes, ears, mouth, limbs, and trunk. Occult sarcoids may appear as areas of alopecia with scaling and crusting. Diagnosis is based upon clinical appearance and biopsy results. Incisional biopsy may stimulate sarcoid growth, and it may be best to not biopsy a suspicious lesion unless the owner is willing to treat resulting sarcoid activity. Numerous topical therapies have been used for treatment of sarcoids. As yet, there does not appear to be a topical drug that has been shown to be completely effective, and therefore topical therapy is not relevant.

Supplemental Readings

Frank LA: Dermatophytosis. *In* Robinson NE (ed): Current Therapy in Equine Medicine, ed 3. Philadelphia, WB Saunders, 1992, pp 698–700.
Kwochka KW: Symptomatic topical therapy of scaling disorders. *In* Griffin GE, Kwochka KW, MacDonald JM (eds): Current Veterinary Dermatology: The Science and Art of Therapy. St. Louis, CV Mosby, 1993, pp 191–202.
Scott DW: Parasitic diseases. *In* Scott DW (ed): Large Animal Dermatology. Philadelphia, WB Saunders, 1988, pp 207–251.

°*Solganal, Schering, Kenilworth, NJ*
†*Cortispray, DVM Pharmaceuticals, Miami, FL; or Dermacool, Allerderm/Virbac, Hurst, TX; or PTD-HC, VRx Products, Division of St. Jon Products, Harbor City, CA*
‡*Relief Spray, DVM Pharmaceuticals, Miami, FL*

°*Preventic LA, Allerderm/Virbac, Ft. Worth, TX; or Expar, Coopers Animal Health, Mundelein, IL; or Duocide, Allerderm/Virbac, Hurst, TX; or SynerKyl Pet Spray, DVM Pharmaceuticals, Miami, FL*

Cryotherapy for Equine Skin Conditions

R. REID HANSON
Auburn, Alabama

Cryotherapy is the controlled use of freezing temperatures to destroy undesirable tissue while doing minimal damage to surrounding healthy tissue. Conditions in which cryotherapy may be indicated include certain skin lesions; ophthalmic, orthopedic, and respiratory tract disorders; and cryoneurectomy. This chapter focuses on the use of cryotherapy for specific skin conditions. One should have a thorough knowledge of the basic principles, freezing agents, cryosurgical units, techniques, and clinical applications before using cryotherapy. Cryotherapy is most useful for small localized skin lesions treated on an outpatient basis.

PRINCIPLES OF CELL DESTRUCTION

Understanding the basic principles of cryotherapy is fundamental to a successful outcome. Cell destruction is best accomplished with rapid freezing, slow thawing, and three freeze-thaw cycles. Cell death is a direct result of ice crystal formation, intracellular fluid and electrolyte disturbances, denaturing of cell membranes, and thermal shock. These factors act dynamically to cause overwhelming cellular pathology. Three major categories of events—immediate, delayed, and late—occur at the cellular level after the application of low temperatures to tissue. Within the immediate phase, there is the abrupt transformation of the intra- and extracellular fluid into ice crystals, which causes dehydration and toxic concentration of electrolytes. Ice crystal formation harms the cell membranes and organelles, causing disruption of their normal function. Freezing denatures proteins and lipoprotein complexes in the cell membranes, leading to cellular swelling and bursting. Other biochemical functions are destroyed by the thermal shock. Cell death is associated with the rate at which tissue is frozen and allowed to thaw. Rapid freezing causes more severe intracellular dehydration but smaller ice crystal formation than with slow freezing. These crystals are physically less disruptive than large ice crystals. The small crystals convert into large crystals if the tissue is allowed to thaw slowly. Therefore, in clinical use, the most effective approach for maximal cellular destruction is to freeze the tissue as rapidly as possible and allow it to thaw slowly, at room temperature, to 0°C.

The delayed phase occurs during the hours following the freeze-thaw cycle. Additional cell death occurs as a result of vascular stasis and endothelial damage. Thrombosis and ischemia produce cell death beyond direct cryogenic damage. In the late phase of cryonecrosis, there is evidence to support an enhanced immune response against tumors from the formation of antibodies and through cell-mediated responses as a result of cryotherapy. Regression of distant lesions following cryotherapy of isolated equine sarcoids and papillomas has been reported.

FREEZING AGENTS

Liquid nitrogen is the most popular freezing agent for cryotherapy. It is a clear, colorless, odorless, nonflammable liquid that produces a temperature of −195.8°C (−320.5°F). Liquid nitrogen can usually be obtained from medical supply companies that sell oxygen. It is easily poured from the vacuum-insulated flask into the cryosurgical unit. Liquid nitrogen can be kept active for a limited time, usually a maximum of 2 to 4 weeks, if the original container is opened only a few times.

Nitrous oxide is the second most popular freezing agent and is most effective for removing tumors less than 3 cm in diameter or for treating superficial skin lesions. Nitrous oxide does, however, require cryosurgical units specifically designed for its use. Applied with probes, it produces a temperature of −89°C (−138°F). Although more expensive on a unit basis than liquid nitrogen, there is minimal waste with nitrous oxide, and therefore greater efficiency. Nitrous oxide is readily available in veterinary hospitals that use gas anesthesia. One large tank can be used for many months because it usually connects directly to the unit rather than being poured, as with liquid nitrogen.

CRYOSURGICAL UNITS

Cryosurgical units deliver their freezing action by spray or probe. Cryoprobes use the Joule-Thompson effect: rapid expansion of gas under pressure provides low temperatures. The probe is held against the tissue to be destroyed. A phase-changing probe is the method used with nitrous oxide. Liquid nitrogen can be applied with a solid contact probe. A great variety of probes is available, each for a different purpose.

Currently, there is a trend toward the use of spray units. Some units look like modified insulated ("thermos") bottles with a spraying tip at the top.* A mixture of liquid and vaporized liquid nitrogen is sprayed directly onto the area to be treated. Different spray devices deliver different mixtures of vapor and liquid. This can vary from 15% vapor and 85% liquid to 55% vapor and 45% liquid. The higher the percentage of liquid in the spray, the lower the temperature and the more potent the freeze. The amount of

---

*The Cryogun, Arista Surgical Supply Co. Inc., New York, NY

cryogen applied is controlled by valves and/or aperture sizes on the spray tips. This technique allows larger and deeper areas to be frozen at a faster rate. Care must be taken to avoid adjacent tissue damage. Freezing too rapidly or too extensively can lead to cryogen runoff, freezing too deeply, or increased lateral spread of freezing before adequate tissue depth is achieved. Protection of healthy tissue is possible through the use of air foam cups with a hole cut in the bottom to fit the lesion's shape, metal or plastic spray cones, and petroleum jelly applied to normal tissue around the periphery of the lesion. Rapid freezing rate may cause poor visibility because of the production of liquid nitrogen vapor. Application precision can be improved by debulking the lesion prior to cryotherapy and by recording the temperature at the margins and base of the lesion by the use of cryosensors or thermocouple needles.

CRYOTHERAPY TECHNIQUES

Patients receiving cryotherapy should have received recent tetanus vaccination. The procedure can usually be performed in the standing horse sedated with xylazine and butorphanol with or without local infiltration of anesthetic. In some cases, the procedure may require general anesthesia. The site requiring treatment should be cleaned and the hair clipped. Core or segment biopsies of the lesion should be taken the day before cryotherapy, if possible. The biopsy site provides a hole for insertion of the cryoprobes. Surgical debulking of skin lesions, where applicable, improves the efficiency of spray freezing by flattening the irregular surface of the lesion. After biopsy or debulking, hemostasis must be achieved by use of a tourniquet, ligature, direct pressure, or packing the wound.

Most tissues are adequately destroyed by two well applied freeze-thaw cycles. However, increased vascularization, cellular density, and large areas of tissue dilute and impede penetration of the freezing agent and the lesions require more freeze-thaw cycles. The area of cryonecrosis that results is in direct relation to the duration of the freeze. Damage to vital structures such as nerves, blood vessels, and tendons underlying the cryolesion can be minimized by sound anatomic and surgical knowledge and cryotherapy experience. The need for cryosensors depends on the size, shape, and location of the lesion, and the experience level of the operator. It is desirable to freeze a margin of 5 to 10 mm of normal tissue around most malignancies.

Postoperatively, there is considerable local edema and swelling, although bandages and antibiotics are rarely necessary. Swelling resolves in a few days but can be accompanied by a serosanguineous discharge caused by transient vasodilation, especially if the area was previously ulcerated. Hemostasis is excellent postoperatively except where larger vessels have been cut preoperatively through debulking or biopsy. The previously frozen tissues begin to separate from healthy tissues at 4 to 7 days and are occasionally associated with discharge. Use of a fly repellent may be indicated. Usually a dry, hard scab forms, which should be allowed to remain as temporary protection for as long as possible. At approximately 4 weeks after cryotherapy, the scab separates, exposing the granulation bed. The exposed granulation bed heals by secondary intention. The time for complete healing depends on the size and depth of the cryolesion but is usually 14 to 21 days after the scab disappears. Scarring is minimal but some depigmentation may occur.

CLINICAL APPLICATION

Cryotherapy has advantages over surgical excision in many situations. Cryotherapy is often superior for removal of large lesions such as sarcoids on the lower portion of the leg where poor skin mobility prevents closure with sutures. Conventional surgical excision often produces excessive blood loss, whereas cryotherapy usually results in minimal hemorrhage. This is particularly effective in old or debilitated patients. After cryotherapy, scarring usually is slight, and the cosmetic effect is good. Selective destruction of diseased or neoplastic skin is possible with little damage to normal tissue. Chances of tumor cells spreading from premalignant lesions are reduced. The delayed phase of cryotherapy may provide an immunotherapeutic effect on malignant neoplasms.

Disadvantages of cryotherapy are also recognized. The surgeon performing cryotherapy needs to be experienced in its use. The necrosis and sloughing of frozen tissue may be visually unpleasant and malodorous for 2 to 3 weeks following treatment. Regrowth of white hair near the cryotherapy site sometimes leaves a cosmetic blemish. If the application is too aggressive, vital structures surrounding the frozen lesion may be damaged. This applies especially to blood vessels, nerves, tendons, ligaments, and joint capsules. Large blood vessels frozen during cryotherapy for tumor destruction may start bleeding 30 to 60 minutes later when postoperative attention has been relaxed, or several hours later when a veterinarian is not present.

Skin conditions amenable to cryotherapy include cutaneous neoplasms, usually sarcoids, squamous cell carcinomas, papillomas, and melanomas; exuberant granulation tissue; habronemiasis; and pythiosis. Sarcoids and squamous cell carcinomas are the two conditions in horses most commonly treated with cryotherapy.

The equine sarcoid, the most common tumor of the horse, is a locally invasive, nonmalignant, fibroblastic tumor of the skin. Young horses have a higher incidence of sarcoids with about one third of these having multiple lesions. No predilection for gender or breed exists, and the most common sites are the lower limbs, axilla, ventral abdominal wall, prepuce, groin, ears, periocular region, and commissure of the mouth. Sarcoids are notoriously difficult to treat and rarely undergo spontaneous regression. Regression of distant lesions has been reported following cryosurgical removal of only a few sarcoids. Unless directly adjacent to vital structures, cryotherapy is the treatment of choice for equine sarcoids. Cryotherapy is one of the most effective treatments to prevent recurrence of sarcoid tumors, with 80 to 90% reported cure rates at 12 months later. Conventional surgical excision with or without electrocautery can be followed by local recurrence in up to 60% of the cases.

Success of sarcoid removal was found to be higher after three, rather than two, freeze-thaw cycles. It may be necessary to repeat cryotherapy to attain a higher rate of success. Large lesions should be surgically debulked before freezing. Debulking the sarcoid followed by pressure bandaging can be done the day before cryosurgery if hemorrhage is anticipated. When treating lesions on the lower limb, freezing of the underlying periosteum and bone should be avoided. Because sarcoids are skin lesions, retention of subcutaneous mobility is a good indication that the deeper tissues are being spared. Around the eye region, care should be taken to avoid excessive freezing and complications of eyelid scarring. Other forms of therapy such as intralesional cisplatin (see below) should be considered for sarcoids in this location. Sarcoids that recur following cryotherapy may be refrozen or frozen in conjunction with other types of therapy.

Cryotherapy is a common form of treatment for tumors of the eye, orbit, nictitating membrane, and conjunctiva. In horses, this form of treatment has been used successfully for early ocular squamous cell carcinoma. Squamous cell carcinoma is a malignant tumor arising from the squamous layer of the epithelium. It is the most common ocular neoplasm in the horse. The healing time can be slow but the cosmetic appearance is usually good. In cattle, cryotherapy reportedly has a 70 to 90% success rate for early stages of ocular squamous cell carcinoma. Radical surgical excision and radiation therapy may be preferred for more extensive lesions.

Squamous cell carcinoma in horses also has a predilection for mucocutaneous junctions, such as the eyelids, lip, nose, vulva, prepuce, and penis. Cryotherapy is a successful form of treatment at these sites, as long as the condition is diagnosed and treated early. Cryotherapy has several advantages over conventional surgical excision or amputa-

tion in treating squamous cell carcinoma of the penis. With cryotherapy, the procedure is relatively simple and quick, there is minimal hemorrhage or infection, and there is a lower recurrence rate. It may also allow the continued use of the stallion. Regardless of the site, squamous cell carcinomas are frequently ulcerated, bleed easily, infiltrate extensively at their base, and slowly metastasize. The prognosis for complete resolution is diminished with locally invasive tumors or in the presence of metastasis to regional lymph nodes.

Although a clinically important form of therapy for specific uses, cryotherapy is not a total replacement for conventional surgery. The appeal of cryotherapy is convenience and cost effectiveness. As improved units are manufactured, with some that are designed especially for veterinary application, the practitioner will find it easier to select the proper cryosurgical apparatus and use it effectively.

Supplemental Readings

Clem MF, DeBowes RM: Cryosurgical applications. *In* White NA, Moore JN (eds): Current Practice of Equine Surgery. Philadelphia, JB Lippincott, 1990, pp 12–16.

Fretz PB, Barber SM: Prospective analysis of cryosurgery as the sole treatment for equine sarcoids. Vet Clin North Am Sm Anim Pract 10(4):847–859, 1980.

Fretz PB, Martin GS, Jacobs KA, McIlwraith CW: Treatment of exuberant granulation tissue in the horse: Evaluation of four methods. Vet Surg 12(3):137–140, 1983.

King TC, Priehs DR, Gum GG, Miller TR: Therapeutic management of ocular squamous cell carcinoma in the horse: 43 cases (1979–1989). Equine Vet J 23:449–452, 1991.

Munroe GA: Cryosurgery in the horse. Equine Vet J 18(1):14–17, 1986.

Cisplatin Treatment for Cutaneous Tumors

ALAIN P. THÉON
Davis, California

The use of systemic chemotherapy in equine oncology is limited because of substantial toxicity and cost. Intratumoral chemotherapy consists of injecting anticancer drugs directly into the tumor and adjacent tumor bed. The intratumoral route of administration results in very high drug concentrations in the tumor and tumor bed, and very low concentrations in surrounding normal tissue and plasma. The high tumor-to-plasma drug concentration ratio achieved results in enhanced antitumor activity with no systemic toxicity. Direct administration of the drug into the gross tumor allows optimal local distribution of drug. By comparison, systemic chemotherapy relies on the blood supply to transport and distribute the drug in the tumor. Intratumoral chemotherapy allows the safe use of high-potency anticancer drugs at a reasonable cost in horses because small amounts of drug are used.

The choice of cisplatin for intratumoral chemotherapy

in the treatment of equine cutaneous tumors is based on its wide spectrum of activity against solid tumors including all cutaneous carcinomas, sarcomas, melanomas and lymphomas; long response duration observed after treatment; and its relatively low cost. Cisplatin or *cis*-diamminedichloroplatinum is a heavy metal compound that inhibits deoxyribonucleic acid (DNA) synthesis by directly binding to DNA, which leads to death of actively dividing cells.

TECHNIQUE OF INTRATUMORAL CHEMOTHERAPY

Drug Formulation

The pharmacokinetic advantage of intratumoral chemotherapy is optimized by increasing the time of drug expo-

TABLE 1.   COMMERCIALLY AVAILABLE SAFETY EQUIPMENT

Drug preparation
    Disposable, plastic-backed absorbent liner
    °Hydrophobic air-venting filter (2 μ)
    Syringes (3 ml) with Luer-Lok fittings
    Syringe connector (2- or 3-way stopcock) with Luer-Lok
       fittings
Protection garb
    Disposable protective gown made of low-permeability fabric
    Disposable high-efficiency respirator
    Chemical splash goggle
    †Talc-free disposable latex gloves (thickness ≥0.009 inch)
Disposal of contaminated materials
    ‡Spill kit
    Sealable plastic bag for cytotoxic waste
    Locking lid, leakproof, plastic canister for cytotoxic waste

°An alcohol-dampened pledget wrapped around the needle and vial top may be used during withdrawal. The pledget should be used when expelling air bubbles from the syringe as well.

†Hands should be washed after glove removal. Large animal OB glove may be used under the latex glove to protect the fore and upper arms from aerosolization.

‡Located in areas where drug is mixed and administered. Chemical inactivation with dilute bleach can be used safely to clean up spills.

sure to cancer cells. This is achieved by use of drug carriers that keep the drug at the site of injection and vasoactive agents that limit drug reabsorption. A number of viscous fluid drug carriers, such as proteinaceous matrices (e.g., collagen implant°) or vegetable oils (e.g., sesame seed and poppy seed oil) have been shown to prolong local exposure of the tumor to high concentrations of cisplatin.

This article presents the clinical data obtained with the use of sesame seed oil as drug carrier. Medical-grade purified sesame seed oil has been chosen because of its good record of safety for intramuscular depot administration in horses, and its low cost and wide availability. Sesame seed oil is stable, neutral, biodegradable with no residue; it produces no local reaction and forms a viscous fluid water-oil emulsion that flows readily through narrow-bore needles (20–25 gauge). It can be sterilized by use of gamma-irradiation or by pasteurization. The emulsifier sorbitan monoleate† may be added to sesame seed oil (1:20 volume) to decrease the fluidity of the mixture. This formulation is useful for highly vascularized tumors such as hamartoma or hemangiosarcoma, because the thick, stable emulsion prevents excessive bleeding from the site of injection.

Epinephrine (Adrenalin, 1:1000) may be added (1:10 volume of final mixture) to cause vasoconstriction and prolong tumor cell exposure to cisplatin. This formulation is useful for melanomas and large fibroblastic ulcerated sarcoids. Great care must be taken with this formulation because it can produce extensive necrosis in the tumor as well as in normal tissue. It should not be used when normal skin in the treatment field must be preserved.

Drug Preparation

The mixture is prepared immediately prior to use; any delay may affect drug potency. Cisplatin is available in vials

of 10 mg powder° upon special request to the manufacturer, or in vials of 25 mg power (cis-platinum[II] diamminedichloride, Sigma Chemical Co., St Louis, MO). The steps for drug mixture of the 10 mg and 25 mg vials are slightly different. The 10 mg vial of cisplatin is reconstituted with 1 ml of sterile water for injection, USP, to obtain a saturated solution of 10 mg of cisplatin per ml; commercial premixed cisplatin solution at a dilution of 1 mg/ml should not be used because it is not potent enough with this technique. One ml of cisplatin in water (10 mg/ml of water) is then mixed with 2 ml of sesame oil. The 25 mg vial of cisplatin is reconstituted with 2.5 ml of sesame oil. A rubber stopper and a cut-out top plastic cap (Aldrich Chemical Co., Milwaukee, WI) must first be fitted on the 25 mg vial, which is not designed for reconstitution and fluid withdrawal. One ml of cisplatin in sesame oil (10 mg/ml of oil) is then mixed with 1 ml of water and 1 ml of sesame oil. The final steps for drug mixing and preparation of the emulsion include (1) attachment of a mixing unit (2- or 3-way connector) to the Luer-Lok syringe containing the diluent, i.e., 2 ml of sesame oil or 1 ml of water and 1 ml of sesame oil; (2) removal of air in the mixing unit by gently pushing the diluent through it (air bubbles disrupt the emulsion); (3) attachment of the syringe containing cisplatin, i.e., 1 ml of cisplatin in water or 1 ml of cisplatin in sesame oil, to the free end of the mixing unit; (4) with both syringes securely fastened, mixture of the contents of the syringes by exchange of the syringe contents, i.e., the pumping method.

Technique of Administration

To administer the drug, the needle mounted on the syringe is inserted into the tissue to the desired depth, and the drug is injected at a constant flow while the needle is withdrawn. The target volume of tissue to be injected should include all visible tumor and a margin of normal tissue of 1 to 2 cm (depending on tumor type and tumor size). Planning the pattern of injections is critical to achieve a uniform dose distribution. Depending on the shape and accessibility of the lesion, the target volume is injected via multiple sites using a parallel-row technique or field-block technique. Because cisplatin does not diffuse in tissues farther than 3 to 5 mm from the site of injection, the rows of injections should be kept 0.6 to 0.8 cm apart. If the injections are farther apart, the dose distribution is not uniform and some areas of the tumor may be underdosed, which results in tumor recurrence. If the injections are too close, the tissue at the site of puncture is exposed to excessive doses of drug, which results in excessive reactions of the neighboring local tissue. Depending on the treatment volume, multiple planes of injections may be needed using parallel or orthogonal axes of injection.

Safety Guidelines

Only personnel properly trained in the handling and use of antineoplastic drugs should be involved in the treatment procedure. Guidelines have been designed to assist all health care professionals who may be exposed to antineoplastic agents. Cisplatin is mutagenic and carcinogenic at

°*Matrix Pharmaceuticals, Menlo Park, CA*
†*Span 80, Sigma Chemical, St. Louis, MO*

°*Platinol, Bristol-Myers Squibb, Princeton, NJ*

Veterinary Medical Teaching Hospital
University of California, Davis

Release Form for Owners of Patients Treated with Cisplatin

Your horse was treated with an intratumoral administration of an anticancer drug mixed with a drug carrier _____ on _____, 19__. Due to the non-detectable levels of drug in the urine and bowel movements, no special safety precautions are needed when handling body wastes. Your next appointment is on _____, 19__

RECOMMENDATIONS

With release of the patient to your care, you are accepting responsibility for the protection of yourself and all other persons who may come in contact with your animal. Please observe the following safety precautions.

1.   Initially, a small amount of drug may leak from the site of injection. If the area around the site of injection must be touched, latex exam gloves should be worn for a period of 3 days following treatment. Hands should be washed after glove removal. Precautions should be taken to minimize aerosol generation during cleaning of the treated area and water hosing should be avoided for a period of 3 days following treatment.

2.   Your horse should not be in direct contact with children or pregnant women for a period of 1 week after each treatment

3.   If your horse must be seen by a veterinarian outside the VMTH, please inform the doctor of the type of treatment your horse has received and the date it was treated or show this form to the doctor prior to the examination.

4.   If your animal should die, please notify us as soon as possible.

SIDE-EFFECTS

1.   The treatment has no effect on tumors and/or metastases outside the area receiving treatment.

2.   The side-effects and complications of the treatment are purely local and relate to the drugs and the actual injection procedure. The following side-effects may be related to this particular treatment:

_____

_____

3.   Antibiotics (systemic and/or topical ointment) and anti-inflammatory drugs may be prescribed after treatment to prevent infection and alleviate pain.

3.   Any clinical signs outside the treated area are not related to the treatment and need to be brought to the immediate attention of your veterinarian.

_____

I have read this form, and the information contained in it has been explained to me. I understand the potential treatment risks and safety precautions that I must follow.

_____   _____
Signature of owner   Date

_____   _____
Signature of Clinician   Date

Figure 1. Sample form for release of horses treated with cisplatin.

low doses and with repeated exposure. Therefore, strict safety rules must be observed concerning preparation, handling, and administration. Good technique is critical to maintain product sterility and avoid contamination of the environment or personnel by accidental exposure to cytotoxic dust or aerosols. Equipment is available that can aid in providing a safe environment for handling cisplatin (Table 1). If a class II containment cabinet is not available, the drug mixture should be prepared on a disposable, plastic-backed absorbent liner in a quiet, low-traffic work area, away from drafts and personnel. Protective clothing is required during and after treatment. A release form should be given to the owner outlining the precautions to be taken after treatment (Fig. 1). Cytotoxic chemical waste must be handled separately from other hospital trash and disposed of in accordance with federal and state regulations. All equipment used for compounding and administration of chemotherapeutic agents should be placed in specific containers for hazardous waste (see Table 1). Treated horses must be prevented from entering the human food chain.

CLINICAL APPLICATIONS OF INTRATUMORAL CHEMOTHERAPY

Treatment Protocol

Tumor dosage is planned to be 1 mg of cisplatin (0.3 ml of mixture) per cubic centimeter of tissue in the target volume, which includes all macroscopic areas of tumor and a margin of normal tissue. Treatments are done on an outpatient basis. Several dose intensity protocols are available. A standard intensity treatment protocol includes four intratumoral chemotherapy treatment sessions at 2-week intervals. A time interval of less than 10 days between treatments may result in an increased risk of local reactions, whereas a time interval of more than 21 days may allow tumor repopulation and result in a loss of therapeutic effect. A high-intensity protocol includes six treatments given as a standard protocol with a 4-week rest, followed by two treatments given also at a 2-week interval. The treatment can be used alone or in combination with other treatment modalities including surgery (Fig. 2), irradiation, and biologic therapy (i.e., immunomodulation).

Intratumoral Cisplatin Chemotherapy Used Alone

For tumors with diameters of 3 to 5 cm, the treatment may be used alone. The treatment field size should remain the same during the course of treatment; the volume of tissue treated should not be decreased if a reduction in tumor size is observed. The indications for intratumoral cisplatin are based on tumor size, tumor type, and location. The most important factor is tumor size. Tumor types responsive to the treatment include squamous cell carcinoma/papilloma, sarcoid, soft tissue sarcoma (neurofibrosarcoma, fibrosarcoma, hemangiosarcoma, schwannoma), melanoma, lymphoma, and hamartoma. The most responsive tumors include fibroblastic ulcerated sarcoids and lymphomas, the least responsive tumors include flat sarcoids and benign and malignant melanomas. The treatment is ideal for tumors in locations where a complete surgical resection would result in a cosmetic or functional deficit.

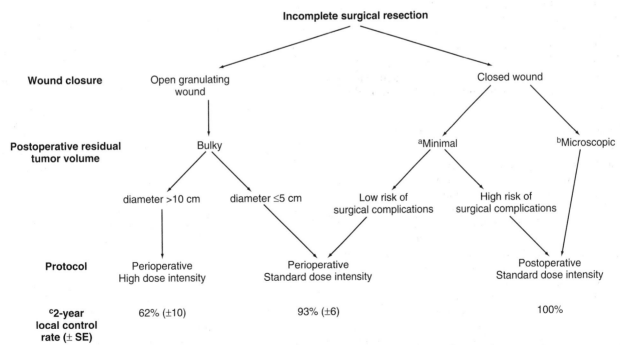

Figure 2. Protocols and results of intratumoral chemotherapy with cisplatin and incomplete surgical resection for treatment of equine cutaneous tumors. ([a]Tumor removed in fragments with no margin of normal tissue; [b]complete removal of gross tumor but histologically positive surgical margins; [c]product limit estimates ± standard error obtained from 98 horses treated at UCD-VMTH followed for a minimum of 2 years.) (Data derived from studies funded by The California Center for Equine Health and Performance.)

The most commonly indicated sites include the face (eyelid, lip, pinna, nose), distal extremities, and male and female genitalia because the treatment is effective and the cosmetic results are excellent.

A treatment with standard dose intensity is used for tumors less than 3 cm in their greatest dimension, corresponding to a volume of tissue equaling approximately 20 cm³. For a given size, tumor response is a function of histologic type and growth rate. For example, fibroblastic ulcerated sarcoids or cutaneous lymphomas are more responsive than indolent melanomas or flat sarcoids. The 2-year relapse-free rates range from 80 to 90% for sarcoids in all locations, 70 to 80% for periorbital carcinomas and 90 to 100% for carcinomas of the genitalia. Previous unsuccessful treatment including cryotherapy or immunotherapy does not affect treatment efficacy. In horses with melanoma arising at the base of the tail, a formulation including epinephrine is most effective but produces substantial tissue necrosis.

In horses with multiple cutaneous lesions such as sarcoids, melanomas, or lymphomas, no spontaneous regression of untreated lesions has been observed to date. In horses with multicentric cutaneous lymphoma, intratumoral cisplatin is used only for the large ulcerated lesions. The treatment protocol includes a 2-week pretreatment course of dexamethasone (a decreasing dose schedule beginning with 50 mg/day) followed by intratumoral cisplatin for the residual tumor masses. In horses with multiple melanomas, intratumoral cisplatin is used only for inoperable lesions. The treatment protocol includes a 2-month pretreatment course of cimetidine (4 mg/kg t.i.d.) to potentially produce cytoreduction, followed by intratumoral cisplatin for the residual tumor mass. For histologically aggressive melanomas, a 2-month prophylactic treatment course of cimetidine (2.5 mg/kg t.i.d.) is recommended after completion of intratumoral cisplatin.

High-dose-intensity treatment is indicated for large (3–5 cm in largest dimension) inoperable tumors or when a combination of surgery and intratumoral cisplatin is not technically or financially feasible. Examples include cutaneous tumors of the face, including periorbital and peribuccal areas; neck; vulva; and distal extremities.

Intratumoral Cisplatin Combined With Surgery

The basis for combining surgery and intratumoral cisplatin chemotherapy is that conservative surgery and adjuvant intratumoral chemotherapy are as effective as radical surgery. The two treatments are complementary; conservative surgery removes the tumor bulk and intratumoral cisplatin eradicates the residual disease. Combined surgery and intratumoral cisplatin is the most effective protocol. In most cases, the cosmetic and functional results of the combination are superior to those of a radical surgery or high-intensity intratumoral cisplatin alone.

Horses with large tumors of any histologic type located on the face, genitalia, distal extremities, perineum, and tail base, where a wide surgical resection would result in a substantial cosmetic and functional deficit, benefit from combined surgery and intratumoral cisplatin. For large lesions, cytoreductive surgery improves the efficacy of the intratumoral cisplatin with no increase in complications.

Depending on tumor location, type of surgical wound (open versus closed), volume of residual tumor (microscopic versus macroscopic), and tumor proliferative activity, several treatment protocols are feasible. A protocol is defined by the timing of the two treatments and the dose intensity of intratumoral cisplatin. The most common combinations revolve around perioperative and postoperative intratumoral cisplatin using the standard dose intensity. Perioperative treatment means that the first administration of cisplatin is done at the time of surgery. Postoperative treatment means that the first administration of cisplatin is done 2 to 3 weeks after surgery when the wound has healed.

For tumors with visible residual disease that cannot be surgically closed and an open wound measuring less than 5 cm in largest diameter, the protocol of choice is perioperative intratumoral cisplatin. No advantage is found in delaying treatment, and excessive delay between incomplete excision and intratumoral cisplatin administration may reduce the efficacy of the treatment because of active tumor regrowth. For larger tumors with an open wound measuring more than 5 cm in largest diameter, perioperative intratumoral cisplatin with a high-dose-intensity protocol or a combination of intratumoral cisplatin and irradiation is recommended.

When primary closure is possible, the choice of perioperative versus postoperative treatment depends on the risk of surgical complications determined by the extent of the surgical resection and location, and the surgical margin status. Surgical margins may be grossly positive when there is macroscopic residual disease, or they may be microscopically positive when tumor cells are observed on histopathologic evaluation of the margins of the resected specimen. Postoperative intratumoral cisplatin is recommended after extensive surgery when there is a high risk of skin wound dehiscence, because of skin tension, or after microscopically incomplete surgical resection in which there is no visible residual disease. The use of intratumoral cisplatin to treat recurrence after surgery is less effective than when planned postoperative treatment is initiated before tumor recurrence. Perioperative intratumoral cisplatin is recommended after incomplete removal of gross tumor, when the margins are grossly positive and when the risk of postoperative complications is low. When the length of the incision is less than 7 cm on the neck or trunk and 5 cm on the eyelid or distal extremities, perioperative intratumoral cisplatin does not increase postoperative morbidity. Studies are ongoing to compare the effects of perioperative and postoperative intratumoral cisplatin on larger incisions.

At the time of surgery and before wound closure, the total extent of tissue involvement, the estimated volume of residual tumor, and the areas of gross tumor in regard to the cutaneous surgical wound and other anatomic landmarks should be well documented to plan the treatment. This is important because the treatment field should remain the same during the course of treatment. The only time that the volume of tissue treated may be decreased (after the second or third treatment) is in the treatment of microscopically incomplete surgical excision.

The overall results of combined surgery and intratumoral cisplatin are excellent (see Fig. 2). In a series of horses with periocular tumors (N = 74, follow-up 2 years or more), treated at the University of California, with surgery (closed wound and minimal residual disease) and either perioperative or postoperative intratumoral cisplatin, the 2-year local control rates were 89% for squamous cell carcinomas and 94% for soft tissue sarcomas (i.e., sarcoids, fibrosarcomas, and neurofibrosarcomas).

Side Effects of Treatment

The effects of treatment are strictly local. All acute reactions including inflammation, swelling, and focal ulceration are self-limiting and resolve quickly. Swelling frequently occurs after treatment of facial lesions. It usually starts 2 to 3 days after each treatment and lasts about 7 to 10 days. Phenylbutazone or flunixin meglumine may be prescribed to minimize discomfort. Focal skin ulceration, usually less than 1-cm diameter, may be observed after the third or fourth treatment. Perioperative intratumoral cisplatin does not appear to compromise the healing of skin, mucosa, or subcutaneous normal tissue. A substantial risk for local infection is present with this treatment technique. Treatment of grossly infected lesions should be postponed until the infection has resolved. Prophylactic systemic antibiotherapy is recommended after each treatment session. Damage to nerve, muscle, or vessels has not been observed. A second course of treatment for recurrent tumor can safely be given without increased local reactions. The cosmetic results are excellent even after treatment of open granulating wounds because the treatment does not produce tissue fibrosis or necrosis and does not affect hair growth and color.

Causes of Treatment Failure

During the course of treatment, tumor clearance is progressive. It is sometimes difficult to evaluate tumor response because changes in tissues during treatment can mimic tumor growth. Edema due to inflammation in normal tissue and the cumulative volume of drug injected can cause enlargement, which can be mistaken for tumor growth.

For treatment of open granulating wounds, granulation tissue may be differentiated from tumor because the former responds to a pressure bandage and is associated with rapid centripetal re-epithelialization. The effects of treatment are objectively evaluated 4 to 6 weeks after the last treatment when most normal tissue reactions have subsided and active tumor growth, if present, can be assessed.

Cisplatin resistance, intrinsic or acquired, does not seem to be clinically significant because less than 2% of all tumor types treated with intratumoral cisplatin at the University of California did not respond initially to treatment, and recurrent tumors are retreated successfully. The analysis of pattern of failures is indicative of the importance of the technique of injection in the overall success of the treatment and may be used as a quality control assessment of the operator's technique in an equine oncology practice. Treatment failures may be classified as marginal recurrence when the tumor grows back at the periphery of the treated field or in-field recurrence when the tumor grows back within the treated field. A marginal recurrence is usually the result of inadequate treatment planning with a field size too small to cover the tumor margins. An in-field recurrence indicates that the technique of injection was improper or the dosage was inadequate.

Supplemental Readings

Théon AP, Pascoe JR, Carlson GP, Krag DN: Intratumoral chemotherapy with cisplatin in oily emulsion for treatment of tumors in horses. J Am Vet Med Assoc 202(2):261–267, 1993.

Théon AP, Pascoe JR, Meagher DM: Perioperative intratumoral administration of cisplatin for treatment of cutaneous tumors in Equidae. J Am Vet Med Assoc 205(8):1170–1176, 1994.

Yodaiken RE, Bennett D: OSHA work-practice guidelines for personnel dealing with cytotoxic (antineoplastic) drugs. Am J Hosp Pharm 43:1193–1204, 1986.

Pruritic Dermatoses

J U L I E   M .   D E L G E R
Columbia, South Carolina

Pruritus in the horse may vary from very mild, with only occasional scratching, rubbing, or chewing, to severe, with serious disfigurement from self-mutilation. Pruritus may be the only abnormality noted with some diseases, or it may be accompanied by varying degrees of alopecia, erythema, or other skin lesions. In many disorders, pruritus follows the formation of lesions, if it develops at all, and resolves when the lesions clear. This chapter is devoted to those conditions in which pruritus is the hallmark of the disease and is often the presenting complaint.

The first step in diagnosis of a pruritic skin disease is obtaining a complete history. The clinician should determine if the pruritus is seasonal or nonseasonal, its duration, the percentage of affected horses on the premises, the number of animals in direct contact with the patient, and if new horses have been introduced to the group. An example of an equine dermatologic history form is provided in Table 1. Once the history is complete, a diagnostic plan can be formulated.

INSECT HYPERSENSITIVITIES

Insect hypersensitivities are the most common causes of pruritic dermatoses in horses. They represent types I and IV hypersensitivity reactions, mainly to salivary antigens of

TABLE 1. EQUINE DERMATOLOGIC HISTORY FORM

1. Lesions seen: ___ itch ___ rash ___ hair loss ___ redness ___ sores ___ loss/gain of skin/hair pigment ___ other (describe) _____

   _____

2. How long have the lesions been present? _____

3. Where were the lesions *first* seen? ___ ears ___ nose ___ face ___ mane ___ neck ___ back ___ trunk ___ legs ___ axillae (armpits) ___ groin ___ tail ___ hooves

4. Have the lesions spread? ___ yes ___ no If so, where? _____

5. Does the horse rub, scratch, or chew? ___ yes ___ no
   If so, where? _____

6. Is the problem seasonal? ___ yes ___ no ___ year round but worse in season.

   Worse in ___ spring ___ summer ___ fall ___ winter

7. What is the horse's primary use? _____

8. How many horses are on the premises? _____
   In direct contact with the patient? _____

9. Are any other horses affected? ___ yes ___ no

10. Do any people in contact with the patient have skin lesions?

    ___ yes ___ no

    If so, what type? _____

11. Last deworming date _____ drug used _____

12. Last vaccination date _____ vaccines given _____

13. Last breeding date/last foaling _____

14. Has the patient been outside of its normal environment?

    ___ yes ___ no

    Where? _____ When? _____

15. Previous treatments _____

16. How effective were these treatments? ___ not ___ very
    ___ somewhat effective

17. Does the patient have any other illness? ___ yes ___ no
    If so, what illness? _____

18. Describe the patient's diet, including any supplements or treats

    _____

biting flies, including *Culicoides* species, stable flies, horn flies, mosquitoes, and horse and deer flies. Pruritus is usually seasonal during warm weather especially in cooler climates. In subtropical regions, pruritis may occur year-round. Disease most often begins in young adults and generally worsens with age. Pruritus is severe, commonly resulting in self-mutilation. Insect hypersensitivities are problems not of a herd, but rather of one or a few individuals within a herd because some horses are genetically predisposed to these allergic diseases. This is an important factor in differentiating hypersensitivity disease from ectoparasitic disease.

Clinical Signs

Clinical signs are variable. Lesions are most commonly distributed dorsally, and there is persistent rubbing of the face, neck, mane, withers, rump, and tailhead. Some horses may roll on the ground to rub their backs. Complete loss of the mane may occur in severely pruritic horses. Alopecia, papules, crusts, and excoriations are present along the dorsum and on the face, especially around the eyes, and on the pinnae. In horses in which pruritus is restricted to the tailhead (pruritus ani), insect hypersensitivity must be differentiated from oxyuriasis and food hypersensitivity. Intensely pruritic horses may lose significant amounts of body weight, because they are constantly distracted from grazing or eating to rub or scratch. These horses are also considered unsafe for riding, because they may suddenly drop to the ground in order to roll and rub their backs and necks.

Ventrally distributed lesions are commonly seen, including alopecia and crusting of the chest, groin, proximal limbs, and intermandibular space. Horses with this distribution of lesions may try to straddle fences, tree stumps, and other objects on which they can rub or scratch their undersides. Some horses have been reported to try to drag their bellies along the ground. In the southeastern United States, especially in Florida, many horses have a combination of dorsal and ventral lesions.

Diagnosis

Differential diagnoses for dorsally distributed lesions include atopy, psoroptic or sarcoptic mange, pediculosis, and dermatophytosis. Differential diagnoses for ventrally distributed pruritic lesions include horn fly dermatitis, cutaneous onchocerciasis, atopy, *Pelodera* or *Strongyloides* dermatitis, and dermatophytosis.

Initial diagnostic procedures should always include skin scrapings and a fungal culture. Psoroptic mange mites, lice, and larval nematodes are usually found in deep skin scrapings, and dermatophytosis may be ruled out by a negative result on fungal culture. A history of routine deworming using ivermectin and of no new additions to the herd or travel outside of the herd by the patient is sufficient to rule out cutaneous onchocerciasis, oxyuriasis, and mange. Skin biopsies may reveal the presence of *Onchocerca* species larvae, *Pelodera* species or *Strongyloides* species larvae, fungal organisms, eosinophilic pustular dermatitis from horn fly bites, or eosinophilic and mononuclear superficial and deep perivascular dermatitis as seen with hypersensitivity diseases. The presence of the latter histopathologic pattern is diagnostic for hypersensitivity disease, but not specific for insect versus other types of hypersensitivity.

Intradermal skin testing is very useful in diagnosing insect hypersensitivity, when it is combined with an appropriate history and clinical presentation. Aqueous extracts of whole insects are injected intradermally and the sites are then evaluated. Intradermal skin testing is best performed by a veterinary dermatologist or a clinician with considerable experience in the performance and interpretation of the test.

Treatment

The best therapy for insect hypersensitivities is avoidance of the offending insect. Separation of horses from cattle is essential in treatment of ventral midline dermatitis caused by horn fly bites, and helps relieve pruritus in horses allergic to horn flies. Stabling of horses during the day prevents blackfly bites. Avoidance of offending insects is most often accomplished by frequent application of insecticidal sprays to the animal. Topically applied insecticides include pyrethrins, permethrins, and organophosphates. Relatively new to the insecticide market is a long-acting permethrin spray for dogs with excellent residual activity.* The author has used this spray on horses every 2 to 3 weeks, with good success. Attachment of an insecticide-impregnated cattle ear tag to the halter also may be helpful.

Hyposensitization based on intradermal skin test results may be effective in some individuals. If avoidance or hyposensitization is not possible or helpful, systemic glucocorticoids are indicated. Prednisone or prednisolone (1 mg/kg p.o. s.i.d.) is administered until the pruritus has resolved, and the dose is then decreased gradually to as low an alternate-day dose as possible.

ATOPY

Atopy is an inherited type I hypersensitivity. Allergens inciting atopic disease include pollens of grasses, weeds, and trees; molds; environmental allergens including dust, dust mites, cotton, wool, and feathers; and insects. In horses, the age of onset is early adulthood. Arabians and Thoroughbreds appear to be predisposed. There is no gender predilection.

Clinical Signs

Clinical signs include pruritus of the legs, neck, ears, face, and ventrum; urticaria that can be chronic or acute, pruritic or nonpruritic; and occasionally respiratory signs typical of chronic obstructive pulmonary disease. Signs may be seasonal or nonseasonal. Horses with both insect allergies and atopy may be difficult to distinguish from horses with only insect hypersensitivities. In the latter group, however, insect avoidance results in clinical resolution, whereas in the former group residual pruritus remains after insect avoidance has been accomplished.

Diagnosis

Differential diagnoses for atopy include insect hypersensitivities, food hypersensitivity, psoroptic or sarcoptic mange, pediculosis, and cutaneous onchocerciasis. Mange and cutaneous onchocerciasis may be ruled out by the history, and pediculosis is easily detected by close physical examination and skin scrapings. Control of biting flies should rule out insect hypersensitivities. Feeding of an elimination diet, discussed later in this chapter, will rule out food hypersensitivity, leaving a diagnosis of atopy.

Intradermal skin testing is currently the most accurate, precise, and reproducible means of determining the allergens to which an animal reacts. This testing should be performed by a veterinary dermatologist or by a clinician with considerable experience in the performance and interpretation of the test. The purpose of the intradermal skin test in atopic individuals is not to confirm the diagnosis, but rather to determine reactivity to individual allergens so that a hyposensitization solution may be formulated.

Serum testing is not recommended as a first choice for atopy diagnosis in any species because of high numbers of false-positive and false-negative reactions. In addition, several reports have indicated an appalling lack of reproducibility in serum testing. If, however, intradermal skin testing is not possible, serum testing and resultant specific immunotherapy are preferable to symptomatic therapy alone.

Therapy

Immunotherapy based on intradermal skin test results may be very effective in atopic horses with skin disease. Horses with pollen and mold allergies manifested as pruritus tend to have better responses to immunotherapy than do horses with an insect component, or urticaria. The author believes that specific immunotherapy based on the results of intradermal testing also may be beneficial in some horses suffering from chronic obstructive pulmonary disease. In addition to specific immunotherapy, some horses may benefit from antihistamine and fatty acid therapy. The most effective antihistamine is hydroxyzine hydrochloride (500–600 mg p.o. b.i.d.). The fatty acid most often used is DermCaps ES* at a dose of four to five capsules orally twice a day. If these therapies are ineffective, systemic glucocorticoids may be used at the dose previously described.

FOOD HYPERSENSITIVITY

Food hypersensitivity is one of the most difficult pruritic dermatoses to diagnose. It is suspected to be mediated by types I, III, and IV hypersensitivity reactions, but the precise pathogenesis is unclear. Virtually any foodstuff may cause hypersensitivity, although foods high in protein are most likely to do so. No age, breed, or sex predilections are reported.

Clinical Signs

Clinical signs include generalized pruritus, pruritus ani, or pruritic urticaria. Papules, plaques, crusts, and excoriations may be seen as secondary lesions, and may be found almost anywhere on the body. The condition is usually nonseasonal, although seasonality may be seen if seasonally available foodstuffs are the offending agents.

Diagnosis

Differential diagnoses for food hypersensitivity include atopy, insect hypersensitivities, oxyuriasis, psoroptic or sarcoptic mange, pediculosis, and cutaneous onchocerciasis. Diagnostic tests should include skin scrapings to rule out lice or psoroptic mange mites. A history of routine deworming with ivermectin rules out sarcoptic mange and cutaneous onchocerciasis. Diligent application of insecticidal sprays rules out insect hypersensitivities. A definitive diagnosis of food hypersensitivity requires the feeding of an elimination diet for 3 to 4 weeks.

The first step in formulation of an effective test diet

---

*Preventic L.A. flea and tick spray for dogs, Virbac, Fort Worth, TX

*DVM Pharmaceuticals, Miami, FL

is taking a complete dietary history, making note of any supplements or treats given in addition to the base diet. All supplements and treats must be discontinued, and the diet changed to, preferably, a hay to which the patient is naive. This test diet is fed for 3 to 4 weeks. If improvement is seen, a tentative diagnosis of food allergy may be made. The former diet should be reinstituted to see if the pruritus recurs. Exacerbation of pruritus with this challenge confirms a diagnosis of food hypersensitivity. At this point, the test diet should be fed again until clinical resolution occurs. Individual ingredients of the former diet should be introduced one at a time, for 1 week each, to determine which ingredient causes the pruritus. If pruritus relapses with feeding of any one ingredient, the test diet should again be fed until clinical resolution, then the provocation testing resumed. The most appropriate therapy is avoidance of the offending foodstuff. Systemic glucocorticoids at the dose given previously may result in some improvement, although food hypersensitivity is usually poorly responsive to steroids.

CUTANEOUS ONCHOCERCIASIS

Onchocerca species are obligate parasites, and the adult nematodes live in connective tissues of horses. Microfilariae are found in the skin, where lesions result from type I or type III hypersensitivity reactions to dead or dying larvae. There are no breed or sex predilections, and affected horses are usually at least 4 years of age. Lesions are nonseasonal, but may worsen in the summer.

Clinical Signs

The face, neck, withers, and ventrum may exhibit focal alopecia, scaling, and crusting. More severe lesions, including plaques, ulceration, exudation, lichenification, and depigmentation may ensue. Chronic lesions may heal by scarring, accompanied by irreversible alopecia and depigmentation.

Diagnosis

Differential diagnoses include horn fly dermatitis, dermatophytosis, atopy, food hypersensitivity, psoroptic or sarcoptic mange, *Pelodera* dermatitis, and trombiculidiasis (chiggers). Skin scrapings help to rule out mange, lice, and chiggers. Horn fly dermatitis may be ruled out if the horses are not kept near cattle. A fungal culture also should be performed as an initial diagnostic test. A definitive diagnosis of cutaneous onchocerciasis may be obtained by demonstrating microfilariae in skin biopsies, accompanied by eosinophilic superficial and deep perivascular or diffuse dermatitis. The tissue sample may be minced and placed in saline for 30 minutes, after which time the saline is examined microscopically for microfilariae that have migrated out of the tissue. This technique, however, merely confirms the presence of microfilariae in the tissue, not that they have caused the dermatitis.

Treatment

Ivermectin (200 μg/kg p.o.) is the therapy of choice for cutaneous onchocerciasis. In fact, the routine use of ivermectin in deworming programs has made cutaneous onchocerciasis an infrequently seen clinical entity in many areas. Other drugs that are effective are levamisole (11 mg/kg p.o. s.i.d. for 7 days), fenbendazole (60 mg/kg p.o. s.i.d. for 5 days), and mebendazole (50 mg/kg p.o. s.i.d. for 5 days). All horses should be concurrently treated with prednisone or prednisolone (1 mg/kg p.o. s.i.d.) during parasiticidal therapy, to prevent severe reactions to the sudden kill-off of the microfilariae.

PEDICULOSIS

Pediculosis (lice infestation) is relatively common. It is seen more often in the winter months, because lice cannot reproduce or even survive high body surface temperatures. Lice are highly host-specific and, in most instances, cannot survive longer than 1 or 2 weeks off the host. Equine lice may be biting (*Damalinia equi*) or sucking (*Hematopinus asini*), feeding on cutaneous debris or blood and other tissue fluids, respectively.

Clinical Signs

Pediculosis is often first seen as pruritus of the neck and mane, with secondary alopecia, scaling, and excoriations. If left untreated, lesions may spread to involve the trunk.

Diagnosis

Differential diagnoses include insect hypersensitivities, psoroptic or sarcoptic mange, fly-bite dermatitis, dermatophytosis, trombiculidiasis, and forage mite infestation. Prolonged insecticidal therapy eliminates insect hypersensitivities and fly-bite dermatitis as well as trombiculidiasis. Chiggers may also be demonstrated in skin scrapings, as will psoroptic mange mites, forage mites, and lice or lice nits. Lice and nits may be seen upon close inspection of the skin and hairs, either with the naked eye or using a magnifying glass. Nits are firmly attached to individual hairs.

Treatment

Therapy with insecticidal sprays 2 weeks apart is usually effective. Care should be taken to thoroughly treat the ears, because this is the most likely site for lice to survive hot weather. Insecticides to be used include pyrethrins, chlorpyrifos, malathion, diazinon, lindane, and coumaphos. Some horses may be sensitive to these chemicals, developing urticaria. In these individuals, two doses of ivermectin (200 μg/kg p.o.) may be given 2 weeks apart. This is most effective against sucking lice, although biting lice also may be sensitive to ivermectin. All tack and grooming implements should be treated likewise with insecticides, because they may act as fomites.

SARCOPTIC MANGE

This highly contagious rare condition is caused by *Sarcoptes scabei* var. *equi*. Lesions are due to the burrowing of mites in the epidermis. Hypersensitivity may play a role in the pathogenesis, because the intensity of pruritus is out of proportion to the numbers of mites and to the degree of skin disease. This is a herd disease and there is no age, breed, or sex predilection.

The intensely pruritic lesions include papules, vesicles, crusts, excoriations, alopecia, and lichenification. These begin on the head and ears, and progress down the neck. Differential diagnoses include psoroptic mange, pediculosis, atopy, and fly-bite dermatitis. Skin scrapings often fail to yield mites or mite eggs; therefore, response to appropriate therapy is considered diagnostic. Skin scrapings are usually positive in cases of psoroptic mange or pediculosis, however. Topical therapies include malathion, diazinon, lindane, coumaphos, and lime sulfur. These must be applied once weekly for 5 to 6 weeks. Ivermectin (200 $\mu g/kg$ p.o. every 2 weeks for three treatments) is effective. All in-contact horses must be treated concurrently. Because sarcoptid mites may survive for several weeks off the host, the housing environment, tack, and grooming implements also should be treated with an appropriate insecticide.

PSOROPTIC MANGE

Psoroptic mange is a highly contagious herd problem that is a common cause of pruritus in the horse. There is no age, breed, or gender predilection. *P. cuniculi* is a cause of otitis externa, the signs of which vary from subclinical to severe pruritus, with head shaking and a lop-eared appearance. *P. equi* usually causes body mange and gives rise to intense pruritus, papules, crusts, scaling, alopecia, excoriations, and lichenification of the ears, mane, and tailhead.

Differential diagnoses include sarcoptic mange, pediculosis, insect hypersensitivities, atopy, and fly-bite dermatitis. Skin scrapings are usually positive for mites, as are examinations of cerumen in cases of otitis externa. Treatment is as described for sarcoptic mange.

OXYURIASIS

This condition is considered to be a disease of poor management, because horses become infected with *Oxyuris equi* by ingesting fecally contaminated material. Oxyuriasis is usually a herd problem, seen most often in stabled horses. Adult worms inhabit the colon and cecum. Gravid females crawl out of the anus and deposit clusters of eggs in a gelatinous "cement" on the perineal skin. It is this gelatinous material that is believed to cause pruritus. The condition exhibits no age, breed, or sex predilection. The hallmark of oxyuriasis is pruritus ani, with a resultant loss of hair at the base of the tail leading to a rat-tail appearance, with or without excoriations. Differential diagnoses include food hypersensitivity, insect hypersensitivities, and pediculosis. Confirmation of the diagnosis is simply made, by pressing the adhesive side of clear tape to the perineal skin, then to a glass slide. Microscopic examination of the slide reveals the operculated eggs characteristic of this parasite.

Therapy with anthelmintics is effective, including ivermectin, thiabendazole, fenbendazole, mebendazole, cambendazole, and pyrantel pamoate. Proper sanitation and prompt disposal of fouled bedding is essential to prevent recurrence.

Supplemental Readings

Greiner EC: Entomologic evaluation of insect hypersensitivity in horses. Vet Clin North Am Large Anim Pract 11:29–41, 1995.
Perris EE: Parasitic dermatoses that cause pruritus in horses. Vet Clin North Am Large Anim Pract 11:11–28, 1995.
Scott DW: Parasitic diseases. *In* Large Animal Dermatology. Philadelphia, WB Saunders, 1988, pp 207–283.
Scott DW: Immunologic diseases. *In* Large Animal Dermatology. Philadelphia, WB Saunders, 1988, pp 284–333.

Dermatologic Conditions Associated With Crusts and Scales

JOHN W. SCHLIPF, JR.
Simpsonville, Kentucky

A crust is a solid accumulation of dried exudate on the surface of skin and is composed of a mixture of serum, cellular debris, and keratin in varying proportions. Dirt and topical medications often become incorporated in the crusts. Examination of crusts can provide diagnostic information about a disease process such as atypical cell morphology or evidence of infectious microorganisms. Scales result from increased exfoliation of the stratum corneum caused by altered epidermal maturation, accelerated keratinization, trauma to the surface of the epithelium, or altered epithelial cohesion.

Skin disorders associated with crusting and scaling are common in the horse and are caused by many different diseases, some of which are listed in Table 1. Crusts and scales may be the primary lesion of the disease (e.g., primary idiopathic seborrhea), or may be a progressional phase secondary to papules, pustules, vesicles, or other primary lesions. Crusting and scaling may be focal (e.g.,

TABLE 1. SKIN DISORDERS ASSOCIATED WITH CRUSTS AND/OR SCALES IN THE HORSE

Dermatophilosis	Toxicoses (selenium, arsenic, iodine)
Bacterial folliculitis	Anhidrosis
Dermatophytosis	Disorders of keratinization
Ectoparasites (lice, mange)	Equine sarcoidosis
Biting flies	Pemphigus foliaceus
Cutaneous onchocerciasis	Vasculitis
Aural plaques	Contact irritant dermatitis
Malnutrition	Insect hypersensitivity
Environmental (heat, cold)	Dietary hypersensitivity
Photosensitization	Drug eruption

linear keratitis) or diffuse (e.g., equine sarcoidosis) and may have infectious (e.g., dermatophytosis) or noninfectious (e.g., pemphigus foliaceus) etiologies. Pruritus may be displayed with crusting and scaling lesions (e.g., insect hypersensitivity); however, many other diseases associated with crusting and scaling do not have pruritus (e.g., dermatophilosis). This chapter is limited to the discussion of six nonpruritic skin conditions associated with crusts and scales: dermatophilosis; bacterial folliculitis; pemphigus foliaceus; equine sarcoidosis; dermatophytosis; and disorders of keratinization.

DERMATOPHILOSIS

Equine dermatophilosis is a common superficial bacterial infection that results in a crusting dermatitis. Dermatophilosis, also referred to as rain scald, rain rot, dew poisoning, and cutaneous streptothricosis, has a worldwide distribution. The causative organism, *Dermatophilus congolensis*, is a gram-positive, non-acid-fast, branching, filamentous aerobic or facultative anaerobic actinomycete. Where it exists in nature is unknown. Attempts at creating the disease using soil samples collected from farms with a high incidence of the disease have been unsuccessful. The actual incidence of the disease depends on geographic location and seasonal weather variations. However, following periods of heavy prolonged rain, incidence often increases.

Several factors are necessary for an infection to develop. Damaged epithelium must exist. This break in skin integrity allows entry of the organism. Exposure to the organism can occur by direct contact or through fomites or insects, including biting and nonbiting flies and ticks. Macerated skin from persistent moisture allows the organism to invade and begin multiplying in viable, noncornified layers of epidermis. Zoospores are formed and germinate, forming a mycelium that proliferates in the living layers of epidermis and hair follicles. The dermis is able to resist infection.

During healing, as the epidermis re-epithelializes, the crusts are lost and the bacteria are usually eliminated. However, the infection may persist as new layers of epidermis are invaded by bacteria from nearby hair follicles. A palisading crust, which is composed of layers of cornified epithelium and suppurative exudate, may develop as a result of reinfection and newly epithelialized tissue. Organisms are quite resistant to drying when present in the scabs, and this ability to survive in crusts despite desiccation probably leads to repeated outbreaks in herd mates.

Clinical Signs

Clinical lesions of papules and pustules are seen in the acute stages. These eventually lead to suppurative crusts and matted hair. When crusts are removed, the underside is moist and exudative. The matted hair has been described as having a "paint brush" appearance. This lesion is not pathognomonic for dermatophilosis, but is strongly suggestive. Areas that are susceptible to moisture damage and trauma are predisposed to developing lesions. Nonpigmented skin may be more susceptible to infection. Lesions of the dorsal midline are very common; however, the limbs and distal muzzle are also affected. Limb involvement may appear similar to that in pastern dermatitis (greasy heel). Dermatophilosis is commonly referred to as *rain scald* because the lesions start over the dorsum and extend ventrally following the course of rain-soaked hair. Often running a hand over the skin may reveal crusts better than visual examination. Chronic infection may lead to alopecia and hyperpigmentation. Crusts associated with chronic infection do not have the moist appearance and discharge of acute lesions. Scale may be present on the surrounding skin.

Diagnosis

Several skin diseases appear clinically similar to dermatophilosis, depending on severity and acuteness of the lesions. Differential diagnoses should include dermatophytosis, bacterial folliculitis, pemphigus foliaceus, and drug eruptions.

Diagnosis is based on clinical signs, a thorough clinical history, physical examination, cytology testing of smears made directly from crusts and emulsified crusts, bacterial and fungal cultures, and histopathology testing. Acute lesions are suppurative, and direct smears from crusts may be examined after staining with methylene blue, Gram's stain, or Giemsa stain. If organisms are not identified on direct smears, an emulsified preparation may be rewarding. The characteristic organisms appear as gram-positive, branching, filamentous bacteria forming parallel rows of cocci, which are described as having a "railroad track" appearance.

Bacterial culture may be unrewarding when incubated under aerobic conditions. Overgrowth with contaminants may prevent accurate diagnosis. Incubating the culture plates in a microaerophilic environment may improve culture results. Acute lesions are better for isolating organisms. Histologic examination of crusts more commonly results in a positive diagnosis of the bacteria's presence than skin alone. Therefore, the skin should not be shaved or scrubbed before biopsy. Biopsies should include crusts and hair follicles, and several samples need to be taken. Characteristic changes are seen on a skin biopsy that help confirm the diagnosis, such as palisading crust and intracellular edema of keratinocytes.

Treatment

Most cases of dermatophilosis are self-limiting and resolve independent of treatment. The most important part of any treatment is eliminating the predisposing factors such as moisture, trauma, and exposure to infected animals. Removing surface scabs and debris can be accomplished using an antiseborrheic shampoo containing tar and sulfur or an antimicrobial shampoo containing povidone-iodine or chlorhexidine. Lesions are often painful, and sedation may be necessary for removing crusts. Daily topical treatment should be continued for 7 to 10 days and then twice a week until lesions resolve. Antibiotics are reserved for use in severe cases and nonresponsive cases. Procaine penicillin (22,000–44,000 IU/kg) is the drug of choice, which is given every 12 hours intramuscularly (IM) for 5 days. The prognosis is good for most cases of dermatophilosis.

BACTERIAL FOLLICULITIS

Inflammation of hair follicles, known as folliculitis, is a common skin disease of horses. This condition is also known as sweating eczema, acne, summer rash, summer scab, saddle scab, heat rash, and heat pox. A seasonal variation exists, with a majority of cases reported in the spring and summer. Sweating and trauma predispose certain regions of the horse to infection, such as under the saddle and tack, and on the distal limbs and cervical region. Shedding and accumulation of hair may predispose the horse to the disease. Horses that are bathed after exercise are less at risk of developing folliculitis. Common bacterial isolates include *Staphylococcus aureus* and *S. intermedius*, *Corynebacterium pseudotuberculosis*, *C. equi*, *Streptococcus zooepidemicus* and *S. equi* may be cultured from some cases. Moisture and trauma allow bacteria to become established in hair follicles.

Clinical Signs

Clinical signs begin as papules associated with hair follicles. These progress to crusts and areas of alopecia. The hair in areas involved is easily epilated. Pruritus is not frequently reported; however, the horse may have pain. Often there is a considerable regional edema associated with the distal limbs when they are involved.

Diagnosis

Differential diagnoses include dermatophytosis, contact allergies, dermatophilosis, and pemphigus foliaceus. Diagnosis is based on the season, history, management, thorough physical examination, cytology testing of impression smears from exudate and epilated hairs, skin biopsies for bacterial and fungal cultures, and histologic examination.

Treatment

Treatment includes eliminating underlying precipitating factors such as poor-fitting tack and inadequate hygiene. Medicated baths with an iodine-based shampoo or chlorhexidine are usually effective in eliminating the bacteria. Systemic antibiotics may be necessary in nonresponsive or severe cases. The potentiated sulfonamides such as trimethoprim/sulfadiazine (30 mg/kg p.o. b.i.d.) are the first choice. Penicillin may be effective in some cases, but many *Staphylococcus* species are resistant to penicillin. If antibiotics are required, selection should be based on culture and sensitivity results. Many cases may be self-limiting and resolve within a few weeks without treatment. The prognosis is good for most cases of bacterial folliculitis.

PEMPHIGUS FOLIACEUS

Autoimmune skin disease in the horse is a rare problem, with pemphigus foliaceus being the most commonly reported form. Autoantibodies that are directed against cell membrane-associated epidermal antigen result in the production of blisters as the intercellular basement membrane is disrupted. No age or sex predilection has been identified; however, Appaloosas appear to be predisposed; there is an overrepresentation of reported cases.

Clinical Signs

Clinical signs include generalized exfoliative dermatitis. Erythematous scaling and pustular dermatitis commonly begin on the face and/or limbs and may become a generalized condition within days to weeks. The primary lesions are vesicles and pustules. However, depending on duration since the onset of signs, there may be a variety of secondary lesions present including crusts, scales, erosions, epidermal collarettes (remnants of blisters or pustules), serum exudation, and marked alopecia. Usually only mild pruritus is reported, but the horse is often in severe pain and demonstrates this discomfort when touched, making clinical evaluation and tissue sampling difficult. Other clinical signs and findings identified during a thorough history and physical examination include lethargy, weight loss, anorexia, pyrexia, an obtunded attitude, ventral and/or limb edema, coronary band erosions, low-grade fever, and in some cases, a positive Nikolsky sign.

Diagnosis

A differential diagnosis list for generalized eruptive dermatitis should include dermatophilosis, dermatophytosis, staphylococcal folliculitis, sarcoidosis, exfoliative eosinophilic dermatitis and stomatitis, drug eruption, external parasite hypersensitivity, and chemical dermatosis. A diagnosis of pemphigus foliaceus is based on results of history, clinical signs, physical examination, laboratory findings, skin biopsies, cultures, and direct immunofluorescence. Histologic evidence for the classic lesion of acantholysis is present and diagnostic in approximately 80% of cases. Direct immunofluorescence is an adjunctive diagnostic tool detecting autoantibodies in the intercellular space in 65 to 70% of cases. Lesion selection is very important when performing direct immunofluorescence. Intact pustules or vesicles are necessary for an accurate diagnosis. The tissue sample is usually preserved in Michel's fixative, but the laboratory performing the test should be contacted for their preference. Fluid aspirated from intact blisters may be examined cytologically for acantholytic epidermal cells. Hematologic and serum biochemistry results are usually normal. Abnormalities that sometimes exist are inconsistent and reflect severity, duration, and secondary complications associated with the disease.

Treatment

Immune-modifying chemotherapeutics are the treatment of choice for pemphigus foliaceus. Treatment can be difficult; however, uncomplicated cases usually respond well to treatment. Young horses less than 1 year old usually respond better to treatment and are more likely to remain in drug-free remission than the adult horse. Immunosuppressive doses of glucocorticoids such as oral prednisone or prednisolone (2.2–4.4 mg/kg daily) are the first choice for treatment. Treatment is continued at this dose until remission is noted, or if there is no clinical response in 10 days, treatment is altered. If the horse responds to treatment and clinical signs abate, the dose of prednisone or prednisolone is gradually reduced by 20% every 2 weeks. This reducing protocol should be continued until a maintenance dose is achieved. The maintenance level is usually a dose 20% higher than the dose at which clinical signs begin to return. Once this dose is achieved, alternate-day therapy should be attempted. If remission of signs persists, attempts should be made to discontinue therapy after 4 to 6 months; however, treatment may be life-long.

If there is little or no response at the lower dose of prednisone or prednisolone, the higher dose should be used. If the response is still unsatisfactory, alternate treatments such as dexamethasone or aurothioglucose (injectable gold salts) may be used. Dexamethasone should be administered orally at a dosage of 0.1 to 0.2 mg/kg daily. Improvement should be noted within 10 days, and if there is improvement, the dose should be decreased as described for prednisone or prednisolone. When using any of the glucocorticoids, the risk of laminitis should always be considered and discussed with the owners.

Aurothioglucose is an alternate therapy that may be attempted if glucocorticoid therapy is unsuccessful. It is administered once weekly until a clinical response is observed. This usually requires 6 to 8 weeks of treatment. Treatment is started at 20 mg intramuscularly (IM), then increased to 40 mg the following week. Treatment is continued at a weekly maintenance dose (1 mg/kg), and once remission occurs, therapy is continued at 1 mg/kg bimonthly, then monthly. If the horse remains in remission after 4 to 6 months of therapy, discontinuing therapy should be considered. Toxicity has not been observed in horses, but a complete hemogram should be performed monthly. The prognosis is fair for drug-free remission.

SARCOIDOSIS

Equine sarcoidosis, also referred to as *generalized granulomatous disease* or *equine histiocytic disease*, possesses many similarities to the human form of the disease. This is a rare disease with unknown etiology. In humans, sarcoidosis is thought to be associated with an atypical response to an undetermined immunologic stimulation. Multiple organ systems may be involved, including gastrointestinal, hepatic, renal, pulmonary, and pancreatic systems. Skin and gastrointestinal tract are generally more commonly affected sites.

Other clinical variations of generalized inflammatory diseases in horses have been recognized and described, including multisystemic eosinophilic epitheliotropic disease, exfoliative eosinophilic dermatitis and stomatitis, eosinophilic gastroenterocolitis and dermatitis, and lymphocytic-plasmacytic enterocolitis. These idiopathic immune disorders often have lesions involving the skin in addition to multiple organ involvement. These disorders differ from equine sarcoidosis mainly by the type of cell infiltrate.

Clinical Signs

With equine sarcoidosis the clinical presentation observed reflects the systems involved. Weight loss, intractable diarrhea, and dermatitis may be present, depending on duration of the disease. An age, sex, or breed predisposition does not appear to exist. Most often, dermatitis is the owner's chief complaint. Clinical signs include scaling, crusting, serum exudation, and alopecia of the head or limbs. Eventually the disease progresses to a generalized exfoliative dermatitis. Cutaneous nodules may be apparent but they are quite rare, and peripheral lymph nodes may be enlarged. With progression of the disease, signs of weight loss, exercise intolerance, diminished appetite, ventral edema, diarrhea, and low-grade fever indicate multiple organ involvement. Laboratory findings may include leukocytosis and hyperfibrinogenemia.

Diagnosis

Diagnosis is based on history, physical examination, clinical signs, ruling out other diseases, bacterial and fungal cultures, and the presence of characteristic histologic changes in skin biopsies. Histopathology observations consist of a superficial dermal infiltrate of epithelial cells and multinucleated histiocytic giant cells and smaller number of neutrophils, lymphocytes, and plasma cells. Similar histologic changes may be seen in other involved tissues. A peripheral circulating eosinophilia is rarely seen, and direct immunofluorescence test results are negative. Differential diagnoses should include other generalized immune-mediated inflammatory diseases, dermatophilosis, dermatophytosis, pemphigus foliaceus, contact dermatitis, drug eruptions, and toxicoses, including those to arsenic or iodine.

Treatment

Treatment results are usually unfavorable. The prognosis is poor, especially if there are signs of weight loss and wasting. Glucocorticoids at immunosuppressive doses daily may be effective (2.2–4.4 mg/kg prednisone or prednisolone or 0.1–0.2 mg/kg dexamethasone). If malabsorption is present, corticosteroid administration should be parenteral. If the horse responds, treatment is required for several weeks to months, and the dosage should be reduced to an every-other-day schedule similar to the protocol described for pemphigus foliaceus. Recrudescence may occur when treatment is discontinued. Spontaneous remission has been reported; however, most horses do not respond well and their clinical signs worsen over several months, eventually requiring euthanasia for humane reasons.

DERMATOPHYTOSIS

Superficial mycotic infections are regularly encountered in equine practice. Dermatophytosis, commonly known as ringworm or girth itch, is a contagious, superficial fungal infection of the skin. *Trichophyton equinum*, *T. verrucosum*, and *T. mentagrophytes* account for most clinical cases of dermatophytosis. *Microsporum canis*, *M. equinum*, and *M. gypseum* are responsible for a small percentage of cases. Numerous other fungi are occasionally associated with a case of ringworm. Ringworm is zoonotic and thus care must be taken to prevent exposure to humans, especially when young children are involved.

Dermatophytosis affects the superficial skin because the organism only survives in nonviable skin. It does not possess the ability to penetrate and invade deeper tissues. These fungi invade actively growing hairs, which leads to the classic expanding lesion because the spread of the organism extends peripherally into growing hairs. Lesions may be very pruritic, and the incubation period varies according to environmental influences of temperature and humidity. Most often it ranges from 1 to 4 weeks.

Many more animals are exposed to ringworm than actually develop clinical disease. Exposure occurs through natural infection or commonly via fomites such as shared tack and grooming equipment. The immune system usually eliminates the organism, preventing infection. Several factors may lead to developing infection. Young animals with an immature naive immune system, an animal with poor nutritional status or secondary debilitating disease, and immunocompromised animals are susceptible. Older animals develop a natural resistance, which reduces the likelihood of infection or decreases severity of infection.

Clinical Signs

Clinical appearance can be quite varied. Usual clinical signs include circular areas of asymmetrical alopecia of varying size, heavy crusts and scales in the hairless areas, and sometimes short broken hair shafts throughout the lesion. Hair growth starts in the center of the lesion and may be present in some of the lesions. Hairless areas may be quite small and irregularly shaped. Papules and pustules may be seen at the periphery of the expanding lesion and are the initial lesions seen. However, pustules quickly progress to crusts and scales, and thus they may not be identified. The typical hairless lesions are commonly found on the head, neck, and thorax, but they may become generalized. As the lesions become more generalized, the epidermis may become hyperplastic. Urticarial plaques sometimes are seen due to hypersensitivity to fungal toxins and allergens. Differential diagnosis should include dermatophilosis, bacterial folliculitis, allergic dermatitis, grease heel, parasitic infection such as *Demodex equi*, selenium toxicosis, plaque form of sarcoids, and patchy shedding.

Diagnosis

Diagnosis is based on results of clinical examination, fungal cultures, microscopic examination of hair follicles, and histologic examination of skin biopsies. Microscopic examination of hair follicles for ectothrix spores produced by dermatophytes aids in diagnosis. However, it may be difficult for the inexperienced examiner to identify hyphae and spores. Often conidia and hyphae are identified in the skin biopsy. Culturing for dermatophytes is performed on dermatophyte test medium (DTM), with a few drops of vitamin B complex added to supply the niacin requirement of *T. equinum*. Hair and scales from the periphery of the lesion should be collected for culture. Phenol red is used as an indicator of pH change. Pathogenic fungi produce an alkaline environment resulting from protein metabolism, and this causes a red color change in the media. However, after 14 days' incubation, nonpathogenic fungi (sapro-

phytes) may produce a similar change in the media. Because of this, color change is not entirely diagnostic of a pathogenic dermatophyte. Dermatophyte test medium is approximately 90% reliable for providing evidence of an infection and identifying the species of fungus present based on microscopic examination. Because *M. canis* rarely causes ringworm in the horse, using a Wood's lamp for diagnosis is of little value.

Treatment

Most cases of ringworm are self-limiting unless there is an immune deficiency or reinfection is occurring. Treatment is intended to decrease the convalescent period, lessen the severity of the disease, and reduce exposure to other animals. Many effective treatment methods are available. Captan° is a rose fungicide that works well; however, it is difficult to obtain and is considered a carcinogen so it is not recommended. Dilute bleach solution (sodium hypochlorite 0.5%) and a 1% chlorhexidine solution are quite safe and efficacious. Thiabendazole as a 5% solution in 90% dimethyl sulfoxide (DMSO) can also be used. Using a plant spray bottle is an effective method of applying medicated solutions to the lesions and surrounding hair. The hair must be thoroughly saturated for the treatment to be effective. Treatment should be done daily for 7 to 10 days, then continued twice-weekly until the lesions resolve and there are no new lesions developing. Oral griseofulvin has not proven efficacious.

Fungi are quite resistant and may persist on tack, blankets, grooming equipment, bedding, and in the environment for more than 1 year. Treatment must include eliminating exposure by cleaning tack and grooming equipment and disinfecting the stall, feed bunk, and bedding. Disinfectants that are effective include 5 to 10% bleach solution, 5% lime sulfur, and 3 to 5% povidone-iodine solution. Removing crusts; maintaining good nutritional status, good hygiene, and exposure to sunlight are important aspects of any treatment protocol. The prognosis is good for complete resolution.

DISORDERS OF KERATINIZATION

Seborrhea has been used to describe crusting and scaling skin associated with keratinization disorders. This is a misnomer because seborrhea by definition means "flow of sebum." Disorders of keratinization may or may not be a problem with production of sebum. With keratinization disorders, there is decreased cell turnover time or increased cohesiveness of cells, leading to accumulation of scaly material on the skin. Disorders of keratinization encompass a wide range of clinical problems from simple dry skin (dandruff) to marked inflamed crusting and scaling skin. Most keratinization disorders are the consequence of a primary skin disease. Examples of primary diseases that lead to keratinization disorders include dermatophytosis, allergic reaction, immune-mediated disorders, nutritional causes, neoplasia such as sarcoids, and external parasites. Primary problems with keratinization are rare and include

---

°Orthocide, Ortho Products, San Francisco, CA

such conditions in horses as primary idiopathic seborrhea (a diagnosis made by exclusion) and mane and tail seborrhea.

Clinical Signs

Typical clinical signs of keratinization disorders depend on the underlying cause and duration of the problem. Scaling, crusting, alopecia, and greasy-feeling hair are usual signs. Pruritus, self-inflicted trauma, inflammation, and secondary bacterial infection may be present. The accumulation of scale, crusts, and bacteria may produce a noticeable foul odor.

Treatment

Treatment should be directed at an underlying cause if it can be identified. Symptomatic treatment includes frequent bathing with an antiseborrheic shampoo such as one containing tar and sulfur. Dry skin responds to emollient shampoos and rinses. Oily skin often improves with benzoyl peroxide.

Specific examples of idiopathic keratinization disorders in the horse include linear keratosis and cannon keratosis. Linear keratosis is recognized in Quarterhorses but has also been described in a Morgan, Standardbred, and Percheron. It is usually seen in young animals less than 5 years old. The disease may be hereditary or developmental (similar to epidermal nevus in humans). The thorax and cervical and pectoral regions are most commonly involved. The signs seen are linear areas of hair loss and accompanying hyperkeratosis. Diagnosis is based on clinical signs and skin biopsy. There is no cure and treatment, if necessary, is only palliative and similar to that for other keratinization disorders. Linear keratosis should be differentiated from linear alopecia, a condition characterized by mural folliculitis, which is therefore less likely to respond to antiseborrheic shampoo.

Cannon keratosis is observed on the hindlimbs over the dorsum of the cannon bone. Scaling, crusting, and alopecia are clinical signs seen. This condition may represent a defect in keratin formation. Antiseborrheic shampoo and topical corticosteroids may be helpful.

Supplemental Readings

Evans AG: Dermatophilosis: Diagnostic approach to nonpruritic, crusting dermatitis in horses. Comp Cont Ed Pract Vet 14:1618–1623, 1992.

Manning T, Sweeney C: Immune-mediated equine skin diseases. Comp Cont Ed Pract Vet 8:979–987, 1986.

Mullowney PC, Fadok VA: Dermatologic diseases of horses: Part II. Bacterial and viral skin diseases. Comp Cont Ed Pract Vet 6:S16–S22, 1984.

Mullowney PC, Fadok VA: Dermatologic diseases of horses: Part III. Fungal skin diseases. Comp Cont Ed Pract Vet 6:S324–S331, 1984.

Scott DW: Unusual immune-mediated skin diseases in the horse. Equine Pract 13(2):10–17, 1991.

Dermatologic Conditions Associated With Oral Lesions

DONNA WALTON ANGARANO
Auburn, Alabama

Oral lesions are an uncommon clinical finding in the horse, the most common being ulceration. The tongue, palate, and buccal mucosa may be affected. Oral ulceration may occur as the single clinical abnormality or in conjunction with other findings. The major causes of oral ulceration include trauma or irritation, toxins, infectious diseases (viral, bacterial, or mycotic), immune-mediated diseases, neoplasia, and ulceration as a consequence of metabolic diseases. Symptomatic therapy of oral ulceration is sometimes helpful when the etiology is unknown. However, in nonresponsive cases, a thorough diagnostic work-up is indicated to determine the specific etiology, prognosis, and therapy.

DIAGNOSIS

Horses with oral disease are often presented with a history of anorexia, painful mastication, ptyalism, and foul mouth odor. A complete history and physical examination are indicated. If there is evidence of systemic disease, a more thorough diagnostic work-up may be indicated based on the clinical signs present.

The mouth and tongue should be examined thoroughly to determine the type, location, and severity of lesions. Chemical sedation may be needed and use of a mouth wedge or speculum may be helpful (see page 139). Depending on the extent of the lesions, the diagnostic work-up may include impression smears, a mucosal biopsy for histopathology and direct immunofluorescence or immunoperoxidase staining, a hemogram, serum biochemical profile, an antinuclear antibody test (ANA), and viral isolation.

TRAUMA AND IRRITATION

The majority of oral lesions in the horse are the result of irritating or traumatic insults. The grinding action of mastication often results in traumatic lesions of the tongue and cheek mucosa. The upper cheek teeth develop sharp edges on the lateral surface, whereas the lower cheek teeth develop sharp edges on the medial or lingual surface (see page 151).

Foreign objects contacted while eating may result in lip or tongue lacerations. These lesions are easily distinguished from other disease processes. Other foreign bodies, in particular grass awns or wooden splinters, may penetrate the oral mucosa and result in fistulous tracts. Anesthesia, contrast radiology, and surgery may be necessary to locate and remove the foreign body.

Chemical irritation of the oral cavity may occur as a result of the horse licking topical agents that have been applied as blisters, from the long-term administration of medications such as trichlorfon paste, or from the ingestion of alkaloid plant toxins. The mucosa tends to heal readily after the source of irritation is removed. Symptomatic therapy using dilute potassium permanganate or povidone-iodine flushes may be helpful.

TOXICITIES

Phenylbutazone and other nonsteroidal anti-inflammatory drugs have been found to cause toxicity in some animals. Signs in susceptible horses generally occur following oral administration and may manifest as ulceration of the gastrointestinal tract. Oral and gastrointestinal ulceration is progressive and can result in death. If suspected, administration of the nonsteroidal anti-inflammatory agents should be stopped immediately. Symptomatic therapy is usually effective.

Cantharidin is a toxin that is found in the tissue of blister beetles (*Epicauta* species). Blister beetles are sometimes clustered in alfalfa and, after the hay is harvested, the beetles are ingested. Cantharidin is a potent irritant, causing vesicle formation, epidermal acantholysis, and ulceration of the skin and oral mucosa. Once absorbed, cantharidin causes systemic toxicity producing severe abdominal pain, hypocalcemia, renal failure, and cardiac abnormalities. The prognosis in affected horses is poor.

Oral lesions associated with mercury poisoning may occur when horses ingest grain treated with mercury-containing preservatives and fungicides or when horses lick mercury-containing blisters. Both organic and inorganic mercury are converted to methylmercury, which causes renal tubular degeneration and necrosis. The prognosis varies with the duration and volume of mercury ingestion.

FUNGAL, BACTERIAL, AND VIRAL STOMATITIS

Stomatitis associated with bacteria or fungal agents is infrequent. In most cases, this probably occurs as a secondary problem in an immunocompromised host. Mycotic stomatitis due to *Candida* species has a typical clinical appearance. It produces a foul-smelling, white coating of the mucosal surface. Antimycotic agents may be helpful, but efforts should be directed toward identifying an underlying cause of immunosuppression.

Oral lesions resulting from viral disease are also uncommon in the horse. Vesicles are the primary lesion and may be seen in the mouth as well as other cutaneous locations. Diagnosis is confirmed by serology and virus isolation. Horsepox has not been seen in the United States, but has been reported as a benign disease in Europe. Equine herpes coital exanthema is a contagious venereal disease. Vesicular and pustular lesions are most prominent in the genital areas but also have been reported to occur in the mouth or on the lips or nostrils.

Vesicular stomatitis is caused by a rhabdovirus. Lesions may occur on the distal extremities, genital areas, muzzle, tongue, and mouth. Vesicles quickly rupture, leaving a painful ulcer. Treatment is usually not necessary, because the disease course is only 1 to 2 weeks. The mechanism of transmission of vesicular stomatitis is not well understood but is thought to be by biting insects or contact with fluid from vesicles. Morbidity is 5 to 10% in affected herds. The virus may affect horses, swine, cattle, goats, sheep, llamas, wild animals, and humans. Of major significance is its clinical similarity to foot-and-mouth disease. Vesicular stomatitis has only been seen in North and South America. Before the outbreak in New Mexico in 1995, it had not been seen in the United States for 10 years. Vesicular stomatitis is a reportable disease.

IMMUNE-MEDIATED DISEASE

Immune-mediated diseases are unusual but should be considered in the horse when oral vesicles or ulcers are present. Pemphigus vulgaris is a rare autoimmune disease. Antibody deposition within the epidermis ultimately results in acantholysis, vesicle formation, and ulceration. Both the oral mucosa and skin may be affected. Impression smears from ulcerated areas may reveal neutrophils and acantholytic cells. Suprabasilar separation may be evident on histologic examination of intact vesicles. Immunosuppressive agents are the primary mode of therapy. Treatment regimens for horses with pemphigus include immunosuppressive doses of prednisolone or prednisone (2 mg/kg per day p.o.). The dose is often divided into a twice-daily dose. A high dosage is continued for 7 to 14 days until the horse's lesions are controlled. The dose is then reduced and changed to an alternate-day schedule as soon as possible. Each horse responds differently, and the dose should be based on the individual patient and not a preconceived schedule. In some cases, oral fatty acid supplementation has allowed a lower dose of glucocorticoids to be used. Aurothioglucose is not initially recommended, but may be used in horses that show adverse reactions to immunosuppressive glucocorticoids. Aurothioglucose (1 mg/kg IM) is administered once weekly for 6 to 10 weeks, until signs are controlled. Maintenance dosages are given once monthly. Treatment of pemphigus is considered to be life-long. The horse must be closely monitored and medications altered based on response. The prognosis is poor.

Bullous pemphigoid is similar to pemphigus vulgaris, with autoantibody deposition resulting in dermal-epidermal separation. Acantholysis is not a feature of bullous pemphigoid. Immunosuppressive therapy, as described earlier, is required. The prognosis is poor.

Systemic lupus erythematosus is a rare multisystemic disease of the horse. A variety of autoantibodies may be produced against several target organs. In addition to oral ulceration, affected horses may have polyarthritis, thrombocytopenia, hemolytic anemia, lymphedema, and proteinuria. Cutaneous lesions include depigmentation, erythema, crusts, and ulceration. Diagnosis is based on the multisystemic findings, a positive antinuclear antibody test (ANA), histopathology of biopsies from skin and oral mucosa, and direct immunofluorescence testing or immunoperoxidase staining. Immunosuppressive agents are the primary mode of therapy. The prognosis is guarded.

A case of equine paraneoplastic bullous stomatitis has been reported. The affected horse developed oral ulceration concurrent with the growth of a cervical mass. Vesicles and ulcers were present on the tongue, buccal mucosa, and lips. Subepidermal clefts and vesicles were observed on histologic examination of oral biopsies. Direct immunofluorescence testing showed intraepidermal staining. The cervical mass was excised and determined to be a hemangiosarcoma. Although the oral lesions had previously failed to resolve with immunosuppressive therapy, they completely regressed following excision of the cervical mass. Using immunoprecipitation with metabolically labeled keratinocytes, serum from the horse was demonstrated to contain antibodies against desmoplakin I and II, the bullous pemphigoid 230 antigen, and a 190-kd antigen that is not characterized. These clinical and laboratory findings are consistent with reported cases of paraneoplastic pemphigus in humans.

Several drugs have been reported to cause drug eruptions in the horse. Although most clinical signs are cutaneous, oral lesions may be seen. Any drug is capable of causing a reaction, and there is no specific reaction associated with any compound. Obtaining a thorough history of current and past medication is important in establishing the diagnosis. The only way to confirm the diagnosis is to withdraw the drug and readminister it after resolution of the lesions. This is not recommended.

Erythema multiforme is an immune-mediated disease of the horse that is associated with drug reactions or a variety of other antigens. The syndrome has multiple cutaneous manifestations. Oral ulceration has not been reported in the horse, but has been seen in other species. Supportive diagnostic findings including individual keratinocyte necrosis (dyskeratotic cells) should be seen on histologic examination of skin or mucosal biopsies. Examination of biopsies from horses with the dermal form of erythema multiforme reveals severe edema of the superficial dermis (gossamer collagen effect).

Both oral and cutaneous lesions may occur in the horse as a result of vasculitis. Equine vasculitis has many etiologies (see page 293). Equine purpura hemorrhagica due to *Streptococcus equi* is the most common cause. Some cases are idiopathic. Edema, necrosis, crusts, and ulceration are most prominent on the distal extremities. Diagnosis is confirmed by examination of skin or mucosa biopsies. Treatment is directed toward removing the underlying cause. Antibiotics and glucocorticoids are often part of the treatment regimen.

Ulcerative stomatitis, dermatitis, and gastrointestinal signs have been seen in horses with graft-versus-host disease. The disease has been reported in foals with combined immunodeficiency syndrome that were treated using fetal hepatic or thymic cells transplants or peripheral blood lymphocytes from unrelated horses.

Equine exfoliative eosinophilic dermatitis and stomatitis is associated with an eosinophilic infiltrate of epithelial tissues. Oral ulceration may be an early sign of the disease. As the disease progresses, horses exhibit severe weight loss, along with oral lesions and generalized cutaneous exfoliation and ulceration. Eosinophilic granulomas are sometimes demonstrated in internal organs. The peripheral eosinophil count is usually normal. Diagnosis is based on histopathology examination outcome. The disease is progressive and the prognosis is poor. An effective therapy has not been found.

OTHER ETIOLOGIES

Several neoplastic diseases including squamous cell carcinoma, fibrosarcoma, malignant melanoma, hemangiosarcoma, and rhabdomyoma have been reported to occur in the equine oral cavity. Although the horse may be presented with clinical signs similar to the previously described diseases, oral examination usually reveals a focal, ulcerated mass. Biopsy is indicated to determine the specific diagnosis, prognosis, and treatment.

Oral ulceration may occur in several metabolic diseases including uremia resulting from renal failure, stress resulting from systemic disease, and photosensitization. The oral lesions are usually secondary and other clinical findings predominate. A thorough history and physical examination often reveal the underlying disease process.

Supplemental Readings

Hennig GE, Steckel RR: Diseases of the oral cavity and esophagus. In Kobluk CN, Ames TR, Geor RJ (eds.): The Horse: Diseases and Clinical Management. Philadelphia, WB Saunders, 1995, pp 287–314.
Herbert KS: Vesicular stomatitis update: Disease appears to be spreading. The Horse 12(8):6–9, 1995
Scott DW: Large Animal Dermatology. Philadelphia, WB Saunders, 1988.
Williams MA, Dowling PM, Angarano DW, Yu AA, DiFranco BJ, Lenz SD, Anhalt GJ: Paraneoplastic bullous stomatitis in a horse. J Am Vet Med Assoc 207:331–334, 1995.

Papillomatosis: Warts and Aural Plaques

M. AMY WILLIAMS
Auburn, Alabama

Equine papillomavirus is a host-specific papovavirus (DNA) that infects the basal cell layer of the epithelium. Papillomatosis refers to the development of benign, papillomavirus-induced proliferative skin tumors that occur in humans and many animal species. The proliferative response induced by equine papillomavirus, squamous papilloma, is self-limiting and usually harmless. Histopathologic evidence supports the existence of two different clinical syndromes of papillomatosis in horses—warts and aural plaques. These two clinical presentations have been suggested to be caused by different types of equine papillomaviruses.

WARTS

Equine warts are small, gray-brown to pink, cauliflower-like growths commonly found on the muzzle and lower face. Other frequent sites for lesions include the nose, commissure of the mouth, periocular tissue, pinna, and distal legs. Occasionally, the penis and vulva are involved. Warts are generally multiple in number, ranging from less than 10 to more than 100, with lesions 5 to 20 mm in size. The lesions commonly develop in young horses, those 6 months to 3 years of age. The incubation period is approximately 60 days. The warts reach maturity after a growth period of 4 to 8 weeks. Spontaneous regression usually occurs in 3 to 4 months following the development of immunity. Warts often become necrotic before regressing. Some cases may persist for as long as 18 months. Persistent warts lasting 2 years or longer, generalized warts, or warts spreading to atypical body locations may suggest an inappropriate immune response in young horses.

Warts are contagious, and transmission can occur directly by intradermal injection or indirectly via fomites. Natural transmission most likely requires traumatized skin, such as abrasions and punctures by plant thorns and barbed wire, and bites from insects. Contact of the damaged skin with viral-contaminated curry combs and brushes, surgical instruments, or feeding insects can lead to infection. The papillomavirus remains fully viable at room temperature for at least 3 weeks and is able to persist for variable periods in the environment. Yearly infection of young stock has been reported on large breeding farms. Lesions found on the penis or vulva can result in transmission of the equine papillomavirus through breeding; therefore, affected individuals should be isolated from the breeding herd. Congenital papillomatosis also occurs, possibly by spread of the virus across the placenta. Congenital lesions are usually found on the lips or other areas of skin and appear soft, rubbery, and darkly pigmented. Disinfection of the premises and equipment with lye, formaldehyde, or povidone-iodine helps decrease spread of the virus. Insecticide repellents may also help reduce transmission through insect vectors.

Diagnosis

Diagnosis is usually based on the clinical appearance, but large growths on the lower limb can resemble verrucous-type sarcoids. The latter is a fibromatous tumor demonstrated to contain bovine papillomavirus DNA by polymerase chain reaction. If the clinical diagnosis is in question, a biopsy specimen should be collected in formalin and submitted for a histologic diagnosis. Histopathologically, biopsy specimens show orthokeratotic hyperkeratosis, papillated epidermal hyperplasia with ballooning degeneration of keratinocytes, and basophilic inclusion bodies of different sizes.

Treatment and Prevention

For the most part, treatment of equine warts is not necessary because warts are harmless and usually regress spontaneously. Management practices should be considered to limit the number of animals infected. To help minimize skin trauma, pasture mowing and the use of insecticides are recommended. To reduce spread of the disease, affected animals should be isolated, and stalls, water buckets, and feed troughs disinfected.

In certain circumstances, however, treatment of warts is desirable. Warts can become irritated by trauma, insects, or secondary bacterial infections, making it painful for the horse to eat, resulting in loss of condition. Myiasis, especially with *Habronema*, is a concern during summer months. Animals with large warts situated in areas that interfere with the bit and other tack often experience pain during riding, which can cause delayed training. Warts are aesthetically unattractive and can present a problem for animals being prepared for critical shows or sales. The time missed in training or attending certain shows and sales can be a serious economic loss for owners.

Table 1 provides a list of treatments that have been reported for equine warts and the current understanding of their efficacy. The routine spontaneous regression of equine warts makes treatment evaluation difficult. The suggestion that removal of a few warts by surgical excision will induce the remaining warts to regress has not been proved true, and the associated stress may even allow lesions to persist longer. Surgical excision and cryosurgery are often recommended, but when large numbers of warts are present, substantial secondary trauma to normal tissue can occur. Release of viral antigens during late-phase tissue necrosis associated with cryosurgery is thought to enhance the host's immune response and may improve the success rate of partial wart removal. Topical caustic or mitosis-modulating compounds have shown some success, but the following precautions are advisable. Topical compounds should be carefully applied with a cotton-tip applicator and adjacent tissue protected with petrolatum. In addition, the horse should be prevented from licking or chewing around the treated area. Except for retinoic acid cream, which is applied daily, all of the topical compounds listed in Table 1 should be applied at 4-day intervals because of the inflammatory response. An intravenous immunostimulant* has had reported success in both prevention and treatment of equine warts. Any treatment for warts that creates an inflammatory response may increase the risk of residual skin depigmentation.

AURAL PLAQUES

Aural plaques differ from warts in their clinical appearance, location, lack of spontaneous regression, and poor response to treatment. These benign ear lesions were formerly called papillary acanthomas and were thought to be the result of chronic irritation from black fly bites. Aural plaques are often incorrectly described by owners as "ear fungus."

Aural plaques are clinically recognized as multiple smooth or raised depigmented plaques located bilaterally on the inner surface of the pinna. The lesions are asymptomatic unless severely irritated by biting flies. Infrequently, lesions may be seen around the anus, penis, and vulva. The location of these lesions suggests that the condition is transmissible by insect bites and during breeding. Unlike equine warts, aural plaques can be found in any horse older than 1 year. They are persistent and rarely undergo spontaneous regression.

Diagnosis of aural plaques is based on clinical appearance. Occasionally, plaques may resemble precancerous stages of squamous cell carcinoma, especially when they are located on genitalia. In these cases, a biopsy specimen should be submitted for histologic diagnosis. Biopsy specimens of aural plaques reveal orthokeratotic hyperkeratosis, papillated epidermal proliferation, and epidermal hypomelanosis.

No successful treatment has been reported for aural

---

*Eq-Stim Immunostimulant (non-viable Propionibacterium acnes suspension), Immunovet, Tampa, FL

TABLE 1. MODES OF THERAPY FOR EQUINE PAPILLOMATOSIS (WARTS)

1. *Most often recommended*
   a. Surgical excision of all lesions
   b. Cryosurgery ($-20°C$)
   c. Radiofrequency hyperthermia (50°C for 30 seconds)
2. *Reported effective but lacking supportive data*
   a. Topical caustic or mitosis modulating compounds
      Trifluoroacetic acid mixture
         25 g anhydrous trifluoroacetic acid, 3 g water, and 20 g glacial acetic acid
      Salicylic acid (25%) with crude castor oil
      Salicylic acid (25%) with podophyllin* (2%) and DMSO
      Podophyllin (50%)
      Podophyllin (20%) with ethyl alcohol (95%)
      Retinoic acid cream (0.1%)
   b. Intra-lesional
      Immunostimulant† (1–2 ml, repeat in 14–30 days)
      Vitamin A
   c. Oral
      Potassium or sodium iodides (8 g P.O. daily, 14–30 days)
   d. Intravenous
      Immunostimulant† (1 ml/115 kg BW, repeat on day 4, 7, and weekly)
3. *Questionable efficacy*
   Autogenous vaccines
4. *Not effective*
   Bovine wart vaccine
5. *Experimental*
   a. Podofilox‡—topical
   b. Cisplatin§—intralesional (see page 372)
   c. Interleukin 2—intralesional

---

*Resin obtained from the roots of *Podophyllum peltatum*
†Eq-Stim Immunostimulant, Immunovet, Tampa, FL
‡One of the active compounds from podophyllin, Oclassen Pharmaceuticals, San Rafael, CA
§Theon AP, et al: J Am Vet Med Assoc 202(2):261–267, 1993

plaques. Irritation of aural plaques can be controlled with regular application of insecticide repellents.

Supplemental Readings

Fadok VA: Overview of equine papular and nodular dermatoses. Vet Clin North Am Equine Pract 11(1):61–74, 1995.
McMullan WC: The skin. *In* Mansmann RA, McAllister ES, Pratt PW (eds): Equine Medicine & Surgery, vol 2, ed 3. Santa Barbara, CA, American Veterinary Publications, 1982, pp 789–883.
Scott DW: Large Animal Dermatology. Philadelphia, WB Saunders, 1988, pp 420–428.
Theilen GH: Papillomatosis (warts). *In* Robinson NE (ed): Current Therapy in Equine Medicine. Philadelphia, WB Saunders, 1983, pp 536–537.

Dermatologic Conditions Associated With Abnormal Pigmentation

ANTHONY A. YU
Portland, Oregon

Melanocytes arise in embryonic life from the neural crest. They are secretory cells that contain pigment-bearing melanosomes, which determine the skin color by their type (I–IV), number, size, and distribution. These pigment granules are transferred into the epidermis and hair follicle cells via their dendritic processes, which interdigitate between the cells of the epidermis, cells of the outer root sheath of the hair follicles, and ducts of the sweat and sebaceous glands. Melanin is derived from the conversion of tyrosine to dihydroxyphenylalanine (dopa) by the copper-containing enzyme tyrosinase. Tyrosinase then oxidizes dopa to dopaquinone, which undergoes a series of oxidative reactions to form either pheomelanin or eumelanin. The synthesis of the two pigment classes and their combination to form intermediates, is genetically dictated. The formation of melanin is influenced by breakdown products of adrenocorticotropic hormone (ACTH) (β-lipoprotein, melanin-stimulating hormone [MSH]), thyroid hormones, glucocorticoids, sex hormones, and ultraviolet (UV) light. The purpose of melanin is to protect against the harmful effects of UV irradiation.

Several disease processes result in focal reduction of pigment at the skin (leukoderma) and at the hair (leukotrichia). These events result either from an absence of the pigment-synthesizing melanocytes or from a failure of melanocytes to produce normal amounts of melanin or to transfer it to adjacent keratinocytes. Leukoderma and leukotrichia may occur independently and may be hereditary or acquired. Acquired hypopigmentation follows damage to the epidermal melanin unit by various insults. In general, most horses tend to have depigmentation following cutaneous injury, whereas other animals tend to become hyperpigmented.

Table 1 lists depigmenting equine disorders with known etiologies. Many of these disorders are described in other chapters within this text. The present chapter describes vitiligo and reticulated and hyperesthetic leukotrichia.

VITILIGO

Vitiligo is an acquired leukoderma hypomelanosis characterized by gradually expanding pale macules that are often symmetrical or segmental in distribution. It is rarely a hereditary disease and, when it is, the onset is delayed. Vitiligo is a depigmenting skin disorder rather than a genetically programmed abnormality in melanin synthesis or transfer (Table 2). Hypotheses to explain the pathogenesis of vitiligo are listed in Table 3. The presence of melanin antibodies in the serum of vitiligo patients coupled with the presence of lymphocytes at the leading edge of the lesion supports the autoimmune hypothesis.

Arabian fading syndrome (pinky syndrome) is an idiopathic leukoderma in Arabian horses, and occasionally other breeds, which has been likened to vitiligo. It is more common in young healthy grays and is characterized by nonpruritic, noninflammatory, round, depigmented macules or patches at mucocutaneous regions of the body

TABLE 1. ACQUIRED SKIN DEPIGMENTATION DISORDERS IN HORSES

Infective
 Dourine (*Trypanosoma equiperdum*)
 Onchocerciasis
 Culicoides bites/hypersensitivity (*Haematobia irritans*)
 Parafilaria multipapillosa infestation
 Aural plaques (verruca plana)
 Coital exanthema (equine herpesvirus [EHV]-3)

Noninfective
 Immunological (systemic and discoid lupus erythematosus)
 Physicochemical
  Cold branding/cryosurgery
  Trauma (pressure wounds [tack, plaster casts], accidents, rope burns)
  Chemical agents
   Blisters
   Rubber toxicity (monobenzyl ether of hydroquinone, mono- or dihydroxyphenol compounds found in bits, cruppers, cheek pieces)
   Local anesthetic with epinephrine (nerve blocks)
  Radiation therapy
 Nutritional
  Copper deficiency
  Vitamin A deficiency
 "Idiopathic" depigmenting disorders
  Vitiligo
  Reticulated leukotrichia
  Hyperesthetic leukotrichia
  Spotted leukotrichia
  Alopecia areata and universalis

TABLE 2. GENETICALLY INFLUENCED SKIN DEPIGMENTATION DISORDERS IN HORSES

	Genetic component
Appaloosa pattern	Vitiligo
Coat greying	Arabian fading syndrome
Lethal white foal disease	Spotted leukotrichia
Piebaldism	Reticulated leukotrichia

391

TABLE 3. HYPOTHESES EXPLAINING THE
PATHOGENESIS OF VITILIGO

1. Chemical, failure of melanocytes to be protected against toxic effects (including free radicals) on melanin precursors
2. Release of toxic factors from peripheral nerves (noted by depigmentation along line of peripheral nerve innervation)
3. Autoimmune
4. Self trauma
5. Nutritional metabolic imbalance

(perioral, periocular, perineal, preputial regions, and hooves) that tend to be permanent. Although no gender predilection has been noted, mares commonly show signs during pregnancy or shortly after foaling potentially as a result of hormonal alterations, and their offspring are more at risk. Stabled animals may be more prone to the condition than those at pasture. Spontaneous resolution of the condition occurs within 1 year in some animals but, more frequently, the condition waxes and wanes and eventually becomes permanent.

Diagnosis is based on history, clinical signs, and a biopsy to help rule out other disorders (see Table 1). An autoimmune pathogenesis may be supported by the detection of circulating antimelanocytic antibodies. Evaluating vitamin A and thyroid levels may be of value considering the report of nine (six male, three female) 2-year-old Spanish Thoroughbreds with depigmentation around the eyes and muzzle, scrotum, perineum, and umbilical areas. Affected individuals were sired by four different stallions and from dams with no previous history of depigmentation. Dermatohistopathology revealed distinct borders between pigmented and depigmented areas with a lack of inflammation. No abnormal laboratory data including plasma copper levels were noted. Further historical evaluation revealed that depigmentation occurred following the administration of thyroprotein-based product over a 2- to 3-month period. As thyroid hormones enhance catabolism of vitamin A to carotene and inhibit anabolism of vitamin A, excessive thyroxine administration may, therefore, lead to a vitamin A deficiency. The lesions resolved after supplementing the diet with 4 to 5 kg of carrots per animal. Repigmentation evolved centripetally with full recovery noted within 1 year and speedier repigmentation in darker individuals. This is in contrast to animals with Arabian fading syndrome, in which only partial recovery is expected. Because supplementation with vitamin A or its carotene precursors was beneficial in the Spanish Thoroughbred horses fed a thyroprotein supplement, a nutritional metabolic imbalance for the depigmentation may directly or indirectly play a role in Arabian fading syndrome. Human vitiligo patients have improved after supplementation with oral L-phenylalanine combined with UVA sunlight irradiation, once again suggesting a nutritional metabolic imbalance of this disorder.

Dietary copper imbalances may cause loss of pigmentation and are diagnosed by plasma copper concentrations significantly below the normal value of 0.7 to 2 ppm in plasma. If plasma copper levels fall outside the reference ranges, measurements of hair copper levels may be of value. Many compounds containing cyanide ions, organic sulfur, or molybdenum form weakly dissociable complexes with copper, thus inactivating the copper component of tyrosinase, resulting in decreased melanin formation. Noticeable repigmentation can be obtained by providing supplemental copper° (0.6 g chelated copper s.i.d.) for 1 month.

RETICULATED AND HYPERESTHETIC LEUKOTRICHIA

Reticulated leukotrichia is recognized in Standardbred, Thoroughbred, and particularly Quarterhorse breeds. The lesions occur predominantly in yearlings and comprise linear crusts arranged in a crosshatch pattern over the back and rump of affected horses. There is no associated pain or pruritus. Crusting is followed by alopecia and a regrowth of permanent leukotrichia and normally pigmented underlying skin.

Hyperesthetic leukotrichia is a less common disorder seen in mature horses with no breed predilections. Originally reported only in Californian horses, it has been anecdotally reported in other states. Sudden onset of extreme cutaneous pain is associated with early vesicular lesions or single to multiple crusts in the later stages. Lesions affect primarily the dorsal midline. Leukotrichia develops as the underlying skin heals. The disease has a 1- to 3-month course, during which the horse cannot bear to be touched or even approached. In some horses, the disease recurs on a regular basis. The horses do not respond to glucocorticoid therapy.

Biopsies from reticulated and hyperesthetic leukotrichia are both characterized by a pronounced band of inflammatory cells at the dermoepidermal junction (interface dermatitis) and apoptotic keratinocytes within the basal layer. Intraepidermal and subepidermal vesicles are observed in some biopsy specimens. Mononuclear cells with a prominent dendritic morphology are plentiful in the inflammatory infiltrate. The dermal findings include superficial edema and pigmentary incontinence.

These two diseases may represent the opposite ends of a spectrum of disorders that may overlap, at least in terms of etiology. Some of the early histologic features suggest a diagnosis of erythema multiforme or possibly fixed-drug eruption. An association has been made between the development of hyperesthetic leukotrichia and the administration of rhinopneumonitis vaccines in about 50% of affected horses. A weaker association also exists between reticulated leukotrichia and rhinopneumonitis vaccination. Clinically the impressionable pain in hyperesthetic leukotrichia resembles that of herpes zoster in humans, and histologically, the similarities between early leukotrichia lesions and those observed in human herpes-infected skin suggest that the dendritic cells found in these skin eruptions may be antigen-presenting cells. The dendritic cells may present viral or drug antigens to cutaneous T cells, which then mount an attack on keratinocytes in the epidermis and in the hair follicle. Current data thus suggest that rhinopneumonitis vaccine is a likely etiology for hyperesthetic and possible reticulated leukotrichia in susceptible horses. The permanent leukotrichia may represent a type of drug reaction in affected horses.

°*Molycu, Schering-Plough Animal Health, Union, NJ*

Because glucocorticoids do not relieve pain in horses, therapy prescribed for treatment of herpes zoster in humans may be useful; that is, acyclovir* for the specific infection and amitriptyline† for the "postherpetic neuralgia." Dosages, cost efficacy, adverse effects, and therapeutic response require further investigation in the horse. A synthetic cyclic analogue of α-MSH stimulates follicular melanogenesis and darkening of the hair coat without adverse effects in dogs. The dose for use in dogs is 1 mg/day for 21 days. This treatment may provide an effective means of therapeutically repigmenting cases of leukotrichia for protection against UV light. In fact, β-lipoprotein, which is thought to be the main pituitary-derived melanocyte stimulating hormone and is two to four times more potent than α-MSH, may prove to be effective in the treatment of both leukotrichia and leukoderma.

Supplemental Readings

Fadok VA: Update on four unusual equine dermatoses. Vet Clin North Am Equine Pract 11(1):105–110, 1995.

Johnson PD, Dawson BV, Dorr RT, Hadley ME, Levine N, Hruby VJ: Coat color darkening in a dog in response to a potent melanotropic peptide. Am J Vet Res 55:1593–1601, 1994.

Mozos E, Novales M, Sierra MA: Focal hypopigmentation in horses resembling Arabian Fading Syndrome. Equine Vet Educ 3(3):122–125, 1991.

Thomsett LR: Pigmentation and pigmentary disorders of the equine skin. Equine Vet Educ 3(3):130–135, 1991.

Scott DW: Disorders of pigmentation and epidermal appendages. *In* Large Animal Dermatology. Philadelphia, WB Saunders, 1988, pp 387–392.

Yager JA, Scott DW: The skin and appendages. *In* Jubb KVF, Kennedy PC, Palmer N (eds): Pathology of Domestic Animals, vol. 1, 4th ed. San Diego, Academic Press, 1993, pp 407–549.

---

*Zovirax, Burroughs Wellcome, Research Triangle Park, NC
†Etrafon, Schering Co., Kenilworth, NJ

Subcutaneous Abscesses Caused by *Corynebacterium pseudotuberculosis*

BRUCE A. SOMERVILLE
MONICA ALEMAN
SHARON J. SPIER
Davis, California

Corynebacterium pseudotuberculosis is a gram-positive pleomorphic facultative intracellular anaerobic rod with worldwide distribution causing ulcerative lymphangitis, external subcutaneous abscesses, as well as internal abscesses in horses. The North American geographic distribution of disease is concentrated in the southwestern United States, but cases of *C. pseudotuberculosis* infection have been reported throughout the southern United States. The portal of entry of this soil-borne organism is thought to be through abrasions or wounds in the skin or mucous membranes. Many insects have been incriminated as vectors for the transmission of the disease to horses including *Haematobia irritans*, *Musca domestica*, *Stomoxys calcitrans*, and *Culicoides*; however, this has not been confirmed by experimental studies.

The regional location of abscesses suggests that ventral midline dermatitis is a predisposing cause of infection. The incidence of disease fluctuates considerably from year to year, presumably because of environmental factors such as rainfall and temperature. The highest number of cases in California is observed in the fall during the dry months of the year, although cases may be seen all year. Most clinical cases are single episodes of infection. In a retrospective study, 9% of the horses had recurrent episodes of infection over subsequent years. No breed or sex predisposition has been documented. Horses of all ages may be affected, although the low incidence of disease in foals younger than 6 months of age suggests possible colostral protection in foals born to mares in endemic areas. A serologic study in young goats demonstrated passive transfer of immunoglobulin, which declined to undetectable levels by 6 months of age. Similar studies have not been undertaken in foals.

CLINICAL SIGNS

External abscesses may occur anywhere on the body, but most frequently develop in the pectoral region and along the ventral midline of the abdomen. Abscesses contain tan, odor-free pus and are usually well-encapsulated. Additional sites for abscess formation are the region of the prepuce, mammary gland, axilla, limbs, and head. Horses may have an abscess involving a single site or involving multiple regions of the body. It is common to observe multiple subcutaneous abscesses coursing along a suspected lymphatic. Clinical signs most frequently associated with external abscesses are edema, fever, and nonhealing wounds. Other clinical signs include lameness, ventral dermatitis, weight loss, depression, anorexia, and mammary gland or preputial swelling. Clinical pathologic abnormalities that may be observed include anemia of chronic disease, leukocytosis with neutrophilia, hyperfibrinogenemia, and hyperproteinemia. These hematologic parameters can occur with either internal or external abscesses but are more consistently observed with internal abscesses.

Abscesses of internal organs or lymph nodes may occur in both the thorax and the abdominal cavity. Clinical signs associated with internal abscesses include fever, weight loss, decreased appetite, pale mucous membranes, and depression. Other signs observed in horses with internal abscesses include colic, presence of external abscesses, ventral edema, ventral dermatitis, ataxia, hematuria due to renal abscesses, nasal discharge due to pulmonary abscesses, and, rarely, abortion.

Because the clinical presentation with both external and internal abscesses due to *C. pseudotuberculosis* is so varied, there are numerous differential diagnoses to consider. The disease should be readily suspected in a horse with the typical ventral midline or pectoral abscesses; however, other common differentials include seromas, hematomas, foreign bodies, tumors, and abscesses due to other bacteria.

PATHOGENESIS

The pathogenesis of *C. pseudotuberculosis* infection in horses is poorly understood. The incubation period is not known. Following entry into the host, the bacteria are phagocytosed but continue to replicate, resulting in phagocytic cell death. Intracellular survival of *C. pseudotuberculosis* has a key role in the formation of abscesses and is possibly mediated by two virulence factors: bacterial cell wall lipids and a phospholipase D (PLD) protein exotoxin. The bacterial cell wall lipids may facilitate survival in macrophages, whereas the PLD exotoxin has profound effects on survival and multiplication within the host. The PLD toxin may directly affect phagocytic cells or inactivate complement and reduce opsonization of the bacteria. The exotoxin also increases vascular permeability, enhancing the spread of infection both locally and via the lymphatics. The subsequent vascular changes permit bacterial spread to additional locations including regional lymph nodes. Humoral and cell-mediated immune responses ultimately develop, clearing the bacterial infection. Recovery generally is complete within 2 to 4 weeks, although rarely horses develop persistent or recurrent infections lasting for more than 1 year.

DIAGNOSIS

The typical clinical presentation of single or multiple maturing pectoral abscesses, with or without ventral midline abscesses, is highly suspicious of *C. pseudotuberculosis* infection. Culture of the characteristic tan or blood-tinged, odorless exudate is diagnostic. Bacteriologic culture of aspirates or draining abscesses readily yields growth of moderate to large numbers of organisms on blood agar in 24 to 48 hours. The colonies appear small, white, and opaque. Gram's stain shows gram-positive pleomorphic rods. The

equine isolates reduce nitrate unlike strains from small ruminants.

Without a positive culture of the bacteria, the practitioner must rely on hematology, clinical chemistry, and serologic testing to support a diagnosis. Hematologic changes are nonspecific and indicative of a chronic inflammatory response. Alterations in serum biochemical profiles may be seen such as increased creatine phosphokinase (CPK), and increased gamma glutamyltransferase (GGT). Increases in liver enzymes may be observed in horses with internal abscesses involving hepatic tissue. Serology testing using the synergistic hemolysis inhibition (SHI) test can be useful in aiding the diagnosis of internal abscesses. The SHI test measures IgG to the exotoxin of *C. pseudotuberculosis* and is available through the California Veterinary Diagnostic Laboratory in Davis, California. Serology testing is generally not helpful for diagnosis of external abscesses and results may be negative early in the course of disease and even at the time of abscess drainage. Positive SHI titers must be interpreted carefully and combined with clinical signs to distinguish active infection from exposure or convalescence. Both published and unpublished data from the University of California suggest that a reciprocal titer of 256 or higher is indicative of active infection. Horses with internal abscesses generally have SHI titers 512 or higher. Titers 8 or less are considered negative, whereas titers between 16 and 128 are considered suspicious or indicative of exposure. Experimental inoculation of horses with a bacterin-toxoid developed from *C. pseudotuberculosis* produced increased SHI titers equivalent to those seen with active infection; however, the protection offered from this bacterin has not been proved to date.

Additional diagnostics for internal abscesses include bacterial isolation from abdominal paracentesis, blood culture, transtracheal lavage, and necropsy.

TREATMENT

The treatment regimen must be individualized for each horse depending on the severity of disease, including the presence of systemic illness such as fever or anorexia, extent of soft tissue inflammation, maturity of the abscess and the ability to successfully establish drainage of pus. Establishing drainage is the most important treatment and ultimately leads to faster resolution and return to athletic performance. The proximity of the fibrous abscess capsule to the skin varies, often being less than 1 cm deep for ventral midline abscesses to more than 10 cm deep under muscle for some pectoral, axillary, or inguinal abscesses. Aspiration and drainage of superficial abscesses are easily performed; however, the use of diagnostic ultrasound is very helpful for localization of deeper abscesses and for judging maturity of the abscess and proximity to the skin. If the abscess is immature or cannot be safely incised, subsequent ultrasound examinations may be necessary to establish the ideal time to lance into the abscess. The abscess contents and lavage solutions such as saline with or without antiseptic should be retrieved and disposed of to prevent further contamination of the immediate environment.

Antimicrobials are indicated for horses with ulcerative lymphangitis of the distal extremities and for horses with internal abscesses. The use of antimicrobials for external abscesses is not necessary in most horses and may prolong the time to resolution. Antimicrobial therapy may be used when signs of systemic illness are present, such as fever, depression, and anorexia, or when extensive cellulitis is present. Horses in which deep abscesses are draining through healthy tissue also may benefit from antimicrobial therapy.

C. pseudotuberculosis is susceptible to most common antimicrobials in vitro, including penicillin, trimethoprim-sulfonamide combinations, tetracycline, cephalosporin, chloramphenicol, erythromycin, and rifampin. Several factors should be considered when choosing an antimicrobial. The intracellular location of the organism, presence of exudate and a thick abscess capsule, and duration of therapy are important, as is the cost of the drug and the convenience of administration. Despite in vitro susceptibility, the nature of the bacteria and the subsequent abscess render certain antimicrobials ineffective for some cases. Trimethoprim/sulfa (5 mg/kg based on the trimethoprim fraction p.o. b.i.d.) and procaine penicillin (20,000 IU/kg IM b.i.d.) are highly effective for external abscesses especially on the ventral midline. Internal abscesses have reportedly responded to procaine penicillin (dose as given earlier), trimethoprim/sulfa (dose as given earlier), potassium penicillin (20,000–40,000 IU/kg IV q.i.d.), as well as erythromycin estolate (15–25 mg/kg p.o. b.i.d. or t.i.d.). Erythromycin has been successfully used for internal abscesses and unresponsive ulcerative lymphangitis, however the duration and cost of therapy have limited its use. Rifampin (2.5–5 mg/kg p.o. b.i.d.) may be used in combination with erythromycin for treatment of internal abscesses. It is not recommended to use rifampin alone because of the rapid development of bacterial resistance.

Antimicrobial therapy for internal abscesses and ulcerative lymphangitis must be continued for a lengthy duration, ranging from 1 to 6 months. Resolution of infection is determined based upon clinical signs, normal clinical pathologic values, and decline in immunoglobulin concentrations. Some horses with very high SHI titers remain seropositive for up to 1 year, because of the 21-day half life of IgG and for other reasons that are unknown. Under such situations one should monitor a steady decline in serum SHI titers to *C. pseudotuberculosis*. The prognosis is excellent for external abscesses (fatality 0.8%), whereas internal abscesses have a more guarded prognosis (fatality 40.5%).

PREVENTION AND CONTROL

Until the exact epidemiology of *C. pseudotuberculosis* is known, one can only suggest that horse owners in endemic areas practice good sanitation and fly control and avoid unnecessary environmental contamination from diseased horses. Presently there is no evidence that diseased horses within a stable should be quarantined, other than paying strict attention to insect control. Proper sanitation, disposal of contaminated bedding, and disinfection may reduce the incidence of new cases. Proper wound care is also important to prevent infection from a contaminated environment.

Research is being performed to develop a protective vaccine for horses. A commercial bacterin-toxoid has been used in small ruminants with success and is approved in some countries. The safety and effectiveness of this product has not been tested in horses. Use of an experimental bacterin-toxoid demonstrated increased SHI titers following two injections; however, the protection remains to be established. The inability to experimentally reproduce the disease as seen in the endemic areas, and the sporadic incidence of disease complicates research efforts.

Supplemental Readings

Aleman M, Spier S, Wilson WD: Retrospective study of *Corynebacterium pseudotuberculosis* infection in horses: 538 cases (1982–1993). Proc 40th Annu Conv Am Assoc Equine Pract, 1994, p 117.
Davis EW: *Corynebacterium pseudotuberculosis* infections in animals. *In* Smith PB (ed): Large Animal Internal Medicine. St. Louis, CV Mosby, 1990, pp 1120–1126.
Judson R, Songer JG: *Corynebacterium pseudotuberculosis*: in vitro susceptibility to 39 antimicrobial agents. Vet Microbiol 27:145–150, 1991.
Knight HD: A serologic method for the detection of *Corynebacterium pseudotuberculosis* infections in horses. Cornell Vet 68:220–237, 1978.
Meirs KC, Ley WB: *Corynebacterium pseudotuberculosis* infection in the horse: Study of 117 clinical cases and consideration of etiopathogenesis. J Am Vet Med Assoc 177:250–253, 1980.
Rumbaugh GE, Smith BP, Carlson GP: Internal abdominal abscesses in the horse: A study of 25 cases. J Am Vet Med Assoc 172:304–309, 1978.
Songer JG, Prescott JF: *Corynebacterium*. In Gyles CL, Thoen CO (eds): Pathogenesis of Bacterial Infections in Animals. Ames, Iowa State University Press, 1993, pp 57–62.

Pythiosis

JOE NEWTON

JOHN SCHUMACHER
Auburn, Alabama

Equine pythiosis is an ulcerative, proliferative, pyogranulomatous disease caused by *Pythium insidiosum* (formerly *Hyphomyces destruens*). Although it is commonly referred to as a fungus, the organism is actually an oomycete belonging to the kingdom Protista, class Oomycetes.

Equine pythiosis has been variously referred to as Florida horse leech, swamp cancer, bursatii, phycomycosis, oomycosis, and hyphomycosis destruens equi. The disease has been reported in horses of all ages in tropical and subtropical areas of the world including Costa Rica, Australia, Brazil, Colombia, Japan, Indonesia, India, and the United States. In the United States, equine pythiosis is most often diagnosed in states bordering the Gulf of Mexico, but the disease has also been sporadically reported from more northern states.

The pathogenesis of equine pythiosis is poorly understood. Organisms in the class Oomycetes are commonly associated with freshwater aquatic environments. *Pythium insidiosum* parasitizes aquatic plants in stagnant water and produces motile zoospores as part of its life cycle. It has been postulated that these motile zoospores are attracted to animal hair and probably gain entry through traumatized skin. This hypothesis has not been proven, however, because all attempts to infect horses with *P. insidiosum* experimentally have been unsuccessful. Following dermal penetration, a severe pyogranulomatous inflammation occurs at the site of entry. Over a period of several weeks, the organism develops within the lesion, causing skin ulceration, proliferation of an extensive granulation tissue bed, and fibrosis.

CLINICAL SIGNS AND GROSS LESIONS

Pythiosis most commonly appears clinically as single large (up to 45 cm) round to oval, ulcerated, proliferative lesions in the skin and subcutaneous tissues of either the legs, ventral thorax and abdomen, or head. Enteric and pulmonary pythiosis has been reported in the horse, but these infections are rare. The infection can extend to bones and joints especially during chronic infections of the lower legs.

Close examination of cutaneous lesions reveals numerous randomly distributed sinus tracts within an inflamed bed of granulation tissue. A thick, sanguinous, mucopurulent exudate fills sinus tracts and covers the wound surface. Contained within sinus tracts are yellowish-gray, irregularly shaped, firm, coral-like bodies (kunkers, leeches) composed of pythium hyphæ, degenerating inflammatory cells, proteinaceous debris, and degenerating blood vessels. Some kunkers can be expressed by digital palpation, whereas other kunkers are firmly attached to the surrounding granulation tissue and resist removal.

Cutaneous lesions are intensely pruritic, and severe lameness is often associated with appendicular lesions. Chronically affected horses are often emaciated.

DIAGNOSIS

Timely diagnosis of equine pythiosis is important to the successful treatment of the disease. Initially, lesions of equine pythiosis can be confused with other skin diseases of horses including cutaneous habronemiasis, basidiobolomycosis, excessive granulation tissue, and certain equine neoplasms such as fibrous sarcoid. Preliminary diagnosis of equine pythiosis is often based on gross appearance, evidence of intense pruritus, lesion location, and presence of draining tracts containing kunkers. Histopathologic examination of biopsy tissues is helpful in diagnosis, but the histologic appearances of equine pythiosis, basidiobolomycosis, and conidiobolomycosis are similar, making histologic diagnosis difficult. Immunohistochemical identification of *P. insidiosum* in tissue section may be helpful in differentiation of *P. insidiosum* from the fungal diseases listed earlier.

Definitive diagnosis of the disease requires culture and identification. The organism grows on a variety of media including Sabouraud dextrose agar, brain-heart infusion agar, corn meal agar, and vegetable extract agar. Small pieces of the lesion or kunkers are placed on the surface of agar, and plates are incubated at a temperature between 34°C and 37°C. Infected tissues or kunkers for culture should not be transported to the laboratory on ice or refrigerated before culture. If the tissues are chilled before culture, the likelihood of growing *P. insidiosum* in the laboratory is greatly reduced. Serologic testing by agar gel immunodiffusion, complement fixation, or enzyme-linked immunosorbent assay is reported to be helpful in diagnosis of equine pythiosis. Because the disease is progressive and because clinical signs and gross lesions are highly suggestive of pythiosis, treatment is often undertaken before there is laboratory confirmation.

TREATMENT

Several treatment regimens for equine pythiosis have been tried with varied success. Surgical excision is the method of choice, provided that the lesion is small and all diseased tissue can be removed. This is often difficult, however, especially when the disease involves the lower legs. Recurrence is common in those cases in which diseased tissue is not completely removed.

Systemic antifungal agents such as amphotericin B have been used alone or in combination with surgery for successful treatment of pythiosis, but the drug's expense and the potential for nephrotoxicity restrict the use of such agents.

Immunotherapy can be coupled with appropriate antibiotic therapy to control secondary bacterial invaders. Immunotherapy is accomplished by use of vaccines prepared with various antigens derived from *P. insidiosum*. At present, there are two vaccines available.

Miller's vaccine, which is prepared from killed, sonicated, whole-cell hyphal antigen of *P. insidiosum*, is administered by subcutaneous injection at weekly intervals for 3 to 5 weeks. Using this vaccine, Miller was able to cure 51% of treated horses. Success rate was increased to almost 100% when immunotherapy was preceded by surgical debridement of lesions. Even extensive lesions not amenable to complete surgical resection responded to vaccination. In a majority of these cases, large lesions were reduced in size and severity and only a few draining tracts remained. These tracts were easily removed surgically. A common reaction to immunotherapy with Miller's vaccine is moderate to severe swelling, pain, and heat at the injection site. Sterile abscesses that may require surgical drainage may also occur at the injection site. The vaccine is usually given in the subcutaneous tissues overlying the pectoral muscles to facilitate drainage of potential abscesses. The vaccine must be kept cold (4°C) but cannot be frozen. The vaccine also loses its effectiveness after 8 weeks of storage, and fresh vaccine must continually be prepared.

The other vaccine, developed by Mendoza, is prepared by precipitating soluble antigen from pythium broth cultures. This vaccine (0.1 ml) is also administered subcutaneously. A second injection of 0.1 ml is given after 1 to 2 weeks if evidence of lesion regression is not obvious. Although response to Mendoza's vaccine is similar to that of Miller's vaccine, the undesirable side effects at the injection site are reduced. This new vaccine is also reported to have a longer shelf life because it retains its potency for more than 18 months at 4°C.

In horses responding to immunotherapy, the first signs indicating positive response usually occur 7 to 21 days after the initial injection and include gradual cessation of pruritus, reduction in amount of exudation from sinus tracts, and stabilization in lesion size. Over the next 5 to 10 days, lesions appear less inflamed and there is gradual reduction of lesion size. As lesions heal over the next 14 to 21 days, kunkers are expelled, sinus tracts close, and there is less exudate on the surface of the lesion. Epithelialization of the granulation tissue bed begins 14 to 21 days following the initial injection of vaccine and continues well after immunotherapy is complete.

In some horses, all of the above indicators of response to immunotherapy are present except for the closure of all sinus tracts. If a few sinus tracts persist and continue to discharge a seropurulent exudate despite continued immunotherapy, surgical removal of these inflamed sinus tracts is necessary.

Successful treatment of equine pythiosis appears to depend on several factors including lesion size, site and duration of lesions, and possibly immunologic status and age of the horse. Mendoza found the most important factor to be duration of the disease. All (7 of 7) of the horses in his study with pythium lesions of 2 weeks' duration or less were cured by immunotherapy. As lesion duration increased cure rate decreased. Horses having pythiosis for 2 or more months usually did not respond well to immunotherapy and were considered to be anergic. In addition, chronic lesions were usually heavily infected with secondary bacterial invaders complicating treatment.

Presently, there is one commercial source for Mendoza's vaccine.* The vaccines may also be made by individual veterinarians for use in their practices, but few private practitioners have laboratories equipped with the instrumentation required to produce the vaccine. Both vaccines are considered experimental by the United States Department of Agriculture and, as such, require permits before the vaccine can be made and shipped (Code of Federal Regulations, Title 9, Parts 101 and 123).

PREVENTION

At present, there are no methods available for the prevention of pythiosis in horses. The use of the immunotherapeutic treatments described earlier as vaccines for the prevention of equine pythiosis has not been investigated but may hold some promise on farms where the disease is a commonly recurring problem.

Supplemental Readings

Fadok VA: Appendicular inflammatory disorders. *In* Robinson NE (ed): Current Therapy in Equine Medicine, ed 3. Philadelphia, WB Saunders, 1992, pp 161–165.

Mendoza L, Villalobos J, Calleja CE, Solis A: Evaluation of two vaccines for the treatment of pythiosis insidiosi in horses. Mycopathologia 119:89–95, 1992.

Miller RI, Campbell RSF: Immunological studies on equine phycomycosis. Aust Vet J 58:227–231, 1982.

Newton JC, Ross PS: Equine pythiosis: An overview of immunotherapy. Comp Cont Ed Pract Vet 15(3):491–493, 1993.

*Bio-Medical Services, Austin, TX

Pastern Dermatitis

KEVIN KISTHARDT
Auburn, Alabama

Scratches and cracked heels are colloquial terms for a dermatitis syndrome that usually involves the plantar/palmar aspects of the pastern and bulbs of the heels but may extend proximally to mid-cannon. In Europe and Australia the syndrome is known as *mud fever* or *mud rash*. A more exudative form of pastern dermatitis is called *grease heel* or *dew poisoning*. In chronic stages mounds of granulation tissue called "grapes" appear on the caudal aspect of the lower limb. Collectively, the different presentations have been termed *equine pastern dermatitis*.

ETIOLOGY AND PATHOGENESIS

The dermatitis is usually preceded by mechanical injury to the stratum corneum layer of the epidermis. Chronically moist conditions, abrasions from plants in pasture or irritants in the soils of tracks or riding arenas, or beddings may be the source of mechanical damage. Ectoparasites such as chorioptic or straw itch mites may also traumatize epithelium. Horses with long hair (i.e., feathers) at the caudal aspect of the fetlock are more likely to develop pastern dermatitis because the long hairs accumulate mud and moisture and are a source of prolonged skin irritation. Alsike clover-induced photosensitization tends to produce lesions in areas of skin that contact moisture, such as the muzzle and lower legs. Pathogens that may invade the injured skin to incite or increase the dermatitis include *Dermatophilus congolensis*, *Staphylococcus* species, dermatophytes, mites, and nematodes such as *Pelodera strongyloides* and larvae of *Strongyloides westeri*.

CLINICAL SIGNS

Clinical signs of pastern dermatitis are variable. Hindlimbs are more often affected and the condition is commonly bilaterally symmetrical. In "scratches," the mildest and most prevalent form, the surface of the pastern is inflamed with scales and crusts and alopecia. Skin may be thickened and painful and some horses may be lame. Horses afflicted with mites may also be pruritic. In more advanced cases known as "grease heel," exudative dermatitis with epidermolysis develops. Horses affected by "grapes," the chronic form of pastern dermatitis, develop excessive granulation tissue that may become cornified.

TREATMENT

Most important in the treatment of pastern dermatitis is creation of a dry environment. If possible, affected horses should be stalled during wet weather conditions and until morning dew has dried. Hair, especially feathers, can be clipped to avoid moisture retention. If the horse cannot be placed in a drier area, lesions can be covered with ointments that create a moisture barrier,* or the lower limbs can be covered with padded, water-repellent bandages that are changed every 24 to 48 hours. An antibiotic-corticosteroid ointment† can be applied to the lesions several times daily, or if the lesions are wrapped, once every 24 to 48 hours. If the lesions are exudative, astringent lotions are applied several times a day for several days under light elastic gauze bandages. Once the lesions are dry, antibacterial-corticosteroid preparations can be applied. Parasite-induced dermatitis can be treated with ivermectin at 2-week intervals for two to three doses, or with topical insecticides such as malathion and coumaphos, or with lime sulfur.

Ichthammol,‡ applied liberally as a topical antibacterial and emollient, can be used effectively under light wraps or without bandages in the milder forms of scratches. A compounded mixture of 30 ml dimethyl sulfoxide (DMSO) and 30 g thiabendazole (TBZ) paste or powder and 0.5 kg sulfa cream has been used to treat pastern dermatitis. Thiabendazole is an anti-inflammatory, antifungal agent and DMSO and sulfa ointment are antibacterial. Investigation into the etiology of pastern dermatitis may be warranted in some cases. This may involve inspection of the housing or riding areas and microscopic examination of slides of skin scrapings. Slides of skin scrapings can be stained with methylene blue, Giemsa or Gram's stain when looking for the typical railroad track appearance of *Dermatophilus congolensis*. Skin scrapings may help identify mites. Bacterial culture may direct selection of topical antibiotics. Identification of dermatophyte-induced pastern dermatitis by fungal culture may prompt early specific treatment with fungicidal ointments.

When dermatitis has progressed to the chronic proliferative stage, surgical removal of granulation tissue is indicated. Proliferative granulation tissue is removed down to the level of the skin under general anesthesia using either electrocautery or an Esmarch bandage to control hemorrhage. Caution should be used to avoid excision of epithelial tissue from wound edges. After 24 hours of pressure bandaging, the surgical wounds can be treated with corticosteroid-antimicrobial ointment under wrap.

Prognosis and healing time of pastern dermatitis depends on the stage of disease at which treatment is begun, and, in some cases, whether an etiologic diagnosis can be made.

---

*Flanders Buttocks Ointment, Flander's, Inc., P.O. Box 39143, Charleston, SC 29407-9143; or Desitin, Pfizer Laboratories, New York, NY
†Panalog ointment, Solvay Animal Health, Mendota Heights, MN; Neo-Synalar, Syntex Laboratories, Palo Alto, CA
‡Ichthammol, The Butler Company, Columbus, OH

Supplemental Readings

Jacobs DE: A Colour Atlas of Equine Parasites. Philadelphia, Lea & Febiger, 1986.

McMullan WC: Scratches. *In* Robinson NE (ed): Current Therapy in Equine Medicine. Philadelphia, WB Saunders, 1983, p 549.
Scott DW: Miscellaneous dermatoses. *In* Scott DW (ed): Large Animal Dermatology. Philadelphia, WB Saunders, 1988, pp 399–410.

Melanomas

K. ANN JEGLUM
West Chester, Pennsylvania

Equine melanomas most commonly occur in gray or white horses at 5 to 6 years of age or older. The Arabian breed is predisposed to developing melanomas, probably because of the high incidence of gray coloring. A male predilection has been reported and also disputed. The most common skin sites are perianal area, tail, male genitalia, ear, eyelid, neck, and limb. The tumors appear black, gray, or amelanotic and are frequently ulcerated. It is common for dermal melanomas to be multicentric. The skin accounts for 66.6% of the overall incidence, and the second most commonly affected site is the eye (i.e., the pigmented tissues of the iris and choroid). Melanomas are locally invasive and can metastasize via lymphatics and blood vessels to regional lymph nodes and distant viscera, including lungs, liver, serosal surfaces, spleen, kidney, brain, bone, and heart. Those occurring in gray horses tend to behave more aggressively.

It has been estimated that 80% of gray horses, of either gender, over 15 years of age develop melanoma. The high incidence of melanoma in gray horses is thought to be related to the pigment changes associated with aging; this can be illustrated in Arabian horses, which are born black. The graying process begins at 2 years and progresses so that the 9-year-old may be white. The loss of pigment begins around the eyes and in the region of the anus at an early age, accounting for the high incidence of melanoma at these sites. The graying is associated with the onset of vitiligo, which is defined as the loss of melanin in the hair follicle (see page 391). This change in melanin metabolism may stimulate new melanoblasts that become malignantly transformed or may stimulate an overproduction in the dermis of the sites that most often develop cutaneous melanoma. These focal areas of hyperpigmentation are not observed in horses of other colors because there is a steady loss of melanin through desquamation of skin and epilation.

Equine melanomas present in three different clinical patterns without distinct histopathologic classification. The majority of melanomas grow slowly over many years without evidence of regional or distant metastases. Repeated treatment, primarily surgical excision, is required because the anatomic site may interfere either with normal functions such as urination, defecation, and coitus, or with application of the saddle, bridle, or halter. The second most common clinical presentation is the malignant transformation of a benign melanoma. Some melanomas are malignant from the onset and commonly metastasize. A histologic grading system has not been developed for the horse, and tumors are interpreted simply as malignant or benign.

BIOLOGY OF MELANOMA RELEVANT TO BIOLOGIC THERAPY

Historically, melanoma has been considered one of the tumors most amenable to immunologic manipulation based on clinicopathologic and basic immunologic observations. Although the features of melanoma described later are based on reports in humans and in animal models, there is no reason to believe that equine melanomas differ. As is the case in the horse, the clinical course of melanoma varies in humans, and includes spontaneous regression and paraneoplastic syndromes of depigmentation associated with prolonged survival of patients with metastases. The latter phenomenon is known as *vitiligo-like cutaneous hypopigmentation,* and has also been observed in association with response to immunotherapy. Histopathologic evidence of lymphoid infiltrates occurs in dysplastic nevi, a preneoplastic lesion, and in melanomas. Both of these features suggest that the immune response is a determinant of the clinical course of melanoma.

Immunotherapy with a variety of biological approaches has been used for several decades. Treatment with nonspecific immunomodulators including microbial agents such as Coley's toxin, bacillus Calmette-Guérin (BCG), and *Corynebacterium parvum* resulted in clinical responses. In an attempt to achieve a more specific antitumor immune response, a variety of tumor cell vaccines have been used, again with antitumor effects observed. More recently, therapy with cytokines, including interferon (IFN) and interleukin-2 (IL-2), monoclonal antibodies against melanoma-associated antigens, and adoptive cellular therapy with lymphokine-activated or tumor-infiltrating cells have shown promising clinical results. Vitiligo-like depigmentation was prognostically significant in patients responding to immunotherapy with BCG, tumor cell vaccines, and IFN and IL-2 combinations. Advances in the immunology of tumor antigens have resulted in the molecular dissection of the T- and B-cell response to antigens, allowing significant refinement in tumor vaccine preparation.

TREATMENT

Several treatment modalities have been used in equine melanoma, including surgical excision, cryosurgery, intralesional BCG, and radiotherapy. Little has been written concerning efficacy of the various approaches. Surgical excision is often made difficult by the anatomic sites that are most commonly affected. Recurrence rates are high. Cryosurgery and radiotherapy have been used, but no reports of results have been compiled. Clearly, there is a need for an alternative treatment of equine melanomas that cannot be removed surgically.

Cimetidine Therapy

Cimetidine has been reported to have antitumor effects in a variety of human and animal tumors, including malignant melanoma. Cimetidine blocks the histamine H_2 receptors on suppressor T cells, thereby potentially inhibiting the activation of T suppressor cells. A preliminary report of use of cimetidine in horses with melanoma showed beneficial effects in the clinical management of progressive, multifocal, benign; and malignant, cutaneous, and abdominal melanomas in six adult gray horses (see Goetz and coworkers in Supplemental Readings). The number and size of melanomas decreased by 40 to 90% in four horses treated with cimetidine alone. Stabilization of progressive disease occurred in five horses. Several interesting clinical observations were made. In five of the six horses, antitumor effects were observed after 3 to 4 months, a finding consistent with responses to treatment with biologic response modifiers. The immunologic cascade necessary to induce tumor responses requires time. This is in contrast to the more immediate effects with cytotoxic drugs. It also raises questions with regard to the timing and duration of treatment. The initial dose of cimetidine in this study was 2.5 mg/kg p.o. t.i.d. for 3 months. The optimal dosage of cimetidine is not established, and high doses may not be necessary, as demonstrated by clinical responses at lower doses. Two horses were treated with combination therapy, surgery, and cimetidine. One horse had complete excision of all melanomas and was treated with adjuvant cimetidine, and the other had surgical debulking followed by cimetidine. Although no new masses have developed 9 months after surgery in one horse, it is difficult to evaluate the role of cimetidine. A rationale for surgical biopsy or excision is to release tumor antigens, possibly allowing a more specific immunologic response.

In another study of 12 horses, four showed a positive response to cimetidine treatment, defined as a decrease in size or number of masses, but none had a greater than 50% reduction (see Hare and coworkers in Supplemental Readings). No differences were observed between responders or nonresponders with regard to signalment, anatomic site, rate of growth, distribution and size of tumors, and dosage and duration of cimetidine or other concurrent medications. These results seem in disparity with the results of Goetz and coworkers and indicate the need for a prospective, well-designed clinical trial to evaluate the efficacy of cimetidine.

Active Specific Immunotherapy

Based on the results obtained with use of tumor vaccines in human melanoma, the author and coworkers initiated a preliminary study in equine melanoma. The autochthonous vaccine is prepared by a method similar to that reported by Peters and coworkers (see Supplemental Readings). The tumor is surgically excised (at least 2×2 cm of tissue), placed immediately in Hank's balanced salt solution with 10% fetal calf serum, and placed on ice. The tumor is dissociated with collagenase into a single-cell suspension and cryopreserved as a whole-cell preparation. Before administration, the vaccine is irradiated to eliminate tumorigenicity. At the time of administration an immunologic adjuvant, Ribigen,° is combined with the cell preparation and injected subcutaneously over regional lymph nodes. The adjuvant is usually only added to the first vaccines because of local reaction. The vaccines are administered every other week for six injections and then every 6 weeks. The researchers decided to use a whole-cell vaccine approach for several reasons. Most importantly, there has been no characterization of equine melanoma antigens equivalent to that done for human melanoma. Therefore, synthetic vaccines are not feasible. In addition the whole-cell vaccine allows whatever component of the cell surface that acts as an antigen to be present in the vaccine.

To date, the researchers have treated 12 horses with follow-up to 2 years. Ten of the 12 had external dermal melanomas. One horse had an intrapelvic mass and another had multiple intra-abdominal masses. Tumors have regressed in 11 of the 12 horses. The most consistent finding reported by owners and veterinarians is significant improvement in the well-being and activity of all the horses treated, particularly in their ability to resume normal work. Although the results in these 12 horses are preliminary and somewhat anecdotal, they have convinced the researchers that this approach is worth further investigation. Because preparation of the vaccine is conducted in the author's laboratory but the vaccine is not administered by researchers, more detailed monitoring and follow-up are being requested in present and future cases.

Supplemental Readings

Goetz TE, Ogilvie GK, Keegan KG, Johnson PJ: Cimetidine for treatment of melanomas in three horses. J Am Vet Med Assoc 196:449–452, 1990.

Goetz TE, Boulton CH, Ogilvie GK: Clinical management of progressive multifocal benign and malignant melanomas of horses with cimetidine. Proc 35th Annu Conv Am Assoc Equine Pract 1989, pp 431–438.

Hare JE, Staempfli HR: Cimetidine for the treatment of melanomas in horses: Efficacy determined by client questionnaire. Equine Pract 16(5):18–21, 1994.

Jeglum KA, Young KM, Barnsley K, Whereat A: Chemotherapy versus chemotherapy with intralymphatic tumor cell vaccine in canine lymphoma. Cancer 61:2042, 1988.

Madewell BR, Theilen GH: Mast cell and melanocytic neoplasms. In Theilen GH, Madewell BR (eds): Veterinary Cancer Medicine, ed 2. Philadelphia, Lea & Febiger, 1987, pp 310–325.

Mastrangelo JJ, Maguire HC Jr, Lattime EC, Berd D: Whole cell vaccines. In DeVita VT, Hellman S, Rosenberg SA (eds): Biological Therapy of Cancer, ed 2. Philadelphia, JB Lippincott, 1995.

Peters LC, Brandhorst JS, Hanna MG: Preparation of immunotherapeutic, autologous tumor cell vaccines from solid tumors. Cancer Res 39:1353–1360, 1979.

°RIBI, Immunochem Research, Hamilton, MT

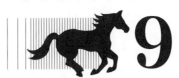
THE RESPIRATORY SYSTEM

Edited by Jean-Pierre Lavoie

Diagnostic Techniques for Upper Airway Diseases

ERIC J. PARENTE
Kennett Square, Pennsylvania

Veterinarians are often asked to examine horses suspected to have upper airway disease. The primary complaint can be epistaxis, nasal discharge, facial swelling or asymmetry, abnormal respiratory noises, or poor performance of undetermined cause. The signalment, a thorough history, and a complete physical examination, including palpation of the larynx and head, form the basis for a list of differential diagnoses, but further diagnostic techniques are usually necessary to establish the ultimate cause of the disorder. Many of the techniques described in this section can be performed easily by most clinicians, but the correct interpretation of the results is more challenging.

ENDOSCOPIC EXAMINATION IN THE STANDING HORSE

This procedure should be performed in all cases of suspected upper airway disease. Most horses tolerate the examination with only a twitch for restraint. Three people are generally required; one restrains the horse, another passes the endoscope, and the third directs the endoscope during the examination. It is preferable not to use sedation because it can dramatically alter the appearance of the larynx and pharynx.

A flexible 1-m fiberoptic endoscope or video endoscope is directed down the ventral meatus toward the pharynx. The video endoscope provides greater clarity to the picture and allows more than one individual to see the image. Because most horses resent initial insertion of the endoscope, it is easier to pass it 30 to 40 cm without hesitation. This distance allows positioning the tip of the endoscope directly in front of the larynx in the average adult horse.

After examination of the pharynx and larynx, slow withdrawal of the endoscope allows visualization of the ethmoid region and nasal passage. Examination through both nasal passages is essential whenever structural deformity is suspected or if no abnormality is identified through the first nasal passage.

The majority of structural abnormalities of the upper respiratory tract (Table 1) can be identified during endoscopy of the standing horse. A systematic approach should be developed to examine all structures. The arytenoid cartilages should appear uniform in size, should move in synchrony, and should abduct symmetrically after swallowing or during nasal occlusion. Unequal maximal abduction of the arytenoids may indicate a grade 3 or 4 laryngeal hemiplegia, or arytenoid chondropathy, if the arytenoid appears

TABLE 1. UPPER RESPIRATORY ABNORMALITIES

Structural	Functional
Arytenoid chondropathy	Alar fold redundancy
Intralaryngeal granulation tissue	Nostril collapse
Lymphoid hyperplasia	Laryngeal hemiplegia
Epiglottitis entrapment	Dorsal displacement of the soft palate
Subepiglottic cysts	
Epiglottic hypoplasia	Pharyngeal collapse
Ethmoid hematoma	Axial deviation of the aryepiglottic folds
Nasopharyngeal cicatrix	
Guttural pouch infection/tympany	Vocal chord deviation
Septal deviations	Epiglottic retroversion
Neoplasia	
Polyp formation	
Paranasal sinus cysts	
Paranasal sinus infection	

enlarged. Fixation of one arytenoid in an abducted position indicates previous "tie-back" (laryngeal prosthesis) surgery.

As an obligate nasal breather, the horse should always have its somewhat convex epiglottis positioned over the soft palate. Fine surface vessels and a corrugated or scalloped edge should be visible on the epiglottis. The surface may be distorted by epiglottic inflammation (see page 407), or epiglottic entrapment. A hypoplastic epiglottis is relatively small or flaccid, blending into the contour of the palate. Although a hypoplastic epiglottis in itself does not present an obstruction, it may be a contributing factor to dorsal displacement of the soft palate during exercise. Subepiglottic cysts are sometimes visible on endoscopic examination. If a cyst is present under the free edge of the palate, a small bulge of the normal tissues may be the only indication of its presence. Cysts often rise above the palate after swallowing.

An asymmetric bulging of the pharynx rostral to the larynx and a history of nasal discharge or epistaxis warrants exploration of the guttural pouches. The flap-like openings are several centimeters rostral and dorsal to the larynx. Entrance can be facilitated by first passing a small biopsy instrument through the biopsy channel of the endoscope and into the guttural pouch. Rotating the endoscope so that the biopsy channel is 180° away from the pharyngeal wall wedges the flap open wider and allows passage of the endoscope into the pouch as the biopsy instrument is withdrawn. The maximal diameter of the endoscope should be 11 mm. Both the medial and lateral compartments should be closely examined for masses and signs of infection or hemorrhage. Familiarity with the vital structures running adjacent to the pouch lining is important.

The ethmoid region can be examined at the caudodorsal extent of the nasal passage. Normally, multiple bulbous-like structures sit within the cavern-like space. An encapsulated mass of abnormal shape and greenish black color is most likely an ethmoid hematoma. Ethmoid hematomas can be large enough to obliterate the entire space and extend around the free edge of the nasal septum to the contralateral side.

Obstruction of the nasal passage is most often a consequence of sinus disease or septal deviations that result in narrowing of the nasal passage and disfigurement of the normal architecture. Less frequently, neoplasia or polyp formation obstructs the nasal passage. Any narrowing of the nasal passage warrants further diagnosis by use of radiographs and possibly sinocentesis. Purulent material from the nasomaxillary opening may pool at the middle meatus and is strongly suggestive of sinusitis.

RADIOGRAPHY

Radiographs are indicated whenever there is a discharge or structural asymmetry within the upper respiratory tract. Sedation is generally required, and a rope halter prevents confounding artifact on the radiographs. The natural air-filled cavities of the paranasal sinuses and the nasal passage provide good contrast for space-occupying lesions. A dorsoventral and lateral projection may be sufficient to delineate most abnormalities. Oblique projections are employed to offset the tooth roots or for greater clarity of a particular

side of the head. The recommended technique is 70 kVp/12 mAs in the adult horse.

Interpretation of skull radiographs is difficult. If a soft tissue density is suspected on the lateral radiograph, a dorsoventral projection should be used to corroborate the finding. Fluid lines are best seen on the lateral projection in the maxillary sinuses and should run parallel to the ground. The absence of a fluid line does not rule out sinusitis, because the fluid may completely occupy the space or the radiographic technique may be incorrect.

Delineation of the caudal pharynx and larynx is much improved with the excellent soft tissue resolution provided by xeroradiography. A technique using 95 kVp/50 mAs is adequate in the average-sized horse. Although disorders such as arytenoid chondrosis, subepiglottic cysts, and other masses can usually be seen with standard radiographs, they are more apparent on xeroradiographs.

CENTESIS

Centesis, which is used to sample fluid from the maxillary or frontal sinuses, can be performed easily in the standing sedated animal with local anesthesia of the sampling site. The site for penetration into the caudomaxillary sinus is 2 to 3 cm dorsal to the facial crest and 2 to 3 cm rostral to the medial canthus of the eye. Very young or miniature horses have a relatively small caudomaxillary sinus, and thus it is easier to enter it via the frontal sinus approximately halfway between midline and the medial canthus, and slightly caudal to the medial canthus. The large communication between the frontal and caudomaxillary sinus permits this approach. The rostral maxillary sinus can be entered 3 cm dorsal to the facial crest and approximately 3 cm caudal to the infraorbital foramen.

The chosen site of penetration is clipped and prepared for aseptic surgery. Several milliliters of anesthetic are placed subcutaneously directly over the site of centesis. A 1-cm incision is made through the skin and underlying tissue, to the bone. A 2-mm trocar-point Steinmann pin attached to a Jacob's chuck is used to drill the hole through the bone. Only 2 to 3 cm of the Steinmann pin should extend from the chuck to ensure that deeper underlying structures are not damaged. Fluid obtained can be submitted for Gram's stain, cytologic examination, and culture. Larger holes can be made to flush through the sinus with polyionic fluids or to take biopsies with Ferris Smith rongeurs.

ENDOSCOPIC EXAMINATION OF THE PARANASAL SINUSES

Endoscopic examination of the paranasal sinuses can be very informative and is much less invasive than the standard exploration of the sinuses through a bone flap when the horse is under general anesthesia. The procedure, which can be performed under local anesthesia in the standing sedated animal, allows diagnostic biopsy and identification of diseased tooth roots.

A 6.35-mm Steinmann pin is used to create the portal for a 4.0-mm arthroscope. The portal for entry into the frontal sinus is 60% of the distance from dorsal midline to the medial canthus and 0.5 cm caudal to the medial canthus. It is most useful for examining the frontal and then the caudomaxillary sinus by advancing the arthroscope through the frontomaxillary opening. A separate portal into the caudomaxillary sinus is necessary to see the sphenopalatine sinus. A third portal is necessary to see the rostral maxillary sinus. These portals are the same as those used for centesis. Anatomic review and practice on a cadaver specimen are recommended to assist in distinguishing normal from abnormal structures.

ENDOSCOPY DURING EXERCISE ON A TREADMILL

Endoscopy during exercise on a treadmill has become essential for the diagnosis of functional upper respiratory abnormalities in performance horses (see Table 1). It has become increasingly clear that conclusions based on the structure of the upper respiratory tract viewed during endoscopy in the standing horse can have little bearing on the respiratory tract's ability to remain patent in the face of large pressure changes that occur during maximal exercise.

To draw useful conclusions from endoscopy during exercise, it is necessary to have a fit horse, a treadmill that has a maximal speed equivalent to that of the horse or that can incline to increase the horse's workload, and a videoendoscopy system with slow-motion playback. Several people are required to ensure the safety of the animal as well as the people involved in the examination.

Several hours are required to complete the examination if the horse is unaccustomed to running on a treadmill. A schooling session accustoms the horse to the basic gaits and shows its ability to run at high speed. This session is followed by a rest period before the actual examination. A heart rate monitor is recommended to ensure that the horse is undergoing maximal exertion with a heart rate of 210 beats/minute or greater.

For the examination, the horse undergoes a short warm-up period through a light walk, trot, and canter. The treadmill is slowed and then stopped once the heart rate returns to a low level. A 6- to 8-inch strip of Velcro is pretaped to the endoscope at the 35- to 40-cm mark. A twitch is placed on the horse and the endoscope is passed into the nares. It is held in place by attaching the Velcro from the endoscope to the matching Velcro piece that was pretaped to the noseband of the halter. The tip of the endoscope should be approximately at the level of the guttural pouch openings. The twitch is removed once the endoscope is

properly positioned, and the operator of the treadmill increases the speed as quickly as possible to begin the test. Some disagreement exists on how fast and how far the horse should go for an accurate performance evaluation. The authors try to reach maximal speed within 1600 m and maintain that speed for up to 1600 m while monitoring heart rate in most racehorses. Because some abnormalities occur very quickly and transiently, video recording and review during slow-motion playback assists in defining the abnormality.

Laryngeal hemiplegia and dorsal displacement of the soft palate are just two of the dynamic abnormalities that can be confirmed by high-speed treadmill endoscopy. Axial deviation of the aryepiglottic folds is another abnormality that can lead to severe inspiratory compromise, is associated with a roarer-like noise, and, on occasion, precedes dorsal displacement of the soft palate. Vocal chord deviation can occur when an arytenoid achieves less than maximal abduction but does not dynamically collapse, or even when both arytenoids do abduct fully. Pharyngeal collapse can occur in a circumferential, primarily dorsoventral or primarily lateral manner, and can also cause a low-pitched roarer-like noise. Epiglottic retroversion, in which the epiglottis is pulled into the glottis with each inspiration, makes a vibrating inspiratory noise. None of these functional abnormalities can be definitely identified in the standing horse.

In conjunction with treadmill endoscopy, flow-volume loops and intratracheal and intrapharyngeal pressure profiles are being used to assess the degree of compromise associated with the many dysfunctions. Because of the specialized equipment required and variability among individuals, these techniques may be more difficult to perform and interpret unless a large sample size of normals is available for comparison.

Supplemental Readings

Ducharme NG, Hackett RP, Ainsworth DM, Erb HN, Shannon KJ: Repeatability and normal values for measurement of pharyngeal and tracheal pressures in exercising horses. Am J Vet Res 55:368–374, 1994.
Ducharme NG, Hackett RP, Fubini SL, Erb HN: The reliability of endoscopic examination in assessment of arytenoid cartilage movement in horses: Part II. Influence of side of examination, reexamination and sedation. Vet Surg 20:180–184, 1991.
Farrow CS: Radiographic examination and interpretation. In Beech J (ed): Equine Respiratory Disorders. Philadelphia, Lea & Febiger, 1991, pp 89–119.
Lumsden JM, Derksen FJ, Stick JA, Robinson NE: Use of flow-volume loops to evaluate upper airway obstruction in exercising Standardbreds. Am J Vet Res 54:766–775, 1993.
Ruggles AJ, Ross MW, Freeman DE: Endoscopic examination of normal paranasal sinuses in horses. Vet Surg 20:418–423, 1991.

Left Recurrent Laryngeal Neuropathy

HOWARD J. SEEHERMAN
North Grafton, Massachusetts

Upper airway obstruction caused by left recurrent laryngeal neuropathy (LRLN) results in an abnormal inspiratory noise during exercise and a variable degree of exercise intolerance in clinically affected horses. This condition has been classified as a motor neuron disease. Affected nerve cell bodies lose their ability to maintain a normal trophic influence on their nerve cell axons, resulting in a distal axonopathy or "dying back" phenomenon. Associated loss of nerve cell function results in neurogenic atrophy of the intrinsic laryngeal muscles innervated by the left recurrent laryngeal nerve. Progressive atrophy primarily affecting the left cricoarytenoideus dorsalis muscle (CAD) leads to impeded left arytenoid cartilage abduction and a decreased capacity of the upper airway to accommodate changes in air flow during exercise. Reduced performance in horses with LRLN has been attributed to exercise intolerance due to "lack of air." Lack of arytenoid abduction during exercise causes a distinctive inspiratory noise referred to as "roaring" or "whistling" and is considered an "unsoundness of wind" in many sport horse events.

In the majority of the cases, the etiology of LRLN remains unknown. In a small percentage of horses, this condition has been associated with trauma to the left recurrent laryngeal nerve, perivascular or perineural injection, guttural pouch mycosis, *Streptococcus equi* abscessation, and lead poisoning. A genetic basis for LRLN as a specific manifestation of a more generalized polyneuropathy has been proposed. Although the exact mechanism of inheritance has not been elucidated, the progeny of clinically affected horses have a much higher incidence of the condition compared with the progeny of clinically unaffected horses. Pathologic changes in the recurrent laryngeal nerve and the CAD muscle consistent with LRLN have been reported in neonates.

The incidence of clinically affected horses with total paralysis appears to be less than 10%. A larger number (70%) exhibit some degree of laryngeal asynchrony. An even larger percentage have palpable atrophy of the CAD muscle or exhibit abnormal conduction velocity based on electrolaryngography. Draft breeds and other large breed horses (>16 hands) appear to have a much higher incidence of LRLN compared with smaller breeds. Complete paralysis of the right arytenoid cartilage is less commonly observed and is usually associated with extravascular injection of irritant drugs damaging the right laryngeal nerve. Bilateral laryngeal neuropathy resulting in severe airway obstruction during exercise has also been observed.

DIAGNOSIS

Diagnosis of LRLN can be made based on a variable combination of presenting signs. These signs include palpable atrophy of the left CAD muscle, abnormal upper airway inspiratory noise during exercise, variable exercise intolerance, and resting endoscopy. Advanced diagnostic tests include endoscopy during exercise on a treadmill, respiratory function testing, exercise testing on a treadmill, and electrolaryngography.

Palpation

Palpation of the muscular process of the arytenoid cartilage represents a quick and reliable method for assessing atrophy of the CAD muscle. This technique is easily performed in the standing awake horse with the examiner positioned at the front of the horse facing forward. The first tracheal space and ventral aspect of the cricoid cartilage are located on the ventral midline just behind the angle of the mandible. Using firm pressure with the index fingers, the dorsal aspect of the body of the thyroid cartilage is located simultaneously on both sides of the neck under the tendon of insertion of the sternomandibularis muscle. The muscular process of the arytenoid cartilage and the thickness of the overlying CAD muscle can be assessed by moving the fingers in a circular manner just dorsal and cranial to the dorsal margin of the thyroid cartilage. The degree of atrophy can be graded from 1 to 4, corresponding to normal, mild, moderate, and severe atrophy. Horses with significant atrophy have a distinct knob or knuckle-like projection on the left side created by the exposed muscular process with minimal overlying muscle.

Inspiratory Noise

The most reliable diagnostic sign in clinically affected horses remains an abnormal upper airway noise associated with the inspiratory phase of respiration during exercise. The inspiratory phase of respiration coincides with the obvious flaring of the nostrils. The severity of the inspiratory noise increases with increased exercise intensity, increased temperature, and exaggerated flexion of the neck. Although an abnormal inspiratory noise is most often associated with LRLN, endoscopy during exercise on a treadmill has implicated vocal fold collapse, aryepiglottic ligament collapse, and dorsal or lateral pharyngeal wall collapse (see page 412) in cases without significant LRLN.

Exercise Intolerance

Sport horses with LRLN may not necessarily show signs of exercise intolerance. Horses participating in the cross-country phase of the 3-day event are the most likely to exhibit exercise intolerance. Significant exercise intolerance due to LRLN is rarely evident in racehorses competing over distances less than 1 mile, despite the presence of an abnormal inspiratory noise. In longer races, exercise intolerance occurs late in the race.

Endoscopy in the Resting Horse

Endoscopic evaluation of the upper airway in at-rest horses reveals a rhythmic increase in abduction of the arytenoid cartilages during inspiration and return to partial abduction during expiration. The magnitude of both asymmetric position and movement of the left arytenoid cartilage relative to the right can be graded on a scale of I to IV. Grade I horses have normal resting position and synchronous abduction during inspiration or breath-holding or following swallowing. Grade II represents normal resting position, asynchronous movement (left slower than right), but full abduction. Grade III horses exhibit a partially adducted position at rest, asynchronous movement, and only partial abduction. Grade IV represents an adducted resting position with no movement during inspiration (Fig. 1A). The most reproducible results are obtained without sedation and with the endoscope introduced from the left side.

Endoscopy During Exercise on a Treadmill

As the horse begins to exercise, the arytenoid cartilages can be seen endoscopically to alternately open and close in synchrony with breathing. With increased exercise intensity and respiratory effort, the arytenoid cartilages are maintained in the fully abducted position throughout the respiratory cycle. Continuous activity of the CAD muscles is required to maintain abduction and oppose the tendency for the arytenoid cartilages to adduct into the airway owing to the increased negative pressure generated in the larynx during inspiration.

Depending on the severity of the axonopathy and the degree of muscle atrophy, LRLN results in a variable ability to maintain the maximally abducted position of the affected arytenoid cartilage during exercise. In severely affected horses (grade IV) the left arytenoid is adducted into the airway during inspiration and passively abducted during

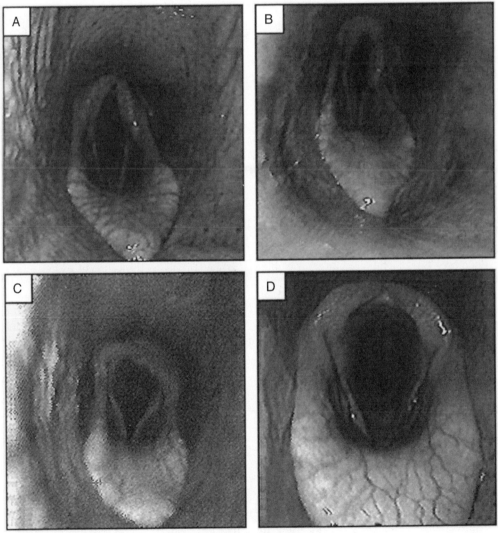

Figure 1. Endoscopic view of LRLN. (A) Resting evaluation; (B) evaluation during treadmill exercise; (C) evaluation during treadmill exercise following prosthetic laryngoplasty showing uncorrected vocal fold collapse; (D) evaluation during treadmill exercise following prosthetic laryngoplasty and bilateral vocal cordectomy showing the improved airway caliber. Magnification of D was increased to better illustrate the appearance of the vocal cordectomy.

expiration. Loss of abduction results in insufficient tension on vocal folds. Increased airway negative pressure results in unilateral or bilateral vocal fold collapse, further obstructing the airway (see Fig. 1B). Horses with severe LRLN alter the normal 1:1 ratio of respiratory frequency to stride frequency during the gallop, to varying patterns of alternating 1:1 and 1:2 ratios, further contributing to poor performance.

Comparisons of the results of endoscopic examination at rest and during exercise indicate that horses with grade I and II classifications are capable of full abduction during exercise. The majority of grade III horses also appear to be capable of partial or full abduction during exercise. Increased neuronal activation during exercise appears to be responsible for this seemingly paradoxical diagnostic dilemma of horses, with incomplete paralysis being more severely affected at rest than during exercise. Clinically affected grade III horses may start exercise with an adequate airway but gradually show progressive adduction of the left arytenoid cartilage, and they exhibit an inability to tense the vocal folds, resulting in an increasing intensity of inspiratory stridor and obstruction as the exercise is continued.

Respiratory Function Testing

Ventilatory alterations in horses with LRLN include an increase in inspiratory impedance (dynamic resistance to flow), increased inspiratory and expiratory trans-upper airway driving pressure, and reduced peak flows, particularly during inhalation. These changes are associated with decreased minute ventilation. Exercising horses with laryngeal hemiplegia also become more hypoxemic, hypercapnic, and acidotic compared with normal horses.

Exercise Testing on a Treadmill

Exercise efficiency has been postulated to decrease in horses with LRLN because of increased metabolic power requirements for breathing used to compensate for inspiratory obstruction. Increased metabolic power required for respiration also decreases total metabolic power available to locomotory muscles. During prolonged exercise, respiratory muscle fatigue due to increased breathing effort may also contribute to decreased performance. Decreased minute ventilation, hypoxemia, and hypercapnia also suggest a reduction in peak aerobic power (oxygen [O_2] peak) in horses with LRLN as a result of reduced flux in the transport steps responsible for delivering oxygen from air to the muscle mitochondria. A significant decrease in O_2 peak represents a severe disadvantage at exercise intensities such as racing because of increased reliance on anaerobic sources to maintain total metabolic power input. Treadmill exercise testing can be used to quantify exercise efficiency and O_2 peak in horses with LRLN by measuring oxygen consumption and lactate production as a function of speed. Performance can also be estimated from exercise test duration. No measurable change in exercise efficiency was detected in a group of Thoroughbred racehorses with high O_2 peak and crossbred horses with low O_2 peak using a reversible local anesthetic model to create grade IV LRLN. These results suggest that the ventilatory alterations caused by LRLN do not result in a measurable increase in the metabolic power required for breathing. However, induced

LRLN did result in a 15% reduction in O_2 peak and a 7% reduction in exercise test duration in the Thoroughbred racehorses. Similar results have been reported in racehorses with LRLN compared with control populations of clinically normal racehorses. In contrast, the nonracing cross-bred horses with induced LRLN did not have a reduction in either O_2 peak or exercise test duration. These results indicate that performance in Thoroughbred racehorses with high O_2 peak appears to be ventilation-limited and is significantly decreased by grade IV LRLN. Performance in sport horses does not appear to be ventilation-limited and in most cases is not affected by LRLN.

Electrolaryngography

Recurrent laryngeal nerve function can be determined by measuring latency (time) and latency rates (velocity) of the thoracolaryngeal reflex (slap test). Increased latency rate in horses with LRLN is the result of demyelination and loss of faster conducting wide-diameter nerve fibers. Latency rates show a high degree of variation in horses with LRLN. Although these measurements demonstrate a high incidence of LRLN, latency rates indicate that the progression of LRLN does not appear to be as rapid as was once thought.

TREATMENT

Treatment of perivascular or perineural injection induced LRLN includes topical dimethyl sulfoxide (DMSO), oral anti-inflammatory drugs, and subcutaneous dilution of the injected material with normal saline. In cases of exercise intolerance, correction of the inspiratory obstruction and reduction of the abnormal inspiratory noise generally requires surgical intervention. Care should be taken to rule out other causes of exercise intolerance such as lameness, lower respiratory disorders, cardiovascular abnormalities, reduced musculoskeletal strength, or thermoregulatory disorders before recommending surgical intervention. Establishing LRLN as the cause of exercise intolerance is especially important in sport horses and in racehorses competing over distances less than 1 mile where athletic performance may not be ventilation-limited. Surgical procedures used to improve upper airway function or to reduce inspiratory noise in horses with LRLN include prosthetic laryngoplasty, vocal fold resection (cordectomy), ventriculectomy, arytenoidectomy, and nerve muscle pedicle grafting. Horses with grade III and grade IV LRLN associated with inspiratory stridor and exercise intolerance are candidates for surgical intervention.

Prosthetic laryngoplasty alone or in combination with cordectomy and or ventriculectomy is the most commonly performed procedure. Respiratory function testing indicates that normal ventilatory parameters can be restored following prosthetic laryngoplasty for LRLN. Success rates for prosthetic laryngoplasty range from 40 to 60% in adult racehorses. Success rates in sport horses and 2-year-old racehorses are considerably higher (80–90%), which is related to the lack of ventilation limitation associated with athletic competition in these groups of horses. Correction of failed prosthetic laryngoplasty is best achieved with a second procedure. Success of subsequent attempts at surgical correction are limited by excessive scar tissue. In these cases, and in cases with arytenoid chondritis, arytenoidectomy is indicated.

Videoendoscopy during maximal exercise in a number of horses with prosthetic laryngoplasty and ventriculectomy has revealed that vocal fold occlusion and inspiratory stridor can still occur if the arytenoid cartilage is not abducted sufficiently at the time of surgery or if the position of the arytenoid changes in the postoperative period (see Fig. 1*C*). Horses in which bilateral chordectomy is performed in association with these other procedures appear to have larger airways (see Fig. 1*D*) and significantly decreased inspiratory stridor even if the arytenoid cartilages remain only partially abducted following surgery. Venticulectomy and cordectomy by themselves do not restore normal ventilation but have been used successfully for noise reduction in draft breeds.

Nerve muscle pedicle (NMP) grafts have recently been introduced as a surgical technique to restore normal upper airway function in horses with LRLN. The surgery involves a NMP created from the first cervical nerve and omohyo-

deus muscle transplanted into the left CAD muscle. In successful cases, normal upper airway function is restored in approximately 1 year. The prolonged time for return of function makes this procedure most suitable for young horses with grade III or IV LRLN or adult sport horses, which have longer athletic careers than racehorses.

Supplemental Readings

Hackett RP, Ducharme NG (eds): Upper airway diseases. *In* Robinson NE (ed): Current Therapy in Equine Medicine, ed 3. Philadelphia, WB Saunders, 1992, pp 265–297.

Morris EA, Seeherman HJ: Evaluation of upper respiratory tract function during strenuous exercise in horses. J Am Vet Med Assoc 196:431–438, 1990.

Russell AP, Slone DE: Performance analysis after prosthetic laryngoplasty and bilateral ventriculectomy for laryngeal hemiplegia in horses: 70 cases (1986–1991). J Am Vet Med Assoc 204:1235–1241, 1994.

Seeherman HJ, Morris E, O'Callaghan MW: Comprehensive clinical evaluation of performance. *In* Auer JA (ed): Equine Surgery. Philadelphia, WB Saunders, 1992, pp 1133–1173.

Seeherman HJ, Ehrlich PJ, Morris E: Physiological versus clinical consequences of left recurrent laryngeal neuropathy (LRLN). Equine Vet J 18[Suppl]:7–12, 1995.

Epiglottitis

ERIC TULLENERS
Kennett Square, Pennsylvania

The mucous membrane of the aryepiglottic fold attaches along the lateral free margins of the epiglottis and is loosely attached on the ventral, lingual, epiglottic surface. There is some redundancy to this mucous membrane, which allows for caudal and dorsal reflection of the epiglottis to help cover the opening to the larynx during swallowing. Inflammation affecting this tissue may result in intermittent or persistent epiglottic entrapment or epiglottitis.

The cause of epiglottitis is not known. Possible predisposing factors include pharyngeal inflammation from respiratory tract infection or inhaled allergens; mucosal irritation initiated by intermittent dorsal displacement of the soft palate, epiglottic entrapment, trauma from ingestion of foreign bodies, or poor quality roughage; inflammation caused by inhalation of track dirt; or nonspecific irritation caused by the stress of race training.

CLINICAL SIGNS AND DIAGNOSIS

Approximately 90% of the horses with epiglottitis are racehorses. Clinical signs include exercise intolerance, respiratory noise, coughing, and, less commonly, dysphagia and dyspnea. Epiglottitis is diagnosed by means of endoscopic examination and is observed as edema, reddening, and thickening of the epiglottis and aryepiglottic fold mucous membrane. Severe swelling and marked discoloration, primarily of the mucosal tissue that attaches loosely to the

lingual surface of the epiglottis, are common, and swelling of the lingual surface causes mild to marked dorsal elevation of the epiglottic axis (Fig. 1). Often, cartilage at the tip of the epiglottis is exposed, and granulation tissue is frequently seen. Chondritis of the epiglottic cartilage can develop and may result in epiglottic deformity during healing (Fig. 2).

In a series of 20 cases of epiglottitis, other commonly encountered endoscopic abnormalities included intermittent or persistent dorsal displacement of the soft palate (75%), dorsal deviation of the epiglottic axis (55%), ulceration or thickening of the free border of the soft palate (40%), exposure of cartilage of the epiglottic tip (40%), and subepiglottic granulation tissue (30%).

TREATMENT

Affected horses should receive enforced rest for a minimum of 7 to 14 days with endoscopic re-evaluation before resuming training of any kind. Antimicrobial medication may be of benefit if there is evidence of infection. Anti-inflammatory medication including nonsteroidal anti-inflammatory drugs, a pharyngeal spray, and systemic corticosteroids have been successful in resolving the epiglottic edema and inflammation. After the initial endoscopic examination, the horse should receive 0.044 mg/kg dexamethasone and 4.4 mg/kg phenylbutazone intravenously (IV). Phenylbutazone is continued (2.2 mg/kg p.o. b.i.d.) for 7

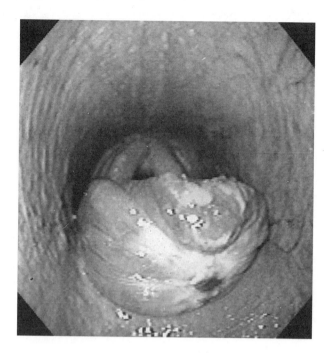

Figure 1. Endoscopic photograph of an 8-year-old Standardbred gelding race-horse with chronic untreated epiglottitis. Notice the marked thickening on the lingual surface of the epiglottis.

to 10 days. Horses with mild inflammatory changes should receive dexamethasone (0.022 mg/kg p.o. s.i.d.) for 3 days and then 0.022 mg/kg p.o., 48 hours later. Horses with more substantial inflammatory changes or ulceration are given a more protracted tapering dose of corticosteroids consisting of prednisone (0.8 mg/kg p.o. s.i.d.) in their morning feed for 7 days. The same dose is then given every other day for three treatments. The dose of prednisone is then reduced to 0.4 mg/kg given every other day for three treatments.

Topical administration of a pharyngeal medication also appears to provide benefit. A 10-French catheter° is advanced into the floor of the nasal passage into the pharynx. Ten to 15 ml of a mixture of furacin, dimethyl sulfoxide (DMSO), glycerin, and prednisolone† can be sprayed slowly through this catheter, watching for swallowing movements, at 12-hour intervals for 7 days. An endoscopic

---

°*Monoject, Division of Sherwood Medical, St. Louis, MO*
†*750 ml (2 mg/ml) of furacin, 250 ml (90 mg/ml) of DMSO, 1000 ml of glycerin (99% solution), 2000 mg of prednisolone, prepared by New Bolton Center Pharmacy, Kennett Square, PA*

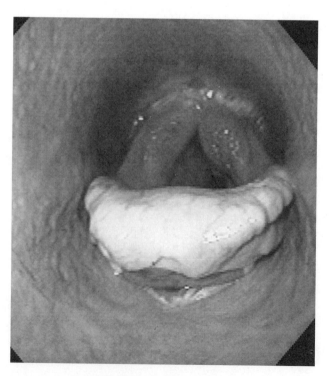

Figure 2. Endoscopic photograph of a 6-year-old Thoroughbred gelding racehorse with chronic untreated epiglottitis. Notice the blunting and deformity of the epiglottic tip, and the extensive thickening, mucosal ulceration, and exposed granulation tissue on the lingual epiglottic surface. This horse also suffered from severe problems with intermittent dorsal displacement of the soft palate, and the free border of the soft palate was extensively ulcerated and fibrotic.

examination should be performed 10 to 14 days after initiating treatment to evaluate the extent of healing and determine if the horse may return to exercise. Additional rest and anti-inflammatory medication may be continued as needed, based on the results of this examination.

PROGNOSIS

Owners must be warned that epiglottitis is a serious, potentially performance-limiting problem in horses used for athletic endeavors. In one report, 50% of 16 racehorses had performance-limiting complications. Epiglottic entrapment may develop in approximately 5% of horses after treatment for epiglottitis. The most serious complication was intermittent or persistent dorsal displacement of the soft palate. Persistent dorsal displacement of the soft palate may develop during healing of epiglottitis as a result of

formation of excessive subepiglottic fibrosis, persistence of granulating mucosal ulcers, or development of epiglottic cartilage deformity that causes epiglottic shortening. These anatomic changes may cause loss of the normal synchrony between the soft palate and the epiglottis or may alter the normal relationship between the free edge of the soft palate and the base of the epiglottis. Epiglottic deformities that may occur include excessive shortening and thickening of the epiglottic tip and thickening of the lingual surface of the epiglottis. Surgical intervention during the acute inflammatory phase of the disease is not recommended because of the potential for increasing scarring and subsequent problems with dorsal displacement of the soft palate.

Supplemental Readings

Hawkins JF, Tulleners EP: Epiglottitis in horses: 20 cases (1988–1993). J Am Vet Med Assoc 205(11):1577–1580, 1994.
Speirs VC, Tulleners EP, Ducharme NG, Hackett RP: Larynx. In Auer JA (ed): Equine Surgery. Philadelphia, WB Saunders, 1992, pp 460–480.

Soft Palate Ulceration

ERIC TULLENERS
Kennett Square, Pennsylvania

Ulceration of the free border of the soft palate is a condition that primarily affects horses used for athletic purposes. The etiology of this condition is unknown, but repeated trauma to the soft palate during exercise is believed to be the primary initiating cause in most horses. Pre-existing inflammation of the pharynx may predispose the soft palate to this condition.

The horse is an obligate nasal breather, and under normal breathing conditions, the V- to U-shaped free border of the soft palate lies in close contact with the base of the ventral, lingual surface of the epiglottis. During high-speed exercise, relatively unsupported soft tissue structures such as the free border of the soft palate undoubtedly experience substantial vibrational forces. Intermittent dorsal displacement of the soft palate (IDDSP) may occur from loss of the normal snug seal between the free border of the soft palate and the base of the epiglottis. Repeated trauma caused by the normal pressure swings or IDDSP may incite the inflammation and ulceration seen on the free border of the soft palate in horses used for athletic purposes. Severe pharyngeal lymphoid hyperplasia can also contribute to inflammatory changes of the mucosa and of the underlying muscle and supportive tissues and, thus, may predispose to ulcer formation.

An important interaction and relationship exist between the redundant mucous membrane of the aryepiglottic fold tissue on the lingual surface of the epiglottis, the base of the epiglottis, and the free border of the soft palate. Epiglottic contour and size, including length, width, and thickness, may therefore also play a role in the development of dorsal displacement of the soft palate and ulcer formation.

CLINICAL EXAMINATION

Horses with soft palate ulceration present with various clinical signs, most of them referable to the coexistent presence of intermittent or persistent IDDSP. Ideally, the horse should be only loosely restrained by a nose twitch or in stocks and examined without sedation or tranquilization. Critical evaluation of the free border of the soft palate should be a routine part of every endoscopic examination. Visible inflammatory changes seen on the free border of the soft palate during routine endoscopic examination occur by far most frequently in horses such as racehorses or 3-day event horses that are subjected to strenuous high-speed exercise. Soft palate function should be evaluated by inducing multiple swallowing movements and by occluding the nasal passages to cause forced inspiration. Most normal horses with an anatomically normal-appearing pharynx and larynx on endoscopic examination only infrequently dorsally displace the soft palate and then usually only fleetingly before they swallow and replace it beneath the epiglottis. Advancing the endoscope into the proximal trachea usually induces coughing and a protective swallowing movement, causing transient dorsal displacement of the soft palate. By withdrawing the endoscope to a position in the rostral pharynx, generally the free border of the soft palate can be briefly examined before the horse swallows, replacing the palate into a normal position ventral to the epiglottis. The free border should be thin and pliable and pink in color (Fig. 1). Early signs of disease include edema and mild reddening, particularly on the midline (Fig. 2). Mild focal ulceration and reddening may progress to more diffuse

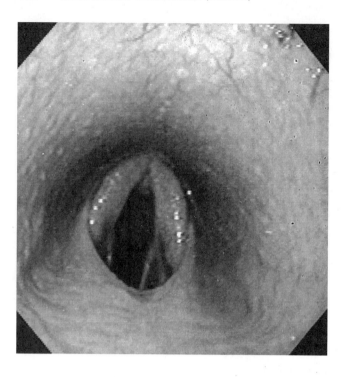

Figure 1. Free border of the soft palate in a 3-year-old Thoroughbred filly racehorse with normal soft palate function. Note the typical U shape and the thin, uniform-appearing margin.

inflammatory changes along the entire free border of the soft palate if left untreated or if the problem with dorsal displacement of the soft palate and/or epiglottic entrapment is particularly severe (Fig. 3). Complete erosion of the soft palate, producing a typical "keyhole" or notched appearance of the central free border, may lead one to believe that the soft palate has been trimmed when, in fact, this merely represents chronic wear-and-tear inflammatory changes (Fig. 4).

TREATMENT

Yearlings and 2- and 3-year-old horses may have extensive residual pharyngeal lymphoid hyperplasia that extends from the roof and walls of the pharynx down onto the soft palate. These inflammatory changes may extend into the submucosa and affect the palatine muscle, as previously described. This situation apparently may exacerbate the problem with IDDSP in some horses. The best treatment

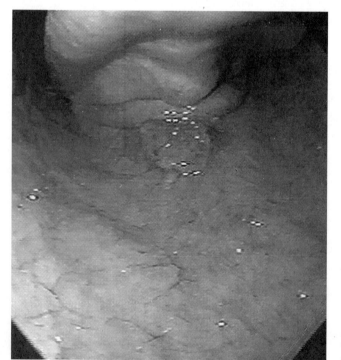

Figure 2. Free border of the soft palate in contact with the lingual surface of the epiglottic base in a 4-year-old Thoroughbred gelding racehorse with a clinical diagnosis of epiglottic entrapment and intermittent dorsal displacement of the soft palate. Note the mild edema at the interface.

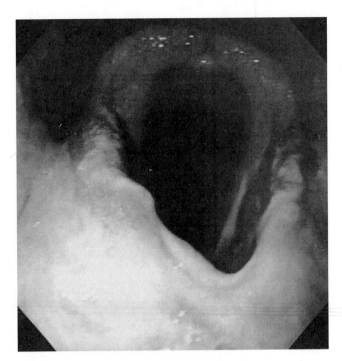

Figure 3. Inflammation, ulceration, and thickening of the free border of the soft palate seen in an 8-year-old Thoroughbred gelding racehorse with persistent dorsal displacement of the soft palate and concomitant badly ulcerated entrapment of the epiglottis by the aryepiglottic folds. This problem was corrected by careful excision of the most severely involved tissue (approximately 10 mm of the free border) of the soft palate and by a central one-third resection of the aryepiglottic folds.

for IDDSP with or without soft palate ulceration in this age group is to take the horse out of work and to treat the upper or lower respiratory tract infections present. Appropriate anti-inflammatory medication and restricted exercise should also be provided until the diffuse pharyngeal inflammation subsides. In some horses this may necessitate eliminating them from training until further pharyngeal maturation occurs.

As the horse gets older, repetitive trauma may lead to extensive ulceration, which, if not allowed to heal, eventually causes a loss of the normal thin, pliable appearance of the soft palate. The result may be infiltration with fibroblasts and deposition of collagen. Therefore, it is important to recognize changes in the free border early on and treat them aggressively while they are still reversible. Enforced rest and anti-inflammatory medication should be provided, ideally allowing complete resolution of visible changes before resuming training. If the horse has an epiglottic entrapment, this should be corrected ideally by axial midline division in most horses. With patience and appropriate

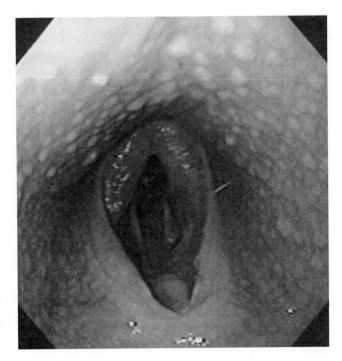

Figure 4. Typical notched "keyhole" appearance of the central free border of the soft palate associated with chronic problems with intermittent dorsal displacement of the soft palate in a 4-year-old Thoroughbred mare racehorse. The central free border has been completely eroded away and is replaced with a white fibrous scar on the margin. This horse was treated successfully with anti-inflammatory and antimicrobial medication and by excision of the granulation tissue mass located on the axial surface of the right arytenoid.

therapy, an impressive amount of progress can be made toward resolving even very serious-appearing inflammatory changes.

Most horses with typical mild-to-moderate inflammatory changes respond well to 10 to 14 days of exercise restricted to hand walking and stall and paddock confinement. Initially, 0.044 mg/kg dexamethasone and 4.4 mg/kg phenylbutazone are given intravenously (IV). Phenylbutazone is continued at a dose of 2.2 mg/kg p.o. b.i.d. for 7 to 10 days. Horses with mild inflammatory changes should be given dexamethasone (0.022 mg/kg p.o. s.i.d.) for 3 days and then 0.022 mg/kg p.o. 48 hours later. Horses with more substantial inflammatory changes or ulceration are given a more protracted tapering dose of corticosteroids consisting of prednisone (0.8 mg/kg p.o. s.i.d.) in their morning feed for 7 days. The same dose is then given every other day for three treatments. The dose of prednisone is then reduced to 0.4 mg/kg given every other day for three treatments.

Topical administration of a pharyngeal medication also appears to provide benefit. Ten to 15 ml of a mixture of furacin, dimethyl sulfoxide (DMSO), glycerin, and prednisolone° can be sprayed slowly, watching for swallowing

°750 ml (2 mg/ml) of furacin, 250 ml (90 mg/ml) of DMSO, 1000 ml of glycerin (99% solution), 2000 mg of prednisolone, prepared by New Bolton Center Pharmacy, Kennett Square, PA

movements into the pharynx, through a 10-French catheter.° This treatment should be performed at 12-hour intervals for 7 days. An endoscopic examination should be performed 10 to 14 days after initiating this treatment to evaluate the extent of healing and to determine if the horse may return to exercise. Additional rest and anti-inflammatory medication may be continued as needed based on the results of this examination.

Horses with severe ulceration and fibrosis of the free border of the soft palate may need to have 5 to 10 mm of this severely thickened tissue sharply excised via laryngotomy if complete resolution does not occur with the previously described medical treatment. Routine laryngotomy aftercare and 4 to 6 weeks of restricted exercise generally result in uneventful healing.

Supplemental Readings

Blythe LL, Cardinet GH III, Meagher DM, Brown MP, Wheat JD: Palatal myositis in horses with dorsal displacement of the soft palate. J Am Vet Med Assoc 183(7):781–785, 1983.
Ducharme NG: Physiology of upper airway obstruction in exercising horses. Proc Am Coll Vet Surg Vet Symp 1993, p 169.
Nickel R, Schummer A, Seiferle E, Sack WO: The viscera of the domestic mammals, ed 2. Berlin, Verlag Paul Parey, 1973, p 73.

°Monoject, Division of Sherwood Medical, St. Louis, MO

Soft Tissue Collapse of the Upper Airway

ERIC J. PARENTE
Kennett Square, Pennsylvania

The pharynx is an intricate system of soft tissue that needs to be malleable enough to move food and water into the esophagus and rigid enough to maintain an open airway under extreme swings in pressures. At times, the system fails, and one of several forms of pharyngeal collapse occurs. A diagnosis of dynamic pharyngeal collapse must be made at speed by endoscopy during exercise on a treadmill (Fig. 1A). Often a "soft"-looking pharynx in a standing animal becomes much more expansive and rigid-appearing during exercise. In the more severely affected cases of pharyngeal collapse, a distinctly abnormal noise originates from the upper respiratory tract (see Fig. 1B). In other cases, pharyngeal collapse may precede another dynamic obstruction of the upper airway, such as dorsal displacement of the soft palate.

DORSAL DISPLACEMENT OF THE SOFT PALATE

Although horses have been treated for this disorder (see Fig. 1C) for many years, its cause remains unknown. The results obtained with different surgical treatments have been extremely variable. This is in part because many horses treated for a suspected displacement problem based on history and endoscopy at rest do not actually displace their palate at speed, but have other problems. Furthermore, displacement of the palate may occur in conjunction with other disorders and for a variety of reasons. More detailed information is available on page 415.

PHARYNGEAL COLLAPSE

Pharyngeal collapse without displacement of the soft palate has been seen in many horses, and probably goes unrecognized unless horses are examined on a treadmill. Pharyngeal collapse usually occurs during inspiration and can be dorsoventral, circumferential, or lateral.

Dorsoventral collapse is most common and the animal is more severely affected during neck flexion. In most cases, collapse does not have a dramatic effect on the horse's performance and is not associated with abnormal noise. Circumferential collapse usually causes greater compro-

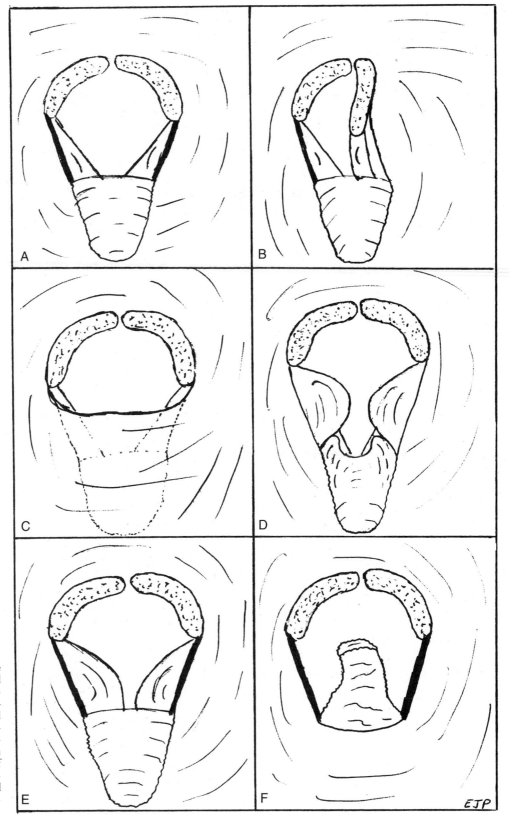

Figure 1. Schematic endoscopic view of the larynx during high-speed exercise. (A) Normal larynx. (B) Dynamic collapse of left arytenoid—laryngeal hemiplegia. (C) Dorsal displacement of the soft palate—epiglottis in dashed lines under the palate. (D) Axial deviation of the aryepiglottic folds—base of epiglottis is rolled up at the attachment to the folds. (E) Vocal cord deviation. (F) Epiglottic retroversion.

mise of respiratory function, but also does not cause a loud abnormal noise. These forms of collapse have been seen in both Standardbreds and Thoroughbreds of all ages.

Lateral wall collapse is more unusual and is seen primarily in Thoroughbreds younger than 2 or older than 5 years of age. An abnormal noise is heard by the owner or trainer even before horses have trained enough to race. No abnormalities are observed during endoscopy of the resting horse. Some horses improve as they mature but others, which are more severely affected, do not. The pressure profiles in the upper airway of severely affected horses are dramatically altered.

Because skeletal muscle is the framework for maintaining pharyngeal stability, training appears crucial in treating horses with all forms of pharyngeal collapse. Each horse needs to be trained as an individual, and horses with pharyngeal collapse seem to do worse when raced frequently. Training frequently is not as detrimental because the distance traveled is shorter, particularly in Thoroughbreds, and the pharyngeal muscles are less fatigued. No surgical or medical treatment is available, although in cases of severe collapse systemic anti-inflammatory drugs are given to reduce the associated inflammation.

AXIAL DEVIATION OF THE ARYEPIGLOTTIC FOLDS

This is seen most commonly in young Thoroughbreds (see Fig. 1D). The problem can be intermittent, and may be dependent upon the frequency of racing. The diagnosis is made only during endoscopy on a treadmill and has a wide range of severity. Mild deviation of one of the two folds is relatively common but is of no clinical significance. It becomes clinically significant when one or both of the aryepiglottic folds impinge on the glottis, and this is associated with a "poor finish" or "stopping." With this degree of severity a "roar"-like noise can be heard by a discerning ear. Axial deviation of the aryepiglottic folds also has been noted in horses with less than full abduction of their arytenoids, and can precede dorsal displacement of the soft palate.

Horses with this disorder appear to benefit from longer periods of time between races, and they often improve with age. Laser resection of the aryepiglottic folds has been used in the few horses that do not respond favorably to more conservative treatment.

VOCAL CORD DEVIATION

This disorder is seen in both Standardbreds and Thoroughbreds of any age, and often in horses older than 3 years of age (see Fig. 1E). It has been associated with less than maximal abduction of the ipsilateral arytenoid, and severe axial deviation of the contralateral aryepiglottic fold. The degree of noise heard is commensurate with the amount of narrowing across the glottis. The diagnosis can be made only by endoscopy during exercise.

Resection of the offending tissue is recommended in most cases. This can be performed endoscopically with a laser or through a standard laryngotomy with a scissors. If the deviation of the vocal cord is a result of poor abduction of the arytenoid, the arytenoid abduction must be improved by use of laryngeal prosthesis ("tie-back" procedure), and the vocal cord may or may not require resection.

EPIGLOTTIC RETROVERSION

This relatively rare abnormality has been seen in both Thoroughbreds and Standardbreds of any age (see Fig. 1F). It creates a loud resonant inspiratory flutter as the epiglottis is sucked up into the airway and retroflexes into the glottis with each inspiration. The problem appears to be associated with a return to training after severe respiratory disease, and the severity of the disorder increases with continued exercise. Endoscopic examination of the standing horse is normal. Epiglottic retroversion appears to be the result of dysfunction of the rostral hyoid muscles because it can be reproduced by local anesthesia in that region. Before this knowledge was obtained, epiglottic augmentation had been attempted in two cases with questionable success. No other attempts at treatment are known to this author.

Supplemental Readings

Ducharme NG: Dynamic pharyngeal collapse. *In* Robinson NE (ed): Current Therapy in Equine Medicine, ed 3. Philadelphia, WB Saunders, 1992, pp 283–285.

Hackett RP, Ducharme NG, Rehder RS: Use of the high-speed treadmill in management of horses with dorsal displacement of the soft palate. Proc 38th Annu Conv Am Assoc Equine Pract, 1992, p 153.

Parente EJ, Martin BB, Tulleners EP, Ross MW: Upper respiratory dysfunctions in horses during high-speed exercise. Proc 40th Annu Conv Am Assoc Equine Pract, 1994, pp 81–82.

Strand E, Staempfli HR: Dynamic collapse of the roof of the nasopharynx as a cause of poor performance in a Standardbred colt. Equine Vet J 25:252–254, 1993.

Intermittent Dorsal Displacement of the Soft Palate

NORM G. DUCHARME

RICHARD P. HACKETT

Ithaca, New York

Dorsal displacement of the soft palate (DDSP) may be either persistent or intermittent. Persistent displacement of the soft palate may be the result of either functional disorders, such as impaired innervation or myopathy of pharyngeal musculature, or anatomic abnormalities, for example, marked epiglottic hypoplasia, subepiglottic or palatine cyst, and subepiglottic cicatrix. This disorder is generally accompanied by dysphagia as evidenced by the discharge of water or chewed feed at the nostrils and by signs of tracheal aspiration of ingesta, that is, coughing and purulent nasal and tracheal exudates. Affected animals are markedly exercise-intolerant and may make snoring or gurgling sounds at rest and during work. In affected horses, palate displacement is readily observed during endoscopic examination at rest, and the free border of the palate does not return to its normal subepiglottic position despite repeated swallows.

In contrast, horses with intermittent displacement of the soft palate are typically normal at rest and light work but may exhibit exercise intolerance and respiratory noise during strenuous exercise. During resting endoscopic examination of the horse at rest, the palate is not displaced or is only transiently displaced. Dysphagia is not a feature of this disorder. Intermittent dorsal displacement of the soft palate has been reported as a common cause of upper airway obstruction in racehorses. It is also observed in show horses as a cause of abnormal noise, leading to lower scoring by judges. Intermittent DDSP rarely occurs at rest, and thus endoscopic surveys have likely underestimated the prevalence of this problem. Of 151 horses presented to the Equine Performance Testing Clinic (EPTC) at Cornell University with complaints of respiratory problems or poor athletic performance, 29 horses (19%) were diagnosed by videoendoscopy and airway pressure profile determinations during exercise on a high-speed treadmill to have DDSP. The prevalence of tongue-ties in racehorses is further evidence that DDSP is at least perceived to be a very common problem.

ETIOPATHOPHYSIOLOGY

Although intermittent DDSP has been recognized since 1949, the cause of this condition is still a mystery. Early hypotheses that this problem was the result of paresis of palatal muscles have not been supported by histopathologic examination. The hypothesis that the soft palate was abnormally long led to treatment of DDSP by resection of the caudal edge of the soft palate (staphylectomy). Elongation of the soft palate is no longer believed to be a factor in DDSP. Factors that lead to or facilitate dislocation at the laryngopalatal junction are (Fig. 1): (1) open-mouth breathing leading to lifting of the soft palate; (2) caudal retraction of the tongue leading to lifting of the soft palate; (3) more negative pressure in the nasopharynx; (4) hypoplastic or flaccid epiglottis; (5) incompetent laryngopalatal seal; (6) increased caudal traction on the larynx; (7) excessive head flexion; and (8) lack of pharyngeal tone associated with unfitness.

In 1981, Cook introduced the "button-hole" theory, which is currently thought to best represent morphologic events associated with soft palate displacement. He described the soft palate in horses as a continuum of soft tissue extending from the hard palate and terminating caudally as the confluence of the palatopharyngeal arches that cover the esophageal orifice. The caudal-free margin of the soft palate and the palatopharyngeal arches together form the intrapharyngeal ostium (i.e., the button-hole), producing an airtight seal around the arytenoid and epiglottic cartilages (the button). Cook theorized that in patients displacing the soft palate dorsally during exercise, the epi-

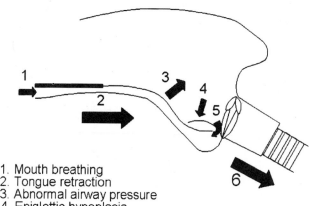

1. Mouth breathing
2. Tongue retraction
3. Abnormal airway pressure
4. Epiglottic hypoplasia
5. Incomplete laryngopalatal seal
6. Laryngeal retraction

Figure 1. Summary of conventional hypothesized causes of DDSP: (1) open-mouth breathing leading to lifting of the soft palate; (2) caudal retraction of the tongue leading to lifting of the soft palate; (3) more negative pressure in the nasopharynx; (4) hypoplastic or flaccid epiglottis; (5) incompetent laryngopalatal seal; and (6) increased caudal traction on the larynx.

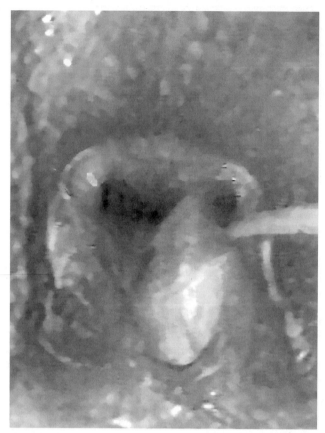

Figure 2. Complete retroversion of the epiglottic cartilage during inspiration in a 3-year-old female Standardbred during treadmill exercise. Note the maintenance of soft palate position despite lack of epiglottic contact.

glottis becomes unhooked from the free edge of the soft palate. This disrupts the normally airtight seal of the intrapharyngeal ostium around the arytenoid and epiglottic cartilages and allows the soft palate to create a functional obstruction of the airway. In support of the hypothesis that DDSP results from an unhooking of the epiglottic cartilage from the soft palate, Linford reported on the association of epiglottic hypoplasia with DDSP.

The authors are unsure of the contribution of the epiglottic cartilage to maintenance of the normal position of the soft palate because of the following observations: (1) many horses without DDSP demonstrate a flaccid epiglottis at rest but have a normal-appearing epiglottic cartilage during exercise. The authors have also seen horses with apparently proper stiffness of the epiglottic cartilage at rest, that during exercise experience epiglottic flaccidity and DDSP. (2) Experimentally, the authors have created extreme flaccidity of the epiglottis leading to its retroversion during inspiration (Fig. 2). The soft palate maintained normal position with no epiglottic contact at all. A recent study suggests that a flaccid and/or hypoplastic epiglottis (and without Teflon* augmentation) did not affect postoperative success in horses undergoing surgical treatment of DDSP.

Teflon paste: Mentor Polytef paste for injection, Mentor O and O, Norwell, MA

CLINICAL PRESENTATION

Horses affected with intermittent DDSP typically have no abnormalities at rest. Clinical signs are nonprogressive and may include exercise intolerance, poor performance, and intermittent noise production at exercise. Dorsal displacement of the soft palate occurs during high-speed exercise, leading to acute breathing difficulty usually referred to as "choking up" or "swallowing the tongue."

A gurgling vibrating noise most obvious on expiration is noted. This gurgling noise has been observed during treadmill videoendoscopy to be caused by vibration of the caudal edge of the soft palate on expiration. Upper airway pressure measurements in horses experiencing soft palate displacement revealed that the tracheal and transpharyngeal pressures increase during expiration, suggesting that DDSP primarily causes an expiratory obstruction. The pharyngeal pressure is greatly diminished on expiration, suggesting a deviation of the air flow into the oropharynx. This is consistent with the open-mouth breathing frequently seen in horses with DDSP.

DIAGNOSIS

The diagnosis of intermittent DDSP is made by correlation of clinical signs and endoscopic observations. The examiner should be aware that some normal horses displace their palate during endoscopic examination, a tendency exaggerated by sedation, excessive restraint, or anxiety. On endoscopy, DDSP is recognized by the lack of a visible epiglottic cartilage and the free edge of a membrane in front of the rima glottidis (Fig. 3). Unlike arytenoepiglottic entrapment, the outline of the epiglottic cartilage is obscured in horses with DDSP. If DDSP is not observed

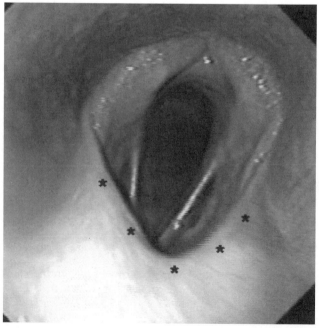

Figure 3. DDSP is recognized by the lack of visible epiglottic cartilage and the free edge of membrane (°) in front of the rima glottidis.

during endoscopic examination of the horse at rest but one suspects that it is occurring during exercise, three specific evaluations are made.

1. Swallowing is induced by touching the larynx with the endoscope and observing if DDSP can be induced. A presumptive diagnosis of DDSP is made if clinical signs of DDSP are present historically and the soft palate displaces dorsally and is maintained in this position for 10 seconds or more, or maintains this position despite multiple attempts to swallow.

2. The external nares are occluded to accentuate the intrapharyngeal inspiratory pressures and induce caudal retraction of the larynx. Again, a presumptive diagnosis can be made if the previously described conditions are met.

3. Because epiglottic hypoplasia and/or flaccidity have been associated with the occurrence of DDSP, the clinician may suspect DDSP if careful examination of the epiglottis reveals abnormality of epiglottic shape, size, and length.

The clinician must remember that diagnosis of DDSP in the resting horse is presumptive. Videoendoscopic examination during exercise on a treadmill has revealed that many horses can have temporary DDSP at rest but not during exercise, and that up to 30% of horses with clinical signs of DDSP have other dynamic abnormalities such as the axial collapse of arytenoepiglottic membrane, intermittent epiglottic entrapment, or pharyngeal collapse.

TREATMENT

Medical Management

Treatment is first directed at modifying or eliminating factors associated with the occurrence of DDSP. Unfit horses should have their level of fitness raised before owners consider surgical treatment. Horses with pharyngeal inflammation should first be treated with systemic (phenylbutazone or flunixin meglumine) and topical anti-inflammatory agents. The latter are usually administered by passing a flexible rubber tube* via the nasal passages into the nasopharynx. The authors use 10 ml once or twice daily of a solution containing 250 ml of glycerine, 50 ml prednisolone† (25 mg/ml), 250 ml dimethyl sulfoxide‡ and 500 ml nitrofurazone.§ Changing the bit to keep the tongue under the bit (i.e., a **W** bit) and tack modifications to decrease head flexion should be investigated.

Two additional procedures appear to be relatively successful in reducing the occurrence of DDSP—the tonguetie and the figure-8 nose band. For the tongue-tie to be effective, it should be placed at the frenulum of the tongue and then secured to the rostral aspect of the interdental space. One of the more effective treatments is use of a figure-8 nose band to prevent opening of the mouth and thus lifting the palate and breaking the laryngopalatal seal.

Some trainers have observed that horses may displace

*8 to 14 French feeding tube, Sovereign feeding tube, Sherwood Medical, St. Louis, MO
†Prednisolone acetate, Steris Laboratory, Phoenix, AZ
‡90% Dimethyl sulfoxide, Domoso, Syntex Animal Health, West Des Moines, IA
§Nitrofurazone, The Butler Company, Columbus, OH

the palate if their concentration is changed by whipping. Some horses also displace their palate as speed is being changed, perhaps also attributable to a change in concentration. These are, of course, very subjective observations but are easy to investigate in an individual horse. Others have reported to the authors that the addition of dietary supplements to calm nervous horses may reduce the occurrence of DDSP.

Surgical Management

Staphylectomy

Staphylectomy (resection of the caudal border of the soft palate) was the first surgical procedure proposed to correct DDSP and was based on the hypothesis of elongation of the soft palate. It is no longer believed that elongation of the soft palate is a significant factor in the etiology of intermittent DDSP. If the button-hole theory is considered, clinicians may conclude that staphylectomy should be harmful to horses with DDSP. This procedure, alone or in combination with other procedures, has nonetheless remained a relatively popular treatment. Proponents of this procedure suggest that stiffening (scarring) of the caudal aspect of the soft palate induced by staphylectomy reduces the likelihood that DDSP will occur and that a shorter palate is less obstructive and will more easily return to a normal subepiglottic position if displacement still occurs.

Under general anesthesia, the horse is placed in dorsal recumbency and a laryngotomy is performed via the cricothyroid ligament. The caudal free edge of the soft palate is identified and a crescent section of the soft palate (1 cm at the midline and tapering to each side) is resected using Satinsky scissors. The cricothyroid membrane is reapposed using number 0 polyglactin 910 in a simple continuous pattern. Closure of the rest of the laryngotomy is optional. Postoperatively, parenteral anti-inflammatory agents are given for 3 days and antibiotics (procaine penicillin G or trimethoprim-sulfamethoxazole) for 5 to 7 days. Training can be resumed in 2 to 3 weeks. Recent reports indicate a success rate of 60% following this procedure.

Complications of soft palate resection can be observed if too large a section of palate is resected. In these cases, the barrier between the oropharynx and nasopharynx is incompetent and food particles enter the nasopharynx. This leads to signs of tracheal or pulmonary aspiration. In addition, if the soft palate is too short, air flow on expiration reaches the ventral surface of the soft palate and leads to displacement.

Strap Muscle Resection

Resection of portions of the ventral strap muscles has been a common surgical treatment for horses with DDSP. This procedure is consistent with the current button-hole theory and has minimal risk of complications. Strap muscle resection attempts to address the problem of caudal traction of the larynx as a cause of laryngopalatal dislocation leading to DDSP. The muscles that are addressed surgically are the sternothyroid, sternohyoid, and omohyoid muscles. Although the best success rate was reported when all three muscles were transected, the need for general anesthesia, and the high incidence of postoperative seromas and incisional infection combined with a similar success rate had led to popularity of resection of only the sternohyoid and sternothyroid muscles.

With the horse standing, and after infiltration of local anesthetic, a 10-cm ventral midline incision is made at the junction of the middle and proximal trachea. The incision is extended through the subcutaneous fascia to expose the sternohyoideus muscle. Using a curved forceps, each sternohyoid muscle is undermined and transected at its proximal section. The section of muscle distal to the transection site is grasped and pulled cranially to enable a distal transection to remove an approximately 15-cm section of muscle. Resection of the sternohyoideus muscles exposes the smaller sternothyroid muscles on the ventral surface of the trachea. A section of each of these muscles is resected in the same fashion. The skin is closed in an appropriate fashion.

If resection of the omohyoid muscles is elected, the horse must be placed in dorsal recumbency under general anesthesia. A 20-cm ventral midline incision is made at the junction of the middle and proximal trachea. The incision is extended through the subcutaneous fascia and the strap muscles exposed. The sternohyoid and sternothyroid muscles are resected as described earlier. A section of the omohyoid is exposed from its medial surface near the sternohyoid extending laterally near the jugular vein. This section of omohyoid is then resected as described for the sternohyoid and sternothyroid muscles. Careful evaluation and ligation of all vessels is made and the subcutaneous tissues and skin are closed after placement of Penrose drains.

Postoperatively, a pressure bandage is applied (if omohyoid resection was made) and anti-inflammatory agents are administered for 3 days and antibiotics for 5 to 7 days. The horse is kept in a stall and is walked daily for 2 weeks. Training can be resumed 2 weeks after surgery. Complications are usually minor in severity and are related to incisional seromas or abscess requiring appropriate drainage. No long-term complications are noted except for the cosmetic defect associated with lack of strap muscle at the operative site. A recent survey indicates a success rate of 59% after surgery.

Combined Staphylectomy and Sternothyroid Muscle Resection

This technique, introduced by Lewellyn, is the authors' current treatment of choice for both Standardbreds and Thoroughbreds with intermittent DDSP. The sternothyroid muscle/tendon resection results in less dead space than the more extensive strap muscle resection and thus less seroma and incisional infection. When performing the staphylectomy, if less than 1 cm of the caudal border of the soft palate is resected, coughing and regurgitation are not postoperative problems. Therefore, the authors see no advantage in performing these procedures in succession rather than at the same anesthetic procedure.

Under general anesthesia, a ventral midline incision is made as in laryngotomy but extending 5 cm more caudally. After extending the incision through the subcutaneous tissue and bluntly dissecting between the paired sternohyoid muscles, dissection is carried laterally to expose the caudolateral border of the thyroid cartilage. The tendon of insertion of the sternothyroid muscle onto the thyroid cartilage is identified and transected. Removal of a section of the muscle and its tendon is optional.

A laryngotomy and staphylectomy is then performed as described earlier. Postoperatively, parenteral anti-inflammatory agents are given for 3 days. Training is often resumed in 2 to 3 days. A recent report indicates a success rate of 60% following this procedure.

Epiglottic Augmentation

This procedure was developed to stiffen the epiglottic cartilage of horses with epiglottic flaccidity leading to DDSP. It has been shown in experimental patients to enhance the thickness and stiffness of the epiglottic cartilage.

Under general anesthesia and after a laryngotomy, the epiglottic cartilage is inverted into the lumen of the larynx, exposing the ventral surface of the epiglottis. Using an injector, 3 to 7 ml of Teflon paste is injected submucosally in three craniocaudal lines. Postoperatively, parenteral anti-inflammatory agents are given for 3 days. Training can resume in 4 to 6 weeks. A recent report indicates a success rate of 60% following this procedure.

Other Surgical Treatments

Considering that no surgical treatment for intermittent DDSP has been entirely satisfactory, investigators continue to seek alternative therapies. Oral palatopharyngoplasty was described in 1992 as a procedure to reduce dorsal billowing of the soft palate. The ventral aspect of the soft palate is stiffened by the transoral resection of an elliptical section of the ventral aspect of the soft palate. This procedure has not been widely adopted owing to its technical difficulty and the potential for serious complication such as oronasopharyngeal fistula.

Supplemental Readings

Anderson LJ: Problems of the equine larynx and pharynx. New Z Vet J 25:387–389, 1977.
Anderson JD, Tulleners EP, Johnston JK, Reeves MJ: Sternothyrohyoideus myectomy or staphylectomy for treatment of intermittent dorsal displacement of the soft palate in racehorses: 209 cases (1986–1991). J Am Vet Med Assoc 206:1909–1912, 1995.
Cook WR: Some observations on form and function of the equine upper airway in health and disease: I. The pharynx. Proc 27th Annu Meet Am Assoc Equine Pract, 1981, pp 355–391.
Tulleners E, Mann P, Raker CW: Epiglottic augmentation in the horse. Vet Surg 19:181–190, 1990.

Sinusitis

SHEILA LAVERTY
St. Hyacinthe, Quebec

JOHN R. PASCOE
Davis, California

Sinusitis may occur from infectious diseases of the respiratory tract or from dental disease, trauma, cysts of the respiratory mucous membrane, ethmoid hematoma, or neoplasia. Inflammatory exudate usually accumulates in the maxillary sinuses but, because of the communication between the sinuses, exudate may accumulate in all sinus cavities. Exudate may accumulate if it is too thick to drain or because there is inflammation, trauma, or expansile masses causing obstruction of the nasomaxillary apertures.

ANATOMY

The sinuses are paired, and those of clinical importance include the frontal, maxillary (rostral and caudal), and conchal (dorsal and ventral) sinuses (Fig. 1). The latter lie within the nasal conchae. The frontal sinus occupies the dorsal aspect of the skull and is confluent with the dorso-conchal sinus (conchofrontal sinus). A large oval communication is present between the frontal sinus and the caudal maxillary sinus (frontomaxillary aperture). Both right and left maxillary sinuses are divided into rostral and caudal compartments by an oblique septum, which is variable in location but usually is about 5 cm behind the rostral end of the facial crest. The ventral part of each maxillary sinus is also divided into medial and lateral spaces by an upright bony plate supporting the infraorbital canal and fused to

the alveoli containing the roots of the cheek teeth. The rostral maxillary sinus communicates with the ventral conchal sinus, which lies medial to it, through the conchomaxillary aperture dorsal to the infraorbital canal. All sinuses drain into the rostral or caudal maxillary sinuses. The latter share a slit-like communication (nasomaxillary opening) with the caudal middle nasal meatus. The nasolacrimal duct runs in the lateral bony wall of the maxillary sinus.

The volume of the maxillary sinus varies directly with the age of the horse, reflecting development, eruption, and rostral migration of the cheek teeth with age. The rostral end of the facial crest is related ventrally to the caudal part of the second cheek tooth in the newborn foal, to the caudal part of the third cheek tooth in the young horse, and to the fourth cheek tooth in the older horse. It is important to realize that the cheek teeth in the young horse occupy most of the sinus space.

CLINICAL SIGNS

Important clinical signs of sinusitis include nasal discharge, halitosis, and facial deformity; and occasionally ocular discharge, abnormal mastication, labored breathing, epistaxis, and sinus fistula. The nasal discharge may be serous, mucoid, purulent, or blood-stained, depending on the cause. Blood-stained nasal discharge may occur with trauma, tumors, ethmoid hematoma, and fungal infections. A fetid odor generally accompanies sinusitis associated with dental disease, neoplasia, and chronic accumulation of inspissated pus in the ventral conchal sinus.

Facial deformity may be caused by inflammation, deformation of the sinus wall by an expanding mass, or accumulation of fluid because of a blocked nasomaxillary aperture. Epiphora may be caused by obstruction of the nasolacrimal duct from trauma or from facial deformity. Masses expanding into the nasal cavity or deformity of the conchal sinuses may cause respiratory distress and may eventually result in nasal septum deviation and occlusion of the contralateral nasal passage. Abnormal mastication is usually related to dental problems.

DIAGNOSIS

Diagnostic procedures include visual examination, sinus percussion, oral cavity examination, evaluation of air flow, endoscopy of the nasal passages, radiography, computed tomography, scintigraphy, sinography, sinocentesis, sinoscopy, biopsy, and exploratory surgery.

Visual examination allows detection of facial deformity

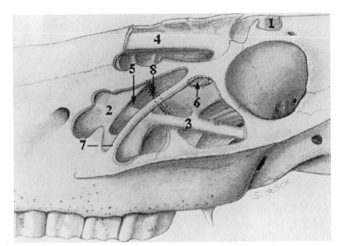

Figure 1. Paranasal sinuses of the horse. 1 = frontal sinus, 2 = rostral maxillary sinus, 3 = caudal maxillary sinus, 4 = dorsal conchal sinus, 5 = ventral conchal sinus, 6 = frontomaxillary opening, 7 = septum between rostral and caudal maxillary sinuses, 8 = nasomaxillary opening. (Reprinted from Budras K-D, Sack WO, Röck S: Anatomy of the Horse: An Illustrated Text. New York, Mosby-Wolfe, 1994, p 31.)

by comparison with the facial contour over the sinus on the opposite side. Diminished resonance may be detected on percussion, with or without auscultation, when fluid or space-occupying lesions are present. Less resonant sound may be heard in normal young horses because the tooth roots occupy proportionately more of the sinus. Failure to detect a change in sound on percussion does not preclude a diagnosis of sinusitis. A thorough oral examination using a buccal speculum should be performed, but a complete examination may be possible only when the horse is anesthetized. Oral examination should include examination of the architecture of the dental arcades, occlusal surface with an infundibular pick, and gingival margins with a perioprobe for gingival recession. Sinusitis of dental origin most frequently involves the third or fourth cheek tooth. Endoscopic oral examination in the anesthetized horse improves observation of the teeth and gingival margins.

Rhinoendoscopy is useful for detection of nasal cavity obstruction from sinus distortion; it is also an aid to rule out other diseases of the upper respiratory tract that may cause similar clinical signs. Patency of the nasomaxillary apertures can be inferred from observation of exudate in the caudal nasal cavity.

Radiography is the most useful commonly available diagnostic procedure to establish the location and extent of sinus disease. Standard radiographic projections include a standing lateral, dorsoventral, and left and right oblique views (D60°L-VLO). Single or multiple air-fluid interfaces may be detected. Frontal sinus opacification is associated with primary sinusitis and rarely presents with sinusitis resulting from dental disease. Radiographic examinations allow identification of affected teeth in only half of the cases because increased radiodensity associated with bone sclerosis and accumulation of material within the sinus cavity often obscure root detail.

Radiographic signs most often associated with dental disease include loss of the lamina dura, periapical lucency, maxillary osteitis, and radicular distortion. Chronic persistent sinusitis in the absence of signs of dental disease or other sinus disease may be caused by inspissated pus in the ventral conchal sinus. Identification of soft tissue density dorsal to the third through fifth cheek teeth on the lateral projection and confined to the ventral conchal sinus (medial to cheek teeth three to five) on dorsoventral projections is consistent with presence of inspissated material in the ventral conchal sinus. Positive contrast paranasal sinography may help establish the location, nature, and extent of pathologic changes not identified on survey radiographs. When available, computed tomographic examination of the sinus cavities and teeth yields more specific anatomic information about the probable cause of sinusitis.

Percutaneous sinus centesis can be performed in the standing horse (see *Current Therapy in Equine Medicine 2*, page 606) using a drill bit, 16-gauge needle, or Steinmann pin mounted in a hand chuck. Care should be taken to avoid damaging sinus structures. Material can be aspirated through a needle, intravenous catheter, or extension tubing attached to a 50-ml syringe. Instillation of 20 to 30 ml of sterile saline before aspiration may facilitate recovery of material in some cases. Sinocentesis samples should be cultured for aerobic and anaerobic bacteria and, if suspected, for fungi. A cytologic examination (including a Gram stain) is performed for detection of bacteria, fungi, inflammatory, and neoplastic cells. Observation of feed material on cytologic examination is indicative of a dental problem.

Sinoscopy is easy to perform in the standing sedated horse. A 4.0-mm 300 arthroscope or flexible endoscope may be used. Sites for insertion of the sinoscope are described on page 402. Sinoscopy allows evaluation of the sinus in a minimally invasive fashion and permits precise biopsy of masses. Blood and exudate should be removed before the examination begins, and sinus irrigation can be performed to improve visualization.

TREATMENT

Primary Sinusitis

Daily lavage with 1 L of warmed saline should be performed, until the discharged solution runs clear. The sinus can be irrigated through a 24-French Foley balloon catheter placed through entry portals in the frontal sinus or rostral maxillary sinus. If fluid does not drain through the nasomaxillary aperture, a drainage portal can be established in the maxillary sinus. The organisms involved are usually *Streptococcus equi* and *Streptococcus zooepidemicus*. Penicillin is usually effective against streptococci and is a logical choice for primary sinusitis while awaiting culture and antibiotic susceptibility results. Appropriately selected antibiotics should be administered for 14 days, and horses should be fed on the ground and turned out to pasture or exercised as soon as possible to encourage drainage.

Inspissated purulent exudate in the ventral conchal sinuses should be suspected when primary bacterial sinusitis does not resolve with sinus irrigation and parenteral administration of antimicrobial drugs. Sinusotomy can be used to remove the inspissated pus from the sinus. Alternatively, conchofrontal sinus trephination and digital perforation of the dorsal wall of the ventral conchal sinus can be used. After irrigation, an endoscope should be inserted to visualize the rostral part of the sinus to ensure complete removal of all exudate.

Dental Disease

Dental disease is the most common cause of chronic sinusitis in horses but is uncommon in horses younger than 4 years of age. Diseases of the cheek teeth leading to sinusitis include fractures, patent infundibulum, displaced teeth, dental malposition, and crown defects. Treatment is directed at removal of the affected tooth or teeth. This is usually accomplished by sinusotomy. In addition, the removal of abnormal mucosa, establishment of good drainage to the nasal cavity through the ventral conchal sinus, irrigation of the sinus, and administration of appropriate systemic antimicrobial drugs are important treatment tenets. Obligate anaerobic bacteria may be involved in tooth root abscesses; therefore, special handling and isolation techniques for culturing anaerobes should be requested. Endodontic therapy such as apicoectomy and retrograde filling of the pulp chamber should be considered when the periodontal ligament is intact. Tooth salvage is preferable to extraction or repulsion because it helps maintain the architecture of the arcade and prevents abnormalities of wear in the opposing arcade.

Antimicrobial administration alone or in combination with sinus lavage may be successfully used in cases of sinusitis when there are financial restrictions; these methods, when repeated, may prolong the life of geriatric horses with problems such as tooth loss or tooth root abscesses.

Trauma

Traumatic events may fracture the bony boundaries of the sinus, resulting in secondary infection of the sinus. Depressed and fractured facial bones may be elevated and stabilized with orthopedic wire. Damage to the nasolacrimal duct may lead to epiphora and chronic sinusitis because of altered lacrimal drainage. Bony sequestra can also lead to chronic sinusitis and should be removed.

Paranasal Sinus Cysts

Sinus cysts are loculated fluid-filled cavities with an epithelial lining that develop in the maxillary sinuses or ventral concha and may extend into the frontal sinus. They occur in young horses, usually those younger than 2 years of age, or in horses older than 9 years of age. The cause of these cysts is not known, but there is usually progressive accumulation of amber-colored fluid with subsequent sinus cavity distortion. Frequently streptococci are isolated from the fluid. Sinocentesis and radiography are usually diagnostic; multiloculated densities, fluid lines, and dental distortion may be evident.

Sinusotomy is indicated, and removal of the cyst by digital dissection and nasomaxillary drainage is necessary to prevent further sinus distortion. The prognosis for recovery is good even with facial distortion, which usually remodels with time. With severe facial and sinus distortion, it may be necessary to remove the nasal septum to alleviate airway obstruction.

Neoplasia

Squamous cell carcinoma is the most common neoplasm, but tumors of any of the sinus tissues may occur. The prognosis is generally poor because invasion of local structures and distortion of the architecture of the nasal cavity are often extensive by the time of presentation. Radical surgery combined with adjunctive chemotherapy or radiation therapy offers the best hope for resolution. Osteomas are benign slow-growing tumors involving the maxillary sinuses of young male horses that carry a favorable prognosis with tumor removal.

Ethmoid Hematoma

Ethmoid hematomas are progressive, locally destructive angiomatous masses of unknown cause. They usually arise from the mucosa of the ethmoid labyrinth but can also arise from the floor of the sinus, and can occur in horses of any age but are more common in horses older than 8 years of age. Altered respiratory noise and a nasal discharge with intermittent unilateral epistaxis are the most common clinical signs. Masses may fill the sinuses and nasal passages, causing abnormal respiratory noise and effort and even choking. The affected ethmoid is usually abnormal on endoscopic examination of the pharynx, although occasionally the mass is present only in the sinus. Large masses are usually removed by curettage through a frontonasal sinusotomy. The origin of the mass is not always visible, and visibility may be poor because of profuse hemorrhage during surgery. Cryosurgery or laser resection may be used on the base of the lesion to avoid hemorrhage.

The mass (<5 cm) may also be removed by repeated photoablations in the standing horse using a Nd:YAG laser. A recurrence rate of 30 to 50% following surgery and lower recurrence rates following laser ablation have been reported. Intralesional injection of 10% formalin has been used successfully for treatment and control of ethmoid hematomas. With endoscopic observation, a catheter is passed through the biopsy channel of the endoscope into the ethmoid mass and advanced toward the base. Ten ml of 10% formalin are injected into the mass; repeated injections can be performed at approximately 10-day intervals until the mass has sloughed.

Fungal Infections

Fungal infections of the sinus cavities are rare but may occur in conjunction with fungal nasal cavity disease. On endoscopic examination of the nasal passages, firm lobulated or nonlobulated masses covered by mucosa are observed. A discrete smooth-walled soft tissue density may be evident on radiographs. Biopsy of the lesion allows a definitive diagnosis. Cryptococcal organisms may be identified by microscopic examination or fungal cultures of aspirates from the affected sinus.

Treatment is aimed at removal of affected tissues and administration of systemic antifungal medication (see page 439), but the prognosis for recovery is guarded.

Supplemental Readings

Behrens E, Schumacher J, Morris E, Shively M: Equine paranasal sinusography. Vet Radiol 32(3):98–104, 1991.

Dyce KM, Sack WO, Wensing CJG: The head and ventral neck of the horse. In Dyce KM, Sack WO, Wensing CJG (eds): Textbook of Veterinary Anatomy. Philadelphia, WB Saunders, 1987, pp 462–487.

Honnas CM, Pascoe JR: Diseases of the paranasal sinuses. In Smith BP (ed): Large Animal Internal Medicine. St. Louis, C.V. Mosby, 1990, pp 555–557.

Schumacher J, Crossland LE: Removal of inspissated purulent exudate from the ventral conchal sinus of three standing horses. J Am Vet Med Assoc 205(9):1312–1314, 1994.

Trotter GW: Paranasal sinuses. Vet Clin North Am Large Anim Pract 9(1):153–169, 1993.

Hemorrhage From the Upper Respiratory Tract

DAVID E. FREEMAN
Urbana, Illinois

Hemorrhage from the upper respiratory tract usually presents as unilateral, less commonly as bilateral, epistaxis that can be categorized loosely as mild, moderate, or severe. Exercise and stress are not required to induce hemorrhage from the upper respiratory tract of horses. The following diseases are grouped according to severity of hemorrhage, although there may be considerable overlap between categories and difficulty in assessing the severity of hemorrhage in many cases.

MILD HEMORRHAGE

Mild hemorrhage can pose a diagnostic challenge, although the volume of blood lost does not cause anemia. Diseases that cause mild hemorrhage also can be difficult to manage and many have life-threatening consequences. Mild hemorrhage tends to be intermittent, almost continuous over a long period of time, and unilateral.

Ethmoid Hematoma

Ethmoid hematoma is a progressive and locally destructive mass of unknown cause. Large hematomas arise from the ethmoidal labyrinth and extend into the nasal passages. Smaller lesions that arise by a stalk from the sinus and are confined to the sinus cavity are less common.

Clinical Signs

Ethmoid hematomas usually occur in horses 6 years of age and older. The most consistent clinical sign is mild, spontaneous, intermittent unilateral epistaxis of variable duration. Large lesions can cause a stertorous respiratory noise at rest and especially at work. Sinus deformity is rare.

Diagnosis

On endoscopic examination, the smooth-walled, greenish-black mass can be seen extending from the ethmoid region into the nasal passage. The hematoma can also be seen on lateral and dorsoventral radiographs as a well-circumscribed density that contrasts with the air in the sinuses.

Treatment

Surgical removal of the entire lesion through a frontonasal flap sinusotomy is the recommended treatment. Currently, laser surgery is being evaluated for treatment of this disease, applied through the nasal passages or through a sinusotomy. Some success has been claimed for intralesional injection of formalin under endoscopic guidance (Jim Schumacher, Texas A & M University, personal communication). The response to surgical treatment is usually good, but recurrence is possible.

Fungal Infections of Sinuses and Nasal Passages

Phycomycosis, cryptococcosis, coccidioidomycosis, aspergillosis, rhinosporidiosis, and mycetomas are rare and sporadic diseases of the nasal passages and paranasal sinuses. Some have a specific geographic distribution. Diagnosis can be made by endoscopy, radiography, and biopsy, and treatment consists of surgical removal, if possible, followed by topical and systemic antifungal agents. These diseases are very difficult to manage and many pose a public health concern. Bacterial infections of the upper respiratory tract rarely cause epistaxis.

Neoplasia

Neoplasms of the nasal passages, sinuses, and guttural pouches are rare and usually are advanced when diagnosis is made. More than 50% of sinus and nasal passage neoplasms are malignant. Squamous cell carcinoma is the most common type, but many others have been reported. A wide age range of horses can be affected. Neoplasia in these sites causes local destruction of bone and soft tissue, leading to facial deformity, dyspnea, weight loss, epistaxis, and anemia of chronic disease. Diagnosis can be based on history, clinical signs, and endoscopic, radiographic, and biopsy findings. Treatment is usually unsuccessful, especially if the lesion is diffuse, but some favorable responses have been obtained with combinations of surgery and radiation therapy for discrete tumors.

Foreign Bodies

Intranasal foreign bodies and concretions are rare in horses, but isolated cases have been reported as causes of mild epistaxis and partial upper airway obstruction. Foreign bodies in the guttural pouch can cause mild to moderate hemorrhage.

MODERATE HEMORRHAGE

Moderate hemorrhage usually causes a single episode of unilateral epistaxis that appears alarming to the owner or handler but rarely causes significant blood loss and anemia. Moderate hemorrhage can be seen in some diseases that also cause severe hemorrhage.

Wounds and Fractures

Blunt injuries to the frontal and nasal bones and sinuses from kicks and other forms of trauma can cause open or closed wounds of the sinuses.

422

Clinical Signs and Diagnosis

Epistaxis and subcutaneous emphysema are common clinical signs of sinus trauma. Severe cases can be dyspneic. Facial deformity may not be seen initially with depression fractures because the skin usually pulls away from the fractured bone and assumes a normal contour; however, facial deformity can become evident as the fracture heals. Unless both sides are involved, the epistaxis is unilateral.

Diagnosis of a depression fracture or sinus trauma can be made on the basis of history, clinical signs, and radiography. Radiographs may not reveal the true extent of bone injury.

Treatment

A conservative approach is used if a cosmetic appearance is not required and if the fracture is mildly displaced. In such cases, 5 to 7 days of topical treatment of a skin wound, stall rest, antibiotics, and nonsteroidal anti-inflammatory drugs are sufficient. Surgical treatment is indicated if the horse has signs of airway obstruction, if the fracture is severe, if the skin is broken, and if a cosmetic result is needed. Treatment involves surgical elevation of depressed bone into a normal position and wiring it in place. The prognosis is usually good, and many fractures heal without a blemish.

Miscellaneous

A stomach tube, endoscope, nasotracheal tube, or other instrument passed through the nasal passage can injure the nasal concha. Injury is most likely to happen during withdrawal of the instrument. Although treatment is not required, hemorrhage inflicted in this manner is disturbing to all concerned.

SEVERE HEMORRHAGE

Severe hemorrhage usually recurs, and blood loss may be sufficient to cause hemorrhagic shock and anemia after one episode.

Guttural Pouch Mycosis

Guttural pouch mycosis is the most common cause of severe epistaxis and is caused by a fungal infection on the roof of the caudal and medial aspects of the guttural pouch. No apparent age, sex, or breed predisposition to this disease is observed. The typical lesion of guttural pouch mycosis is a diphtheritic membrane that is closely attached to underlying tissue; it can vary in size. Epistaxis is caused by fungal erosion of the wall of the internal carotid artery in approximately 70% of cases and the external carotid artery and its continuation, the maxillary artery, in the remainder.

Clinical Signs

Epistaxis is severe, and usually bouts of hemorrhage recur over a period of weeks before fatal hemorrhage occurs. Approximately 60% of horses with guttural pouch mycosis and hemorrhage die from this complication. The epistaxis is usually bilateral, but it is more severe on the affected side, and blood can continue to drain from the guttural pouch and nostril for up to 1 week after active hemorrhage ceases. Some cases are complicated by dysphagia, which is the second most common clinical sign of the disease and is extremely difficult to manage. Other neurologic disorders can also complicate the condition.

Diagnosis

On endoscopy, blood can be seen draining from the pharyngeal orifice on the affected side, but it is also possible for blood from other parts of the respiratory tract to enter the guttural pouch and drain from there into the pharynx. For this reason, the interior of the guttural pouch must be examined with the endoscope to demonstrate the typical mycotic lesion.

Treatment

The problem with medical treatment of guttural pouch mycosis is a uniformly inconsistent response. Even when successful, medical treatment is too slow to prevent several bouts of hemorrhage.

Surgical treatment is recommended in all horses with hemorrhage caused by guttural pouch mycosis. A prompt diagnosis is of great importance to prevent delay in referral that can lead to additional hemorrhage and render the horse a poor candidate for general anesthesia and surgery. Support of extracellular fluid volume through use of intravenous fluids or blood transfusions is rarely needed after the first bout of hemorrhage but may be required after subsequent bouts. Balloon catheter techniques have proved to be successful for preventing hemorrhage from the affected arteries, and the procedure should be done as soon as possible. If the guttural pouch is full of blood and the affected artery cannot be identified, all arteries in the guttural pouch should be occluded by a balloon catheter, without risk of complications. Blindness does not occur after balloon catheter occlusion of the affected arteries. The mycotic lesion usually regresses rapidly after the affected artery has been occluded. Medical treatment other than supportive efforts is, therefore, not used after surgery.

Rupture of the Longus Capitis Muscle

The longus capitis muscle is one of the ventral straight muscles of the head, and it inserts onto the basisphenoid bone at the base of the skull. Rupture at the site of insertion occurs during a traumatic episode that probably involves hyperextension of the head and neck. Most horses have a history of falling over backward.

Clinical Signs

The severity of hemorrhage varies from moderate to severe so that the clinical presentation of the disease can closely resemble guttural pouch mycosis, with the exception of a history of recent trauma. Neurologic signs can occur as well.

Diagnosis

Diagnosis is based on results of endoscopic examination, combined with radiology and ultrasound examination. On endoscopy, the roof of the pharynx is collapsed, especially on the affected side, and blood can be seen draining from the pharyngeal orifice of the guttural pouch. With the endoscope in the guttural pouch, the caudal aspect of the guttural pouch and the arteries appear normal, but blood, a hematoma, and disruption of the muscle can be seen in the more rostral aspect of the guttural pouch. The lesion can be seen best by complete retroflexion of the endoscope. Similar but milder lesions are evident in the other guttural pouch.

Radiographs reveal a soft tissue density on the roof of the guttural pouch impinging on the radiolucent outline of the guttural pouch cavity. It may also be possible to see a fragment of bone that has fractured off the site of muscle insertion. Ultrasound examination can determine more completely the extent of hemorrhage. It may be possible to see blood dissecting through the retropharyngeal tissues and even extending through fascial planes along the ventral aspect of the neck. Blood accumulation in these areas can be severe enough to obstruct the upper respiratory tract.

Treatment

Hemorrhage caused by rupture of the ventral straight muscles is managed conservatively. Broad-spectrum antibiotics are administered over a period of 5 to 7 days to prevent infection of the hematoma at the site of muscle rupture. Administration of dimethyl sulfoxide (DMSO, 10% solution, 1 g/kg IV slowly once a day for 1 to 3 days)

or dexamethasone (0.08 mg/kg IV) may be considered in the presence of severe ataxia. These horses are also given stall rest for 4 to 6 weeks. They should be observed closely for signs of hemorrhage or dyspnea or for exacerbation of neurologic problems. It is important in these horses to limit the range of extension of the head and neck so that repeated tearing of the damaged tissues is prevented.

The prognosis for complete recovery is fair to good in horses without neurologic signs. Horses with ataxia have a poorer prognosis but can improve with time. Subsequent bouts of hemorrhage can cause retropharyngeal swelling and death from pharyngeal collapse and asphyxia.

Supplemental Readings

Freeman DE: Paranasal sinuses. *In* Beech J (ed): Equine Respiratory Disorders. Philadelphia, Lea & Febiger, 1991, pp 275–303.

Freeman DE: Guttural pouches. *In* Beech J (ed): Equine Respiratory Disorders. Philadelphia, Lea & Febiger, 1991, pp 305–330.

Greet TRC: Outcome of treatment in 35 cases of guttural pouch mycosis. Equine Vet J 19:483–487, 1987.

Sweeney CR, Freeman DE, Sweeney RW, Rubin JL, Maxson AD: Hemorrhage into the guttural pouch (auditory tube diverticulum) associated with rupture of the longus capitis muscle in three horses. J Am Vet Med Assoc 202:1129–1131, 1993.

Tracheal Collapse

MARCEL MARCOUX
St. Hyacinthe, Quebec

The equine trachea is a flexible membranous and cartilaginous tube that extends from the outlet of the larynx to the level of the fifth or sixth intercostal space where it bifurcates into the right and left bronchi. The thoracic part of the trachea lies in the cranial and middle parts of the mediastinum. In the trachea, there are 48 to 60 cartilaginous plates that are bent to form incomplete hoops with the transversely oriented tracheal muscle attached dorsally to the inner surfaces of these plates.

Tracheal collapse results in airway obstruction owing to collapse of the cartilaginous rings or of the soft tissues of the trachea. It can be congenital or acquired. When congenital, the collapse is due to a lack of rigidity of the cartilaginous rings with resultant dorsoventral flattening of the trachea. Acquired collapse can be caused by external trauma in the cervical region, chondrodysplasia, peritracheal tumors, abscesses, or bone callus consequent to fractured ribs. Both congenital and acquired collapse can be located in the cervical or thoracic portion of the trachea.

In dogs, tracheal collapse has been classified as follows (Fig. 1):

Grade I. The trachea is nearly normal. The trachealis muscle is slightly pendulous but the tracheal cartilages maintain a **C** shape. The tracheal lumen is reduced by approximately 25%.

Grade II. The trachealis muscle is widened and pendulous.

The tracheal cartilages are partially flattened and the tracheal lumen is reduced by approximately 50%.

Grade III. The trachealis muscle is almost in contact with the ventral surface of the tracheal cartilages. The tracheal cartilages are nearly flat, and the ends may be palpated on physical examination. The tracheal lumen is reduced by approximately 75%.

Grade IV. The tracheal muscle is lying on the ventral surface of the tracheal cartilages. The tracheal cartilages are flattened and may invert dorsally. The tracheal lumen is essentially obliterated.

CLINICAL SIGNS

Congenital tracheal collapse is usually manifested in the first few days or weeks of life. With mild collapses (grades I and II), foals may only present a poor weight gain and poor general condition. Adult horses with grades I and II tracheal collapse may manifest exercise intolerance without abnormal respiratory noises.

Clinical signs of congenital or acquired tracheal collapse are, in severe cases (grades III and IV), exercise intolerance and respiratory stridor. Tachypnea and stridorous breathing are often present. When a large part of the trachea is involved, as with congenital collapse, inspiratory and expiratory respiratory distress and a goose-honk cough are pres-

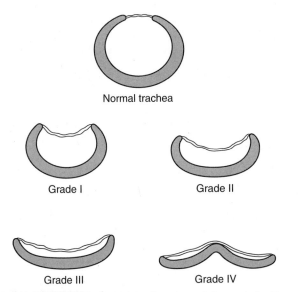

Figure 1. Classification of tracheal collapse reported in animals. (Reproduced with permission from Tangner CH, Hobson HP: A retrospective study of 20 surgically managed cases of collapsed trachea. Vet Surg 11: 146–149, 1982.)

ent and are usually more prominent when the head is elevated. When the collapse is localized, the respiratory distress and abnormal sounds are usually worse on inspiration.

Tracheal deformity may be noted on palpation of the tracheal rings in the cervical region, especially in the adult horse. Palpation of the trachea may also reveal an abnormal vibration at the site of collapse or, by accentuating the collapse, may worsen the clinical signs. Auscultation usually reveals harsh sounds or respiratory stridor, which is best heard over the area of obstruction. Crackles or wheezes may be heard over the lung regions.

In true emergencies, exaggerated flaring of the nares is noticed with vigorous breathing movements of the abdominal and thoracic areas. The animal can become violent in these cases and can present some danger for the environment. The presence of blood at the nostrils is suggestive of pulmonary edema, which can cause death rapidly if the airway obstruction is not relieved.

DIAGNOSIS

Although clinical signs, palpation, and auscultation of the cervical trachea may be diagnostic, endoscopic examination is generally necessary to identify the site and severity of the collapse. Horses with labored breathing or with clinical signs of hypoxemia should be treated by pharyngeal insufflation of oxygen, or tracheotomy distal to the site of collapse, before endoscopic examination. Endoscopy should be then performed rapidly and with minimal restraint. In foals, a small-diameter endoscope (8 mm) is used. In certain cases, passage of the endoscope is impeded by the tracheal collapse. Dorsoventral flattening is often seen, but triangular and key-hole types of deformation also have been reported. When only partial collapse is present, endo-

scopic identification and gradation are difficult, and the lesion can be missed.

Because most lesions have a dorsoventral flattening pattern, a radiograph taken in a lateral position may allow localization of the site and extent of the lesion. Normally, a uniform tracheal diameter is present over the entire length of the trachea. Radiographic examination may also identify the cause of the collapse.

TREATMENT

If the collapse is severe and is located in the cervical region, an emergency tracheotomy can be performed distal to the lesion. Because tracheal surgery may cause tracheal collapse, a suitable surgical technique must be respected. The tracheotomy can be performed by a method of incision or by a method of excision (Fig. 2). With the incision technique, the annular ligament is transversely incised in a two-step procedure using a scalpel. The incision is started at the 3 o'clock position and proceeds toward the sagittal plane and is similarly repeated at the other side starting at 9 o'clock. This technique helps to avoid incision of the carotid sheath or the esophagus, which runs parallel to the trachea.

With the excision technique, a tracheal stoma is created by removal of a semicircular portion of cartilage out of two adjacent rings. A maximum of 50% of the width of each ring should be resected; otherwise, collapse of the tracheal ring may occur. A scalpel blade is used to penetrate a cartilage ring in the center of its width and a quarter of its circumference is incised; then the procedure is repeated on the other ring, joining the two incisions. A Backhaus clamp is used to secure the piece of trachea partly resected, and the same procedure is performed on the opposite side.

The incision technique is used in foals and mature horses when a tracheotomy is needed for a few days only. When using the excision technique in the foal, special care should be taken to avoid exceeding 50% of the width of the cartilage ring. When needed, a surgical procedure has been described for the horse, in which the skin is sutured di-

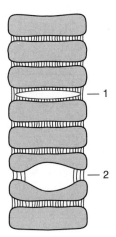

Figure 2. Tracheostomy performed by incision of the intra-annular ligament (1) or by partial excision of two adjacent tracheal rings (2).

rectly to the cartilage rings to form a permanent tracheotomy.

A variety of tracheal tubes are manufactured, but self-retaining tubes° are more popular because they do not require skin sutures for security. More recently, soft malleable tubes† that can also be employed for general anesthesia are used, but they need to be secured to the skin. In an emergency, a segment of a stomach tube, garden hose, or cut barrel of a 50-ml syringe can temporarily provide a patent airway. For temporary relief of an obstruction in dyspneic and violent horses, the passage of a length of tubing like a nasogastric tube from a nostril to the trachea, thus bypassing the obstruction, can be lifesaving and make the animal much more manageable.

When deciding on a treatment for tracheal collapse, it is important to determine the length of the collapse, its loca-

tion, whether there is soft tissue collapse alone or cartilage collapse as well. A soft tissue collapse associated with pneumonia may heal completely after medical treatment consisting of rest, antibiotics, and anti-inflammatory agents. If cartilaginous tracheal ring deformity is the source of the collapse, various surgical treatments have been reported for use in the horse. Overall, localized lesions involving only a few cartilaginous rings can be treated surgically, whereas collapse involving larger segments often has a very poor prognosis.

Supplemental Readings

Honnas CM: Diseases of the trachea. In Colahan PT, Mayhew IG, Merritt AM, Moore JN (eds): Equine Medicine & Surgery, ed 4, vol 1. Wheaton, IL, American Veterinary Publications, 1991, pp 424–429.

Pascoe JR: Tracheotomy and tracheostomy. In White NA, Moore JN (eds): Current Practice of Equine Surgery. Philadelphia, JB Lippincott, 1990, pp 261–264.

Rose RS, Hodgson DR: Tracheal stenosis. In Rose RS, Hodgson DR (eds): Manual of Equine Practice. Philadelphia, WB Saunders, 1993, pp 156–157.

°*Hauptner Instruments, Solingen, Germany*
†*Bivona Inc, Gary, IN*

Lower Airway Inflammation in Young Performance Horses

LAURENT VIEL
Guelph, Ontario

Lower airway inflammation is a common and often unrecognized cause of exercise intolerance in young performing horses. Clinicians tend to believe that chronic obstructive pulmonary disease (COPD) or heaves is a respiratory condition restricted to the older horse, generally one over 6 years of age. However, a body of evidence is growing that demonstrates that airway inflammatory reactions due to environmental insults, such as moldy hay, dusty bedding, and infectious agents, are responsible for comparable, less chronic respiratory disorders in young performing horses.

Inflammation is the body's response to injury by various insults such as infectious agents, parasites, and trauma. This inflammation is usually a beneficial reaction that defends the animal from microinvaders. However, inflammation can act as a double-edged sword and can be harmful if it occurs excessively or is not self-limiting. This overreaction seems to happen in equine small airway disease due to environmental allergens, chemicals, and even some respiratory viral infections. Chronic obstructive pulmonary disease (heaves) exemplifies a self-perpetuating neutrophilic inflammation of the small airways leading to excess mucus production (purulent nasal discharges), bronchospasm (auscultable wheezes), and/or airway hyperresponsiveness and irritability (coughing). Inflammatory cells identified in this syndrome of inflammatory small airway disease are depicted in Figure 1.

Lower airway inflammation in young performing horses may be divided into mast cell–mediated airway disease,

neutrophil-associated airway disease, granulomatous lung disease, and respiratory viral infection. Bronchoalveolar lavage (BAL), a sensitive method to characterize the airway cell population, can be used to aid in differentiating the various forms of inflammatory airway diseases.

MAST CELL–MEDIATED AIRWAY DISEASE

Horses with this disease exhibit immunologic reactions characteristic of type I hypersensitivity. Typically, these are young horses showing a gradual decline in their training and racing performance. These horses have an intermittent cough while standing in the box stall and at the beginning of training session, and have often been treated for 1 or more weeks with broad-spectrum antibiotics with little or no success.

On clinical examination, resting respiratory rate is usually within the normal range, but it is common to observe a prolonged return to normal respiratory rate after exercise. Chest auscultation reveals increased bronchial sounds over the dorsal area of both lung fields. During rebreathing in a plastic bag, wheezes can be detected but crackles are seldom heard. Lung field percussion may be hyper-resonant and expanded dorsally and caudally. On endoscopic examination, the trachea contains either a moderate amount of clear mucoid secretions, indicative of a mast cell inflammatory process, or mucopurulent secretions, indica-

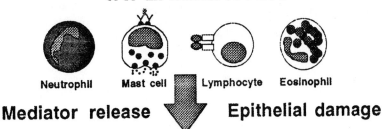

Figure 1. Effects of inflammatory cells involved in airway disease of the horse.

tive of an eosinophilic inflammatory process. The bronchi become irritated because of the passage of the endoscope and the horse coughs excessively, leading to observable mucosal hyperemia, edema, and bronchoconstriction.

The BAL fluid recovered in these cases is abundant and clear in appearance, with no flocculent debris present, and the cytologic analysis may indicate a significant increase in the mast cell population with very few eosinophils or a significant increase in the mast cell population and a significant increase in eosinophils (Table 1). The clinical significance of the two different inflammatory processes is that the horse with mast cells as the predominant inflammatory cell may be successfully treated with a mast cell stabilizer such as sodium cromoglycate, whereas in the latter case the addition of corticosteroids to control the eosinophilic inflammation of the airways is necessary. Sodium cromoglycate° can be administered by a metered-dose inhaler (MDI) using a face mask.† The recommended dosage is 10 to 12 puffs (1 mg/puff) daily before exercise for 2 to 3 weeks, then on alternate days for as long as needed. The suggested withdrawal time is 24 hours. If corticosteroid administration is deemed necessary, oral prednisone (300 mg b.i.d. for 1 week, 300 mg s.i.d. 1 week, then 300 mg s.i.d. on alternate days as long as needed) can be used.

°*Intal, Fisons, Rochester, NY*
†*Equine Aeromask, Canadian Monaghan Ltd., Ontario, Canada*

NEUTROPHIL-ASSOCIATED AIRWAY DISEASE

The neutrophil-associated airway disease affecting young performing horses is identical to the inflammatory process observed in COPD (heaves) except that the disease is in its early stage. The disease is often referred to as type III hypersensitivity; however, there is no evidence at the present time demonstrating that complement-regulated immune complexes (Arthus reaction) are deposited in the equine airways.

The history of reduced performance and the clinical findings in young racing horses suffering from neutrophil-associated airway disease are similar to those of horses with mast cell-mediated airway disease. Occasional mucopurulent nasal discharge is observed and, using a rebreathing bag, chest auscultation may reveal the presence of wheezes and crackles over the lung field. Endoscopically the secretions are whitish in color, and small pinpoint plaques of mucopurulent debris can easily be visualized in the bronchi. The airway mucosa is edematous, hyperemic, and hyperreactive to the passage of the endoscope.

BAL fluid samples have suspended flocculent debris and a markedly elevated total cell count where polymorphonuclear cells account for a large proportion of the cell population (see Table 1). It is not unusual to observe a neutrophilic inflammatory reaction in horses with chronic exercise-induced pulmonary hemorrhage, and blood may

TABLE 1.   BRONCHOALVEOLAR LAVAGE FLUID CELL DIFFERENTIAL COUNTS EXPRESSED AS A PERCENTAGE OF 400 CELLS COUNTED FOR THE FOUR TYPES OF CASES (MEAN ± S.D.)

Group	n	Macrophages	Lymphocytes	Neutrophils	Mast Cells	Eosinophils	Epithelial Cells
Normal	11	60.1 ± 1.4	36.7 ± 1.6	2.2 ± 0.4	0.4 ± 0.1	0.03 ± 0.03	0.4 ± 0.1
Type I	6	57.0 ± 12	35.0 ± 13	2.4 ± 2.7	3.9 ± 2.8	0.8 ± 0.5	1.5 ± 2.7
Type I	5	55.6 ± 8.6	26.0 ± 3.6	0.9 ± 0.7	1.5 ± 0.8	13.3 ± 7.6	0.6 ± 1.4
Type III	6	26.7 ± 5.9	36.4 ± 8.7	28.0 ± 11.2	3.3 ± 0.8	1.8 ± 1.0	3.7 ± 0.5
Type IV	5	30.6 ± 9.7	57.6 ± 13.0	7.6 ± 7.0	4.0 ± 2.7	0.3 ± 0.7	—

be responsible for maintaining the momentum of continued airway inflammation in some of these cases.

Oral prednisone (300 mg b.i.d. for 1 week, 300 mg s.i.d. for 1 week, then 300 mg s.i.d. on alternate days as long as needed) can be administered to control lower airway inflammation. Very likely, without appropriate treatment and environmental management, the disease progresses to the lung lesions typically described for heaves.

GRANULOMATOUS LUNG DISORDERS

Although granulomatous lung disease is uncommon in horses, repetitive injections of the immunostimulant, such as mycobacterium cell wall extract, may produce an inflammatory process resembling type IV immune mediated hypersensitivity. Affected race horses develop clinical signs resembling acute viral infections, namely, markedly elevated body temperature, rapid respiratory rate, and occasionally loss of appetite. On auscultation, increased bronchial sounds over the entire lung field are the main feature. Chest radiography reveals the presence of severe diffuse interstitial pattern. Cytologic features of the BAL are marked increase in the total cell counts, particularly lymphocytes and alveolar macrophages as well as numerous multinucleated cells. Histology examination of a lung biopsy clearly demonstrates an active inflammatory reaction with multiple granuloma formations throughout the alveolar structure of the lung parenchyma.

The therapeutic response to corticosteroids (oral prednisone, 400 mg b.i.d. for 1 week, 300 mg b.i.d. for 1 week, 300 mg s.i.d. for 1 week, then 300 mg s.i.d. on alternate days for 2 weeks) is variable and related to the number and size of the granuloma. Characteristically, the horse is unresponsive to antibiotic therapy, and the benefit from antipyretic medication is usually of short duration. Because of the widespread nature of the pulmonary inflammation, the prognosis is very guarded to poor because the healing process leads to pulmonary fibrosis.

RESPIRATORY VIRAL INFECTION

Historically, trainers and owners of 2- and 3-year-old horses observe a sudden decline in training performance, which is reported to be of no more than 5 to 7 days in duration. Commonly the complaint is associated with several horses in the stable presenting with acute episodes of coughing not necessarily associated with feeding.

On physical examination, the vital signs are within the normal range but horses have a serous nasal discharge and enlarged submandibular lymph nodes. Chest auscultation reveals a marked increase in bronchial sounds throughout the entire lung field. Cough is easily elicited during the rebreathing bag procedure.

Endoscopic examination of the trachea and large bronchi is characterized by a markedly hyperemic mucosa, plaques of clear mucus more abundant in the tracheal puddle, and induction of spastic cough while passing the endoscope in the bronchial area. Cytology examination of the BAL initially shows a massive exfoliation of mucosal epithelial cells accompanied by numerous free cilia and detached ciliated tufts from the cytoplasm of the columnar epithelial cells. In addition, the total number of alveolar macrophages and lymphocytes is elevated. Horses that continue to have a persistent cough and poor training performance 3 to 4 weeks following the primary viral insult may have a BAL cytology examination revealing an active inflammatory process with mast cells as the major player, similar to a type I hypersensitivity reaction.

Respiratory viral infection can be suspected based on the clinical signs and the changes in BAL fluid cytology examination described above. Viral culture or serology examination of paired serum samples allows confirmation of the diagnosis. Affected horses should be rested for 14 to 21 days, then training can be resumed with the concurrent administration of sodium cromoglycate (10–12 puffs, 1 mg/puff, s.i.d. before exercise for 2–3 weeks, then on alternate days). Interestingly, the administration of sodium cromoglycate in these horses has a significant impact in reducing or abating the clinical signs of cough. This sensitivity or hyperresponsiveness of the airways with viral infections has been demonstrated to persist as long as 8 weeks from the beginning of the infection. It is, therefore, highly rational to recommend a minimum of 2 to 3 weeks' rest to allow the epithelial airway lining to regenerate coupled with the administration of sodium cromoglycate to stabilize mast cells.

CONCLUSIONS

Equine small airway disease is the result of multiple interrelated factors. Rapid symptomatic relief of the air flow obstruction (bronchospasm) may be achieved by bronchodilator administration. On the other hand, many other factors contributing to air flow obstruction, such as airway inflammation and edema, need to be a major focus of therapeutic strategies for more appropriate and long-term management.

Supplemental Readings

Derksen FJ, Robinson NE, Armstrong PJ, Stick JA, Slocombe RF: Airway reactivity in ponies with recurrent airway obstruction (heaves). J Appl Physiol 58:598–604, 1985.

Hare JE, Viel L, O'Byrne PM, Conlon PD: Effect of sodium cromoglycate on light racehorses with elevated metachromatic cell numbers on bronchoalveolar lavage and reduced exercise tolerance. J Vet Pharmacol Therap 17:237–244, 1994.

Hoffman AM: Small airway inflammatory disease in equids. Proc 13th ACVIM Forum, 1995, pp 754–757.

Viel L, Hare JE: Bronchoalveolar lavage in domestic animals: Clinical usefulness. 12th Vet Resp Symp, Comp Resp Soc Symp Proc, 1993.

Inhalation Therapy for the Treatment of Lower Airway Disease

East Lansing, Michigan

Lower airway diseases of horses may be caused by viral, bacterial, or fungal infections; allergens; aspiration; inhalation of toxic agents; and autoimmune reactions. The lung has a stereotypical response to these injuries, and inflammation and bronchospasm are characteristic of all of these conditions. Thus, therapeutic interventions in cases of equine lung diseases often include elimination of offending agents, control of inflammation, and bronchodilator therapy. In human medicine, anti-inflammatory and bronchodilator therapy is best achieved by inhalation. Other therapeutic modalities such as antibacterial therapy are best achieved using the oral or systemic routes. Therefore, in this chapter, the author discusses the rationale for and application of bronchodilator and anti-inflammatory therapy in the horse.

CHARACTERISTICS OF THERAPEUTIC AEROSOLS

The clinical efficacy of therapeutic aerosols is mainly determined by the dose of aerosol deposited in the lower respiratory tract and the distribution of that dose within the lung. Dose and distribution of an aerosol in turn are determined by patient characteristics such as size and shape of the airways; pattern of breathing, including tidal volume and flow rates; and particle characteristics such as size, shape, and chemistry.

The characteristics of equine airways and pattern of breathing lend themselves very well to inhalation therapy. The large tidal volume and high flow rate of resting horses are ideally suited for effective inhalation therapy. In addition, the horse is an obligate nasal breather and cannot mouth breathe to bypass an inhalation device placed on the nose. In horses with lower airway disease, airway narrowing influences the drug dose deposited and the distribution of that dose within the lung. For example, in horses with recurrent airway obstruction (heaves), pulmonary function tests suggest that aerosols are deposited primarily in the central airways. As therapy progresses and bronchodilation is achieved in the central airways, deposition of therapeutic aerosols may occur deeper within the lung. Early in therapy higher doses of bronchodilator agents may be needed to achieve clinical objectives in these cases, and drug doses may be reduced as therapy progresses.

The dose of drug delivered to the lower respiratory tract is also a function of aerosol characteristics, primarily the size of the aerosol produced and the number of particles available (mass). The finer aerosols distribute to more peripheral airways, but because of their smaller size contain less drug. Large-particle aerosols contain more drug, but are deposited in more proximal airways. It is generally accepted that aerosols with a mass median aerodynamic diameter of less than 5 μ produce the best therapeutic results. Larger particles deposit in delivery devices or the upper airway, and nebulizers that primarily produce large aerosol particles are likely to be ineffective. The aerosol mass produced varies greatly among nebulizers and, therefore, it is important to know the aerosol characteristic of the aerosol delivery system to be used.

AEROSOL DELIVERY DEVICES

Devices available in equine medicine for inhalation therapy include jet nebulizers, ultrasonic nebulizers, and pressurized canisters for use in metered-dose inhalers. Jet and ultrasonic nebulizers have been available to veterinarians for many years, but they have not enjoyed widespread clinical use. These devices are generally large, cumbersome, inefficient, and slow, requiring horses to wear uncomfortable masks for 20 minutes or longer (Table 1). However, development of new delivery devices has made inhalation therapy for horses a practical alternative to systemic or oral administration of therapeutic agents. The Aero-Mask, which consists of a valved mask and spacer, has been used to deliver fenoterol, a β_2-agonist bronchodilator, to horses with heaves. A commercially available metered-dose inhaler is attached to the spacer, and aerosol is delivered in this device. The advantages of a valved spacer are that delivery of the aerosol using the metered-dose inhaler does not have to be coordinated with the horse's breathing and that the characteristics of the therapeutic

TABLE 1. RADIOAEROSOL DEPOSITION IN EQUIDS

Aerosol Generator	Subject	Mean Deposition (%)	Reference
Jet	Foals	1.33	Viel and Tesarowski
Jet	Foals	0.32	Viel and Tesarowski
Jet	Foals	0.78	Viel and Tesarowski
Ultrasonic	Foals	0.27	Viel and Tesarowski
Ultrasonic	Foals	0.32	Viel and Tesarowski
Aero-Mask	Pony	6.12	Viel and Tesarowski
Hand-held, metered-dose inhaler	Horse	23.3	Geor and Johnston

TABLE 2. DRUGS USED FOR INHALATION THERAPY IN THE HORSE

Class	Drug	Device	Disease Condition	Dose	Reference
β_2-agonist	Fenoterol	Aero-Mask	RAO	2–3 µg/kg	Tesarowski, et al
	Pirbuterol	HHMDI	RAO	1–2 µg/kg	Derksen, et al
	Albuterol	HHMDI	RAO	1–2 µg/kg	Derksen, et al
	Terbutaline	Ultrasonic nebulizer	RAO	20 µg/kg	Murphy, et al
Anticholinergic	Ipratropium bromide	Ultrasonic nebulizer	RAO	2–3 µg/kg	Robinson, et al
Corticosteroid	Beclomethasone	Aero-Mask	RAO	3750 µg b.i.d.	Ammann, et al
Mast cell stabilizer	Sodium cromoglycate	Jet nebulizer	SAD	200 mg b.i.d.	Hare, et al
	Sodium cromoglycate	Ultrasonic nebulizer	RAO	80 mg s.i.d.	Thompson and McPherson

HHMDI = hand-held metered-dose inhaler; RAO = recurrent airway obstruction (heaves); SAD = small airway disease

aerosol are improved. In studies with radiolabeled fenoterol, it was demonstrated that, using this system, significantly more aerosol was deposited in the lung (6.12%) than using jet or ultrasonic nebulizers (<1.5%) (see Table 1).

A hand-held metered-dose aerosol delivery device that is inserted directly into a nostril has been demonstrated to deliver aerosol throughout all lung fields, with minimal deposition in the nasal cavity, oral pharynx, and trachea. The dose of aerosol delivered into the midthoracic region was 23.3%, making this device the most efficient method to date for delivery of therapeutic aerosols into the equine lung.

In summary, several devices may be used to deliver therapeutic aerosols into the equine lung. The efficacy of these devices is markedly dissimilar and, therefore, the clinician needs to pay close attention to the characteristics of the delivery device used. The fraction of aerosol deposited in the lung ranges from a low of less than 1.5% for jet nebulizers to a high of 23.3% for the hand-held metered-dose inhaler. Therefore, when determining dosing schedules, the clinician should carefully consider the performance of the delivery device to be used. Even within the individual horse, when using identical equipment, progression of therapy and lessening of airway obstruction may allow the clinician to use lower doses of therapeutic agents, because these agents become deposited deeper within the lung. Thus, dose ranges given in Table 2 for therapeutic aerosols are guidelines only, and aerosolized therapeutic agents should be administered to effect.

BRONCHODILATOR AND ANTI-INFLAMMATORY THERAPY

The major classes of therapeutic agents administered by inhalation are (1) parasympatholytic agents (ipratropium bromide); (2) β_2-adrenergic agonists (fenoterol, pirbuterol, albuterol); (3) mast cell stabilizing drugs (sodium cromoglycate); and (4) corticosteroids (beclomethasone).

Anticholinergic Agents

Anticholinergic agents like ipratropium bromide° cause bronchodilation by blockade of M_3-muscarinic receptors on smooth muscle. Ipratropium bromide's quaternary structure discourages absorption of compound from the respiratory tract after aerosol administration. In addition, and unlike other parasympatholytic agents, ipratropium bromide does not inhibit mucociliary clearance. In horses with heaves, aerosol ipratropium bromide, administered using an ultrasonic nebulizer at a dose of 2 to 3 µg/mg, causes significant bronchodilation lasting from 4 to 6 hours. The onset of bronchodilation following treatment with ipratropium bromide is slightly slower than after β_2-adrenoceptor agonists, but the effects tend to last longer. It has been suggested that there may be advantages to combining anticholinergics and β_2-agonists in therapeutic protocols.

β_2-Adrenergic Agonists

β_2-adrenoceptor agonist bronchodilators affect bronchial smooth muscle directly by binding to β_2-adrenoceptors. Receptor activation results in increased intracellular cyclic adenosine monophosphate (AMP). β_2-agonists generally have a rapid onset of action (within 5 minutes). Fenoterol° at a dose of 2 to 4 µg/kg is an effective bronchodilator in horses with heaves, but the duration of action of this compound has not been studied in horses with this condition. Pirbuterol† and albuterol‡ at a dose of 1 to 2 µg/kg cause similarly effective bronchodilation, and the duration of action is approximately 1 hour. Administration of β_2-receptor agonists by inhalation has significant advantages over oral or systemic administration of the same compounds. Oral and systemic administration at therapeutic doses results in side effects, including trembling, sweating, tachycardia, and excitement. These side effects are not observed in horses receiving therapeutic doses by aerosol. However, with pirbuterol and albuterol, doses exceeding 6 µg/kg cause side effects related to administration of β_2-adrenoceptor agonists even when drugs are delivered by inhalation.

As mentioned earlier, when determining aerosol bronchodilator dosing, the delivery device to be used must be considered. Doses for fenoterol, albuterol, and pirbuterol were derived using relatively effective delivery devices (Aero-Mask or a, hand-held metered-dose inhaler device). In contrast, the dose recommended for terbutaline is 20 µg/kg, but this dose was determined using an ultrasonic

---

°Atrovent, Boehringer Ingelheim Canada Ltd., Burlington, Ontario, Canada

°Berotec, Boehringer Ingelheim Canada Ltd., Burlington, Ontario, Canada
†Maxair, 3M Pharmaceuticals, St. Paul, MN
‡Ventolin, Glaxo Wellcome, Research Triangle Park, NC

nebulizer, plastic tubing, and face mask. Thus, the differences in recommended doses between terbutaline and the other β_2-agonists are more likely to be primarily a function of delivery device than of drug potency. Bronchodilation achieved with terbutaline has been reported to last as long as 6 hours.

Mast Cell Stabilizing Drugs

Sodium cromoglycate* is reported to inhibit degranulation of mast cells and release of proinflammatory mediators. Although the role of mast cells in inflammatory airway disease of horses has not been established, inhalation of sodium cromoglycate 20 to 30 minutes before antigen inhalation challenge prevents the induction of airway obstruction in horses with heaves. The recommended dose is 80 mg s.i.d. when delivered using an ultrasonic nebulizer. After four consecutive daily treatments, clinical signs of heaves are ameliorated for a mean of 24.3 days. Sodium cromoglycate (200 mg) nebulized using the Aero-Mask was reported to be effective in the treatment of small airway disease in a population of young racehorses. Thus, sodium cromoglycate may be useful in the prophylaxis and management of airway inflammation in horses with various lung diseases.

Corticosteroids

Inhaled corticosteroid therapy has revolutionized the treatment of asthma in human medicine. Long-term, low-dose aerosol corticosteroid therapy is possible because systemic side effects are avoided. Reducing airway inflammation in asthma in this way reduces clinical signs, minimizes the need for bronchodilator therapy, and suppresses airway hyper-responsiveness. A single dose of triamcinolone acetonide (0.09 mg/kg IM) has been reported to improve pulmonary function in horses with heaves for 2 to 3 weeks. Concerns about systemic side effects of corticosteroid therapy, especially using potent corticosteroids such as triamcinolone acetonide, prevent the widespread use of this effective therapeutic modality. Inhalation therapy using corticosteroids may be a useful alternative. It has been reported that aerosol administration of beclomethasone* by use of an Aero-Mask (3750 μg/horse) b.i.d. for 2 weeks improves pulmonary function in horses with heaves. Dose titration studies and long-term efficacy studies need to be done in a variety of equine inflammatory lung diseases before specific therapeutic regimens can be recommended. However, it is likely that low-dose inhalation corticosteroid therapy in the horse may prove useful in the treatment and prevention of inflammatory conditions of the horse lung.

Supplemental Readings

Ammann VJ, Lavoie JP, Vrins AA: Effects of beclomethasone diproprionate in horses with chronic obstructive pulmonary disease (COPD). Proc 13th Annu Vet Med Forum, Am Coll Vet Intern Med, 1995, p 1037.

Derksen FJ, Robinson NE, Berney CE: Aerosol pirbuterol: Bronchodilator activity and side effects in ponies with recurrent airway obstruction (heaves). Equine Vet J 24:107–112, 1992.

Dolovich M: Lung dose, distribution, and clinical response to therapeutic aerosols. Aerosol Science Technology 18:230–240, 1993.

Geor R, Johnston G: Deposition of radiolabelled aerosols within the equine respiratory tract. Proc 12th Vet Resp Symp, Comp Resp Soc, University of Pennsylvania, 1993.

Hare JE, Viel L, O'Byrne PM, Conlon PD: Effect of sodium cromoglycate on light racehorses with elevated metachromatic cell numbers on bronchoalveolar lavage and reduced exercise tolerance. J Vet Pharmacol Ther 17:237–244, 1994.

Hoffman AM: Inhaled medication for small airway disease in horses. Proc 13th ACVIM Forum, 1995, pp 758–760.

Lapointe J-M, Lavoie J-P, Vrins AA: Effects of triamcinolone acetonide on pulmonary function and bronchoalveolar lavage cytologic features in horses with chronic obstructive pulmonary disease. Am J Vet Res 54:1310–1316, 1993.

Murphy JR, McPherson EA, Dixon PM: Chronic obstructive pulmonary disease (COPD): Effects of bronchodilator drugs on normal and affected horses. Equine Vet J 12:10–14, 1980.

Robinson NE, Derksen FJ, Berney C, Goossens L: The airway response of horses with recurrent airway obstruction (heaves) to aerosol administration of ipratropium bromide. Equine Vet J 25:299–303, 1993.

Tesarowski DB, Viel L, McDonell WN, Newhouse MT: The rapid and effective administration of a β_2-agonist to horses with heaves using a compact inhalation device and metered-dose inhalers. Can Vet J 35:170–173, 1994.

Thomson JR, McPherson EA: Prophylactic effects of sodium cromoglycate on chronic obstructive pulmonary disease in the horse. Equine Vet J 13:243–246, 1981.

Viel L, Tesarowski D: Radioaerosol deposition in equids. Proc 40th Annu Conv Am Assoc Equine Pract, 1994, pp 93–94.

---

*Intal, Fisons, Rochester, NY

*Beclovent, Allen Hanburys, Research Triangle Park, NC

Chronic Obstructive Pulmonary Disease

JEAN-PIERRE LAVOIE
St. Hyacinthe, Quebec

Chronic obstructive pulmonary disease (COPD), also known as heaves, broken wind, emphysema, chronic bronchitis, bronchiolitis, and recurrent airway obstruction, is a common condition of horses in cold climates. Most of the names for the condition refer to the end stage of this disease, which is characterized by labored breathing and a typical double expiratory effort. The terms *lower respiratory tract inflammation* and *lower airway disease* are often used in the early stages of the disease because signs of airway obstruction are not evident.

Equine COPD is an inflammatory condition of the lower airways, characterized by the presence of bronchospasm, mucus plugs, and pathologic changes of the bronchiolar walls leading to terminal airway obstruction. Owing to the large total cross-sectional area of the small airways, clinical signs are observed in the resting horse only when obstruction affects a large number of small airways. No gender or breed predisposition is apparent, and the incidence increases with age. The hereditary nature of equine COPD is not clear, although some family lines appear to be more predisposed.

CLINICAL SIGNS

Horses in the early stages of COPD are alert and afebrile and may be exercise-intolerant or may present with an occasional cough at the onset of exercise or when eating. The frequency and severity of the coughing episodes increase as the disease progresses to finally become paroxysmal bouts of deep nonproductive coughs. In severe cases, an increased respiratory rate, flared nostrils, and double expiratory effort may also be present. Emaciation and a "heave line" caused by hypertrophy of the external abdominal oblique muscles may develop. The appearance and severity of the clinical signs tend to wax and wane. The duration of the attacks varies from days to weeks, and some horses are asymptomatic between attacks.

Auscultation during normal tidal breathing is often unremarkable. Auscultation of the thorax during forced breathing, induced by use of a rebreathing bag, by obstruction of the nostrils, or by exercise, may reveal wheezes throughout the lung fields and expiratory crackles that are more intense at the periphery of the lungs. In advanced cases, wheezing can be heard in the trachea and throughout the lung fields, although there may be areas with decreased bronchovesicular sounds because air flow to such regions is totally obstructed. Percussion of the thorax may reveal hyper-resonance of the ventral and caudal borders of the lung fields caused by air trapping.

During endoscopic examination of the respiratory tract, a large amount of mucus may be present in the trachea, and hyperemia and edema of the lower airways may be noted. Radiographic examination of the thorax is often unremarkable but may reveal an increased bronchointerstitial pattern.

ETIOPATHOLOGY

The etiopathology of equine COPD is unknown but it is likely to be multifactorial, leading to lower airway inflammation. Exposure to dusty feed and bedding usually precedes the appearance of the clinical signs. A hypersensitivity reaction to specific antigens (allergic-type reaction), a nonspecific hyper-reactivity reaction, or merely an inflammatory response induced by dust may be associated with the disease. Two molds, *Aspergillus fumigatus* and *Faenia rectivirgula*, have been most commonly implicated as inciting allergens. Close contact between horses and chickens also has been associated with clinical signs closely resembling equine COPD.

The development of COPD may follow a viral respiratory infection. Infectious diseases may induce hypersensitivity- and hyper-reactivity-type reactions by damaging airway epithelium and altering immune responses and mucociliary clearance. In addition, once airway inflammation is established, any foreign element reaching the lower airways may contribute to the continuance of lower airway inflammation.

DIAGNOSIS

The diagnosis of COPD in advanced cases is based on the presence of a chronic cough or labored breathing in an otherwise healthy animal, and the exclusion of other conditions, mainly infectious diseases, affecting the lower airways. In equine COPD, the complete blood count usually remains within normal limits in the absence of concurrent infection.

In the early stages, cytologic evaluation of a bronchoalveolar lavage (BAL) may be necessary to confirm the presence of lower airway inflammation. The most common change, which allows differentiation from horses without lower airway inflammation, is a neutrophilia (neutrophils >10–15%) in the BAL fluid. There is not a good correlation, however, between the severity of the clinical signs observed, degree of neutrophilia in BAL fluid, and prognosis. Cytologic examination of transtracheal washes or tracheal aspirates also reveals neutrophilia, but it is of a lesser value for the diagnosis of COPD, because it evaluates both small and large airways. The presence of bacteria in tracheal aspirates in the absence of other signs of infection most likely represents a secondary colonization of the large airways in COPD-afflicted horses caused by decreased mucociliary clearance.

Arterial blood gas analysis provides an easy way to assess the degree of respiratory dysfunction of severely affected horses with COPD and evaluate their response to therapy. Arterial blood may be obtained from various arteries; the facial artery of horses can easily be reached using a 22-gauge needle and a 1-ml heparinized plastic syringe. If the arterial sample is maintained at room temperature, PaO_2 can be determined accurately for up to 20 minutes after collection time. Glass syringes are more cumbersome to use but allow adequate determination of PaO_2 for up to 2 hours when blood is kept on ice. The PaO_2 values of resting COPD-afflicted horses usually are under 80 mm Hg and may be as low as 40 mm Hg in horses with labored breathing at rest.

Field evaluation of respiratory function is difficult and is limited to the measurement of the maximal variation of intrathoracic esophageal pressures. The esophageal pressure is used to estimate the increased variation in intrapleural pressures required to maintain air flow in the presence of obstructed airways. The measurement can be performed using a commercially available esophageal catheter linked to a portable physiological recorder.* The usefulness of this technique in clinical practice is limited, however, because significant changes in intrathoracic esophageal pressures

---

*Venti-Graph, Boehringer Ingelheim Animal Health, Burlington, ON, Canada

are detected only when obvious clinical signs of respiratory diseases are present.

Lung biopsy may be used for the diagnosis of equine COPD because there is good correlation between the histologic changes on lung biopsy and the severity of clinical signs. Biopsy can be performed at the seventh or eighth intercostal space, approximately 8 cm above the humeroradial joint. However, owing to the uncommon but severe bleeding that may occur with this procedure, routine lung biopsy for the diagnosis of COPD is not recommended. Bronchial biopsy under endoscopic guidance is well tolerated in horses but correlates poorly with the results of transcutaneous lung biopsies.[*]

At the present time, intradermal mold antigen testing and the evaluation of serum antibody titers against common environmental antigens appear to be of questionable value in the investigation of equine COPD.

EVALUATION OF REVERSIBILITY

The reversibility of the airway obstruction is used to predict the response to therapy. Different protocols have been proposed, but evaluation of breathing difficulty and thoracic auscultation before and after the administration of atropine[†] (0.01–0.02 mg/kg IV), an anticholinergic agent, is most commonly used. Respiratory function should be evaluated before and when tachycardia has developed in response to the atropine administration (approximately 30 minutes). Although generally well tolerated, paralytic ileus and severe abdominal pain can develop following atropine administration, especially in horses with severely compromised airway function. Because of these side effects and because most horses with COPD markedly improve with therapy, the routine administration of atropine for diagnostic purpose is not recommended.

SEDATION OF COPD-AFFECTED HORSES

Drugs used for sedation of COPD-affected horses with severe labored breathing should, minimize respiratory depression or, ideally, improve respiratory function. Alpha$_2$ adrenergic agonist agents, such as xylazine[‡] (0.03–0.05 mg/kg IV) and detomidine[§] (10–30 μg/kg IV) may be preferred, because they cause bronchodilation. Care should be taken, however, to keep the head and neck in a horizontal plane because these agents also relax upper airways and increase upper airway resistance. Combinations of α$_2$-adrenergic agonist agents and butorphanol[‖] (20–30 μg/kg IV) are usually well tolerated in horses with COPD. However, because these agents can transiently worsen hypoxemia, they should be used only if sedation is mandatory.

---

[*]*DW Wilson, personal communication*
[†]*Atropine sulfate, M.T.C. Pharmaceuticals, Cambridge, ON, Canada*
[‡]*Rompun, Bayer, Agricultural Division, Animal Health, Etoboke, ON, Canada*
[§]*Dormosedan, SmithKline Beecham, Animal Health, Mississauga, ON, Canada*
[‖]*Torbugesic, Ayers Laboratories, Montreal, QC, Canada*

TREATMENT

The treatment of COPD aims at (1) preventing further exposure to dust; (2) decreasing inflammation of the lower airways; and (3) providing symptomatic relief.

Environmental Changes

Decreased exposure to dust is essential for the long-term control of equine COPD (see Current Therapy in Equine Medicine 3, p 310). Drugs administered to horses with COPD have only transitory effects if strict dust control measures are not applied. The reversal of clinical signs of COPD following strict environmental changes may take up to 3 to 4 weeks. The remission time correlates with age of the horse, duration of airway obstruction, and severity of illness. Horses kept permanently outdoors and fed grass or good quality hay usually remain free of clinical signs. Horses do well when kept outdoors even in very cold conditions, as long as they have access to enough food, fresh water from a heated waterer, and shelter. Horses with labored breathing caused by chicken hypersensitivity pneumonitis become clinically normal when removed from their environment for 48 hours.

The replacement of hay and straw by less dusty feedstuff and bedding can induce clinical remission in stabled horses. Pelleted hay, hay silage, and hydroponic hay are well tolerated and dust-free. Hay soaked in water for at least 2 hours before feeding may control COPD in some horses, although it is less efficacious and is cumbersome. Wood shavings, shredded paper, peanut kernels, and peat moss are good substitutes for straw. Stabling horses away from straw and hay dust, removing the horse from the stable when cleaning the box stalls, and watering the aisles before sweeping all decrease the amount of dust. Proper ventilation is also important, although identifying the proper ventilation system that minimizes dust is problematic. Dust inhaled during exercise may contain large amounts of particles, including fungal spores, that may contribute to airway inflammation. It has been recently shown that appropriate wetting of riding surfaces allows control of air pollution.

Corticosteroids

Corticosteroids (Table 1) are the most effective treatment for the control of equine COPD. A delay of up to 4 days can be expected between the initiation of therapy and the maximal clinical response, although some improvement may be observed within a few hours of drug administration. Long-acting corticosteroids and those with potent anti-inflammatory effects are more likely to be associated with detrimental reactions such as laminitis, infections, and Cushing-like syndrome with signs of muscle wasting, dry hair coat, polydipsia, and polyuria. Drug selection depends on the severity of the clinical signs and the ability to improve the environment of the horse. The minimal effective dose should be used and the prolonged administration of corticosteroids should be avoided.

The administration of corticosteroids for a period of 2 to 4 weeks is usually required for the control of equine COPD. For a severe attack, dexamethasone[*] or isoflu-

---

[*]*Azium, Schering-Plough Animal Health, Pointe Claire, QC, Canada*

TABLE 1. MEDICATIONS RECOMMENDED FOR THE TREATMENT OF EQUINE RESPIRATORY DISEASES

MEDICATION	DOSAGE
Bronchodilators	
Clenbuterol	0.8 to 3.2 μg/kg p.o. b.i.d.
	0.8 μg/kg IV
Terbutaline sulfate	0.02 to 0.06 mg/kg p.o. b.i.d.
Aminophylline	5 to 10 mg/kg orally or IV b.i.d.
Corticosteroids	
Dexamethasone	20 mg° orally IV or IM daily for 2 days; dose is then administered on alternate days and tapered to 5 mg over five to six treatments
Isoflupredone acetate	10–14 mg° IM daily for 5 days; dose is then administered on alternate days and tapered over a period of 10 to 20 days
Prednisone	400–800 mg° orally or IM administered daily for 1 week; dose is then tapered and administered on alternate days
Triamcinolone acetonide	20–40 mg° IM
Expectorants and Mucolytic Agents	
Potassium iodide	2–20 g° p.o. once daily
Dembrexine	0.3–0.5 mg/kg p.o. b.i.d.
Overhydration (isotonic saline solution)	30 L° IV over a 3-hour period once daily for one to three treatments

See page 430 for the dosages of drugs administered by inhalation
°The usual dose for a horse that weighs 450–500 kg

predone acetate° usually provides fast relief. Oral prednisone† or prednisolone is less potent and less toxic and is useful when long-term maintenance therapy is required. Triamcinolone acetonide‡ is used in horses when treatment cannot be administered daily. Although clinical improvement may last more than 3 months in some cases, the effect of triamcinolone is often less than 5 weeks, in the absence of improvement in the horse's environment. Triamcinolone is administered at no less than 3-month intervals to reduce the risk of laminitis.

The administration of corticosteroids by inhalation allows a maximal concentration of drug at the effector sites and minimizes side effects. Beclomethasone dipropionate§ (3500 μg/500 kg b.i.d.) in a metered dose inhaler administered by inhalation using a mask‖ is very effective in controlling the clinical signs of COPD. A clinical improvement in respiratory function is observed within 4 treatment days but lasts less than 1 week after treatment is discontinued if no concurrent dust control is instigated. After 2 weeks of treatment, beclomethasone may be administered once daily, and the dose is gradually tapered until the minimal effective dosage is found.

Bronchodilators

Bronchodilators are used to relieve the obstruction of small airways caused by airway smooth muscle contraction. Administration of bronchodilators should be combined with strict environmental dust control or corticosteroid administration because inflammation of the lower airways may progress despite the improvement of clinical signs observed with bronchodilator therapy. Bronchodilators are particularly helpful when immediate relief of clinical signs is required, owing to their rapid onset of action. The administration of bronchodilators may transiently worsen hypoxemia before an elevation in PaO$_2$ is observed. The agents most commonly used are β-agonist and xanthine derivatives.

Clenbuterol,° a β_2-adrenergic agonist, has bronchodilator effects and increases mucociliary transport. Side effects such as tachycardia and sweating are rarely seen with lower oral doses, but are more frequent with intravenous administration. The clinical efficacy of clenbuterol, at the lower recommended dosage (0.8 μg/kg b.i.d.) is inconsistent, if exposure to dusty hay and bedding is maintained. With higher dosages (up to 3.2 μg/kg), its efficacy improves, but so do the frequency and severity of side effects. Terbutaline sulfate† is another β_2-adrenergic agonist that may be used orally or by inhalation in countries where clenbuterol is not available. Fenoterol, albuterol, and pirbuterol are other β_2-agonist agents with potent bronchodilator effects (see p 430) that can be administered by inhalation. Following inhalation of β_2-agonists, bronchodilation is rapid with minimal side effects but lasts only 1 hour, thus requiring frequent drug administration. The use of sympathomimetic agents such as ephedrine, which stimulate both α and β receptors, has decreased because of the availability of more specific β-adrenergic agonists.

Aminophylline‡ is a xanthine derivative and is used as a bronchodilator in horses. In addition to bronchodilation, it enhances mucociliary clearance, respiratory drive, and contractility of the diaphragm, and modulates immune function. Side effects such as excitability, tachycardia, muscular tremors, and sweating may be observed. Because of its low therapeutic index, the use of aminophylline and other salts of theophylline may be preferred in cases when relief of bronchodilation is not achieved with other therapeutic agents or in horses with hypoventilation.

Because of their potentially severe side effects systemically administered anticholinergic drugs are generally not indicated for the treatment of COPD. Ipratropium bromide can be safely administered by aerosol; its duration of effect is 4 hours (see p 430).

Expectorant, Mucolytic, and Mucokinetic Agents

Expectorants increase pulmonary secretion, whereas mucolytic agents loosen secretions. The term *mucokinetic agent* may be preferred because it indicates that the therapy is aimed at increasing the clearance of the respiratory tract secretions. Although the administration of mucokinetic agents may help loosen the secretions in the large airways, the evidence of their efficacy in improving the clinical signs of COPD is sparse. Clenbuterol, because

°*Predef 2X, Upjohn Company Animal Health, Orangeville, ON, Canada*
†*Apo-Prednisone Tablets USP, Apotex, Toronto, ON, Canada*
‡*Kenalog, Westwood-Squibb, Montreal, QC, Canada*
§*Becloforte, Glaxo Canada, Mississauga, ON, Canada*
‖*Equine Aeromask, Canadian Monaghan Limited, London, ON, Canada*

°*Ventipulmin, Boehringer Ingelheim Animal Health, Burlington, ON, Canada*
†*Bricanyl, AstraPharma, Mississauga, ON, Canada*
‡*Aminophylline Tablets USP, Cyanamid Canada, Montreal, QC, Canada*

of its bronchodilator and mucokinetic properties, may be preferred to clear mucus from the airways. Dembrexine* and potassium iodide also improve clearance of bronchial secretions. Potassium iodide should be administered with caution to COPD-affected horses because it is irritating for the respiratory tract and can induce or worsen bronchospasm.

Overhydration by the massive administration of isotonic saline solution combined with bronchodilators or mucokinetic agents may be occasionally associated with clinical remission in horses whose condition is refractory to other modes of therapy. The proposed beneficial effects of this treatment are improved mucus transport and removal of mucous plugs related to the liquefaction of excessively viscous mucus. This treatment should be administered with caution because a number of side effects including dyspnea and colic have been observed.

Antitussive agents should not be administered to horses with COPD because cough is a mechanism essential for the clearance of respiratory secretions.

OTHER AGENTS

Sodium cromoglycate is most effective when administered to asymptomatic COPD-susceptible horses before exposure to dust, but a favorable response can also be observed in symptomatic animals. The mechanism of action of sodium cromoglycate is unknown but may include stabilization of inflammatory cells and a local effect on nerve endings. The prophylactic administration of sodium cromoglycate (80 mg s.i.d. for 4 days) by inhalation to horses in clinical remission from COPD prevented the appearance of clinical signs for up to 3 weeks after they were introduced to a dusty environment. The administration of sodium cromoglycate by use of a dose-metered inhaler† and a treatment mask facilitated drug administration and therefore decreased treatment failure due to inadequate drug administration.

Histamine has a number of effects on the respiratory system, such as increased mucus secretion, plasma extravasation leading to airway mucosal edema, and smooth muscle contraction, but its role in equine COPD is ill-defined. Antihistamines, which block the histamine H_1-receptor, have been used for the treatment of equine COPD, although there is little evidence of their efficacy.

Humoral and cellular immunity have a pivotal role in the pathogenesis of equine COPD. The clinical efficacy of immunostimulant agents is therefore being investigated. Levamisole, an anthelmintic that also has immunopotentiating properties, has been used for the treatment of COPD in horses. Anecdotal reports suggest that the response to therapy was inconsistent, and severe side effects, including death, occurred. Various bacterial wall extracts are available for the treatment of infectious respiratory diseases in horses, but their efficacy in equine COPD remains to be determined.

Currently available nonsteroidal anti-inflammatory drugs (NSAIDs) are of little use in the treatment of equine COPD. Antimicrobials should be administered to horses with COPD in the presence of a fever, leukocytosis, and hyperfibrinogenemia, which are suggestive of a concurrent bacterial infection.

COPD IN PREGNANT MARES

Pregnant COPD-afflicted mares usually deliver normal foals although anecdotal observations suggest that severely affected mares may have prolonged pregnancy and give birth to low-body-weight foals. The chronic hypoxemia and debilitated condition of severely affected mares could contribute to fetal growth retardation, leading to prematurity and low birth weight. The severity of the clinical signs of COPD improves during pregnancy in some mares.

Little information is available on the effects of drugs and COPD on perinatal risk in mares. In people and experimental animals, theophylline and corticosteroids may be associated with an increased incidence of prematurity and low birth weight. Therefore the decision to treat pregnant mares requires that the potential benefits of therapy be weighed against the possible hazards for the fetus and the mare. Therapy should also depend on the severity of the disease and the ability to control environmental air quality. Theophylline and β_2-adrenergic agonists administered systemically decrease uterine contraction, and their administration should be stopped before the anticipated date of foaling. Anecdotal field experience suggests that β_2-adrenergic agonists and corticosteroids are usually well tolerated in pregnant mares. Inhaled medications are preferred, because their low systemic availability limits the effects on the fetus.

PREVENTION

Equine COPD can be prevented by controlling the air quality of the environment mainly by preventing exposure to dusty hay and straw. Because strong circumstantial evidence links equine COPD to respiratory viral infections, proper vaccination against influenza and rhinopneumonitis may help prevent the disease. In addition, preventing exposure to hay and straw dust during an episode of viral infection, proper medical management of the condition, and rest are mandatory.

Supplemental Readings

Dixon PM: Respiratory mucociliary clearance in the horse in health and disease, and its pharmacological modification. Vet Rec 131:229–235, 1992.

Lavoie JP: Chronic diseases of the respiratory tract. Compend Cont Educ Pract Vet 16:1597–1601, 1994.

Mansmann RA, Osburn BI, Wheat JD, Frick O: Chicken hypersensitivity pneumonitis in horses. J Am Vet Med Assoc 166:673–677, 1975.

Paradis MR: Chronic obstructive pulmonary disease. Compend Cont Educ Pract Vet 12:1651–1654, 1990.

Thomson JR, McPherson EA: Effects of environmental control on pulmonary function of horses affected with chronic obstructive pulmonary disease. Equine Vet J 16:35–38, 1984.

Sputolysin, Boehringer Ingelheim Animal Health, Burlington, ON, Canada
†*Intal, Fisons Corporation, Pickering, ON, Canada*

Summer Pasture–Associated Obstructive Pulmonary Disease

JOHANNA L. WATSON
Davis, California

The classic presentation of obstructive pulmonary disease in the horses is a chronic condition, chronic obstructive pulmonary disease (COPD), usually associated with stabling and exposure to hay and straw. Summer pasture-associated obstructive pulmonary disease is a syndrome of obstructed respiration following exposure to specific pastures during the summer months. Most reported cases of summer pasture-associated obstructive pulmonary disease are from the southeastern United States and Great Britain. Treatment for these animals involves moving them indoors and feeding them hay.

Another form of this syndrome has been reported with increased frequency from southern California with what appears to be an alfalfa hay-associated obstructive pulmonary disease. Horses in different environments fed the same type of hay develop an obstructive respiratory pattern that can be reversed by simply removing the offending lots of hay.

ETIOPATHOGENESIS

The etiology of summer pasture-associated obstructive pulmonary disease is unknown. This condition has been attributed to fungal species in southeastern United States, and it is thought to be related to seasonal pollens in Great Britain. There are three hypotheses that could explain the clinical and pathologic findings in this disease: (1) allergic lung disease (i.e., type I hypersensitivity); (2) antigenic stimulation (i.e., type III or IV hypersensitivity); and (3) an ingested pneumotoxin. The rapid reversal of clinical signs with no treatment other than environmental management suggests that this disease is most likely an allergy or type I hypersensitivity. The pathogenesis of this syndrome is not well understood, but bronchoconstriction and excessive respiratory mucus production are routinely observed. The large-scale influx of neutrophils into the airways is a hallmark of this syndrome, just as it is in COPD. Any number or combination of mediators can be implicated to explain these common clinicopathologic findings.

HISTORY AND CLINICAL SIGNS

This condition occurs most commonly in adult horses older than 8 years of age during the summer months of June through September. Those affected have exposure to pasture for some period each day. Although in many cases the respiratory difficulty experienced during the summer months resolves in the winter, some horses also show classic symptoms of COPD when stabled in the winter. Horses that are asymptomatic during the winter may be affected again the following summer.

Clinical signs may include tachypnea, increased expiratory effort, nasal discharge, and cough. Exercise intolerance is common, and severely affected horses may exhibit anorexia and weight loss. Thoracic auscultation findings vary from end-expiratory wheezes in the caudodorsal lung fields to generalized wheezes and crackles. These animals are not routinely febrile.

DIAGNOSIS

Diagnosis of summer pasture-associated obstructive pulmonary disease involves documentation of airway obstruction in the absence of infection. The hemogram commonly shows a mature neutrophilia as the only abnormality. Airway cytology testing also reflects a neutrophilia, which usually consists of nondegenerate cells. Bacteria may be recovered from the respiratory secretions of some affected horses with this syndrome. Recovered bacteria are likely to be present owing to decreased clearance of mucus and dead inflammatory cells from the obstructed airway, especially if the animal is not febrile and does not exhibit an elevated fibrinogen. Samples for cytologic examination can be obtained by transtracheal aspirate or bronchoalveolar lavage. Transtracheal aspirate is a superior sample for culture, allowing the clinician to identify secondary bacterial infection, and the procedure is less invasive than bronchoalveolar lavage. Some horses with severe respiratory compromise may not tolerate bronchoalveolar lavage.

Diagnosis of obstructive respiratory disease is best done with pulmonary function testing, but this is not practical in most cases. However, an atropine response test can be performed in combination with blood gas analysis to determine if the airway obstruction is reversible. Atropine* (5–7 mg/450kg IV) provides rapid relief of bronchoconstriction in most of these horses. A dramatic reduction in respiratory rate as well as an increase in the depth of respiration and elevation in PaO_2 can be seen. If there is no improvement in pulmonary function following atropine, significant interstitial disease may be present and the prognosis is poor.

Endoscopy often reveals copious tenacious mucus in the airways. Radiography may be useful to rule out other types of pulmonary disease. Thoracic radiographs of horses with summer pasture-associated obstructive pulmonary disease may show a mild to moderate interstitial or bronchointerstitial pattern, and severely affected individuals may show pulmonary overinflation.

*Atropine, Elkins-Sinn, Cherry Hill, NJ

Allergen intradermal skin testing and the measurement of circulating allergen-specific IgE are available for use in the horse. If the pasture- or season- or forage-associated obstructive pulmonary disease is a type I hypersensitivity, the allergens responsible for the disease may be used for hyposensitization. Because it is still unclear whether any of these conditions is driven by allergy, hyposensitization cannot be routinely recommended.

TREATMENT

The therapeutic goals are to (1) remove the bronchoconstricting agents from the environment; (2) treat the airway inflammation; and (3) achieve bronchodilation. The first goal is accomplished through environmental change or management. Horses affected on a particular pasture can be moved indoors to a well-ventilated stall. Horses that are affected on an alfalfa hay diet, regardless of surroundings, need to have the offending hay replaced with hay cubes or pellets that can be moistened to reduce dust. Although these horses may recover with environmental management alone, it is advisable to add anti-inflammatory and bronchodilator therapy to a treatment plan.

Corticosteroids are the anti-inflammatory drug of choice for summer pasture- or forage-associated obstructive pulmonary diseases. Dexamethasone* and prednisone† have both been used effectively in the horse to treat this condition. For the moderate to severely affected horse it is advisable to initiate treatment with dexamethasone because it is more potent than prednisone and has a longer duration of action. Treatment should be initiated with 20 to 40 mg/450-kg horse, divided twice a day. Dexamethasone can be administered by the oral (p.o.), intramuscular (IM), or intravenous (IV) routes. A decremental dose schedule should be followed over a 7- to 14-day period, terminating at 5 to 10 mg/450-kg horse every other day. Prednisone can be used in a similar treatment regimen, starting at a dose of 1 mg/kg orally twice daily. If both environmental and medical management are implemented, pasture- or forage-associated obstructive pulmonary disease can usually

*Dexamethasone, Schering-Plough Animal Health, Kenilworth, NJ
†Prednisone, Roxane Laboratories, Columbus, OH

be resolved, or brought into remission, within 2 to 3 weeks. For this reason, longer-acting corticosteroids are not necessary and are therefore not recommended.

There are three classes of bronchodilators available for the treatment of horses, β₂-adrenergic agonists, methylxanthines, and parasympatholytics. There are no bronchodilators, except atropine, labeled for use in the horse in the United States. Beta₂-adrenergic agonists like clenbuterol* and terbutaline† are clinically reported to be variably effective in the horse. Clenbuterol is not approved for use in the United States, but in other countries it is administered at 0.8 to 1.6 µg/kg (p.o. or IV b.i.d.). Terbutaline is administered at 0.03 to 0.08 mg/kg (p.o. or IV b.i.d.). Methylxanthines include the drugs theophylline and aminophylline‡ and are variably effective bronchodilators in the horse. Therapeutic drug levels tend to be close to levels that cause toxic side effects in the horse.

Ideally, therapeutic drug monitoring should be run on cases treated repeatedly with methylxanthines, keeping the serum level below 15 µg/ml. This author recommends a dose range for aminophylline of 3 to 5 mg/kg twice daily. If effective bronchodilation is not achieved at this dose level, combination therapy with a β₂-adrenergic agonist is recommended. Parasympatholytic drugs like atropine are very effective but have associated gastrointestinal side effects that make them unacceptable for repeated dosing unless they are administered by inhalation.

Suggested Readings

Beadle RE: Summer pasture-associated obstructive pulmonary disease. *In* Robinson NE (ed): Current Therapy in Equine Medicine. Philadelphia, WB Saunders, 1983, pp 512–516.
Beech J: Chronic obstructive pulmonary disease. Vet Clin North Am Equine Pract 7(1):79–91, 1991.
Dixon PM, McGorum B: Pasture-associated seasonal respiratory disease in two horses. Vet Rec 126:9–12, 1990.
Seahorn TL: Summer pasture-associated obstructive pulmonary disease. Proc 11th Annu Forum Am Coll Vet Intern Med, 1993, pp 605–606.
Seahorn TL, Beadle RE: Summer pasture-associated obstructive pulmonary disease in horses: 21 cases (1983–1991). J Am Vet Med Assoc 202:779–782, 1993.

*Ventipulmin, Boehringer Ingelheim Animal Health, Burlington, ON, Canada
†Terbutaline, Geigy Pharmaceuticals, Ardsley, NY
‡Aminophylline, West-Ward Pharmaceuticals, Eatontown, NJ

Equine Interstitial Pneumonia

ANDRÉ VRINS
St. Hyacinthe, Quebec

Equine interstitial pneumonia (EIP) comprises an ill-defined group of pulmonary disorders characterized by diffuse inflammation of the alveolar walls and interstitial tissues. It leads to life-threatening respiratory distress due to hypoxemia, which results from a progressive limitation of oxygen transfer from air to blood.

A juvenile (see page 609) and an adult form of the disease have been reported. The juvenile form appears as an acute respiratory distress syndrome in foals aged from 1 to 8 months. Adult horses with EIP have clinical signs resembling those of chronic obstructive pulmonary disease. Equine interstitial pneumonia has a high mortality rate in both age groups, despite intensive medical treatment.

Infectious and toxic or chemical agents or allergic factors have been suggested as possible causes of EIP. It has been speculated that EIP may have different etiologies in different age groups. Viral and bacterial components have been frequently suspected in foals, and a hypersensitivity/toxic reaction has been proposed in adults. In most cases, however, a specific cause cannot be identified.

CLINICAL SIGNS

Fever, cough, severe dyspnea, cyanosis, and a restrictive breathing pattern are common findings in horses afflicted with EIP. Although foals are usually presented with an acute onset of clinical signs rapidly leading to death, there may be a progressive deterioration of respiratory function leading to death, especially in adult horses. Some horses may also slowly improve with time. More than one foal is often affected on the premises. Thoracic auscultation reveals loud bronchial sounds over the large airways, the peripheral areas of the lung being remarkably quiet considering the increased respiratory effort.

DIAGNOSIS

Infectious bronchopneumonia and chronic obstructive pulmonary disease are the main differential diagnoses to consider in foals and adult horses, respectively. Although a preliminary diagnosis of EIP can usually be made based on the clinical signs (acute onset, restrictive pattern of breathing, cyanosis, and hyperthermia), a complete blood count, thoracic radiographs, transtracheal wash, microbial analysis, and lung biopsy are necessary to make a definite diagnosis in most cases.

The neutrophilic leukocytosis and hyperfibrinogenemia commonly found with EIP may help to differentiate the condition from chronic obstructive pulmonary disease (COPD), but are also a feature of infectious bronchopneumonias. Radiographic examination of the thorax is of paramount importance for a definitive diagnosis. It shows extensive, diffusely distributed interstitial (Fig. 1) and bronchointerstitial pulmonary patterns. This is in sharp contrast to the cranioventral lesions generally observed in infectious bronchopneumonias and the usual absence of radiographic lesions with COPD. Transtracheal wash microbial analysis may give variable results. Material having undergone phagocytosis observed microscopically may be useful to elucidate suspected cases of mineral oil aspiration pneumonia or silicosis. Negative results of a Gram's-stained smear and bacterial culture of tracheal aspirate reinforce the clinical suspicion of EIP in foals.

Histologic examination of lung biopsy specimens may be the only method of documenting the type of the pulmonary disorder involved and should be considered to complete the work-up of a suspected EIP case. The disease is characterized by acute alveolar wall necrosis with the accumulation of a serofibrinous exudate and desquamation of type I pneumocytes. Proliferation of type II pneumocytes, intra-

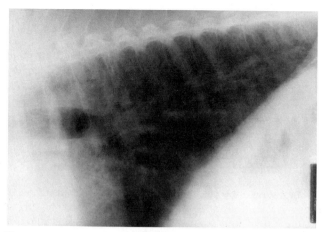

Figure 1. Lateral thoracic radiograph of a 4-month-old foal showing the diffuse interstitial pattern typical of equine interstitial pneumonia.

alveolar accumulation of various mononuclear cells, and interstitial fibrosis may also be present in chronic cases.

TREATMENT

Early and aggressive therapy is required to improve the prognosis. Parenteral corticosteroids can be useful in the treatment to reduce the inflammatory response, especially when administered early. The administration of dexamethasone° (0.1 mg/kg IM, q24h) followed by prednisolone† (1–2 mg/kg p.o. q24h) or inhaled beclomethasone‡ (8 μg/kg q12h) may be considered. Dimethyl sulfoxide§ (0.5–1 g/kg diluted in a 10% solution IV, once daily for 2–3 days) or methyl sulfonyl methane (15–20 mg/kg, p.o. q24h) may be useful for their reported potent anti-inflammatory activity, although their efficacy in acute lung injury still needs to be demonstrated. Antimicrobial treatment and supportive care are also indicated, particularly in foals. Initially, broad-spectrum antibiotics such as sodium penicillin‖ (20,000 IU/kg IV or IM q6h) combined with gentamicin¶ (2–3 mg/kg IV or IM q8–12h) or a trimethoprim-sulfonamide combination# (15–20 mg/kg p.o. IV or IM q12h) are indicated especially in foals. The continuation of therapy and the choice of antibiotics should be based on patients' responses to therapy and on culture and sensitivity results.

Air conditioning can help to control the body temperature and reduce the effort involved in breathing. Hypoxemia ($PaO_2 < 60$ mm Hg), cyanosis, or severe respiratory distress dictate the need for pharyngeal insufflation of oxygen (5 L/min in foals; 10 L/min in adults). At this time it is not known whether bronchodilators may be useful. Although clenbuterol°° (0.8 μg/kg p.o. or by nebulizer q12h) is used in such circumstances, clinicians should keep in

°*Dexamethasone sodium phosphate injection, Austin, Joliette, QC, Canada*
†*Delta-Cortef, Upjohn, Orangeville, ON, Canada*
‡*Becloforte, Glaxo, St-Laurent, QC, Canada*
§*Domoso solution, Syntex, Mississauga, ON, Canada*
‖*Penicillin G sodium, Wyeth-Ayerst, Ville St-Laurent, QC, Canada*
¶*Gentocin, Schering-Plough, Pointe-Claire, QC, Canada*
#*Trivetrin, Coopers, Ajax, ON, Canada*
°°*Ventipulmin, Boehringer, Burlington, ON, Canada*

mind that exacerbation of ventilation-perfusion mismatch and more profound hypoxemia are common complications of bronchodilator therapy. To objectively evaluate the response to therapy, it may be useful to obtain serial blood gas analyses and chest radiographs.

PROGNOSIS

This condition carries a guarded-to-poor prognosis, and although most foals do not respond well to therapy, some ultimately respond to early and aggressive therapy. Further epidemiologic and pathologic studies of EIP are necessary to improve understanding of this disease and eventually lead to its prevention.

Supplemental Readings

Buergelt CD, Hines SA, Cantor G, Stirk A, Wilson JH: A retrospective study of proliferative interstitial lung disease of horses in Florida. Vet Pathol 23:750–756, 1986.
Kelly DF, Newsholme SJ, Baker JR, Ricketts SW: Diffuse alveolar damage in the horse. Equine Vet J 27:76–78, 1995.
Lakritz J, Wilson W, Berry CR, Schrenzel MD, Carlson GP, Madigan JE: Bronchointerstitial pneumonia and respiratory distress in young horses: Clinical, clinicopathologic, radiographic, and pathological findings in 23 cases (1984–1989). J Vet Intern Med 7:277–288, 1993.
Prescott JF, Wilcock BP, Carman PS, Hoffman AM: Sporadic, severe bronchointerstitial pneumonia of foals. Can Vet J 32:421–425, 1991.
Winder C, Ehrensperger F, Hermann M, Howald B, von Fellenberg R: Interstitial pneumonia in the horse: Two unusual cases. Equine Vet J 20:298–301, 1988.

Fungal Diseases of the Lower Respiratory Tract

CORINNE R. SWEENEY
Kennett Square, Pennsylvania

Fungi are ubiquitous in nature, and constant aerosol exposure of respiratory tissue is inevitable. In most samples of stable air, over 90% of particles visible under a light microscope are spores of fungi or actinomycetes. Pulmonary disease due to fungi is caused by inhalation because sporular diameter is sufficiently small to allow penetration into the distal airways and alveoli. Except for pathogenic fungi such as *Coccidioides immitis* and *Histoplasma capsulatum,* tissue invasion usually occurs only in the immunocompromised host, although on occasion the normal individual may be afflicted. Important predisposing factors include defects in neutrophil function and the presence of devitalized tissue. Geographic location is probably important in determining disease incidence.

Fungal pathogens that generally infect only equine patients with abnormal host defenses to infection are called "opportunistic fungi" and include *Aspergillus* species, *Candida* species, *Cryptococcus neoformans,* and the Phycomycetes (*Mucor; Rhizopus*). In vitro studies support the critical role of phagocytic cells in host defense against opportunistic fungi. For example, in the immunocompromised patient, such as a horse with myelomonocytic leukemia, *Aspergillus* species may produce a fulminant invasive pulmonary infection.

In a survey of approximately 34 horses with fungal pneumonias diagnosed at postmortem examination at the George Widener Hospital, University of Pennsylvania, horses had a serious primary problem such as enterocolitis, peritonitis, nephritis, endotoxemia, or septicemia. Approximately one third of the horses had either laminitis or disseminated intravascular coagulation, which is an indication of the severity of their primary disease. Many horses showed no clinical signs of respiratory disease, and the

diagnosis of fungal pneumonia was made solely by postmortem examination. In 19 horses, the histologic lesions were identified or suggestive of *Aspergillus*. Most horses had been on antimicrobial therapy for a varying length of time for their primary problem.

Cases of histoplasmosis and coccidioidomycosis have been described in horses. Signs often did not indicate a primary lung infection, despite lung pathology. Clinical signs include fever, depression, nasal discharge, dyspnea, tachypnea, abnormal lung sounds, and weight loss.

DIAGNOSIS

Clinicians must be careful in attributing significance to the presence of fungal elements in a transtracheal aspirate or the isolation of fungus from these samples. Fungal hyphae are often present either free or in large mononuclear cells in tracheal aspirate from healthy horses. Bronchoalveolar lavage (BAL) offers another sample of the lungs that may aid in the diagnosis of fungal pneumonia. To be significant cytologically, the fungal elements in either the tracheal aspirate or BAL should be present in large numbers and should be involved in the inflammatory process within the lung. Identification of fungus in repeated sampling from a patient may be significant. If fungal pneumonia is suspected, a percutaneous lung biopsy may confirm the diagnosis. However, because the lesions, although multiple and diffuse, are usually small in size and not detectable by ultrasound examination, a biopsy may not sample an affected site. The biopsy sample can be examined cytologically, histologically, and by culture.

In patients with suspected *Aspergillus* infection, careful examination of the nose and paranasal sinuses may be rewarding. In human beings, biopsy of a nasal erosion or ulcer that reveals organisms histologically is highly predictive of concomitant or future invasive pulmonary aspergillosis. Serology testing in horses is not helpful, because normal horses as well as those with chronic obstructive pulmonary disease can have titers to *Aspergillus*.

Clinical signs suggestive of pulmonary aspergillosis may include coughing and hemoptysis. Many horses show no definitive signs of respiratory tract disease. Radiographs of affected patients may reveal virtually any infiltrative pattern. Although miliary patterns are seen, the most common initial radiographic finding is reported to be a patchy bronchopneumonia. Multiple focal sites are common, and lesions tend to be peripheral in distribution.

TREATMENT

Because most equine cases of fungal pneumonia occur as a consequence of a severe primary disease (e.g., enterocolitis, liver failure, and sometimes neoplasia), which is often responsible for the death of the horse, few clinical data are available on treatment regimens. The drug of choice depends on the opportunistic fungus involved. Specific antifungal agents currently being used in the horse include fluconazole, itraconazole, ketoconazole, and amphotericin B. Data on the use of these agents in the horse are a combination of observation of positive clinical response (fluconazole, itraconazole, and amphotericin B), isolated measurements of serum levels in clinical cases (fluconazole), pharmacokinetic studies in the horse (ketoconazole), or extrapolation from other species (fluconazole, itraconazole, and amphotericin B).

Fluconazole,° at a dose of 4 mg/kg p.o. s.i.d., has been successfully used to treat a foal with systemic candidiasis and a horse with fungal keratitis. It is less effective in humans with *Aspergillus* pneumonia than in patients with pulmonary or disseminated coccidioidomycosis, systemic candidiasis, or cryptococcal meningitis.

Itraconazole† is an effective drug against *Aspergillus* and is well absorbed orally in most species. Oral itraconazole has been used successfully in horses to treat a case of vertebral coccidioidomycosis at a dosage of 2.6 mg/kg b.i.d. and nasal aspergillosis at 3 mg/kg b.i.d. Ketoconazole‡ administered orally at 30 mg/kg b.i.d. is poorly absorbed in horses despite acidification. Therefore, the clinical usefulness of ketoconazole in horses is questionable.

°Diflucan, Pfizer, New York, NY
†Sporanox, Janssen Pharmaceutica, Piscataway, NJ
‡ Nizoral, Janssen Pharmaceutica, Piscataway, NJ

Pneumonia caused by *Aspergillus* has been successfully treated with intravenous amphotericin B° using the following regimen: day 1, 0.3 mg/kg body weight; day 2, 0.4 mg/kg body weight; day 3, 0.5 mg/kg body weight; day 4, no drug; day 5, 0.5 mg/kg body weight. This dose is given every 2 days for 1 month. Another regimen used to treat a foal with systemic candidiasis was to start at 0.1 mg of amphotericin B/kg of body weight and increase the dose by 0.1 mg/kg for the next 4 days up a final dose of 0.5 mg/kg used daily. Renal function must be monitored carefully and the drug stopped for 5 days if signs of renal dysfunction are apparent. Successful treatment of a horse with histoplasmosis has been reported using the following dosage regimen of intravenous amphotericin B: 0.3, 0.45, and 0.6 mg/kg on days 1, 2, and 3 respectively, 4 days without treatment, then doses of 0.6 mg/kg every other day until a total cumulative dose of 6.75 mg/kg of amphotericin B has been administered. For each dosage, amphotericin B was mixed in 1 L of 5% dextrose in water and administered over 1 hour via a 14-gauge 5-inch intravenous catheter. Side effects included transient polyuria and polydypsia during the fourth week, an intermittent fever during the first 2 weeks, and lethargy lasting 18 to 24 hours after every treatment.

PREVENTION

Prevention of invasive fungal pneumonia is difficult. Avoidance of large inhaled inocula is impossible in horses because of their environmental conditions. Horses that are recumbent for long periods inhale even greater numbers of spores, even in well-ventilated stables. Improving ventilation and minimizing exposure to inspired spores is most beneficial. Although air filters are sometimes placed in stables, they are frequently inadequate for the size of the stable and are inadequately maintained. Negative ionizers may enhance killing of airborne bacteria but do little to lower levels of fungal spores from moldy hay. At present, the most important method of disease prevention is decreasing environmental exposure, prompt effective treatment of predisposing illnesses, and possibly judicious avoidance of overuse of corticosteroids and broad-spectrum antibiotics.

Supplemental Readings

Heit MC, Riviere JE: Antifungal therapy: Ketoconazole and other azole derivatives. Comp Cont Ed Pract Vet 17:21–31, 1995.
Slocombe RF, Slauson DO: Invasive pulmonary aspergillosis of horses: An association with acute enteritis. Vet Pathol 25:277–281, 1988.
Williamson LH: Review of systemic antifungal therapy in horses. Proc 13th Am Coll Vet Intern Med Forum, 1995, pp 761–764.

°Fungizone Intravenous, ER Squibb & Sons, Princeton, NJ

Exercise-Induced Pulmonary Hemorrhage

JOHN R. PASCOE
Davis, California

Exercise-induced pulmonary hemorrhage (EIPH) is characterized by the presence of blood in the airways after exertion. Most commonly associated with competitive racing and training, EIPH also occurs in horses used for other activities including jumping, polo, barrel racing, roping, and pulling competitions. Current evidence suggests that EIPH most likely results from disruption of pulmonary capillaries as a consequence of high transmural vascular pressures, a reflection of the high cardiac outputs associated with strenuous exercise in horses.

The lungs of horses that have had repetitive episodes of EIPH are characterized by a constellation of morphologic changes—bilateral parenchymal staining of the dorsal caudal regions of the caudal lung lobes, small airway disease, bronchial arterial neovascularization, interstitial fibrosis, and hemosiderophage sequestration in the interstitium and air spaces. Lungs of horses examined after treadmill exercise have electron microscopic evidence of vascular disruption with loss of red cells into alveoli and interstitial spaces, and interstitial edema.

Instillation of autologous blood into the airways results in inflammation, and thus it is likely that repeated episodes of hemorrhage coupled with inhaled airway irritants initiate development of small airway disease. Interstitial fibrosis and bronchial arterial neovascularization of affected lung regions are repair processes that occur in response to inflammation and repeated insult to the lung parenchyma. Once neovascularization occurs, it is likely that these developing vessels also contribute to subsequent episodes of EIPH. Considering that anastomoses exist between the bronchial and pulmonary circulations, it is probable that the interrelationships between the two circulations in the pathogenesis of EIPH are considerably more complex than described. Reasons for the distribution of lesions are less clear but most likely reflect differences in regional architecture such as the apparently increased distribution of bronchial arterial vessels to the dorsocaudal region of the lung as well as the consequences of regional differential diaphragmatic excursion.

CLINICAL SIGNS

Despite the extensive nature of the pathologic changes in some horses, there are often no clinical signs of lung disease associated with EIPH detectable on routine physical examination. About 5% of affected horses have epistaxis evident either at the end of an event or after being allowed to lower their head during cooling out. Because there are other causes of epistaxis, endoscopic examination of the airways is warranted to determine the source of bleeding.

There is no doubt that the performance of some horses is affected by EIPH, but many horses with EIPH appear to perform without impediment. No reliable indicator of a potential performance-limiting effect of EIPH has been identified. Endoscopic scoring of the amount of blood present within airways is not correlated with indices of performance. Loss of form is often ascribed to EIPH because it is a diagnosis that can be readily made, which unfortunately often precludes further evaluation of the performance problem. The author's belief is that performance problems should not be attributed to EIPH until all other potential causes of impaired performance have been ruled out.

DIAGNOSIS

Diagnosis of EIPH is made by endoscopic observation of airway blood that cannot be attributed to other anatomic locations such as the nasal passage, paranasal sinuses, guttural pouches, pharynx, or oral cavity, or by identification of hemosiderophages in washings of airway secretions collected by tracheal aspiration or bronchoalveolar lavage. Airway endoscopy is commonly performed in racehorses 30 to 90 minutes after exercise to establish whether EIPH has occurred. In North America, identification of pulmonary hemorrhage is used as justification in many racing jurisdictions for pre-race administration of medication, particularly furosemide,* in an attempt to prevent EIPH.

Thoracic radiography is of value for detection of concurrent pulmonary disease, such as pulmonary abscess, pleural effusion, and pneumonia, but it is a relatively insensitive technique for detection of EIPH. Airway and pulmonary vascular scintigraphy can be used to assess where morphologic changes associated with EIPH have resulted in regional alterations in ventilation and perfusion.

Thoracic ultrasound can also be used to detect changes in the dorsocaudal lung fields associated with EIPH. Specific abnormalities in the hematologic or biochemical profile have not been identified in horses with EIPH that do not have other concurrent disease. Likewise, abnormalities in hemostatic tests that are normally available from diagnostic laboratory services have not been identified. The significance of changes in platelet aggregability that have been identified in some horses with EIPH is unclear.

Considering that most horses have cytologic evidence of erythrocytes or hemosiderophages in their respiratory

---

*Lasix, Hoechst-Roussel, Somerville, NJ

secretions after exercise, it is probably not surprising that the effect of EIPH on performance is unclear.

TREATMENT

If in fact the initiating events leading to EIPH are a consequence of functional and structural inequalities, pragmatic strategies for therapeutic intervention seem unrealistic. Nevertheless, a number of management and therapeutic approaches are practiced daily in North America in a concerted effort to reduce or prevent EIPH. Unfortunately, there is little scientific justification for these approaches, and their continued use is a source of seemingly endless controversy that pits proponents of permitted race-day medication against those who argue for medication-free racing.

Furosemide

Without doubt, furosemide is the most popular drug administered for prevention of EIPH. In states where race-day furosemide administration is permitted, the dose and time of pre-race administration are usually regulated; permitted doses vary from 250 to 500 mg administered 1 to 4 hours before racing. Furosemide's initial use was based on the presumption that EIPH resulted from pulmonary edema. Although horses with EIPH do not have clinical evidence of pulmonary edema, recent electron microscopic findings have confirmed the presence of interstitial edema; presumably this fluid is being cleared as rapidly as it is formed. Furosemide does attenuate pulmonary vascular pressures in resting and exercised horses. The effect of furosemide on left atrial pressure in exercising horses is unknown, but 250 mg furosemide administered intravenously 4 hours before exertion attenuates pulmonary capillary wedge pressure; and thus it is likely that pulmonary capillary pressure is also attenuated. If stress failure of pulmonary capillaries is an important antecedent event in EIPH, reductions in pulmonary capillary pressure should be beneficial in reducing EIPH.

Inhaled and intravenous furosemide improves lung function in ponies with constricted airways for at least 4 hours after administration. It is conceivable that if horses with small airway disease, EIPH, or both problems experience bronchospasm during exertion, pre-race administration of furosemide may be beneficial in improving lung function. However, it is unlikely that furosemide would enhance lung function in horses with normal airway smooth muscle tone.

Furosemide does not prevent EIPH in more than 50% of the horses to which it is administered, but there is some evidence to suggest that furosemide may reduce the severity of EIPH in individual horses. The effect of furosemide on racing times is still contentious. Some reports indicate no effect of furosemide on racing times of normal horses and horses with EIPH, whereas other reports indicate that the racing times of horses with EIPH and of geldings without EIPH improve after furosemide administration. Differences in methodology confound comparison of these studies. Probably no other topic has polarized racing interests and none is discussed with more passion and supported with more invective and anecdotal evidence than the continuing debate of furosemide's role in the treatment of EIPH.

Other Medications

The efficacy of a small number of other drugs including bronchodilators, conjugated estrogens, coagulants, disodium cromoglycate, antifibrinolytics, and feed additives such as hesperidin-citrus bioflavonoids has been evaluated. These compounds, as well as the use of water vapor therapy, have been largely ineffective in preventing EIPH. Numerous other compounds claiming efficacy abound in tack shops and at race tracks; even superficial investigation reveals that there is no scientific basis for these claims, which at best are substantiated by favorable anecdotes.

MANAGEMENT

The role of individual horse and stable management in reducing or preventing EIPH has not been vigorously explored. The association of small airway disease with EIPH and the apparently high prevalence of small airway disease based on observations of mucopus in the airways of many racehorses in training intuitively suggest that measures designed to improve air quality and ventilation in stables should be further studied. Implementation of beneficial changes may be difficult given the corporate management of most race tracks in North America.

Pre-race management practices such as withholding food and water for variable times before racing or breezing are common in North America. To the author's knowledge, the efficacy of these practices in the management of horses with EIPH is unknown; however, limited observation suggests no differences in the frequency of EIPH between these horses and those allowed access to feed and water until race time.

If stress failure of pulmonary capillaries is the initiating event in EIPH, then factors that mitigate rises in vascular pressure or decreases in alveolar pressure could conceivably prevent EIPH or reduce the severity of individual episodes. Such strategies include identification and correction of causes of airway obstruction, particularly dynamic upper airway obstruction, and perhaps training techniques that improve circulatory efficiency by perhaps improving contractility of the left ventricle without increasing left atrial pressure. Methods for increasing the structural integrity of the blood gas barrier are not intuitively obvious and would most likely compromise gas exchange. It is not known when maturation of the equine lung occurs and if lung development and, in particular, vascular wall strength can be enhanced without increasing the thickness of the blood gas barrier by selectively training horses so that critical transmural pressures are approached but not exceeded during this period of development. Others may argue that the phenomenon of EIPH is merely a manifestation of a system that, no matter how finely tuned by training, is likely to fail under conditions of strenuous exercise because it is only at those extremes that system limits are tested. In fact, it appears that EIPH is not unique to horses, and observations of EIPH in racing greyhounds and elite human athletes suggest that it may indeed be a consequence of circulatory function exceeding the structural capacity of the lungs in strenuously exercising individuals. Thus, efforts may more appropriately be focused on limiting the sequelae such as small airway disease through appropriately targeted management, therapy, and convalescence when indicated.

Supplemental Readings

McKane SA, Canfield PJ, Rose RJ: Equine bronchoalveolar lavage cytology: Survey of Thoroughbred racehorses in training. Aust Vet J 70:401–404, 1993.

Manohar M: Pulmonary vascular pressures of strenuously exercising Thoroughbreds after administration of flunixin meglumine and furosemide. Am J Vet Res 55:1308–1312, 1994.

Sweeney CR, Soma LR, Maxson AD, Thompson JE Holcombe SJ, Spencer PA: Effects of furosemide on the racing times of Thoroughbreds. Am J Vet Res 51:772–778, 1990.

West JB, Mathieu-Costello O: Stress failure of pulmonary capillaries as a mechanism for exercise induced pulmonary haemorrhage in the horse. Equine Vet J 26:441–447, 1994.

Viral Respiratory Disease

ANN A. CULLINANE
Johnstown, Ireland

Viral respiratory disease is of major economic importance to the horse industry worldwide. In racehorses and other performance horses the economic significance frequently exceeds the cost of treatment of the disease. Subclinical infections may result in less than optimal athletic performance, and relatively mild disease may result in loss of training days at a crucial time during the racing or competition season. Immunosuppression resulting from virus infection may increase a horse's susceptibility to secondary infection and prolong the recovery phase. Certain conditions such as the neurologic form of equine herpesvirus (EHV) disease may oblige a trainer or horse owner to close the stable temporarily. Equine influenza epidemics have frequently led to the cancellation of race meetings and other equestrian events. Outbreaks of equine viral arteritis (EVA) have, on occasion, led to trade restrictions.

Diagnosis of respiratory viral disease usually requires laboratory confirmation to establish unequivocally whether a horse has been exposed to virus and, if so, to identify the virus. In the absence of antiviral drugs, veterinarians rely heavily on vaccination, rapid diagnosis, and good management to prevent and control equine viral disease. Many new products have recently been introduced to the market, and additional strains of virus and improved adjuvants have been incorporated into existing products. Veterinarians and equine virologists need to monitor the immunologic response to these products and to evaluate their performance in the face of virus challenge under field conditions.

Veterinarians may need to educate their clients to minimize the threat of viral disease by providing good-quality hay and bedding and by attention to ventilation and stable hygiene. Virucidal disinfectants, such as peroxygen compounds,* chlorine-based products, and detergent iodophors should be used. The importance of having a separate premises, preferably staffed by someone who is not in contact with infected horses, in which to isolate recent arrivals or sick horses cannot be overemphasized. Veterinarians should, if necessary, assist their clients in developing a systematic approach to monitoring their horses for early signs of virus infection. It may be beneficial in a larger

stable for the stable staff to record their horses' temperature, preferably twice daily, appetite, performance and general behavior along with signs of respiratory disease in a "cough book" for inspection each day. Some veterinarians now incorporate regular serologic monitoring of their horses for respiratory viruses in their management program. Larger stables usually screen approximately 25% of their horses each week. Thus, each horse is screened on a monthly basis. Although this type of routine screening is costly, it is of great assistance in the early detection of subclinical virus infection. It also allows a veterinarian to determine when individual horses require a booster vaccination against equine influenza.

Trainers need to be primed to notify their veterinarian immediately when a virus infection is suspected. Affected horses should be isolated, and clinical examination should include the collection of a clotted blood for serologic examination and a nasopharyngeal swab and heparinized blood for virus isolation. The latter need to be kept cold but not frozen and transported to the laboratory as quickly as possible.

When virus infection is confirmed, a decision should be made on whether to close the stable temporarily and rest all the horses. Such a decision is based on the virus involved, the size of the stable, the time of year, and the severity of the infection. If the stable is not closed a horse identified as, or even suspected of, having viral disease should be isolated. Although antibacterial drugs to control secondary infections and supportive therapy such as bronchodilators, mucolytics, and immune stimulants may be of assistance in certain cases, the most important element of a successful recovery program is adequate rest. Return to work of the individual horse should be based on clinical evaluation including endoscopic examination, results of biochemistry and hematology tests, and the trainers' own assessment of the horse. Return of the entire stable to full work should ideally be based on virologic examination because it is important to ensure that there is no evidence of persistent active infection. Horses that return to full work before they have adequately recovered may be predisposed to lower airway disease, epistaxis, and increased sensitivity to respiratory allergens.

---

*Virkon, Antec International Ltd, Sudbury, Suffolk, UK

EQUINE HERPESVIRUSES

The equine herpesviruses, of which there are five genetically and antigenically distinct types have a worldwide distribution. Equine herpesvirus type 1 (EHV-1), a respiratory pathogen, is primarily associated with abortion and more rarely with neurologic disease. Equine herpesvirus type 2 (EHV-2) can be isolated from the majority of horses and has never been conclusively linked to any particular disease syndrome. Similarly, the role of equine herpesvirus 5 (EHV-5) as a pathogen has to be established. Equine herpesvirus type 3 (EHV-3) causes coital exanthema and is primarily transmitted by the venereal route. Equine herpesvirus type 4 (EHV-4) is a major cause of respiratory disease and is associated with sporadic abortion. EHV-1 and EHV-4 are antigenically cross-reactive but can be distinguished unequivocally by restriction endonuclease analysis of their deoxyribonucleic acid (DNA). Like all herpesviruses, equine herpesviruses have the ability to establish a latent infection and to reactivate during the lifetime of the host. A horse experiencing reactivation may show no clinical signs and may fail to mount a detectable antibody response but may shed virus and serve as a source of infection for its cohorts. Reactivation has been associated with the administration of therapeutic doses of corticosteroids and common stress factors such as pain, transport over long distances, and even vaccination against other viruses.

Clinical Signs

Clinical equine herpesvirus respiratory disease is characterized by a transient rise in temperature, inappetance, lethargy, edema of the hindlimbs, pharyngitis, a serous nasal discharge that may become mucopurulent if there is a secondary bacterial infection, and enlargement of the submandibular and retropharyngeal lymph nodes. Coughing is not a major feature of the disease, but affected horses may cough occasionally. Clinical disease is most frequently observed in young animals and is particularly prevalent in yearlings. Routine serologic screening of racing stables coupled with virologic testing during disease outbreaks has demonstrated that the majority of infections in older horses are subclinical or so mild that they frequently go unnoticed by the horse's handlers. The rate of virus spread varies with the age of the horses, the environment, the training program, and the type of virus. EHV-1 is a less common cause of respiratory disease in racehorses and performance horses than EHV-4, but it is a more virulent virus and tends to spread more rapidly. An outbreak of EHV-4 disease may last several months in a large stable with different horses being exposed each week. The slow rate of spread coupled with the often subclinical nature of the disease result in a particularly frustrating problem for trainers. This is exacerbated by the fact that the loss of performance frequently appears to be disproportionate to the severity of the disease. It has been demonstrated that EHV-1 infection results in long-term nonspecific immunosuppression, which may increase the horse's susceptibility to other infectious agents. The recovery period after herpesvirus infections is often prolonged by rhinovirus infection and low-grade tracheitis and bronchitis resulting from secondary bacterial infection.

Respiratory herpesvirus infections may be further complicated by abortion or neurologic disease. Sporadic abortion due to EHV-1 or EHV-4 and multiple abortions due to EHV-1 frequently occur on mixed premises where racehorses, sport horses, ponies, or young stock may serve as a source of infection for brood mares. Abortion may also result from reactivation of latent virus infection. The majority of mares abort during the last third of the gestation period without showing premonitory signs. However, abortions have been recorded as early as 4 months' gestation, and it is not uncommon for the foal to be carried to term and born alive. Such foals are usually weak and jaundiced and they suffer acute respiratory distress. They can survive for several days, during which they serve as a source of virus for their cohorts. Aborted fetuses are also heavily contaminated with virus, and "abortion storms" frequently result when a mare aborts in a field in the company of other pregnant mares.

The neurologic syndrome associated with EHV-1 is uncommon but occurs sporadically in all countries with a significant horse population. The clinical signs, which are acute in onset, vary considerably from mild incoordination to quadriplegia. They usually manifest several days after the respiratory disease, by which time pyrexia associated with the initial exposure to virus has abated and the horse's appetite is usually normal. The most common signs are hindlimb ataxia, atony of the bladder with incontinence, testicular swelling and prolapse of the penis of stallions, and loss of tone of the tail. Horses of all ages and types are susceptible to the neurologic form of EHV-1 disease, but foals appear to be most resistant. However, foals exposed to virus during an outbreak may develop uveitis, iritis, hypopyon, pneumonia, colic, and diarrhea.

Diagnosis

Many EHV-1 and EHV-4 outbreaks that contribute to loss of performance in racehorses and sporthorses are subclinical or so mild that they may go unnoticed in the absence of systematic monitoring, which includes the taking of temperatures twice daily and regular serological screening. Antibody against these viruses can be measured by the complement fixation test (CFT) or the serum neutralization test (SNT). Levels of complement fixing antibodies decline more rapidly than those of serum neutralizing antibodies and are therefore a better indication of recent exposure to virus. Antibody titers usually peak 10 to 14 days after exposure to virus and tend to return to their original level within 3 months. Examination of single samples from a representative number of horses in a stable may be useful in reaching a tentative diagnosis, because significant titers indicate exposure to virus by natural infection or by vaccination at some time. It is, however, preferable to examine paired serum samples collected 10 to 14 days apart because seroconversion, which is a fourfold or greater rise in antibody titer, is indicative of recent exposure to virus. In the absence of a history of recent vaccination, it is indicative of recent virus challenge.

Because of their close antigenic relatedness, infection with EHV-1 and EHV-4 cannot be differentiated using the CFT, and therefore efforts should always be made to isolate the virus. Nasopharyngeal swabs and 20 ml of heparinized blood should be collected from horses in the acute stage of the disease.

Equine herpesvirus abortion cannot be confirmed serologically, and diagnosis is routinely based on postmortem examination of the fetus. All cases of abortion, stillbirth, or foal death within 14 days of birth should be treated as suspect and the fetus or foal submitted to a diagnostic center where postmortem examination routinely includes histopathologic examination for the presence of intranuclear inclusion bodies and virus isolation from selected tissues, usually lung, liver, spleen, adrenal gland, and thymus. Some laboratories employ immunofluorescence for rapid initial diagnosis of viral infection. If the fetus has been partially eaten by predators, remaining tissue should be submitted for virus isolation because the virus can survive for several weeks in a moist environment. If the postmortem examination is carried out by the veterinarian on the farm, formalin-fixed and frozen tissue should be submitted for histopathology examination as well as tissue in virus-transport medium for virus isolation. EHV-1 infection in a neonatal foal can be confirmed by isolation of virus from heparinized blood or from a nasopharyngeal swab. The presence of maternal antibodies may complicate the interpretation of serologic results.

The possibility of EHV-1 infection should always be considered when there is an acute onset of neurologic signs, particularly hindlimb ataxia. Because these signs do not usually become manifest until about 10 days after exposure to virus, the majority of horses suffering from the neurologic form of EHV-1 disease have high antibody titers. However, although the examination of a single serum sample may be a useful diagnostic aid, a minority of horses are slow to show seroconversion, and it is always advisable to examine a second sample from horses that initially present with a low titer. Diagnosis can usually be confirmed by isolating virus from nasopharyngeal swabs or from heparinized blood, a minimum of 20 ml per horse. If horses die or require euthanasia, a diagnosis is based on pathologic investigation and isolation of virus from brain or spinal cord.

Management and Control

In recent years there has been a major increase in the number of vaccines marketed as protecting horses against equine herpesvirus respiratory disease. The majority of these products contain EHV-1 and EHV-4, and many also contain equine influenza viruses. Natural immunity resulting from EHV-1 and EHV-4 respiratory disease does not appear to be strongly protective, and horses can be reinfected 3 months after exposure. However, repeated exposure does eventually elicit a protective response, and the use of some of these vaccines at strategic times during a training program may well reduce clinical signs and virus shedding. This in turn shortens the recovery period and the build-up of virus in a stable. Many veterinarians choose a more intensive vaccination regimen than that recommended by the vaccine manufacturers. Veterinarians who vaccinate every 3 months or at even shorter intervals against herpesvirus should use a vaccine that contains only herpesvirus because it is rarely necessary to vaccinate with such frequency against influenza. Trainers are frequently disappointed by the poor antibody response elicited by

these vaccines as measured by the CFT and the SNT. However, protection against equine herpesvirus does not appear to correlate with humoral immunity and the performance of vaccines in the face of natural virus challenge, and the merits of different vaccination regimens remain to be assessed.

Management of equine herpesvirus respiratory disease depends on rapid diagnosis, isolation, rest, and a gradual return to work. An overly hasty return to work can result in the reactivation of latent virus or in the horse succumbing to other infectious agents. In the case of horses in a large racing or performance stable suffering from EHV-4, closure of the stable is rarely advisable on economic grounds. Because of the slow rate of virus spread, some horses may continue to perform at an optimal level while others require isolation and rest. It is, however, preferable for stables with horses suffering from EHV-1 to close temporarily because overexertion of infected horses could precipitate the neurologic form of the disease. However, because the majority of outbreaks of EHV-1 respiratory disease are very mild, as in EHV-4 infection, many horses in an infected stable often continue to perform well, and do not show incoordination or other neurologic signs, it can be difficult to persuade a trainer to close a stable. Because of the abortogenic potential of the virus it is strongly advisable not to allow a filly from the stable to visit a stud farm for covering or to transport horses in the company of breeding stock.

Prevention of equine herpesvirus abortion depends on vaccination and good management. Vaccines should be used in accordance with the manufacturers' instructions; most products need to be administered at regular intervals during every pregnancy. Although vaccination breakdown has at some time been recorded in most large breeding populations, abortion is less common in vaccinated mares. If an abortion does occur on premises with a vaccination policy, it is less likely to precipitate an abortion storm. In some countries, only vaccines that contain EHV-1 but not EHV-4 are currently licensed to be marketed as an aid to prevent abortion. When available, veterinarians should choose a vaccine containing both EHV-1 and EHV-4, because the latter is occasionally associated with abortion.

Pregnant mares should be segregated from other horses. If this is not possible, all horses in contact with the brood mares should be vaccinated. Efforts should be made to minimize stress to mares in the latter stages of pregnancy.

If herpesvirus abortion occurs, every precaution should be taken to reduce the spread of the virus among the horses on the infected premises. The mare that aborted should be placed in isolation, as should her cohorts, if any. To reduce the risk to other stud farms, all pregnant mares should remain on the infected premises until they foal, and no other horses should leave the premises for 1 month from the date of the last abortion. The efficacy of vaccines containing EHV-1 in protecting against the neurologic form of the disease has not been demonstrated. Because it has been suggested that this condition may result from an inflammatory response to virus antigen and antibody complexes, vaccination in the face of the disease is not recommended by the manufacturers.

No horses should be allowed on or off premises where equine herpesvirus paralysis has been confirmed. Horses should be segregated into small groups and direct contact between the groups should be prevented. Handlers should be advised to disinfect or change their clothing between groups, and whenever possible a separate handler should be assigned to the groups that show no serologic and virologic evidence of infection. These measures are usually sufficient to limit the spread of virus between groups. Horses should not be allowed to move from the premises or resume training until it is free of serologic or virologic evidence of active virus infection. Clinically recovered horses are frequently viremic for several weeks and play a major role in prolonging the restrictions on movement. The wisdom of the administration of immunosuppressive doses of corticosteroids on the basis that this may prevent immune-mediated vasculitis is questionable, because even therapeutic doses can stimulate reactivation of latent virus. Acyclovir° is useful in the treatment of the ocular infections suffered by foals during outbreaks of EHV-1.

EQUINE INFLUENZA

Equine influenza is caused by two discrete subtypes of influenza A virus, which differ in the antigenicity of the surface proteins hemagglutinin (H) and neuraminidase (N). They are designated A/equine 1/H7N7 and A/equine 2/H3N8. Influenza viruses are identified by their place and year of isolation. Thus, A/equine 1/H7N7 and A/equine 2/H3N8 are represented by the prototype virus strains A/equine 1/Prague/56 and A/equine 2/Miami/63. Equine influenza viruses are subject to antigenic drift, and H3N8 variants that gave rise to disease epizootics include A/equine 2/Kentucky/81, A/equine 2/Fontainbleau/79, and A/equine 2/Suffolk/89.

Influenza continues to be one of the major epizootic diseases of the horse. Epizootics are most likely to occur when the virus is introduced to an immunologically naive population, as illustrated by the devastating epizootics in South Africa (1986), India (1987), and China (1989). However, antigenic variation and failure to vaccinate contribute to epizootics in partially immune populations, and in 1989 to 1990 a widespread epizootic occurred in Europe, affecting both unvaccinated and, to a lesser extent, vaccinated horses. All of these epizootics were caused by H3N8 viruses. These viruses are endemic in Europe and North America, where they cause persistent problems. Influenza has not yet been reported in Australia or New Zealand. H7N7 viruses are more antigenically stable and less pathogenic than H3N8 viruses. Although there is some evidence to suggest that they persist, they do not appear to have caused widespread problems for more than a decade.

No evidence exists of a carrier state, and influenza virus must keep circulating in the population to be maintained. Epizootics frequently start at large congregations of horses such as shows, race meetings, or sales. Influenza is contracted by inhalation and is extremely contagious. The persistent dry cough releases large quantities of virus particles into the atmosphere, and horses sharing the same air space can be infected within hours of the introduction of

°*Zovirax eye ointment 3%, Glaxo-Wellcome Plc, London, UK*

an affected horse. The virus may also be carried on the wind and infect horses on neighboring premises.

Clinical Signs

The incubation period is short (1–5 days), the onset of disease is sudden, and the spread is explosive. Morbidity of up to 100% is not uncommon in an immunologically naive population. The first clinical sign is a dramatic elevation in body temperature (up to 41°C) followed rapidly by a dry hacking cough and a serous nasal discharge. Other clinical signs are inappetance, muscular soreness, depression, limb edema, and enlarged submandibular lymph nodes. Secondary bacterial infection is common and can cause bronchopneumonia. H3N8 viruses are more pneumotropic than H7N7 viruses and have on occasion been associated with myocarditis.

The severity of the clinical disease is strongly influenced by the immune status of the horse at the time of exposure. Infection of regularly vaccinated horses or horses that have experienced a natural infection during the previous 12 months may be subclinical or may result in a mild form of the disease. The spread of virus among horses in such a group is slower, and clinical signs may be limited to a slight elevation of temperature, occasional cough, mild rhinitis, and loss of performance in some horses. The horses are less likely to succumb to secondary bacterial infection, and those with high levels of antibody at the time of virus exposure may continue to perform well. Stress such as severe physical exertion and environmental conditions are also major factors in determining the outcome of virus challenge.

Diagnosis

A presumptive diagnosis can frequently be made based on the high morbidity, explosive spread, severe pyrexia, and characteristic dry deep cough. However, in a vaccinated population the clinical signs of influenza may bear a close resemblance to those associated with equine herpesvirus, equine rhinovirus, or some bacterial infections. A definitive diagnosis can be made by isolating the virus from nasopharyngeal swabs or by the detection of a fourfold or greater rise in antibody titer in paired sera collected 10 to 14 days apart. The hemagglutination inhibition (HI) test is most commonly used to detect seroconversion. Nasopharyngeal swabs should be collected during the acute stage of infection. An enzyme-linked immunosorbent assay (ELISA) kit for detection of influenza antigens in nasal secretions is available. It is simple to use and can be useful for making a rapid tentative diagnosis. However, it is advisable to confirm the diagnosis by more conventional methods. Virus isolation is essential for ongoing strain surveillance, which has implications for vaccine development.

Management and Control

Equine influenza can be effectively controlled by vaccination. Young horses that have never been vaccinated or that are at an early stage in their vaccination career are much more susceptible than older horses in the same environment that have been vaccinated regularly for several years. Similarly, racing stables that vaccinate their horses every 4 to 6 months suffer less during an epizootic than stables that vaccinate annually. Young horses should be vaccinated at least twice a year, and it is advisable to monitor horses serologically to ensure that they have responded well to vaccination and that their antibody titers are at a protective level. Because some serologic tests, particularly the HI test, vary between laboratories, the veterinarian should establish what level of antibody their clinical virologist considers to be protective. Horses with low antibody titers frequently introduce virus into a stable. If there are sufficient numbers of such horses coughing in a stable, the virus may be amplified to such an extent that even horses with high titers succumb to challenge.

A minority of horses respond poorly to vaccination. Regular serologic screening not only indicates the appropriate vaccination intervals for a stable, which varies with the age of the horses and the product used, but also identifies the poor responders, which require additional boosters.

On stud farms it is important to ensure a good supply of colostral antibodies to protect the foals. Thus, mares should be vaccinated during late pregnancy. Maternal antibodies interfere with the response to vaccination, and foals should not be vaccinated until they have been weaned. Although it is preferable to monitor antibody level decline by serologic testing, levels have usually declined to a negligible range by 6 months of age.

Current influenza vaccines contain either whole inactivated virus or subunit viral antigens. The majority contain H7N7 and H3N8 strains. The inherent mutability of influenza virus has made it very difficult to develop safe live vaccines, but the inactivated products are occasionally upgraded by the inclusion of recent antigenic variants and improved adjuvants. Experimental studies suggest that vaccines containing immune stimulating complexes (ISCOMS) stimulate a more durable response than vaccines containing more conventional adjuvants.

In the event of an influenza epizootic in a naive population, it is usually necessary to cancel equestrian events to decrease the build-up of virus, the severity of the disease, and the chronic sequelae. Similarly, in the event of an outbreak in an individual stable, it is often advisable for the trainer to close the stable and rest all the horses for 2 weeks or more depending on the severity of the clinical signs, the vaccination status of the horses, and the number of horses in training. Unlike EHV-4 and equine rhinovirus, influenza virus is highly contagious, spreads rapidly, and does not appear to persist in a stable. Resting the horses decreases virus shedding, minimizes the clinical signs, and shortens the recovery period.

The standard recommendation for the management of equine influenza is 1 week of complete rest for every day of elevated temperature followed by a very gradual return to full work. It is routine to reserve antibacterial therapy for those horses that suffer secondary bacterial infection in stables with a policy of regular vaccination. However, where horses are poorly protected against influenza, antibiotics may be administered during the acute stage of viral disease to prevent secondary bacterial infections. Anti-inflammatory drugs may be indicated in horses with high fever, particularly pregnant mares.

EQUINE RHINOVIRUS

Equine rhinoviruses belong to the same genus as human rhinoviruses, the common cold viruses. They are prevalent worldwide and are spread by aerosol and by direct contact. Three equine rhinoviruses have been identified, of which equine rhinovirus type 1 (ERV-1) is the most clinically significant. Most large training stables with young horses experience problems with rhinovirus infections during the first half of the year, particularly at times of stress.

Clinical Signs

Clinical disease is most common in young horses. Symptoms associated with ERV-1 infection include pyrexia, pharyngitis, inappetance, and nasal discharge. Repeated exposure stimulates a protective immunity, and infections in older horses are usually subclinical. However, both clinical and subclinical infections can contribute to a loss of performance.

Diagnosis

Rhinoviruses have been isolated from nasal secretions, blood, saliva, urine, and other bodily fluids. However, isolation can be difficult, and serologic testing is particularly useful in the diagnosis of ERV infections. Serum neutralizing antibodies can persist for years, but antibodies detected by the CFT usually decline to their original level within 3 months of virus exposure. Paired serum samples should be collected 10 to 14 days apart to detect seroconversions. Because infection is often subclinical, routine serologic screening is most useful in alerting the trainer to a rhinovirus problem.

Control and Management

Equine rhinovirus can spread slowly, and as with EHV-4 an outbreak in a large racing stable may occur over many months. Thus, closure of the stable and resting of all the horses is rarely necessary or practical. Older horses frequently perform well during an outbreak. Isolation and rest of infected horses is important. None of the vaccines currently available contains ERV.

EQUINE ARTERITIS VIRUS

Despite serologic evidence of an almost worldwide distribution, outbreaks of clinical disease associated with equine arteritis virus (EAV) are uncommon. Many strains of EAV appear to be of low pathogenicity. Serologic surveys have demonstrated that EAV infection is more prevalent in Standardbreds than in Thoroughbreds. The reason for this is unknown, and experimental challenge studies have failed to demonstrate an increased susceptibility among Standardbreds.

Although the virus is spread by the respiratory route and to a lesser extent by fomites, venereal spread plays a pivotal role in the epidemiology of the disease. EAV is usually introduced into a susceptible population by a carrier stallion. Testosterone plays an essential role in the establishment and maintenance of the carrier state. Although some stallions exposed to EAV may shed virus for only weeks or months, up to 60% become long-term shedders of EAV. They may remain persistently infected for many years, perhaps permanently. The virus localizes in the accessory sex glands, particularly the ampulla of the vas deferens, and is shed constantly in the sperm-rich fraction of the semen. Mares infected by either the respiratory or venereal route may shed virus for up to 1 month in all bodily fluids, but there is no evidence of a carrier state in mares.

Clinical Signs

The majority of infections are subclinical. Clinical signs of arteritis are variable and range from mild pyrexia to the most severe form of natural infection described in 1953 in Bucyrus, Ohio, where 31 out of 60 mares aborted. Typical cases present with depression, inappetance, ocular and nasal discharge, conjunctivitis (pinkeye), stiffness of gait, edema of the scrotum of stallions and of the mammary gland of mares, limb edema, palpebral edema, edema of the orbital fossa, urticarial rashes, and edematous plaques. Less frequently, respiratory distress, coughing, diarrhea, ataxia, photophobia, and opacity of the cornea are observed. Abortion may occur in mares in mid- to late gestation and may not be associated with any other clinical abnormality. Sporadic mortality has been reported in very young foals, but the majority of horses make uneventful clinical recoveries.

Diagnosis

A diagnosis of equine viral arteritis (EVA) can be confirmed by the isolation of virus from nasopharyngeal swabs, semen, urine, buffy coats, and fetal tissues. Serologic diagnosis can be made on the basis of a rise in antibody titer of four-fold or greater. This requires the collection of paired blood samples usually 14 to 28 days apart. Although ELISA tests have been developed, the SNT is currently the serologic test of choice for the measurement of antibodies against EAV, and efforts are currently being made to standardize this test internationally.

Shedder stallions are always seropositive, but not all seropositive stallions are shedders. Test mating or virus isolation from whole ejaculates of semen can be employed to determine the shedding status of a putative carrier stallion. Test mating should be carried out in isolation. The stallion is bred twice a day on two consecutive days to two seronegative mares whose antibody titers against EAV are measured not less than 28 days after the last service. If either mare has seroconversion, the stallion is a shedder.

Control and Management

Because carrier stallions are frequently the source of virus and venereal transmission is followed by lateral spread of virus via the respiratory route, breeding stock should be segregated as far as possible from racehorses and performance horses. All unvaccinated stallions and teasers should be serologically tested before introduction to the breeding pool and at the beginning of each breeding season. The carrier status of seropositive horses should be established, and carriers should not be used for breeding. Only semen collected from horses that have been shown not to be shedders of EAV should be used for artificial insemination. Ideally, all mares should be serologically tested before breeding. A barren mare with stable or falling titers is not considered to represent a risk to other horses, including the working stallion. However, if it is not possible to ascertain when an unvaccinated seropositive pregnant mare was exposed to virus, she should be isolated until she has foaled.

A modified live vaccine° is used in EAV control programs in Kentucky and New York. This vaccine is considered safe for use in stallions and in barren mares but is not recommended for use in pregnant mares or in young foals. Although it does not prevent virus infection, multiplication, or shedding, it appears to protect horses against clinical disease.

This vaccine is not available in the European Community (EC) but an inactivated vaccine,† the efficacy of which has not yet been fully evaluated, is available for use in all horses in the United Kingdom. Its use is restricted to stallions in Ireland.

Arteritis is a notifiable disease in some countries but many others rely on voluntary codes of practice for the control of the disease. Restriction of movement is the basis of all effective control programs. Movement on and off infected premises should cease until there is no longer serologic or virologic evidence of active infection. Horses on the premises should be segregated on the basis of serologic and clinical examination into separated areas with, if possible, different handlers. All breeding should cease. It is particularly important to isolate healthy seronegative stallions from all other stock, which will minimize the risk of them being exposed to virus and possibly becoming permanent venereal shedders. Adequate rest, with supportive therapy if appropriate, allows the majority of horses to make a speedy recovery. In outbreaks of arteritis in training stables, some infected horses have won races approximately 1 month after exposure to virus.

Supplemental Readings

Allen GP, Bryans JT: Molecular epizootiology, pathogenesis, and prophylaxis of equine herpesvirus-1 infections. Prog Vet Microbiol Immunol 2:78–144, 1986.

McCartan CG, Russell MM, Wood JLN, Mumford JA: Clinical, serological and virological characteristics of an outbreak of paresis and neonatal foal disease due to equine herpesvirus-1 on a stud farm. Vet Rec 136:7–12, 1995.

Mumford J, and Woods J: WHO/OIE meeting: Consultation on newly emerging strains of equine influenza. Vaccine 11:1172–1175, 1993.

Timoney PJ, McCollum WH: Equine viral arteritis—epidemiology and control. Equine Vet Sci 8:54–59, 1988.

°*Arvac, Fort Dodge Laboratories, Fort Dodge, IA*
†*Artivac, Fort Dodge Finisklin Industrial Estate, Sligo, Ireland*

Bacterial Pleuropneumonia

M. KEITH CHAFFIN

G. KENT CARTER
College Station, Texas

In cases of bacterial pleuropneumonia, bacteria colonize the lung resulting in pneumonia and/or pulmonary abscessation, followed by extension to the pleural space and accumulation of pleural effusion (pleuritis or pleurisy). Although pleural effusion has many causes, parapneumonic effusion (i.e., effusion that develops in association with pneumonia or lung abscesses) is most common. The true incidence of pleuropneumonia is unknown, but horses of any age, breed, gender, or occupation may be affected.

Because bacterial pleuropneumonia usually results when the lung's defense mechanisms are suppressed or overwhelmed, stress, long-distance transport, or strenuous exercise often precede pleuropneumonia. Racehorses are thought to be at higher risk because they are frequently transported; they are in close contact with a transient population of horses, strenuously exercised, and kept in poorly ventilated housing. It has been suggested that the presence of blood in the airways of horses with exercise-induced pulmonary hemorrhage (EIPH) may favor bacterial colonization. Aspiration of dust and dirt while racing may also contribute to development of pleuropneumonia in racehorses.

Most cases of pleuropneumonia are associated with bacterial infection; however, fungal pneumonia can occasionally result in parapneumonic effusion. Most bacterial isolates are opportunistic organisms that gain access to the lung via inhalation, aspiration, or hematogenous spread. Anaerobic bacteria are frequently involved in the pathogenesis of severe cases of pleuropneumonia. Microbial synergy may exist in vivo between aerobic and anaerobic bacteria, thus mutually amplifying bacterial growth and the pathogenic effects of each.

The evolution of parapneumonic effusion occurs in three stages. During the first or exudative stage, increased capillary permeability of the inflamed lung and contiguous visceral pleura leads to rapid outpouring of sterile, protein-rich fluid into the pleural space. In this stage, the parapneumonic effusion is considered uncomplicated. When recognized in this early stage, appropriate antimicrobial therapy may result in resolution of the pleural effusion. During the second or fibrinopurulent stage, bacteria invade the pleural fluid and multiply, resulting in voluminous pleural fluid that contains many neutrophils, bacteria, and cellular debris. At this stage, the parapneumonic effusion is considered complicated and requires drainage. Fibrin is deposited on the pleural surfaces, resulting in loculation of the fluid. Impaired lymphatic drainage further favors accumulation of pleural fluid. The third or organization stage is characterized by continued fibrin deposition until an inelastic fibrous membrane called the "pleural peel" is formed, which encases the lung and limits lung expansion.

Pleural empyema may also arise in the absence of an associated pneumonic process. Thoracic puncture wounds, esophageal rupture, and "primary pleuritis" are common examples. The clinical signs and treatment of these conditions are often similar to that described here for pleuropneumonia.

CLINICAL SIGNS

Clinical signs of pleuropneumonia are highly variable and may include any combination of the following: lethargy, anorexia, fever, nasal discharge, cough, exercise intolerance, respiratory distress, flared nostrils, weight loss, and sternal edema. Many acutely affected horses exhibit pleurodynia (pleural pain), evident as pawing; stiff gait; abducted elbows; and reluctance to move, lie down, or cough. Pleurodynia may be detected as a painful response when digital pressure is applied to the intercostal spaces. Some horses with pleurodynia exhibit shallow guarded respirations and decreased excursion of the thoracic wall during inspiration. Pleurodynia may easily be misdiagnosed as colic, exertional rhabdomyolysis or laminitis. In the subacute to chronic stages of pleuropneumonia, pleurodynia often becomes less evident.

Nasal discharge may vary from absent to copious and from serous to mucohemorrhagic or mucopurulent. The presence of coughing is also variable; because of pleurodynia, affected horses frequently are reluctant to cough, and when they do, they have a guarded soft cough. Putrid odor to the breath is usually associated with anaerobic infection. Respiratory distress is related to the volume of fluid accumulated in the pleural space and the severity of the pneumonia. Mucous membrane color and the degree of scleral injection is variable and reflects the degree of systemic toxemia. Weight loss is often present in chronically affected horses.

DIAGNOSIS

Auscultation

In horses with pleural effusion, thoracic auscultation reveals attenuated to absent lung sounds over the ventral thorax. A rebreathing bag is often necessary to appreciate attenuation of lung sounds. Over the dorsal lung fields, sounds may be normal or intensified; crackles and wheezes may be audible in some horses. Voluminous pleural effusion may obscure all lung sounds. Friction rubs are usually only audible in the peracute stages; they may change rapidly in location and character, and often disappear as pleural inflammation subsides or pleural effusion accumulates. Thoracic percussion usually delineates a horizontal line on the thorax with resonant sounds dorsally and dull sounds ventrally. Loculated pockets of pleural fluid or pulmonary lesions may produce focal areas of dullness.

Hematology

Results of hematologic and serum biochemical testing are nonspecific for pleuropneumonia. In chronic stages, often there is anemia, hyperproteinemia, decreased albumin:globulin ratio and hyperfibrinogenemia. Leukopenia (neutropenia) often is present in peracute stages, and normal-to-high leukocyte counts often are present in subacute and chronic stages.

Ultrasonography

Thoracic ultrasonography permits the clinician to localize and characterize pleural effusion, fibrin, and loculae, and detect pulmonary atelectasis, consolidation, abscessation, and necrosis. Either sector or linear array scanners can be successfully used to image the equine thorax; a 3.5- to 5.0-MHz transducer is preferred. Pleural effusion is detected as hypoechoic to anechoic fluid between the parietal pleural surface and the lung. Fibrin appears as filamentous strands floating in the effusion. Loculated pockets of fluid may be imaged in some horses. The presence of small (<1 mm) bright echoes (gas echoes) swirling in pleural fluid is associated with anaerobic infection. The lack of ultrasonographically visible gas echoes does not rule out anaerobic infection. Atelectatic lung appears sonolucent and appears as a wedge of tissue floating in the pleural fluid. Consolidated lung varies from dimples of the pleural surface to large, wedge-shaped areas of sonolucent lung. Peripheral lung abscesses appear as sonolucent areas that may be encapsulated.

Radiography

Radiographs of horses with pleural effusion demonstrate a ventral soft tissue opacity that obscures the diaphragmatic and cardiac shadow. It is most efficient to reserve radiography until the pleural effusion has been drained; radiographs should then be obtained to identify deep pulmonary abscesses or enlarged mediastinal lymph nodes.

Culture and Cytology

Airway specimens should be collected and submitted for cytology and aerobic and anaerobic culture testing. Transtracheal aspiration is preferred so as to avoid contamination from the upper airway; however, other procedures using transendoscopic guarded brushes and catheters have been described. In horses with pleuropneumonia, bronchoalveolar lavage is probably not the diagnostic procedure of choice because only a limited segment of the lung is sampled, and thus the diseased region may be missed. Specimens should be stained with Wright's or Diff-Quik stain for cytologic examination and with Gram's stain to characterize the bacterial population and dictate initial antimicrobial therapy.

Thoracocentesis should be performed to collect pleural fluid samples for analysis. Ultrasonographic examination helps to localize the appropriate site for thoracocentesis. If ultrasound equipment is unavailable, thoracocentesis usually yields fluid samples when performed at a site just above the costochondral junction of intercostal spaces 7 and 8 on the left hemithorax and spaces 6 and 7 on the right hemithorax. Aliquots of pleural fluid from each hemithorax should be collected in ethylenediaminetetra-acetic acid (EDTA) tubes for cytologic examination, cell counts, protein concentration, and Gram's stain. Other aliquots should be collected in sterile containers or in transport media and submitted for aerobic and anaerobic bacterial cultures.

Normal equine pleural fluid is clear to light yellow, sterile, odorless, and has a protein concentration less than 4.7 g/dl and nucleated cell count less than 10,000/μl. Parapneumonic effusion typically is exudative, cloudy, yellow to red, has an elevated nucleated cell count and protein concentration, and contains more than 90% neutrophils, many of which are degenerative. Bacteria may be cytologically visible both intra- and extracellularly. Fluid with a putrid odor indicates necrosis and suggests anaerobic infection. Cytologic examination and Gram's stain allow assessment of the presence of septic inflammation and classification of the types of bacteria present.

In some cases, biochemical analysis of pleural fluid can help determine the need for drainage. Low pH (<7.1) and low glucose concentration (<40 mg/dl) have been consistent features of septic parapneumonic effusion in horses with pleuropneumonia.

TREATMENT

The treatment of pleuropneumonia varies widely depending on the severity and duration of the disease process; the causative organisms; presence, character, and volume of pleural effusion; extent of fibrin deposition; and development of sequelae. Mildly affected horses that are diagnosed early may respond to conservative therapy with antimicrobials and supportive care. Severely affected horses may require prolonged thoracic drainage, pleural lavage, and, in some cases, thoracotomy. Initial management includes selection of appropriate antimicrobial agents and determination of the need for pleural drainage.

Antimicrobial Therapy

Antimicrobials should ultimately be selected based on results of culture and susceptibility testing of pleural fluid and transtracheal aspirates. Before obtaining these results, selection of antimicrobials should be based on results from Gram's stain of pleural fluid and airway specimens, and/or knowledge of the prevalence and susceptibility patterns of bacteria frequently isolated from affected horses. Polymicrobial and mixed aerobic/anaerobic infections are common; thus, antimicrobial regimens with a broad spectrum of activity are indicated. Species of *Streptococcus*, particularly *S. zooepidemicus* are the most common aerobic isolates; other common aerobic isolates include *Pasteurella* species, *Escherichia coli*, *Enterobacter* species, *Klebsiella* species, *Pseudomonas* species, *Actinobacillus equuli*, and *Bordetella bronchiseptica*. The most common anaerobic isolate is *Bacteroides* species; other common anaerobic isolates include *Clostridium, Peptostreptococcus, Eubacterium,* and *Fusobacterium* species.

Antimicrobials commonly used for initial therapy include penicillins, cephalosporins, aminoglycosides, and potentiated sulfonamides. Antimicrobials effective against anaerobic bacteria should also be administered to horses with suspected anaerobic infection. Foul-smelling breath and sonographically visible "gas echoes" in the pleural effusion have been associated with anaerobic infection; however, absence of these findings does not rule out anaerobic infection. Most anaerobic bacteria are susceptible to penicillin; however, *Bacteroides fragilis* is capable of producing β-lactamases that render it resistant to penicillin. Metronidazole is effective against most anaerobic isolates, including *B. fragilis,* and should be considered in horses suspected or confirmed to have anaerobic infection. As culture and susceptibility results become available, the antimicrobial regimen should be modified as needed. Duration of antimicrobial therapy is frequently long-term, ranging from 2 to 24 weeks, depending upon the horse's clinical response and the development of sequelae.

In the initial stages of therapy, it may be advantageous to administer antimicrobials intravenously to achieve higher peak serum concentrations. Later in the course of treatment, it is frequently most practical to change to orally-administered antimicrobials when results of susceptibility testing indicate that it is appropriate. Intrapleural administration of antimicrobials has not been adequately evaluated in horses with pleuropneumonia; if used intrapleurally, antimicrobials should always be used as an adjunct to systemic administration.

Drainage

Drainage of pleural effusion results in removal of exudate and debris from the pleural space and allows for re-expansion of the lung. Decisions regarding pleural drainage are based on classification of the pleural fluid as a complicated or uncomplicated parapneumonic effusion. Uncomplicated effusions are those that resolve with antimicrobial therapy, whereas complicated effusions require drainage in addition to antimicrobial therapy for resolution. Indications of a complicated parapneumonic effusion and the necessity for pleural drainage include a poor response to conservative therapy and the presence of pleural fluid with one or more of the following characteristics: sufficient volume to cause respiratory distress, empyematous character, putrid odor, cytologically visible bacteria, positive culture results, glucose concentration less than 40 mg/dl, pH less than 7.1 or lactate dehydrogenase (LDH) concentration greater than 1000 IU/L. When empyema is present and bacteria are cytologically visible in the pleural fluid, pleural drainage is obviously indicated. In some horses, the need for drainage is less obvious, and culture results or biochemical analyses may be necessary to make a decision. Pleural drainage should be initiated as early in the disease course as possible because deposition of fibrin results in loculation that can hinder drainage.

Pleural drainage can be accomplished with either intermittent thoracocentesis or indwelling chest tubes. Intermittent thoracocentesis should be considered in horses with small volumes of pleural fluid that do not have a putrid odor or contain thick cellular debris. Teat cannulas or small (12–20 French) chest tubes are temporarily inserted as needed to remove accumulated fluid.

Indwelling chest tubes permit frequent or continual drainage. Indwelling chest tubes may be required in one or both hemithoraces, depending on the patency of the mediastinum and the extent of fluid loculation. Ultrasonographic examination allows selection of the most appropriate site for tube placement. The site should be clipped and aseptically prepared. Ten ml of local anesthetic is deposited into the subcutaneous tissue and intercostal muscles at the selected site. A stab incision is made through the skin. A large-bore (24–32 French) chest tube° is inserted through the skin, intercostal muscles, and parietal pleura into the pleural space. Subcutaneous tunneling of the chest tube is not recommended. A moderate amount of force is required to punch the tube through the intercostal muscle and parietal pleura; caution should be exercised to avoid punching the tube into the underlying lung. When the pleural cavity is entered, a distinct release of pressure is felt. As the trocar is removed, drainage starts immediately. The tube should be secured to the skin with sutures to prevent inadvertent removal. Either a nonlubricated condom with the tip snipped off or a Heimlich valve† should be secured to the tube to allow unidirectional drainage. The unidirectional valve should be monitored closely to ensure proper function. As an alternative to continuous drainage, indwelling tubes can be plugged and periodically drained as needed via a Heimlich valve.

Pleural fluid should be allowed to drain passively; suction often results in obstruction of the drainage portals with fibrin. The chest tube should be replaced when it becomes nonfunctional or removed when ultrasonography indicates cessation of pleural fluid accumulation. Multiple loculae of pleural fluid may necessitate multiple chest tubes. Potential complications from indwelling tubes include local cellulitis, subcutaneous infection, and pneumothorax. Careful monitoring is necessary to detect complications and initiate appropriate therapy.

Lavage

In horses with thick, viscous pleural fluid, pleural lavage may help remove fibrin, debris, and necrotic tissue, and may dilute fluid to facilitate drainage. Lavage is most effective in subacute stages before loculated pockets of effusion develop. Loculation often prevents adequate lavage of the entire pleural cavity; however, pleural lavage may help break down fibrous adhesions and establish communication between loculae. Large loculae can be sonographically located and individually lavaged through small chest tubes. Care must be exercised that infused fluid is communicating with the drainage tube. Pleural lavage can be performed by infusing fluid in a dorsally positioned tube and draining it through a ventrally positioned tube; alternatively, fluid may be infused and drained through the same tube. Five to 10 L of sterile, warm isotonic solution such as lactated Ringer's solution or saline is infused into each affected hemithorax by gravity flow. After infusion, the chest tube is reconnected to a unidirectional valve and the lavage fluid is allowed to drain.

°Trocar catheter, Deknatel, Fall River, MA
†Becton Dickinson, Lincoln Park, NJ

Pleural lavage is contraindicated in patients with bronchopleural communications. Coughing and drainage of lavage fluid from the nares during infusion of lavage fluid suggests the presence of a bronchopleural fistula. In such cases, lavage should be discontinued to prevent spread of septic, pleural debris up the airways and into normal areas of the lung.

Surgical intervention is indicated for chronically affected horses in which long-term medical therapy fails to completely resolve the thoracic infection. Proper case selection is critical. Indications for thoracotomy include a focal pocket of necrotic debris that is localized to one hemithorax or is walled off from the remainder of the ipsilateral hemithorax. Before surgical therapy, it is critical that the patient's systemic condition be stabilized and that the thorax be no longer diffusely infected. Thoracotomy and rib resection allow exposure for manual débridement and removal of necrotic debris and facilitate thorough lavage of the pleural cavity.

Supportive Care

Supportive care is a critical component of therapy for horses with pleuropneumonia. Supplemental fluid therapy should be administered as needed to correct dehydration, provide maintenance fluid requirements, and replace fluid losses into the pleural space. Phenylbutazone* (2.2–4.4 mg/kg IV or p.o. b.i.d.) or flunixin meglumine† (0.25–1.0 mg/kg IV, s.i.d.–t.i.d.) is usually indicated to minimize inflammation, oppose endotoxemia, and decrease pain. Provision of stall rest, fresh water, and good nutritional support are important. Strict rest for a minimum of 3 to 5 months is critical following recovery from pleuropneumonia.

Thorough and frequent monitoring of the patient's condition is critical to assess response to therapy, dictate alterations in the therapeutic plan, and detect complications. Frequent sonographic reassessment of the thorax is critical for assessing changes in location, character, and amount of pleural fluid, fibrin, debris, and abscessation. Common complications of pleuropneumonia include laminitis, endotoxemia, thrombophlebitis, pneumothorax, and pleural or pulmonary abscesses. Signs of pneumothorax can be absent, subtle, or severe and include tachypnea, lethargy, and respiratory distress. Radiography or ultrasonography detect free air in the dorsal thorax. Abscesses in the cranial mediastinal region may result in tachycardia, pointing of a forelimb, jugular vein distension, forelimb and pectoral edema, spontaneous jugular thrombosis, and auscultable caudal displacement of the heart. Less common complications of pleuropneumonia include bronchopleural fistulas, pericarditis, and immune-mediated hemolytic anemia or thrombocytopenia.

---

*Butazolidin, Coopers's Animal Health, Kansas City, MO
†Banamine, Schering-Plough, Kenilworth, NJ

PROGNOSIS

Prognosis for survival and return to normal athletic function is related to the severity and duration of the disease process and the development of complications. In general, when an early diagnosis is made and aggressive therapy is provided, the prognosis for survival is good for most horses with pleuropneumonia. Retrospective studies show survival rates ranging from 38 to 95%. Many of the nonsurvivors are horses that either succumb in the acute stages of the disease or are euthanized owing to complications or economic considerations. Depending on the value of the horse, the expense of long-term therapy frequently dictates the owner's commitment to therapy. Length and expense of treatment vary greatly, as does the final capacity for athletic function. There is some evidence that horses with anaerobic infection have a poorer prognosis for survival than those without anaerobic infection.

Because the expense of long-term therapy can be substantial, owners of athletic horses, particularly those without value as breeding animals, frequently base their therapeutic decisions on the patient's prognosis for return to full athletic function. In a study reported in the early 1980s, only 42% of surviving horses returned to their previous level of performance. More recent studies show an improved prognosis for athletic function. In one study, all horses without sonographically visible pulmonary consolidation returned to or surpassed their previous level of racing performance, suggesting that sonographic assessment has important prognostic merit. In another recent study of Thoroughbred racehorses, 61% raced after recovery and, of these, 56% won races. Horses requiring pleural drainage via indwelling chest tubes did not have a poorer prognosis for return to racing than horses that did not require pleural drainage. The development of sequelae, such as abscessation, cranial thoracic masses, or bronchopleural fistulas, was associated with a poorer prognosis for return to racing.

Supplemental Readings

Chaffin MK, Carter GK: Equine bacterial pleuropneumonia. Part I. Epidemiology, pathophysiology, and bacterial isolates. Comp Cont Ed Pract Vet 15:1642–1650, 1993.
Chaffin MK, Carter GK, Byars TD: Equine bacterial pleuropneumonia. Part III. Treatment, sequelae, and prognosis. Comp Cont Ed Pract Vet 16:1585—1589, 1994.
Chaffin MK, Carter GK, Relford RL: Equine bacterial pleuropneumonia. Part II. Clinical signs and diagnostic evaluation. Comp Cont Ed Pract Vet 16:362–378, 1994.
Raphel CF, Beech J: Pleuritis secondary to pneumonia or lung abscessation in 90 horses. J Am Vet Med Assoc 181:808–810, 1982.
Sweeney CR, Divers TJ, Benson CE: Anaerobic bacteria in 21 horses with pleuropneumonia. J Am Vet Med Assoc 187:721–724, 1985.

Lung Abscesses in Mature Horses

JEAN-PIERRE LAVOIE
St. Hyacinthe, Quebec

Lung abscesses are collections of pus within necrotic portions of the lung and are most commonly caused by bacteria. Lung abscesses that develop in the absence of concomitant apparent medical problems are called primary lung abscesses. The incidence of primary lung abscesses in mature horses is low. Secondary abscesses are more common and follow aspiration pneumonia, generalized infection, neoplasia, thoracic trauma, chronic obstructive pulmonary disease, and thromboembolism. Ruptured lung abscesses are considered to be a common cause of pleuropneumonia.

CLINICAL FINDINGS

Clinical signs associated with primary lung abscesses are often indistinguishable from those of bronchopneumonia. Coughing, exercise intolerance, lethargy, fever, polypnea, tachycardia, and labored breathing are the most common findings. In horses with secondary lung abscesses, the major clinical signs are often related to the primary disease. Auscultation of the thorax commonly reveals crackles and wheezes, especially when breathing is accentuated by use of a rebreathing bag. Localized silent areas may be detected on lung auscultation, and percussion of the thorax may reveal dullness at the site of the abscess.

DIAGNOSIS

Lung abscesses should be suspected in horses with clinical signs suggestive of bacterial pneumonia that respond poorly to antimicrobial administration, and in the presence of localized silent areas on pulmonary auscultation or localized zones of dullness on thoracic percussion.

Hyperfibrinogenemia is a consistent finding in horses with lung abscesses. Neutrophilia, which may be profound, is common in the early stages of the disease but may be absent in the later stages. An anemia of chronic disease and hyperproteinemia due to hyperglobulinemia are also common findings.

Lung abscesses extending to the surface of the lung can be diagnosed on ultrasonography. The use of 3.5- and 5.0-MHz transducers is preferred. The abscesses appear as thick-walled pockets that contain material of variable echogenicity. Thoracic radiographs are usually required to confirm the diagnosis of lung abscesses. Abscesses appear on radiographs as multiple nodular opacities or large cavitary lesions in which a gas-fluid interface may be visible.

TREATMENT

The successful treatment of lung abscesses requires the administration of antimicrobials, rest, and supportive therapy. Antimicrobials should be efficacious against the bacterial species present and should penetrate abscesses. Antimicrobial selection should therefore be based on the results of aerobic and anaerobic bacterial cultures and sensitivity. Samples submitted for bacterial culture can be obtained from tracheal washes or aspiration of the abscesses. Antimicrobials may be selected based on the culture results of tracheal washes; there is usually an excellent correlation between the bacteria isolated from the trachea and lung abscesses. Abscesses should be aspirated only in cases refractory to medical therapy or when drainage of the abscesses is performed because of the inherent risk of damaging adjacent vital structures or propagating infection. Gram's stain results are helpful to orient the antimicrobial selection, until culture and sensitivity results are reported.

Lipid-soluble antimicrobials such as rifampin, erythromycin, chloramphenicol, and quinilone antimicrobials penetrate abscesses well. Side effects, cost of therapy, or spectrum of antimicrobial activity limit the use of erythromycin, chloramphenicol, and quinilone for first-line therapy in adult horses. Rifampin should not be used alone, because bacteria may develop resistance rapidly, as a one-step process. The successful treatment of lung abscesses may also be achieved by the use of other antimicrobials, if the bacterial species involved are sensitive to them and if the antimicrobials are administered at a proper dosage and for a sufficient period of time. The duration of antimicrobial administration is usually a minimum 4 weeks or until clinical signs have improved, and plasma fibrinogen and neutrophil counts return to normal limits.

Veterinarians dealing with lung abscesses rarely have the opportunity to initiate therapy based on sensitivity results. Therefore, empirical therapy should be directed at the bacterial species most commonly isolated from lung abscesses in horses. In primary lung abscesses, *Streptococcus zooepidemicus* is most commonly implicated in mature horses. *Actinobacillus species* (also called *Pasteurella* species), *Streptococcus equi* and a number of other bacterial species may be recovered in these cases. Penicillin G administration alone or in combination with rifampin* (5–10 mg/kg b.i.d. p.o.) is preferred for empirical therapy in adult horses with primary lung abscesses, because of the efficacy against β-hemolytic streptococci. The intravenous administration of penicillin G† (40,000 IU/kg q.i.d.) may be fol-

*Rofact, ICN Canada Ltd, Montreal, PQ, Canada
†Penicillin G sodium, Wyeth-Ayerst, Montreal, PQ, Canada

lowed by intramuscular procaine penicillin° (20,000 IU/kg b.i.d.) administration when there is clinical evidence of response to therapy. Penicillin G may be combined with gentamicin† (2.2 mg/kg IV t.i.d.) in severe cases because polymicrobial infection may be present. The administration of metronidazole‡ (15 mg/kg p.o. q.i.d.) is recommended when an anaerobic bacterial infection is suggested by the presence of foul-smelling breath, hyperechogenicity of pus within the abscess, or positive bacteriologic test results. In secondary lung abscesses, a wide range of aerobic and anaerobic bacteria are commonly recovered, and therefore broad-spectrum antimicrobials, such as a combination of penicillin-gentamicin and metronidazole, is preferred.

Drainage of the abscess is rarely indicated because most patients respond to conservative therapy. Drainage is recommended for nonresponsive patients with a large solitary abscess that is well circumscribed and adherent to the adjacent parietal pleura. The site for insertion of the thoracotomy tube§ is selected with ultrasonographic guidance. The skin is surgically prepared and anesthetized by the subcutaneous injection of lidocaine.‖ The catheter is inserted at the cranial aspect of the rib and advanced until the abscess is penetrated. The contents of the abscess are aspirated using a 60-ml syringe and submitted for cytologic examination and bacterial culture and sensitivity. Antibiotics may be administered into the abscess. Lavage of the

abscess should be avoided, because it may propagate the infection to adjacent tissues if the abscess is not completely walled off.

The period of rest recommended before returning the horse to training usually varies between 3 and 6 months. Ideally, repeated radiographic evaluations should be performed, and the horse may be returned to exercise 1 month following the disappearance of the radiographically visible pulmonary lesions. Supportive therapy such as administration of nonsteroidal anti-inflammatory drugs, fluid therapy, and bronchodilators may be indicated in individual cases. Treatment of associated primary disease is also required with secondary lung abscess.

PROGNOSIS

Most horses with primary lung abscesses survive the infection with proper therapy. The outcome for secondary lung abscesses varies according to the initiating problems. Horses with lung abscesses that respond to therapy usually return to their intended use and may perform successfully.

Supplemental Readings

Byars TD, Dainis CM, Seltzer KL, Rantanen NW: Cranial thoracic masses in the horse: A sequel to pleuropneumonia. Equine Vet J 23:22–24, 1991.

Lavoie J-P, Fiset L, Laverty S: Review of 40 cases of lung abscesses in foals and adult horses. Equine Vet J 26:348–352, 1994.

Mair TS, Lane JG: Pneumonia, lung abscesses and pleuritis in adult horses: A review of 51 cases. Equine Vet J 21:175–180, 1989.

Raphel CF, Beech J: Pleuritis secondary to pneumonia or lung abscessation in 90 horses. J Am Vet Med Assoc 181:808–810, 1982.

°*Ethacilin, Rogar STB Inc., Montreal, PQ, Canada*
†*Gentocin, Schering-Plough Animal Health, Pointe-Claire, PQ, Canada*
‡*Flagyl, Searle Pharmaceuticals, Chicago, IL*
§*24 French, Argyle trocar catheter, Sherwood Medical Industries, St. Louis, MO*
‖*Lidocaine 2%, Austin, Joliette, PQ, Canada*

Antimicrobial Drug Selection for Lower Airway Infection

JOHN F. PRESCOTT
Guelph, Ontario

GENERAL CONSIDERATIONS

Effective treatment of lower airway infections depends on use of antimicrobial drugs to which microorganisms are sensitive for sufficient time to allow return to normal function without damage to the host. Antimicrobial susceptibility should be determined wherever possible, but initial therapy is usually empirical and is based on knowledge of the agents likely to be present and their historical susceptibility (Tables 1 and 2). Transtracheal wash and tracheal aspiration, using a fiberoptic bronchoscope with a guarded catheter brush, prevent contamination by pharyngeal microflora and are, therefore, ideal means of obtaining infectious material from the lung for cytology testing, Gram's stain, and culture.

The route of administration may be parenteral (IV, IM) or oral (Table 3). Where appropriate, oral administration is the preferred route of administration of some antimicrobial drugs (see Table 3) because of ease of administration to horses and, if drugs are administered over a long time, the avoidance of repeated injection of large volumes of sometimes painful drugs intramuscularly. Parenteral administration of drugs often results in higher tissue concentrations than oral administration and should be used in initiation of treatment, especially in severe infections. The expanded large bowel of the horse makes the horse particularly susceptible to severe colitis, which is most likely of clostridial origin, induced by broad-spectrum antibiotics with activity against anaerobes. For this reason, such drugs (e.g., ampicillin) should not be administered orally to

TABLE 1. IN VITRO PERCENTAGE SUSCEPTIBILITY OF SELECTED EQUINE CLINICAL AEROBIC BACTERIAL ISOLATES
(1992–1994, ONTARIO VETERINARY COLLEGE)

Isolate	Number	AMI	AMO	AMP	CFF	CEF	CPL	CR	CIP	ENR	ERY	GEN	PEN	RIF	TET	TIC	TCA	TRI
Actinobacillus equuli	28	93	100	43	96	100	93	86	100	100	0	89	54	0	89	86	100	89
Actinobacillus suis	22	82	82	68	86	68	100	96	100	96	5	86	68	0	91	91	100	91
Bordetella bronchiseptica	5	80	100	0	60	0	20	80	100	80	0	40	0	0	100	20	40	10
Escherichia coli	56	100	64	46	84	91	36	61	100	100	0	86	0	0	36	45	73	38
Klebsiella pneumoniae	13	92	83	8	92	92	75	83	100	100	8	83	0	0	83	8	75	75
Pseudomonas aeruginosa	7	100	0	0	0	14	0	0	100	86	0	71	0	0	0	57	86	29
Rhodococcus equi	13	85	92	77	15	8	23	77	92	85	54	85	0	85	77	31	31	69
Staphylococcus aureus	25	100	88	28	68	4	88	92	96	96	76	80	24	96	88	96	96	72
Streptococcus zooepidemicus	69	14	96	92	89	92	94	84	84	89	81	23	95	87	74	93	90	70

*AMI, amikacin; AMO, amoxicillin-clavulanate; AMP, ampicillin; CFF, ceftiofur; CEF, ceftizoxime; CPL, cephalothin; CR, chloramphenicol; CIP, ciprofloxacin; ENR, enrofloxacin; ERY, erythromycin; GEN, gentamicin; PEN, penicillin G; RIF, rifampin; TET, tetracycline; TIC, ticarcillin-clavulanate; TRI, trimethoprim-sulfamethoxazole.

TABLE 2. ANTIMICROBIAL DRUGS OF CHOICE FOR TREATMENT OF EQUINE LOWER RESPIRATORY TRACT INFECTIONS

Disease Process	Organism	First Choice	Alternate Choices
Foal pneumonia			
Neonatal	*Actinobacillus* sp.	Ceftiofur[b] + aminoglycoside[a]	Trimethoprim-sulfamethoxazole; ticarcillin-clavulanate
	E. coli	Ceftiofur[b] + aminoglycoside[a]	Cefotaxime[b] + aminoglycoside[a]
	K. pneumoniae	Ceftiofur[b] + aminoglycoside[a]	Cefotaxime + aminoglycoside[a]
Older foals			
Bordetellosis	*B. bronchiseptica*	Ceftiofur ± aminoglycoside	Chloramphenicol
Undifferentiated distal respiratory tract infection	*S. zooepidemicus*	Penicillin G (± trimethoprim-sulfamethoxazole)	Trimethoprim-sulfamethoxazole; erythromycin; ceftiofur
Pneumocystosis	*P. carinii*	Trimethoprim-sulfamethoxazole	Trimethoprim with dapsone[c]
Rhodococcal	*R. equi*	Erythromycin-rifampin	Trimethoprim-sulfamethoxazole; ampicillin-gentamicin; vancomycin[d]
Adult pneumonia/lung abscess	*S. zooepidemicus*	Penicillin G ± aminoglycoside[a]	Trimethoprim-sulfamethoxazole + penicillin G; erythromycin ± rifampin
	S. pneumoniae	Penicillin G	Trimethoprim-sulfamethoxazole + penicillin G; erythromycin
Strangles/aspiration	*S. equi*	Penicillin G	Trimethoprim-sulfamethoxazole + penicillin G; erythromycin
	Mixed opportunist aerobes[e]	Ceftiofur ± aminoglycoside[a]	Penicillin G + aminoglycoside;[a] chloramphenicol
Pleuropneumonia	*S. zooepidemicus*	Penicillin G + aminoglycoside	Trimethoprim-sulfamethoxazole; chloramphenicol
	Mixed opportunist aerobes	Ceftiofur + aminoglycoside[a]	Penicillin G + aminoglycoside; chloramphenicol
	Mixed aerobes/anaerobes[f]	Ceftiofur[b] + aminoglycoside[a] + metronidazole	Chloramphenicol; penicillin G + aminoglycosides + metronidazole
	Mycoplasma felis	Tetracycline	Enrofloxacin[f]; chloramphenicol

[a]Aminoglycoside, gentamicin or amikacin
[b]Alternates are ceftizoxime, cefuroxime
[c]Empirical therapy: trimethoprim 10 mg/kg b.i.d., dapsone 100 mg/kg s.i.d.
[d]Empirical therapy: 4 mg/kg IV t.i.d. diluted in >200 ml 5% dextrose over 2 hours
[e]Mixture of 2 or more of e.g., *Actinobacillus* sp., *E. coli*, *Klebsiella* sp, *S. zooepidemicus*
[f]Mixture of e (above) with e.g., *Bacteroides fragilis*, *Clostridium* sp., *Fusobacterium* sp., or *Porphyromonas* sp.

TABLE 3. COMMON ANTIMICROBIAL DRUG DOSAGES IN HORSES FOR LOWER RESPIRATORY TRACT INFECTIONS; NOT ALL HAVE BEEN APPROVED FOR USE IN HORSES

Drug	Dose (mg/kg)	Frequency	Route
Amikacin sulfate[1]	20	b.i.d.	IV, IM
Ampicillin sodium[2]	10–20	t.i.d.	IV, IM
Ampicillin-sulbactam[3]	3.3 (sulbactam)	s.i.d.	IM (see text for caution in use)
Cefotaxime[4]	20–40 (foals only)	q.i.d.	IV
Ceftiofur[5]	2.2	s.i.d./b.i.d.	IM
Ceftizoxime[6]	50	q.i.d.	IV
Cefuroxime[7]	30	t.i.d.	IV
Chloramphenicol palmitate[8]	25–50	q.i.d.	p.o.
Ciprofloxacin[9]	5	b.i.d.	IV
Enrofloxacin[10]	4	b.i.d. (empirical)	p.o.
Erythromycin estolate[11]	2.5	t.i.d.	p.o.
Gentamicin sulfate[12]	6.6	s.i.d.	IV, IM
Metronidazole[13]	15	q.i.d.	p.o. (IV, 0.5% solution)
Penicillin G (Na, K)	20,000–40,000 IU	q.i.d.	IV
Procaine[14]	20,000 IU/kg	b.i.d	IM
Rifampin[15]	10	s.i.d.	p.o.
Ticarcillin-clavulanate[16]	50 (ticarcillin) (foals only)	q.i.d.	IV
Trimethoprim-sulfonamide[17]	4–5 (trimethoprim) 24–30 (combined)	b.i.d.	p.o.

[1]Ami-Glyde V, Fort Dodge Laboratories, Fort Dodge, IA
[2]Amp-Equine, SmithKline Beecham, Exton, PA
[3]Synergistin, Pfizer, Lee's Summit, MO
[4]Claforan, Hoechst-Roussel, Somerville, NJ
[5]Naxcel, Upjohn, Kalamazoo, MI
[6]Cefizox, Fujiwara, Deerfield, IL
[7]Zinacef, Glaxo Wellcome, Research Triangle Park, NC
[8]Anacetin, Bio-ceutic Laboratories, St. Joseph, MO
[9]Cipro, Bayer, Shawnee Mission, KS

[10]Baytril, Bayer, Shawnee Mission, KS
[11]Ilosone Liquid, Dista Lilly, Indianapolis, IN
[12]Gentocin, Schering-Plough, Kenilworth, NJ
[13]Flagyl, Searle Pharmaceuticals, Chicago, IL
[14]Pfi-Pen, Pfizer, Lee's Summit, MO
[15]Rifadin, Marion Merrill Dow, Kansas City, MO
[16]Timentin, SmithKline Beecham, Exton, PA
[17]Tribrissen, Glaxo Wellcome, Research Triangle Park, NC

horses, and some drugs with anti-anaerobe activity such as lincomycin, which because of its lipophilic character is also partially excreted in the bile after parenteral administration should never be administered by any route. For this reason as well, extra-label use of newer cephalosporins, of β-lactamase inhibitors (clavulanic acid, sulbactam), and of carbapenems (e.g., imipenem) should be done with caution and is not recommended. Despite these precautions, severe colitis in adults has occasionally followed administration of most antibiotics. Foals seem to be less susceptible to antibiotic-induced colitis than adult horses.

Nebulization of poorly locally absorbed antibiotics with high local activity, such as gentamicin, seems to have no advantage over parenteral administration because most antimicrobial drugs are required to penetrate into inflamed and consolidated pneumonic tissue, not just to act at the level of the bronchi and bronchioles. In addition, many antimicrobial preparations are not designed for nebulization and are irritants in the respiratory tract, and their therapeutic dose by this route is not established.

In the case of intracellular microorganisms, such as *Rhodococcus equi*, lipophilic drugs such as erythromycin and rifampin, which penetrate macrophages well, give clinically far superior results to drugs such as beta-lactams and aminoglycosides, which, despite often usefully low minimum inhibitory concentrations in vitro, penetrate macrophages poorly. With this exception, however, relatively poor tissue distribution of drugs such as beta-lactams is often balanced by potent antimicrobial activity so that the drug may be equal in effect to a drug such as trimethoprim-sulfamethoxazole, which is better distributed but which has lower antibacterial activity.

Combination chemotherapy is well established in *R. equi* pneumonia (see Table 2) and with trimethoprim-sulfamethoxazole use. In some cases, penicillin G in aqueous solution is used in combination with trimethoprim-sulfamethoxazole as an empirical treatment in the absence of antimicrobial susceptibility results (see Table 2). Such a combination is not expected to be synergistic or additive in its effect but rather is expected to provide relatively broad-spectrum activity against aerobic bacteria, including those relatively few strains of *Streptococcus zooepidemicus* that may be penicillin G–resistant. Procaine penicillin perhaps should not be used in combination with trimethoprim-sulfonamide, because procaine is rapidly hydrolyzed into para-aminobenzoic acid, which inhibits the actions of sulfonamides. Nevertheless, clinical experience is that this combination has been beneficial. Combination of penicillin G, ampicillin, or ceftiofur with an aminoglycoside (amikacin, gentamicin) (see Table 2) most likely gives additive or synergistic effects against mixed aerobic bacterial pathogens such as S. zooepidemicus and Enterobacteriaceae (*Escherichia coli, Klebsiella pneumoniae*) (except penicillin G and possibly ampicillin for Enterobacteriaceae, see Table 1) and can be recommended for empirical therapy in serious infections.

Duration of treatment should continue for at least 48 to 72 hours after return to clinical normality and should be considerably longer in the case of serious infections, including pleuropneumonia and pulmonary abscess. In the case of *R. equi* infection, treatment of foals should be until

thoracic radiographs and plasma fibrinogen levels are normal, which may take several (4–9) weeks. Antibiotics instilled intrabronchially when a draining bronchus is identified may be of additional value as adjunctive single treatments, for example, after sampling.

INDIVIDUAL INFECTIONS AND DRUGS

Neonatal Pneumonias

Neonatal pneumonia is usually caused by organisms acquired from the intestine (see Table 2) and may involve mixed infections, including those from streptococci. The treatment of neonatal pneumonia should include broad-spectrum bactericidal drugs, which may be in combination (see Table 2). Aminoglycosides, however, should be used in combination for the shortest time required because of their nephrotoxic effects, although limited nephrotoxicity may occur if animals are adequately hydrated with IV fluids. Monitoring for peak and trough concentrations is recommended or dosage should be modified on the basis of serum creatinine concentration if aminoglycosides are used for more than 5 to 7 days. Dosage of foals with gentamicin at 6.6 mg/kg s.i.d. may reduce nephrotoxicity and enhance effectiveness compared with the traditional dose of 2.2 mg/kg t.i.d. Substantial clinical evidence exists from human medicine that once-daily dosing of aminoglycosides is both more efficacious than three-times-daily dosing and is also less nephrotoxic. Further study will show whether 6.6 mg/kg s.i.d. is preferred to 2.2 mg/kg t.i.d.

Use of fluoroquinolones in foals is largely empirical and should probably be reserved for foals for which alternative drugs are not available. Preliminary studies suggest that enrofloxacin causes cartilage damage in foals.

Older Foals
Bordetellosis

The primary role of *Bordetella bronchiseptica* in bronchopneumonia in foals is not clearly established because it is both relatively uncommon and usually isolated with other pathogens. It appears resistant to commonly used antibiotics (see Table 1), but suitable drugs for empirical therapy may include ceftiofur combined with amikacin.

Undifferentiated Distal Respiratory Tract Infection

Undifferentiated distal respiratory tract infection (bronchitis, bronchiolitis) of foals is commonly caused by S. zooepidemicus, which in some cases are found with other bacteria such as *Actinobacillus* species, B. bronchiseptica, or nonhemolytic streptococci. Because of in vitro-determined resistance of some isolates to either penicillin G or trimethoprim-sulfamethoxazole, empirical treatment with trimethoprim-sulfamethoxazole administered orally for 10 to 21 days in combination with parenteral penicillin G, ampicillin, or sulbactam-ampicillin administered IM for 7 days has appeared to provide broader antibacterial effects than with either class of drug alone. Alternative treatments may include erythromycin, ceftiofur, rifampin, or their combination.

Pneumocystosis

Although uncommon, infection with *Pneumocystis carinii* is increasingly recognized in foals. The standard treatment is with trimethoprim-sulfamethoxazole, although in human patients fewer side effects have been seen with trimethoprim and dapsone.

Rhodococcus equi *Pneumonia*

The standard treatment for *R. equi* pneumonia in foals is the combination of erythromycin and rifampin, which are drugs that penetrate macrophages well. These drugs must be used in combination largely to reduce the risk of development of chromosomal forms of resistance but also because the combination is synergistic. Dosage of the estolate form of erythromycin is suggested to be 25 mg/kg t.i.d. Recent pharmacokinetic studies suggested that the less expensive phosphate and stearate salts are better absorbed than the estolate or ethylsuccinate forms. The phosphate or stearate forms of erythromycin may be used for twice-daily oral dosing (at 37.5 mg/kg b.i.d.), although there is no experience with the diarrhea-inducing potential of this dose. A dosage of rifampin 5 to 10 mg/kg s.i.d. gives serum concentrations exceeding the minimum inhibitory concentration (MIC) of the organism. Despite use of this combination, resistant strains may emerge. Alternatives to erythromycin-rifampin recommended for foals include trimethoprim-sulfamethoxazole and, least satisfactorily clinically, ampicillin and gentamicin in combination.

In experimentally infected mice, the use of erythromycin alone in *R. equi* infections was only of marginal benefit. Other drugs such as vancomycin, imipenem, and minocycline (with and without rifampin) are more effective than the erythromycin-rifampin combination in mice. No beneficial effect occurred with ciprofloxacin in mice, despite low MIC. The efficacy and safety of these agents in foals with *R. equi* infection have not been determined.

Adult Pneumonia and Pulmonary Abscess

Most adult lung infections and abscessation involve *S. zooepidemicus*, the major bacterial pathogen of the respiratory tract (see Table 2). For empirical therapy in the absence of culture and susceptibility results, the drug of choice is penicillin G, which can be combined with an aminoglycoside (gentamicin, amikacin); the advantage of the combination is not only that it is synergistic against *S. zooepidemicus* but also that it gives coverage against gram-negative aerobic pathogens that may be present (see Table 1). Gentamicin should not be used for more than 5 to 7 days without monitoring for therapeutic drug levels or serum creatinine concentration. In horses with pneumonia, clinical response usually is evident within 48 hours. Therefore, one strategy in treatment in the absence of results of bacterial susceptibility tests is to treat with penicillin and gentamicin for 5 days and then to change treatment to trimethoprim-sulfamethoxazole administered orally if further antimicrobial drug treatment is judged to be necessary. An alternative drug for subsequent oral treatment is erythromycin. Some have found that administration of 15 mg/kg b.i.d. for 1 to 2 days before increasing to 25 mg/kg t.i.d. reduces the diarrhea that sometimes accompanies immediate use of the higher dose. A similar approach may be used in the presence of lung abscesses, although the clinical signs of response to therapy are often delayed, and the duration of therapy generally exceeds 4 weeks.

Ceftiofur is another alternative first-choice drug for empirical treatment of adult pneumonia or lung abscess, particularly when infection with gram-negative aerobes is suspected. Combination with an aminoglycoside is recommended for serious infections for the reasons described earlier. Although suitable for the treatment of *S. zooepidemicus* and nonenteric gram-negative pathogens at the approved dosage of 2.2 mg/kg b.i.d. of ceftiofur, this dose is low based on the relationship between serum concentrations and minimal inhibitory concentrations of some Enterobacteriaceae, and a dosage of 4.4 mg/kg b.i.d. may be recommended in empirical treatment of serious infections when Enterobacteriaceae are involved.

Pleuropneumonia

Bacterial pleuropneumonia is a pneumonic process that progresses from the lung parenchyma to involve the adjacent pleura, producing a rapidly developing pleural effusion that may initially be sterile. Bacterial invasion from the lung produces the fibrinopurulent stage followed by fibrin organization, which limits extension of the infection but may make drainage difficult. *S. zooepidemicus*, aerobic gram-negative opportunists, and anaerobic bacteria (see Table 2) are commonly implicated. Drugs of choice in empirical treatment without bacterial culture results are those recommended for bacterial pneumonias and lung abscess in adults (penicillin G with aminoglycoside, ceftiofur with aminoglycoside) with the addition of an antibiotic effective against anaerobic bacteria. Anaerobic sensitivity testing is often unavailable. Anaerobes are resistant to aminoglycosides but, although many anaerobes are sensitive to penicillin G or ceftiofur, some, such as *Bacteroides fragilis,* are β-lactamase producers. Metronidazole and chloramphenicol are efficacious against anaerobic bacteria when administered orally and are therefore recommended as additional treatment for established pleuropneumonia. Some horses receiving metronidazole develop anorexia and depression. Once clinical resolution has occurred, antibacterial treatment can be changed to orally administrable drugs based on culture and sensitivity test results. Oral administration of a fluoroquinolone or of chloramphenicol should be effective against *Mycoplasma felis*, which has an etiologic role in some cases of pleuropneumonia.

Supplemental Readings

Ewing PJ, Burrows G, MacAllister C, Clarke C: Comparison of oral erythromycin formulations in the horse using pharmacokinetic profiles. J Vet Pharm Therap 17:17–23, 1994.

Folz SD, Hanson BJ, Griffin AK, Dinvald LL, Swerczek TW, Walker RD, Foreman JH: Treatment of respiratory infections in horses with ceftiofur sodium. Equine Vet J 24:300–304, 1992.

Giguere S, Sweeney RW, Belanger M: Pharmacokinetics of enrofloxacin in adult horses and concentration of the drug in serum, body fluids, and endometrial tissues after repeated intragastrically administered doses. Am J Vet Res 57:1025–1030, 1996.

Godber LM, Walker WD, Stein G, Hauptman JG, Derksen FJ: Pharmacokinetics, nephrotoxicosis, and in vitro antibacterial activity associated with single versus multiple (three times daily) gentamicin treatments in horses. Am J Vet Res 56:613–618, 1995.

Hoffman AM, Viel L, Prescott JF: Microbiologic changes during antimicrobial treatment and rate of relapse of distal respiratory tract infections in foals. Am J Vet Res 54:608–614, 1993.

Sweeney CR, Holcombe SJ, Barningham SC, Beech J: Aerobic and anaerobic bacterial isolates from horses with pneumonia or pleuropneumonia and antimicrobial susceptibility patterns of the aerobes. J Am Vet Med Assoc 198:839–842, 1991.

Sweeney RW, Sweeney CR, Weiher J: Clinical use of metronidazole in horses: 200 cases (1984–1989). J Am Vet Med Assoc 198:1045–1048, 1991.

Acute Equine Respiratory Syndrome

DAVID R. HODGSON

JENNIFER L. HODGSON
Camden, Australia

In September 1994, a fatal, previously unrecorded syndrome of acute respiratory disease occurred in horses in Queensland, Australia. The disease, caused by a *Morbillivirus* (rinderpest and measles also belong to this genus), resulted in the death of 14 of 21 affected horses over 2 weeks. This virus was also implicated in the death of the animals' trainer and illness in another employee of the trainer. Both individuals suffered an influenza-like illness with the trainer dying after 6 days of intensive therapy. This is the first report of a new morbilliviral infection affecting horses and humans; in fact, it is the first report of a new *Morbillivirus* infection in humans since the tenth century, when measles was described. Subsequent serosurveillance involving 90 people and about 1600 horses indicate that the virus has not spread. Although remaining confined to a small area, the implications from this outbreak are significant. The syndrome shared clinical signs of two diseases exotic to Australia—African horse sickness and equine influenza. More than 1 week elapsed between the death of the first horse and notification of the appropriate state quarantine and exotic disease authorities. Therefore, if the agent causing the disease had been particularly contagious, the potential for spread of such a pathogen throughout the horse and possibly human populations was great. An added effect of the outbreak was the interruption of horse movements into and out of the state of Queensland, cancellation of several race meetings, and days lost to training as facilities were closed temporarily.

ETIOLOGY

A virus from the genus *Morbillivirus* was isolated in tissue culture from the spleen and lung of two of the horses dying in Queensland. To demonstrate that the virus was the causative agent of the respiratory disease syndrome, homogenates of the spleen and lung were inoculated into two recipient horses intravenously and via nasal aerosol. Both horses showed signs of the syndrome in 6 and 10 days, respectively, with both being killed after 2 days of severe illness. In addition, purified virus from tissue culture was inoculated into two other horses and also caused the syndrome. All inoculated horses showed characteristic histologic manifestations, and viral nucleocapsids were identified by electron microscopy in the lungs of all recipient horses. Virus was also isolated from samples of the deceased human's kidney. Spread is thought to have been the result of direct contact with infected horses or contaminated tack.

CLINICAL SIGNS

The incubation period for the disease was variable, up to 10 days. In horses inoculated with purified virus it was shorter, 3 to 4 days. Affected horses had signs of an acute respiratory disease syndrome with death usually occurring 1 to 3 days after onset of clinical signs. Most horses were inappetent and febrile (up to 41°C) and had shallow respirations, patchy sweating, and nasal discharge varying from clear to serosanguineous. The sclerae were at times jaundiced and the mucous membranes injected with a cyanotic margin. Dependent edema, ataxia, and head pressing were noted in some horses before death. Samples obtained for hematologic and serum biochemical analyses from a small number of horses revealed no characteristic abnormalities. Horses affected in the initial period of the outbreak often died in extremis, producing voluminous frothy nasal discharge in the terminal period.

PATHOLOGIC FINDINGS

At necropsy, the significant manifestations were restricted to the lower respiratory tract. Severe pulmonary edema and congestion were observed, and the airways were filled with stable foam, which was often blood-stained. Subcutaneous edema was seen in several horses. Microscopically, acute interstitial pneumonia was observed with associated proteinaceous alveolar edema, hemorrhage, alveolar thrombosis and necrosis, and necrosis of small blood vessels. Disseminated intravascular coagulation was common. Changes were most accentuated in horses showing severe clinical signs and a short course of disease. An important feature of the disease was the presence of syncytial giant cells found in blood vessel walls. Syncytial giant cells are common in *Morbillivirus* infections.

DIAGNOSIS

Methods used for making the original diagnosis are described above. A serum neutralization test and indirect fluorescent antibody test have been developed subsequent to the outbreak for detection of specific antibody in horses and humans. A number of affected horses had seroconversion before death, whereas those that did not were likely to have died before sufficient time had passed for seroconversion. The horse trainer had seroconversion before his death, as did the surviving stable hand. An additional seven horses within the stable complex also had seroconversion before they were killed. Despite quite extensive serosurveillance, there is no evidence of spread of the virus outside the affected trainer's stables.

Differential diagnosis of this syndrome included African horse sickness, equine influenza, equine viral arteritis, the equine encephalitides, *Hantavirus* infection, several bacterial diseases (including anthrax, *Pasteurella* species infection, pneumonic plague), and effects of a variety of toxins (such as paraquat, monesin, heavy metals, and mycotoxins). All these agents were ruled out on the basis of clinical signs and laboratory testing.

TREATMENT

No known treatment exists for this infection, as is the case with nearly all viral infections. In addition, because

this disease was unexpected, no means of immunoprophylaxis was available. Control of subsequent outbreaks would best be performed by containment, early identification of the infectious agent, quarantine, and disinfection. In addition, the virus has an apparent limited capacity for spread, which will aid containment.

CONCLUSION

Several important implications can be drawn from the emergence of this new form of viral respiratory disease. The virus has the capacity to cross-infect species, in this case affecting horses and humans. Such characteristics of any potentially fatal disease raise several equine and public health problems. Furthermore, the reservoir host of the virus, and thus the source of infection, is yet to be determined, as is the infectivity of the virus for other domestic and wild animal species. An additional case of equine morbillivirus infection occurred in August 1994. This was an isolated case, remote from the initial outbreak. Seroconversion has been reported in bats. The significance of this finding is unknown. Therefore, until many of these issues are resolved, the overall significance of the outbreak in Queensland remains to be determined. However, if outbreaks of this disease occur again, rapid diagnosis and containment of the virus will be contingent on the vigilance of attending veterinarians suspecting the syndrome and ensuring that appropriate health and quarantine officials are notified.

Supplemental Readings

Murray K, Selleck P, Hooper P, Hyatt A, Gould A, Gleeson L, Westbury H, Hiley L, Selvey L, Rodwell B, Ketterer P: A morbillivirus that caused fatal disease in horses and humans. Science 268:94–97, 1995.
Murray K, Byrne N: Solving the horse virus mystery. Today's Life Science 5:56, 1995.

Smoke Inhalation

TINA KEMPER
Yorba Linda, California

Severe inhalation injury is most likely to occur when horses are trapped within an enclosed burning structure with minimal access to fresh air. Inhalation injury may be compounded by burns, which significantly decreases survival rates. Pulmonary damage from inhalation injury is a result of the decreased oxygen content of the inspired air and exposure to various noxious gases and particulate matter. The presence of noxious gases such as carbon monoxide and cyanide is dependent upon the type of material that is burning. Pulmonary edema results from direct damage to the pulmonary epithelium as well as increased microvascular permeability resulting from an influx of inflammatory cells such as neutrophils, with the subsequent release of

proteolytic enzymes and oxygen free radicals. Superheated air is often cooled by the time it reaches the lower respiratory tract but may cause severe pharyngeal edema and inflammation, leading to upper airway obstruction and asphyxia. Diffuse tracheobronchial mucosal sloughing can lead to the formation of pseudomembranous casts, which may also cause partial or complete airway obstruction (Fig. 1).

CLINICAL SIGNS

Clinical signs may vary depending upon the severity of the injury and the time elapsed before examination. Horses

ination and bacterial culture and sensitivity testing. As the dome of the diaphragm extends to the sixth rib on expiration, horses with wounds caudal to this or with deep penetration should have an abdominal paracentesis performed to detect abdominal cavity visceral perforation. Cytologic examination may reveal peritonitis and the presence of feed material. The detection of mixed bacterial species on Gram's stain confirms visceral perforation. Thoracoscopy could be used when a foreign body is believed to be present in the dorsal thoracic cavity but is not visualized on ultrasonographic or radiographic examination.

TREATMENT

Emergency Treatment of Thoracic Trauma

Initial immediate care should be directed at the reestablishment of effective alveolar ventilation and treatment of shock, if present. Most tranquilizers and sedatives may cause respiratory depression and therefore should be avoided. In horses with a sucking chest wound, in which air rushes into the pleural space on inspiration and exits on expiration, ventilation can be immediately improved by covering the wound. This restores the integrity of the chest wall and allows some ventilation of the lung on the ipsilateral side. Monitoring of the cardiovascular system is important in the presence of continuing hemorrhage. When the horse's condition is stable, ancillary examination and treatment can be performed.

Thoracic Wound Care

Standard wound care is performed. Thoracic wounds may be treated under local anesthesia in the standing horse. Intercostal nerve blocks with long-acting local anesthetics such as 0.5% bupivacaine hydrochloride with epinephrine° (1:200,000) may be used and subsequently facilitate the control of postoperative pain. Two to three ml of bupivacaine hydrochloride should be injected immediately caudal to the involved ribs. Wounds should be inspected for the presence of foreign bodies, hemorrhage, fractured ribs, and traumatized lung or diaphragm. The wound should be enlarged if necessary to perform a thorough exploration. All sources of hemorrhage should be identified and ligated. Vigorous wound lavage and suction of blood accumulated in the thorax should be performed during surgery. If a large foreign body is present in the wound, complications should be anticipated with its removal, such as a deterioration of respiratory function or hemorrhage. In such cases, removal should be performed under general anesthesia with positive-pressure ventilation. It is important that the animal's condition be stabilized before the induction of anesthesia, and ideally the air should be evacuated from the thorax.

Penetrating thoracic wounds should be sutured whenever possible. The pleural cavity should be evacuated of air when suturing is complete. If the animal is under general anesthesia, the last suture is tightened on expiration. The repair of large thoracic wall defects is problematic, and a

---

°*Marcaine, Breon Laboratories, New York, NY*

primary muscle flap, diaphragmatic advancement (which may be advanced to the thirteenth intercostal space), or closure with prosthetic meshes can be attempted.

When the wounds cannot be sutured they should be packed and an airtight seal formed. The choice of dressing depends on the size of the defect, but moist dressings or petrolatum or betadine ointment on dry sponges are necessary to achieve an effective seal. A stent bandage may be placed over the wound using sterile material held in place with cotton tape laced through loops of nonabsorbable suture material around the wound. A bandage around the thorax may be used to hold the packing in place. Broad-spectrum antibiotic administration is indicated prophylactically in horses with penetrating thoracic trauma to attempt to avoid thoracic empyema. Tetanus prophylaxis is also indicated.

Pneumothorax

Pneumothorax should be treated if the horse exhibits respiratory distress. In horses with pneumothorax without respiratory distress there is a gradual resorption of the air. Tension pneumothorax is an emergency and requires immediate correction. If hypoxemia (PaO_2 <80 mm Hg) is present or the horse has labored breathing, nasal insufflation of oxygen (15 L/min) should be performed. After the wounds have been sealed, pneumothorax may be treated by carefully inserting a large-gauge needle or teat cannula into the dorsal thoracic cavity just in front of ribs 12 to 15 to avoid the vessels running on the caudal surfaces of the latter. Local anesthesia facilitates the procedure. A 60-ml syringe and three-way stopcock may be used. If a stopcock is not available, tubing can be used to connect the cannula and syringe. This tubing can be clamped while the syringe is emptied. However, because of the large volume of the pleural space, this procedure may be tedious. A suction device may also be attached to the needle or syringe to speed up the process. Evacuation may need to be repeated because of continuing air leaks from the wound.

When there is a large continuing air leak, continuous suction should be applied through a thoracostomy tube° or a small stomach tube. Problems with the thoracostomy tube are rare, but broad-spectrum antibiotics are indicated as long as it is in place. The tube must have a valve or seal to prevent air from re-entering the pleural space. A container of water may function as a valve by immersing the free end of the tube in the water. With each expiration, the accumulated air is expelled through the tube under water, and bubbles are seen. On inspiration, the water seals the tube. When the bubbles cease to appear, the lung has re-expanded. A Heimlich valve† attached to the thoracostomy tube can also be used and has the advantage of allowing the horse to be mobile. In referral centers, when an animal is distressed because of a large continuing air leak, suction may be applied to the thoracostomy tube either through a three-bottle suction system or a commercial equivalent.‡ A suction pressure of no more than 20 cm of water has been recommended to avoid re-expansion

---

°*Argyle trocar catheter, Sherwood Medical Industries, St. Louis, MO*
†*Heimlich chest drainage valve, Bard-Parker, Division of Becton Dickinson, Rutherford, NJ*
‡*Pleur-Evac, Deknatel, Pfizer, Fall River, MA*

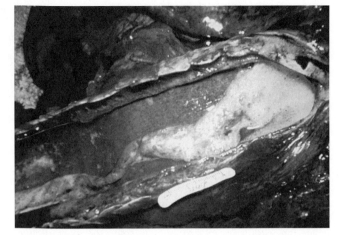

Figure 1. Fibrin cast within the tracheal lumen after inhalation injury.

suffering from inhalation injury often exude a very strong smoky odor and may be covered with soot. Cutaneous burns may be present, or only the hair may be scorched. The heart rate, respiratory rate, and temperature may be within normal limits or marked tachycardia, tachypnea, dyspnea, stridor, and fever may be present. The horse may have a soft cough or may have severe paroxysmal coughing episodes, which may lead to agitation or distress. Pulmonary auscultation findings can vary from normal bronchovesicular sounds to severe crackles and wheezes. The absence of bronchovesicular and adventitious sounds in the presence of labored breathing and minimal air flow detectable at the nares may indicate severe pulmonary edema or, in certain cases, upper airway obstruction. Pulmonary edema may become so severe that foam exudes from both nostrils. Cyanosis is recognized clinically when the PaO_2 falls below 40 mm Hg, but the mucous membranes may be muddy with a prolonged capillary refill time. Carbon monoxide poisoning can be difficult to determine by physical examination results alone but may be suspected if the mucous membranes are bright red. Dehydration and shock may be present, and the animal may exhibit ataxia, weakness, and collapse.

DIAGNOSIS

A diagnosis of inhalation injury is usually made from the history as well as the results of physical examination. Clinical signs of smoke inhalation may not be evident upon initial examination, because pulmonary edema and congestion as well as laryngotracheal damage may not occur for 2 to 3 days with certain types of injury. If inhalation injury is suspected but cannot be confirmed by observations on physical examination, endoscopy can be performed to visualize laryngeal edema, mucosal sloughing, and black carbon particle deposition in the upper airway.

Further diagnostic tests can help determine the severity of the inhalation injury. A complete blood count and plasma fibrinogen determination should be performed to ascertain the degree of dehydration and to rule out secondary bacterial bronchopneumonia. The magnitude of hypoxemia and hypercapnea determined by arterial blood gas analysis indi-

cates the extent of respiratory compromise. Serum electrolytes should be measured, because electrolyte imbalances may occur, especially if cutaneous burns are present. Organ dysfunction can result from poor tissue oxygenation, and thus periodic evaluation of serum chemistry test results is indicated. If bacterial bronchopneumonia is suspected, a transtracheal aspirate allows samples to be taken for bacterial culture and determination of antibiotic sensitivity. Thoracic radiography should be used, when possible, to evaluate the extent of pulmonary infiltrations such as pulmonary edema and bronchopneumonia. However, in acute illness, radiographic findings may not indicate the extent of lung dysfunction, and physical examination findings may correlate more accurately with the severity of the injury.

THERAPY

Therapeutic goals should be directed at alleviating bronchoconstriction, maintaining arterial oxygen tension within normal limits, minimizing pulmonary edema, and managing subsequent bronchopneumonia and organ failure.

Even short-term oxygen therapy (15 minutes to 1 hour) at the scene of the fire can be extremely beneficial for decreasing the half life of carbon monoxide in the blood. Oxygen can be nasally insufflated using a transportable E tank with a pressure regulator, flow meter, and tubing. Flow rates of 5 to 15 L/minute can be used in an attempt to increase PaO_2 in hypoxemic horses and to displace carbon monoxide from hemoglobin. If oxygen therapy is to be given for longer periods, the oxygen should be humidified. In the case of severe airway injury with epithelial sloughing and pseudomembranous cast formation, oxygen insufflation may not be sufficient to improve tissue oxygenation. If the pseudomembranous casts are large enough to create upper airway obstruction, a tracheostomy may be necessary to allow for removal of the large fibrin casts. One of the disadvantages of a tracheostomy is that it eliminates the ability of the horse to produce an effective cough to aid in removal of accumulated debris. If primary laryngospasm is suspected and there is minimal nasal and upper airway swelling, ventilation may be improved by use of an endotracheal tube or clean nasogastric tube passed through the nose into the trachea.

Cough suppressants may be necessary to reduce the paroxysmal coughing, which may cause further dyspnea and distress. Butorphanol° (0.025 to 0.05 mg/kg IV) is effective for cough suppression and causes minimal side effects. Bronchodilators such as aminophylline† (5–10 mg/kg p.o. q12h), terbutaline sulfate‡ (0.02–0.08 mg/kg p.o. q12h) or clenbuterol§ (0.8 μg/kg p.o. q12h) should be used early in the course of inhalation injury to alleviate bronchospasm. The excitatory effects of aminophylline may be seen even when recommended doses are used if drug clearance is impaired.

Nonsteroidal anti-inflammatory drugs (NSAIDs) such as

°*Torbugesic, Fort Dodge Laboratories, Fort Dodge, IA*
†*Aminophylline, West-Ward Pharmaceutical Corp., Eatontown, NJ*
‡*Brethine, Ciba-Geigy, Ardsley, NY*
§*Ventipulmin, Boehringer Ingelheim Ltd., Burlington, Ontario, Canada*

flunixin meglumine° or phenylbutazone† may be used for pain control and anti-inflammatory effects. Care must be used when determining dosages for both the bronchodilators and NSAIDS, because toxic levels may be reached even when the lower dosages are used owing to the poor tissue perfusion and decreased oxygenation associated with severe injury.

Diuretics such as furosemide‡ (0.5 to 2 mg/kg IV or IM q12h) are important to decrease the amount of pulmonary interstitial fluid and alveolar edema. Intravenous fluids are important for cardiovascular support in cases in which shock is present, even if the patient is being treated concurrently with diuretics for pulmonary edema. Survival rates may be improved when early fluid therapy is instituted, as long as the animal is not overhydrated.

The use of corticosteroids is controversial. Glucocorticoids may decrease mortality rates by increasing cell and lysosomal membrane stability and enhancing capillary wall integrity, thereby reducing pulmonary edema. However, steroids that have strong mineralocorticoid activity may increase mortality rates owing to the retention of sodium and the potential to exacerbate pulmonary edema. In addition, corticosteroids should not be administered in horses with cutaneous burns because of the increased potential for the development of sepsis consequent to the immunosuppressive effects of the corticosteroids and the lack of an intact skin barrier. Therefore, the use of corticosteroids such as dexamethasone sodium phosphate§ (0.05–0.1 mg/kg q12–24h for the first 12–36 hours) should be reserved for cases of severe inhalation injury and pulmonary edema but without cutaneous burns.

Antibiotic use is also controversial. Bacterial bronchopneumonia may be a potential sequela to inhalation injury and should be treated accordingly if it occurs. In human medicine, the prophylactic use of antibiotics is discouraged because of the development of resistant strains of bacteria, but this has not been demonstrated to be a problem in horses. If corticosteroids are used, broad-spectrum antibiotics such as trimethoprim/sulfa‖ (5 mg of the trimethoprim fraction/kg p.o. q8h) should be given concurrently.

Nebulization can be used to moisten secretions or deliver medications such as bronchodilators or mucolytics. Nebulization can be delivered via a face mask or directly into a tracheostomy by using an ultrasonic nebulizer attached to an oxygen tank. Experimental studies have shown that the combination of nebulized heparin¶ (10,000 units) along with 3 ml of 90%DMSO° improved survival rates in sheep suffering from inhalation injury by decreasing the production of pseudomembranous casts and decreasing microvascular permeability. Nebulization should be performed every 4 to 6 hours for 15 to 30 minutes. This may not be practical for field cases, in which case intravenous dimethyl sulfoxide (DMSO) (10% solution) at 0.5 g to 1 g/kg q24h for 3 to 5 days may provide some benefit, although no controlled studies are available on the efficacy or potential harm of this type of treatment. The carrier potential of DMSO should be taken into consideration, because the patients are frequently treated with a number of medications, the toxicity of which may be enhanced when used in combination with DMSO.

Other supportive care should be given as needed. Even when cutaneous burns are not present, the cornea may suffer thermal damage and require topical therapy with lubricants or antibacterial ointments or solutions. Organ dysfunction can be a major problem associated with poor tissue oxygenation and perfusion. Each medication that the horse is receiving should be critically evaluated for its continued need so that unnecessary medications can be discontinued to minimize drug-induced organ dysfunction in the compromised patient.

PROGNOSIS

The recovery time for victims of smoke inhalation varies with the severity of the injury. In general, 2 to 6 months may be required before the animal can be returned to partial work. Horses that have suffered from inhalation injury may be more prone to episodes of irritant-induced bronchoconstriction. Efforts should be made, therefore, to reduce environmental dust, molds, and irritants. If bronchoconstriction persists after recovery, a bronchodilator may be used as needed. Depending upon the type of inhalation injury, prognosis for return to prior exercise ability is good if the horse survives the initial insult.

Supplemental Readings

Brown M, Desai M, Traber LD, Herndon DN, Traber DL: Dimethylsulfoxide with heparin in the treatment of smoke inhalation injury. J Burn Care Rehab 9:22–25, 1988.
Geor RJ, Ames TR: Smoke inhalation injury in horses. Comp Cont Ed Pract Vet 13:1162–1169, 1991.
Isago T, Noshima S, Traber LD, Herndon DN, Traber DL: Analysis of pulmonary microvascular permeability after smoke inhalation. J Appl Physiol 71:1403–1408, 1991.
Kemper T, Spier S, Barratt-Boyes SM, Hoffman R: Treatment of smoke inhalation in five horses. J Am Vet Med Assoc 202:91–94, 1993.
Zawacki BE, Jung RC, Joyce J, Rinson E: Smoke, burns, and the natural history of inhalation injury in fire victims: A correlation of experimental and clinical data. Ann Surg 185:100–110, 1977.

°Banamine, Schering-Plough, Kenilworth, NJ
†Phenylbutazone, Victor Medical, Irvine, CA
‡Lasix, Hoechst-Roussel, Somerville, NJ
§Dexamethasone sodium phosphate, Steris Laboratories, Phoenix, AZ
‖Trimethoprim sulfamethoxazole (DS), Viterine Pharmaceuticals, Springfield Gardens, NY
¶Heparin sodium, Fugisawa, Deerfield, IL

°Domoso, Syntex Agribusiness, West Des Moines, IA

Thoracic Trauma

SHEILA LAVERTY
St. Hyacinthe, Quebec

Thoracic trauma may be blunt or penetrating. Blunt thoracic trauma occurs in the newborn foal and may be caused by pressure in the pelvic cavity during difficult parturition in primiparous mares or in association with retention of the elbow. The most common cause of equine penetrating thoracic trauma is collision with an object. Problems encountered in animals with thoracic trauma include respiratory difficulty, pneumothorax, hemorrhage, hemothorax, shock, fractured ribs, flail chest, and, less commonly, diaphragmatic hernia or abdominal cavity penetration.

Pneumothorax is the presence of air in the pleural space and is caused by a defect in the thoracic wall, airways, or lung. Pneumothorax leads to pulmonary collapse and prevents normal lung expansion during inspiration. Tension pneumothorax occurs when there is a flap of soft tissue that acts as a one-way valve, allowing air to enter the pleural space on inspiration but preventing its exit on expiration. There is a progressive increase in intrathoracic pressure, which causes lung compression and respiratory failure. Hemothorax most commonly results from lacerated intercostal arteries or pulmonary parenchyma. Pneumothorax or hemothorax may be unilateral or bilateral depending on whether the mediastinum is intact. A flail chest occurs when two or more ribs are fractured at more than one site, creating a free-floating segment of the thoracic wall. The flail segment moves in a direction opposite the ipsilateral wall during respiration (paradoxical respiration). Because it takes considerable trauma to create a flail chest, there are often serious underlying pulmonary contusions.

The prognosis for penetrating thoracic wounds in which no vital structure is involved and no foreign body is present is good if treated early. Concurrent extrathoracic injury decreases prospects of a good prognosis.

CLINICAL SIGNS

The clinical signs of thoracic trauma are variable and depend on the systems involved and the severity of the trauma. Palpation allows detection of subcutaneous emphysema, edema, hematomas, or fractured ribs. Large penetrating wounds are easily identifiable. A small wound with attendant subcutaneous emphysema should increase the index of suspicion of thoracic penetration. Edema over the thoracic cage may be present in both blunt and penetrating injury. The rate, pattern, and depth of respiration should be evaluated immediately. Fractured ribs cause splinting of the thorax, resulting in shallow respiration because of pain. Pneumothorax or hemothorax causes rapid superficial respiration, which may progress to deep labored breathing. Animals with tension pneumothorax are recognized by the development of respiratory distress, which may be rapid in onset. Tachycardia, weak pulse, and pale mucous membranes may indicate the presence of severe and possibly ongoing hemorrhage from the large thoracic vessels or the heart. Colic and signs of shock may also indicate concurrent abdominal cavity and viscus perforation.

When pneumothorax is present, decreased breath sounds are present on thoracic auscultation and increased resonance on percussion dorsally. A fluid line is detected on percussion of the ventral thorax when hemothorax is present; decreased vesicular sounds may be heard. Subcutaneous emphysema, which is present with most penetrating thoracic wounds, can make interpretation of auscultation findings difficult.

DIAGNOSIS

Thoracic wounds should be thoroughly explored for the presence of a foreign body. In the case of penetrating trauma, the offending object should be inspected to determine whether foreign material remains in the wound.

Fractured ribs are often missed during clinical examination of newborn foals. The cranial ribs are more commonly fractured in the area of the costochondral junction. The sharp ends of the fractured ribs and edema may be palpated. When the foal is carefully placed in dorsal recumbency, asymmetry of the cranial thorax is observed.

In animals with pneumothorax, radiographs may reveal unilateral or bilateral retraction of the lung fields from the vertebral column. Fractured ribs may be detected; however, if the fracture is not displaced it may be missed on radiographic examination, especially in young foals. A diagnosis of diaphragmatic hernia is confirmed by the observation of viscera in the thoracic cavity on radiography or ultrasonographic examination.

Ultrasonographic examination may provide additional information, but the presence of subcutaneous emphysema around the wound may limit its usefulness. A sudden change in reverberation artifacts as the transducer passes from free air dorsally to aerated lung ventrally may be visualized in the presence of pneumothorax. The surface of normal aerated lung is recognized by its characteristic artifact and its movement during respiration. In the presence of pneumothorax, this movement is diminished. A fluid line on ultrasonographic examination indicates possible presence of hemothorax. Foreign bodies in the wound or thorax may also be identified.

A complete blood count should be performed and repeated to determine the degree of blood loss. If possible, arterial blood samples should be obtained to evaluate the degree of hypoxemia in horses with labored breathing. Thoracocentesis (see later) confirms the diagnosis of pneumothorax and hemothorax by the aspiration of a volume of air or blood, respectively, from the pleura. The aspirated fluid should be submitted for cytology.

pulmonary edema. In humans, the latter is a fatal condition, predisposing factors for which include a large pneumothorax present for more than 24 hours or rapid pulmonary re-expansion. The disadvantage of continuous suction systems is that they require constant monitoring.

Hemothorax

Pulmonary re-expansion in a horse with pneumothorax may arrest hemorrhage from the low-pressure pulmonary parenchymal vascular system. When penetrating thoracic wounds are present, evacuation of blood from the pleural space is indicated to avoid thoracic empyema. Thoracocentesis for hemothorax evacuation is performed in the ventral thorax, cranial to ribs six and seven above the lateral thoracic vein. A technique similar to that used for pneumothorax evacuation is used. This should be performed under ultrasonographic guidance to avoid cardiac penetration. Prophylactic broad-spectrum antibiotic administration is advisable because blood is an excellent culture medium.

Management of Rib Fractures

In penetrating trauma cases, surgical fixation of rib fractures is usually unnecessary. It is usually sufficient to remove the fracture fragments and rongeur sharp points that could traumatize the lung parenchyma. Analgesics such as flunixin meglumine* (1 mg/kg b.i.d., IV or IM) should be used for a few days because the pain associated with rib fractures leads to chest splinting, with reduced ventilation and cough reflex. This may predispose to the development of pneumonia.

In horses with flail chest, underlying pulmonary contusion is an additional problem. The contused lung may become edematous following crystalloid solution administration, and the latter should be avoided in these cases. When possible an attempt should be made to surgically stabilize the flail chest by fixation of the ribs to an external thoracic splint or by the use of internal fixation.

Fractured ribs in postpartum foals are usually of no

Banamine, Schering Plough, Kenilworth, NJ

clinical significance; however, they can lead to pneumothorax, hemothorax, and laceration of the heart or diaphragm. Neonatal foals with medical problems should always be checked for this condition and, if it is detected, foals should be handled with care to avoid creating secondary injuries.

Management of Diaphragmatic Hernia

This condition can be confusing because the animal may present with hemothorax, hemoperitoneum, respiratory difficulty, and colic, or none of these symptoms. If possible, repair should be delayed to allow fibrosis of the hernia ring. Surgical repair by suturing or implantation of prosthetic meshes is indicated through a ventral midline laparotomy for ventral diaphragmatic hernias or through a rib resection for dorsal hernias.

Management of Axillary Wounds

Particular problems associated with axillary wounds include severe hemorrhage from large vessels in the area and brachial plexus injury. The wounds often undergo dehiscence after suturing. Horses should be confined until the wound is healed. Subcutaneous emphysema is a common problem with these wounds and is usually resorbed with time. However, some horses develop pneumothorax in the days or weeks following injury. They may develop respiratory distress and require immediate evacuation of pleural air and, in certain cases, continuous suction. Therefore, these horses should be monitored until the wound has healed. They also may develop pneumomediastinum and pneumoperitoneum, which is not clinically significant.

Supplemental Readings

Freeman DE: Standing surgery of the neck and thorax. Vet Clin North Am 7:603–626, 1991.
Jean D, Laverty S, Halley J, Hannigan D, Léveillé R: Thoracic trauma in newborn foals. Proc ACVIM, 1996, page 75.
Laverty S, Lavoie J-P, Pascoe JR, Ducharme N: Penetrating wounds of the thorax in 15 horses. Equine Vet J 28:220–224, 1996.
Speirs VC, Boulton CH: Lower respiratory system. In Auer JA (ed): Equine Surgery. Philadelphia, WB Saunders, 1992, pp 496–506.

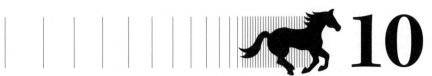

THE URINARY SYSTEM
Edited by Harold C. Schott II

Examination of the Urinary System

ELIZABETH A. CARR
Davis, California

HISTORY AND PHYSICAL EXAMINATION

To begin the evaluation of a horse with urinary tract disease, a complete history should be collected and a thorough physical examination should be performed. Important historical information includes duration and type of clinical signs, number of horses affected, diet, medications administered, and response to treatment. Water intake and urinary output should also be assessed. For example, owners may mistake pollakiuria, frequent urination, for polyuria, increased urine production, and distinction between the two is helpful in forming a diagnostic plan. Pollakiuria is frequently seen in females during estrus or with cystic calculi or cystitis in both sexes. In contrast, polyuria more commonly accompanies renal disease, pituitary adenoma, behavioral problems such as psychogenic water drinking or salt eating, diabetes insipidus, or diabetes mellitus. Astute owners may note increased thirst following exercise or a change in urine appearance, such as a clearer stream, to support polydipsia and polyuria.

Water intake can be determined over a 24-hour period by turning off automatic watering devices and providing a known volume of water to the horse. Water intake may vary widely with environmental conditions, level of activity, and diet so that repeated measurements over several 24-hour periods may be more rewarding in documenting average daily water consumption. Horses stabled in a cool climate and fed a large amount of the diet as a concentrate may drink 15 to 20 L daily, whereas horses exercising in hot climates have been recorded to drink as much as 90 L

daily. Urine output, which should range between 5 and 15 L in a horse with normal renal function, is more difficult to determine. Urine collection harnesses can be applied for 24-hour urine collections; alternately, indwelling Foley catheters attached to a collection apparatus can be used to quantify urine output. Although these methods are fairly well tolerated by horses used for research, they have limited application to the clinical patient.

The most common presenting complaints for horses with urinary tract disease are weight loss and abnormal urination. Other clinical signs vary with the etiology and location of the problem and may include fever, anorexia, depression, ventral edema, oral ulceration, excessive dental tartar, colic, or scalding of the perineum or hind legs. Although lumbar pain and hindlimb lameness have been attributed to urinary tract disease, a musculoskeletal problem is the usual cause of these clinical signs. A decrease in performance may be an early presenting complaint for renal disease, but poor performance is more likely a result of the mild anemia and lethargy that accompany uremia rather than a consequence of renal pain.

In addition to a thorough physical examination, rectal palpation should be included in the evaluation of all horses with suspected urinary tract disease. The bladder should be palpated to determine size, wall thickness, and presence of cystic calculi or mural masses. If the bladder is full, palpation should be performed again following bladder catheterization or voiding. The caudal pole of the left kidney can be palpated for size and texture. The ureters are generally not palpable unless enlarged or obstructed by disease, but the retroperitoneal course of the ureters in the dorsal abdomen and the trigone should be palpated to determine if ureters can be detected. In mares, palpation of the distal ureters through the vaginal wall may be more rewarding. Dilation of a ureter may occur with pyelonephritis or ureteral calculi. The reproductive tract should also be palpated to assess whether a reproductive problem could be a possible cause of the clinical signs.

HEMATOLOGY AND SERUM BIOCHEMISTRY

Results of a complete blood count revealing an elevated white blood cell count and elevated total protein or fibrinogen concentration support an inflammatory or infectious disease process. Mild anemia, indicated by a packed cell volume of 20 to 30%, consequent to decreased erythropoietin production and a shortened red blood cell lifespan, may be found in horses with chronic renal failure.

Blood urea nitrogen (BUN) and serum creatinine concentrations are the most commonly utilized indices of renal function, specifically glomerular filtration rate (GFR). It is important to remember that increases in BUN and creatinine do not occur until the majority of nephrons, generally about 75%, become nonfunctional. For example, complete loss of function of one kidney does not result in increases in BUN or creatinine as long as contralateral renal function remains normal. Thus, these parameters are not very useful in evaluating early or minor changes in GFR. Once elevated, however, small increases in BUN and creatinine are more sensitive indicators of further deterioration in GFR because a doubling of BUN or creatinine can be interpreted as a 50% decline in remaining renal function.

Azotemia may also be pre- or postrenal in origin. Pre-renal azotemia is a result of decreased renal perfusion; postrenal azotemia is a result of obstruction of the urinary tract. Thus, interpretation of serum chemistry test results should be made in light of hydration status of the patient and other presenting signs. Although specific threshold values for BUN and creatinine that differentiate renal disease from pre-renal azotemia do not exist, measures of urine concentration (see later) or the urine-to-serum creatinine ratio can provide useful information. Urine-to-serum creatinine ratios in excess of 50:1 (reflecting concentrated urine) are expected in horses with pre-renal azotemia, whereas ratios less than 37:1 were reported in a group of horses determined to have primary renal disease. Creatinine is a charged molecule that is less membrane-permeable than urea; therefore, acute changes in renal function are more accurately reflected by changes in creatinine than in BUN, and the increase in creatinine is proportionately greater than the rise in BUN. This has led to use of the BUN-to-creatinine ratio to differentiate pre-renal azotemia or acute renal failure from chronic renal failure. With acute renal compromise, a BUN-to-creatinine ratio of less than 10:1 is expected, whereas the ratio should exceed 15:1 in cases of chronic renal failure. Although the BUN-to-creatinine ratio may be useful to consider, the values are not always reliable, especially with chronic renal failure in which BUN may vary considerably with dietary protein intake.

In addition to BUN and creatinine, serum electrolyte, protein (albumin and globulin) and glucose concentrations, and muscle enzyme activities should be included in the laboratory data base. Hypochloremia is the most consistent electrolyte abnormality seen in horses with polyuric renal failure. Hyponatremia has been variably reported in horses with renal disease and is most commonly found with urinary tract disruption and uroperitoneum. Serum potassium concentration is usually normal but may be elevated in cases of acute renal failure or uroperitoneum. Calcium and phosphorus concentrations vary in horses with renal disease. Hypercalcemia and hypophosphatemia are often found in horses with chronic renal failure, especially when fed alfalfa hay, whereas hypocalcemia and hyperphosphatemia are more common with acute renal failure. With protein-losing glomerulopathies, albumin tends to be lost to a greater extent than globulin, owing to the former's lower molecular weight. Although low total protein and albumin concentrations can be found accompanying chronic renal disease in many species, horses appear more refractory to development of hypoproteinemia and the nephrotic syndrome. In fact, some patients have an increase in globulin concentration that suggests chronic antigenic stimulation associated with glomerulonephritis, pyelonephritis, neoplasia, or amyloidosis. Hyperglycemia (blood glucose >175–200 mg/dl) resulting from stress, exercise, sepsis, pituitary adenoma, or diabetes mellitus may result in glucosuria. In cases for which pigmenturia is a complaint, muscle enzyme activities are helpful in differentiating myoglobinuria from hematuria or hemoglobinuria.

URINALYSIS

Urinalysis should be performed in all horses suspected of having urinary tract disease. Urine can be collected midstream during voiding, by urethral catheterization, or by cystocentesis in foals. Color, clarity, odor, viscosity, and specific gravity should be evaluated at the time of collection. Normal equine urine is pale yellow to deep tan in color and is often turbid owing to large amounts of calcium carbonate crystals and mucus. It is not uncommon for urine appearance to change during urination, especially toward the end of micturition when more crystals tend to be voided. If pigmenturia or hematuria is present, noting the timing and duration of discolored urine passage may be helpful in localizing the source. Pigmenturia throughout urination is most consistent with myonecrosis or a bladder or kidney lesion, whereas passage of discolored urine at the start or end of urination is more commonly seen with lesions of the urethra or accessory sex glands.

Urine specific gravity is a measure of the number of particles in urine, and is a useful estimate of urine concentration. In response to water deprivation, a horse with normal renal function should be able to produce concentrated urine with a specific gravity between 1.025 and 1.050. In contrast, foals typically have urine that is more dilute than serum (i.e., hyposthenuria or a specific gravity <1.008) consequent to a high-volume milk diet. Although the constant polyuria decreases their ability to generate a large osmotic gradient in the medullary interstitium, foals can produce urine with a specific gravity higher than 1.030 when dehydrated. With renal disease, the ability to produce either concentrated (specific gravity >1.025) or dilute (specific gravity <1.008) urine is lost. Thus, horses with chronic renal failure typically manifest isosthenuria, which is production of urine that has an osmolality similar to that of serum (specific gravity of 1.008–1.014).

In horses presented with dehydration or shock resulting from a number of problems, urine specific gravity is helpful in differentiating pre-renal from renal azotemia. A high urine specific gravity (>1.035) supports pre-renal azotemia, whereas failure to concentrate urine in the face of dehydration supports a diagnosis of renal disease. It should be emphasized that specific gravity measurement is most valid in the first urine sample voided after fluid therapy is initiated, because successful fluid therapy leads to production of dilute urine. Other disorders that may result in a decreased ability to concentrate urine in the face of dehydration include pituitary or hypothalamic diseases leading to central diabetes insipidus, septicemia or endotoxemia, washout of the medullary interstitium, or nephrogenic diabetes insipidus.

The pH of equine urine is usually alkaline (7.5–9.0). High-intensity exercise or bacteriuria can result in acidic pH. The latter can further result in an ammonia odor to the sample owing to breakdown of urea by bacteria with urease activity. Production of more dilute urine generally results in a decrease in urine pH toward the neutral value. Commercially available urine reagent strips can yield false-positive results for protein when alkaline samples are tested. Thus, proteinuria is better assessed by performing the semiquantitative sulfosalicylic acid precipitation test or by specific quantification with a colorimetric assay, as for cerebrospinal fluid, and by comparing the result with urine creatinine concentration in the form of a urine protein-to-creatinine ratio. Although not well documented in horses, a value above 1.0, which is the threshold value for proteinuria used in small animal patients, appears appropriate for use in horses at this time.

Proteinuria may occur with glomerular disease, bacteriuria, or pyuria, or transiently following exercise. Normal equine urine should not contain glucose. Glucosuria may accompany hyperglycemia associated with the causes described earlier or with administration of dextrose-containing fluids or parenteral nutrition products. In addition, glucosuria may accompany sedation with α_2-agonists or exogenous corticosteroid administration. When glucosuria is detected in the absence of hyperglycemia, primary tubular dysfunction should be suspected. A positive result for blood on a urine reagent strip can result from the presence of hemoglobin, myoglobin, or intact red blood cells in the urine sample. Evaluation of serum for hemolysis and of urine sediment for red blood cells (RBCs), combined with an ammonium sulfate precipitation test to detect myoglobin, can be rewarding in differentiating between these pigments.

Urine sediment should be evaluated for cells, casts, and bacteria within 30 to 60 minutes after collection. Fewer than 5 RBCs per high-power field (hpf) can be seen in an atraumatically collected urine sample. Increases in the number of urinary RBCs/hpf can result from inflammation, infection, toxemia, neoplasia, or exercise. Pyuria (>5 white blood cells/hpf) is seen most commonly with infectious or inflammatory disorders. Casts are molds of protein and cells that form in tubular lumens and subsequently pass into the bladder. They are rare in normal equine urine but may be found with inflammatory or infectious processes. Casts are relatively unstable in alkaline urine; thus, evaluation of urine sediment should be performed as soon as possible after collection to ensure accurate assessment. Normal equine urine should have few to no bacteria. The absence of bacteria on sediment evaluation does not rule out their presence, however, and bacterial culture of urine collected by catheterization or cystocentesis, in foals, should be performed in suspected cases of pyelonephritis or cystitis.

Equine urine is rich in crystals. The majority of these are calcium carbonate crystals of variable size, but triple phosphate crystals and an occasional calcium oxalate crystal can also be seen in normal equine urine. In some samples, addition of a few drops of a 10% acetic acid solution may be necessary to dissolve crystals for accurate assessment of urine sediment.

Gamma glutamyl transferase (GGT) is an enzyme located in the brush border of epithelial cells lining renal tubules. The presence of GGT activity in urine arises from proximal renal tubular cell turnover, and the activity increases with renal tubular damage and sloughing of epithelium into the tubular lumen. Values for urine GGT activity are expressed as a ratio to urine creatinine concentration, with a value higher than 25 considered abnormal.

$$\frac{\text{urinary GGT activity}}{(\text{uCr} \times 0.01)}$$

Use of this ratio in equine urine appears to be a sensitive indicator of tubular damage and has been advocated for use as an early indicator of tubular damage, as well as an aid for monitoring horses on nephrotoxic drug therapy. Unfortunately, elevated urine GGT-to-creatinine ratios can be found with dehydration and after the initial dose or two of nephrotoxic medications. Thus, although results may reflect renal tubular damage, in practical situations the ratio has been deemed too sensitive and currently is not used as much as when the test was originally described.

FRACTIONAL CLEARANCE OF ELECTROLYTES

Fractional clearance of electrolytes is used to evaluate the secretory or reabsorptive function of renal tubules. Fractional clearances are expressed as a percentage of endogenous creatinine clearance:

$$\text{Fractional clearance A} = \frac{[\text{urine A}] \times [\text{plasma creatinine}]}{[\text{plasma A}] \times [\text{urine creatinine}]} \times 100$$

The equine kidneys function to reabsorb more than 99% of filtered sodium, whereas little potassium is conserved. Thus, normal fractional clearance values are less than 1% for sodium and 15 to 65% for potassium (Table 1). Increases in fractional clearance values, specifically for sodium and phosphorus, are early indicators of renal tubular damage. However, fractional sodium clearance can be artifactually increased in horses receiving intravenous polyionic solutions.

TABLE 1. FRACTIONAL CLEARANCES OF ELECTROLYTES IN HORSES

Electrolyte	Normal Ranges
Na^+	0.02–1.00
Cl^-	0.04–1.60
K^+	15–65[a]
PO_4^-	0.00–0.50[b]
Ca^{++}	0.00–6.72[c]

[a]Fractional clearance of K^+ may exceed upper limit on high K^+ diets.
[b]Fractional clearance of PO_4^- exceeding 4% suggests excessive intake.
[c]Fractional clearance of Ca^{++} should exceed 2.5% with adequate intake.

WATER DEPRIVATION

Water deprivation is a simple test used to determine whether hyposthenuric polyuria is due to a behavioral problem such as psychogenic polydipsia or the result of central or nephrogenic diabetes insipidus. A water deprivation test should not be performed in an animal that is clinically dehydrated or azotemic. A baseline urinalysis, from a sample collected by catheterization to empty the bladder at the start of the test, and measurement of serum BUN and creatinine concentrations and body weight should be performed before removal of food and water. Urine specific gravity and weight loss are measured after 12 hours, usually overnight, and 24 hours. The test should be stopped when urine specific gravity reaches 1.025 or greater, there is a loss of 5% of body weight, or evidence of dehydration becomes apparent. With long-standing psychogenic polydipsia, affected horses may not be able to fully concentrate urine owing to washout of the medullary interstitial osmotic gradient. It is of little benefit to extend the test period beyond 24 hours in such patients. However, affected horses should respond to water deprivation more favorably, by producing urine with a higher specific gravity, after a period of partial water deprivation during which daily water intake is restricted to 40 ml/kg for several days. This should allow time for restoration of the medullary interstitial osmotic gradient. Horses with central or nephrogenic diabetes insipidus cannot concentrate urine in response to a water deprivation test. When these problems are suspected, patients should be monitored every 4 to 6 hours because significant dehydration may ensue within 6 hours of water deprivation.

ENDOSCOPY

Endoscopy of the urinary tract is a useful diagnostic aid in patients presenting with abnormal urination. In addition, it can be used to determine whether a patient has two functional kidneys when one kidney cannot be imaged during ultrasonographic examination. A flexible endoscope with an outside diameter of 12 mm or less and a minimal length of 1 m is adequate for examination of the urethra and bladder of an adult horse of either sex. Cold sterilization of the endoscope should be performed before endoscopy of the lower urinary tract. Tranquilization of the patient is recommended, and the distal end of the penis or the vulva should be thoroughly cleansed. The endoscope is passed in a manner identical to that for a catheter, with the air control intermittently used to inflate the urethra or bladder. Normal urethral mucosa is pale pink with longitudinal folds. When dilated with air, the mucosa flattens and may appear more red than normal, and a prominent vascular pattern may be apparent. Passage of a catheter before endoscopy for sample collection or to empty the bladder can result in mild irritation and erythema of the urethral mucosa. These should not be interpreted as abnormal findings. The regions of the ischial arch where the urethra begins to widen into the ampullar portion, and of the colliculus seminalis in the roof of the pelvic urethra just distal to the urethral sphincter, should be closely examined because these are common sites of posturination or postbreeding hemorrhage in the gelding or stallion. Subsequent passage of the endoscope through the urethral sphincter coupled with air distension allows evaluation of the bladder for presence of calculi, inflammation, or masses. Viewing the ureteral openings in the dorsal aspect of the trigone can help determine the source of hematuria or pyuria. A small volume of urine should pass from each ureteral opening asynchronously, approximately once each minute. Ureteral catheterization to obtain urine samples from each kidney can be performed by passing a sterile polyethylene catheter via the biopsy channel of the endoscope. In addition, biopsy of masses in the bladder or urethra can be performed.

ULTRASONOGRAPHY, RADIOGRAPHY, AND NUCLEAR SCINTIGRAPHY

Ultrasonographic examination of the urinary tract can be performed transrectally or transabdominally. Imaging the bladder is best performed transrectally using a 5 MHz probe. It is important to remember the character of equine urine while imaging the bladder because it is an inhomogeneous, echogenic fluid due to the presence of mucus and crystals. Presence of a cystic calculus can be confirmed, because calculi have a highly echogenic surface and produce an acoustic shadow. Similarly, masses in the bladder wall may be both imaged and palpated during the examination.

The right kidney is triangular or horseshoe-shaped and is best imaged transabdominally via the dorsolateral extent of the last two to three intercostal spaces. The left kidney is bean-shaped and lies deep to the spleen in the left paralumbar fossa. Because the left kidney is deeper than the right kidney, it can be difficult to image completely, and it is best examined with a 2.5 or 3 MHz probe. The size and shape of both kidneys, architecture, and echogenecity of the parenchyma should be assessed. In acute renal failure, the kidneys are normal to increased in size; however, the corticomedullary junction may be indistinct. Chronic renal failure may result in kidneys that are smaller and more echogenic than normal. Cystic or mineralized areas within renal parenchyma may be associated with chronic renal disease or congenital anomalies. Calculi within the renal pelvis generally cast an acoustic shadow and can result in hydronephrosis of the affected kidney. Occasionally, one or both kidneys cannot be imaged owing to presence of gas-filled bowel between kidney and abdominal wall. Re-examination at a later time is generally required for successful imaging in such cases.

Radiography is rarely used in evaluation of urinary tract disease in the horse. Diagnostic radiographs of the urinary tract usually can only be obtained in foals or miniature horses. Excretory urography is useful if the clinician suspects a nonfunctional kidney or seeks to identify hypoplastic kidneys or ectopic ureters. The procedure is infrequently used and requires general anesthesia. Retrograde contrast studies can be used in foals suspected of having a ruptured bladder. The technique may also assist in identifying strictures or masses in the urethra or bladder; however, endoscopy is a more useful tool for diagnosing these problems.

Nuclear scintigraphic imaging can be used to assess renal anatomy and to provide a qualitative assessment of renal function. Indications for renal scintigraphy are to document the presence of a functional kidney when multiple ultrasonographic examinations have been complicated by interfering bowel or when unilateral nephrectomy is being considered. The former question may be more easily answered by observation of urine flow from the ureteral openings during cystoscopy. Renal scintigraphic studies have used technetium 99m (^{99m}Tc) tagged to the radiopharmaceutical's glucoheptanate (GH), which is taken up by the proximal tubular epithelial cells to provide anatomic detail, or diethylenetriaminopentaacetic acid (DTPA), which is similar to inulin in that it is neither secreted nor reabsorbed after filtration and provides qualitative functional information. The radiopharmaceutical ^{99m}Tc-DTPA may also be used to measure GFR without use of an external gamma camera. The procedure requires intravenous injection of the radiopharmaceutical followed by collection of multiple blood samples over time to produce an elimination curve.

RENAL BIOPSY

Renal biopsy can be useful in determining the region of the nephron affected, the type of lesion, and the chronicity and severity of disease. Although a relatively safe procedure when performed with ultrasonographic guidance, it has inherent risks, including subcapsular hemorrhage and hematuria and, less commonly, penetration of bowel. With the horse sedated and restrained in a stocks, penetration of the needle* into the renal parenchyma can be imaged ultrasonographically by triangulating the ultrasound beam with the biopsy instrument and the kidney. As an alternative, the site and depth of the biopsy can be determined by ultrasonographic imaging immediately before the biopsy. The tissue collected should be placed in formalin for histopathologic evaluation. If desired, additional samples can be collected for bacterial culture and for immunofluorescent testing, which requires tissue storage in Michel's medium.

Although renal biopsy results should, in theory, provide useful information to characterize the renal disease, they more often document the presence of chronic disease for

which the inciting cause cannot be detected unless it can be associated with a historic event or if immunofluorescent testing is pursued. This limitation can be attributed to the fact that 75% or more of nephron function is typically lost before onset of clinical signs. Pathologic lesions are widespread at this point, and involvement of all nephron segments as well as the interstitium leads to an interpretation of end-stage kidney disease. In the occasional case, the results may aid in separating infectious (pyelonephritis) or congenital (renal dysplasia) from nonspecific causes of renal failure. Although such results would assist in the therapeutic approach to these patients, the limitations and risks of renal biopsy should be considered before performing this diagnostic technique in horses with chronic renal failure.

MEASUREMENT OF GLOMERULAR FILTRATION RATE

Glomerular filtration rate is a measure of functional renal mass. Reductions in GFR can occur with primary renal disease, decreased renal perfusion, or obstructive renal disease. Several diagnostic tests are available for estimation of GFR. As already mentioned, serum BUN and creatinine concentrations begin to increase when approximately 75% of functional renal mass becomes compromised. Other more sensitive measures of changes in GFR include endogenous and exogenous creatinine clearances, inulin clearance, sodium sulfanilate clearance, and ^{99m}Tc-DTPA clearance. Performance of these tests requires timed urine collections, repeated blood sampling, and specialized laboratory assays. Thus, these tests have limited clinical use and are primarily used as research tools.

URETHRAL PRESSURE PROFILES

Cystometrography and urethral pressure profiles are used to evaluate detrusor and urethral muscle function. Both techniques involve measurement of intraluminal pressure during inflation of the bladder or urethra through a catheter. These techniques have been useful for diagnosis of myogenic and neurogenic disorders of the bladder and urethra in dogs and humans. The technique has been performed experimentally in normal female horses and ponies, but there is little information about use of these techniques in clinical cases.

Supplemental Readings

Grossman BS, Brobst DF, Kramer JW, Bayly WM, Reed SM: Urinary indices for differentiation of prerenal azotemia and renal azotemia in horses. J Am Vet Med Assoc 180:284–288, 1982.
Kohn CW, Chew DJ: Laboratory diagnosis and characterization of renal disease in horses. Vet Clin North Am Equine Pract 3:585–615, 1987.
Matthews HK, Andrews FM, Daniel GB, Jacobs WR: Measuring renal function in horses. Vet Med 88:349, 1993.
Sullins KE, Traub-Dargatz JL: Endoscopic anatomy of the equine urinary tract. Comp Cont Ed Pract Vet 6(11):S663–S668, 1984.
Traub-Dargatz JL, McKinnon AO: Adjunctive methods of examination of the urogenital tract. Vet Clin North Am Equine Pract 4(3):339–358, 1988.

*Tru-cut biopsy needle, Baxter Healthcare Co., Deerfield, IL.

Acute Renal Failure

RAYMOND J. GEOR
Guelph, Ontario

Acute renal failure (ARF) can be defined as an abrupt and sustained decrease in glomerular filtration rate resulting in azotemia and disturbances in fluid, electrolyte, and acid-base homeostasis. Acute renal failure may occur because of decreased renal perfusion (pre-renal failure), primary renal dysfunction (intrinsic failure), or obstruction of urine flow (post-renal failure). In horses, ARF is usually pre-renal or renal in origin and is most commonly the result of hemodynamic or nephrotoxic insults. With the exception of bladder rupture in the neonate (see page 494), post-renal failure is rare. Identification and correction of the cause of ARF is important because renal dysfunction is frequently reversible in the early stages of failure, whereas established ARF often requires extensive supportive care and carries a guarded prognosis. By identifying patients at increased risk and attempting to interrupt the cycle of events leading to ARF, it may be possible to reduce the incidence of this condition.

ETIOLOGY

The most common cause of reversible increases in blood urea nitrogen (BUN) and creatinine concentrations is pre-renal failure associated with conditions that result in a decrease in cardiac output or an increase in renal vascular resistance, or both (Table 1). For example, the hemodynamic changes accompanying acute enterocolitis, severe colic, acute blood loss, or prolonged exercise lead to reductions in renal blood flow (RBF), glomerular filtration rate (GFR), and urine output. These changes may lead to azotemia and retention of water and electrolytes. If the decrements in RBF and GFR are severe and prolonged, ischemic injury to the renal tubules and interstitium may occur, resulting in intrinsic renal dysfunction.

Acute tubular necrosis, consequent to ischemia or nephrotoxin exposure, is the most common cause of intrin-sic renal failure in horses. Important nephrotoxins include aminoglycoside antibiotics and nonsteroidal anti-inflammatory drugs (NSAIDs). Less commonly, acute tubular necrosis may develop consequent to exposure to endogenous pigments (myoglobin or hemoglobin), heavy metals (mercury-containing counterirritants), or vitamin D or K_3 (Table 2). Acute immune-mediated glomerulonephritis, interstitial nephritis associated with embolic or ascending renal infections, or renal microvascular injury (hemolytic uremic-like syndrome) are other causes of intrinsic renal failure.

Use of aminoglycoside antibiotics, particularly gentamicin, may lead to development of acute tubular necrosis in horses. Toxicity is the result of damage to proximal tubular epithelial cells, mediated through impaired cell organelle function (see page 476). Administration of other potentially nephrotoxic drugs (NSAIDs) or furosemide, which may exacerbate hypovolemia, can increase the risk of aminoglycoside nephrotoxicity. Although NSAIDs are more likely to damage the gastrointestinal tract than the kidneys, ARF has been reported as a complication of administering either high doses of phenylbutazone (4–8 g/day) or routine doses to dehydrated patients (see page 724).

Myoglobinuria and hemoglobinuria have both been associated with development of ARF in the horse (pigment nephropathy). Myoglobinuric nephrosis can occur as a result of exertional rhabdomyolysis, heat stroke, or extensive crush injuries. Causes of intravascular hemolysis and hemoglobinuria include incompatible blood transfusion, immune-mediated hemolytic anemia, fulminant hepatic failure, and toxicosis from ingestion of onions (*Allium* species) or withered red maple leaves (*Acer rubrum*). Although the mechanism of pigment-induced renal injury remains incompletely understood, increased hydroxyl radical formation, a reaction catalyzed by ferrous iron compounds, and tubular obstruction by casts of heme proteins, are likely to be contributing factors. Concurrent hypovolemia usually potentiates the development of acute tubular necrosis and acute renal failure.

TABLE 1. PRERENAL CAUSES OF ACUTE RENAL FAILURE

I. Decreased cardiac output
   A. Congestive heart failure
   B. Pericardial disease (tamponade)
II. Hypovolemia
   A. Gastrointestinal losses (enterocolitis)
   B. Acute blood loss
   C. Exercise-associated sweat losses
III. Volume redistribution (decrease in effective blood volume)
   A. Pleural or peritoneal effusion
   B. Rhabdomyolysis and muscle swelling
   C. Hypoalbuminemia
IV. Altered vascular resistance
   A. Sepsis and endotoxemia

PATHOPHYSIOLOGY

The kidneys are particularly susceptible to ischemic and toxic injury because of their unique anatomic and physiologic features. Although the kidneys receive approximately 20% of the cardiac output, only about 10 to 20% of total RBF reaches the medulla via the vasa recta. This low medullary blood flow is necessary for a functional countercurrent mechanism, but creates a large corticomedullary oxygen gradient and renders the renal medulla relatively hypoxic and highly susceptible to ischemic injury. Conversely, the renal cortex receives 80 to 90% of total RBF and is particularly susceptible to toxicant exposure. Nephrotoxins that are either secreted or reabsorbed by

TABLE 2.   CAUSES OF ACUTE RENAL FAILURE DUE TO PARENCHYMAL KIDNEY DISEASE

I. Acute tubular necrosis
  A. Nephrotoxins
    1. Antibiotic agents (aminoglycosides, tetracyclines, polymixin B, sulfonamides, cephalosporins)
    2. Heavy metals (mercury, arsenic, gold, lead)
    3. Endogenous substances (myoglobin, hemoglobin)
    4. Miscellaneous (nonsteroidal anti-inflammatory drugs [NSAIDs], vitamin D, vitamin K_3-menadione sodium bisulfite, cantharidin, acorns)
  B. Ischemia
    1. Hypovolemia
    2. Sepsis
    3. Endotoxemia
    4. Hemorrhage/blood loss
    5. Renal infarction
    6. NSAID administration
II. Abnormalities of hemostasis
  A. Renal thrombosis
  B. Vasculitis (purpura hemorrhagica)
  C. Hemolytic-uremic syndrome
III. Abnormalities of the glomeruli
  A. Immune-mediated glomerulonephritis (equine infectious anemia)
  B. Postinfectious glomerulonephritis (*Streptococcus equi*, *Leptospirosis pomona*, herpes virus)
IV. Acute interstitial nephritis
  A. Infection-related (gram-negative sepsis, acute pyelonephritis)
  B. Drug-related (NSAID toxicity)

proximal tubular epithelial cells such as aminoglycoside antibiotics may accumulate in large concentrations in these cells and lead to cellular dysfunction or necrosis.

Acute renal failure is described as having three distinct phases: (1) induction, (2) maintenance, and (3) recovery. The induction phase lasts from onset of the renal insult by decreased perfusion or nephrotoxin exposure to development of decreased urinary concentrating ability and azotemia. Prompt therapeutic intervention during the induction phase, particularly for hemodynamically mediated ARF, has the greatest potential to prevent significant renal damage. The maintenance phase develops when 65 to 75% of nephrons have been damaged, resulting in a sustained decrease in GFR and tubular function. The recovery phase of ARF is associated with resolution of azotemia and a return of concentrating ability. In addition to repair of some of the damaged nephrons during the recovery phase, remaining functional nephrons often hypertrophy to compensate for the reduction in nephron numbers.

CLINICAL SIGNS

In the majority of horses with ARF, clinical signs are usually referable to the primary problem, such as acute colic or enterocolitis, rather than to renal dysfunction. In general, the clinical manifestations of ARF reflect the systemic effects of toxic substances usually excreted in the urine (uremia); urinary tract dysfunction; and derangements of fluid, electrolyte, and acid-base balance. The predominant clinical signs of uremia in horses are depression and anorexia. Signs of encephalopathy may occur in horses with severe azotemia.

Although oliguria is considered to be the hallmark of ARF, urine production in horses with ARF is variable. Oliguria frequently occurs in the early stages of hemodynamically mediated ARF, but anuria is rare. Nonoliguric ARF or polyuric ARF may also occur with exposure to nephrotoxins, and polyuria is common during the recovery phase of ARF. The magnitude of azotemia tends to be lower in nonoliguric ARF than oliguric ARF, possibly indicating less severe injury in nonoliguric ARF. Similarly, nonoliguric ARF is associated with a more favorable prognosis compared with oliguric ARF. In the clinical situation, affected patients are initially treated with large volumes of intravenous fluids for the primary disease such as enterocolitis or colic, and oliguria progresses to polyuria. When significant renal damage has been sustained, persistence of oliguric ARF is usually recognized by failure to produce a significant volume of urine in response to fluid therapy, along with minimal change in the degree of azotemia over the initial day of treatment. If these patients are not carefully monitored, fluid retention may lead to development of subcutaneous and pulmonary edema. Soft feces due to fluid retention may also be observed in patients with oliguric ARF.

Other clinical signs can include dehydration, tachycardia, hyperemic mucous membranes, pyrexia, mild colic, and laminitis. Transrectal palpation may indicate enlargement of the left kidney; however, this assessment is subjective, and normal kidney size does not rule out ARF. Horses with oliguric renal failure can have perirenal edema that may be detected via palpation per rectum or ultrasonographic examination.

DIAGNOSIS

Diagnosis of ARF in horses is based on history, clinical signs, and results of urinalysis and serum biochemical analyses. Increases in BUN and creatinine concentrations are frequently the initial findings that suggest compromised renal function. If azotemia is identified in horses with conditions such as enterocolitis, severe colic, or acute blood loss, it is important to differentiate whether azotemia is predominantly attributable to pre-renal failure or intrinsic renal damage. With pre-renal failure, volume repletion restores renal function, and the magnitude of azotemia should decrease by 50% or more during the initial day of treatment. In contrast, with intrinsic renal failure, fluid therapy usually does not lead to prompt resolution of azotemia. Assessment of urine specific gravity before initiation of fluid therapy is helpful in differentiating pre-renal from renal failure. Because normally functioning kidneys maximally conserve salt and water in response to a transient decrease in RBF, urine specific gravity is typically greater than 1.035 (and may reach 1.050–1.060) with pre-renal failure, whereas urine produced by horses with intrinsic ARF is often dilute (specific gravity <1.020) due to compromised concentrating ability. Additional measures that can be used to differentiate pre-renal failure from intrinsic ARF include fractional sodium clearance (see page 469) and the ratios of urine to serum creatinine and urine to serum osmolality. Intrinsic ARF can be inferred if: (1) the fractional sodium clearance is greater than 1.0%; (2) the ratio of urine creatinine to serum creatinine is less than 37 (normal >50); or (3) the ratio of urine osmolality to serum osmolality is less than 1.7 (normal >2.5). One problem with these laboratory assessments is that they are affected by fluid therapy. Thus, application is limited to use on urine samples collected before initiation of fluid therapy or the first urine sample voided after fluid therapy has been started.

In the clinical situation, assessment of the response to fluid therapy is the most practical way to differentiate pre-renal failure from intrinsic renal failure. Azotemia caused by pre-renal failure should resolve quickly with replacement of fluid deficits and restoration of renal perfusion. Although pre-renal failure and intrinsic ARF are often described as two separate entities, the distinction between the two is probably less clear, and it is likely that some renal damage occurs in horses with pre-renal failure. However, because of the considerable renal reserve capacity, renal damage associated with most conditions resulting in transient renal hypoperfusion rarely affects case progression or outcome.

Electrolyte Anomalies

The most common electrolyte abnormalities in horses with ARF, particularly those with polyuric renal failure, are mild hyponatremia and hypochloremia. Serum potassium concentrations are variable; horses with oliguric or anuric ARF may be hyperkalemic, whereas those with polyuric ARF, particularly anorectic patients, may be normokalemic or hypokalemic. With post-renal failure, especially when complicated by uroperitoneum, hyponatremia and hypochloremia are usually more severe and hyperkalemia is commonly found. Hypocalcemia and hyperphosphatemia may be additional findings with ARF. Affected horses often have a degree of metabolic acidosis, especially when ARF is associated with primary problems such as enterocolitis or severe colic.

Urinalysis

As described earlier, measures of urinary concentrating ability (specific gravity or osmolality) are helpful in assessing development of intrinsic renal failure. Other abnormal urinalysis results can be sensitive indicators of renal damage. This is especially true for changes in urine sediment such as increased numbers of erythrocytes and leukocytes or presence of casts. Proteinuria and glucosuria may be additional findings with glomerular or tubular damage. Enzymuria, specifically the ratio of urinary gamma glutamyl transferase (GGT) activity to urinary creatinine (uCr) concentration (see page 469), has been touted to be a sensitive indicator of renal tubular damage. As GGT is too large to be filtered by the normal glomerulus and is present in large amounts in the brush border of proximal tubular epithelial cells, a urinary GGT/(uCr × 0.01) value greater than 25 has been considered to be indicative of renal tubular disease. Measurement of urinary GGT activity has been advocated for early detection of aminoglycoside-induced renal disease (see page 476). However, this ratio may be falsely elevated in sick horses through a decrease in creatinine excretion consequent to a reduction of GFR.

Other Tests

Renal ultrasonography using a 3- or 5-MHz sector probe can provide useful information regarding renal size and structure. Other abnormalities such as perirenal edema, cystic cavities, or calculi may be demonstrated by ultrasonographic examination. Percutaneous biopsy of the kidneys is possible in the standing horse, but the technique is not without complications including perirenal hematoma formation, hematuria, and hemoperitoneum, and should be reserved for cases in which microscopic examination of renal tissue is necessary for prognostic information. Identification of a renal mass or other abnormality of renal structure on ultrasonographic examination is an indication for renal biopsy. Ultrasonographic guidance and use of a spring-loaded biopsy instrument* may lessen the risk of complications.

TREATMENT

The approach to therapy is similar regardless of whether ARF is due to ischemic or nephrotoxic renal injury. Initial treatment includes administration of intravenous fluids to improve renal perfusion, correct metabolic disturbances, and induce diuresis. In horses with pre-renal failure that are at high risk for development of intrinsic ARF, the goal is to prevent or interrupt the pathophysiologic events leading to development of intrinsic renal damage. The primary disease process resulting in pre-renal failure must also be identified and appropriately treated.

Ideally, administration of nephrotoxic drugs should be discontinued. However, in situations when continued administration of aminoglycoside antibiotics or NSAIDs is necessary, alterations in dosing regimens may lessen the risk of renal injury. With regard to the aminoglycosides, monitoring serum drug concentrations allows the clinician to individualize dosage regimes. For example, the risk of nephrotoxicity with aminoglycosides increases when trough concentrations remain higher than 2 μg/ml for gentamicin or higher than 5 μg/ml for amikacin. Serum trough concentrations can be reduced below these values by increasing the dosage interval. Alternatively, the nephrotoxic effects of the aminoglycosides may be minimized by once-daily dosing (see page 476).

Fluid Administration

Blood samples for biochemical and acid-base analyses should be submitted before initiation of therapy. In addition, packed cell volume, plasma total solids, and body weight should be determined. Although frequently overlooked, daily recording of body weight is perhaps the best measure of fluid balance in horses with fluid losses and renal dysfunction. Deficit fluid requirements should be replaced over the first 6 to 12 hours of treatment. Physiologic saline (0.9% NaCl solution) is the fluid of choice unless hypernatremia is present, in which case a 0.45% NaCl/2.5% dextrose solution should be used. The amount of fluid required can be calculated by multiplying the estimated dehydration (%) by body weight (kg). For exam-

---

Temno Soft Tissue Biopsy Needle, ProAct Limited, State College, PA

ple, a 500-kg horse that is 8% dehydrated requires 40 L $(0.08 \times 500 = 40)$. In horses with pre-renal failure, RBF, GFR, and urine output should return to normal after correction of the fluid deficit. Although the majority of horses with some degree of intrinsic ARF increase urine production in response to fluid therapy, a few patients may remain oliguric after correction of fluid deficits, and these horses must be closely monitored for signs of overhydration. Ideally, central venous pressure, for which normal values are less than 8 cm H_2O, is monitored in patients with oliguric ARF. However, daily measurement of body weight, packed cell volume, and plasma total solids; auscultation of the lungs for sounds consistent with pulmonary edema; and observation for the development of dependent edema are more practical means to assess hydration state.

With the exception of horses with severe oliguric ARF or post-renal failure, serum potassium concentration is usually within normal limits, and specific therapy intended to lower serum potassium concentration is not required. However, in select cases, recognition and treatment of hyperkalemia is essential because increases in serum potassium concentrations to 6.5 to 7.0 mEq/L have the potential to induce cardiac arrhythmias including bradycardia, atrial standstill, and ventricular tachycardia. Moderate hyperkalemia usually resolves in response to administration of potassium-free fluids and improved urine flow. Horses with severe hyperkalemia (>7.0 mEq/L) and cardiac arrhythmias should be treated with agents such as sodium bicarbonate (1–2 mEq/kg IV over 5–15 minutes) or calcium gluconate (0.5 ml/kg of a 10% solution by slow IV injection) that decrease serum potassium concentration or counteract the effects of hyperkalemia on cardiac conduction, respectively.

Diuretics and Vasodilators

If oliguria persists after rehydration, treatment with diuretics or vasodilators may be attempted. Mannitol (0.25–1.0 g/kg as a 20% solution administered IV over 15 to 20 minutes), furosemide (1.0–2.0 mg/kg IV q.i.d.), or dopamine (3–5 μg/kg per minute IV, in a 5% dextrose solution) have been advocated for treatment of oliguric ARF. As an osmotic diuretic, mannitol decreases cell swelling, increases tubular flow, and helps to prevent tubular obstruction or collapse. Mannitol may also improve RBF and GFR by vasodilatory effects, which are mediated via prostaglandin synthesis or by inducing release of atrial natriuretic peptide. The use of an osmotic diuretic agent is contraindicated in an overhydrated patient because the associated increase in intravascular volume may precipitate pulmonary edema. Furosemide is a potent diuretic agent that acts by blocking the $Na^+/K^+/2Cl^-$ cotransporter in the ascending limb of the loop of Henle. However, furosemide must be filtered at the glomerulus to exert its action in the tubule; consequently, patients with intrinsic ARF and marked decreases in GFR may respond poorly to furosemide administration. When there is a response to furosemide, patients require close observation for exacerbations of volume depletion, which potentiates an ischemic or toxic insult. For example, furosemide administration has been demonstrated to exacerbate gentamicin toxicity and probably should be avoided in patients with ARF caused by aminoglycoside usage. Dopamine is a potent renal vasodilating agent that acts via specific dopamine receptors on renal arterioles. It is best administered with an infusion pump through a separate intravenous line. Addition of 120 mg of dopamine to 1 L of 0.9% NaCl or 5% dextrose results in a dopamine concentration of 120 μg/ml. A 500-kg horse requires 12.5 ml of this solution per minute for a desired infusion rate of 3 μg/kg per minute. Although this recommended infusion rate has minimal effects on systemic hemodynamics, dopamine can induce arrhythmias. Therefore, heart rate and rhythm should be monitored regularly during infusion. Administration of furosemide in combination with dopamine appears to be more effective in increasing RBF and inducing diuresis than the use of either agent alone.

Dialysis

If use of fluid therapy and one or more of these agents fail to re-establish urine flow, peritoneal dialysis may be used as a means of short-term support to allow time for nephron repair and hypertrophy. Peritoneal dialysis may also be warranted in horses with aminoglycoside-induced ARF if plasma concentrations of the drug remain elevated after discontinuation of therapy. Hemodialysis is not available for adult horses but has been used in the treatment of acute renal failure in neonatal foals. Both of these dialysis procedures are best accomplished at 24-hour referral centers or teaching hospitals.

Maintaining Hydration

Once volume deficits have been corrected and diuresis has been established, fluid therapy should be tailored to provide for maintenance requirements. The author uses 55 to 60 ml/kg per day (or 1 L/hr to a 400– to 500-kg horse) as an estimate of daily fluid requirements for adult horses. However, during the polyuric recovery phase of ARF, urine volume and urinary electrolyte losses can be increased, and maintenance fluid requirements may be two to three times greater than those of healthy horses. Potassium supplementation (20–40 mEq of KCl added to each liter of IV fluids) may be necessary, particularly for anorectic patients. An estimate of the volume of ongoing fluid losses for the primary disease process such as enterocolitis should also be included in the daily plan for fluid administration. Polyionic fluids such as lactated Ringer's solution should be utilized once electrolyte and acid-base alterations have been corrected.

Nutritional Support

Protracted ARF and anorexia lead to a catabolic state, and affected patients may require nutritional support. Enteral feeding via a nasogastric tube (see Current Therapy in Equine Medicine 3: page 724) is the most economical method of nutritional support. Adding dextrose to intravenous fluids (5–10% solution) may provide some nutritional support, but the calories provided will not meet minimum daily requirements.

Patient Monitoring

Frequent patient monitoring is essential to assess response to therapy. The minimal data collected on a daily basis should include clinical assessment, body weight, packed cell volume, plasma total solids, serum concentrations of creatinine and electrolytes, and volume of fluid administered. Intravenous fluid therapy should be continued until the horse is eating and drinking normally and there has been a substantial decrease (>75%) in creatinine concentration. The volume of fluids administered should be reduced gradually over a 2- to 3-day period before discontinuing fluid therapy. It is important to monitor the patient's hydration status during this period. The serum creatinine concentration should be measured again 2 to 3 days after fluid therapy is discontinued.

PROGNOSIS

The prognosis for ARF in the horse depends on the underlying cause, duration of renal failure, response to initial treatment, and development of secondary complications such as laminitis, thrombophlebitis, and diarrhea. Regardless of the cause, the duration of renal failure before initiation of therapy is the most important determinant of prognosis. Early interruption of the pathophysiologic events that lead to ARF provides the best chance of preventing permanent renal dysfunction. Horses with hemodynamically mediated ARF resulting from conditions such as diarrhea, endotoxemia, hemolytic crises, and myopathy usually have a good prognosis for full recovery of renal function, provided that appropriate therapy is instituted and the primary problem can be corrected. The expected response to therapy in patients with pre-renal failure (serum creatinine typically <5 mg/dl) is rapid resolution of azotemia over the initial day or two of treatment. Patients

with a favorable prognosis for recovery from intrinsic ARF (serum creatinine may range from 5 to 15 mg/dl) have a more gradual decline in serum creatinine concentration over a 3- to 7-day period. When oliguric ARF persists over the initial 24 to 48 hours of treatment, the prognosis is poor even with dialysis. Uremia in these cases is usually severe (creatinine often >15 mg/dl) and the incidence of secondary complications such as generalized edema and laminitis is high.

Nephrotoxic ARF, other than that induced by heavy metal toxicity, has a more favorable prognosis than ARF consequent to ischemia, because tubular basement membranes are more likely to remain intact following nephrotoxicant-induced injury, and ARF is usually nonoliguric.

Supplemental Readings

Bayly WM, Brobst DF, Elfers RS, Reed SM: Serum and urinary biochemistry and enzyme changes in ponies with acute renal failure. Cornell Vet 76:306–316, 1986.

Divers TJ, Whitlock RH, Byars TD, Leitch M, Crowell WA: Acute renal failure in six horses resulting from hemodynamic causes. Equine Vet J 19:178–184, 1987.

Maxie G, Van Dreumel T, MacMaster D, Baird J: Menadione (vitamin K3) toxicity in six horses. Can Vet J 33:756–757, 1992.

Rossier Y, Divers TJ, Sweeney RW: Variations in urinary gamma glutamyl transferase/urinary creatinine ratio in horses with or without pleuropneumonia treated with gentamicin. Equine Vet J 27:217–220, 1995.

Schmitz DG: Toxic nephropathy in horses. Comp Cont Ed Pract Vet 10:104–111, 1988.

Schuh JCL, Ross C, Meschter C: Concurrent mercuric blister and dimethyl sulphoxide (DMSO) application as a cause of mercury toxicity in two horses. Equine Vet J 20:68–71, 1988.

Aminoglycoside Dosing

RAYMOND J. GEOR
Guelph, Ontario

The aminoglycoside antibiotics remain a cornerstone of treatment for gram-negative bacterial infections in horses. They are generally used in combination with a β-lactam agent to produce a synergistic broad-spectrum bactericidal effect. Increased use of aminoglycoside antibiotics in equine practice has been accompanied by greater recognition and concern for development of aminoglycoside-induced nephrotoxicity. As a consequence, there has been a great deal of investigation of the pharmacokinetics of the aminoglycoside antibiotics to improve dosing regimens to both maximize antibacterial activity and minimize the risk for nephrotoxicity.

Conventional aminoglycoside dosing regimens were designed to achieve peak serum drug concentrations in the range of two to three times the minimum inhibitory concentration (MIC) for the bacterial isolate recovered. In addition, the dosing interval was designed so that drug concentrations ("trough" concentrations) had declined well below toxic thresholds before administration of the next

dose. These goals were met by administering the drug twice a day or three times a day. Unfortunately, because of a wide range of clearance times between horses, serum drug concentrations are highly variable with this conventional dosing regimen. Consequently, the only way to ensure both adequate antibacterial activity and a low risk of nephrotoxicity has been measurement of peak and trough serum drug concentrations. More recently, recognition that less frequent administration of aminoglycoside antibiotics lowers the risk of nephrotoxicity while preserving or perhaps enhancing antibacterial activity has provided a rationale for administration of a full day's amount of an aminoglycoside in a single dose rather than as divided doses. This dosing regimen appears to be a practical alternative to measurement of serum drug concentrations in the majority of sick horses.

The recommended conventional dosing regimens (Table 1) for gentamicin and amikacin, the aminoglycoside antibiotics most commonly used in equine practice, are based

TABLE 1. CONVENTIONAL DOSING REGIMENS FOR
GENTAMICIN AND AMIKACIN IN HORSES

Drug	Dose/Dosing Interval	Target Serum Concentrations	
		Peak	*Trough*
Gentamicin			
Adults	2.2 mg/kg, q8h	8–10 µg/ml	<1 µg/ml
Foals°	3.3 mg/kg, q12h	8–10 µg/ml	<1 µg/ml
Amikacin			
Adults	6.6 mg/kg, q8h	>15 µg/ml	1–3 µg/ml
Foals°	6.6 mg/kg, q8h	>15 µg/ml	1–3 µg/ml

°For neonatal foals, these recommended doses are appropriate for initial dosing, but dosage regimens should be individualized and adjusted based on measured peak and trough serum drug concentrations.

on pharmacokinetic data from healthy animals. Large interindividual and age-related variations exist in the volume of distribution and clearance of these drugs in healthy subjects and even more so in diseased animals. As an example, longer clearance times for gentamicin and amikacin occur in premature foals and in full-term foals with hypoxia, azotemia, and septicemia, probably the result of renal hypoperfusion and decreases in glomerular filtration rate. Alterations in extracellular fluid (ECF) volume associated with conditions such as dehydration, endotoxemia or sepsis, peritoneal or pleural effusion, or the higher percentage of total body water in neonatal foals, changes the volume of distribution and thereby affects peak serum concentrations. Because the outcome of treatment of susceptible infections is correlated with the peak serum concentration of the aminoglycoside used, dosing regimens that fail to achieve adequate peak concentrations may result in treatment failure.

The aminoglycoside antibiotics are not metabolized and are cleared almost exclusively by renal excretion. Thus, longer clearance times with disease states affecting renal perfusion and glomerular filtration may increase the risk of aminoglycoside-induced nephrotoxicity. In this context, measuring peak and trough serum drug concentrations is the best way to determine appropriate dosing regimens for critically ill equine patients. Adjustments usually involve an increase in both the amount of drug administered per dose and the time interval between doses.

Although individualization of dosing regimens may optimize therapeutic efficacy and reduce nephrotoxicity, such monitoring is expensive and not often available in general equine practice. In this context, administration of the total daily dose of the aminoglycoside as a single bolus evolved as a way to ensure high peak serum concentrations and allow adequate time for drug clearance and thus reach the appropriate trough concentrations. In fact, once-daily dosing may provide additional therapeutic advantages over conventional dosing regimens. Two pharmacologic properties of the aminoglycoside antibiotics, concentration-dependent killing and the post-antibiotic effect (PAE), may contribute to the effectiveness of a once-daily dosing regimen. The PAE, defined as persistent suppression of bacterial growth following exposure to an effective antibiotic, allows for less frequent dosing because maintenance of serum drug concentrations in excess of the MIC for an entire

dose interval is not necessary. Further, the PAE is also concentration-dependent, with a higher aminoglycoside concentration resulting in a longer PAE. Achievement of high peak serum concentrations of the aminoglycoside is the major determinant of aminoglycoside antibacterial efficacy. This finding reflects the importance of concentration-dependent killing by aminoglycoside antibiotics, which contrasts with the time-dependent action of β-lactam antibiotics.

Aminoglycoside-induced renal toxicity results from accumulation of these agents within the renal cortex. After filtration at the glomerulus, aminoglycoside antibiotics bind to phospholipids on the brush border of proximal tubular cells and are subsequently reabsorbed. Accumulation of aminoglycosides in proximal tubular cells interferes with lysosomal, mitochondrial, and sodium/potassium/adenosinetriphosphatase($Na^+/K^+/ATPase$) function. Binding to the brush border is saturable so that sustained exposure of proximal tubular cells to the drug, as can occur with multiple daily dosing regimens, results in greater accumulation of the drug and increased nephrotoxicity. Therefore, a once-daily dosing regimen that results in high peak concentrations and low trough concentrations in serum may maintain, or even improve, therapeutic efficacy and attenuate the risk of nephrotoxicosis.

ONCE-DAILY DOSING

Studies in horses have provided evidence to support the use of once-daily aminoglycoside dosing. Once-daily dosing with gentamicin (6.6–8.8 mg/kg) in adult horses produced peak serum drug concentrations approximately three times higher than those measured after conventional dosing (2.2 mg/kg). Similarly, drug concentrations in synovial and peritoneal fluids are two to three times higher than those achieved with conventional dosing. At this time, there are no published reports of once-daily dosing of amikacin to horses; however, empirical evidence suggests that this drug can also be safely administered at a dose of 15 to 20 mg/kg s.i.d.

Clinical studies in sick horses are needed to further evaluate the efficacy of once-daily aminoglycoside dosing. However, once-daily dosing should result in higher tissue concentrations, more effective and prolonged bacterial killing, and a lower risk of nephrotoxicosis. Further advantages of once-daily dosing include convenience, improved compliance, and reduced cost. It should be emphasized that aminoglycoside dosing regimens cannot be completely standardized. When selecting an aminoglycoside dosing regimen, attention must be paid to the site of infection, the susceptibility of the pathogen, the severity of illness, and the patient's renal function. For example, the aminoglycoside antibiotics are poorly distributed to the lung and may not be the most appropriate antimicrobial selection for treatment of pulmonary infections. Further, because neutrophil activity appears to be an important component of the PAE, use of the once-daily dosing regimen in neutropenic patients may not be advisable, particularly if the aminoglycoside is not combined with a β-lactam antibiotic. When aminoglycoside antibiotics are needed in patients with compromised renal function, monitoring serum drug concentrations (especially trough concentrations) remains the best safeguard against exacerbating renal damage.

MONITORING RENAL FUNCTION

All patients receiving aminoglycoside therapy for more than 5 days should be monitored for evidence of nephrotoxicity, and the impact of concurrent risk factors should be minimized. Adequate hydration should be maintained and other nephrotoxic agents, particularly the nonsteroidal anti-inflammatory drugs, should be used at the lowest effective dose or avoided altogether. To monitor for aminoglycoside nephrotoxicity, serum creatinine concentration should be measured every 3 to 5 days during treatment. If renal dysfunction is indicated by a 0.3 mg/dl or greater increase in serum creatinine concentration, consideration should be given to discontinuing therapy or increasing the dosing interval. Ideally, trough serum drug concentrations should be serially monitored to adjust the dosing interval.

Increases in serum creatinine are a late manifestation of aminoglycoside-induced nephrotoxicity. A more sensitive method for monitoring nephrotoxicity is serial urinalysis. Changes in urine sediment, enzymuria, mild proteinuria, glucosuria, and decreased concentrating ability may develop several days before an increase in serum creatinine concentration. An increase in the ratio of urinary gamma glutamyl transferase (GGT) activity to urinary creatinine (uCr) concentration (see page 469) reflects damage to the brush border of proximal tubular epithelial cells and a urinary GGT/(uCr × 0.01) value higher than 25 has been suggested to be an early indicator of nephrotoxicity. In four of five research ponies administered toxic doses of gentamicin (20 mg/kg IV q8h), urinary GGT/(uCr × 0.01) values exceeded 100 2 to 4 days before increases in serum creatinine were detected. Further, considerable variation between ponies was observed. The findings of this study illustrate several important points with regard to monitoring for aminoglycoside-induced nephrotoxicity in equine patients: (1) the risk of nephrotoxicity varies considerably between horses; (2) urinary changes precede increases in serum Cr concentration by several days; and (3) minor increases in the urinary GGT to urinary creatinine ratio should be interpreted with caution.

Supplemental Readings

Doherty TJ, Novotny MJ, Desjardins MR, Kretzschmar B: Gentamicin concentrations in body fluids of adult horses following high-dose administration. Proc 40th Annu Conv Am Assoc Equine Pract, 1994, pp 113–114.

Godber LM, Walker RD, Stein GE, Hauptman JG, Derksen FJ: Pharmacokinetics, nephrotoxicosis, and in vitro antibacterial activity associated with single versus multiple (three times) daily gentamicin treatments in horses. Am J Vet Res 56:613–618, 1995.

Green, SL, Conlon PD: Clinical pharmacokinetics of amikacin in hypoxic premature foals. Equine Vet J 25:276–280, 1993.

Green SL, Conlon PD, Mama K, Baird JD: Effects of hypoxia and azotaemia on the pharmacokinetics of amikacin in neonatal foals. Equine Vet J 24:475–479, 1992.

Hinchcliff KW, McGuirk SM, MacWilliams PS: Gentamicin nephrotoxicity. Proc 33rd Annu Conv Am Assoc Equine Pract, 1987, pp 67–75.

Magdesian KG, Hogan PM, Brumbaugh G, Bernard WW, Chaffin MK, Cohen ND: Pharmacokinetics of gentamicin administered once daily by the intravenous and intramuscular routes. Proc 40th Annu Conv Am Assoc Equine Pract, 1994, pp 115–116.

Chronic Renal Failure

A. BRUCE KING
Pullman, Washington

HAROLD C. SCHOTT II
East Lansing, Michigan

Chronic renal failure is a well recognized but infrequently diagnosed syndrome in the horse. One widely cited abattoir study revealed that 16% of horses examined had glomerular lesions on light microscopy, and 36% exhibited deposits of immunoglobulin and/or complement on immunofluorescent testing. Although these findings suggest that up to one third of horses may have renal disease, only one of the horses in this survey exhibited signs of chronic renal failure. This disparity can be attributed to a large renal reserve capacity because clinical signs of chronic renal failure do not become apparent until two thirds to three fourths of functional nephrons have been lost.

ETIOLOGY

Disorders of the kidneys leading to chronic renal failure may be congenital or acquired. In patients younger than 5 years of age lacking a history of an event that may have been complicated by acute renal failure, congenital renal disorders should be suspected. These may include renal agenesis, dysplasia, hypoplasia, polycystic kidney disease, and hydronephrosis (see page 492). Although each of these congenital abnormalities is occasionally recognized, acquired disorders are the more common cause of chronic renal failure in horses.

Acquired disease may be a consequence of tubular or glomerular damage. Tubulointerstitial disease usually occurs as a sequela to an episode of acute tubular necrosis. Renal ischemia and nephrotoxic compounds are the mechanisms of damage. Hypovolemia associated with acute blood loss, colic, diarrhea, or sepsis can lead to renal hypoperfusion and ischemic damage. Aminoglycoside antibiotics, nonsteroidal anti-inflammatory drugs, vitamin D, vitamin K_3, and heavy metals such as mercury are all potentially nephrotoxic. Intravascular hemolysis or rhabdomyolysis can also lead to acute tubular damage consequent to the nephrotoxic effects of hemoglobin or myoglobin. In addition, severe tubulointerstitial disease culminating in chronic renal failure may develop consequent to ascending urinary tract infection, resulting in bilateral pyelonephritis or bilateral obstructive disease with ureteroliths or nephroliths (see page 482).

Although administration of nephrotoxic agents is commonly implicated as a cause of tubular damage leading to chronic renal failure, immune-mediated glomerular injury appears to be the more common initiating cause in horses. Glomerular injury is typically the result of deposition of circulating immune complexes along the glomerular basement membrane and in the mesangium. In rare cases, glomerulonephritis may be attributed to a true autoimmune disorder in which antibodies directed against the glomerular basement membrane are produced. Both immune mechanisms lead to complement activation, leukotaxis, and lysosomal degranulation that damages the glomerular capillaries and leads to glomerulosclerosis. Thickening of the filtration barrier leads to a progressive decline in glomerular filtration rate and development of azotemia. Although streptococcal antigens have frequently been incriminated, equine infectious anemia virus is the only antigen that has been experimentally demonstrated to be associated with development of glomerulonephritis in horses. Renal amyloidosis is an unusual cause of glomerulopathy and is somewhat unique to horses hyperimmunized for serum production. Another acquired cause of chronic renal failure is renal neoplasia. Although rare in the horse, the most common primary renal neoplasm is renal cell carcinoma, which is usually a unilateral lesion that does not result in azotemia.

CLINICAL SIGNS

Chronic weight loss is the most common presenting complaint for horses with chronic renal failure. Lethargy, rough hair coat, partial anorexia, ventral edema, polyuria and polydipsia, and poor athletic performance also are frequent owner concerns. Deterioration of body condition and lethargy may be attributable to several factors. As the magnitude of azotemia increases, clinical signs of uremia develop. An increase in the concentration of nitrogenous wastes in blood can have a direct central appetite suppressant effect that can lead to partial or complete anorexia. In the later stages of uremia, urea may be converted to ammonia by oral bacteria and may lead to oral ulceration, uremic halitosis, and excessive dental tartar formation. Uremic gastroenteritis may further lead to a mild to moderate

protein-losing enteropathy. Severely affected animals may develop soft feces. Alterations in the integrity of the highly anionic glomerular filtration barrier can also lead to loss of protein, predominantly albumin, in the urine. In some cases, protein loss may be great enough to lead to a decline in plasma protein concentration; however, horses appear to be more refractory to development of severe proteinuria, hypoproteinemia, and the nephrotic syndrome than small animal veterinary patients with chronic renal failure. In some cases with a normal total plasma protein concentration, an increase in globulin concentration offsets mild hypoalbuminemia, whereas in other cases hyperglobulinemia may result in an increase in total plasma protein concentration. A decrease in the albumin-to-globulin ratio is found in these horses. Most importantly, the combined effects of uremia with or without severe proteinuria place the affected patient in a catabolic state in which body mass declines as body reserves are tapped to meet basal energy requirements.

Mild ventral edema is a common but inconsistent finding in horses with chronic renal failure and may be attributable to three factors: decreased oncotic pressure, increased vascular permeability, and increased hydrostatic pressure. An albumin concentration below 1.0 to 1.5 g/dl is generally required before plasma oncotic pressure is significantly reduced. Because this degree of hypoalbuminemia is a rare finding in horses with chronic renal failure, uremic vasculitis causing increased vascular permeability may be a more important factor contributing to development of edema in patients without hypoalbuminemia. Further, chronic renal insufficiency can lead to renal hypoxia and hypoperfusion, which are stimuli for renal juxtaglomerular cells to release renin. Activation of the renin-angiotensin system tends to elevate hydrostatic pressure and contributes to edema formation. Unlike small animal and human patients, alterations in blood pressure in horses with chronic renal failure have not been documented.

Polyuria and polydipsia are variable findings in horses with chronic renal failure. The degree of polyuria and polydipsia is theoretically related to the degree of tubulointerstitial damage; however, the degree of polyuria does not appear to be correlated with the magnitude of azotemia in clinical cases. Typically, polyuria with chronic renal failure is not as severe as with diabetes insipidus or psychogenic water drinking such that it may not be observed by an owner. The wide variation in water intake in normal horses and common use of automatic waterers and large stock tanks further make polydipsia less apparent to owners.

An early complaint for horses with chronic renal failure may be decreased performance. Poor performance is most likely related to mild anemia, packed cell volume of 20 to 30%, and lethargy. In fact, administration of genetically engineered erythropoietin to human patients awaiting renal transplantation has been one of the most significant advances in management of chronic renal failure in people because it has improved exercise capacity and decreased morbidity associated with the uremic syndrome. This observation suggests that mild exercise can have a positive impact during the early stages of chronic renal failure in horses.

DIAGNOSIS

A diagnosis of chronic renal failure is established when persistent isosthenuria accompanies azotemia and typical clinical signs. Results of rectal palpation of the left kidney may be normal or may suggest a smaller than normal kidney. Rarely, the kidneys and ureters may be enlarged if obstructed by uroliths or if infection or neoplasia is present. Common clinicopathologic findings accompanying chronic renal failure include a mild normocytic, normochromic anemia; variable hypoalbuminemia and hypoproteinemia; mild hyponatremia and hypochloremia; hypercalcemia and hypophosphatemia; and a low plasma bicarbonate concentration. As suggested earlier, a non-regenerative anemia is related, in part, to a deficient supply of the renally secreted glycoprotein, erythropoietin. However, reduced erythrocyte lifespan may be a more significant factor contributing to anemia. Normally, the equine erythrocyte has a lifespan of 150 to 155 days. In the uremic patient, lifespan is shortened because excessive nitrogenous waste products alter protective mechanisms of the red cell membrane. These less resilient cells are more likely to be removed from the circulation by the reticuloendothelial system.

Electrolyte alterations are a consequence of the loss of tubular function. Because sodium, chloride, bicarbonate, and phosphate are conserved by renal tubules, chronic renal failure may be accompanied by excessive urinary loss of these electrolytes and a degree of metabolic acidosis unless hypochloremia becomes severe, allowing metabolic alkalosis to develop. Although fractional electrolyte clearance values (see page 469) may remain within normal ranges or may increase only slightly in horses with chronic renal failure, significant daily urinary loss of electrolytes may still occur. As an example, consider a horse with chronic renal failure with serum creatinine and sodium concentrations of 5.0 mg/dl and 130 mEq/L, respectively. If the horse is producing 30 L of urine daily with respective creatinine and sodium concentrations of 50 mg/dl and 13 mEq/L, the fractional clearance of sodium is 1.0% with a daily urinary sodium loss of 390 mEq. An increase in urinary sodium concentration to 26 mEq/L owing to a further decrease in tubular reabsorption would result in an increase in fractional sodium clearance to 2% but would represent an additional 390 mEq of daily sodium loss in the urine. The latter value would approach about 3% of the exchangeable sodium content of the body and would require an additional 20 to 25 g of daily salt intake to accommodate this loss. This example illustrates the importance of providing adequate access to salt, in addition to water, to horses with chronic renal failure.

Hypercalcemia is a unique finding in horses with chronic renal failure, and the magnitude of hypercalcemia is dependent on the amount of calcium in the diet. Hypercalcemia is not the result of hyperparathyroidism because parathormone concentrations in horses with chronic renal failure appear to be decreased. Because the equine kidney is an important route of calcium excretion (via calcium carbonate crystals), impaired tubular function in the face of continued intestinal absorption results in calcium accumulation in blood. This simplified explanation is supported by the similar development of hypercalcemia following experimental bilateral nephrectomy in ponies.

The influence of dietary calcium can be demonstrated by changing the type of hay fed to horses with chronic renal failure. Patients with serum calcium concentrations exceeding 20 mg/dl on a predominantly alfalfa diet can have their serum calcium concentrations return to the normal range within a couple of days after changing the diet to grass hay. It remains unknown whether the presence of hypercalcemia in horses with chronic renal failure is associated with exacerbation of the renal disease or tissue mineralization.

Urinalysis in horses with chronic renal failure typically reveals persistent isosthenuria with a urine specific gravity of 1.008 to 1.014. In an exceptional case with significant proteinuria, this value may increase to 1.020 to 1.025. The amount of crystals and mucus is much reduced owing to the dilute nature of the urine. Generally, urine sediment is free of red cells, leukocytes, casts, and bacteria except in cases of pyelonephritis. Bacterial culture of an appropriately collected urine sample should be performed in all cases because pyelonephritis is not always accompanied by obvious urine sediment abnormalities.

Additional diagnostic tests include renal ultrasonography to evaluate kidney size and to look for cysts or nephroliths. Horses with chronic renal failure typically have slightly smaller kidneys that are more echogenic than normal because of sclerosis and possible tissue mineralization. Renal biopsy using ultrasonographic guidance may be performed to document the presence of renal disease. Unfortunately, because most horses are presented for evaluation in the later stages of disease, biopsy results typically reveal glomerular, tubular, and interstitial lesions consistent with end-stage kidney disease. Rarely do the lesions provide information about the inciting cause of the renal disease, unless immunofluorescent testing is pursued. The latter requires placing a sample in Michel's fixative, in addition to a second sample placed in formalin for routine histopathology examination. In some cases, renal biopsy results supporting pyelonephritis or a congenital anomaly (dysplasia) as the cause of chronic renal failure are useful in developing a therapeutic plan.

Assessment of the severity of renal disease can be performed at many levels of sophistication. The magnitude of azotemia is the most readily available parameter, but it is a relatively insensitive and variable measure. Azotemia becomes apparent only after 75% or more of renal function has been lost. Further, the degree of azotemia may vary with nonrenal factors such as diet, body mass, and hydration. In general, serum creatinine concentration is a more reliable measure than urea nitrogen concentration. Serum creatinine concentrations in the range of 10 to 12 mg/dl indicate a marked decline in renal function, and values exceeding 15 mg/dl are consistent with a grave prognosis. Although measurement of glomerular filtration rate is more time-consuming and technically demanding, it provides a more accurate quantitative assessment of renal function (see page 471).

TREATMENT

Once significant renal disease becomes established, an irreversible decline in glomerular filtration rate and progression of renal failure generally ensue. Thus, management of the equine patient afflicted with chronic renal failure involves palliative efforts to minimize further loss of renal function. The goals are management to prevent complicating conditions such as a lack of water or salt availability, to discontinue administration of nephrotoxic agents, and to provide a palatable diet to stimulate the appetite and minimize further weight loss. Intravenous fluid therapy to cause diuresis is of much greater benefit in cases with acute, reversible renal failure but may also be of benefit to the patient that suffers a sudden exacerbation of chronic renal failure. Intravenous fluid therapy must be administered cautiously to patients with chronic renal failure because significant pulmonary edema may develop in patients with transient oliguria or anuria.

Supportive therapy may include supplementation of sodium chloride (50–75 g/day p.o.), possibly in combination with sodium bicarbonate (50–150 g/day p.o.) when serum bicarbonate concentration is consistently below 20 mEq/L. Supplemental electrolytes may need to be added to bran mashes or administered as pastes because horses may not ingest adequate amounts from licking a salt block. If electrolyte supplementation aggravates ventral edema, the amount should be decreased. Substituting high-calcium and high-protein feed sources such as alfalfa hay with good-quality grass hay and carbohydrates such as corn and oats may help control hypercalcemia and the level of azotemia. Ideally, the hay and grain should contain less than 10% crude protein, which is an adequate but not excessive amount and should maintain the blood urea nitrogen (BUN)-to-creatinine ratio within a target range of between 10:1 and 15:1. Although advocated in the past, a lower protein diet does not appear to be of benefit in slowing progression of renal failure. It is important to provide unlimited access to fresh water and to encourage adequate energy intake by feeding a variety of palatable feeds. In fact, if appetite for grass hay deteriorates, it is preferable to offer less ideal feeds such as alfalfa hay or increased amounts of concentrate to meet energy requirements and lessen the degree of wasting. Administration of B vitamins or anabolic steroids for their touted appetite-stimulating effects may be of benefit in some animals. Although dietary fat supplementation may provide a dense source of calories, it must be approached judiciously because some uremic patients may develop hyperlipidemia as a result of reduced triglyceride utilization. Further, hyperlipidemia is associated with progressive loss of renal function in dogs. Subcutaneous injections of heparin at 40 to 100 IU/kg twice daily may stimulate lipoprotein lipase and reduce plasma triglyceride concentrations. Edema is usually not a significant problem, and, unless it interferes with ambulation, it should be tolerated rather than treated with diuretic agents, which may be ineffective or may lead to further electrolyte wastage.

Specific treatment for chronic renal failure such as renal transplantation is not available for horses. An exception is with pyelonephritis (see page 482) in which specific antibiotic treatment is warranted. The progressive renal injury that occurs in chronic renal failure is associated with continued damage to tubular and glomerular membranes mediated by ongoing activation of the inflammatory cascade. Although not supported by experimental data in the horse,

treatment with anti-oxidant medications and free radical scavengers could, in theory, be of benefit.

Interest has arisen in the role of dietary fatty acids as precursors of eicosanoids. Specifically, dietary supplementation with sources rich in omega-3-fatty acids (linolenic acid), as compared to omega-6-fatty acids (linoleic acid), appears to decrease generation of more damaging fatty acid metabolites during activation of the inflammatory cascade. In horses, dietary supplementation with omega-3-fatty acids in the form of linseed oil has been effective at ameliorating the effects of endotoxin in in vitro studies; supplementation with menhaden oil, another rich source of omega-3-fatty acids, slowed the progression of renal failure in dogs. Unfortunately, the in vivo effects of endotoxin were not ameliorated by feeding linseed oil in preliminary equine studies, and the possible benefits of feeding omega-3-fatty acids to horses with chronic renal failure are unknown at this time.

Although administration of corticosteroids or nonsteroidal anti-inflammatory drugs also limits the inflammatory response, their negative effects on renal blood flow outweigh the possible beneficial effects, and they are not recommended in the treatment of chronic renal failure in horses. Administration of synthetic prostaglandin-E analogues is another treatment that, in theory, could increase renal blood flow and ameliorate progression of chronic renal failure. However, no data are available to support use of these treatments at this time.

PROGNOSIS

Most horses diagnosed with chronic renal failure are exhibiting obvious weight loss and other clinical signs at the time of presentation. Because of the progressive and irreversible nature of the renal disease, the long-term prognosis is grave. However, the short-term prognosis for non-oliguric patients may be more favorable. Some horses with chronic renal failure may maintain serum creatinine concentrations between 3 and 6 mg/dl for months with minimal deterioration, whereas other horses with similar laboratory data may lose weight rapidly. Prediction of which cases will deteriorate more rapidly is difficult, but a recent history and initial ability to counteract weight loss with improved management are useful indicators. Laboratory analysis of blood samples at 2- to 4-week intervals to follow the degree of azotemia and serum electrolyte alterations may be useful in monitoring disease progression. Extrapolation of the decline of the reciprocal of serum creatinine (1/Cr) over time has been used in some cases to estimate disease progression. However, this calculation assumes a constant rate of decline in remaining renal function and, when applied to many human patients and to a few equine patients the authors have studied, the technique has been unrewarding because the course of disease is not constant or predictable. In general, animals that are eating well and maintaining reasonable body condition carry the best short-term prognosis and may still be able to perform a limited amount of work. Their utility as breeding animals may be reduced because azotemia and cachexia can reduce the chance for normal conception and gestation. The goal in each case is to monitor the horse closely in order to be able to provide euthanasia before the patient reaches a state of uremic decompensation.

Supplemental Readings

Divers TJ: Chronic renal failure in horses. Comp Cont Ed Pract Vet 5:S310–S317, 1983.

Divers TJ: Management of chronic renal failure in the horse. Proc 31st Annu Conv Am Assoc Equine Pract, 1985, pp 679–681.
Klahr S, Schreiner G, Ichikawa I: The progression of renal disease. N Engl J Med 318:1657–1666, 1988.
Koterba AM, Coffman JR: Acute and chronic renal disease in the horse. Comp Cont Ed Pract Vet 3:S461–S469, 1981.
Tennant B, Kaneko JJ, Lowe JE, Tasker JB: Chronic renal failure in the horse. Proc 23rd Annu Conv Am Assoc Equine Pract, 1978, pp 293–297.

Dysuria

BRAD R. JACKMAN
Oakdale, California

HAROLD C. SCHOTT II
East Lansing, Michigan

URETHRITIS, CYSTITIS, AND PYELONEPHRITIS

Bacterial infections of the urinary tract appear to be uncommon in horses. As in other species, ascending urinary tract infections (UTIs) are most common, although septic nephritis may be an occasional consequence of septicemia, especially in neonatal foals. Because of their shorter urethra, mares are at greater risk for UTIs than geldings or stallions, especially when they are used as breeding animals.

Urethritis

Bacterial urethritis has been described as a cause of hematuria, hemospermia, and/or stranguria in geldings and stallions. However, with the exception of traumatic, parasitic, or neoplastic conditions involving the distal urethra, the authors are unaware of documented cases of primary bacterial urethritis. Bacterial infections of accessory sex glands or the prepuce may also cause dysuria. Preputial infections can occur as a consequence of trauma, presence of a foreign body, habronemiasis, or neoplasia. Owners present affected horses for a malodorous swollen sheath. Examination of the penis and sheath, in combination with biopsy of abnormal tissue, allows diagnosis of the primary problem. Occasionally, an older gelding may develop recurrent sheath swelling and/or infection that cannot be attributed to a primary disease process. The pathogenesis of this problem is unknown, although fat accumulation, poor hygiene, and inactivity may be contributing factors. Treatment involves repeated sheath cleaning, application of topical anti-inflammatory and antibacterial ointments and, when more severe involvement occurs, systemic antibiotic administration.

Cystitis

Bacterial cystitis is usually a complication of urolithiasis, bladder neoplasia, bladder paralysis, or an anatomic defect of the bladder such as a persistent urachal remnant. Dysuria may be manifested by pollakiuria, stranguria, hematuria, and/or pyuria. Scalding and accumulation of urine crystals may be observed on the perineum of affected mares or on the front of the hindlimbs of affected male horses. These findings should not be confused with normal estrus activity in an occasional mare. Diagnostic evaluation includes physical and rectal examinations and collection of a urine sample for urinalysis and quantitative bacterial culture. Although the bladder is usually felt to be normal during rectal palpation, endoscopic examination of the bladder may be helpful in assessing mucosal damage due to cystitis. Because normal equine urine is rich in mucus and crystalloid material, gross examination may be unrewarding, but sediment examination may reveal increased numbers of white blood cells (>10 leukocytes per high power field) and presence of bacteria (>20 organisms per high power field) in some, but not all, cases of cystitis. Quantitative culture results exceeding 10,000 organisms/ml in a urine sample collected by midstream catch or urethral catheterization are diagnostic for bacterial cystitis. For best results, urine sediment should be evaluated within 30 minutes of collection and samples for culture should be cooled during transport because bacterial numbers may increase in samples left at room temperature. Organisms that may be recovered on culture include *Escherichia coli* and species of *Proteus, Klebsiella, Enterobacter, Corynebacterium, Streptococcus, Staphylococcus,* and *Pseudomonas,* and isolation of more than one organism is not uncommon.

Treatment

Successful treatment of bacterial cystitis requires correction of predisposing problems such as urolithiasis and administration of systemic antibiotics. Selection of an antibiotic is ideally based on the results of sensitivity testing of isolated organisms, and the initial course of treatment should not be less than 1 week. A trimethoprim/sulfonamide combination, ampicillin, penicillin and an aminoglycoside, or ceftiofur are initial alternatives. If clinical signs return after treatment is discontinued, a urine culture should be repeated and longer term treatment instituted. In such cases, ease of administration and cost are additional considerations for antibiotic selection. For example, trimethoprim/sulfonamide combinations and the penicillins are excreted via the kidneys and concentrated in urine. Although sensitivity testing may indicate resistance, these agents may have effective antimicrobial activity against the causative agents because of the high concentrations achieved in urine. Metabolism of the antibiotic should also be considered. As an example, sulfamethoxazole is largely metabolized to inactive products prior to urinary excretion, whereas sulfadiazine is excreted largely unchanged in urine. Next, addition of 50 to 75 g salt to the diet or provision of warm water during cold weather may increase water intake and urine production, which are of benefit in cases of bacterial cystitis. Urinary acidifying agents including ammonium chloride (20 mg/kg per day p.o.) and vitamin C (2 g/kg per day p.o.) have also been administered to horses, but use of these agents at these doses has not produced a consistent decrease in urine pH. Use of ammonium chloride at a dose of 520 mg/kg per day p.o. or ammonium sulfate at 175 mg/kg per day p.o. was successful in reducing urine pH to below 6.0 in a limited number of horses. At these doses, the medications were unpalatable and had to be administered by dose syringe. Adding grain to the diet is another simple way to decrease urine pH, although the decline is modest and urine pH typically remains higher than 7.0.

Upper Urinary Tract Infections

Upper urinary tract infections involving the kidneys and ureters are rare in horses. The course of the distal segment of the ureters in the dorsal bladder wall creates a physical barrier to vesiculoureteral reflux, which is a prerequisite for ascending pyelonephritis. Problems that interfere with this barrier and increase the risk for upper UTI include ectopic ureter or bladder distension as may occur with bladder paralysis, urethral obstruction, or pregnancy. Because the kidneys are highly vascular organs, septic nephritis may develop in association with septicemia in neonatal or adult horses. Unless renal involvement is extensive, the upper UTI may go undetected but could lead to development of nephrolithiasis or chronic renal failure months or years later.

In addition to dysuria, horses with upper UTIs generally have other clinical signs including fever, weight loss, anorexia, and depression. Upper UTI is often accompanied by stone formation, which may lead to nephrolithiasis and ureterolithiasis and signs of obstruction. In an occasional case, small uroliths may travel down the ureter and lead to urethral obstruction and renal colic as the presenting complaint. As for cystitis, diagnostic evaluation includes physical and rectal examinations, urinalysis, and a quantitative urine culture. In addition to the organisms listed earlier, organisms such as *Actinobacillus equuli*, *Streptococcus equi*, *Rhodococcus equi*, or *Salmonella* species can also be isolated from cases of hematogenous septic nephritis. In horses with upper UTIs, a complete blood count and serum biochemistry profile should be performed to assess the systemic inflammatory response and renal function. Cystoscopy, including watching for urine flow from each ureteral opening, and ultrasonographic imaging of the bladder, ureters, and kidneys are helpful adjunctive diagnostic procedures. Ureteral catheterization by passing polyethylene tubing via the biopsy channel of the endoscope or by use of an 8- to 10-French polypropylene catheter, which can be passed blindly in mares, may allow collection of urine samples from each ureter to distinguish unilateral from bilateral disease.

Treatment

Treatment for upper UTIs includes a prolonged course of appropriate systemic antibiotics and, in select cases with unilateral disease, surgical removal of the affected kidney and ureter. Although treatment successes are rare, poor outcomes are likely to be related to failure to diagnose an upper UTI until relatively late in the disease course.

OBSTRUCTIVE DISEASE OF THE URINARY TRACT

The majority of cases of obstructive urinary tract disease in the horse occur consequent to urolithiasis. Trauma, urethral strictures, urinary tract displacement, and neoplasia are other causes. From 1970 to 1989, urolithiasis was responsible for 0.11% of equine admissions to 22 veterinary teaching hospitals and accounted for 7.8% of diagnoses of urinary tract disease. Male horses, especially geldings, were predisposed to urolithiasis, but breed and age predispositions have not been described.

Uroliths are most commonly found in the urinary bladder, although they may also develop in the kidneys, ureters, and urethra. Two basic forms of uroliths are described, both of which are primarily composed of calcium carbonate. The more common form is a yellow-green, spiculated stone that can be easily fragmented. Less commonly, uroliths are gray-white, smooth stones that are more resistant to fragmentation. The latter form generally contains a greater amount of phosphate.

Factors contributing to urolith formation include supersaturation of urine, prolonged transit time, and reduced inhibition of crystal growth. In general, two steps are required for calculus formation: (1) nucleation or formation of a nidus around desquamated epithelial cells, leukocytes, or necrotic tissue; and (2) crystal growth. Because supersaturation with calcium carbonate crystals is a normal finding in equine urine, the relatively low incidence of urolithiasis is somewhat surprising. However, equine urine is rich in mucus, which acts as a natural inhibitor of stone formation. Tissue damage from various causes is likely to be the most important factor for the development of uroliths in horses. As an example, nephroliths may form in the renal medulla or pelvis consequent to papillary necrosis accompanying phenylbutazone toxicity. Similarly, adherence and accumulation of crystalloid material occurs rapidly at sites of mucosal irritation in the bladder.

Nephrolithiasis and Ureterolithiasis

Although renal and ureteral calculi are rarely described, their occurrence should not be overlooked. In a review of 68 horses with urolithiasis, 25% had uroliths in the kidneys and ureters and a few horses with cystic calculi also had calculi in the upper urinary tract. Nephroliths may develop around a nidus associated with a variety of renal diseases including pyelonephritis, tubular necrosis, or papillary necrosis. It has been speculated that racehorses may be at greater risk of developing renal calculi because of the common use of nonsteroidal anti-inflammatory drugs in these athletes.

Horses with nephroliths or ureteroliths may remain asymptomatic until bilateral obstructive disease leads to development of acute or chronic renal failure. When clinical signs are present, they tend to be nonspecific. Presenting complaints may include poor performance, lethargy, inappetence, and weight loss. In an occasional horse, obstruction may lead to more acute signs of colic, dysuria, and hematuria. Rectal palpation may reveal an enlarged kidney or ureter, and ureteral calculi may be palpable in an enlarged ureter.

Diagnosis of renal and ureteral calculi is usually made during ultrasonographic examination. Although ultrasonographic imaging may provide information regarding the presence, number, and location of calculi, small stones can be missed despite complete examination. Other ultrasonographic findings to support upper tract lithiasis in affected horses include dilation of the renal pelvis or proximal ureter and, in long-standing cases, hydronephrosis. Although azotemia generally accompanies bilateral disease, horses with unilateral disease often maintain normal renal function. Because infection often accompanies urolithiasis in horses, a quantitative urine culture should be performed in all affected patients.

Treatment

Few reports have been presented on successful management of horses with renal and ureteral calculi. Removal of the calculus, which is limited to horses with unilateral disease, has been the only means of effective treatment. Nephrectomy is the preferred technique for management of unilateral renal calculi. The approach involves a dorsal flank incision, rib resection, and blunt retroperitoneal dissection to expose the kidney. Although nephrotomy through a similar approach has also been described for stone removal in horses, the procedure is technically more challenging and of limited benefit because function of the affected kidney is often minimal. Ureteral calculi have been removed by ureterolithectomy via both ventral celiotomy and paralumbar approaches. A basket stone dislodger,* introduced through a vestibulourethral approach and guided by rectal palpation, has also been used for removal of distal ureteral calculi in the mare. Although ureterolithectomy is the only option for bilateral ureterolithiasis, surgical removal of the affected kidney and ureter is the procedure of choice with unilateral disease because it minimizes the possibility of recurrence. Furthermore, removal of the affected kidney and ureter should eliminate associated upper urinary tract infection.

Cystic Calculi

Cystic calculi are the most commonly recognized form of urolithiasis. No age or breed predilection is recognized, but the incidence is greater in males, especially geldings. Cystic calculi are thought to be relatively rare in mares due to their short, distensible urethra. Cystoliths are typically

---

*Dormia Stone Dislodger, V. Mueller, Division of American Hospital Supply, McGaw Park, IL

flattened sphere-shaped stones with a spiculated surface, but smooth calculi or accumulation of a crystalloid sludge, termed *sabulous urolithiasis*, can also occur. The latter form usually develops as a result of bladder paralysis.

Dysuria consequent to cystic urolithiasis may be manifested as hematuria, stranguria, pollakiuria, and pyuria. Hematuria may be more apparent after exercise. An affected male horse may demonstrate stranguria by repeatedly dropping its penis and posturing to urinate, but little or no urine may be voided. An affected mare may also repeatedly posture to urinate and demonstrate winking; these signs could be confused with estrus activity. Less common signs may include urine scalding, an irritable attitude, recurrent colic, and loss of condition.

The diagnosis of cystic calculi is usually made by palpation of the bladder per rectum. Bladder uroliths are usually large enough to be easily detected; however, if the bladder is distended, it may have to be catheterized to facilitate palpation of the stone. Bladder catheterization further allows assessment of urethral patency and collection of samples for urinalysis and quantitative culture. A complete blood count and serum biochemical profile should be performed to document whether anemia, inflammation, and/or azotemia have developed. Cystoscopic examination is helpful in assessing the severity of damage to the bladder mucosa and asymmetry in appearance or function of the ureteral openings. Because it is not uncommon for calculi to be in multiple sites of the urinary system, thorough evaluation of the upper urinary tract is warranted in cases of cystic urolithiasis.

Treatment

Several surgical options exist for management of cystic calculi. The size of the calculus, gender of the horse, and surgeon's preference play a role in treatment selection. The preferred technique in males, especially for larger stones, is laparocystotomy through a ventral midline or paramedian incision with the horse placed in dorsal recumbency under general anesthesia. For removal of smaller cystoliths, a perineal urethrotomy can be performed in the standing male horse following the use of local or epidural anesthesia. The urethra is catheterized to facilitate its identification and an incision is made at the level of the ischial arch. After the urethra has been incised, forceps are used to grasp and remove the calculus, and the bladder is lavaged free of remaining debris. Removal of larger calculi may be attempted via this approach by using a lithotribe to crush the urolith into smaller fragments. The urethral incision can be closed but is usually allowed to heal by second intention. Although perineal urethrostomy can be performed at little expense and avoids the risks of general anesthesia, complications including urethral trauma and stricture formation may occur. The distensible urethra of the mare allows retrieval of cystic calculi via the urethra in most cases. Using sedation and epidural anesthesia, the stone can be removed intact with forceps or by direct grasping if the surgeon has small hands. A spiculated urolith may be crushed to ease removal. Spiculated stones or urolith fragments can further be manipulated into a sterile plastic bag or palpation sleeve to lessen trauma to the urethral mucosa during removal. If necessary, the urethral lumen can also be enlarged by performing a sphincterotomy in the dorsal aspect of the urethra. Electrohydraulic lithotripsy has also been used in male and female horses for treatment of cystic calculi. This procedure uses a hydraulic shock wave to fragment the calculus. Although this method of stone fragmentation is less traumatic than use of a lithotribe, expense of the equipment has limited its use.

Following surgical removal of cystoliths, systemic antibiotics are administered for a minimum of 1 week. Interestingly, in a case review, material from the centers of calculi yielded positive bacterial cultures in more than 50% of uroliths examined, whereas positive quantitative urine culture results were infrequent. As for cystitis, antibiotic selection should be based on sensitivity testing of isolates recovered. If culture results are negative, a sulfonamide that is concentrated in an active form in the urine (e.g., sulfadiazine) is an appropriate selection. In a recent report, clinical signs of urolithiasis recurred in 12 of 29 horses (41%) and recurrence rate was suspected to be higher following removal by perineal urethrotomy, in comparison to laparocystotomy. In an attempt to prevent recurrence, use of urinary acidifiers, as described under cystitis, has been recommended but benefits of their use have not been well documented. A perhaps more important consideration for decreasing the chance of recurrence may be to modify the diet to decrease calcium excretion. Changing the diet from a high-calcium hay such as alfalfa to grass or oat hay would decrease calcium intake and should decrease urinary calcium excretion because fecal calcium excretion is relatively constant in horses. Although this dietary change should decrease total calcium excretion, it may also decrease urinary nitrogen excretion and daily urine volume. The latter changes could enhance supersaturation of urine. Another factor affecting urinary calcium excretion is dietary cation-anion balance (DCAB), because a lower DCAB has been associated with an increase in urinary calcium concentration. A lower DCAB is usually achieved by increasing the amount of grain in the diet or changing to a poorer quality hay. Thus, specific dietary recommendations to minimize the chance for cystolith recurrence cannot be made without further investigation of the factors affecting urinary calcium excretion. At the least, however, dietary supplements containing calcium should be avoided in horses with urolithiasis.

Urethral Calculi

Urethral calculi are a problem of male horses. In the absence of urethral mucosal damage or stricture formation, urethroliths are usually small cystoliths that are passed into the urethra. Thus, most urethroliths initially lodge where the urethra narrows as it passes over the ischial arch. They may slowly pass more distally until complete obstruction results in signs of renal colic.

An obstructing urethral calculus should be considered in male horses that show colic signs along with frequent posturing to urinate. Occasionally, blood may be seen on the end of the urethra. Palpation of the penis may reveal repeated urethral contractions and a firm mass in the urethra. Rectal palpation reveals a distended bladder that is turgid, unlike the flaccid bladder distension in cases of bladder paralysis. If bladder rupture occurs, colic signs are replaced by progressive depression and anorexia, consequent to the development of electrolyte alterations and azotemia. The diagnosis is confirmed by passage of a urinary catheter that is obstructed by the urethrolith, or by endoscopic examination of the urethra. When bladder rupture is suspected, it can be confirmed by measuring a two-fold or greater increase in peritoneal fluid creatinine concentration in comparison with serum creatinine concentration.

Treatment

Calculi lodged at the ischial arch can be removed through a perineal urethrotomy. Passage of a catheter into the bladder, if not performed before surgery, is necessary to ensure a patent urinary tract after stone removal. The urethrotomy is allowed to heal by second intention, and temporary use of an indwelling bladder catheter is usually not necessary. Calculi lodged in the distal urethra can often be removed in a sedated horse by gentle crushing of the urolith with a hand or forceps. When the calculus is lodged distal to the ischial arch and cannot be palpated in the distal portion of the penis, general anesthesia and positioning the horse in dorsal recumbency is generally required for surgical removal of the stone. The urethra may be closed or it may be allowed to heal by second intention. Urethral trauma is an obvious consequence of obstruction with a urethral calculus, but the mucosal damage typically resolves without serious complications. A follow-up endoscopic examination of the urethra allows assessment of possible stricture formation. Further treatment includes administration of antibiotic and anti-inflammatory agents until dysuria resolves.

Bladder Displacement

Displacement of the urinary bladder is a rare cause of obstruction and dysuria. In the mare, bladder displacements include extrusion through a tear in the floor of the vagina or a true prolapse with eversion of the bladder. Urethral obstruction may also occur with vaginal or uterine prolapse. In the male horse, scrotal herniation of the bladder has been described, but this type of bladder displacement is extremely rare.

Bladder displacements are typically a consequence of repeated abdominal contractions and/or straining. Thus, they are most commonly associated with parturition and, to a lesser extent, with colic. Perineal lacerations, consequent to trauma or foaling, may lead to extrusion, whereas excessive straining without laceration leads to prolapse or eversion. Because the bladder turns inside out with the latter problem, the diagnosis is established by recognizing the appearance of the bladder mucosa and ureteral openings. Eversion does not always result in obstruction.

In cases of urethral obstruction, a catheter should be passed into the bladder before correction of the displacement. In the absence of obstruction, extrusions are corrected during repair of the perineal or vaginal laceration. A course of broad-spectrum antibiotics and an anti-inflammatory agent should be instituted because pelvic abscess and peritonitis are potential complications. In horses with bladder prolapse, application of hypertonic dextrose or saline solutions to the everted mucosa may decrease edema before manual replacement. Urethral sphincterotomy may be needed to replace the bladder and, in some cases, reduction via laparotomy may be necessary because the filling of the everted bladder by the colon complicates manual reduction.

Supplemental Readings

Boyd WL, Bishop LM: Pyelonephritis of cattle and horses. J Am Vet Med Assoc 90:154–162, 1937.

DeBowes RM: Surgical management of urolithiasis. Vet Clin North Am Equine Pract 4:461–471, 1988.

Ehnen SJ, Divers TJ, Gillete D, Reef VB: Obstructive nephrolithiasis and ureterolithiasis associated with chronic renal failure in horses: Eight cases (1981–1987). J Am Vet Med Assoc 197:249–253, 1990.

Holt PE, Pearson H: Urolithiasis in the horse—A review of 13 cases. Equine Vet J 16(1):31–34, 1984.

Laverty S, Pascoe JR, Ling GV, Lavoie JP, Ruby AL: Urolithiasis in 68 horses. Vet Surg 21(1):56–62, 1992.

Nouws JFM, Firth EC, Vree TB, Baakman M: Pharmacokinetics and renal clearance of sulfamethazine, sulfamerazine, and sulfadiazine and their N_4-acetyl and hydroxy metabolites in horses. Am J Vet Res 48:392–402, 1987.

Remillard RL, Modransky PD, Welker FH, Thatcher CD: Dietary management of cystic calculi in a horse. J Equine Vet Sci 12(6):359–363, 1992.

Vaughn JT: Equine urogenital system. In Jennings PB (ed): The Practice of Large Animal Surgery, ed 2. Philadelphia, WB Saunders, 1984, pp 1136–1137.

Polyuria

CHRISTOPHER M. BROWN
Ames, Iowa

NORMAL BODY WATER DISTRIBUTION AND BALANCE

The body of an adult horse is about two-thirds water, which is distributed in three compartments: intracellular, interstitial, and intravascular. The latter two represent components of extracellular fluid. Body water is derived from two major sources: that which is ingested as liquid water or a component in solid feed, and that which is produced by metabolic activity. Water is lost from the body by four major routes: in urine, in feces, across the skin, and across the respiratory tract. More than 75% of water loss occurs in feces, and urinary output adds fine control to total body water homeostasis. Water intake is dependent upon diet, work load, and environmental temperature and can range from 15 to 20 L/day to more than 90 L/day.

In a normal horse, glomerular filtration rate exceeds 1,000 L/day—a value 10 times greater than the total extracellular fluid volume. However, 99% of this water is reabsorbed in the renal tubules and collecting ducts. Urine output varies between 5 and 15 L/day, and urine specific gravity ranges from 1.020 to 1.050, with a mean of about 1.035. Urine that is isosmotic with plasma has a specific gravity of 1.008 to 1.014; in hyposthenuria, with urine more dilute than plasma, specific gravity is less than 1.008. Newborn foals typically produce hyposthenuric urine compared to adults owing to the high volume of milk ingested, which may approach 20% of their body weight daily. Because foals experience this constant volume diuresis, they do not develop much of a medullary osmotic gradient and are less able to concentrate their urine in response to water deprivation. As a result, foals are at greater risk, compared with adult horses, of developing more severe dehydration and acute renal failure when affected with conditions such as diarrhea.

POLYURIA

Establishing that a horse is producing more urine than normal is often difficult, especially in horses kept at pasture. Owners may report that a horse is passing more urine than normal when in fact it is the frequency of urination that has increased, pollakiuria, rather than the volume. Pollakiuria occurs with conditions such as cystitis or during estrus in the mare. Close observation of a horse in a stall, combined with documentation of excessive water consumption, is often necessary to establish a diagnosis of polyuria.

The major causes of polyuria in the horse include chronic renal failure, pituitary adenoma, and psychogenic polydipsia. Less common causes include excessive salt consumption, central and nephrogenic diabetes insipidus, diabetes mellitus due to pancreatic insufficiency, sepsis or endotoxemia, and iatrogenic causes such as sedation with α_2-adrenergic agonists, corticosteroid therapy, or diuretic usage.

Figure 1 outlines an approach that can be used to evaluate horses with suspected polyuria. As mentioned earlier, it is sometimes difficult to determine that a horse is producing an excessive amount of urine. Horses stabled in stalls bedded with straw are difficult to evaluate because excessive urine may not be obvious to the casual observer. For those bedded on shavings or sawdust, excessively wet bedding may be easier to recognize, but this is a subjective impression. In an occasional horse, polyuria may be so severe that urine may flow from the stall into the barn aisle. When there is doubt as to whether a horse is polyuric, it may be necessary to collect urine over a 12- or 24-hour period. For geldings and stallions, a collecting device can be constructed by cutting off the bottom of a large plastic bottle, which is then padded and fitted over the prepuce. The opening of the bottle is covered with a rubber tube and clip, and urine can be removed every few hours. In mares, an indwelling Foley catheter can be placed in the bladder or a urine collection harness can be applied. For both sexes, the animal should be tied so that it cannot lie down and interfere with the collection process.

Renal Failure

In horses with acute renal failure, there is usually a transient period of anuria or oliguria. If these horses sur-

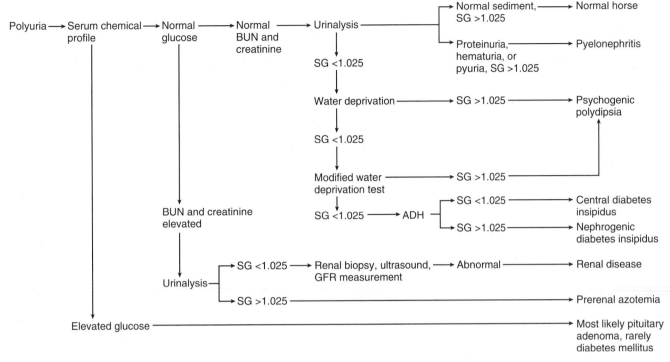

Figure 1. Approach to the horse with polyuria. Adapted from Roussel A, Carter K: Polydipsia and polyuria. *In* Brown CM (ed): Problems in Equine Medicine. Philadelphia, Lea & Febiger, 1989, p 153.

vive the peracute phase of renal disease, tubular damage results in a subsequent period during which impaired concentrating ability results in polydipsia and polyuria. These persist until tubular repair has occurred. Horses recovering from acute renal failure should be provided with adequate water, salt, and a low nitrogen (protein) and calcium diet. Such a diet can be achieved by feeding grass hay and corn or nonlegume pasture. Repair of tubules and return of concentrating ability may take 4 to 6 weeks. Although these animals appear to have normal renal function after this recovery period, a permanent reduction in total renal function is likely to persist because most animals can maintain apparently normal health with only about 25 to 50% of nephrons functioning.

Chronic renal failure may develop consequent to damage from nephrotoxins. In addition, immune-mediated mechanisms, chronic infections, and nephrolithiasis may also give rise to chronic renal failure. In addition, the condition of horses that do not recover from the renal damage occurring with acute ischemia from hypovolemic or endotoxic shock may also progress to chronic renal failure. Signs are variable and include polyuria and polydipsia in some but not all cases. Most exhibit weight loss and some have ventral edema. Affected horses tend to have poor athletic performance. A variable degree of azotemia is present, and urinalysis reveals isosthenuria, with a urine specific gravity of 1.008 to 1.014.

Pituitary Adenoma (see also page 499)

Pituitary adenomas are common in older horses and may lead to polyuria by several mechanisms. First, polyuria may be a consequence of actions of hormones derived from proopiomelanocortin, most specifically adrenocorticotro-

phin (ACTH). Hyperadrenocorticism resulting from excessive ACTH activity leads to hyperglycemia, which may exceed the renal tubular threshold for reabsorption. The resultant glucosuria leads to an osmotic diuresis. Although commonly implicated as the cause of polyuria in horses with pituitary adenomas, glucosuria was found in only one of five affected horses in a clinical report. A second mechanism implicated in the development of polyuria is antagonism of the action of antidiuretic hormone (ADH) on the collecting ducts by cortisol. Although commonly cited as the mechanism of polyuria in canine hyperadrenocorticism, experimental evidence to support this mechanism is lacking in both dogs and horses. Furthermore, there is considerable species heterogeneity in the effects of corticoids on ADH activity. As an example, corticoids actually potentiate the effect of ADH and lead to a decrease in urine output in humans. Growth of the adenoma may lead to impingement on the posterior pituitary and hypothalamic nuclei. The latter are located immediately dorsal to the pituitary gland and are the sites of ADH storage and production, respectively. Decreased ADH production and release results in a partial central diabetes insipidus as a third mechanism for polyuria. Central diabetes insipidus, however, is not likely to be the primary cause of polyuria in all cases because some affected horses can usually concentrate their urine when deprived of water. Consequently, the polydipsia and polyuria seen in many, but not all, horses with pituitary adenomas is likely to be a combined effect of several mechanisms.

In addition to polydipsia and polyuria, animals with pituitary adenoma may show weight loss, lethargy, laminitis, a potbelly appearance, and recurrent infections. However, the most consistent clinical sign is hirsutism. Diagnosis is based on the presence of the excessive hair growth, one or more of the other clinical signs, and supportive laboratory data. In addition to hyperglycemia, neutrophilia, lymphopenia, and mild anemia are often present. Serum activity of hepatic enzymes may also be elevated. Confirmation of the diagnosis may be made by assaying serum cortisol concentration and its suppression in response to administration of dexamethasone. Treatment with serotonin antagonists such as cyproheptadine or dopamine agonists such as bromocriptine or pergolide may modify the clinical signs, but do not effect a cure as the pituitary lesion continues to slowly grow.

Psychogenic Polydipsia

Psychogenic polydipsia is probably the most common cause of polyuria and polydipsia in adult horses. Anecdotally, it is reported to be more common in southern states during periods of high temperature and humidity. It appears to be a stable vice that reflects boredom in affected horses. Typically, psychogenic polydipsia results in more dramatic polyuria than either renal failure or pituitary adenoma. Horses exhibiting this behavior are usually in good body condition and are not azotemic.

The diagnosis of psychogenic polydipsia/polyuria is made by exclusion (see Table 1). In early cases, water deprivation for 12 to 24 hours is usually sufficient to demonstrate urine-concentrating ability. Specific gravity should exceed 1.025 after 24 hours of water deprivation. In cases in which there has been long-standing polyuria, medullary washout occurs, and the osmotic gradient between the lumen of the collecting tubule and the medullary interstitium is lost. In these cases ADH activity may not lead to a substantial increase in urine specific gravity. Consequently, in horses with suspected psychogenic polydipsia and polyuria of several weeks' duration that fail to concentrate their urine after 24 hours of water deprivation, a modified water deprivation test should be tried. This is performed by restricting water intake to approximately 40 ml/kg per day for 3 to 4 days. By the end of this period, urine specific gravity should exceed 1.025 in a horse that has had medullary washout.

Management of these horses is empirical. Because it is a condition diagnosed by exclusion, once one has established that the animal is not suffering from a significant renal or metabolic disease, it is safe to consider restricting water intake to meet maintenance, work, and environmental requirements of the horse. In addition, steps should be taken to improve the attitude of the horse by reducing boredom. Increasing the amount of exercise or turning the horse out to pasture are possible options, as are providing a companion or toys in the stall. In addition, increasing the frequency of feedings or the amount of roughage in the diet may increase the time spent eating and thereby reduce the habitual drinking.

Other Causes of Polyuria

Polyuria may occasionally be associated with excessive salt consumption, which is suspected to be another psychogenic or behavioral problem. Affected horses usually have an increased fractional sodium clearance. This problem can be controlled by reducing the amount of salt available to these horses.

Horses are occasionally afflicted with diabetes insipidus, which can be central or nephrogenic in origin. Central diabetes insipidus results from failure in production, transport, or release of ADH, as was described earlier as a possible contributing factor to the polyuria accompanying a pituitary adenoma. With central diabetes insipidus, horses have only a limited ability to concentrate their urine in response to water deprivation. Azotemia is not apparent and the remainder of the urinalysis results are normal. The condition has been reported in association with viral encephalomyelitis and as an idiopathic condition. Because the kidneys are normal with central diabetes insipidus, affected horses respond to parenteral administration of ADH. A suggested regimen for an adult horse is administration of 60 IU of ADH every 6 hours in combination with monitoring urine specific gravity. Horses that fail to concentrate their urine in response to ADH therapy may have nephrogenic diabetes insipidus, in which ADH production is normal, but the collecting ducts are insensitive to its effects. Nephrogenic diabetes insipidus can be a hereditary disorder in humans, and a similar hereditary disease has been described in sibling Thoroughbred colts.

Polydipsia and polyuria have also been reported as clinical signs in some horses with sepsis or endotoxemia, although other clinical signs such as fever, abdominal pain, and weight loss predominate. The mechanism is unclear but may be a consequence of endotoxin-induced prostaglandin production. Prostaglandin E_2 is a potent renal vasodilating agent in laboratory animals, and it also antagonizes the effects of ADH on the collecting ducts. Perhaps some horses with chronic gram-negative bacterial infections such as peritonitis or pleuritis may have low-grade or intermittent endotoxemia as a mechanism for polyuria, similar to the polyuria observed with canine pyometra. Furthermore, polyuria may be iatrogenically induced. The most obvious iatrogenic cause is fluid therapy for which polyuria is a desired response. Polyuria has also been observed with exogenous corticoid administration, although as for pituitary adenomas the mechanism remains unclear. People and dogs appear to experience a potent thirst response to exogenous corticoids; thus, polydipsia may be an important cause of the polyuria observed. In horses on chronic dexamethasone treatment for immune-mediated disorders, profound glucosuria (2–3 g/dl) may be observed and may lead to an osmotic diuresis in these patients. A transient diuresis or polyuria accompanies sedation with the α_2-adrenergic agonists xylazine and detomidine. Although these agents cause hyperglycemia and occasional glucosuria, a more likely mechanism for the transient polyuria is the existence of α_2-adrenoreceptors on collecting duct epithelial cells. Activation of these receptors is another mechanism by which ADH actions can be antagonized.

Supplemental Readings

Brown CM: Equine nephrology. *In* Grunsell CSG, Hill FWG, Raw M-E (eds): Veterinary Annual, issue 26. Bristol, Scientechnia, 1986, pp 1–16.
Roussel AJ, Carter GK: Polyuria and polydipsia. *In* Brown CM (ed.): Problems in Equine Medicine. Philadelphia, Lea & Febiger, 1989, pp 150–160.
Schott HC, Bayly WM, Reed SM, Brobst DF: Nephrogenic diabetes insipidus in sibling colts. J Vet Intern Med 7:68–72, 1993.

Hematuria

HAROLD C. SCHOTT II
East Lansing, Michigan

Hematuria can be the presenting complaint for a variety of disorders of the urinary tract. The problems causing hematuria can range from relatively minor disorders to more severe disease processes that may result in life-threatening hemorrhage. Hematuria throughout urination is consistent with hemorrhage from the kidneys, ureters, or bladder, whereas hematuria at the beginning or end of urination may be associated with lesions in the distal or proximal urethra, respectively. A thorough diagnostic evaluation including physical examination, rectal palpation, analyses of blood and urine, endoscopy, and ultrasonography is usually rewarding in establishing the source and cause of urinary tract hemorrhage.

CYSTITIS AND PYELONEPHRITIS

Urinary tract infection, although relatively uncommon in horses, may result in hematuria. With infection of the upper urinary tract, partial anorexia, weight loss, and fever may be additional presenting complaints, whereas horses with cystitis generally manifest stranguria or pollakiuria.

Diagnostic evaluation should include the list detailed earlier along with submission of a urine sample for bacterial culture. Occasionally, horses may have an anatomic bladder defect or bladder paralysis, which predisposes them to cystitis. Treatment consists of appropriate antimicrobial therapy as well as addressing predisposing causes (see Dysuria, p. 482, for further discussion).

UROLITHIASIS

The presence of uroliths at any level of the urinary tract may cause mucosal irritation and hemorrhage, resulting in hematuria. Typically, affected horses also show signs of renal colic or painful urination indicated by stranguria or pollakiuria, especially with uroliths in the bladder or urethra. Rectal examination, passage of a urinary catheter, cystoscopy, or ultrasonography are generally rewarding in establishing the diagnosis. Furthermore, urolithiasis can be accompanied by urinary tract infection, and thus all horses with urolithiasis should additionally be evaluated for infection. Successful treatment consists of appropriate antimicrobial therapy and surgical removal of the urethral or bladder stones, although recurrence is possible. Nephroliths and ureteroliths carry a more guarded prognosis, especially with bilateral disease resulting in chronic renal failure. Nephrectomy may be an effective treatment option in horses with unilateral disease (see Dysuria for further discussion).

URINARY TRACT NEOPLASIA

Neoplasia of the kidneys, ureters, bladder, and urethra may result in hematuria. Renal cell carcinoma and squamous cell carcinoma have been the neoplasms most frequently reported to affect the upper and lower urinary tract, respectively. Physical, rectal, laboratory, cystoscopic, and ultrasonographic examinations are usually rewarding in detecting the neoplasm. Treatment is usually unsuccessful unless a benign neoplasm can be removed by unilateral nephrectomy or a squamous cell carcinoma can be removed by partial resection of the bladder or penis. Neoplasms affecting the distal urethra, which are usually squamous cell carcinoma or sarcoid, may also be amenable to surgical resection in combination with local application of antineoplastic agents.

DRUG TOXICITY

Nephrotoxicity, particularly that resulting from administration of nonsteroidal anti-inflammatory drugs, especially phenylbutazone, may result in moderate to severe hematuria. The historical or current use of nephrotoxic medications supports this diagnosis, and discontinuation of the nephrotoxic agent and supportive care are the appropriate treatments.

URETHRAL DEFECTS

Although a recognized cause of hemospermia in stallions, defects or tears of the proximal urethra at the level of the ischial arch are a more recently described cause of hematuria in geldings. Because the defects are difficult to detect without use of high-resolution videoendoscopic equipment, it is likely that lesions may have been missed in previous reports of urethral bleeding. Consequently, hematuria has been attributed to urethritis or hemorrhage from "varicosities" of the urethral vasculature. Because the vasculature underlying the urethral mucosa becomes quite prominent when the urethra is distended with air during endoscopic examination, especially in the proximal urethra, it is easy to suspect that hemorrhage can arise from an apparent urethritis or urethral varicosity.

Urethral defects or tears typically result in hematuria at the end of urination, in association with urethral contraction. Affected horses generally void a normal volume of urine that is not discolored. At the end of urination, affected geldings have a series of urethral contractions that result in passage of squirts of bright red blood. Occasionally, a smaller amount of darker blood may be passed at the start of urination. In most instances, the condition does not appear painful or result in pollakiuria. Interestingly, the majority of affected geldings have been Quarterhorses or Quarterhorse crosses that have been free of other complaints. Treatment with antibiotics for a suspected cystitis or urethritis has routinely been unsuccessful, although hematuria has resolved spontaneously in some cases.

Examination of affected horses is often unremarkable. In comparison, horses with hematuria due to neoplasms involving the distal urethra or penis are usually presented with additional complaints such as pollakiuria, a foul odor to the sheath, or presence of a mass in the sheath or on the penis. With urethral defects, laboratory analysis of blood reveals normal renal function, although mild anemia can be an occasional finding. Urine samples collected in midstream or by bladder catheterization appear grossly normal. Urinalysis may have normal results or there may be an increased number of red blood cells on sediment examination, a finding that also results in a positive reagent strip result for blood. Bacterial culture of urine yields negative results.

The diagnosis is made via endoscopic examination of the urethra, during which a lesion is typically seen along the dorsocaudal aspect of the urethra at the level of the ischial arch (Fig. 1). With hematuria of several weeks' duration, the lesion appears as a fistula communicating with the vasculature of the corpus spongiosum penis, the cavernous vascular tissue surrounding the urethra. External palpation of the urethra in this area is usually unremarkable but can assist in localizing the lesion because external digital palpation can be seen via the endoscope as movements of the urethra.

Although the pathophysiology of this condition remains unclear, it has been speculated that the defect is the result of a "blowout" of the corpus spongiosum penis into the urethral lumen. Contraction of the bulbospongiosus muscle during ejaculation causes a dramatic increase in pressure in the corpus spongiosum penis, which is essentially a closed vascular space during ejaculation. The bulbospongiosus muscle also undergoes a series of contractions to empty the urethra of urine at the end of urination; thus, the defect into the urethra may develop by a similar mechanism in geldings. Once the lesion has been created, it is maintained by bleeding at the end of each urination, and the surrounding mucosa heals by formation of a fistula into the overlying vascular tissue. An explanation for the consistent location along the dorsocaudal aspect of the urethra at the level of the ischial arch has not been documented but may be related to the anatomy of the musculature supporting the base of the penis and an enlargement of the corpus spongiosum penis in this area. Furthermore, there is a narrowing of the lumen of the urethra at the distal extent of the ampullar portion of the urethra, which may also contribute to the location of the defects. An anatomic predisposition in Quarterhorses has not been documented but could be proposed, based on an apparent increased risk in this breed.

Because hematuria may resolve spontaneously in some affected geldings, no treatment may be initially required. If hematuria persists for more than a month or if significant anemia develops, a temporary subischial urethrotomy has been successful in a number of affected geldings. With sedation and epidural or local anesthesia, a vertical incision is made down to a catheter that has been placed in the urethra. The surgical wound requires several weeks to heal, and moderate hemorrhage from the corpus spongiosum penis is apparent for the first few days after surgery. Additional treatment consists of local wound care and prophylactic antibiotic treatment, typically a trimethoprim/sulfonamide combination, for 7 to 10 days. Hematuria should resolve within a week following this procedure. Treatment by incising into the corpus spongiosum penis but not into the urethral lumen has been successfully employed. This treatment option provides support for the "blowout" etiology and lessens the risk of urethral stricture formation.

IDIOPATHIC RENAL HEMATURIA AND RENAL VASCULAR ANOMALIES

Macroscopic hematuria, often accompanied by passage of blood clots and development of life-threatening anemia, has been observed in a limited number of adult horses. A similar condition of severe and recurrent renal hemorrhage, unassociated with trauma or other obvious causes of hemorrhage, has been described as idiopathic renal hematuria or benign essential hematuria in humans and dogs. In these species, hematuria is more commonly a unilateral than a bilateral problem, similar to that which has been observed in the few affected horses. The pathophysiology remains poorly understood, but in humans the macroscopic hematuria has been associated with immune-mediated glomerular damage caused by acute postinfectious glomerulonephritis, membranoproliferative glomerulonephritis, and IgA nephropathy or Berger's disease. In other instances, a vascular anomaly has been detected. Although hematuria has been recognized with systemic disease in horses, patients affected with idiopathic renal hematuria appear to have spontaneous, severe hematuria

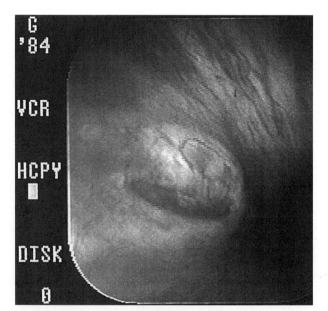

Figure 1. Urethral defect in a gelding that resulted in hematuria at the end of urination. Dorsocaudal aspect of urethra is to the left.

in the absence of other signs of disease. Urinary tract infection or lithiasis has not been detected, and the magnitude of hematuria has resulted in death or the need for repeated blood transfusions in several horses.

The diagnosis of idiopathic renal hematuria is made by exclusion of systemic disease, alterations in hemostasis, and other causes of hematuria. Physical examination may reveal tachycardia, tachypnea, and pale membranes consistent with acute blood loss. Rectal palpation may reveal an enlarged, irregular bladder owing to the presence of blood clots. Azotemia has not been detected, and urinalysis typically shows only hematuria and proteinuria. Endoscopic examination is important to document that hematuria is originating from the upper urinary tract. Blood clots can be seen exiting the ureters in affected horses. Endoscopy also helps determine whether hemorrhage is unilateral or bilateral. Repeated examinations may be required to answer the latter question. Ultrasonographic imaging may be within normal limits or may reveal loss of parenchymal detail (i.e., loss of the corticomedullary junction). Ultrasonographic imaging is necessary to rule out nephrolithiasis or ureterolithiasis and may occasionally reveal a distended vascular space or renal vascular anomaly as the cause of hematuria. Renal biopsy may assist in documenting immunologic glomerular injury, but the significance of such results is not well understood at this time.

Treatment for idiopathic hematuria consists of supportive care for acute blood loss, including blood transfusions. The condition may be self-limiting in some patients, and thus treatment is warranted. With severe and recurrent hematuria of unilateral renal origin or when a vascular anomaly is detected on ultrasonographic imaging, a nephrectomy may be indicated.

EXERCISE-ASSOCIATED HEMATURIA

Exercise is accompanied by increased filtration of red blood cells and protein across the glomerular barrier in a high percentage of human and equine athletes. Typically, the hematuria is microscopic, but occasionally gross discoloration of urine may be observed. Gross hematuria may more commonly be a consequence of bladder erosions, which may be traumatically induced by the abdominal contents pounding the bladder against the pelvis during exercise. Detection of focal bladder erosions or ulcers with a contrecoup distribution and a history of emptying the bladder immediately before the exercise bout are characteristic for this problem. A diagnosis of exercise-associated

hematuria should be one of exclusion after diagnostic evaluation has ruled out other causes of hematuria, such as presence of a cystolith.

PIGMENTURIA ASSOCIATED WITH SYSTEMIC DISEASE

With any systemic disease that may lead to alterations in hemostasis or vascular permeability, hematuria or hemoglobinuria may develop. Discolored urine has the potential to be accompanied by a degree of nephrotoxicity because of interaction of iron ions of the heme molecules with proximal tubular epithelial cells. With transient pigmenturia, as with exercise-associated hematuria, changes in renal function may not be apparent, but with more severe disease processes and hemolysis, acute renal failure may develop. In people, development of acute renal failure in association with diseases complicated by coagulopathies and disseminated intravascular coagulation has been termed the *hemolytic-uremic syndrome*. The syndrome is recognized more commonly in infants and children than in adults. A similar syndrome has been described in a limited number of horses. Similarly, hemolysis and hemoglobinuria may be recognized with liver disease or immune-mediated hemolytic anemias consequent to infection with *Streptococcus equi* or to drug treatments. Conditions accompanied by extensive rhabdomyolyis may also result in pigmenturia. Assessment of muscle enzyme activity in these cases is usually rewarding in establishing myoglobin as the most likely cause of pigmenturia.

Supplemental Readings

Behm RJ, Berg IE: Hematuria caused by renal medullary crest necrosis in a horse. Comp Cont Ed Pract Vet 9:698–703, 1987.
Fischer AT, Spier S, Carlson GP, Hackett RP: Neoplasia of the urinary bladder as a cause of hematuria. J Am Vet Med Assoc 186(12):1294–1296, 1985.
Kaufman AC, Barsanti JA, Selcer BA: Benign essential hematuria in dogs. Comp Cont Ed Pract Vet 16:1317–1323, 1994.
Lloyd KCK, Wheat JD, Ryan AM, Matthews M: Ulceration in the proximal portion of the urethra as a cause of hematuria in horses: Four cases (1978–1985). J Am Vet Med Assoc 194:1324–1326, 1989.
Morris CF, Robertson JL, Mann PC, Clark S, Divers TJ: Hemolytic uremic-like syndrome in two horses. J Am Vet Med Assoc 191:1453–1454, 1987.
Schott HC, Hines MT: Severe urinary tract hemorrhage in two horses [Letter to editor]. J Am Vet Med Assoc 204:1320, 1994.
Schott HC, Hodgson DR, Bayly WM: Haematuria, pigmenturia and proteinuria in exercising horses. Equine Vet J 27:67–72, 1995.
Schumacher J, Varner DD, Schmitz DG, Blanchard TL: Urethral defects in geldings with hematuria and stallions with hemospermia. Vet Surg 24:250–254, 1995.

Congenital Disorders of the Urinary Tract

HAROLD C. SCHOTT II
East Lansing, Michigan

JOHN K. PRINGLE
Charlottetown, Prince Edward Island

RENAL AGENESIS, HYPOPLASIA, AND DYSPLASIA

Renal agenesis may be unilateral or bilateral. Although unilateral anomalies have been more frequently described, they may simply reflect the incompatibility of bilateral agenesis with postnatal life. Unilateral defects may be incidental findings in otherwise healthy horses or may be detected during examination of the reproductive tract, because most are associated with anomalies of the latter system. Although there is no information to suggest a hereditary basis in horses, renal agenesis can be a familial disorder in other species, and thus it may be advisable to discourage repeated matings if this anomaly is detected.

Renal hypoplasia is diagnosed when one kidney is at least 50% smaller than normal or when the total renal mass is decreased by more than one third. The anomaly may be confused with renal dysplasia, the term used to describe disorganized development of renal tissue resulting from anomalous differentation, intrauterine ureteral obstruction, fetal viral infection, or exposure to teratogenic agents. Unilateral renal hypoplasia is usually accompanied by contralateral hypertrophy and normal renal function, whereas bilateral hypoplasia or dysplasia generally leads to chronic renal failure before 5 years of age.

POLYCYSTIC KIDNEY DISEASE

One or more renal cysts are occasionally discovered as incidental findings on necropsy examination. The cysts may arise from any portion of the nephron but are more commonly observed in the cortex than in the medulla. Renal cysts vary in size from microscopic to as large as the organ itself. Routinely, renal cysts have a clear to slightly opaque wall and a thin, clear fluid content. Polycystic kidney disease is a disorder in which numerous variably sized cysts are found throughout the cortex and medulla. Cysts of the bile duct and pancreas may also be observed with polycystic kidney disease, and both conditions have been described in stillbirths in many species. There are two major types of polycystic kidney disease in people: (1) a rare congenital or infantile form that may be found in stillborns and is inherited as an autosomal recessive trait; and (2) a more common adult form inherited as an autosomal dominant trait that leads to renal insufficiency in later life. In horses, the condition has been reported in stillborn foals as well as in a few adult horses. Although a genetic cause has also been proposed in some domestic animal species, patterns of inheritance have not been established.

VASCULAR ANOMALIES

Anomalies of the vascular supply to the equine kidneys are rare but may result in hematuria or ureteric obstruction and hydronephrosis. If an abnormality can be detected via ultrasonographic examination or if hematuria is observed from only one of the ureters during cystoscopic examination, unilateral nephrectomy may be a successful treatment option when azotemia is not apparent.

URETERAL AND BLADDER DEFECTS

Retroperitoneal accumulation of urine and uroperitoneum have been described in foals with ureteral and bladder defects. The cause of these defects is not known, but a smooth margin to the defects combined with a lack of appreciable inflammation suggests anomalous development rather than a traumatic etiology. Ureteral defects may be unilateral or bilateral but have been limited to the proximal one third of the ureter. Bladder defects are found in the dorsal or ventral bladder wall and are clinically indistinguishable from ruptured bladders, except perhaps during surgical repair. These defects have typically been detected during exploratory celiotomy after a diagnosis of uroperitoneum has been made. Ureteral catheterization and injection of methylene blue via a cystotomy may allow localization of ureteral defects. Surgical correction can be performed by suturing the ureteral defect around an indwelling catheter. Treatment of bladder defects is identical to that for bladder rupture (see page 494).

Anomalous fusion of the bladder to the inner umbilical ring may occur with absence of the urachus. This malformation precludes normal contraction and evacuation of the bladder, and a markedly enlarged bladder may develop. Surgical separation of the bladder from the umbilical ring may restore normal anatomic and functional integrity of the bladder.

ECTOPIC URETER

Ectopic ureter is a developmental anomaly in which a ureter terminates at a site other than the trigone of the bladder. The ectopic ureter may open into the urethra, vagina, or another part of the reproductive tract. Incontinence from birth in the absence of neurologic deficits is a hallmark of most horses with ectopic ureters. The condition has no apparent breed predilection and has been diagnosed more often in females than in males. It is unclear as to whether there is a true sex predilection or whether incontinence and perineal urine scalding are more easily recognized in females. Unless secondary complications such as urinary tract infection or hydronephrosis and pyelonephritis complicate the anomaly, there are usually no other clinical abnormalities, and growth is unaffected.

The aberrant openings of the ureters can be observed in females via vaginal speculum examination, in the case of entry into the genital tract, or by endoscopy if the ureters enter the bladder or urethra aberrantly (Fig. 1). Cystoscopic examination should focus on the neck of the bladder where, in normal horses, both ureter openings can be seen in the dorsal wall of the trigone area. To assist in localizing the aberrant openings, dyes such as indigo carmine (0.25 mg/kg IV) or sodium fluorescein (10 mg/kg IV) can be administered during the examination. Alternatively, contrast excretory urography can be used to diagnose ectopic ureter, but this technique may not be as helpful in localizing the site of entry of the aberrant ureter. Because both urinary tract infection and hydronephrosis are possible complications, further evaluation of affected horses should include urinalysis and urine culture.

Without surgical intervention, incontinence persists and hydronephrosis, if not already present, is likely to develop. With unilateral ectopic ureter, treatment options include unilateral nephrectomy or reimplantation of the ureter by ureterovesicular anastomosis. In a review of 11 cases of ectopic ureter, three of six horses treated by ureterovesicular anastomosis survived longer than 1 year, whereas all three horses treated by unilateral nephrectomy had a long-term survival. Bilateral ectopic ureters appear to carry a poorer prognosis, and surgical treatment is limited to ureterovesicular anastomosis.

RECTOURETHRAL AND RECTOVAGINAL FISTULAS

If the urorectal fold fails to completely separate the primitive hindgut from the urogenital sinus, a rectourethral fistula may be found in the colt or a rectovaginal fistula or a persistent cloaca may be found in the filly. These anomalies are rare in horses and, when present, are usually accompanied by atresia ani and other anomalies including agenesis of the coccygeal vertebrae and tail, scoliosis, adherence of the tail to the anal sphincter area, angular limb deformities, and microphthalmia. Evidence for a fistula is provided when fecal material is passed from the vagina or urethra. Some affected horses may be candidates for surgical correction of the defects, but they should not be used as breeding animals because these defects have a hereditary basis in other species.

PATENT URACHUS

The urachus is the conduit through which fetal urine passes from the bladder to the allantoic cavity. Normally, the urachus closes at the time of parturition, but incomplete closure is the most common malformation of the urinary bladder and it occurs more commonly in foals than in other domestic species. A greater than average length of partial torsion of the umbilical cord has been suggested to cause tension on the attachment of the umbilical cord to the body wall. The result is dilation of the urachus and subsequent failure to close at birth. With patent urachus, the umbilicus is moist from birth and urine leaks in drips or as a stream during micturition. It is important to distinguish a nonseptic patent urachus from infection of the umbilicus, which may also result in patent urachus within a few hours to days after birth. The former has been referred to as a congenital problem and the latter an acquired patent urachus, but both may be observed from the time of birth. Neither is a life-threatening condition but local sepsis is often accompanied by more severe illness, including septicemia or infection at other sites (commonly joints).

The congenital patent urachus has traditionally been

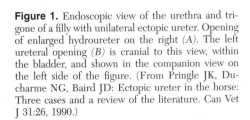

Figure 1. Endoscopic view of the urethra and trigone of a filly with unilateral ectopic ureter. Opening of enlarged hydroureter on the right (*A*). The left ureteral opening (*B*) is cranial to this view, within the bladder, and shown in the companion view on the left side of the figure. (From Pringle JK, Ducharme NG, Baird JD: Ectopic ureter in the horse: Three cases and a review of the literature. Can Vet J 31:26, 1990.)

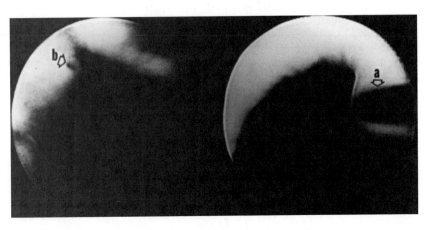

treated with frequent (two to four times daily) chemical cauterization with swabs dipped in a 90% phenol or a Lugol's iodine solution or with silver nitrate applicators. Because cauterizing agents desiccate and irritate tissue, predisposing it to infection, the rationale for this treatment approach has been questioned. Consequently, in the absence of apparent infection, no treatment may be specifically indicated but affected foals are routinely placed on prophylactic antibiotics. With an acquired patency accompanied by local infection or septicemia, broad-spectrum systemic antimicrobial therapy is indicated and resolution of the umbilical infection is accompanied by closure of the urachus. Chemical cauterization is contraindicated with local sepsis because it may lead to urachal rupture and uroperitoneum. If no decrease in urine leakage from the urachus is observed after a few days of medical therapy or if ultrasonographic examination reveals abnormalities of multiple structures within the umbilicus, surgical explora-tion and resection of the affected urachus and umbilical vessels are generally performed.

Supplemental Readings

Andrews FM, Rosol TJ, Kohn CW, Reed SM, DiBartola SP: Bilateral renal hypoplasia in four young horses. J Am Vet Med Assoc 189:209–212, 1986.

Blikslager AT, Green EM: Ectopic ureters in horses. Comp Cont Ed Pract Vet 14:802–807, 1992.

Divers TJ, Byars TD, Spirito M: Correction of bilateral ureteral defects in a foal. J Am Vet Med Assoc 192:384–386, 1988.

Pringle JK, Ducharme NG, Baird JD: Ectopic ureter in the horse: Three cases and a review of the literature. Can Vet J 31:26–30, 1990.

Ramsay G, Rothwell TLW, Gibson KT, Moore JD, Rose RJ: Polycystic kidneys in an adult horse. Equine Vet J 19:243–244, 1987.

Sullins KE, McIlwraith CW, Yovich JV, MacHarg MA, Fessler J: Ectopic ureter managed by unilateral nephrectomy in two female horses. Equine Vet J 20:463–466, 1988.

Zicker SC, Marty GD, Carlson GP, Madigan JE, Smith JM, Goetzman BW: Bilateral renal dysplasia with nephron hypoplasia in a foal. J Am Vet Med Assoc 196:2001–2005, 1990.

Miscellaneous Disorders of the Urinary Tract

JOHN K. PRINGLE
Charlottetown, Prince Edward Island

HAROLD C. SCHOTT II
East Lansing, Michigan

UROPERITONEUM

Uroperitoneum may accompany a number of disorders that result in disruption of the urinary tract. In addition to the ureteral and bladder defects described earlier, trau-matic bladder rupture may occur in either the mare or foal during parturition. Although the classic bladder rupture involves traumatic disruption of a full bladder during delivery of a male foal (predisposed by a longer urethra), the condition has also been observed in fillies and foals with a patent urachus. On occasion, septic omphalitis may also lead to urachal leakage or rupture. If this complication occurs within the abdomen, signs compatible with uroperi-toneum develop. If urine also leaks into the abdominal musculature and subcutaneous tissues, a rather rapid onset of swelling of the ventral abdominal wall may be observed. There also have been reports of redevelopment of uroperi-toneum in the months, or even years, following prior blad-der surgery.

Clinical Signs

Clinical signs of uroperitoneum include tachycardia, tachypnea, and progressive abdominal distension. As the metabolic alterations associated with uroperitoneum ensue, nonspecific signs including inappetence, depression, and colic or diarrhea may be observed. In an occasional foal, accumulation of a large volume of urine in the abdomen may lead to severe respiratory embarrassment. Despite presence of a leak in the collecting system, affected foals may void normal streams of urine, but they more often repeatedly assume the stance for urination and appear to strain. The latter signs may be confused with colic.

Laboratory Findings

Uroperitoneum leads to a number of clinicopathologic abnormalities including azotemia (postrenal), hypona-tremia, hypochloremia, hyperkalemia, and variable changes in acid-base status. Because the peritoneum allows fairly free exchange of uncharged or small molecules, azotemia and electrolyte abnormalities develop as urine, which is poor in Na^+ and Cl^- but rich in K^+, accumulates in the abdomen and effectively expands extracellular fluid vol-ume. It is important to assess the severity of metabolic alterations because hyperkalemia can lead to cardiac ar-rhythmias, especially when combined with the effects of general anesthetics such as halothane.

Diagnosis

A diagnosis of uroperitoneum should be suspected on the basis of signalment and clinical signs; however, it is best confirmed by either demonstration of a defect in the bladder wall or urachus or documentation of the presence of urine in the abdomen. The former can be pursued via transurethral contrast radiographic techniques or, under field conditions, auscultation of air escaping into the abdominal cavity while air is injected through a bladder catheter. More commonly, the diagnosis is confirmed by demonstrating a two-fold or greater increase in creatinine concentration in abdominal fluid, in comparison with serum. Measurement of the abdominal fluid-to-serum creatinine ratio is more accurate than the same ratio for urea nitrogen because urea, being a small uncharged molecule, is more freely permeable across the peritoneal membrane. When uroperitoneum is accompanied by signs of septicemia in neonatal foals, it is important to realize that external palpation is an insensitive method to detect umbilical problems in foals, in comparison with other large animal species. In suspect cases, ultrasonographic examination is helpful in detecting the presence of free abdominal fluid as well as evidence of infection of umbilical structures.

Treatment

Treatment of uroperitoneum involves surgical closure of the tear or defect. Before surgery, however, supportive care including intravenous administration of several liters of 0.9% NaC1 is often necessary to correct metabolic alterations. If abdominal distension is a significant problem, uroperitoneum can be temporarily corrected via drainage with a teat cannula or small-diameter (12–16 French) trocar catheter. Thus, surgical correction should be considered an elective procedure to be performed after metabolic alterations have been addressed. In combination with surgery, placement of a temporary indwelling bladder catheter, via the urethra, may also be of benefit, especially when the surgical repair is incomplete or there is a greater risk of having complications owing to the size of the tear or condition of the bladder wall. Broad-spectrum antibiotic treatment, such as intravenous penicillin G and an aminoglycoside, are recommended for 7 to 10 days following surgical repair. The prognosis is usually favorable as long as signs of sepsis are not apparent.

URINARY INCONTINENCE

Incontinence has been described with a number of disorders in horses including cystitis, urolithiasis, bladder paralysis, ectopic ureter, vaginal injuries or polyps, and hypoestrogenism. Horses with incontinence may have intermittent or continuous dribbling of urine unrelated to micturition. Mares tend to be at increased risk owing to the combination of a short urethra with an increased likelihood of acquiring lower urinary tract abnormalities during breeding or parturition. In mares, urine scalding and dermatitis of the medial aspects of both hind legs may accompany incontinence, whereas soiling of the dorsal aspect of the hind legs and ventral abdomen can be observed in males. In both sexes a strong urine odor may be present. Incontinence is typically exacerbated by factors that increase intra-abdominal pressure; in fact, it is often first observed during exercise or in association with coughing. Occasionally, owners confuse the frequent urination observed during estrus with incontinence. Although mares in estrus may accumulate urine crystals on the perineal area, their bladders are usually small rather than distended.

Etiology

Cystitis may be a primary cause of incontinence in some horses but more often is a secondary problem consequent to incontinence or bladder paralysis. Regardless of the cause of incontinence, urinalysis and bacterial culture of urine should be performed in all cases to assist in selection of appropriate antimicrobial treatment. Urolithiasis can cause signs of incontinence in some affected horses. However, it is not a predictable feature of the disease, whereas persistent hematuria, often in the absence of inflammatory cells in urine, is the major clinical abnormality.

Bladder paralysis in the face of ongoing urine production leads to bladder distension and overflow of urine. Horses with incontinence due to bladder paralysis may have other neurologic signs including hindlimb ataxia and atrophy or loss of tail or anal tone. When trauma, equine protozoal myelitis (EPM), equine herpesvirus 1 (EHV-1) myeloencephalitis, or aberrant parasite migration cause spinal cord disease cranial to the sacral region (with sacral spinal cord segments remaining intact), upper motor neuron dysfunction results in a spastic or automatic bladder. Conscious voiding is lost, but the detrusor muscle can be activated once the bladder is filled beyond a threshold volume. Rectal palpation reveals a moderately enlarged bladder. When these neurologic diseases or others, including cauda equina neuritis, sorghum or Sudan grass toxicity, or sacral fractures, involve the lower motor neurons of the pelvic region, detrusor function is lost and the bladder becomes greatly distended and atonic, yet can easily be expressed via rectal manipulation. Incomplete emptying or complete paralysis may lead to accumulation of urine sediment in the ventral aspect of the bladder, which may lead to mucosal irritation and further stretching of the distended bladder. In geldings, excessive sediment accumulation and bladder paralysis appear to occasionally develop without associated neurologic deficits. This condition has been termed *sabulous urolithiasis* and its recognition has led to the suggestion of a myogenic form of bladder paralysis. The excessive sediment in affected horses can also be confused with a mass in the bladder or bladder wall.

Vaginal malformations, such as postfoaling strictures or polyps, have been associated with incontinence, possibly by impairing function of the external urethral sphincter, or by causing urine accumulation in the vagina. Whereas hypoestrogenism is a common cause of incontinence in companion animals, there has been only one well-documented case of estrogen-responsive incontinence in an aged pony mare. Therefore, other causes of incontinence should be ruled out before considering this diagnosis.

Evaluation

Horses with urinary incontinence can be evaluated objectively by cystometrography and urethral pressure profilometry. These diagnostic tests measure intravesicular pressure and urethral pressures, respectively. Although comparison of these pressures in horses with bladder paralysis to those of normal horses allows documentation of the nature of the bladder paralysis, the prognostic value of these pressure measurements appears limited at this time.

Treatment

Specific treatment of incontinence is dependent on the underlying cause. Incontinence attributable to cystitis, urolithiasis, ectopic ureter, or vaginal malformations can be alleviated by appropriate antibiotic treatment and corrective surgery. Treatment for specific neurologic diseases should also be instituted when such diagnoses are established. With incontinence due to bladder paralysis, regardless of whether or not it is associated with a specific neurologic disease, repeated manual expression or catheterization to empty the bladder may be of benefit. This procedure is performed in an attempt to allow recovery of detrusor function and is most helpful in acutely affected cases. Surgical removal of the sabulous material in geldings via perineal urethrotomy or cystotomy has also been attempted. Results have generally been poor, and cystotomy is no longer recommended because of difficulties in evacuating the material without contaminating the peritoneal cavity. Perineal urethrotomy, combined with irrigation of large volumes of fluid, seems to be the most effective way of removing this material. However, improvement is often only temporary, and surgery is not routinely performed on these cases.

In horses with bladder distension in which some detrusor activity is apparent, medical treatment may be of benefit. The α-adrenergic antagonist phenoxybenzamine may be given (0.7 mg/kg p.o. q6h) to decrease urethral tone, thereby facilitating bladder emptying. Bethanechol chloride is a parasympathomimetic agent that has been used to stimulate detrusor muscle activity. The dose ranges from 0.025 to 0.075 mg/kg SC or 0.2 to 0.4 mg/kg p.o. t.i.d. or q.i.d. Because bethanecol treatment produces varying results, clinicians should start with the lowest dose and subsequently increase the amount administered if improvement is not apparent in 24 to 48 hours.

Antibiotics are a common adjunct treatment for incontinence and are especially important when indwelling or regular catheterization is used to combat persistent distension. Incontinence due to hypoestrogenism has been successfully treated with 2 mg of estradiol cypionate (ECP) every other day in one pony mare. Because withdrawal of the ECP treatment resulted in recurrence of incontinence within a few days, responsive horses may need prolonged treatment.

Prognosis

The prognosis for recovery of bladder function in horses with incontinence is generally poor, unless the problem can be attributed to a specific neurologic disease such as EHV-1 or EPM. Because of the potential return of detrusor muscle function and automaticity, incontinence caused by upper motor neuron disease carries, in theory, a more favorable prognosis than that caused by lower motor neuron deficits or myogenic dysfunction. In practice, all forms of incontinence associated with bladder paralysis carry a guarded to poor prognosis for improvement. Consequently, owners of affected horses should be advised to clean the perineal area daily to prevent excessive urine scalding. Because bladder distension predisposes to sabulous urolithiasis and ascending urinary tract infection, it is advisable to maintain affected horses on an intermittent or continuous antibiotic prophylaxis. Once-daily administration of a sulfonamide antibiotic preparation, which is concentrated in urine, may be a practical and economic approach, unless a resistant pathogen is isolated on bacterial culture of a urine sample.

RENAL TUBULAR ACIDOSIS

Renal tubular acidosis (RTA) is an uncommon disorder of renal tubular acidification of urine that has been described in a limited number of horses. Two types of RTA occur in horses: Type 1 is failure of distal tubular epithelial cells to secrete hydrogen ions against a pH gradient; and type 2 is wasting of bicarbonate by proximal tubular cells. Inciting causes of the tubular defects may include autoimmune diseases, drug reactions, pyelonephritis, or obstructive disorders. Although a hereditary form has been suggested, a foal produced from a mare and stallion affected with type 1 RTA did not have renal tubular acidosis.

Clinical signs are related to the degree of metabolic acidosis associated with the disorder and can range from mild weakness and anorexia to profound depression and ataxia. Other complaints may include weight loss or mild abdominal pain. The disorder may also be detected as an incidental laboratory finding on examination for other problems.

Clinicopathologic evaluation characteristically reveals hyperchloremia (up to 120 mEq/L) and metabolic acidosis (blood pH as low as 7.0 with a HCO_3^- concentration of 7 to 10 mEq/L). Hypokalemia may also be present. Urine usually remains alkaline despite acidemia, indicative of an inability to retain HCO_3^-. Replacement of lost HCO_3^-, in part by chloride ions, leads to hyperchloremia. An important diagnostic criterion for RTA is recurrence of the metabolic derangements after withdrawal of therapy.

Both types of RTA affecting horses appear to resolve with supportive therapy including intravenous fluids supplemented with sodium bicarbonate to correct the base deficit. Potassium chloride may also be added to the fluids or administered via nasogastric intubation to replace potassium deficits. The amount of HCO_3^- to administer is calculated by the formula:

$$0.3 \times [BW\ (kg)] \times [base\ deficit]$$

Once the metabolic acidosis has been corrected, the horse can be managed successfully with oral supplementation of sodium bicarbonate (baking soda) at 150 g b.i.d. to t.i.d. Bicarbonate therapy may need to be continued for an extended period (12–24 months) or for the life of the horse, depending on persistence of the tubular defect. With type 2 RTA, massive HCO_3^- wasting is less responsive to bicarbonate supplementation. In people, thiazide diuretics may be administered to increase HCO_3^- reabsorption in the distal tubules, but such treatment has not been attempted in horses.

NEOPLASIA OF THE URINARY TRACT

Neoplasia is a rare disorder of the equine urinary tract. However, because it may affect all levels of the urinary tract, presenting complaints vary from anorexia and weight loss to hematuria with or without stranguria. Lesions of the distal penis may result in a swollen or malodorous sheath, in addition to producing dysuria.

The most common neoplasm affecting the equine kidney is renal cell carcinoma. This benign tumor is most effectively treated by unilateral nephrectomy, provided that function of the contralateral kidney is normal. Other neoplastic disorders of the upper urinary tract include renal adenocarcinoma, nephroblastoma, or metastatic lymphoma or melanoma. These may be suspected when an enlarged kidney is palpated on rectal examination.

The most common neoplasm affecting the bladder and urethra is squamous cell carcinoma. Transitional cell carcinoma, leiomyoma, and leiomyosarcoma have also been described as causes of hematuria and stranguria. Although surgical resection of the affected portion of the bladder or penis may be curative, it only results in temporary improvement if the neoplastic tissue cannot be completely excised. The penis and prepuce may also be affected by sarcoids or melanomas. Treatment of these neoplasms is discussed elsewhere in this text (see pages 370, 372, and 399).

Supplemental Readings

Brown PJ, Holt PE: Primary renal cell carcinoma in four horses. Equine Vet J 17:473–477, 1985.

Fischer AT, Spier S, Carlson GP, Hackett RP: Neoplasia of the urinary bladder as a cause of hematuria. J Am Vet Med Assoc 186:1294–1296, 1985.

Hackett RP: Rupture of the urinary bladder in neonatal foals. Comp Cont Ed Pract Vet 6:S488–S494, 1984.

Holt PE, Mair TS: Ten cases of bladder paralysis associated with sabulous urolithiasis in horses. Vet Rec 127:108–110, 1990.

Johnson PJ, Goetz TE, Baker GJ, Foreman JH: Treatment of two mares with obstructive (vaginal) urinary outflow incontinence. J Am Vet Med Assoc 191:973–975, 1987.

Madison JB: Estrogen-responsive urinary incontinence in an aged pony mare. Comp Cont Ed Pract Vet 6:S390–S392, 1984.

Reef VB, Collatos C, Spencer PA, Orsini JA, Sepesy LM: Clinical, ultrasonographic, and surgical findings in foals with umbilical remnant infections. J Am Vet Med Assoc 195:69–72, 1989.

Richardson DW, Kohn CW: Uroperitoneum in the foal. J Am Vet Med Assoc 182:267–271, 1983.

Trotter GW, Miller D, Parks A, Arden W: Type II renal tubular acidosis in a mare. J Am Vet Med Assoc 188:1050–1051, 1986.

Ziemer EL, Parker HR, Carlson GP, Smith BP: Clinical features and treatment of renal tubular acidosis in two horses. J Am Vet Med Assoc 190:294–296, 1987.

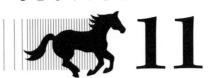
THE ENDOCRINE SYSTEM

Edited by Noël Dybdal

Pituitary Pars Intermedia Dysfunction (Equine Cushing's-like Disease)

NOËL DYBDAL
San Francisco, California

So-called adenomas of the pituitary pars intermedia in the horse, which are associated with the clinical syndrome of equine Cushing's-like disease (ECD), were first described more than 40 years ago. Although this early description of the enlarged pars intermedia as an adenoma has been widely embraced, it has now been shown that the condition actually results from loss of normal inhibitory control. This results in the classic endocrine processes of hypertrophy, hyperplasia, and, rarely, eventual adenoma formation.

The initial lesion is not in the pituitary. Pituitary enlargement begins when, for reasons unknown at this time, there is a decrease or loss of the neurotransmitter dopamine in the innervation of the pars intermedia. The function of melanotropes in the pars intermedia is normally inhibited when dopamine released from nerve endings extending from the hypothalamus activates type 2 dopaminergic receptors. Loss of inhibition is followed by increased synthesis and secretion of the proopiomelanocortin (POMC)-derived peptides. In the melanocyte, the POMC-derived peptides are primarily α-melanophore-stimulating hormone (MSH) and β-endorphin (END). Over time there is hypertrophy and hyperplasia of the pars intermedia resulting from this loss of normal dopaminergic inhibition. In most cases of ECD the pars intermedia is enlarged because of hypertrophy and hyperplasia, a physiologic response that becomes pathologic. In some cases, the process may progress to the point that adenomas develop, but this late event is the exception rather than the rule.

In ECD, the hyperplasia of melanotropes results in a dramatic increase in POMC synthesis with release of large amounts of α-MSH- and β-END-related peptides together with comparatively small and inconsistent amounts of adrenocorticotrophic hormone (ACTH). The end result of this increase in secretion of POMC-derived peptides is a slight elevation in plasma corticosteroid concentrations but, more importantly, the loss of the circadian pattern of corticosteroid secretion. Adrenocortical hypertrophy and hyperplasia are present in a large percentage of horses with ECD; however, resting plasma cortisol levels are rarely elevated and response to ACTH stimulation is rarely abnormal. The alteration in POMC-derived hormones contributes to adrenal dysfunction by at least two mechanisms. First, the release of ACTH in ECD, although small compared to that of the other POMC-derived peptides, is still much larger than that observed in normal horses and is sufficient to stimulate adrenal steroidogenesis. Second, other POMC-derived peptides can potentiate the actions of ACTH; MSH- and β-END-related peptides produce a six-fold increase in the steroidogenic properties of ACTH. Therefore a relatively small increase in ACTH levels, coupled with a large increase in potentiating peptides (e.g., MSH and beta-END), contributes to melanotrope-mediated adrenal dysfunction.

Two observations are difficult to understand and are somewhat paradoxical. First, many horses with adrenocortical enlargement exhibit a normal response to administration of exogenous ACTH (ACTH stimulation test). Second, a small number of horses with ECD do not have adrenocortical enlargement despite elevations of the POMC-derived peptides. There is no significant correlation between pituitary and adrenal weight in horses with ECD.

CLINICAL SIGNS

At the time of diagnosis, the average age of horses with ECD is 20 years, with a range from 7 to 42 years. The majority of horses (>85%) are older than 15 years of age at the time of diagnosis. A gender or breed predilection is not apparent in horses, but ponies have a very high incidence of the disease after the age of 15 years.

The clinical signs most consistently observed are hirsutism and abnormal hair coat shedding patterns, polyuria, polydipsia, and hyperhidrosis. Periodontal abscesses, laminitis, sinusitis, sole abscesses, and pneumonia are also seen with frequency in horses with ECD.

The most commonly recognized clinical sign is hirsutism. The pathogenesis of hirsutism is unknown. It does not appear to be the result of increased adrenal androgen production or hypothalamic compression resulting from pituitary enlargement. Hirsutism develops months to years after pituitary pars intermedia dysfunction has actually begun. The long, thick, frequently curly, hair coat is often preceded by years of subtle coat variations including retention of sparse long hair in the jugular groove of the neck or on the legs for an extended time following shedding in the spring. Some horses with early ECD develop transient alopecia when shedding, which is most commonly confined to the head. In some cases, the only sign of hirsutism is a very dense, impressive winter coat that comes in slightly earlier and sheds out slightly later or slower than the winter coats of stablemates kept under similar conditions.

Polyuria and polydipsia are common in horses with ECD. These related conditions are not solely the result of hypercortisolism, which has been suggested in the literature. The multifactorial etiology of these conditions has not been systematically investigated in the ECD horse. The complex pathogenesis probably includes a decrease in antidiuretic hormone production owing to damage of the pars nervosa by the enlarged pars intermedia, coupled with osmotic diuresis resulting from hyperglycemia, which is usually present in ECD horses with polyuria and polydipsia. Cortisol is also reported to cause an increase in glomerular filtration rate. The primary cortisol disruption in the ECD horse is loss of circadian rhythmicity (leading to increased 24-hour cortisol secretion), but there is no significant increase in plasma cortisol concentration at any time and thus it is difficult to know if there is a cortisol-mediated effect on glomerular filtration rate (GFR).

Hyperhidrosis is present intermittently in many horses with ECD. The mechanism of this dysfunction has not been determined, but it does represent a management challenge. In hirsute ECD-affected horses with hyperhidrosis, hair must be clipped over the body so that horses do not stand with wet coats for long periods of time. Appropriate blanketing must be provided, particularly in the winter. Occasional ECD-affected horses have intermittent problems with anhidrosis. The mechanism is not known, but these horses should be kept cool by sponging or showering, if environmental conditions necessitate.

The presenting complaint for horses with ECD is frequently not directly related to the pituitary dysfunction. Evidence to suggest pituitary dysfunction is often revealed by careful history taking and physical examination. Presentation of horses with ECD for weight loss or debilitation is common. These horses can generally be divided into two groups. In the first, debilitated horses have severe gastrointestinal parasitism and dental abnormalities, including severe wavemouth, excessive dental points, and missing teeth with concomitant overgrowth of opposing teeth. The horses in this group frequently respond very well to deworming, dentistry, and appropriate diet. In the second, debilitated animals have severe intercurrent disease problems, which frequently respond poorly to therapy. Horses with ECD without intercurrent nutritional or disease problems generally maintain adequate body weight or are overweight. Decreased muscle mass and tone can give an appearance of decreased weight even in horses carrying excess body fat, as evidenced by bulges over the eyes.

EVALUATION OF PARS INTERMEDIA FUNCTION

Clinical evaluation should include, in addition to thorough history-taking and physical examination, a complete blood count (CBC), clinical chemistry panel, and urinalysis. Generally, if there are no intercurrent disease problems, CBC and chemistry test results are within normal ranges. A relative neutrophila and lymphopenia may be present in some cases. If there is a clinical history of abnormal hair shedding patterns, polyuria, polydipsia, laminitis without clear cause, hyperglycemia, or glucosuria, further testing is indicated. The overnight dexamethasone suppression test is safe and efficient (Table 1). In horses with hyperglycemia, insulin concentration should be evaluated together with measurement of blood glucose. If plasma insulin concentration is high in the presence of a persistently elevated blood glucose concentration, a presumptive diagnosis of ECD can be made. If plasma insulin concentration is low in the presence of a persistently elevated blood glucose concentration, the differential diagnoses should include

TABLE 1. DEXAMETHASONE SUPPRESSION TEST

Overnight protocol—Begin test between 4 and 6 PM

1. Draw pre-dexamethasone blood sample between 4 and 6 PM
2. Administer dexamethasone, 40 µg/kg (2 mg/100 lbs) intramuscularly
3. Draw post-dexamethasone blood sample between 10 AM and noon the following day (approximately 19 hours after dexamethasone administration).

Interpretation of results—Normal horses have a pre-dexamethasone plasma cortisol concentration >2 µg/dl (20 ng/ml) and post-dexamethasone plasma cortisol concentration of ≤1 µg/dl (10 ng/ml).

Any higher post-dexamethasone concentration is diagnostic of ECD. Results must not be interpreted by evaluating the percentage change in cortisol concentration following dexamethasone administration.

Before performing the test, check with the clinical laboratory regarding preferred methods of sample handling.

ECD with secondary pancreatic β cell "burnout" or primary pancreatic disease. The latter is very rare and usually is a result of abscess or damage resulting from strongyle migration. Measurement of any plasma hormone concentration such as ACTH, MSH, β-endorphin, or cortisol at a single point is not a recommended approach to confirmation of a diagnosis of ECD. Basing a diagnosis of any endocrine disorder on a single measurement leads to a high rate of both false-negative and false-positive results.

TREATMENT

All ECD-affected horses must be managed with excellent husbandry practices. Deworming, particularly if the horse is kept in a group or allowed to graze a common pasture, must be done at least every 8 weeks because these horses appear to be severely compromised in their natural immunity to gastrointestinal parasites. Teeth should be checked at least every 6 months or more frequently if chronic dental problems dictate. A routine vaccination program is recommended. The author has not seen clinical evidence of dysfunction in ability to mount a humoral immune response. If the animal is hirsute, regular clipping of the hair over the body is recommended, even in the winter. Appropriate blanketing and protection from the elements must be provided. A higher incidence of pneumonia is found in unclipped ECD horses than in clipped ECD horses.

These horses should not be allowed to become obese. Conversely, if they are poor keepers, their calorie intake can be increased by adding vegetable oil and rice bran to their diet. Older horses can often benefit from being fed a pelleted or meal-type feed, with hay provided only for entertainment. Care should be taken with grain.

Even minor sole abscesses should be treated as potentially life-threatening and approached aggressively. Periodic CBC and chemistry evaluations are recommended to ensure no significant change in the horse's metabolic state. Owners can also regularly monitor glucose status by use of urine glucose dipsticks.

In the ECD-affected horse in which CBC and chemistry test results are within normal limits, and there is no evidence of chronic or recurrent laminitis, sole abscesses, intercurrent infection or, decreased ability to perform, no specific medical treatment is recommended. In the ECD-affected horse in which significant metabolic abnormalities are present or clinical signs indicate serious complications, the treatment of choice is pergolide mesylate,* a type-2 dopaminergic receptor agonist. The melanotrope possesses type-2 dopaminergic receptors and is highly responsive to this drug. Pergolide has no activity at type-1 dopaminergic receptors and thus does not affect cells with these receptors, such as the vascular endothelium of the feet. Although controlled dose range finding trials have not been performed to establish the correct dose in the horse with ECD, there is substantial anecdotal evidence to support the use of 0.5 to 2 mg per day per adult horse. Horses are

generally started at 0.5 mg/day, and the horse is reassessed at 4 to 8 weeks by means of the dexamethasone suppression test and measurement of blood glucose concentration if hyperglycemia was pre-existing in the horse. If these parameters are normal, the horse is maintained for life on pergolide. If the parameters are not normal, the dose is increased in 0.25 mg increments with periodic reassessment of dexamethasone suppression and blood glucose concentration. The majority of horses respond to doses in the 0.75 to 1.25 mg/horse range. Clinical improvement is usually seen within 6 weeks and includes shedding of the abnormal hair coat. Attempts to find the lowest effective dose are important for at least two reasons. The drug is expensive and, because it is replacement therapy for dopamine in the pituitary, it must be given for the life of the horse. The loss of dopamine in horses with ECD may be considered somewhat analogous to the loss of dopamine that occurs with Parkinson's disease in humans. Parkinsonian patients eventually become resistant to dopamine therapy. It is not known if resistance may arise with time in horses with ECD, but minimizing the dose of pergolide may help to delay the onset of resistance and allow the option of attempting to override resistance by increasing the dose.

Cyproheptidine has also been used to treat horses with ECD primarily because of its anti-serotonin effects. Although there have been anecdotal reports from owners and veterinarians of clinical improvement in horses with ECD, several controlled treatment trials at the University of California, Davis have yielded inconsistent evidence of a therapeutic benefit of this drug. Serotonin appears to play little if any role in the pathogenesis of ECD. These observations taken together suggest that if cyproheptidine is functional in the treatment of ECD, its effect is indirect, possibly at some peripheral target. The recommended dose is 0.25 mg/kg per day given once in the morning. No undesirable side effects have been reported. The margin of safety is high; the recommended dose has safely been doubled and given twice daily in several cases.

Further investigation into the pathogenesis of ECD may lead to additional therapeutic approaches in the future. At this time, further investigation into the appropriate use of pergolide and possible mechanism of action of cyproheptidine also seems warranted.

Supplemental Readings

Beech J: Tumors of the pituitary gland (pars intermedia). *In* Robinson NE (ed): Current Therapy in Equine Medicine, ed 2. Philadelphia, WB Saunders, pp 182–185.

Dybdal NO: Endocrine disorders. *In* Smith BP (ed): Large Animal Internal Medicine, ed 2. St. Louis, MO, C.V. Mosby, 1996, pp 1296–1306.

Dybdal NO, Hargreaves KH, Madigan JE, Gribble DH, Kennedy PC, Stabenfeldt GH: Diagnostic testing for pituitary pars intermedia dysfunction in horses. J Am Vet Med Assoc 204:627–632, 1994.

Millington WR, Dybdal NO, Dawson R, Manzini C, Mueller GP: Equine Cushing's disease: Differential regulation of β-endorphin processing in tumors of the intermediate pituitary. Endocrinology 123:1598–1604, 1988.

Orth DN, Holscher MA, Wilson MG, Nicholson WE, Plue RE, Mount CD: Equine Cushing's disease: Plasma immunoreactive proopiolipomelanocortin peptide and cortisol levels basally and in response to diagnostic tests. Endocrinology 110:1430–1441, 1982.

---

*Permax, Athena Neurosciences, South San Francisco, CA

Thyroid Disease (Dysfunction)

NAT T. MESSER IV
Columbia, Missouri

Thyroid dysfunction in horses is an uncommon and poorly understood endocrine abnormality that has been associated with various clinical disorders. Hypothyroidism accounts for the majority of cases seen in horses. Primary hypothyroidism is due to inadequate production of thyroxine (T_4) or triiodothyronine (T_3) from the thyroid gland. Thyroid dysfunction also occurs because of suppression of thyroid-stimulating hormone (TSH) release or inadequate conversion of T_4 to T_3 in peripheral tissues caused by certain nonthyroidal factors. Phenylbutazone administration, high-energy diets, high-protein diets, diets high in zinc and copper, glucocorticoid administration, food deprivation, and ingestion of endophyte-infected fescue grass have all been shown to cause low levels of thyroid hormones in euthyroid horses. With the latter types of thyroid dysfunction, the thyroid gland itself is normal and capable of responding to stimulation with either TSH or thyrotropin-releasing hormone (TRH). Most cases of apparent thyroid dysfunction are diagnosed on the basis of simply detecting low resting levels of T_4 or T_3 in serum. Stimulation tests, using either TSH or TRH, are used infrequently in horses because of the expense and limited availability of the stimulating hormones. Validated assays for equine TSH are not readily available for routine testing. For these reasons, naturally occurring thyroid dysfunction in adult horses has been difficult to characterize.

CLINICAL SIGNS

Inadequate levels of thyroid hormones induced by surgical thyroidectomy in horses are reported to result in retarded growth; increased sensitivity to cold; delayed shedding of the hair coat; edema in the hind legs; a coarse, thickened appearance of the face; a decrease in feed consumption and decrease in body weight gains. The clinical signs caused by surgical thyroidectomy are considerably different from those typically associated with hypothyroidism in clinical practice (e.g., obesity, "cresty" necks, and chronic laminitis). Although horses with these clinical signs may have low resting levels of T_4 or T_3, careful evaluation of the endocrine system may reveal other endocrine abnormalities that account for the thyroid dysfunction, such as high circulating levels of cortisol owing to pituitary pars intermedia dysfunction (see page 499). Further evaluation of the history may indicate the presence of nonthyroidal factors that cause low thyroid hormone levels.

In adult horses, hypothyroidism has been associated with alopecia, anhidrosis, episodic rhabdomyolysis, exercise intolerance, laminitis, and infertility in mares. In most cases, the diagnosis was based on measurement of resting levels of T_4 or T_3, occasionally combined with administration of TSH or TRH. It seems as though many horses receive thyroid hormone supplementation for such problems, despite what appears to be a low incidence of primary hypothyroidism in horses. The effects of thyroid supplementation in euthyroid horses have yet to be determined and supplementation should therefore be used with caution. Such supplementation may compound the problem in horses with low thyroid hormone levels due to nonthyroidal factors.

In foals, hypothyroidism is manifested as two entities. One manifestation of hypothyroidism in neonatal foals is that of a hypometabolic state characterized by incoordination, poor suckling and righting reflexes, hypothermia, and goiter presumably caused by intake of excessive iodine or goitrogenic plants by the dam during gestation and accompanied by low serum levels of thyroid hormone. Another manifestation occurs as a geographically specific syndrome in western Canada in foals that have low levels of thyroid hormones and fail to respond to TSH stimulation. These foals have a consistent pattern of musculoskeletal lesions including mandibular prognathia, flexural deformities of the front legs, ruptured digital extensor tendons, and incompletely ossified carpal and tarsal bones. In most reported cases or studies in foals, hypothyroidism has been based on measurement of serum levels of T_4 or T_3, occasionally along with either TSH or TRH stimulation. It is also possible that certain developmental abnormalities, such as disturbances in endochondral ossification, may become clinically apparent weeks or months subsequent to the period of time during which serum levels of thyroid hormones are low.

EVALUATION OF THYROID DYSFUNCTION

Measurements of T_4 and T_3 and the response to TSH and TRH stimulation tests are the current means of diagnosing equine thyroid dysfunction. Protocols for both TSH and TRH stimulation tests are available for the horse. After a baseline blood sample is drawn for determination of T_4 and T_3, either TSH (5 IU) or TRH (0.5–1.0 mg) is administered intravenously. Blood is then collected at 2 and 4 hours. If the thyroid is normal, T_3 increases at least twofold at 2 hours and T_4 increases at least two-fold at 4 hours following the administration of either TSH or TRH. Currently, TSH is not available and TRH is not approved for use in horses; therefore, the equine clinician must rely on measurement of T_4 and T_3 as the primary means of assessing thyroid function. These tests alone are frequently unreliable in differentiating euthyroid and hypothyroid horses because of the many nonthyroidal factors affecting thyroid hormone levels. It has been shown that even TSH stimulation did not clearly differentiate euthyroid from hypothyroid horses when nonthyroidal factors were affecting thyroid function. It is important to consider these factors carefully when interpreting the results of thyroid hormone assays in horses. Until thyroid function is more thoroughly understood in the horse, a diagnosis of thyroid disease based upon T_4 and T_3 levels alone may lead one in the pursuit of nonexistent disease. Validated methods for measuring fT_4, fT_3, rT_3, and TSH need to be developed for more widespread use to further define the clinical significance of equine thyroid dysfunction.

TREATMENT

When it is discovered that a horse has low resting levels of thyroid hormones, clinical signs that are suggestive of hypothyroidism, and known nonthyroidal factors affecting equine thyroid function have been ruled out, thyroid hormone supplementation should be considered. It must be remembered that thyroid hormone supplementation is of no benefit, and it may be detrimental, in horses with low serum T_4 and T_3 caused by certain nonthyroidal factors. Thyroid hormone supplementation in horses consists of administering either L-thyroxine at 20 μg/kg p.o. once daily or iodinated casein, which contains approximately 1% T_4 (50 mg of T_4 per 5 g iodinated casein), once daily p.o. Therapy can be evaluated from the clinical response by the horse as well as from monitored levels of T_4 and T_3. It must be kept in mind that many problems associated with low levels of thyroid hormones have multifactorial causes, and what appears to be a favorable response to thyroid hormone supplementation may actually be spontaneous resolution of another problem.

Supplemental Readings

Beech J: Evaluation of thyroid, adrenal, and pituitary function. Vet Clin North Am Equine Pract 3(3):649–660, 1987.
Harris P, Marlin D, Gray J: Equine thyroid function tests: A preliminary investigation. Br Vet J 148:71–80, 1992.
Irvine CHG: Hypothyroidism in the foal. Equine Vet J 16:302–306, 1984.
Lowe JE, Baldwin BH, Foote RH, Hillman RB, Kallfelz FA: Equine hypothyroidism: The long term effects of thyroidectomy on metabolism and growth in mares and stallions. Cornell Vet 64:276–295, 1974.
Messer NT, Ganjam VK, Nachreiner RF, Krause GF: Effect of dexamethasone administration on serum thyroid hormone concentrations in clinically normal horses. J Am Vet Med Assoc 206:63–66, 1995.
Messer NT, Johnson PJ, Refsal KR, Nachreiner RF, Ganjam VK, Krause GF: Effect of food deprivation on serum iodothyronine and cortisol concentrations in healthy adult horses. Am J Vet Res 56:116–121, 1995.
Sojka JE: Factors which affect serum T_3 and T_4 levels in horses. Equine Pract 15:15–19, 1993.
Sojka JE, Johnson MA, Bottoms GD: Serum triiodothyronine, total thyroxine, and free thyroxine concentrations in horses. Am J Vet Res 54:52–55, 1993.

12

REPRODUCTION

Edited by Mats H. T. Troedsson

Breeding Soundness Examination of the Mare

SCOTT MADILL

MATS H. T. TROEDSSON
St. Paul, Minnesota

The successful brood mare needs to be a reliable producer of viable foals. To achieve this, she needs to have regular ovulatory estrous cycles, mate, conceive, maintain pregnancy, give birth, and rear the foal. The veterinary assessment of her potential in this regard constitutes the breeding soundness examination. Clients may request a breeding soundness examination as a prepurchase assessment of future breeding performance, or for an infertile mare.

THE PREPURCHASE EXAMINATION

Recommended standards for the breeding soundness examination of mares for sale have been established in many countries by professional veterinary associations or by equine and reproductive interest groups. These standards are very similar, and clinicians are urged to familiarize themselves with those applying in their area. Familiarity with regulations regarding export and interstate transport requirements is also useful.

The breeding soundness examination requires patience, thoroughness, attention to detail, and excellent recordkeeping. The aim of the examination is to determine whether the animal has defects that may potentially prevent it from conceiving, maintaining pregnancy to term, and delivering and rearing a viable foal. The findings of the examination need to be interpreted in the light of these aims. Where limitations are placed on the examination by facilities, personnel, or the nature of the horse being examined, these should be stated, with the involved circumstances, in the examination report. Like all prepurchase examinations, the veterinarian should think carefully about conflict of interest and consider declining to examine a horse for a buyer when the seller is a regular client. Any procedure to be performed on the mare needs to be agreed to by the current owner (i.e., the vendor).

The ideal examination consists of (1) identification; (2) history; (3) a general physical examination; and (4) a detailed examination of the reproductive organs. In practice, the history is frequently deleted. This is because the veterinarian is usually acting for the prospective buyer and therefore is not familiar with the mare in question and is at the mercy of the seller in obtaining an accurate history of past breeding performance, prior use, and medications. As such, the veterinarian, unless also the regular stud veterinarian, should not certify such information as factual. A separate form for history and medication may be provided that can be filled out and signed by the vendor.

The use of printed examination forms acts as a prompt to prevent inadvertent omissions and aids accurate recordkeeping. Date, time, duration, and place of examination should be included, and if insufficient space is available to record all findings and recommendations, additional sheets should be attached.

Identification

An accurate thorough identification should include both a written description and a drawing. Information required includes sex, height, color, and the presence and location of white markings, whorls, permanent scars, and brands or tatoos. Brands and tatoos should be described as they appear on the animal at the time of the examination, not as what they are supposed to be on proffered registration papers. Photographs taken by a camera that marks date and time on the image may be used as an adjunct. Age should be estimated by examination of the teeth (see page 146).

History

In all cases the veterinarian should try to establish the current status of the mare, whether she is pregnant or has foaled and her last breeding date. This information may be obtained when setting up the appointment so the likely depth of examination can be discussed with the buyer and cleared with the vendor beforehand. When used, a complete history sheet should contain information on general medical history, past use, and detailed reproductive history. The type of information collected is set out in the section on examination of the infertile mare.

General Physical Examination

If possible, the mare should be observed while loose in a yard or stall and while being caught. Vices or handling difficulties observed during the examination should be recorded and are especially valuable in assessing suitability for a novice owner. The mare should be examined from all sides at a distance to assess overall conformation and balance. Unless he or she is a breed expert, it is not for the veterinarian to assess type for breed; that is a decision the prospective owner should have ascertained on the advice of a recognized breed judge. However, defects of conformation should be noted. In combination with the distance examination, palpation should be used to assess body condition. A further aim of the distance examination is to determine weak areas of the animal that should be targeted in the subsequent palpation and limb examinations. The symmetry of the pelvis should be particularly noted. A general physical examination, including body temperature, heart rate, and respiration should be performed. Inspection of the teeth aims to detect abnormalities of occlusion or wear that may impair feed intake or mastication and is done at the time of age estimation. A guide to visual acuity can be obtained by observing the horse while it is being caught or by turning it loose in a yard. The eyes should be examined with a menace response, bright focused light, and ophthalmoscopically. Superficial lymph nodes should be palpated and auscultation of the upper airways, thorax, and abdomen performed. Each limb is examined by close inspection, palpation, flexion, and hoof tester application. Particular attention should be paid to the feet for evidence of laminitis and, if necessary, permission should be obtained to remove shoes. The horse is observed at a walk and trot, while turning in both directions, and backing. Flexion tests and other techniques such as wedge testing for navicular syndrome are performed as needed. The desirability of ancillary tests, such as radiography, to further assess the significance of abnormal findings should be discussed with the buyer.

Detailed Reproductive Examination

It is prudent that all mares be considered pregnant until proved otherwise on the basis of breeding history and a rectal palpation or ultrasound examination. The mare should be adequately restrained for her own safety and that of personnel. The tail should be bandaged or placed in a rectal sleeve secured by tape and held out of the way by an assistant or tied with a cord passed around the neck and tied near the withers.

Perineal Inspection

Before performing a rectal palpation, the conformation of the perineum should be assessed. The vulva should be close to vertical (<10% cranial slope) and approximately 75% of its length below the level of the pubis. The lips of the vulva should be examined for scarring, fibrosis, tumor formation especially in gray mares, herpesvirus infection (coital exanthema), and the presence of any discharges there or crusted on the tail or thighs. The presence of Caslick vulvoplasty should be noted. The lips of the vulva should then be parted to examine for aspiration of air, which indicates compromise of the important vestibulovaginal seal. The clitoris should be everted and examined for size and, if required, swabs taken from the central sinus to be cultured for contagious equine metritis.

Rectal Palpation

Personal preference dictates whether an ovary, the uterus, or the cervix is located first. For current purposes the cervix will be the starting point. The cervix is palpated against the pubis and is assessed for length, diameter, and tone. The region of the uterine bifurcation is palpated for the presence of pregnancy, which determines the subsequent course of the breeding soundness examination and vigor of further palpation. Diameter and tone of the horns are recorded together with dilations and the presence of fluid accumulation. Endometrial folds are assessed by gentle compression between thumb and fingers and slipping them as the hand is moved cranially. The ovary is usually easily found by opening the hand from the tip of the uterine horn with the palm directed dorsolaterally. The ovulation fossa is located ventromedially. The dimensions of the ovary and the size and location of ovarian structures are determined. The hand is swept back along the uterine horn and the process repeated for the opposite horn and ovary. The uterine body is palpated by gentle compression against the pelvic floor. The pelvis should be palpated for evidence of callus formation from old fractures that may interfere with normal delivery.

Ultrasonography

The next step is an ultrasound examination. Ultrasound is the standard technique in stud farm medicine and should be part of the minimal breeding soundness examination whenever possible. Measurements of uterine size and ovarian structures are made using the machine's inbuilt calipers rather than estimates from palpation; but the two should be in reasonable agreement and, if not, the source of discrepancy identified. The presence of abnormalities, such as intraluminal fluid or endometrial cysts, should be recorded. It is recommended that the examination be recorded in its entirety on videotape; alternatively, selected features such as pregnancy, ovarian structures, or uterine anomalies can be placed on hard copy (printer/photograph), if the equipment is available. In any case of pregnancy, the examination should include assessment of fetal viability, and twin pregnancy should be ruled out.

Speculum Examination of the Vagina

Overt contamination of the vulva and perineum should be removed by washing with a mild disinfectant soap followed by thorough rinsing, and the area dried. A single-use or sterilized speculum is lightly coated with a sterile, water-soluble lubricant and introduced into the vagina. During passage a further assessment of the competence of the vestibulovaginal sphincter can be made based on resistance to passage of the speculum through this region. When examining maiden mares, the clinician should be alert to the possibility of imperforate hymen, which is often suggested by mucometra on palpation or ultrasound of the uterus, and excessive resistance should be investigated visually and manually before continuing. The vagina is assessed for color, moistness, and the presence of discharges; the cervix for position in the cranial vaginal wall, degree of relaxation, color, and moistness. These assessments should be made quickly following speculum introduction because air contact alters the findings. During estrus a small quantity of clear fluid may be pooled on the floor of the cranial vault, and this should not be confused with urine pooling. If doubt exists, the appearance of the cervix, normal estrous versus inflamed, appearance and odor of recovered fluid, and the results of endometrial cytology examination can be used to differentiate the two situations. Presence of cervical lacerations may not always be detected on speculum examination. The dorsal vaginal wall should be examined for evidence of rectovaginal fistulation and the walls of vagina and vestibule for lacerations, abscesses, varicosities, and gland dilations that are usually insignificant. Rectovaginal fistulation is often more easily appreciated on digital palpation.

Endometrial Culture

Sampling for endometrial culture and cytology tests is performed next. A swab sample may be taken from the endometrium either through the speculum already in place or by manual introduction based on clinician preference. In the latter case it is preferable to complete sampling before performing detailed digital palpation to avoid contamination of samples. From a strictly medical viewpoint, endometrial culture is probably unnecessary in many mares with no evidence of infection. However, the small risk of missing a diagnosis and the legal implications mean that it should be part of the purchase examination of all mares. The danger of misdiagnosing an infection based on the growth of a few insignificant contaminants is well recognized, and a culture should be performed in conjunction with an assessment of endometrial cytology.

Endometrial culture should be taken during estrus if possible, because false-negative culture results may occur when samples are obtained during diestrus. If the breeding soundness examination is performed during diestrus, a culture sample obtained from an endometrial biopsy specimen is more reliable than a sample obtained from an intrauterine swab.

Endometrial Cytology

Cytology smears can be made from debris collected in the cap of many guarded swabs, a second swab may be taken specifically for cytology, or a low-volume lavage may be performed. The obtained sample is smeared on a microscopic slide and stained.* A good correlation exists between the presence of polymorphonuclear neutrophils (PMNs) and the isolation of bacteria. Generally, only if the cytology shows evidence of inflammation should culture growth be considered significant. Although several different criteria have been suggested, there is currently no standard method to interpret endometrial cytology. Clinical judgment should be employed. The ratio of PMNs to epithelial cells appears to be superior to PMNs per microscopic field. A result should always be considered positive if more than 1 PMN is found per 10 epithelial cells.

Examination of concurrent cytology prevents the error of false-negative culture results being made. Evidence of inflammation on cytologic examination in the absence of organism growth should alert the clinician to seek other explanations, such as intermittent urine pooling and repeat sampling using different culture conditions. Samples should be obtained during estrus for the same reasons as for endometrial cultures.

Manual Vaginal Examination

Digital palpation of the vestibule, vagina, and cervix is performed next. The technique permits another assessment of vestibulovaginal sphincter tone; is more sensitive than speculum examination for the detection of small defects in the dorsal vaginal wall resulting from foaling injuries; and is necessary to detect defects in the cervix resulting from lacerations, scarring, and adhesions. It may also be combined with rectal palpation in the assessment of perineal body defects.

Endometrial Biopsy

All purchase examinations should include an endometrial biopsy. As with culture, it is in many situations (for example, in most cyclic maiden mares) superfluous, but is included "to be on the safe side." Biopsy should be strongly recommended to the buyer as part of the breeding soundness examination of aged and barren mares and those with palpable or ultrasonically detected abnormalities of the uterus, such as thinning of the wall or extensive cyst formation.

Samples may be obtained at any stage of the estrous cycle as long as the person that evaluates the biopsy is informed of the stage of the cycle. Diestrual samples are preferred by most laboratories because normal changes during estrus make the interpretation more difficult. Following manual removal of feces from the rectum, the perineal region is thoroughly cleansed, and the biopsy instrument† is passed into the vagina and through the cervix with closed jaws, guarded in a gloved hand. The operator's hand is withdrawn from the vagina and intro-

---

*Diff-Quik, American Scientific Products, McGaw Park, IL.
†Equine uterine biopsy forcep, Pilling, Fort Washingtion, DE.

duced into the rectum. The tip of the biopsy instrument is identified per rectum and guided to an appropriate position for sampling. The instrument is opened with the jaws located horizontally, and a piece of the endometrium is pushed into the jaws. The jaws are closed, the biopsy forceps quickly turned 90°, and the instrument withdrawn from the uterus. The tissue specimen should be approximately 0.5 cm by 2 cm. If uterine abnormalities have been detected on rectal palpation or ultrasonography, the specimen should be taken from this location. In the absence of abnormal findings, specimens should be obtained from the ventral aspect of the base of one of the uterine horns. Although most studies suggest that one biopsy is diagnostic for the condition of the entire uterus, two biopsies, one from each horn, have been recommended by others. The specimens should be transferred into a fixative, 10% formalin or Bouin's solution, and transported to a laboratory for preparation and staining with hematoxylin and eosin.

Histopathologic interpretation of the biopsy includes the presence and degree of inflammatory cell infiltration, periglandular fibrosis, cystic glandular dilation, lymphatic lacunae, and endometrial atrophy. Based on pathologic findings, the biopsy will be classified into a four-category system. Category I indicates a normal endometrium with a 60 to 90% predicted ability of the mare to become pregnant and deliver a live foal. Mares with an endometrial biopsy classified as category IIA have only mild endometrial pathology and can be expected to have a 40 to 60% foaling rate. Moderate endometrial pathology is classified as category IIB. Mares with a category IIB uterus can only be expected to have a 10 to 40% chance to carry a foal to term. A category III biopsy involves severe endometrial pathology with less than 10% chance of the mare carrying a foal to term. Laboratory results should be interpreted with care by the clinician. Clinical judgment as to the responsiveness to therapy of a specific endometrial lesion, the age of the mare, and other clinical findings should be considered. Inflammatory lesions are generally responsive to therapy and a new biopsy following treatment should be recommended before a final classification of the mare is done. Degenerative lesions are less responsive to therapy and carry a poor prognosis (see page 517).

Mammary Glands

If not examined during the general physical examination, the udder should be inspected and palpated. Assessment of function is only obtainable in lactating mares, but all mares should be checked for normal conformation and evidence of mastitis, fibrosis, and neoplasia.

Conclusions

This completes the breeding soundness examination in most cases. The recommendation of the clinician as to suitability for breeding purposes should be based on the results of the entire examination. All findings and their possible implications are carefully discussed with the client. Those mares in which the above examination has revealed findings that should be further investigated by use of endoscopic or bimanual examination of the uterus are unlikely to be recommended as suitable for breeding purposes. Performance horses retired to breeding are unlikely to be perfectly "sound of limb." A mare with a mild to moderate permanent lameness from injury can be a productive brood mare for many years, whereas a similar mare whose lameness is a result of chronic laminitis is a poor risk. Similarly,

---

TABLE 1. HISTORICAL INFORMATION TO BE COLLECTED DURING INVESTIGATION OF THE INFERTILE MARE

Signalment
  Animal name, age, breed, and sex
Presenting complaint
General history
- What was the mare previously used for (how long ago and how long for)?
- Is she currently used for anything other than breeding (when, intensity, duration)?
- Does she currently have any medical problems?
- What medical problems has she had in the past (when and how treated)?
- Has she ever had abdominal surgery?
- What medication has she received in the last 3 months?
- Where and how is she housed?
- What is she fed (any supplements)?
- Vaccinations (what and when)?
- Parasite control programs?

Reproductive management
- What date this season did breeding attempts commence?
- Were lights or GnRH used to hasten the onset of cyclic activity?
- Were hormones (e.g., altrenogest) used to control her cycles?
- Where was she bred (home, sent to stud, trailergate)?
- How was she bred (paddock, hand service, fresh AI, chilled AI, frozen AI)?
- How was heat determined?
- How was time of ovulation determined?
- When was she bred relative to estrus/ovulation?

Stallion
- Number of mares bred this season
- Number pregnant (calculate pregnancy rate)
- Average cycles/conception
- How many conceived around the time this mare was bred?

Mare—general
- How long has the mare been infertile?
- Number of seasons at stud
- Number of foals delivered
- In the years she did not foal did she not conceive or did she abort (stage)?
- Dystocias and how relieved
- Reproductive surgeries

Mare—this season
- Current reproductive status
- Last breeding date
- Pregnancy examination results
- Number of cycles
- Length of cycles (regular or irregular)
- Number of cycles bred
- Number of breedings/cycle
- Previous diagnostic work (what, when, and results)
- Treatments given (what, when, who, and results)

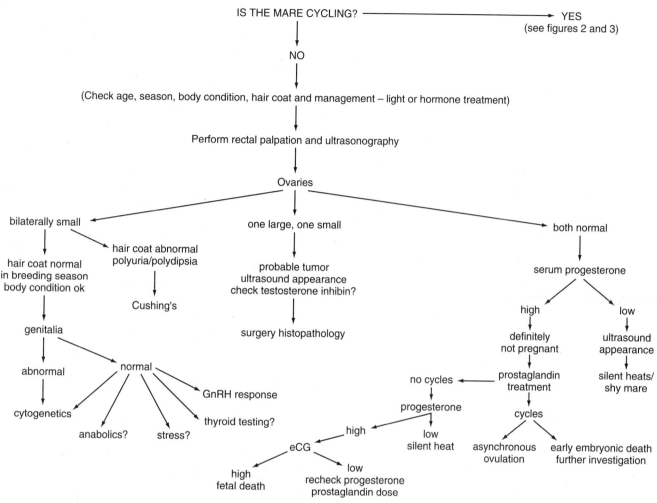

Figure 1. Differential diagnosis of the anestrous mare.

a quiet blind mare in a carefully managed environment can make a long-term producer. These animals need assessment on a case-by-case basis with their shortcomings and the likely, but possibly unpredictable, progression and outcome of their condition pointed out to the client.

If during the course of the examination a problem or combination of problems is uncovered that is so severe as to rule the mare unsatisfactory, the examination may be terminated at that point with the agreement of the client.

INVESTIGATION OF THE INFERTILE MARE

In many ways this examination is modeled after that for prepurchase. However, whereas prepurchase tends to be a process of exhaustion, with all recommended tests being performed on all mares, a mare with infertility should be subjected to an investigation based on hypothetico-deductive reasoning.

History

The examination starts with a thorough history-taking. This is similar in all mares, but along the way the clinician begins to form hypotheses that direct more questions to certain areas and subsequently shape the rest of the examination. The history should include the signalment, presenting complaint, a general history, and a detailed reproductive history, which may be subdivided into management aspects, a check of stallion fertility, and the mare herself (Table 1). The quality of this information depends on how long the client has owned the animal and what records are kept.

Physical and Initial Reproductive Examination

Following the history, or in conjunction with it, a limited physical examination is performed to obtain a general impression of the animal including its body condition, coat, and attitude. Abnormalities noted or suspicions raised on this limited examination should lead to a more complete general physical examination. The examiner then generally proceeds to the initial portions of the detailed reproductive examination described earlier, including examination of perineal conformation, presence of vulval discharge, rectal palpation, ultrasonography, and vaginoscopy. All mares presented for infertility should receive this basic examination.

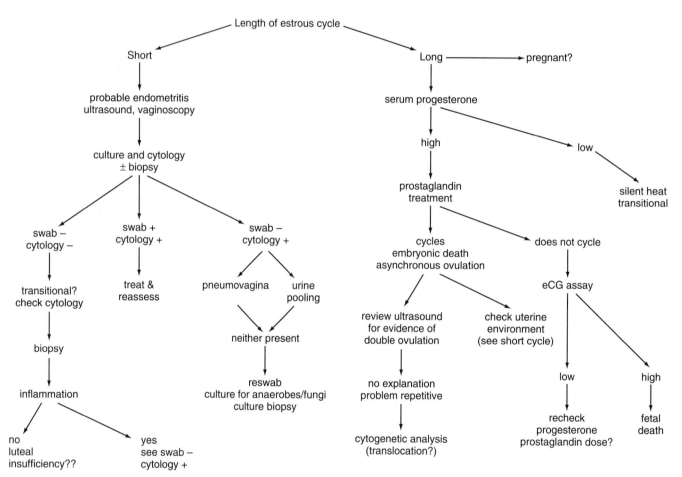

Figure 2. Differential diagnosis of infertility in the mare with abnormal estrous cycle length.

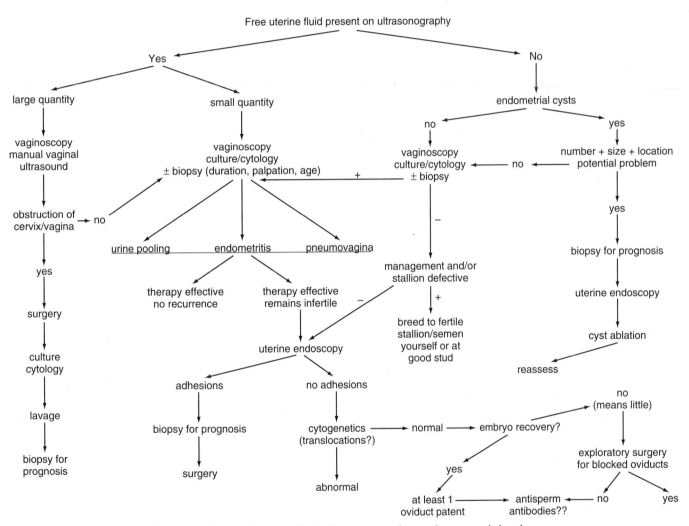

Figure 3. Differential diagnosis of infertility in mares with normal estrous cycle length.

Most also receive a culture and cytology examination, but some may just receive a biopsy; for example, in a mare barren for several years and of low economic value, a grade III biopsy result and its poor prognosis may be the most useful service the clinician can provide to the owner by permitting clients to cut their losses, rather than pursuing repeated cultures, corrective surgery, and medical treatment.

From this point the examination branches out depending on the results of history, physical examination, and initial tests. For example, the duration of the problem is important. A young mare that has foaled this season but has failed to conceive on three subsequent cycles, and has fluid in her uterus on ultrasound examination, should receive an endometrial culture and cytologic examination but is unlikely to warrant a biopsy. In contrast, a mare with similar findings that has not conceived for three seasons needs a biopsy.

Sample algorithms are presented in Figures 1 to 3. These present one starting point for classification that is not applicable in all cases, and the clinician must make adjustments. Similarly, there is frequently overlap, with many diagnoses appearing in several of the trees. For example, mares experiencing early embryonic death be-cause of a hostile uterine environment may present with shortened, normal, or prolonged cycle lengths depending on the time of death and degree of endometrial inflammation; or a mare with mucometra/pyometra may well have an abnormal cycle length.

Supplemental Readings

Anderson GF: Purchase examination of the performance horse. *In* Robinson NE (ed): Current Therapy in Equine Medicine, ed 3. Philadelphia, WB Saunders, 1992, pp 68–71.

Doig PA, Waelchli RO: Endometrial biopsy. *In* McKinnon AO, Voss JL (eds): Equine Reproduction. Philadelphia, Lea & Febiger, 1993, pp 225–233.

Ginther OJ: Ultrasonic Imaging and Reproductive Events in the Mare. Cross Plains, WI, Equiservices, 1986.

Kenney RM: Cyclic and pathologic changes of the mare endometrium as detected by biopsy, with a note on early embryonic death. J Am Vet Med Assoc 172:241–262, 1978.

Ricketts SW, Alonso S: Assessment of the breeding prognosis of mares using paired endometrial biopsy techniques. Equine Vet J 23:185–188, 1991.

Wingfield Digby NJ, Ricketts SW: Results of concurrent bacteriological and cytological examinations of the endometrium of mares in routine stud farm practice 1978–1981. J Reprod Fertil 32[Suppl]:181–185, 1982.

Diseases of the External Genitalia

MATS H.T. TROEDSSON
St. Paul, Minnesota

DISEASES OF THE VULVA

The constrictor muscles of the vulva close the vulvar lips, functioning as a seal and forming the first protective barrier between the external environment and the uterus. The vulvar lips should meet evenly and be in a vertical position with a cranial-to-caudal slope of no more than 10° from the vertical. Less than one third of the vulvar opening should be located above the ischial arch of the pelvis to form an effective protective barrier. Abnormal perineal conformation results in the compromise of the vulvar seal, predisposing to aspiration of air and fecal material into the vestibule.

Diagnosis

Visual examination of the vulva and the perineal region reveals conformational abnormalities or inflammatory processes. A scoring system was developed by Pascoe (1979) to evaluate the mare's perineal conformation based on the effective length and the angle of declination of the vulva. The system uses the Caslick index, which equals the distance (cm) between the dorsal commissure and the pelvic floor multiplied by the degrees of declination of the vulvar lips. Mares with a Caslick index higher than 150 experienced lower than normal pregnancy rates. It was suggested that all mares with a Caslick index of more than 100 should undergo reconstructive surgery.

Abnormal Perineal Conformation

Several predisposing factors contribute to abnormal perineal conformation. Mares with a flat croup, elevated tail head, sunken anus, or underdeveloped vulvar lips are more likely to have poor perineal conformation. Abnormal conformation may also be caused by perineal trauma resulting from dystocia. Poor physical condition, advanced age, and parity all contribute to abnormal perineal conformation. Visceroptosis may contribute to an abnormal conformation of the perineum, as the abdominal and pelvic organs relax and sink in older mares. The diagnosis is made upon visual examination of the perineal region and the use of Caslick index.

Several surgical procedures to correct abnormal perineal conformation have been described. These include Caslick vulvoplasty, perineal body reconstruction, and perineal body transection. The reader is referred to a surgery textbook for a review of these techniques.

Perineal Lacerations

Most perineal lacerations occur as a result of dystocia. Minor injuries to the perineum do not require surgery, but those that compromise the perineal seal affect fertility unless they are surgically corrected.

Clinical Signs and Diagnosis

Perineal lacerations result from dystocia, and have been classified into first-, second-, and third-degree lacerations. First-degree perineal lacerations involve the vestibular mucosa and vulvar skin. Second-degree perineal lacerations involve the entire wall of the dorsal vestibule including the perineum. Third-degree perineal lacerations extend through the dorsal vestibule, perineal body, ventral rectum, and anal sphincter.

Treatment

Most first-degree lacerations require no surgery other than Caslick vulvoplasty if the dorsal commissure of the vulva is involved. Second-degree lacerations may result in a faulty perineal conformation that can predispose the mare to pneumovagina. Immediate surgery is, in most cases, not necessary. The surgical procedure performed is determined by the character and degree of the perineal abnormality. Minor second-degree lacerations heal without surgery. When the injury involves enough of the perineal body to cause the dorsal aspect of the vulva to descend cranially, resulting in an altered angle of declination of the vulva, perineal body construction should be considered. Surgical repair of third-degree perineal lacerations should not be attempted until at least 4 weeks after injury. Several surgical procedures have been described, and the reader is referred to a surgery textbook for description of these techniques. Mares with third-degree lacerations should be given systemic antibacterial therapy for 5 to 7 days, and the clinician should ensure that the mare's tetanus prophylaxis status is current.

Coital Exanthema

Coital exanthema is a sexually transmitted disease caused by equine herpesvirus-3 (EHV-3). The disease is manifested by the appearance of multiple papules, pustules, and erosions on the vulvar mucosa and the perineal skin. Fertility is not affected by coital exanthema.

Clinical Signs and Diagnosis

Lesions appear typically within 1 week of sexual contact with an infectious stallion or contaminated equipment. Initial lesions consisting of multiple papules 2 to 3 mm in diameter progress rapidly to pustules and ulcers (5 to 10 mm in diameter). The lesions are painful to touch. The ulcers heal spontaneously within 2 to 3 weeks, unless the condition is complicated by secondary bacterial infection. After complete healing of the lesions, unpigmented spots are left as evidence of previous infection. Lesions located at sites other than the genitalia are rare but may occasionally be found on the lips and nasal mucosa. Signs of systemic disease are uncommon in horses with coital exanthema but may occur if a bacterial infection is present. Secondary bacterial infection is characterized by a mucopurulent exudate and a prolonged healing process. Coital exanthema is diagnosed by the presence of typical lesions. In addition, intranuclear inclusion bodies may be found in epithelial cells on cytologic smears.

Treatment

The lesions heal spontaneously. Sexual rest for 3 weeks or until the lesions are completely healed is recommended to prevent further spread of the disease. Coital exanthema cannot be transmitted after the ulcers are healed. Topical treatment with antibiotics may prevent a secondary bacterial infection. No vaccine is available for EHV-3.

Dourine

Dourine is a sexually transmitted chronic infection in equids, caused by the protozoa *Trypanosoma equiperdum*. The disease has been eradicated from North America and western Europe, but still occurs in parts of Eastern Europe, Central and South America, the Middle East, and Africa.

Clinical Signs and Diagnosis

After an incubation time of several weeks, clinical signs of fever and systemic illness slowly develop over a long period of time. Early clinical signs include mild fever, genital edema, and a mucopurulent vaginal discharge. Following these initial signs, typical cutaneous raised plaques (2–10 mm in diameter) can be observed at the external genitalia. The genital signs may be followed by systemic disease with high mortality.

Dourine is diagnosed based on the typical clinical signs and by identification of *T. equiperdum* from vaginal discharge. Several serologic tests have been described for the diagnosis of dourine. The complement fixation test appears to be the most reliable.

Treatment

Treatment of horses with dourine using quinapyrine sulfate has been reported. Isolation of suspected horses, serologic screening with subsequent culling of positive-testing animals is the preferred method to control disease outbreaks of dourine.

DISEASES OF THE VAGINA

Although extremely dilatable, the vaginal lumen is collapsed dorsoventrally under normal conditions. The collapsed lumen helps to form an effective protective barrier. Aspiration of air or urine pooling results in distension of the lumen, which predisposes to vaginitis and chronic recurrent endometritis.

Diagnosis

Mares with pneumovagina or urovagina often have a history of chronic recurrent endometritis and subfertility. Frequently the perineal conformation is poor. Evaluation of Caslick index, monitoring for aspiration of air following gentle separation of the vulvar lips, and vaginoscopy aid in the diagnosis of vaginal abnormalities. Videoendoscopic examination may be useful in the examination of the cranial aspect of the vestibulovaginal transverse fold. Determination of pH and cytology testing and culture of vaginal secretions can be used to determine the origin and contribution of inflammation to accumulated vaginal fluid.

Urovagina or Urine Pooling

The normal cranial equine vagina rises approximately 10 degrees dorsally from the horizontal plane. If the slope of the vagina changes to cranioventral, the vaginal fornix falls below the pelvic floor, pulling the urethral orifice cranial to the ischium. As a result, urine cannot be completely voided through the caudal vagina and vulvar lips and a backflow of urine occurs, forming a pool in the anterior portion of the vagina. Mares with urine pooling are often subfertile. Factors that predispose to urovagina include abnormal perineal conformation, pneumovagina, obstetric trauma, urethral sphincter paralysis, advanced age and parity, and visceroptosis. If urine is present in the cranial vagina at the time of ejaculation, semen is mixed with urine, which is toxic to spermatozoa. Urine can also enter the uterus when the cervix is relaxed during estrus. This may cause irritation to the endometrium, resulting in chronic endometritis.

Diagnosis

In typical cases of urovagina, an accumulation of urine at the vaginal fornix can be visualized during a vaginoscopic examination. The condition can be intermittent, with mares being more likely to pool urine during estrus than during diestrus. Hormonal changes during estrus result in relaxation and edema of the mare's reproductive tract. This may cause a cranial displacement of the tract, resulting in a cranioventral slope of the vagina. During diestrus, the increased tone and absence of edema may change the vaginal slope back to craniodorsal. The potential for urine pooling during estrus should always be suspected in mares with a cranially tilted vagina, even if no urine is present at the time of examination. Ultrasonographic examination of the vagina and the uterus can be used to detect fluid in the cranial vagina and in the uterine body.

Treatment

Treatment of urovagina is directed toward correcting the underlying cause of the disease. Several surgical procedures have been described to correct urine pooling. The cause and severity of the disease determine if vaginoplasty, urethral extension, or perineal body transection (perineoplasty) should be performed. Vaginoplasty or caudal relocation of the transverse fold may be performed in mares with mild vaginal slope and conformational abnormalities. The procedure is not suitable for mares with a severe vaginal cranioventral slope. These mares require a urethral extension. Perineal body transection should be considered in mares suffering from urine pooling caused by a severely deformed perineal conformation.

A complete breeding soundness evaluation should always precede surgical treatments. In addition to the importance of a correct diagnosis of predisposing factors to the disease, an endometrial biopsy serves as a valuable prognostic tool to determine future fertility. The prognosis for fertility depends on the underlying cause of the condition and the severity of endometrial degenerative pathology found on biopsy.

Pneumovagina

Aspiration of air and contaminating microorganisms into the vagina may progress into vaginitis, cervicitis, and chronic endometritis. Poor perineal conformation, poor physical condition, and relaxation of the pelvic ligaments during estrus predispose to pneumovagina.

Clinical Signs and Diagnosis

Aspiration of air may be heard upon manual separation of the vulvar labia and during exercise. Signs of inflammation in the vaginal mucous membranes are frequently observed upon vaginoscopic examination.

Treatment

Treatment of pneumovagina should be directed toward surgically correcting defective perineal conformation. Mares with pneumovagina require a Caslick operation to close the dorsal vulva. This may cause practical problems in the periparturient mare and during natural breeding. An episiotomy should be performed close to parturition. Mares with episiotomies may aspirate air between breedings. This can be prevented by closing the vulva with staples without resecting labial tissue, until ovulation is detected.

The prognosis for future reproductive performance following treatment is good if the condition is unaccompanied by endometrial fibrosis and degeneration.

Vaginitis

Vaginitis is rare in the mare. It may be seen as a consequence of dystocia, pneumovagina, urine pooling, or endometritis. Rectovaginal fistulas frequently lead to vaginitis. The most common causative agents of vaginitis are those commonly cultured from the mare's uterus, and include *Streptococcus zooepidemicus* and *Escherichia coli*. Necrotic vaginitis can develop as a result of secondary infection of traumatic lesions by clostridial or gram-negative anaerobes.

Clinical Signs and Diagnosis

Mares with vaginitis often display moderate amounts of vaginal mucopurulent discharge. Edema and hyperemia of the vaginal mucous membranes can be observed on vaginoscopy. Culture of vaginal exudate determines the causative organism.

Treatment

The treatment of vaginitis should include eliminating predisposing factors. Mild cases recover spontaneously. Vaginal douches with dilute solutions of antiseptics or antibiotics may be tried in severe or persistent cases. Necrotic vaginitis requires aggressive treatment with systemic antibiotics and anti-inflammatory drugs. The prognosis for mild vaginitis is good, but necrotic vaginitis may result in vaginal adhesions and stenosis.

Varicose Veins

Varicose veins are frequently observed during vaginoscopic examination of older mares. In most cases the condition goes undetected in the absence of clinical signs. Some mares with vaginal varicose veins exhibit vaginal hemorrhage, which may be of great concern to the owner. A thorough clinical examination of the reproductive tract is necessary to determine the origin of the bleeding.

Diagnosis

Varicose veins are best detected with vaginoscopy. However, if present only at the cranial aspect of the vestibulovaginal transverse fold, fiber endoscopic examination may be beneficial. Clinical signs associated with vaginal varicose veins vary from no signs to persistent and profuse vaginal hemorrhage. The bleeding may be spontaneous, or more commonly it is associated with breeding or is seen in the periparturient period. Vaginal hemorrhage from varicose veins must be differentiated from mating-induced vaginal trauma and premature separation of the placenta in periparturient mares.

Treatment

Most mares with vaginal varicose veins do not require treatment. If vaginal bleeding from ruptured veins is severe, surgical correction with ligation of the veins may be necessary. Although the short-term prognosis following surgery is good, the condition often recurs.

Vaginal Trauma

The vagina may be traumatized as a result of dystocia, human mutilation (sadism), or breeding accidents. The consequences of mild cases of vaginal trauma are often limited to vaginitis that resolves spontaneously. However, if the trauma involves a large portion of the vagina and vestibule or if a full-thickness tear into the peritoneum occurs, the condition requires immediate attention.

Clinical Signs and Diagnosis

Mares with vaginal mucosal lacerations following dystocia often exhibit external signs of genital trauma. A swollen vagina, vaginal discharge, and tenesmus that either is constant or is associated with urination or defecation are common signs associated with vaginal trauma. With breeding accidents, vaginal hemorrhage and blood on the stallion's penis can be observed following dismounting. Speculum examination of the vagina and gentle digital examination confirms the diagnosis and is helpful in assessing the severity of the lesion.

Treatment

Vaginal trauma that involves only the mucosa does not require treatment. If the lesion fails to resolve spontaneously, treatment should be similar to that for vaginitis. Surgical repair of vaginal lacerations is not necessary. If the trauma is excessive, or involves both mucosa and submucosa, local treatment with an antibiotic-based ointment that contains corticosteroids may prevent the formation of adhesions and vaginal stenosis. Vaginal tears resulting from breeding accidents should be carefully examined for depth and tissue involvement. If the lesion involves only the retroperitoneum, systemic broad-spectrum antibiotics and repeated vaginal douches may control secondary infections. The laceration should not be closed, and good drainage of the lesion should be maintained to prevent abscessation. Frequently, breeding-induced vaginal lacerations are of full thickness and involve the peritoneum. If the penis penetrates the peritoneum, the pressure against the glans disappears, which in most cases prevents ejaculation. However, with or without ejaculation, bacterial contamination of the peritoneum results in acute peritonitis. If possible, local treatment of the laceration should be avoided to prevent further contamination of the peritoneum. Treatment should be focused on the peritonitis. Caslick vulvoplasty

should be considered if further contamination of the vagina is likely. Treatment with broad-spectrum antibiotics, anti-inflammatory drugs, and aggressive abdominal lavage with normal saline or lactated Ringer's solution should be employed. The close monitoring of complete blood counts and abdominal fluid analysis aid in the decision on the necessary duration of treatment and frequency of abdominal lavage.

Although penile penetration into the peritoneum is serious, rapid detection and onset of therapy often result in complete recovery. Breeding injuries can be prevented by the use of a breeding roll when mares are bred to a stallion with a large penis. Artificial insemination should be considered if allowed by the particular breed registry.

DISEASES OF THE CERVIX

The equine cervix is a relatively weak protective barrier compared with that in other species because of its dilatability during estrus and parturition and the lack of obstructing cervical rings and longitudinally arranged folds. Nevertheless, the cervix must be considered to be the most important external barrier against an ascending uterine contamination during the luteal phase. The production of sticky mucus together with contractions of thick layers of circular muscle, which are rich in elastic fibers, are responsible for sealing the lumen during diestrus and pregnancy.

Diagnosis

The cervix can be palpated per rectum and per vagina. Abnormalities can be visualized on speculum examination of the cervix. Normal variations of cervical consistency and appearance during the estrous cycle must be considered when evaluating the cervix for abnormalities. High blood concentrations of progesterone (i.e., during diestrus and pregnancy) is associated with a tight, closed, dry, and pale cervix. In the absence of progesterone and in the presence of estrogen (i.e., during estrus) the cervix is relaxed and open and appears moist and pink upon vaginoscopic examination.

Cervical Lacerations

Cervical lacerations are most often seen following dystocia. Tearing of the fibromuscular layer of the cervix may occur without mucosal laceration. Cervical lacerations can result in adhesions and a nonpatent cervix, or in a failure to seal the uterus during diestrus. If cervical adhesions are formed in combination with uterine inflammation, pyometra may be the result. Failure of the cervix to adequately close often results in chronic endometritis and subfertilty.

Clinical Signs and Diagnosis

Cervical lacerations can be diagnosed by vaginoscopy and digital palpation of the cervix. The extent of the laceration cannot adequately be evaluated on vaginoscopic examination. A digital examination of the entire circumference of the cervix is necessary to locate the extent of the laceration. Full-thickness lacerations and those that involve the internal os carry a worse prognosis than partial-thickness lacerations or involvement of only the external os. Evaluation of the ability of the cervix to close adequately is best performed in the presence of high blood progesterone concentrations. Cervical lacerations may be diagnosed immediately after parturition, but excessive cervical dilation may often limit the ability to make a diagnosis at that time. Re-examination a few days later is recommended if cervical laceration is suspected.

Treatment

If the cervical laceration is detected shortly after parturition, antimicrobial ointment should be applied frequently to the lesion, and early signs of adhesions should be broken down until the tissue is healed. The treatment may prevent the formation of adhesions.

If the laceration results in an incompetent cervix, it should be corrected surgically during diestrus. A two- to three-layer closure of the laceration is recommended. Although some authors recommend surgery after foal heat, most mares undergo surgical correction after complete healing of the initial injury. Surgery should be followed by 4 to 6 weeks of healing before breeding. Evaluation of an endometrial biopsy is recommended before surgery to ensure that the mare's reproductive performance is not compromised by other uterine pathology. A single-layer closure of the cervical tear 2 to 3 days after breeding and ovulation can be used when lacerations are detected during a prebreeding examination or insemination. Although surgical repair of cervical lacerations has been reported to result in a high rate of subsequent pregnancies, the condition is likely to recur at the time of parturition, and surgery may have to be repeated after each foaling. Embryo transfer should be considered if allowed by the breed registry.

Cervical Adhesions

Trauma to the cervix in association with parturition or mating may cause cervical adhesions. Adhesions can also be formed as a result of uterine therapy with irritating agents or as a result of cervicitis.

Clinical Signs and Diagnosis

Reproductive performance is reduced by cervical adhesions. The adhesions may completely or partially occlude the lumen. In addition to interference with deposition of sperm in the uterus, cervical occlusion also prevents intraluminal fluid from being expelled from the uterus. Mares with cervical adhesions and concurrent endometritis often develop pyometra. Adhesions can also be formed between the external os of the cervix and the vaginal wall. This is commonly seen following cervical lacerations associated with dystocia. These adhesions may prevent the cervix from closing adequately, resulting in repeated or persistent uterine contamination.

Diagnosis of cervical adhesions can be made by speculum examination and manual palpation of the cervix per vagina. An accurate assessment of the extent and involvement of the lesion is necessary before prognostic and therapeutic decisions can be made.

Treatment

Cervical adhesions can be broken down manually or can be cut by long-handled scissors. Daily manual breakdown is often necessary, and an antimicrobial ointment that contains corticosteroids should be administered to prevent the formation of new adhesions. The prognosis for reproductive performance depends on the severity of the lesion.

Cervicitis

Inflammation of the cervix is often the result of endometritis, vaginitis, or possibly trauma (see Cervical Laceration and Adhesions). Cervicitis may result in a failure of the cervix to close sufficiently, which predisposes the horse to recurrent endometritis and pregnancy failure.

Vaginoscopic examination reveals a dark red to purple, edematous and dilated cervical mucosa. Other findings depend on the primary cause of the disease, and may include signs of cervical lacerations, endometritis, vaginitis, or urovagina. Treatment of cervicitis should be directed toward the primary problem (see Endometritis, Vaginitis, Cervical Lacerations and Adhesions).

Supplemental Readings

Aanes WA: Cervical laceration(s). *In* McKinnon AO, Voss JL (eds): Equine Reproduction. Philadelphia, Lea & Febiger, 1993, pp 444–449.

Easley J: Correction of vesiculovaginal reflux. *In* McKinnon AO, Voss JL (eds): Equine Reproduction. Philadelphia, Lea & Febiger, 1993, pp 428–436.

Pascoe RR: Observations on the length and angle of declination of the vulva and its relation to fertility in the mare. J Reprod Fertil 27[Suppl]:299–305, 1979.

Roberts SJ: Other infectious diseases of the genital organs of mares. *In* Veterinary Obstetrics and Genital Diseases (Theriogenology), ed 3. Woodstock, VT, SJ Roberts, 1986, pp 618–619.

Trotter GW: Surgical diseases of the caudal reproductive tract. *In* Auer JA (ed): Equine Surgery. Philadelphia, WB Saunders, 1992, pp 730–750.

Diseases of the Uterus

MATS H. T. TROEDSSON
St. Paul, Minnesota

The uterus consists of the endometrium, the myometrium, and the perimetrium. Diseases of the uterus most often involve the endometrium, with endometritis and endometrial cysts being most frequently diagnosed. However, a functional defect of the myometrium has been shown to be involved in the persistent endometritis complex. Other diseases of the myometrium include leiomyoma and periparturient atony resulting in dystocia.

DIAGNOSIS

Rectal palpation of the uterus should be performed to note its position, size, tone, and presence of abnormalities. Digital palpation of the endometrium for the detection of uterine tears is possible after parturition but has to be performed with care, because the uterine wall can be very fragile at that time. Vaginoscopy should be used to detect uterine discharge through the cervix. Transrectal ultrasonography confirms most palpable findings, and in addition gives information on the presence and quality of even a small amount of intraluminal fluid, endometrial cysts, uterine neoplasia, abscesses, and hematoma. Endometrial cytology samples should be obtained when the mare is in estrus and aids in the diagnosis of active endometritis. Collection of endometrial cytology samples can be achieved by the use of a swab or by a uterine flush with subsequent centrifugation of the sample. An endometrial culture sample is often obtained in conjunction with a cytology sample and identifies any microorganisms causing endometritis (see Breeding Soundness Examination p 505). Endometrial biopsy provides important information on the condition of the endometrium, and identifies inflammatory as well as degenerative pathology of the endometrium. Endometrial biopsies have also been used to predict fertility with a high rate of accuracy (i.e., the mare's ability to conceive, maintain the pregnancy, and deliver a live foal at term). Hysterendoscopy has been used to diagnose uterine disease but is limited by cost and its practical considerations. The procedure is helpful in some clinical situations such as uterine adhesions and to evaluate macroscopic endometrial quality. In addition, hysterendoscopy can be used to retrieve foreign bodies such as endometrial swabs from the uterus and to perform endometrial laser surgery.

ENDOMETRITIS

Inflammation of the uterus is a well-recognized cause of reduced fertility in broodmares. Based on etiology and pathophysiology, endometritis in the mare may be divided into (1) sexually transmitted diseases, (2) chronic uterine infection, (3) persistent mating-induced endometritis, and (4) chronic degenerative endometritis.

Sexually Transmitted Diseases

Contagious equine metritis (CEM) caused by *Taylorella equigenitalis*, is a true sexually transmitted disease resulting in endometritis in the mare. The first outbreak of CEM was reported on stud farms in England and Ireland in 1977. CEM has since been diagnosed in most European countries, Japan, and the United States. Two separate outbreaks occurred in Kentucky and Missouri during 1978 and 1979. Both outbreaks originated from infected carrier stallions imported from Europe. Vigorous control measures prevented further spread of the disease, and the United States is currently free from CEM. Because the disease is associated with great economic losses, import regulation and required quarantine of imported horses from countries that are not pronounced to be free from CEM are still in effect in the United States. Most countries with CEM present in their equine population have established a control program with screening of breeding animals to prevent the disease from being spread.

In addition to CEM, genital infection with *Pseudomonas aeruginosa* and *Klebsiella pneumoniae* have been suggested to be sexually transmitted in horses. In contrast to the high pathogenicity of *T. equigenitalis*, the consequences of exposure to *P. aeruginosa* and *K. pneumoniae* are determined by individual host susceptibility and the pathogenicity of the particular bacterial strain involved. Endometritis caused by *P. aeruginosa* and *K. pneumoniae* are discussed under the section on chronic uterine infection.

Clinical Signs and Diagnosis

T. equigenitalis is a gram-negative microaerophilic coccobacillus previously named *Haemophilus equigenitalis*. Infected stallions are asymptomatic carriers of the disease. Mares bred to an infected stallion typically develop clinical signs within 2 to 10 days after mating. Characteristic signs of CEM consist of endometritis, vaginitis, and cervicitis with a copious mucopurulent discharge. The exudate contains a large number of polymorphonuclear neutrophils (PMNs). A shortened luteal phase caused by prostaglandin ($PGF_2\alpha$) release associated with the acute uterine inflammation is commonly seen in infected mares. The acute endometritis causes a temporary but marked decrease in conception rates, and although many mares recover spontaneously from the disease and may become pregnant later during the season, the seasonal pregnancy rate is typically severely affected by CEM. An overall decrease in the seasonal conception rate from 80% to 40% was reported from a farm in England with an outbreak of CEM. Some mares do not show any clinical signs of CEM other than a temporary reduction in fertility. Mares that recover from the acute endometritis can still be infectious, with the microorganism persisting in the genital tract for several months or longer. The clitoral sinuses and fossa are preferred locations of persistent infection in nonclinical carrier mares.

Diagnosis of CEM is based on clinical signs and the isolation of *T. equigenitalis* from the genital tract. Culture samples should be taken from the endometrium, cervix, clitoral fossa, and sinuses. Samples from the endometrium should be collected during estrus. Samples from the clitoral sinuses and fossa can be obtained at any stage of the cycle. The clinician needs to strictly follow a protocol when handling specimens, to ensure successful and accurate bacteriologic diagnosis of CEM. Samples should be placed in Amies media with charcoal or Stewart's media and be kept refrigerated until delivered to the laboratory. At the laboratory, the samples should be transferred to a chocolate agar medium, and incubated in 5 to 10% carbon dioxide at 37°C. *T. equigenitalis* grows in culture within 48 to 72 hours in mares showing clinical signs, but organisms isolated from carrier mares grow more slowly. Selective media containing antibiotics have been used to suppress the outgrowth of *T. equigenitalis* by contaminants, and media containing streptomycin is often used. However, strains of *T. equigenitalis* that are sensitive to streptomycin have been reported, and thus it is necessary to also culture samples in streptomycin-free media.

A technique to detect the presence of *T. equigenitalis* using polymerase chain reaction (PCR) was recently reported. This method is considerably more sensitive when compared with culture assays. It was concluded from the study that many horses that carry *T. equigenitalis* may go undetected with current culture techniques.

Several serologic tests that detect circulating antibodies against *T. equigenitalis* have been described. Although complement fixation tests can be successfully used to diagnose CEM in acutely infected mares, serologic tests have limited value in chronic carrier states.

Treatment and Prevention

Mares with CEM should be treated with intrauterine infusions of antibiotics based on sensitivity tests, in combination with local treatments of the clitoral fossa and sinuses. *T. equigenitalis* is sensitive to several antibiotics. Daily intrauterine infusions of 5 to 10 million units of penicillin for 5 to 7 days can eliminate *T. equigenitalis* from the uterus. For best result, treatment should be initiated when the mare is in estrus and should be combined with intrauterine lavage if inflammatory debris or intraluminal fluids are present. Cleansing of the vulva and clitoris daily for 5 days with a 4% chlorhexidine solution followed by packing of the clitoris with a chlorhexidine or nitrofurazone ointment has been recommended. Mares that are still culture positive for *T. equigenitalis* following treatment should have clitoral sinusectomy performed.

No effective vaccine is available for CEM. The spread of CEM on stud farms in endemic countries is best prevented by implementation of strict hygiene, use of disposable and sterile equipment and supplies, screening of breeding stallions before the breeding season, and the use of artificial insemination, if allowed by the breed registry. Import restrictions and regulations in countries free from CEM will prevent outbreaks of the disease. Currently, the United States requires all horses imported from countries with CEM to be quarantined. Sinusectomy is required

on all mares with intact sinuses. Negative samples for *T. equigenitalis* obtained on three different occasions at intervals of no less than 7 days apart are required from the endometrium, the cervix, the urethral fossa, and the clitoral fossa. At least one set of samples should be collected at the time of estrus. Pregnant mares are kept in quarantine throughout pregnancy. Three negative postpartum culture samples, 7 days apart, are required before the mares are released from quarantine. Imported stallions stay in quarantine for a minimum of 45 days. Three negative samples for *T. equigenitalis* from the prepuce, urethral fossa, and urethra are required. In addition, the stallion has to test breed three mares that demonstrate negative culture results for *T. equigenitalis* on three different occasions with the samples obtained 7 days apart. CEM has not been diagnosed in the United States since 1979.

Chronic Uterine Infection

Uterine infections caused by *Streptococcus zooepidemicus* and *Escherichia coli* are often the result of contamination of the uterus by fecal and genital flora. Although the uterus is well protected from external contamination by physical barriers consisting of the vulva, vestibule, vagina, and cervix, any compromise of these areas may predispose the mare to a recurrent or chronic uterine infection. In contrast to the high morbidity of CEM, the pathophysiology of infections with *S. zooepidemicus* and *E. coli* is complex and involves active participation of all facets of the mare's uterine defense mechanisms. Mares with a functional uterine defense are capable of eliminating a bacterial contamination from the uterus within 36 to 48 hours. These mares are classified as resistant to chronic uterine infection. Mares that fail to clear the uterus from a bacterial contamination are classified as susceptible to chronic uterine infection and are believed to have a compromised uterine defense. Susceptibility to chronic endometritis is common in older and multiparous mares and is a major cause of equine infertility. Susceptible mares often develop a persistent endometritis after breeding, and may even become contaminated spontaneously when the mare is in estrus. During estrus, the strength of the external barriers decreases as the vulva and cervix relax. This is normally compensated for by strengthened uterine defense mechanisms. In susceptible mares, the impaired uterine defense may allow the normal genital flora to contaminate the uterus and develop into persistent endometritis.

Clinical Signs and Diagnosis

Mares with endometritis may exhibit vaginal discharge during estrus. A small amount of exudate is often observed at the ventral vulvar commissure after rectal examination as a combined result of induced myometrial activity and manual pressure on the uterus and vagina. Speculum examination per vagina may demonstrate the presence of exudate in the vagina. Variable amounts of cloudy or purulent exudate can often be observed passing out of the cervical os. Endometritis should be suspected in mares with ultrasonographic evidence of intraluminal uterine fluid. The presence of inflammation in the uterus causes release of $PGF_2\alpha$. The endogenous prostaglandins are luteolytic, resulting in a shortened estrous cycle in mares with endometritis. Because endometritis is a leading cause of subfertility in the mare, it should always be a differential diagnosis for pregnancy failure following breeding to a fertile stallion. Endometritis is not associated with systemic illness in the mare.

The diagnosis of endometritis is confirmed by a positive bacterial or fungal endometrial culture in association with the presence of PMNs in the uterus. The bacterial culture should be taken during estrus, and should always be combined with uterine cytology examination to be reliable. Interpretation of endometrial culture and cytology test results is discussed under Breeding Soundness Examination, page 505. *S. zooepidemicus*, *E. coli*, *P. aeruginosa*, and *K. pneumoniae* are the most common bacteria cultured from mares with endometritis. Anaerobic microorganisms, such as *Bacteroides fragilis*, have been suggested to cause endometritis. Yeast (i.e., *Candida* species) or fungal infections (i.e., *Aspergillus* species) can also be cultured from the endometrium and may be the result of repeated intrauterine treatment with broad-spectrum antibiotics.

The presence of inflammatory cells on an endometrial biopsy serve as evidence of endometritis. A culture from the biopsy specimen before histologic preparation can determine the causative organism.

Treatment

The first therapeutic concern should be to correct the predisposing causes, such as a breakdown of external genital barriers. This may be accomplished by use of Caslicks vulvoplasty, urethral extension, cervical repair, and other techniques. Antibiotics may be administered by either local or systemic routes. Advantages of local antibiotic therapy are that high and predictable levels of antibiotics can reach the site of infection. Most cases of endometritis involve only the uterine lumen and the superficial layers of the endometrium. This is in contrast to the postpartum metritis complex, discussed under the section on dystocia and retained fetal membranes (see pages 552 and 560). Thorough cleansing of the perineal region, with special attention to the clitoral fossa, is necessary to avoid contamination of the tract during local treatments. Systemic therapy with antimicrobials may be considered in horses in which recontamination of the uterus is of great concern. Systemic treatment should be performed when an endometrial biopsy suggests a deep endometrial infection. Systemic treatment with a combination of ciprofloxacin (2.5 g/day) and probenecid (1 g/day) have been reported to be effective against *Pseudomonas* infections in the uterus (W. Zent, personal communication). Antibiotic therapy should be selected based on results of sensitivity tests. Although a few pharmacokinetics studies on intrauterine antibiotic therapy have been conducted, therapeutic guidelines are mainly based on clinical observations (Table 1). Most antibiotics do not function well in the presence of inflammatory debris. Therefore, if free fluid and inflammatory debris are present in the uterine lumen, the uterus should be lavaged with a buffered saline solution or lactated Ringer's solution before treatment. Aminoglycosides may be irritating to the endometrium, and some authors recommend that these drugs be adequately diluted and buffered in an equal volume of 7.5% sodium bicarbonate solution before use. The volume of fluid used for antibiotic therapy is dependent on the size of the uterus. If a low volume of antimicrobial solution is used to infuse the uterus, the antibiotics may not be distributed throughout the entire lumen. Excessive volumes will only result in expulsion of the drug from the uterus. A total volume of 30 to 60 ml is usually sufficient. Daily treatments for 4 to 6 days during estrus are recommended.

Yeast or fungal infections are often the result of extensive use of antibiotics in the uterus. These infections are difficult to treat and may cause permanent damage to the endometrium. No controlled clinical reports are in the literature on the treatment of genital yeast and fungal infections in the mare. Irrigation of the uterus with dilute povidone-iodine solution (1 to 2%), vinegar (<5%), or

TABLE 1. RECOMMENDED DOSES FOR INTRAUTERINE ANTIBIOTICS THERAPY IN THE MARE*

Antibiotics	Dose	Comments
Amikacin sulfate	2 g	Gram-negative spectrum; buffer with equal volume of 7.5% bicarbonate
Carbenicillin	6 g	*Pseudomonas*
Gentamicin sulfate	1–2 g	Gram-negative spectrum; buffer with equal volume of 7.5% bicarbonate
Kanamycin sulfate	1–2 g	*E. coli*
Neomycin sulfate	3–4 g	*E. coli*
Penicillin	5 million units	*S. zooepidemicus*
Polymyxin B	1 million units	*Pseudomonas*
Ticarcillin	6 g	Broad spectrum
Ticarcillin/clavulanic acid	6 g/200 mg	Broad spectrum
Ceftiofur	1 g	Broad spectrum (*S. zooepidemicus*)
Antimycotics		
Nystatin	500,000 units	Dissolve in 30 ml 0.9% saline solution; daily for 7 to 10 days
Clotrimazole	500 mg	Suspension or cream; daily for 1 week
Vinegar	2%	20 ml wine vinegar to 1 L of 0.9% saline solution; used as uterine lavage

*Parts adapted from Asbury AC, Lyle SK: *In* Equine Reproduction, McKinnon AO, Voss JL (eds): Philadelphia, Lea & Febiger, 1993, p 381; Neely DP: *In* Equine Reproduction, Veterinary Learning Systems, 1983, p. 40; and Zent W: personal communication.

dilute acetic acid has been tried by clinicians with varying results. Specific antifungal drugs that have been used for intrauterine treatments in the mare are listed in Table 1. An intrinsic problem with uterine yeast and fungal infections is the sustained therapeutic duration that is required for successful treatment. Several weeks of daily treatments may not be cost-effective.

Clinical reports of alternative treatments of chronic endometritis include intrauterine infusions with a variety of disinfectants, irritants, autologous or heterologous blood plasma, colostrum, filtrates of bacterial toxins, and systemic treatments with immunostimulants. Most of these treatments have not been tested in controlled studies and are controversial. Before using a controversial or new treatment of chronic endometritis, the clinician has to ensure that infusion of a chemical into the uterus does not cause additional and even irreversible damage to the endometrium. It is the author's opinion that most cases of endometritis benefit from effectively removing inflammatory debris and tissue-destructive agents along with the causative organism from the uterus rather than adding more potentially damaging chemicals into the uterine lumen. Repeated daily treatments with intrauterine plasma infusions were shown to be beneficial in cases with recurrent endometritis in mares that were highly susceptible to chronic endometritis. It was believed that the addition of complement from blood plasma would enhance the phagocytic capacity of PMNs. This treatment has failed to demonstrate efficacy in controlled experiments, but these studies used a protocol of single rather than repeated infusions of plasma. If intrauterine plasma infusions are used, they have to be prepared antiseptically and with heparin solutions rather than a chelator of calcium as anticoagulants in order not to inactivate complement.

Hormone therapy has been used as an adjunct treatment of endometritis. Uterine defense mechanisms, including PMN phagocytosis, intraluminal concentrations of immunoglobulins, and physical clearance mechanisms, are suppressed during diestrus and enhanced during estrus. Manipulation of the estrous cycle to provide multiple estrus periods and short periods of progesterone influence may aid in the treatment of endometritis. Most commonly, luteolysis is induced with exogenous prostaglandins as soon as the corpus luteum is responsive (approximately 5 days after ovulation). Although estrogen therapy has been shown to help ovariectomized mares to effectively clear the uterus of inoculated bacteria, it is questionable if additional exogenous estrogen during estrus is beneficial in an intact mare.

Persistent Mating-induced Endometritis

A transient and probably physiologic postmating endometritis occurs as a result of intrauterine deposition of semen. The opportunity for uterine contamination during breeding is great despite all protective physical barriers. In addition, recent studies strongly suggest that spermatozoa rather than bacteria induce a uterine inflammatory response following mating. After fertilization has taken place, the fertilized egg remains in the oviduct for 5 days. The conceptus then descends into the uterine lumen, where the presence of bacteria and inflammatory products may be incompatible with the survival of the embryo. The uterus must thus be able to spontaneously clear uterine

contamination of microorganisms and inflammatory products within the first 5 days after conception. Although uterine clearance is easily accomplished by resistant mares, susceptible mares often fail to clear the uterus within the required time. Local components of the uterine defense mechanisms are responsible for the rapid clearance of an infection. Although a local immunosuppression of the endometrium has been suggested to be responsible for susceptibility to chronic uterine inflammation, research demonstrates that an impaired physical clearance is the main factor involved in susceptibility to a persistent endometritis. Studies using radioactive-labeled microspheres and scintigraphy to assess uterine clearance demonstrated a delayed and dysfunctional uterine clearance in susceptible mares (Fig. 1). Although the resistant mares cleared microspheres from the uterus within 24 hours, susceptible mares retained microspheres within the uterine lumen up to 96 hours after inoculation. Using electromyographic (EMG) registration of myometrial activity, it was later shown that the impaired uterine physical clearance in susceptible mares is caused by a dysfunctional myometrial activity in response to intrauterine contamination (Fig. 2).

Clinical Signs and Diagnosis

Persistent postmating endometritis is most common in older multiparous mares. Mares susceptible to persistent postmating endometritis often have a history of recurrent bacterial endometritis. They may accumulate fluid in the uterine lumen when in estrus. Palpation may reveal that the uterus is abnormally flaccid for the stage of the estrous cycle, and most susceptible mares have visceroptosis resulting in the uterus being pulled over the pelvic brim into an abdominal position. The position of the uterus could negatively affect uterine clearance via the cervix. Mares that repeatedly fail to conceive after being bred to a fertile stallion should be suspected of having postmating endometritis.

An accurate diagnosis of postmating endometritis can be difficult to make in individual cases. It must be kept in mind that a postmating endometritis normally occurs dur-

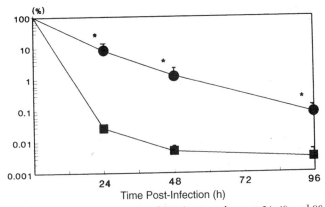

Figure 1. Intrauterine retention of (^{51}Cr) microspheres at 24, 48, and 96 hours after inoculation in mares susceptible (●) and resistant (■) to persistent endometritis. Susceptible mares were significantly different from resistant mares at all times ($P <0.0001$). (From Troedsson MHT, Liu IKM: Uterine clearance of non-antigenic markers (^{51}Cr) in response to a bacterial challenge in mares potentially susceptible and resistant to chronic uterine infection. J Reprod Fertil 44[Suppl]:283, 1991).

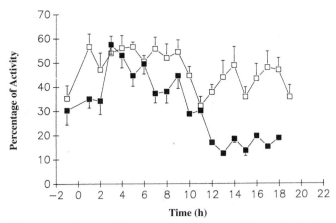

Figure 2. Total uterine electrical activity following an intrauterine bacterial challenge in mares susceptible (■) and resistant (□) to persistent endometritis. Resistant mares showed more uterine activity than did susceptible mares (P <0.001). Susceptible mares had delayed onset of uterine activity followed by a sharp decline of activity. (From Troedsson MHT, Liu IKM, Ing M, Pascoe J, Thurmond MJ: Multiple site electromyographic recordings of uterine activity following an intrauterine bacterial challenge in mares susceptible and resistant to chronic uterine infection. J Reprod Fertil 99:307, 1993).

ing the first 24 to 36 hours after breeding. A presumptive diagnosis is based on the mare's reproductive history, clinical signs, and the presence of intraluminal fluid for more than 20 hours after mating. A shortened estrous cycle following breeding is suggestive of persistent postmating endometritis. The diagnostic value of endometrial biopsies to identify mares that were susceptible to persistent endometritis has been investigated. It was concluded that mares without endometrial pathology (Kenney category 1) generally were resistant to persistent inflammation, whereas mares with severe endometrial pathology (category 3) were likely, although not absolutely certain, to be susceptible. It was not possible to predict the persistent postbreeding endometritis in mares with endometrial biopsies classified as category 2a or 2b.

Treatment

Although treatment of sexually transmitted diseases and chronic uterine infection should be directed against the microbial agent that causes the disease, treatment of mares that are susceptible to persistent mating-induced endometritis should be aimed at assisting the uterus to physically clear contaminants and inflammatory products.

Before breeding a mare that is susceptible to persistent postmating endometritis, the reproductive tract has to be free from predisposing factors and current infection. This can be achieved by surgical corrections of breakdown of the external barriers and treatment of an existing bacterial or fungal endometritis. The uterus should be confirmed free from infection, based on culture and cytology test results.

Uterine lavage with large volumes of fluid 6 to 24 hours after each breeding effectively aids the mare to clear inflammatory products from the uterus in good time to allow embryonal survival. Following thorough cleansing of the perineum, a 30-French, 80-cm-long flushing catheter with

a 75-ml balloon cuff* is introduced through the cervix. Once the cuff is located in the uterus, it is inflated until it effectively seals the internal cervical os. A total of 1 L of buffered saline solution or lactated Ringer's solution is infused into the uterus. Following brief transrectal massage of the uterus to ensure an even distribution of fluid in both horns, the fluid should be recovered in a bottle that allows visual examination. The lavage should be repeated until the recovered fluid is clear. A cloudy fluid is indicative of inflammatory debris. Measurement of the recovered fluid volume or ultrasonographic examination of the uterus ensures that all fluid has been recovered. This is important, because the mare has an impaired ability to spontaneously clear the uterus. Uterine lavage should be performed after each mating to be effective.

The use of drugs to stimulate myometrial contractions can also assist in the clearance of inflammatory fluid from the uterus. The administration of oxytocin (20 IU IM) at 4 to 8 hours after mating effectively clears the uterus. $PGF_2\alpha$ has also been demonstrated to increase myometrial activity and assist in clearing the uterine lumen of contaminating products. Studies of the duration of myometrial activity following administration of oxytocin and $PGF_2\alpha$ show that 20 IU of oxytocin causes 1 hour of increased myometrial activity, and 10 mg of $PGF_2\alpha$ causes 5 hours of increased activity. Both drugs also affected the oviductal smooth muscles in a similar way. Consideration of the duration of the effect of oxytocin and prostaglandins on both myometrial and oviductal activity should be made before these hormones are used in postmating treatments. It appears that the efficacy and safety aspects favor oxytocin over prostaglandins. A combination of postmating uterine lavage and oxytocin treatment is preferred by some practitioners.

Chronic Degenerative Endometritis

Degenerative changes of the endometrium may result from repeated inflammation, but they have also been observed in older mares without known history of endometritis. This suggests that degenerative fibrosis of the endometrium may be a process of aging.

Clinical Signs and Diagnosis

Mares with endometrial fibrotic degeneration of the endometrium are typically older and often multiparous mares. Their ability to conceive and carry a foal to term is compromised. Diagnosis is confirmed on endometrial biopsy.

Treatment and Prognosis

Several treatments have been suggested for degenerative fibrosis of the endometrium, but consistent results have not been reported. Mechanical and chemical irritation of the endometrium have been used. Uterine curettage caused improvement in 80% of mares with chronic degenerative endometritis in one study. Concerns that mechanical trauma to the endometrium may produce more scar tissue than repair have limited the popularity of the method. Intrauterine infusion of kerosene was believed to improve fertility in mares with chronic degenerative changes to their endometrium. However, there are no controlled studies to show the effectiveness of this treat-

---

*Bivona, Gary, IN

ment. Infusion of dimethyl sulfoxide (DMSO) into the uterine lumen was shown to improve fibrosis in mares with chronic degenerative endometritis. Others were not able to repeat these results.

The list of treatments for chronic degenerative endometritis is indicative of the difficulties that face clinicians who attempt to successfully treat these mares. Regardless of treatment, the prognosis for reproduction is poor.

PYOMETRA

Pyometra is characterized by an accumulation of purulent exudate in the uterine lumen. The etiology of pyometra in the mare is not completely clear. It may result from trauma to the cervix with subsequent obstruction and bacterial contamination. Cervical adhesions as a result of uterine therapy with irritating agents or as a result of cervicitis may also lead to pyometra if the sealed uterus is contaminated by bacteria. Some mares develop pyometra without any apparent functional or physical occlusion of the cervix. Impaired uterine clearance in mares susceptible to persistent or chronic endometritis may predispose mares to pyometra. The author has diagnosed cases of pyometra as a result of retained endometrial culture swabs. Mares with pyometra often have a prolonged luteal phase with sustained elevations in progesterone. However, increased progesterone is not believed to have the same significance for etiology of equine pyometra as it does in the bitch and the queen. The prolonged luteal phase in mares with pyometra is rather a result of inflammatory destruction of the endometrium, prohibiting synthesis and release of PGF$_2\alpha$.

Clinical Signs and Diagnosis

Mares with pyometra rarely show clinical signs of systemic disease. Although mares with large amounts (50 to 60 L) of exudate in the uterus may become anorectic and exhibit some signs of systemic illness when the uterus becomes distended with pus, others show no concurrent clinical signs. Hematologic changes are minimal and nondiagnostic. Ovulatory intervals may be shortened, normal, or prolonged in mares with pyometra.

Only mares with cervical patency have observable discharge. In brood mares, pyometra is frequently diagnosed during a breeding soundness evaluation for infertility. In mares that are kept for purposes other than breeding, the diagnosis is often incidental during routine reproductive examination.

The diagnosis of pyometra is made by palpation and ultrasonographic examination of the uterus per rectum. The uterus has uniformly enlarged horns, and its consistency can range from thin-walled and atonic to more commonly thick-walled and doughy. Pyometra may be mistaken for an 80- to 120-day pregnancy upon rectal palpation. Transrectal ultrasonography and determination of hormone concentrations can be used to distinguish between these. In contrast to the anechoic or hypoechoic allantoic fluid that is seen in the uterus during pregnancy, intraluminal fluid in mares with pyometra is hyperechogenic because of inflammatory cells. Determination of serum estrogen or equine chorionic gonadotropin (eCG) concentration may also be helpful to confirm or rule out pregnancy at this stage. Both hormones should be elevated if the mare is pregnant.

Bacteria can be cultured from some but not all cases of pyometra. The same bacterial flora that is found in mares with endometritis can be expected.

Treatment and Prognosis

Mares with a consistently small or moderate amount of exudate in the uterus may·not require treatment, unless they are going to be used for breeding in the future. Brood mares and mares with a large accumulation of exudate in the uterus should have their uteri drained through the cervix. If cervical obstruction is present, adhesions should be removed and cervical patency ensured. A tube should be inserted with utmost care through the cervix into the uterus. The uterine wall may be fragile in mares with a large distended uterus. A small amount of exudate can be drained rapidly, but emptying of large quantities of fluid from the uterus can cause signs of shock, and should therefore be performed slowly. The amount of exudate varies from less than 1 L to more than 60 L of thick milky fluid, or in some cases serosanguinous fluid. Following drainage, the uterus should be lavaged with saline or lactated Ringer's solution. The uterine lavage can be repeated until the quality of the recovered fluid has improved and continued daily until the uterus stays empty and the uterine size approaches normal. If the cervix remains patent between treatments, the administration of oxytocin (20 IU IM) or PGF$_2\alpha$ (10 mg IM) helps the uterus to reduce its size and expel freshly formed fluid. In addition, PGF$_2\alpha$ also lyses a corpus luteum if present. An endometrial biopsy provides a prognosis for future fertility. Generally, the prognosis for reproductive performance is poor in cases of chronic pyometra. The prolonged distension of the uterus often causes a permanent failure of the uterine clearance mechanisms. In addition, chronic cervical adhesions tend to recur. Degenerative changes to the endometrium are usually permanent. The severity of histopathologic findings on an endometrial biopsy from mares with pyometra often correlates with clinical and endocrine observations of the estrous cycle. Mares with shortened or normal cycles can be expected to have pathologic changes in their endometrium limited to signs of inflammation. Mares with a prolonged luteal phase often have severe degenerative changes with widespread fibrosis and atrophy of the endometrium. Mares with continuous luteal phase have almost complete endometrial destruction. These mares are considered to be sterile. Hysterectomy should be considered in mares with chronic pyometra that are not intended for breeding. Although hysterectomy in mares is more difficult than in bitches, the technique can be performed successfully. Uterine drainage and treatment with antimicrobials, until the uterus is empty and close to normal size, greatly facilitate surgery and reduce the chance of peritonitis. An alternative to hysterectomy in nonbreeding animals is to empty the uterus at regular intervals.

ENDOMETRIAL CYSTS

Endometrial cysts originate from either endometrial glands or obstructed lymphatics. Glandular cysts are less than 10 mm in diameter and are believed to be the result of periglandular fibrosis. Lymphatic cysts can reach several centimeters in diameter and may be palpated as enlargements in the uterus. The etiology of lymphatic cysts remains unclear. The prevalence of endometrial lymphatic cysts was reported to be 27% of all mares, and was much higher in mares older than 11 years of age. It has been associated with both normal and abnormal uterine pathology test results.

Clinical Signs and Diagnosis

The relationship between endometrial cysts and subfertility is controversial. Endometrial cysts have been associated with lower conception rates and a higher incidence of fetal loss, but it is not clear if the cysts interfere with fertility or if they just are more common in mares with endometrial pathology of other causes. Both subfertility and endometrial cysts tend to increase with age, but each may occur independently. It has been proposed that large endometrial cysts are capable of preventing normal migration of the embryo, restricting the ability of the embryonic vesicle to prevent luteolysis after day 10. In addition, some authors suggest that endometrial cysts that are located at the base of one uterine horn may interfere with absorption of nutrients. However, large endometrial cysts are often observed in pregnant mares with normal pregnancies. A study involving just under 300 mares concluded that the presence, number, diameter, or volume of endometrial cysts had no effect on establishing or maintaining pregnancy.

Transrectal ultrasonography is the best method to detect endometrial cysts. Additional diagnostic tools include direct view of the cysts through hysterendoscopy and palpation of large cysts per rectum. Endometrial cysts can easily be mistaken for an early pregnancy. Mistakes are best avoided by scanning the uterus for detection of cysts before breeding, with the location and size of all detected cysts recorded in detail. Embryonic vesicles grow in a predictable pattern (2.5 to 3 mm/day up to day 17). The growth rate of endometrial cysts is not known but the size appears to remain constant or increases very slowly. Particular care must be taken when twin pregnancy is suspected. The clinician has to be absolutely sure that one vesicle is not actually a cyst before twin reduction is attempted.

Treatment

Endometrial cysts do not require treatment unless they are suspected to interfere with pregnancy. Several treatment options have been reported. Needle aspiration, mechanical rupture of the cyst with endoscopic biopsy instruments, uterine curettage, or intrauterine infusion of hypertonic saline solution have all been suggested to effectively remove cysts. However, the value of these treatments may be questioned, because the cysts often recur following treatment. Successful obliteration of endometrial cysts using endoscopic-guided laser surgery has been reported in the literature. Laser surgery permanently removes cysts, but the long-term effect on fertility has not yet been critically evaluated.

VENTRAL SACCULATION OF THE UTERINE WALL

Partial dilation of the ventral uterine wall at the base of one uterine horn has been described as a result of myometrial atony. The endometrium over the sacculated area has atrophied with a focal loss of glands. The site of sacculation is identical to the site of embryonic fixation and implantation.

Clinical Signs and Diagnosis

Ventral uterine sacculation is seen in aged multiparous mares. Because of its location and susceptibility to persistent postmating endometritis, infertility is often associated with the condition. The sacculation can be palpated per rectum, ventrally at the base of one of the uterine horns. The condition may be mistaken for an early pregnancy by inexperienced clinicians. Transrectal ultrasonographic examination of the tract may reveal accumulation of fluid during estrus.

Treatment

Repeated oxytocin therapy or uterine lavages with hot saline (40–45°C) temporarily increases uterine tone. Long-term benefit of this treatment is questionable. Postmating uterine lavage has been used to prevent the accumulation of fluid, mating-induced debris, and inflammatory products from the uterus. Although this treatment may prevent fluid accumulation in the uterus, it does not restore long-term myometrial tone or improve endometrial atrophy.

NEOPLASIA

Uterine neoplasia is rare in the mare; leiomyoma is most commonly diagnosed. Leiomyomas consist of interwoven bundles of smooth muscle cells. They may be palpated as multiple or more often solitary masses in the uterine lumen or wall. Leiomyomas are usually pedunculated, but may also be attached to a broad area of the uterine wall. If pedunculated, they can be removed with a surgical snare through the cervix.

Other tumors that have been reported in the mare's uterus include fibroma, leiomyosarcoma, adenocarcinoma, lymphosarcoma, and botryoid rhabdomyosarcoma.

ADHESIONS

Uterine adhesions are often associated with other uterine pathology. Adhesions may result from trauma from dystocia or intrauterine therapy with irritating chemicals. The adhesions may cause infertility if they interfere with embryo migration during early pregnancy or if they obstruct effective uterine clearance. Complete uterine adhesions can predispose to pyometra if they are associated with a uterine infection.

Clinical Signs and Diagnosis

Incomplete uterine adhesions may not be diagnosed until they interfere with normal pregnancy. If fluid accumulates in the uterus proximal to an adhesion, it can be diagnosed by ultrasonographic examination. However, most adhesions are observed during a hysterendoscopic examination of the uterus. The adhesions may completely obstruct the uterine lumen or they may be incomplete.

Treatment

Uterine adhesions can be broken down with a uterine biopsy instrument while visualized by hysterendoscopy. Videoendoscopic-guided laser surgery is probably the preferred method to treat the adhesions.

Supplemental Readings

Hughes JP, Stabenfeldt GH, Kindahl H, Kennedy PC, Edquist L-E, Neely DP, Schalm OW: Pyometra in the mare. J Reprod Fertil 27[Suppl]:321–329, 1979.

Kenney RM, Ganjam VK: Selected pathological changes of the mare uterus and ovary. J Reprod Fertil 23[Suppl]:335–339, 1975.

LeBlanc MM: Recurrent endometritis: Is oxytocin the answer? Proc 40th Annu Meet Am Assoc Equine Pract, 1994, pp 17–18.

Powell DG: Contagious equine metritis. In Morrow DA (ed): Current Therapy in Reproduction 2. Philadelphia, WB Saunders, 1986, pp 786–792.

Santschi EM, Adams SB, Robertson JT, DeBowes RM, Mitten LA, Sojka JE: Ovariohysterectomy in six mares. Vet Surg 24:165–171, 1995.

Troedsson MHT: Uterine defense mechanisms in the mare. Arch STD/HIV Res 8:259–270, 1994.

Troedsson MHT, Liu IKM: Uterine clearance of non-antigenic markers (^{51}Cr) in response to a bacterial challenge in mares potentially susceptible and resistant to chronic uterine infections. J Reprod Fertil 44[Suppl]:283–288, 1991.

Troedsson MHT, Liu IKM, Ing M, Pascoe J, Thurmond M: Multiple site electromyography recordings of uterine activity following an intrauterine bacterial challenge in mares susceptible and resistant to chronic uterine infection. J Reprod Fertil 99:307–313, 1993.

Troedsson MHT, Scott MA, Liu IKM: Comparative treatment of mares susceptible to chronic uterine infection. Am J Vet Res 56:468–472, 1996.

Diseases of the Ovary

MATS H.T. TROEDSSON

JANE A. BARBER
St. Paul, Minnesota

Equine ovaries are suspended within the abdominal cavity by the mesovarium, which is part of the broad ligament. The anatomy of the equine ovary differs significantly from that in other species. In the ovary of the adult mare, the medulla is superficial and the cortex, which contains the oocytes and follicles, is located in the interior of the ovary. The germinal epithelium of the cortex reaches the surface only at the ovulation fossa. This is the only area from which ovulation occurs. Although follicles easily can be palpated per rectum, the corpus luteum does not protrude above the surface of the ovary as in other species, and it may be difficult to detect on rectal palpation.

Ovarian abnormalities and diseases may cause temporary or permanent infertility. For the purpose of this chapter, ovarian diseases are divided into abnormal small ovaries, abnormal large ovaries, and other ovarian abnormalities.

DIAGNOSIS

A complete and accurate history of the mare's reproductive performance, estrous cycles, and behavior should always be obtained. Mares with ovarian abnormalities may exhibit stallion-like behavior, lack of estrus, irregular estrus, or persistent estrus. Examination of the reproductive tract should include vaginoscopy, rectal palpation, and transrectal ultrasonography. The appearance of the mucous membranes of the vagina and the cervix reflects changes during both the estrous cycle and in anestrus. Following visual evaluation of the mare's external genitalia, rectal palpation and transrectal ultrasonographic examination of the ovaries should be performed. Size, location, and follicular and luteal activity of the ovaries should be evaluated. The presence of an ovary smaller than 2 cm or larger than 10 cm suggests an ovarian abnormality and should be further investigated. Parovarian cysts and remnants of the mesonephric duct are commonly found on mares' ovaries. They are clinically insignificant but should not be confused with follicular activity on ultrasonographic examination. A thorough rectal palpation of the ovaries distinguishes these findings. The ovulation fossa should be palpable on normal ovaries. All observations, normal or abnormal, should be recorded for comparison at future examinations. Repeated serial examinations are useful to observe progressive changes in ovarian activity.

Peripheral blood hormonal profiles add important information on ovarian cyclic activity and specific ovarian pathology. Elevated serum progesterone concentrations confirm the presence of active luteal tissue in nonpregnant mares. Analysis of baseline and gonadotropin-releasing hormone (GnRH)-stimulated concentrations of estrogens, luteinizing hormone (LH), and follicle stimulating hormone (FSH) may be helpful in cases in which endocrine dysfunction is suspected to cause ovarian inactivity. A blood sample for karyotyping should be obtained from mares with suspected chromosomal abnormalities.

ABNORMALLY SMALL OVARIES

The most common causes of bilaterally small ovaries in the mare are (1) severe malnutrition, (2) hypothalamopituitary dysfunction, (3) immaturity, (4) seasonal anestrus, (5) advanced age, (6) use of anabolic steroids, and (7) gonadal dysgenesis.

Severe Malnutrition

Poor nutrition, particularly in lactating mares, severe weight loss, and chronic disease may affect the release of GnRH from the hypothalamus. GnRH stimulation of the anterior pituitary gland is essential for the release of gonadotropins that regulate ovarian activity.

Clinical Signs and Diagnosis

Physical examination reveals a mare in poor body condition. The ovaries palpate as small, hard, and inactive bodies. The uterus feels flaccid, and the cervix is typically relaxed or has slight tone. These findings should be confirmed by transrectal ultrasonography. Small nonpalpable "follicles" 5 to 10 mm in diameter can occasionally be found on inactive ovaries. These structures do not indicate ovarian activity and they do not produce hormones. The diagnosis is based on clinical signs and serum progesterone concentrations less than 1 ng/ml.

Treatment

Correction of the underlying condition and improving the nutrition will, in time, overcome ovarian inactivity due to malnutrition.

Hypothalamopituitary Dysfunction

Specific pituitary abnormalities are rare in the horse, but ovarian inactivity caused by adenomatous hyperplasia or neoplasia of the intermediate pituitary (Cushing's syndrome) has been reported. The mechanism for the dysfunction of the hypothalamopituitary-gonadal axis in mares with Cushing's syndrome is not clear but may be similar to that observed in women with this condition. Elevated concentration of adrenocorticotropic hormone (ACTH) released from the pituitary gland results in an increased adrenal androgen secretion. Increased blood concentrations of androgens may adversely affect the development of ovarian follicles via negative feedback on the hypothalamopituitary-gonadal axis. Secondary pituitary inactivity can also occur in emaciated horses and as a temporary condition during transition between seasonal anestrus and the breeding season.

Clinical Signs and Diagnosis

Mares with ovarian inactivity as a result of adenomatous hyperplasia or neoplasia of the pituitary have classic signs of Cushing's syndrome such as long curly hair coat, potbelly, polyuria, polydipsia, and hyperhidrosis. In addition, these mares have small inactive ovaries and a flaccid reproductive tract.

The diagnosis of hypothalamic-pituitary-gonadal dysfunction is based on clinical signs and endocrine testing. Cushing's syndrome can be diagnosed with a dexamethasone suppression test (see *Current Therapy in Equine Medicine 2*, pages 183–184). Determination of blood concentrations of gonadotropins and ovarian hormones and results of GnRH stimulation tests may be helpful in diagnosing a primary hypothalamopituitary dysfunction.

Treatment

Correcting the underlying cause of the hypothalamopituitary-gonadal dysfunction re-establishes normal ovarian activity. If a primary dysfunction of the hypothalamopituitary-gonadal axis is diagnosed, supplemental hormone therapy (i.e., GnRH) may be helpful. The clinician has to be aware of the complex feedback mechanisms involved in the hypothalamopituitary-gonadal axis and also must consider the possibility of downregulation of receptors when pharmacologic doses of GnRH are used. Mares with Cushing's syndrome are often older mares, and the prognosis for reproductive function is poor.

Immaturity

The average age at which mares reach puberty is 18 months with a wide range from 10 to 24 months. Diagnosis of ovarian inactivity or limited follicular activity in fillies younger than 2 years of age should, therefore, be made with caution. Fillies younger than 2 years old with inactive ovaries accompanied by a flaccid and relaxed reproductive tract may still be too young to cycle and should be re-examined at a later time. The condition has to be differentiated from gonadal dysgenesis. Karyotyping to rule out gonadal dysgenesis may be indicated if puberty is delayed beyond 24 months. As most parents are aware, immature development and puberty is most successfully treated with time.

Seasonal Anestrus

Mares are seasonal polyestrous, long-day breeders. Approximately 80% of all mares have a normal anestrus period during the late fall and winter months. The duration of seasonal anestrus is approximately 6 months with some variation, depending on changes in photoperiod and body condition of the mare. Typically, mares in the Northern Hemisphere cease to have ovarian activity in October and November and start their cyclic activity in April. Most mares exhibit a period of irregular estrus, accompanied by follicular activity without ovulation during the spring. The mechanism of seasonal anestrus and transition into the breeding season is described in *Current Therapy in Equine Medicine 2*, pages 491–494.

Clinical Signs and Diagnosis

The detection of inactive ovaries or limited follicular activity (<20 mm in diameter) in the absence of luteal tissue during the winter and early spring suggests seasonal anestrus rather than ovarian pathology. The reproductive tract of seasonally anestral mares palpates as flaccid and thin, and the mare's behavior in the presence of a stallion varies from passive avoidance to receptivity. Reproductive soundness examinations during this time have to be interpreted with caution because seasonal reproductive inactivity may mask ovarian inactivity of other origin. Interpretation of an endometrial biopsy for uterine pathology may be difficult in seasonal anestral mares. The histopathologic findings are characterized by low glandular density during this time. Diagnosis is based on time of the year, findings on rectal palpation, ultrasonographic examination of the reproductive tract, and repeated serum progesterone concentrations <1 ng/ml.

Treatment

The condition is physiologic and does not need to be treated in most mares. However, many breed registries have assigned January 1 as the arbitrary birth date of all foals born in the Northern Hemisphere (June 1 in the Southern Hemisphere). An imposed artificial breeding season during the winter and early spring may require treatment of seasonally anestral mares. Adding artificial light at sunset to achieve a total of 16 hours of daylight results in cyclic ovarian activity within 60 days. Treatment with continuous release or subcutaneous pulses of native GnRH* (10 μg/hour) or twice-daily injections of a GnRH agonist† (10 μg sq b.i.d.) results in follicular growth and ovulation in anestral mares. The management and treatment of breeding mares early during the year is not within the topic of this chapter, but has been described in detail elsewhere (see *Current Therapy in Equine Medicine 2*, p. 493).

Advanced Age

The effect of age on ovarian follicular activity is not well documented. Examination of pony mares at slaughterhouses shows that many mares older than 20 years are still reproductively active but that some mares have reached ovarian senescence. Ovarian dysfunction in aged mares is manifested by delayed initiation of the ovulatory season and failure of ovulation. Mares older than 19 years ovulate for the first time each year 2 weeks later than young mares. Some aged mares fail to ovulate throughout the entire season. In addition to ovulatory failure, a report revealed an increased rate of defective oocytes in aged mares, which further compromises fertility.

Clinical Signs and Diagnosis

Clinical signs of anovulation due to age are similar to those exhibited by seasonally anestral mares. The ovaries are small and firm with no or limited follicular activity, and the reproductive tract is flaccid with pale, dry mucous membranes. Serum progesterone concentrations are less than 1 ng/ml. Aged mares with ovarian inactivity may show estrous behavior similar to that of seasonal anestral mares. The condition may, therefore, go undetected in mares that are being mated on the basis of estrous behavior alone. Because older mares may have a delayed seasonal onset of ovarian activity, mares with inactive ovaries during the early part of the breeding season need to be re-examined before a diagnosis of permanent ovarian inactivity can be confirmed.

Treatment

Currently no treatment is available for age-related ovarian inactivity. A delayed onset of the ovulatory season may affect the seasonal conception rate negatively, because fewer cycles are available for mating. Older mares, therefore, benefit from an artificial light regimen starting 60 to 90 days before the breeding season. Treatment of age-related ovarian inactivity with exogenous GnRH has been discouraging. However, too few mares have been treated to evaluate the effectiveness of the treatment.

---

*Lutrelef, Ferring Laboratories, Ridgewood, NJ
†Buserelin, Hoechst-Roussel AgriVet, Somerville, NJ

Use of Anabolic Steroids

Anabolic steroids are derivates from androgens that have been altered to provide high anabolic activity with minimal androgenic side effects. The androgenic potency is variable among preparations. A dose- and drug-dependent suppression of gonadotropin secretion and ovarian activity has been well documented.

Clinical Signs and Diagnosis

Mares that are treated with low doses of anabolic steroids may show clinical signs of abnormal or stallion-like sexual behavior, such as increased aggressiveness towards other horses and mounting of other estral mares. Ovarian activity ceases when higher doses are administered. Treated mares have small firm ovaries, a flaccid reproductive tract, and serum progesterone concentrations less than 1 ng/ml. Prolonged treatment of prepubertal mares with anabolic steroids results in hypertrophy of the clitoris.

Treatment and Prognosis

Ovarian inactivity persists for some time after discontinuation of anabolic steroids, but pituitary and ovarian function eventually returns to normal in most mares. The abnormal sexual behavior may persist for longer periods of time. Anabolic steroids are not recommended in mares intended for breeding.

Gonadal Dysgenesis

Sexual determination and development occur in a deliberate manner. Initiation of gonad formation requires only one X or one Y chromosome. However, completion of normal gonadal development requires that germ cells in the ovary have precisely two X chromosomes, and that those in the testis have one Y and no more than one X chromosome. A signal from the Y chromosome, named the testis determining factor (TDF), converts undifferentiated gonads into testes. Absence of the signal results in ovary formation. The TDF has recently been identified as a small gene, SRY (*Sex-determining Region of the Y*), with a conserved core of less than 250 nucleotide bases.

The role of SRY in sex determination is not analogous to a simple "on-off" switch in which the mere presence of the SRY gene results in male sex determination. Evidently, many genes are required in the pathway leading to testis formation. The SRY gene on the Y chromosome is believed to initiate a series of steps, involving other autosomal or X-linked genes, that ultimately culminates in male sex determination. Abnormalities such as sex reversal syndrome can result when any of these genes is prevented from functioning in an XY embryo or is gratuitously induced in an XX embryo. Pathway errors can occur if there is mosaicism for Y-bearing cell lines, transfer of the SRY-containing portion of the Y chromosome to the X chromosome, or mutation of any gene in the pathway.

Clinical Signs and Diagnosis

Chromosomal abnormalities are believed to exist in all breeds of horses, because they have been reported in a variety of draft, Warmblood, light, pony, and Miniature horse breeds. A survey suggests that the prevalence of sex chromosomal abnormalities in mares selected for breeding

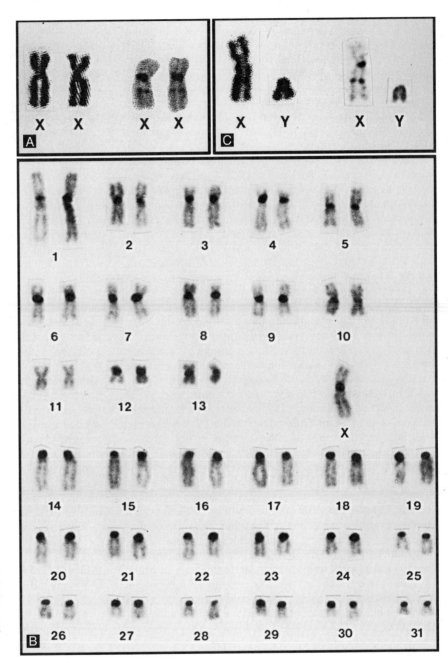

Figure 1. Conventional or C-banded karyotype of a mare demonstrating (A) normal 64,XX sex chromosomes, (B) a single X chromosome as seen in 63,X monosomy, and (C) single X and Y chromosomes as seen in 64,XY sex reversal syndrome. (From Buoen LC, et al: Sterility associated with an XO karyotype in a Miniature Horse mare. Equine Vet J 25(2):164–165, 1993.)

is less than 3%. A chromosomal abnormality can be suspected if the mare: (1) never has been able to become pregnant; (2) does not exhibit normal estrous cycles; and (3) has small, inactive ovaries regardless of seasonal influence. One study showed that more than half (52%) of infertile mares with abnormal reproductive organs have chromosomal anomalies. This contrasts sharply with the 2% incidence of chromosomal abnormality reported for infertile stallions. Typically, mares with chromosomal abnormalities have irregular or absent estrous cycles, and when teased by a stallion, may reject, show indifference, or allow mounting. Owners may perceive affected mares as lacking estrous behavior.

Definitive diagnosis of a chromosomal abnormality is made by karyotyping and cytogenetic analysis of chromosomes from cultured cells arrested in metaphase of mitosis (Fig. 1). For clinical diagnosis, lymphocytes obtained from a heparinized blood sample are generally used.

Types of Chromosomal Abnormalities

Chromosomal abnormalities are either numeric or structural in nature. A numeric abnormality can be a missing (monosomy) or extra (trisomy) chromosome. Structural anomalies include inversions, reciprocal translocations, centric fusions, and partial deletions. With respect to the reproductive system, primary infertility typically involves aneuploidy of the sex chromosomes. The diploid chromosome number of the domestic horse is 64. The mare normally has 31 autosomal pairs and two sex chromosomes, both of which are X (annotated 64,XX).

X Monosomy. The most common karyotypic abnormality associated with primary infertility and gonadal dysgenesis in the mare is X monosomy (63,X or 63,XO) in which one of the sex chromosomes is lacking (see Fig. 1). X monosomy conditions account for almost half of the karyotypic abnormalities observed in infertile mares (Table 1). The X monosomy karyotype is analogous to that seen in human cases of Turner's syndrome. Patients affected with Turner's syndrome have vestigial gonads, underdeveloped genitalia, and an assortment of somatic abnormalities such as short stature, webbing of the neck, a shield-like chest, and skeletal, cardiac, and renal abnormalities. X monosomy mares are frequently undersized, and have irregular or absent estrous cycles; small, firm ovaries lacking follicular development; and a small flaccid reproductive tract. With the exception of small stature, X monosomy mares do not exhibit phenotypic autosomal anomalies. External genitalia appear normal; the vulva may be small but does not preclude introduction or insertion of a vaginal tube speculum, and there is no clitoral enlargement. Among mares with X monosomy and gonadal dysgenesis, about 15% are mosaics (63,X/64,XX or 63,X/64,XY) having a second cell line with structurally normal sex chromosomes. Although the occasional Turner's syndrome individual is fertile, mares with X monosomy, even mosaics, should be considered effectively sterile. To date, no compelling evidence substantiates a heritable component to X monosomy in the mare.

XY Sex Reversal. The second most common chromosomal abnormality observed (approximately 40% of abnormal karyotypes) in infertile mares is 64,XY sex reversal syndrome in which the phenotypic sex does not coincide with the chromosomal sex (see Fig. 1 and Table 1). Although 64,XY mares are generally considered to be infertile, rare cases of fertility have been reported among them. Phenotypic expression in sex reversal syndrome is highly variable, ranging from the completely feminine mare with a relatively normal reproductive tract, to a greatly masculinized mare with female external genitalia, aplasia of the uterus and cervix, and gonads with histologic characteristics of both ovaries and testes (testicular feminization). Many XY mares have gonadal dysgenesis, and like X monosomal mares, have small, inactive ovaries and flaccid cervix and uterus. Unlike X monosomy, sex reversal syndrome is heritable. Pedigree analysis suggests that there are two modes

of inheritance: (1) female transmission of an X-linked recessive or an autosomal sex-limited gene, and (2) male transmission of a variably expressed Y chromosomal genetic mutation or an autosomal sex-limited dominant gene. In one study of 69 stallions, the normal secondary progeny sex ratio was approximately 53 male : 47 female. However, in every pedigree in which XY mares were diagnosed, the secondary progeny sex ratios deviated significantly from normal. Pedigree analysis in combination with cytogenetic screening aids in eliminating XY sex reversal syndrome in the mare.

Other Chromosome Anomalies. Together, X monosomies and 64 XY sex reversals account for approximately 80% of karyotypic abnormalities in infertile mares. Other karyotypic abnormalities associated with primary infertility and gonadal dysgenesis in the mare include 64,XX,delXp and 65,XXX (see Table 1). In 64,XXdelXp, a portion of the short (p) arm of one of the X chromosomes is deleted. Affected mares are phenotypically similar to X monosomy mares. Although many 64,XX,delXp mares have nonfunctional ovaries and are completely infertile, some affected mares occasionally develop follicles and ovulate but fail to conceive, and some have conceived and produced live foals. X trisomies (65,XXX) have an extra X chromosome. Although X trisomy is often a fertile karyotype in the human, no reports of fertility for this karyotype in the mare have been published.

Chromosomal abnormalities are occasionally found in subfertile, barren mares that appear normal and have produced foals. If other causes of subfertility can be ruled out, karyotyping should be considered. Balanced translocations occur when portions of chromosomes are rearranged without any loss or gain of genetic material. Affected mares produce chromosomally unbalanced gametes, which leads to lowered fertility.

ABNORMALLY ENLARGED OVARIES

The most common causes of unilaterally or bilaterally enlarged ovaries in the mare are (1) tumors, (2) hematoma, (3) pregnancy, and (4) anovulatory follicles.

Ovarian Tumors

In accordance with the World Health Organization (WHO) classification of ovarian neoplasms, the majority of equine ovarian tumors can be categorized as (1) sex cord-stromal tumors, (2) epithelial tumors, or (3) germ cell tumors.

Sex Cord-stromal Tumors

The *granulosa cell tumor* (or *granulosa-theca cell tumor*) is by far the most common ovarian neoplasm in the mare. It is usually benign, although malignant equine granulosa cell tumors have been reported. The tumor is hormonally active and typically unilateral, and the contralateral ovary is almost always inactive. Granulosa cell tumors have been reported in all breeds and in neonates and maiden, barren, and pregnant mares.

Clinical Signs and Diagnosis. Mares with granulosa cell tumors may exhibit one of three types of behavior: (1)

TABLE 1. KARYOTYPES OF 59 MARES WITH CHROMOSOMAL ABNORMALITY

Karyotype	Number	%
64XY	25	42.4
63XO	18	30.5
63XO/64XX	6	10.2
65XXX	4	6.8
63XO/64XY	1	1.7
63XO/64XX/64XY	1	1.7
64XX + fragment	1	1.7
64X,iso(Xp)	1	1.7
63XO/64X,del(Xq)	1	1.7
63XO/64XX/65XXX	1	1.7
Total	59	100

From Zhang TQ, Buoen LC, Weber AF, Ruth GR: Variety of cytogenetic anomalies diagnosed in 240 infertile equines. Proc 12th Int Cong Anim Reprod 4:1939–1941, 1992.

prolonged anestrus, (2) persistent or intermittent estrous behavior (nymphomania), or (3) stallion-like behavior. Mares with stallion-like behavior often have elevated serum testosterone concentrations (>100 pg/ml). In addition to masculinized behavior, these mares may develop a crested neck, heavy muscling of the forelegs and chest, and clitoral hypertrophy.

On rectal palpation and ultrasound examination, the affected ovary is found enlarged and often multicystic, although single cysts and solid masses have been reported (Fig. 2). The contralateral ovary is small and inactive. The ovary is devoid of both significant follicular activity and corpora lutea. Regression of the contralateral ovary is believed to be the result of a suppression of pituitary FSH secretion by inhibin, which is secreted by the tumor. Inhibin has been shown to be synthesized by granulosa cell tumors, and serum concentrations are elevated in most affected mares.

Diagnosis of a granulosa cell tumor is based on clinical signs, rectal palpation and ultrasonography, and determination of serum hormone concentrations. A unilaterally enlarged ovary in the presence of a small inactive opposite ovary is suggestive of a granulosa cell tumor if it is found during the physiologic breeding season. (One must keep in mind that any type of unilateral ovarian enlargement is associated with an inactive opposite ovary during seasonal anestrus). Serum inhibin is elevated in 87% and testosterone in 54% of affected mares. Although serum progesterone concentration alone is a poor diagnostic sign for granulosa cell tumors, it is almost consistently less than 1 ng/ml in affected mares.

Determination of serum concentrations of inhibin, testosterone, and progesterone are useful adjuncts for diagnosis of granulosa cell tumors.

Treatment and Prognosis. Granulosa cell tumors are treated by surgical removal of the affected ovary. Follicular activity and ovulation in the remaining ovary can be expected to return in an average of 6 to 8 months, with a range of 2 to 16 months, following surgery. The mare resumes normal estrous cycles and fertility.

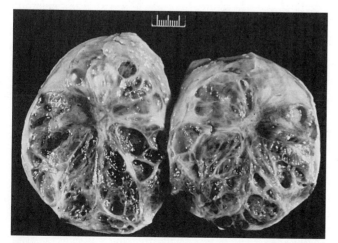

Figure 2. Cut surface of a granulosa cell tumor removed from a mare. The tumorous ovary is enlarged and multicystic. The contralateral ovary was inactive but resumed normal cyclic activity during a subsequent breeding season.

Epithelial Tumors

Cystadenomas are rare benign ovarian tumors that arise from the surface epithelium of the ovulation fossa. The tumor is unilateral and the contralateral ovary is normal. Cystadenomas are not considered to be hormonally active, but elevated serum testosterone concentrations have occasionally been reported in affected mares.

Clinical Signs and Diagnosis. Mares with cystadenomas cycle normally from the opposite ovary, and may even become pregnant. Rectal palpation and ultrasonography reveal the presence of one normal ovary and one enlarged multicystic ovary, which may be similar to that of a granulosa cell tumor.

Diagnosis of cystadenoma is based on the results of rectal palpation and ultrasonography. Hormone assays for inhibin, testosterone, and progesterone may differentiate a cystadenoma from a granulosa cell tumor. In contrast to mares with granulosa cell tumors, mares with cystadenomas are unlikely to have elevated serum concentrations of inhibin or testosterone. Serum progesterone concentrations are rarely higher than 1 ng/ml in mares with granulosa cell tumors, but they may be elevated in mares with cystadenomas if they are in diestrus.

Treatment. Although cystadenomas are benign tumors without any effect on normal cyclicity, they should be surgically removed if diagnosed. The prognosis for reproductive performance is excellent.

Germ Cell Tumors

Dysgerminomas and teratomas are rare ovarian tumors of germ cell origin. Dysgerminomas are analogues to testicular seminomas in stallions. Both tumors are unilateral and hormonally inactive, allowing the contralateral ovary to function normally.

Clinical Signs and Diagnosis. Dysgerminomas have been diagnosed in young mares with recurrent episodes of colic and rapid weight loss. They are malignant and often metastasize to the peritoneal abdomen and thoracic cavity. A unilaterally enlarged, multicystic ovary or abdominal mass is the typical finding on rectal palpation and ultrasonographic examination. Two cases of hypertrophic osteopathy have been reported in mares with dysgerminomas.

Teratomas are benign tumors of germ cell origin. The neoplasm may arise from all three germinal layers. The affected ovary is cystic and may contain bone, cartilage, teeth, hair, muscle, and nerves. Teratomas do not generally cause clinical signs and are often diagnosed in association with a routine examination of the reproductive tract.

Treatment. Surgical removal is recommended for both dysgerminomas and teratomas. Although the prognosis for mares with teratomas is good, it is usually poor for mares diagnosed with dysgerminoma. Thoracic radiography and abdominocentesis may be helpful for assessment of metastasis in suspect mares.

Other less common ovarian neoplasms in the mare include cystadenocarcinomas, hemangiomas, lymphosarcomas, and melanomas.

Hematoma

Ovarian hematoma is a common cause of ovarian enlargement in the mare. Hematomas are believed to originate from excessive hemorrhage into a follicle at the time of ovulation. The condition is quite similar to that of hemorrhagic follicles (see Anovulatory Follicles). Hematomas, however, are considered to originate from a normal fertile ovulation.

Clinical Signs and Diagnosis. Ovarian hematomas are often larger than 10 cm in diameter and can reach a diameter of 40 cm or more. They are unilateral and do not interfere with the normal estrous cycle. The lifespan of the luteal tissue in the hematoma is similar to that from a normal ovulation. On ultrasonographic examination, hematomas appear similar to a corpus hemorrhagicum, but larger.

The diagnosis is made upon rectal palpation and ultrasonography of the affected ovary. Ovarian hematomas can be differentiated from other forms of ovarian enlargement in that they are unilateral, they display an ultrasonographic image similar to a corpus hemorrhagicum, and the opposite ovary is normal. Hormone analysis may be used to differentiate the condition from a granulosa cell tumor.

Treatment and Prognosis. Ovarian hematomas generally regress in size without treatment over a period of several weeks. Occasionally, the hematoma may become large enough to persist for several months. The condition may result in the destruction of normal ovarian tissue, rendering the affected ovary nonfunctional. However, the contralateral ovary remains functional, ensuring normal cyclic activity.

Pregnancy

Secondary corpora lutea are formed during the production of equine chorionic gonadotropin (eCG), starting approximately at day 40. Regression of these supplementary corpora lutea begins between days 160 and 180 of gestation. Multiple corpora lutea may significantly enlarge the mare's ovaries, and they have been mistaken for ovarian pathology.

Clinical Signs and Diagnosis. Ovarian enlargement in pregnant mares is commonly bilateral. In addition to enlarged ovaries, pregnant mares may show stallion-like behavior in connection with increased testosterone production by the fetus (regardless of fetal sex) during midgestation. It is essential to rule out pregnancy as a cause of enlarged ovaries when presented with a mare with stallion-like behavior, elevated serum testosterone concentrations (>100 ng/ml), and enlarged ovaries.

Pregnancy at this stage is diagnosed by rectal palpation and ultrasonographic examination, or increased serum concentrations of eCG and estrogens.

Anovulatory Follicles

Cystic ovarian disease, as described in cows, does not occur in the mare. Different kinds of anovulatory or persistent follicles have been described in the mare. Autumn follicles are large fluid-filled ovarian structures most frequently found during fall transition to winter anestrus. They contain blood with liquid or gelatinous consistency. A similar condition of hemorrhagic follicles has been found to occur during the breeding season. Ginther reported that vascular accidents in association with failure of ovulation or at the time of follicular evacuation can result in the formation of a hemorrhagic follicle. He suggested that the amount of follicular fluid at the site of follicular evacuation determines the timing of coagulation. The mechanism of delayed coagulation in association with evacuation of follicular fluid is not known. However, follicular fluid in other species has anticoagulant properties.

Persistent follicles as a result of ovulation failure are common findings during the transitional period into the breeding season. They are rarely seen during the breeding season.

Clinical Signs and Diagnosis

Hemorrhagic follicles palpate as large follicular structures (>6 cm in diameter). Ultrasonographic examination reveals free-floating echogenic material that swirls during ballotement of the enlarged follicle. Over time, fibrinous bands form, and the structure gives the impression of a gelatinous consistency. Hemorrhagic follicles regress over time and are often not detectable after 1 month.

Diagnosis of anovulatory follicles and hemorrhagic follicles should be based on ultrasonographic findings, the season, and reproductive history of the mare.

Treatment

Anovulatory follicles regress spontaneously over time. They are generally nonresponsive to treatment with human chorionic gonadotropin. Hemorrhagic follicles that produce progesterone can be treated with $PGF_2\alpha$ in order to lyse the luteal tissue and bring the mare into estrus.

OTHER OVARIAN ABNORMALITIES

Persistent Luteal Activity

Prolonged or persistent luteal activity is characterized by a prolongation of luteal activity in nonpregnant mares beyond 14 to 16 days of diestrus. Besides pregnancy, it is the most common cause of failure to exhibit estrus during the breeding season. Persistent luteal activity may be caused by (1) ovulation late in diestrus, resulting in an additional corpus luteum that is immature at the time of $PGF_2\alpha$ secretion and therefore nonresponsive to prostaglandin; (2) embryonic loss after the recognition of pregnancy; (3) pharmacologic inhibition of $PGF_2\alpha$ release from the endometrium (by nonsteroidal anti-inflammatory drugs); (4) inadequate release of $PGF_2\alpha$ from the endometrium at day 14 to 15 postovulation; and (5) inability of the endometrium to synthesize and secrete $PGF_2\alpha$ as a result of severe uterine pathology (i.e., pyometra).

Clinical Signs and Diagnosis

Persistent luteal activity is reported to occur in up to 25% of estrous cycles with a mean duration of 63 days (range 35–95 days). Mares with persistent luteal activity have a tight cervix and good uterine tone, and they fail to show estrous behavior as a result of elevated serum progesterone concentrations. If the mare was bred, her condition may be confused with pregnancy. Because persistent luteal activity often remains for 2 to 3 months, failure to detect the condition can result in the loss of an entire breeding season. Confirming the presence or absence of an embryonic vesicle by the use of ultrasonography helps differentiate persistent luteal activity from pregnancy.

Diagnosis is based on clinical signs, detection of ovarian luteal tissue on rectal palpation or transrectal ultrasonography, and serum progesterone concentrations higher than 1 ng/ml.

Treatment

Persistent luteal activity is effectively treated by the administration of exogenous prostaglandins ($PGF_2\alpha$) or synthetic prostaglandins.

Parovarian Cysts

The term *parovarian cysts* is used to describe cysts located around the ovary. They originate from the mesonephric tubules and ducts. Parovarian cysts are common findings in the mare. They are located in the mesovarium near the ovary, sometimes reaching a size of more than 5 cm. The cysts have no effect on the reproductive cycle or fertility, but they may be confused with an ovarian follicle on ultrasonography. Concurrent rectal palpation of the ovaries helps to differentiate the two structures.

Epithelial Inclusion Cysts

Inclusion cysts of the surface epithelium may, if present in large numbers, obstruct ovulation and may even destroy much of the ovarian parenchyma. In advanced cases of epithelial inclusion cysts, the affected ovary is nonfunctional. If the ovary still produces follicles, subfertility may be seen as a result of blocked ovulation. The definitive diagnosis is made by histopathology examination. Removal of the ovary is indicated when the inclusion cysts affect fertility.

Supplemental Readings

Carnevale EM, Ginther OJ: Reproductive function in old mares. Proc 40th Annu Conv Am Assoc Equine Pract, 1994, p 15.

Dybdal NO: Endocrine disorders: Hypothalamus and pituitary gland. *In* Smith BP (ed): Large Animal Internal Medicine. St. Louis, C.V. Mosby, 1990, pp 1296–1300.

Ginther OJ: Reproductive Biology of the Mare, ed 2. Cross Plains, WI, Equiservices, 1992, pp 217–230.

Halnan CRE: Equine cytogenetics in infertility and clinical practice. *In* Halnan CRE (ed): Cytogenetics of Animals. Wallingford, Oxon, UK, CAB International, 1989, pp 185–203.

Jubb KVF, Kennedy PC, Palmer N: The female genital system. *In* Pathology of Domestic Animals, vol 3, ed 3. New York, Academic Press, 1985, pp 305–407.

McCue PM: Equine granulosa cell tumors. Proc 38th Annu Conv Am Assoc Equine Pract, 1992, pp 587–593.

Nie GJ, Momont HW, Buoen L: A survey of sex chromosome abnormalities in 204 mares selected for breeding. J Equine Vet Sci 13(8):456–459, 1993.

Rossdale PD: Exogenous control of the breeding season. *In* Robinson NE (ed): Current Therapy in Equine Medicine, ed 2. Philadelphia, W.B. Saunders, 1987, pp 493–494.

Trommerhausem Bowling A, Millon L, Hughes JP: An update of chromosomal abnormalities in mares. J Reprod Fertil 35[Suppl]:149–155, 1987.

Vanderwall DK, Woods GL: Age-related subfertility in the mare. Proc 36th Annu Conv Am Assoc Equine Pract, 1990, pp 85–89.

Zhang TQ, Buoen LC, Weber AF, Ruth GR: Variety of cytogenetic anomalies diagnosed in 240 infertile equines. Proc 12th Int Cong Anim Reprod 4:1939–1941, 1992.

Early Pregnancy Loss in Mares: Applications for Progestin Therapy

BARRY A. BALL

PETER F. DAELS

Ithaca, New York

Progesterone is clearly an essential hormone during pregnancy in mares; however, there remains considerable debate regarding the use of exogenous progestins for the prevention of pregnancy loss in mares. Currently, the use of exogenous progestins in pregnant mares is widespread, and a rational method for selection of mares for progestin therapy is lacking. In many cases, progestin supplementation does not appear warranted and may even be counterproductive. However, there is a growing body of evidence that progestin supplementation may be useful under specific circumstances. Rational application of progestin therapy requires some consideration of mechanisms that may lead to pregnancy failure and the relationship of these mechanisms to progesterone.

During the first 120 days of gestation, progesterone is produced by the primary corpus luteum (CL). After 40 days of gestation, progesterone production by the primary CL is supplemented with progesterone produced by secondary CLs. Luteal production of progesterone persists through approximately day 100 to day 210 of gestation. Beginning around day 50 to 70 of gestation, there is a measurable production of progestogen by the placenta, and the placenta is the only source of progestogen during the second half of gestation in the mare. Placental progesterone is rapidly metabolized to 5α-pregnanes in the placenta. These 5α-metabolites cannot be measured by most conventional progesterone assays. Therefore, after midgestation in the mare, the circulating progesterone concentration is low and does not accurately reflect progesterone production by the fetoplacental unit. In broad terms, one can consider that before 150 days of gestation the progesterone concentrations measured by the available assays reflect progesterone production by the maternal CLs. After 150 days of gestation, progesterone concentrations represent only 1 to 5% of the total progestogens and are an unreliable parameter for assessment of placental progesterone production.

POTENTIAL MECHANISMS RESULTING IN INADEQUATE PROGESTERONE

It has been suggested that pregnancy failure may be related to low or reduced luteal progesterone production through a number of mechanisms: (1) primary luteal insufficiency; (2) luteolysis due to uterine inflammation (endometritis) and release of prostaglandin $F_2\alpha$; (3) failure of the embryo to prevent luteolysis and return to estrus; (4) luteolysis due to systemic endotoxemia; and (5) stress. Our ability to relate detected pregnancy loss to one of these potential mechanisms is limited, and this limitation complicates our rational application of exogenous progestin therapy.

Although luteal insufficiency or inadequate production of progesterone by the CL has been proposed as a cause of early pregnancy failure, there is limited evidence to support primary luteal insufficiency as a cause of early pregnancy loss in mares. In other species, there remains considerable controversy concerning the importance of luteal insufficiency in early pregnancy loss. Ginther (1992) examined characteristics of embryonic losses in 21 mares. Embryonic losses that occurred before day 20 appeared to be related to endometritis and premature luteolysis in most cases. Embryonic losses that occurred between days 20 and 40 of pregnancy were associated with a decline in progesterone preceding embryonic death in 25% of cases, and it was suggested that these losses could have been the result of luteal insufficiency. Irvine and coworkers (1990) examined serum progesterone concentrations in 179 mares between 17 and 42 days of gestation and found only one mare in which detected embryonic loss was associated with a preceding decline in progesterone concentration.

Uterine-induced luteolysis is reasonably well documented as a cause of early pregnancy loss in mares. Uterine inflammation with subsequent release of prostaglandin $F_2\alpha$, and a shortened diestrous interval appears to be a frequent cause of pregnancy loss. Many of the embryo losses resulting from endometritis appear to occur prior to Day 20. Frequently, embryonic losses associated with endometritis are preceded by the appearance of endometrial edema or intraluminal free fluid, and this finding may provide clinical evidence of the cause of such losses. When endometritis due to uterine infection is present, progestin supplementation is contraindicated because it may exacerbate the problem. If progestin therapy is continued long enough, it may result in pyometra and permanent damage to the uterus.

Pregnancy failure related to failure of maternal recognition of pregnancy is also relatively difficult to document in mares. Although maternal recognition of pregnancy can be disrupted experimentally and results in luteolysis and return to estrus, there is only one report to date to support

spontaneous failure of maternal recognition of pregnancy as a cause for embryonic loss in mares. It is possible that conceptuses that are retarded in development may not adequately signal their presence in the uterus and therefore may not prevent luteolysis. Such small-for-age conceptuses do appear to be lost with higher frequency than normally sized conceptuses.

During the first 2 months of gestation, endotoxin-induced $PGF_2\alpha$ secretion results in pregnancy failure due to regression of the maternal CLs, the main source of progesterone at this stage. Although other factors, such as bacteremia and fever, can also have detrimental effects on fetal survival, the experimental data suggest that progestin supplementation is very effective in the prevention of pregnancy loss in mares in which endotoxemia is suspected. Later in gestation, endotoxin-induced luteolysis is not the main reason for pregnancy failure because the fetoplacental unit is capable of supporting pregnancy in the absence of the maternal ovaries. However, clinical experience suggests that endotoxemia and systemic illness is occasionally associated with pregnancy failure. It is possible that prolonged exposure of the gravid uterus to high levels of $PGF_2\alpha$, as may be the case during endotoxemia, culminates in myometrial contractions and abortion. Results of recent studies suggest that the potential detrimental effect of $PGF_2\alpha$ on the gravid uterus can be blocked by increasing progesterone levels. Exogenous progesterone (300 mg/day) or altrenogest* (44 mg/day) administered to pregnant mares at 4 months of gestation significantly reduced the incidence of abortion following 5 daily $PGF_2\alpha$ injections. These observations suggest that progesterone or altrenogest supplementation may be useful in the prevention of pregnancy failure in systemically ill mares. It is noteworthy that progestin supplementation was terminated after the last $PGF_2\alpha$ injection, and this did not appear to compromise pregnancy. Thus, there do not appear to be residual effects of $PGF_2\alpha$ on pregnancy, and treatment may only need to be applied when an acute risk is present. In contrast, pregnant mares exposed to endotoxin early in gestation need to be maintained on progestins until either a new CL has developed or the fetoplacental unit is capable of maintaining adequate progesterone levels.

Stress related to conditions such as transport, disease, climate, social separation, or nutrition has long been proposed as a potential cause of pregnancy loss in mares. Anecdotal reports have indicated that stress may depress progesterone concentrations and result in pregnancy loss. However, in a controlled study, transport of pregnant mares (third or fifth week of gestation) for 9 hours resulted in elevated cortisol and transiently increased progesterone concentrations with no detectable effect on embryonic survival. Therefore, the relationship between stress and reduced progesterone concentrations remains unclear.

EVALUATION OF CIRCULATING PROGESTERONE CONCENTRATIONS

Evaluation of serum progesterone concentrations during early pregnancy in the mare requires an understanding of

---

Regu-Mate; Hoechst-Roussel AgriVet, Somerville, NJ

the variability in these values both within and between mares. It is also important that reference values be available for the particular laboratory that will conduct the assay. In general, at least two daily samples should be evaluated for serum progesterone concentration before a diagnosis of adequate progesterone concentration is made. The absolute concentration of progesterone needed to maintain pregnancy remains poorly defined, although it has been suggested that concentrations greater than 2.0 ng/ml should be present during early pregnancy. In the authors' laboratory, they have occasionally observed progesterone concentrations as low as 1 ng/ml for up to 4 days without loss of pregnancy. Because the practitioner may be presented with a mare that has a suspected impending pregnancy loss based on previous history or clinical findings, it may not be possible to wait for several days for results from a diagnostic laboratory before initiating progestin therapy. Altrenogest does not cross-react with most progesterone assays and allows the measurement of concentrations of endogenous progesterone while the mare is being supplemented with progestins. Thus it is possible to start progestin therapy and monitor endogenous progesterone during treatment. However, one should be aware that altrenogest therapy has been demonstrated to reduce luteal production of progesterone to some degree in pregnant mares. When progestin supplementation will be terminated before adequate fetoplacental progestogen production is present, endogenous progesterone levels should be measured to ensure adequate luteal progesterone production.

In addition to measurement of progesterone concentrations, transrectal ultrasonography may also be used in diagnosis of impending pregnancy loss. Based on ultrasonographic evidence, it has been suggested that failure of fixation or dislodgement of the embryonic vesicle after day 18 may be indicative of low progesterone and a possible impending embryonic loss. Similar observations were made later around 30 to 40 days of gestation when declining progesterone concentrations were induced experimentally. In a few mares, dislodgment and movement of the 40-day-old conceptus were observed for 1 to 2 days before expulsion of the fetus. Ultrasonographic examination indicated that the fetus was viable, suggesting that perhaps progestin supplementation could have been effective in preventing fetal death at this stage. The embryo can survive for several days following a luteolytic dose of $PGF_2\alpha$ on day 12. When progestin administration was started on day 16 in these mares, the vesicle continued to develop normally, provided that the vesicle was still viable on the first day of treatment. This leaves the clinician up to 48 hours to confirm the presence of a conceptus and initiate progestin therapy after an incident that may have induced luteolysis or in mares in which progesterone insufficiency is suspected because of uterine edema. Routine use of ultrasonography has demonstrated that uterine edema is likely to be the first sign of failing luteal function, before pregnancy loss, and thus may be a good criterion for initiation of progestin supplementation. However, one needs to keep in mind that the etiology of luteal failure may include pathologic development of the conceptus or endometritis resulting from infection. Thus re-examina-tion of the pregnancy following initiation of progestin therapy is critical.

PRODUCTS FOR PROGESTIN SUPPLEMENTATION

A number of progestins on the market have been used to supplement endogenous progesterone in mares. These include but are not limited to melgestrol acetate,[*] norgestomet implants,[†] hydroxyprogesterone caproate,[‡] acetoxyprogesterone,[§] and medroxyprogesterone acetate.[‖] Although there are anecdotal reports of the use of some of these synthetic progestins to suppress estrus or maintain pregnancy, there are very few reports of controlled studies to evaluate their use in the mare. Species-specific differences in bioactivity exist, and it is ill-advised to select these products based on their effectiveness in other species. For example, although previously reported as being effective for maintenance of pregnancy, the authors have recently demonstrated that medroxyprogesterone acetate, acetoxyprogesterone, and progesterone-estradiol benzoate implants[¶] are ineffective for the maintenance of pregnancy. Because of the lack of safety and efficacy studies for these preparations in the mare, products not tested in horses should be avoided for use in pregnancy maintenance in favor of products that have been adequately tested for effectiveness and safety in mares.

Currently, two preparations are available for supplementation of progesterone during pregnancy in the mare: injectable progesterone (typically in an oil vehicle such as sesame oil) and the synthetic oral progestin, altrenogest. Although neither of these preparations has been approved for use in pregnancy maintenance, there is adequate data to establish dosages effective for maintenance of pregnancy in the absence of endogenous progesterone. Altrenogest is typically used at 22 mg p.o. s.i.d. Progesterone in oil is typically used at 150 and 300 mg IM s.i.d. Lower dosages or less frequent administration of progesterone may not adequately elevate progesterone concentrations for pregnancy maintenance.

A long-acting form of progesterone has considerable advantage for long-term administration in pregnant mares. Previously, repository progesterone (propylene glycol base) was available in the United States and provided adequate progesterone concentrations when administered at 4-day intervals. Unfortunately, this form of progesterone is no longer available. The authors have evaluated the effectiveness of a microencapsulated progesterone[#] for maintenance of pregnancy in mares. This preparation consists of a sustained release form of progesterone in poly (DL-lactide) microspheres. When administered in dosages of 1.5 or 2.25 g at 10-day intervals, pregnancy was maintained in mares without an endogenous source of progesterone. This product is not currently available to practitioners.

---

[*]*Ovaban, Schering-Plough Animal Health, Kenilworth, NJ*
[†]*Synchro-mate-B, Rhone Merieux, Athens, GA*
[‡]*Prodox 250, Legere Pharmaceuticals, Scottsdale, AZ*
[§]*Gestafortin, Bayer, Leverkusen, Germany*
[‖]*Depo-Provera, The Upjohn Company, Kalamazoo, MI*
[¶]*Synovex S (200 mg progesterone and 20 mg estradiol benzoate), Syntex Animal Health, West Des Moines, IA*
[#]*Lutamate, Thorn Biosciences, Lexington, KY*

TIMING AND DURATION OF PROGESTIN SUPPLEMENTATION

The time of initiation of progestin administration to pregnant mares is also an important consideration. Sometimes initiation of progestin administration to pregnant mares is recommended after a positive diagnosis of pregnancy by ultrasonography around day 14. It should be considered, however, that this may be too late in mares that may have luteal insufficiency or premature luteolysis resulting from endometritis. Therefore, beginning progestin therapy earlier, on day 4 after ovulation, may have potential benefit in some mares. Research conducted in the authors' laboratory indicates that progestin can be administered beginning as early as the day of ovulation without adversely affecting conception rate and early embryonic development.

Although it has been suggested that progestin therapy be continued for most of gestation, many of the potential benefits of supplemental progestin are limited to the first 100 to 120 days of pregnancy. After 100 to 120 days, placental progesterone production is adequate to maintain pregnancy, villous placentation is reasonably well established, and the conceptus is less dependent on secretion of uterine milk (histotroph) for its growth and development. Therefore, continuation of progestin therapy beyond 120 days probably has limited benefits. When supplemental progestin is stopped after 3 to 4 months of pregnancy, it may be prudent to reduce the dosage by 50% for 10 to 14 days rather than abruptly discontinuing supplemental therapy. However, the authors have not observed pregnancy failure associated with the abrupt discontinuation of progestin therapy.

ADVERSE EFFECTS OF PROGESTIN SUPPLEMENTATION

Casual use of progestin supplementation can have detrimental effects on reproductive function. Mares that are receiving exogenous progestin do not return to estrus if pregnancy loss is not detected. Therefore, monitoring of pregnancy status during treatment is indicated. Progesterone has long been known to suppress phagocytosis by uterine neutrophils and clearance of material from the uterus. Therefore, if a mare with a residual endometritis is treated with progestin, there is an increased risk of a prolonged and exacerbated endometritis during treatment with progestin. In extreme cases, this can result in pyometra and severe damage to the endometrium. The effect of prolonged treatment with injectable progesterone on the reproductive performance of the mare's offspring has not been studied. However, administration of altrenogest (44 mg/day) from day 20 to 325 to pregnant mares did not appear to have significant effects on the reproductive activity of their offspring.

Supplemental Readings

Ball BA: Embryonic death in mares. In McKinnon AO, Voss JL (eds): Equine Reproduction. Philadelphia, Lea & Febiger, 1993, pp 517–531.
Ball BA, Miller PG, Daels PF: Influence of exogenous progesterone on early embryonic development in the mare. Theriogenology 38:1055–1063, 1992.
Ball BA, Wilker C, Daels PF, Burns PJ: Use of progesterone in microspheres for maintenance of pregnancy in mares. Am J Vet Res 53:1294–1297, 1992.
Daels PF, Besognet B, Hansen B, Odensvik K, Kindahl H: Efficacy of treatments to prevent abortion in pregnant mares at risk. Proc 40th Annu Meet Am Assoc Equine Pract 40:31–32, 1994.
Daels PF, Stabenfeldt GH, Hughes JP, Odensvik K, Kindahl H: Evaluation of progesterone deficiency as a cause of fetal death in mares with experimentally induced endotoxemia. Am J Vet Res 52:282–288, 1991.
Daels PF, Stabenfeldt GH, Kindahl H, Hughes JP: Prostaglandin release and luteolysis associated with physiological and pathological conditions of the reproductive cycle of the mare: A review. Equine Vet J 8[Suppl]:29–34, 1989.
Ginther OJ: Reproductive Biology of the Mare: Basic and Applied Aspects. Cross Plains, WI: Equiservices, 1992, pp 525–529.
Irvine CHG, Sutton P, Turner JE, Mennick PE: Changes in plasma progesterone concentrations from Days 17 to 42 of gestation in mares maintaining or losing pregnancy. Equine Vet J 22:104–106, 1990.
Squires EL: Progestin. In McKinnon AO, Voss JL (eds): Equine Reproduction. Philadelphia, Lea & Febiger, 1993, pp 311–318.
Wilker C, Daels PF, Burns PJ, Ball BA: Progesterone therapy during early pregnancy in the mare. Proc 37th Annu Meet Am Assoc Equine Pract, 1991, pp 161–172.

Abortion

MATS H. T. TROEDSSON
St. Paul, Minnesota

Abortion° refers to pregnancy loss after the completion of organogenesis. The rate of abortion after pregnancy diagnosis at 50 days of gestation has been estimated to be 8 to 15% in horses. Fetal death may result in abortion or retention of the fetus in the uterine lumen with subsequent fetal maceration or mummification. After 80 days, the maintenance of pregnancy does not require a functional corpus luteum, because the fetus and placenta produce progestogens. Fetal death after this time causes an immediate loss of the fetal contribution to pregnancy maintenance, resulting in the expulsion of a relatively nonautolyzed fetus. Mummification of the fetus occurs when fetal fluids are

°Portions of this chapter are adapted from Troedsson MHT, McCue PM: Pregnancy loss. In Smith BP (ed): Large Animal Internal Medicine, ed 2. St Louis, C.V. Mosby, (with permission) 1996.

reabsorbed and its membranes remain in the uterus indefinitely. This is rare in mares but may occur as a consequence of twin pregnancy with unequal placentation in which a great disparity exists in the size of the twins. If one twin occupies only a small portion of one uterine horn, it will die early during the pregnancy as a result of insufficient placental support. Mummification of the dead twin fetus may occur if the intact fetoplacental unit of the viable twin maintains pregnancy. The mummified twin is expelled with the abortion or birth of the other twin. Rare cases of mummified singleton fetuses have been reported. In a recent report, a case of a retained mummified singleton fetus was associated with progesterone supplementation of the mare throughout gestation.

DIAGNOSIS

A definitive diagnosis is reached in 50 to 60% of equine abortions. The generally low diagnostic success rate is a result of the complexity of the disease complex. Abortion involves diseases in the maternal, placental, and fetal compartments individually or together, and all of these compartments have to be examined thoroughly. In addition, a "triad" of determinants for animal disease has to be considered: (1) the presence of a pathogenic organism, (2) the environment in which a host lives, and (3) the susceptibility of the host to the disease. To enhance diagnostic success, information and samples must be collected from the fetus, placenta, dam, and herd mates. A thorough history should be obtained, including the gestational age of the fetus; reproductive, medical, and vaccination history of the dam and other individuals in the herd; new arrivals to the herd and contacts with other herds; potential causes of maternal stress; possible access to toxins and poisonous plants; and sources of nutrition.

A physical examination that includes all body systems should be performed on the dam. Samples should be collected from the uterus for culture and cytology testing. Examination of the reproductive system should include palpation and ultrasonography of the reproductive tract per rectum, speculum examination of the vagina, and digital examination of the cervix. Paired serum samples 2 weeks apart from the dam and other mares in the herd may also help demonstrate activity of an infectious agent. Demonstration of a significant rise in titer between acute and convalescent serum samples suggests a recent exposure to an agent, but presence of antibodies does not necessarily indicate that the agent caused the abortion.

For optimal diagnostic efficiency, the entire aborted fetus and placenta should be submitted to a diagnostic laboratory for necropsy. If this cannot be done, a prompt necropsy should be performed and collection of fetal, placental, and maternal samples should be submitted to a diagnostic laboratory (Table 1).

A systematic necropsy must be performed on the aborted fetus. Fetal age and development may be assessed by measuring crown-rump length, hair patterns, and color. Meconium staining of the skin suggests intrauterine fetal distress. Condition of the fetus, including degree of autolysis, should be noted. Histopathologic samples should be immersed in a volume of 10% formalin (or Bouin's fixative) equivalent to 10 times the volume of tissue. Samples for culture, virus isolation, and fluorescent antibody tests should be submitted on ice in separate sterile containers. A sample of stomach contents should be aseptically collected for culture. Fetal heart blood may be collected for serologic evaluation. The late-term fetus is immunologically competent, and high titers may indicate activity of a pathogenic agent. Serology of fetal fluids can be useful both in detecting a nonspecific active fetal immune response (total IgG) and for titers against a specific antigen.

The fetal membranes should be examined for size, weight, degree of autolysis, condition, and completeness. Samples of placental tissue, especially abnormal areas, should be collected for histology, impression smears, bacterial culture, virus isolation, and fluorescent antibody tests. The placenta should be examined for its integrity, lesions, and distribution of chorionic villi. The normal equine placenta is everted following expulsion, with the allantoic surface presented outward and chorioallantois ruptured at the site of the cervical star. Blood should be collected from the free end of the cord. The allantoic surface should be examined for abnormalities such as multiple allantoic pouches that may indicate compromised fetal circulation. The chorionic surface of the placenta should be examined for lesions and distribution of chorionic villi. Areas of avillous chorion are normally observed in association with the cervical star, narrow folds over large vessels, and areas opposing endometrial cups. Absence of chorionic villi over a circumscribed area is characteristic of twins and represents the region where two placentas were in contact. The region of the placenta adjacent to the cervix should be examined for loss of chorionic villi and the presence of inflammatory exudate, which is a hallmark of ascending infection.

All aborted fetuses and placental tissues should be han-

TABLE 1. TISSUE SAMPLES FROM THE MARE, PLACENTA, AND ABORTED FETUS TO BE SUBMITTED FOR DIAGNOSING THE CAUSE OF ABORTION

Source	Preservation Method	
	Chilled/Frozen	*Fixed**
Fetus	Lung, liver, kidney, spleen, thymus, skeletal muscle, heart, heart blood, stomach contents	Lung, liver, kidney, spleen, thymus, skeletal muscle, heart, adrenal gland, lymph node, brain
Placenta	Allantochorion, allantoamnion, amniotic fluid, cord blood	Allantochorion, allantoamnion
Dam/herd	Paired serum samples, uterine swabs	

°10% formalin or Bouin's fixative.

dled with care, and tissues that are not submitted to a diagnostic laboratory should be burned or buried. Dams that have aborted should be isolated from the remainder of the herd.

CAUSES OF ABORTION

Infectious

Equine Herpesvirus

The most commonly diagnosed infectious cause of abortion in horses is equine herpesvirus 1 (EHV-1; formerly EHV-1, subtype 1). This respiratory virus can cause abortion, perinatal foal mortality, rhinopneumonitis, and neurologic disease (Table 2). Although equine herpesvirus 4 (EHV-4; formerly EHV-1, subtype 2) is considered to be confined to the respiratory tract, sporadic cases of abortion have been reported during EHV-4 outbreaks. Clinical signs and fetal lesions of abortion caused by EHV-1 and EHV-4 are clinically indistinguishable.

Clinical Signs and Diagnosis. Abortion resulting from EHV-1 usually occurs after 7 months of gestation and has been reported to account for up to 15% of all diagnosed abortions. Recent reports suggest a less important role of equine herpesvirus in equine abortions, with only 3% of all abortions in central Kentucky being caused by equine herpesvirus. Increased awareness of the disease and preventive measures may have resulted in the decline. Although epidemic abortions occur, losses may be confined to only a few mares in a herd.

EHV-1 is transmitted through inhalation of the virus. Following respiratory infection, EHV-1 causes an episode of viremia and infects the fetus via transplacental migration of virus-bearing leukocytes. Respiratory clinical signs of infected mares may be severe, mild, or subclinical. The time between infection and abortion varies greatly, with 14 to 120 days reported in one study. The virus infects several fetal organs including the lung and the liver. In addition, evidence of uterine endothelial lesions in some cases suggests a possible alternative maternal contribution to the pathogenesis of herpesvirus abortion. Abortion occurs as a result of a rapid separation of the placenta, causing suffocation of the fetus. Near-term fetuses may be born alive and die within days because of overwhelming respiratory pathology. Aborting mares clear the virus quickly from the reproductive tract, and subsequent fertility is often not affected by the disease.

TABLE 2. SELECTED EQUINE HERPESVIRUSES OF IMPORTANCE FOR EQUINE REPRODUCTION*

Virus	Name	Clinical Features
EHV-1	Equine rhinopneumonitis virus Equine abortion virus (equine herpesvirus-1, subtype 1)	Respiratory infections Abortions Neonatal disease
EHV-3		Coital exanthema
EHV-4	Equine rhinopneumonitis virus (equine herpesvirus-1, subtype 2)	Respiratory infections Abortions, sporadic (rare)

*In part adapted from Ostlund EN: Update on infectious diseases. Vet Clin North Am 9(2):283–294, 1993.

Abortions occur suddenly without maternal clinical signs. The aborted fetus is fresh with minimal signs of autolysis. Increased fluid in the thoracic and abdominal cavities, congestion and edema of the lungs, an enlarged liver with small (approximately 1 mm) necrotic, yellow-white lesions, subcutaneous edema, and icterus are commonly found gross lesions in the fetus. Histologically, the most characteristic lesion is areas of necrosis in lymphoid tissue, liver, adrenal cortex, and the lung, with large intranuclear eosinophilic inclusion bodies. In addition, a hyperplastic necrotizing bronchiolitis is often found. The lesions in an individual fetus may involve only a few of the targeted tissues. The placenta may be normal or edematous, with no specific microscopic lesions.

Laboratory diagnostics include (1) fluorescent antibody staining of fetal tissue, (2) virus isolation from aborted fetuses, (3) virus isolation from maternal whole blood, (4) presence of viral inclusion bodies in liver, lung, and thymus, and (5) fetal serology. Equine fetuses have been found to be capable of producing antibodies to EHV-1 at 200 days gestation. Maternal serology testing is of limited diagnostic value because mares may abort several weeks following infection. The rise in serologic titer may have disappeared at the time of the abortion.

Treatment and Prevention. Several vaccines against herpesvirus infections are available. Effective killed vaccines for abortion should contain antigenic strains of both EHV-1 1P and EHV-1 1B. Vaccination is typically recommended in the fifth, seventh, and ninth month of pregnancy. The vaccine is not fully protective, and abortion may occur in vaccinated mares. However, consistent vaccination of pregnant mares should be expected to decrease the incidence of abortion storms as well as sporadic abortions in a herd. Because the time between actual infection and abortion may be long, some clinicians recommend vaccination every 2 months throughout the pregnancy. To maximize the effectiveness of a vaccination program it needs to be combined with a management strategy that minimizes exposure of mares to the virus and that prevents activation of a latent viral infection. All horses, young, adult, nonpregnant, and pregnant, should be vaccinated to restrict shedding of the virus. Unnecessary stress, such as transportation and overcrowding, should be avoided as far as possible. Pregnant mares should be kept separate from other horses on the farm. Newly arrived horses should not be mixed with pregnant mares on the farm. Newcomers should be isolated from the resident population for 3 weeks, over which time they should be monitored daily for signs of respiratory disease. If possible, pregnant mares should be divided into small groups.

Following an incident of abortion, the entire fetus and fetal membranes should be placed in a plastic bag and transported away from the area without contaminating the surrounding environment. The stall in which the mare aborted should be disinfected with a phenolic or iodinophoric compound, and the bedding should be prevented from contaminating other areas on the farm.

All pregnant mares on an infected farm should remain on the farm until they have foaled. No horse should leave the farm until 3 to 4 weeks after the last abortion.

Equine Infectious Anemia

Equine infectious anemia (EIA) is caused by a retrovirus that is transmitted by biting insects and mechanical vectors.

Foals from asymptomatic carriers of the disease are born free of infection and are seronegative before colostrum intake.

Clinical Signs and Diagnosis. Infected mares may abort during any stage of gestation. Abortions are often associated with weight loss or febrile episodes accompanied with high virus titers in the mare. A direct causal relationship between EIA and abortion has not been established.

Infected mares are diagnosed serologically. Agar gel immunodiffusion (Coggins test) and a competitive enzyme-linked immunosorbent assay (ELISA) are both approved for diagnosis of EIA.

Prevention and Control. The disease is regulated by federal and state control measures in the United States. The incidence of EIA has decreased since control measures were instituted in 1972, but the disease has not been eradicated from the country.

Equine Viral Arteritis

Equine viral arteritis (EVA) was first recognized as a cause of abortion in the 1950s, with abortion occurring in up to half of all infected mares. Few cases of EVA-induced abortion were reported between 1953 and 1984. A renewed interest in the disease has followed a 1984 epidemic of Thoroughbreds in Kentucky, although a low incidence of EVA abortions has been reported after 1984.

Clinical Signs and Diagnosis. The virus can be transmitted among horses as an aerosol or venereally to mares by infected stallions. Asymptomatic infected stallions have been suggested to play an important role in the transmission of the disease. Clinical signs of the disease include moderate to severe depression, fever, conjunctivitis, nasal discharge, and generalized vascular necrosis resulting in edema of the hindlimbs. Abortions have been observed from 3 months to the end of gestation. Abortion may occur 3 to 8 weeks after exposure as a result of placental detachment or anoxia of the endometrium resulting from compression of myometrial vessels by edema. There are often no obvious fetal or placental lesions. Aborted fetuses may be partly autolyzed. Vascular lesions may be observed in the placenta and expelled fetuses.

Diagnosis of EVA abortion is based on isolation of virus from fetal tissues and the placenta. Virus neutralization in sera from infected mares may confirm the cause of abortion. Paired samples at 21- to 28-day intervals should be obtained from aborting mares.

Prevention and Control. Control measures including isolation of newly arrived horses, regulation of traffic to and from the farm, and dividing pregnant mares into smaller groups should be implemented on breeding farms. Most specific control programs for EVA focus on identification of carrier stallions and vaccination of all high-risk breeding stallions at least 4 weeks prior to the onset of the breeding season. Stallions should be screened for serologic titers to EVA and, if positive, should undergo tests for semen virus isolation. Stallions that are confirmed semen shedders should be bred only to seropositive mares (either from natural infection or vaccination). Seronegative mares should be vaccinated no less than 3 weeks before being bred. Following breeding, all recently vaccinated mares should be kept apart from other seronegative mares for a period of 3 weeks.

A modified live vaccine that has been demonstrated to be safe and effective in stallions and nonpregnant mares is available on the market. The vaccine is not recommended to be used in pregnant mares, especially during the last 2 months of gestation. Foals born to immunized mares are protected against the disease for 2 to 6 months through passive transfer of antibodies in the colostrum. The passively acquired immunity has been found to interfere with vaccination with the modified live EVA vaccine.

Placentitis

Bacterial and fungal abortions in mares are primarily caused by ascending infections through the cervix, causing placentitis and subsequent fetal infection. In a retrospective study of more than 3000 aborted equine fetuses in Kentucky between 1986 and 1991, placentitis was the leading cause of reproductive loss. Bacterial organisms most commonly cultured from aborted fetuses include *Streptococcus* species, *Escherichia coli*, *Pseudomonas* species, *Klebsiella* species, *Staphylococcus* species, and *Leptospira* species. A nocardioform actinomycete was also found in the Kentucky study to be an important cause of placentitis. The most frequently recovered fungus is *Aspergillus* species.

Clinical Signs and Diagnosis. Mares that abort from placentitis often show clinical signs of pending abortion before the actual pregnancy termination. Premature udder development and vaginal discharge are common signs of pending abortion due to placentitis. Transrectal ultrasonography may show edema of the allantochorion and separation from the endometrium in an area close to the cervix. The space between the endometrium and the separated allantochorion is often filled with varying amounts of hyperechoic fluid.

The cause of abortion in infected mares is not clear. Fetal death from septicemia or insufficient placental support cannot explain all abortions from placentitis. Hormonal mechanisms associated with placental separation and uterine endocrine disturbances have been suggested as possible provocative mechanisms. The gross lesions of the fetus are not specific. An increased amount of fluid in the thoracic and abdominal cavities and an enlarged liver are frequently observed in aborted fetuses. Placental lesions are most severe on the chorionic surface at an area from opposite the cervix ("cervical star") to the body of the placenta. The affected area is edematous, thickened, and discolored or brown with a mucoid or fibronecrotic exudate on the surface (Fig. 1). Lesions are well demarcated from the rest of the chorionic surface. Microorganisms can be isolated from the placenta and several fetal organs, most consistently from the stomach.

Treatment. Pregnant mares with clinical signs of placentitis such as vaginal discharge or premature udder development should be treated with systemic broad-spectrum antimicrobials and anti-inflammatory drugs (see Prepartum Conditions, page 541). Treatments that cause uterine quiescence should also be considered. Altrenogest° (0.44 mg/ kg s.i.d. p.o.), isoxsuprine† (0.4–0.6 mg/kg IM b.i.d.), and

---

°Regu-Mate, Hoechst-Roussel, AgriVet, Somerville, NJ
†Duphaspasmin, Solvay Animal Health, Mendota Heights, MN

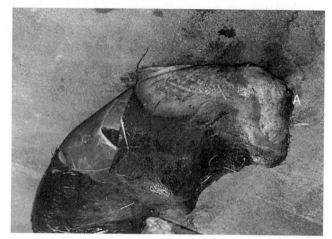

Figure 1. Abortion due to placentitis of a 10-month-old fetus. The mare had premature separation of the placenta with the dead fetus delivered in an intact allantochorion. Note the well-demarcated lesions at an area adjacent to the cervical star (A). The chorion has lost its villi, and is edematous, thickened, and discolored.

clenbuterol* (0.8 μg/kg IM or IV) have been used. Unfortunately, the disease process has often progressed too far for treatments to be effective once obvious clinical signs are observed. Transrectal ultrasonography in susceptible mares may allow for early detection of the disease with potentially improved treatment results.

Although most mares are capable of conceiving and successfully carrying a foal to term in subsequent breedings, reproductive performance may be negatively affected following placentitis. One study found an approximately 10% increase from previous seasons in conception failure and pregnancy losses following placentitis. This report emphasizes the importance of prompt treatment of mares following abortion due to placentitis. Treatments for endometritis, such as uterine lavage and intrauterine infusions of appropriate antibiotics, should also be implemented.

Leptospirosis

Until recently, leptospirosis has only occasionally been reported to cause equine abortions. Over the past few years, however, equine abortions caused by leptospirosis have been more frequently reported, and it was recently identified as a significant cause of equine abortion in Kentucky. The most common isolated serovar in the Kentucky study was *Leptospira* serovar *pomona*, but *Leptospira* serovar *grippotyphosa* was also identified from aborted fetuses. Serovars *hardjo*, *bratislava*, and *icterohemorrhagiae* have also been associated with sporadic abortions.

Clinical Signs and Diagnosis. Abortions have been observed from 6 months of gestation up to full term. Stillbirths and neonatal death of foals have been reported. Infected mares may show systemic signs over a period of 3 to 4 days, with mild depression, elevated temperature, anorexia, and slight icterus. Abortions occur weeks after the acute infection. Aborted foals could be icteric and may show some autolysis.

The diagnosis of leptospira abortion is based on isolation

of the organism, immunofluorescence staining, and serology testing. Bacteriologic isolation and staining of *Leptospira* species is difficult, and the diagnosis is often made based on serologic tests (microscopic agglutination test [MA] ELISA). Mares often have high leptospiral titers at the time of abortion. A rising titer associated with abortion is considered to be diagnostic.

Treatment and Prevention. Aborting mares should be isolated and the stalls should be disinfected, as for any other cause of infectious abortion. Infected mares may be treated with streptomycin (10 mg/kg b.i.d.), penicillin (10–15,000 IU/kg b.i.d.), or oxytetracycline (5–10 mg/kg) for a period of 1 week. Potassium penicillin G (20,000 IU/kg IV q.i.d.) has been used to treat mares with rising titers in late gestation. No vaccines against leptospirosis are available for horses.

Equine Ehrlichial Abortion

Ehrlichia risticii is a known cause of colitis in horses (Potomac horse fever). The disease is seasonal with a peak occurring when insect activity is high. An arthropod vector has been suggested as a transmitter of the disease, but the mode of transmission is not completely understood. Clinical signs of acute ehrlichial colitis may include one or more of the following signs: fever, depression, anorexia, ileus colic, diarrhea, and laminitis. Mild and subclinical forms of the disease are common. In addition, *E. risticii* has been associated with equine abortions. A recent study showed that mares experimentally infected with *E. risticii* at 100 to 160 days of pregnancy aborted their fetuses between 6 and 8 months of gestation. Histopathologic examination of the aborted fetuses supported *E. risticii* as a causative agent, and the organism was also cultured from some of the fetuses. However, the incidence of naturally occurring ehrlichial abortion is not known.

Clinical Signs and Diagnosis. Mares that were infected with *E. risticii* developed characteristic signs of colitis from which they recovered. When mares aborted 2 to 3 months later, they showed signs of both maternal and fetal pathology. Abortions were associated with placentitis and retained fetal membranes. Consistent histopathologic findings of aborted fetuses included colitis, periportal hepatitis, and hyperplasia and necrosis of lymphoid organs.

Diagnosis of equine ehrlichial abortion should be based on clinical signs; typical histopathologic lesions of the fetus; and culture of the organism from the colon, mesenteric lymph nodes, spleen, liver, and bone marrow. The diagnosis can be confirmed by identifying small amount of rickettsia by the use of polymerase chain reaction (PCR).

Treatment and Prevention. Commercial vaccines against ehrlichiosis are available. However, vaccination does not result in complete protection against disease, and the protective effect of vaccines on abortion is unknown.

Treatment with oxytetracycline (6.6 mg/kg IV s.i.d.) for up to 5 days in pregnant mares with clinical signs of acute ehrlichial colitis may prevent or reduce the incidence of abortion.

Endotoxemia

Gram-negative septicemia and endotoxemia associated with intestinal disorders that alter the integrity of the mucosal barrier, such as intestinal obstructions, acute enteritis,

---

*Ventipulmin, Boehringer Ingelheim Animal Health, St. Joseph, MO

colitis, and grain overload, result in the release of vasoactive metabolites including PGF$_2\alpha$. Endogenous release of PGF$_2\alpha$ during an episode of experimental endotoxemia has been shown to cause abortion in pregnant mares. The equine pregnancy is dependent on ovarian sources of progesterone for the first 80 days of gestation. After this time the fetoplacental unit takes over progesterone production that is necessary for maintenance of the pregnancy. Endogenous release of PGF$_2\alpha$ results in luteolysis and abortion during the first 2 months of pregnancy. However, it has been suggested that elevated concentrations of prostaglandins over a period of 2 to 3 days in midgestational mares also may cause abortion. The study was limited to mares between 82 and 152 days of gestation, and the effect of chronic prostaglandin release on more advanced pregnancies was not investigated.

Clinical Signs and Diagnosis. Mares aborting from endogenous release of endotoxin have had a recent experience of stress induced by endotoxemic shock or gram-negative endotoxemia. Pregnancy loss at early stages of gestation may go undetected unless fetal membranes or parts can be found in the stall. Abortions during later stages of the pregnancy may be observed as vaginal discharge or the detection of an expelled fetus. Pregnant mares showing signs of endotoxemia should always be examined for pregnancy status following the recovery of the disease.

Treatment and Prevention. Progestogen supplementation to pregnant mares is discussed in detail in the chapter on application for progestin therapy, page 531. Daily administration of altrenogest (0.44 mg/kg p.o.) has been shown to effectively prevent experimental endotoxin-induced abortion. If treated while the pregnancy still is corpus luteum (CL)-dependent (approximately before day 80), analysis of serum progesterone concentrations following the acute episode of the disease help to decide if the supplementation needs to continue. Serum progesterone concentrations less than 1 ng/ml indicate the loss of active luteal tissue, and supplemental progestogen treatment should continue until the fetoplacental unit positively is responsible for maintenance of the pregnancy. For practical reasons, supplementation until day 100 is commonly recommended. Serum progesterone concentrations higher than 1 ng/ml are compatible with functional luteal tissue, and the treatment can be discontinued.

Treatments with flunixin meglumine or other prostaglandin inhibitors have not been proved to effectively prevent endotoxin-induced fetal losses, unless administered prior to clinical signs.

Noninfectious

Twin Pregnancy

The most common noninfectious cause of equine abortion is twin pregnancy. The mechanism of twin pregnancies has been studied intensively and described in detail elsewhere. Twin pregnancies occur in most horse breeds. They are believed to be more common in Thoroughbreds and are rarely observed in pony breeds. Double ovulation occurs at a rate of approximately 20% of all ovulations with some breed, age, and seasonal variations. Half of these ovulations result in twin pregnancies. Depending on whether the embryos are fixed bilaterally or unilaterally in

the uterine horns, spontaneous reduction may occur. Both twins can be expected to survive beyond 40 days if fixation is bilateral, whereas reduction of one twin occurs in more than 80% of cases in which embryo fixation is unilateral.

The high abortion rate and negative consequences associated with twin pregnancies in the mare are related to the type of placentation in equids. The equine placenta is diffuse, and it covers the entire endometrial surface. Inability of the uterus to support two fetuses to term owing to insufficient placental support often results in abortion. Termination of pregnancy can occur at any stage of gestation, but is most common after 7 months. Even if twins are carried to term, the combined birth weight of the two fetuses rarely exceeds the normal birth weight of a singleton foal. The markedly smaller size of twins is the result of the reduced placental areas in twin pregnancies.

Three distributions of twins are possible in the uterus. (1) One twin occupies the uterine body and one horn, and possesses approximately 70% of the functional surface area. Where the two chorions are in contact, there is usually a degree of invagination of the smaller one into the larger one. This is the most common type of twin pregnancy. It often results in abortion or stillbirth of one or both twins in late gestation. (2) The villous surface area is equally divided between the twins, each of which occupies one horn and half of the body. The twins may be aborted or born alive, but weak and undersized. (3) A great disparity of villous surface area exists, with the chorion of one twin almost totally excluding the other by occupying the uterine body, one horn, and most of the other horn. The smaller twin dies relatively early in gestation with the other twin usually born alive.

Clinical Signs and Diagnosis. Mares aborting from twin pregnancies commonly show all the characteristic signs of impending parturition (i.e., udder development, relaxation of sacrosciatic ligaments, and relaxation of external genitalia). In addition to the two aborted fetuses, placental lesions bear evidence of twin pregnancy. A circumscribed area where the two placentas were in contact displays a complete absence of chorionic villi. This is seen as a smooth noncharacteristic area of the otherwise velvet-like chorion (Fig. 2). One fetus often shows more advanced signs of autolysis, indicating that it died first. The smaller fetus is more likely to die before the larger one, but the opposite situation may occur in as often as 20% of all twin abortions.

Treatment and Prevention. Management of twin pregnancies is described in detail in *Current Therapy of Equine Medicine 3*, page 657. Early pregnancy diagnosis using ultrasonography allows for highly successful manual reduction of one twin if done before day 25 of pregnancy. This technique has significantly reduced the incidence of abortion caused by twin pregnancies. Other methods of twin reduction have also been described. Ultrasound-guided fetal heart puncture with an intracardiac injection of a potassium chloride solution through the maternal abdominal wall results in cardiac arrest. When performed between 70 and 170 days of gestation, approximately 40% of the mares can be expected to give birth to a single live foal. Restricting the diet has been suggested to be effective for converting a twin pregnancy to a singleton. This method needs to be further investigated before it can be recom-

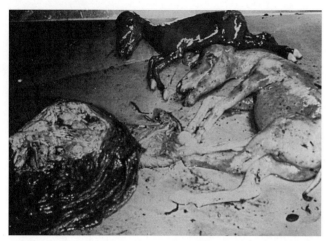

Figure 2. Twin abortion at 7 months of gestation from a Warmblood mare. The larger of the twins occupied the uterine body and one horn, depriving the smaller twin of sufficient placental surface area. The smaller twin shows more advanced signs of autolysis, indicating that it died first. Note the area where the two placentas were in contact. The absence of chorionic villi is seen as a smooth, well-circumscribed area of the otherwise velvet-like chorion.

mended. Transvaginal ultrasound-guided aspiration of allantoic fluid has been described as a means of pregnancy termination. Further studies of this interesting method to reduce twins will be necessary. If reduction of one twin is not an option, the pregnancy can be terminated by the use of $PGF_2\alpha$. This prevents complications associated with late twin abortions (i.e., dystocia and future subfertility).

Placental Abnormalities

Pregnancy losses are significantly higher in mares with extensive endometrial fibrosis, as seen on an endometrial biopsy, compared with mares without uterine pathology. An association also appears between severe endometrial fibrosis and a history of abortion. The mechanism of abortion in mares with widespread endometrial fibrosis has not been critically investigated. Histopathologic examination of the reproductive tract of mares with endometrial fibrosis postpartum showed that fibrosis and atrophy of the endometrium was associated with abnormal chorionic areas. This suggests an inadequate placental exchange and support of the growing fetus as a cause of abortion.

Body pregnancy is rare and is diagnosed by placental evidence of a fetus that has been restricted to the uterine body rather than the body and one uterine horn. Limited placentation restricts fetal growth, and abortion may occur when the nutritional demands of the fetus no longer can be met.

Excessive variations from normal length of the umbilical cord (about 84 cm in Thoroughbreds) have been associated with death of the fetus and subsequent abortion. Increased length may result in torsion of the cord.

Abnormal shortening of the umbilical cord may cause premature rupture of the cord before parturition. The rupture usually occurs near the abdominal wall, resulting in fetal asphyxiation.

Diagnosis and Treatment. Clinical aspects of diagnosis and treatment of degenerative fibrotic endometritis is

discussed on page 521. Diagnosis of endometrial fibrosis is based on histopathologic evaluation of an endometrial biopsy. No documented effective treatment is available for degenerative fibrotic endometritis.

Diagnosis of umbilical cord abnormalities is based on clinical findings of the aborted fetus. Only when the torsion is accompanied by signs of vascular obstruction (i.e., localized edema and discoloration) should it be diagnosed as a cause of abortion. Twisting of the umbilical cord is common and does not result in fetal death.

Body pregnancies may be diagnosed early in gestation by rectal palpation and ultrasonography. Because of the increased risk for abortion, confirmed body pregnancies should be terminated and the mare bred back during the same season.

Other noninfectious causes of large animal abortion include genetic or chromosomal factors, inadequate nutrition, vitamin or mineral deficiencies, ingestion of poisonous plants or other toxins, hormonal factors, environmental factors, physical factors, and certain medications.

PREVENTION OF ABORTION

Mares at risk of abortion should be carefully examined for reproductive soundness before breeding. Abnormal perineal conformation and the presence of chronic uterine infection can predispose to fetoplacental infection during pregnancy. Extensive endometrial fibrosis seen on a uterine biopsy indicates a high risk for abortion. Vaccination of mares against infectious agents that cause abortion should always be considered, especially if mares are kept in a susceptible herd.

Progesterone supplementation is widely used in pregnant mares in an attempt to prevent abortion. Research has clearly demonstrated the value of progesterone supplementation in mares with a loss of luteal activity resulting from endogenous prostaglandin release (i.e., endotoxemia). Practical experience suggests that fetal loss can be prevented in mares without clinical signs of disease. Repeated attempts to document a primary luteal deficiency in the mare have failed. Serum progesterone concentrations seem to decline as a result of fetal loss rather than being a cause of abortion. Regardless, mares with a history of fetal loss often are administered progesterone supplementation with good results. If supplementation is initiated, it is not necessary to keep mares on progesterone beyond 100 days of gestation. Furthermore, fetal viability needs to be examined regularly during the course of treatment, because exogenous progesterone may cause retention of a nonviable fetus. Management of high-risk pregnancies is discussed under perinatology (page 541).

Supplemental Readings

Acland HM: Abortion in mares. *In* McKinnon AO, Voss JL (eds): Equine Reproduction, Philadelphia, Lea & Febiger, 1993, pp 554–562.

Daels PF, Besognet B, Hansen B, Odensvik K, Kindahl H: Efficacy of treatments to prevent abortion in pregnant mares at risk. Proc 40th Annu Conv Am Assoc Equine Pract 1994, pp 31–34.

Donahue JM, Smith BJ, Redmon K, Donahue JK: Diagnosis and prevalence of leptospira infection in aborted and stillborn horses. J Vet Diagn Invest 3:148–151, 1991.

Long MT, Goetz TE, Kakoma I, Whiteley HE, Lock T: Evidence for fetal infectivity and abortion caused by *Ehrlichia risticii*. Proc 38th Annu Conv Am Assoc Equine Pract, 1992, pp 571–578.

Macpherson ML, Homco LD, Varner DD, Blanchard TL, Harms PG, Cohen ND, Flanagan MN, Forrest DF: Transvaginal ultrasound guided allocentesis for pregnancy elimination in the mare. Biol Reprod (Monograph series 1), 215–223, 1995.

Miller RB: Evaluation of the equine and bovine placenta: Lesions vs nonlesions. Proc Soc Therio, 1993, pp 39–44.

Ostlund EN: The equine herpesviruses. Vet Clin North Am Equine Pract 9(2):283–294, 1993.

Roberts SJ: Veterinary Obstetrics and Genital Diseases (Theriogenology), ed 3. North Pomfret, VT, SJ Roberts, 1986, pp 162–180.

Timoney PJ, McCollum WH: Equine viral arteritis. Vet Clin North Am Equine Pract 9(2):295–309, 1993.

Whitwell KE: Infective placentitis in the mare. Proc 5th Int Conf Equine Infect Dis, 1989, pp 172–180.

Prepartum Conditions

ELIZABETH M. SANTSCHI
St. Paul, Minnesota

Prepartum conditions that affect pregnancy outcome can primarily affect either the mare or conceptus (i.e., the fetus and placenta). Pregnancies affected by conditions that can result in death or disability to the mare or fetus are designated as high risk. A list of the most common conditions that can result in high-risk pregnancy is presented in Table 1. The best outcome of these pregnancies is survival of both the mare and the fetus, but this result cannot always be achieved. Therapy for the wide range of conditions occurring during pregnancy is dictated by the specific condition, owners' wishes, and achievable goals of the pregnancy. Early identification of high-risk pregnancy is sometimes difficult but is essential to the successful treatment of many disorders.

IDENTIFICATION OF PREPARTUM DISORDERS

Prepartum disorders of the mare are usually easily recognized, but identification of conditions affecting the fetus and placenta is more difficult. Important information about the health of the mare and fetus is obtained by taking a good history, performing a physical examination, performing selected laboratory tests of maternal blood and mammary secretions, and by imaging the uterus and its contents by transabdominal ultrasound. The extent of maternal insult can often be estimated, but fetal compromise is difficult to detect and quantify because of the inability to directly access the conceptus and a lack of established normal data.

History

Important historical information can be gathered from both present and past pregnancies. From the present pregnancy, the results of diagnostic tests such as uterine culture, cytology, and biopsy performed before breeding can provide valuable information, as can the results of rectal and ultrasound examinations. The determination of accurate breeding dates is also imperative. The consumption of endophyte-infested fescue forage; exposure to equine herpesvirus-1 (EHV-1), equine viral arteritis (EVA), leptospirosis, or *Ehrlichia risticii*; and medications administered during pregnancy should also be determined.

If the mare has previously delivered a high-risk foal, the present pregnancy should be monitored very closely. Results of a previous pregnancy that indicate the potential for problems in the present pregnancy include: abortion, dystocia, twins, or delivery by hysterotomy. Additional causes for concern include producing a foal that was small for gestational age, was septic, or had failure of passive transfer or neonatal isoerythrolysis.

Physical Examination

The physical examination of the late-term pregnant mare differs from that for nonpregnant horses only in the examination of the reproductive tract. All other systems should be examined thoroughly; however, the gastrointestinal and cardiopulmonary systems have the greatest effect on the pregnancy and should receive the most attention. The evaluation of the reproductive tract should include inspection of perineal conformation, a speculum examination of the cervix, palpation of the vagina and cervix, and palpation of the uterus per rectum. After noting the perineal conformation, the speculum examination of the cervix should be performed, noting cervical position, color, and the presence of the cervical plug or discharge. For the first 10 months of gestation, the cervix is firm and closed and appears pale pink with a cervical mucous plug. The presence of a bloody or purulent uterine discharge is abnormal. In normal mares during the last month of gestation, the cervix can lose the

TABLE 1. CONDITIONS CAUSING HIGH-RISK PREGNANCY

Maternal Conditions	Conceptal Conditions
Colic	Placentitis
Endotoxemia	Twins
Abdominal tunic hernias	Hydrops
Dystocia (pelvic/uterine abnormalities)	Prolonged gestation
Malnutrition	Dystocia (fetal abnormalities)
Uterine inadequacy	Fescue toxicity
Hypogalactia	Congenital abnormalities
Uterine torsion	Umbilical abnormalities
Hyperlipemia	

mucous plug and soften. This is normal in the absence of other signs of intrauterine disease. Palpation of the vagina and cervix should be performed if the speculum examination indicates a potential abnormality. The vaginal walls should be tacky and closely adherent as a result of the elevated progesterone concentrations. In the first 10 months of gestation, the cervix should be firm and closed. In the last month, the cervical softening can be sufficient to admit a closed hand and allow palpation of the placenta. This is normal, but palpation should be very limited to avoid cervical stimulation that can cause the release of prostaglandins that can affect uterine motility.

The rectal examination determines cervical and uterine tone and detects pelvic or uterine masses and fetal movement. The fetus should be palpable directly or by ballotement after 200 days of gestation, and movement indicates viability. Changes in the tone of the uterus or a reduction of uterine fluid suggest a need for further fetal evaluation. Excessive uterine fluid results in an inability to palpate the fetus and suggests hydrops of the fetal membranes.

The mammary gland should be included in the evaluation of the reproductive tract, because it can suggest uterine and intrauterine pathology. The mammary gland develops during the last month of gestation, with most of the development occurring immediately before parturition. Mammary gland development is individual, and some mares develop a mammary gland overnight. The major abnormality seen in the mammary gland is the development of premature lactation. The presence of mammary secretions in the mammary gland collecting system is normal a few days before parturition, but the volume should be small. Collection of small amounts of thick dried secretion (wax) around the teat orifice is also normal. When milk streams from a pregnant mare's udder, it is considered premature lactation. Premature lactation is significant for two reasons: it suggests a placental insult, and, if occurring just prior to parturition, it can result in the loss of colostrum essential in the transfer of passive immunity to the foal.

Laboratory Analysis

The appropriate laboratory tests should be performed to determine the health status of the pregnant mare. These tests include complete blood counts, serum chemistries, serum titers, blood gases, and cytology and cultures. In addition, some laboratory investigations are helpful in the evaluation of fetal and placental health.

Various hormones have been measured in maternal serum or plasma in an attempt to detect fetal compromise. Progestogens have received the most attention, but the studies performed have provided conflicting results. Confusion arises because there are several progestogen compounds present in maternal and fetal blood and because there are several techniques available to measure these substances, making comparison between laboratories difficult. It appears that early (<308 days of gestation) increases in progestogen concentration suggest placental damage and that low (<2 ng/ml) or rapidly decreasing progestogen concentrations in late pregnancy suggest fetal compromise. However, therapeutic decisions should not be made on the basis of one sample. Because of normal diurnal and individual variation, a single sample can give misleading results.

The best information can be obtained from serial sampling of serum or plasma to describe the trends of progestogen production. Concentrations of conjugated estrogens such as estrone sulfate have also been measured in the maternal serum of mares with high-risk pregnancy in late gestation, but they are not useful in detecting fetal compromise.

Measurement of the concentrations of sodium, potassium, and calcium in mammary secretions of normal mares before foaling can provide information about fetal maturity. Approximately 1 week before parturition, sodium concentrations are at relatively high levels in mammary secretions, and potassium and calcium are at low levels. Between 2 and 3 days before parturition, the sodium level drops and the potassium level rises, and thus the potassium level becomes greater than the sodium (i.e., there is a sodium-potassium inversion). In addition, in the few hours before parturition, the calcium level in the mammary secretion rises abruptly. Analysis of these electrolytes in high-risk equine pregnancies can be helpful in providing information about fetal maturity. All electrolyte levels should be measured, because placental pathology can elevate mammary secretion calcium in the absence of fetal maturity. In pregnancies with placental pathology and elevated concentrations of calcium in mammary secretions, the sodium-potassium inversion in mammary secretions should occur before a fetus is considered mature. Occasionally, a sodium-potassium inversion can occur before fetal maturity, and thus it is essential to use the mammary secretion electrolyte data in conjunction with gestation length and other clinical parameters before fetal maturity is estimated.

MATERNAL PREPARTUM CONDITIONS

Colic and Endotoxemia

Colic is the most common condition that affects the pregnant brood mare. The vast majority of these colics resolve with minimal treatment and pose little risk to the mare or fetus. Colic episodes that require surgery, occur repeatedly over a few days, or result in severe endotoxemia have a much more significant effect on survival of the mare and foal.

Approximately 18% of pregnancies in mares with colic that require surgery for diagnostic or therapeutic reasons result in abortion. About half of these abortions occur long after the colic episode and are thought to be unrelated to the surgery or colic. However, about 9% of the mares abort in the perioperative period, and these abortions are presumed to be related to the colic or its treatment. Abortions are often associated with arterial hypoxia (PaO$_2$ <80 mm Hg) when surgery occurs in the last 60 days of gestation. Abortions also occur in mares showing signs of endotoxemia, whether or not surgery and anesthesia were part of the treatment. The best methods for avoiding abortion in mares with colic are to determine the need for surgery as early as possible, keep the operative time as short as possible, and maintain arterial oxygenation above 80 to 100 mm Hg during surgery. Treatment of endotoxemia is also critical and requires the use of fluids and anti-inflammatory drugs such as flunixin meglumine.

Experimental administration of endotoxin has resulted in luteolysis and abortion in pregnant mares at less than 60 days of gestation because of endogenous prostaglandin release. Pregnancy was maintained in these mares given endotoxin when altrenogest was administered. Administration of supplemental progestogens to mares in early pregnancy that show clinical signs of endotoxemia is recommended until progestogen production by the corpus luteum is established.

Uterine Torsions

Uterine torsions also cause colic-like symptoms. One clinical sign that suggests a uterine torsion instead of a gastrointestinal lesion is that mares with uterine torsions often continue to pass feces. The diagnosis of uterine torsion is made by palpation of the uterus per rectum. The ovary on the side away from the torsion assumes a midline position, and the ovarian suspensory and broad ligaments can be palpated as a tight horizontal band dorsal to the uterus. Treatment of uterine torsions can be performed by rolling under anesthesia, by surgery through a flank incision usually with the mare standing, or via a ventral midline approach with the mare in dorsal recumbency. The rolling procedure is performed using a board placed in the flank to hold the fetus in position, and the mare is rolled in the direction of the torsion to "catch up" with her uterus. During surgery torsion of the uterus can be corrected manually. Fetal survival after uterine torsion is probably less reliant on the method of correction than early diagnosis and correction.

Abdominal Tunic Ruptures

Ruptures of the abdominal tunic can occur in the muscular or tendinous portions. Mares with ruptures of the abdominal tunic have pain and varying degrees of edema of the ventral abdomen. Prepubic tendon ruptures are diagnosed by an abnormal positioning of the pelvis and mammary gland. The tuber coxae is tipped up and the tuber ischii tipped down. The mammary gland is displaced because of the loss of the caudal attachment of the abdominal wall. When the tendon is totally ruptured, the likelihood of carrying the foal to term and saving the mare is very low. If the mare's life is important but subsequent fertility is not, the fetus should be aborted and delivered with assistance. Abortion risks further damage to the abdominal tunic, but maintaining the pregnancy also is very risky for the mare. Some owners choose to continue with the pregnancy despite the poor prognosis; stall confinement, anti-inflammatory drugs, and abdominal supports can be used. Parturition should be induced when the fetus is ready for birth.

Partial damage to the prepubic tendon can sometimes be managed successfully. These mares have pain and ventral edema, but do not have a tipped pelvis or mammary gland. Sometimes the prepubic tendon appears stretched, and there is an extreme distance between the umbilicus and the base of the mammary gland. Such mares should be stall-confined and given anti-inflammatory drugs as needed. Abdominal supports should be used if they appear to provide benefit. If used, supports should be of stout construction, either heavy canvas or leather, and padded over the back and on the ventral abdomen. Tape supports usually stretch and are of questionable benefit. Delivery should be induced or mares should have attended foalings, because they may not be able to provide sufficient abdominal contraction to deliver the foal quickly. Carrying future pregnancies to term is unwise, but embryo transfer may be an option if future reproductive capability is essential.

Mares with ruptures of the muscular support of the abdomen also exhibit edema and pain, but the swelling is asymmetrical. Mares with large muscular tears usually require euthanasia owing to pain from either the muscle damage or from colic. These muscular hernias tend to entrap bowel and cause an abdominal crisis. Surgery to correct the hernia in the acute stages is usually unsuccessful because the hernial margin is not strong enough to hold suture. Small muscular tears can be managed successfully using stall rest, abdominal supports, and anti-inflammatory drugs. If a mare with a small hernia carries her fetus to term, occasionally the hernia can be surgically repaired after parturition and the mare may have further successful gestations.

Pelvic Abnormalities

Pelvic abnormalities that cause high-risk pregnancy are those that can impede parturition. The most common cause is healed pelvic fractures with callus that reduces the pelvic internal diameter. Occasionally, a tumor, granuloma, or hydronephrotic kidney also result in a reduction of pelvic or caudal abdominal diameter and impede fetal delivery. These mares should have their fetuses delivered by hysterotomy, and the decision to perform a hysterectomy should be made before parturition begins. Using breeding dates and mammary secretion electrolytes, the hysterotomy can be performed at term, and excellent fetal viability can be anticipated.

Hyperlipemia

Hyperlipemia describes the condition of elevated serum triglycerides. The triglycerides enter the circulation when a state of negative energy balance exists. The clinical signs of hyperlipemia include anorexia, dullness, diarrhea, and lethargy. Hyperlipemia occurs most often in pregnant pony mares, but it also occurs in miniature horses and donkeys, and rarely in light horses. In ponies, hyperlipemia can be a primary disease associated with obesity, pregnancy, lactation, or stress. In horses or miniature horses, hyperlipemia is a secondary complication to a condition that results in a negative energy balance. Hyperlipemia is not a common condition, but it results in a high mortality rate in pregnant ponies.

The most important treatment of hyperlipemia is nutritional support, and enteral support is preferable. Horses that will not eat can be fed via nasogastric tube, using either commercial enteral diets or a gruel of soaked pellets. In addition, insulin can be used to prevent further mobilization of peripheral adipose tissue, and heparin has been advocated to promote the peripheral utilization of triglycerides.

PLACENTAL PREPARTUM CONDITIONS

Placental conditions such as infective placentitis, premature placental separation, placental insufficiency, and hydrops of the fetal membranes are the most common causes of equine high-risk pregnancy. The health of the fetus is most commonly at risk in placental conditions. However, hydrops can result in maternal death, and infective placentitis can result in uterine damage that can impact a mare's future reproductive capability.

Placentitis

The placenta of the equine fetus can be infected by bacteria and fungi. These agents affect the placenta by interfering with the exchange of nutrients and waste products. The placenta is also a very active endocrinologic organ, and insult to the placenta can damage those functions that are vital to fetal survival. Most cases of bacterial placentitis are diagnosed in the last 60 days of gestation. Mares with infective placentitis can abort without premonitory signs, but they often exhibit premature lactation and vulvar discharge. Bacterial placentitis is more common than fungal placentitis. The route of infection is probably the cervix, and infection is presumed to occur most commonly during the pregnancy. The diagnosis of placentitis is made by observing cervical discharge and an inflamed cervix. Transrectal ultrasound can also be used to image the caudal uterus and placenta to determine placental thickness, presence of fluid between the uterus and placenta, and placental detachment.

Treatment of bacterial placentitis should include antimicrobials, anti-inflammatory drugs, and stall rest. The antimicrobial chosen should be based on a culture of the uterine discharge. Systemic administration of antimicrobials is the preferred method for therapy, although local administration through the cervix has also been used. Little information is available on the appropriate antimicrobials for the treatment of bacterial placentitis. Both combinations of penicillin (potassium penicillin, 22,000 IU/kg, IV q.i.d.) and gentamicin (6.6 mg/kg IV s.i.d.) or trimethoprim/sulfa (30 mg/kg p.o. b.i.d.) have been effective in clinical cases. The antimicrobials should be continued for a minimum of 1 week after the resolution of clinical signs.

Anti-inflammatory drugs appear to have a beneficial effect on mares with placentitis. The uterus can produce prostaglandins in response to infection, and increases in uterine prostaglandins have been associated with premature delivery and reduced fetal survival. Prostaglandins are potent mediators of uterine motility, and a quiet endometrium is thought to be essential to pregnancy maintenance. Either flunixin meglumine (1 mg/kg IV b.i.d.) or phenylbutazone (4.4 mg/kg p.o. s.i.d.) can be used as a prostaglandin-synthetase inhibitor in pregnant mares. Some concerns have been expressed about inducing fetal pulmonary hypertension or reducing the effectiveness of uterine contractions during parturition with the use of nonsteroidal anti-inflammatory drug, but this concern has not been supported in clinical cases. It is probably wise, however, to only use nonsteroidal anti-inflammatory drugs as necessary while clinical signs persist. Stall rest is also thought to have a beneficial effect on mares with active uterine inflammation. Bed rest in women has a calming effect on uterine motility, and stall rest in mares may have a similar beneficial effect.

Fungal placentitis can occur in mares and is most commonly caused by *Aspergillus* species. Treatment of fungal placentitis is similar to that for bacterial placentitis. The use of antimicrobials is optional but is encouraged if there appears to be a secondary bacterial component to the infection. The use of human antifungal vaginal suppositories placed in the uterus may have a beneficial effect.

Hydrops of the Fetal Membranes

Hydrops is the accumulation of excessive fluid within the amnionic or allantoic cavity. This condition is uncommon in mares and occurs most often in the allantoic cavity. Clinical signs include abortion or respiratory distress and abdominal enlargement. If the mare is in the process of aborting, treatment is directed at facilitating the expulsion of the fetus and treating the hypovolemia that can occur after delivery. If the mare presents in respiratory distress or abdominal distension, the diagnosis is made by physical examination. The fetus should be detectable either by direct palpation or by ballottement after 200 days. Mares with fetuses affected by hydrops have large fluid-filled uteri for the stage of gestation, and the fetus cannot be palpated. The abdomens of these mares appear rounded, and they can appear to have difficulty breathing, especially when lying down. Transabdominal ultrasound can be used to detect the presence of excessive fluid or multiple fetuses.

The pregnancy of a mare with hydrops should be aborted. These mares are at great risk for rupture of the abdominal tunic and subsequent death. The viability of fetuses affected by hydrops of the fetal membranes is very poor, because they often have other abnormalities. When parturition is induced, it should be assisted because uterine inertia is common. If possible, the uterine fluid should be removed during stage-1 labor using a sterile nasogastric tube. The fluid should be removed over several minutes to reduce the insult to the mare's cardiovascular system by a rapid removal of the large amount of fluid. Hypovolemic shock should be anticipated and prophylactic intravenous fluid therapy started before induction. After parturition, retained placenta and delayed uterine involution are common and should be treated as necessary.

Premature Placental Separation

Premature placental separation occurs either acutely at parturition ("red-bag") or chronically during late gestation. Acute placental separation can result in fetal asphyxia and death and is an emergency. Acute placental separation is apparent during second-stage labor; the intact red velvety allantochorion appears at the vulvar lips instead of the glistening white amnion. When this occurs, the fetus and placenta are moving as a unit. Because of the mare's diffuse placentation, this means the placenta is sliding out intact, no gas exchange is occurring, and the fetus is suffocating. The allantochorion should be ruptured and the fetus delivered immediately. Appropriate therapy for neonatal asphyxia should follow.

Chronic placental separation occurs more insidiously during late gestation. The placenta detaches from the endometrium and causes premature lactation. This occurs most frequently at the cervical star, and the cervix softens and opens. The endometrial surface of the allantochorion can be palpated and the separation detected. Deciding on treatment for chronic placental detachment is difficult; there is currently no good way to determine the extent of fetal insult. Fetal heart rates and measurement of sodium and potassium in the mammary secretions can provide valuable information about fetal maturity and viability. Induction should be done with caution, and only when the mammary secretion electrolyte test results indicate maturity and extreme fetal distress is suspected. Most mares should be stall-confined and closely monitored. The use of supplemental progesterone should be considered. Antimicrobials should be used if an infection is suspected, and anti-inflammatory drugs may be beneficial to decrease uterine inflammation and irritability.

Use of Supplemental Progestogens

Whenever high-risk pregnancies are treated, the use of supplemental progestogens is often considered. Very few conditions are the result of low production of progestogens. A possible exception is mares that undergo luteolysis after the natural release of prostaglandins; experimental studies have demonstrated pregnancy maintenance when supplemental progestogens are administered to mares that lack a functional corpus luteum. There is no question that supplemental progestogens are overused in equine practice; the detrimental effect of such therapy is unknown. Progestogens are progestational; their use has been associated with a calming of the uterus, and experience suggests that there are beneficial effects of the use of supplemental progestogens even if the mare has normal circulating endogenous progestogen levels. Each clinician must decide the appropriate use of supplemental progestogens; the author has found them useful in mares with colic, endotoxemia, uterine torsions, placentitis, and premature placental separation. Two forms of exogenous progestogen are available—oral altrenogest and injectable progesterone. The oral product is expensive and some have questioned its efficacy, but it does not interfere with assay of endogenous progestogens. The injectable product can be hard to obtain and causes muscle soreness when given daily, as is recommended.

FETAL PREPARTUM CONDITIONS

Conditions such as prolonged gestation; twinning; congenital abnormalities; and infectious diseases such as EHV-1, leptospirosis, and *E. risticii* infection affect the fetus. These conditions can also adversely affect the health of the dam because of their ability to damage the reproductive tract during parturition.

Prolonged Gestation

The wide range of the length of normal gestation in mares (320–350 days) requires that the diagnosis of prolonged gestation be made only after the pregnancy persists after 350 days of gestation. At that time, transabdominal ultrasound should be performed to check for twins and to estimate fetal size. It is uncommon for a foal born after a long gestation to be very large; usually these foals are small to normal-sized. Induction is often contemplated but is uncommonly indicated in these cases and should not be performed until the gestation is at least 365 days in length.

The pathogenesis of prolonged gestation is not known. A period of embryonic rest of up to 30 days early in gestation has been suggested based on palpation of a small uterus in early gestation and a delay in the secretion of pregnant mare serum gonadotropin (PMSG). If this is true, waiting for spontaneous delivery is the best treatment and should be used in mares with prolonged gestation if a small uterus was detected at 30 to 60 days of gestation. An alternative explanation for prolonged gestation is that there is an interruption in the normal sequence of events that initiate parturition. Induction may be appropriate in these mares but should be performed cautiously. The use of dexamethasone as an induction agent may be appropriate in mares lacking a history of apparent embryonic rest, those with normal-sized fetuses, and those with an apparent failure to complete gestation. To induce parturition with dexamethasone, the length of gestation should be at least 365 days. Dexamethasone (100 mg IV s.i.d.) is given over 5 days. The mares usually foal within 2 to 7 days after beginning treatment.

Steroids have been shown to be important in the final stages of fetal maturation in some species. The mechanism of fetal maturation is poorly understood in horses, but exogenous dexamethasone may "turn on" the last phase of maturity. In contrast to its effect in ruminants, therapeutic doses of dexamethasone (20–40 mg/day) do not induce parturition or cause abortion at any stage of gestation in the mare. Because of the other possible actions of dexamethosone, the steroid should be used cautiously as an induction agent in mares with pre-existing medical conditions such as laminitis.

Twins

Twin pregnancy can become apparent in late gestation as a consequence of the fetuses' competition for the endometrial surface. Abortion without premonitory signs can occur, but often the mare begins to lactate prematurely, and the cervix softens. Transabdominal ultrasound establishes the diagnosis and presence of fetal viability. If one fetus is dead, treatment is usually futile, but treatment includes the use of nonsteroidal anti-inflammatory drugs, progesterone, and stall rest. These mares should be closely monitored for signs of parturition to facilitate delivery of the fetuses.

Infection

Infectious agents that primarily affect the fetus and can cause high-risk pregnancy include EHV-1, leptospirosis, and *E. risticii* infection, which is the agent that causes Potomac horse fever. Foals infected with EHV-1 can be aborted or born compromised at term. There is no treatment for EHV-1, only prevention by vaccination.

Leptospira pomona has been associated with equine abortion. Abortions caused by leptospiral organisms usually occur without any premonitory signs. Because the agent lives in the environment and is excreted in urine, pregnant mares in contact with the aborting mare, the aborted conceptus, or the same environment should have a *Leptospira* titer determined. Mares with high titers may benefit from treatment with penicillin (40,000 IU/kg IV q.i.d.) or oxytetracycline (5 to 10 mg/kg b.i.d.) for 7 to 10 days.

Another agent that is suspected to cause abortion after natural exposure is *E. risticii*; experimental infection has resulted in abortion of infected fetuses. *E. risticii* causes diarrhea most commonly, although subclinical infection is also common. The diagnosis is established by demonstrating a rising serum titer to *E. risticii*. If *E. risticii* is suspected to be a cause of abortion, pregnant mares can be treated with oxytetracycline in an attempt to eliminate the infection.

INDUCTION OF PARTURITION IN A HIGH-RISK PREGNANCY

The preferred method of induction of parturition for the majority of mares regardless of the primary condition is the use of low-dose oxytocin (15–30 IU IV, see page 548). After administration of the first dose, the mare should be placed in a large, clean stall and left alone. She should be allowed to lie down and get up at will, because this helps with proper fetal positioning. Proper positioning of the fetus should be determined before the mare begins strenuous labor. A high-risk mare may have a compromised abdominal press, and it may be necessary to provide traction on the fetus during second-stage labor. Proper cervical dilation should be established before traction is applied. The dose of oxytocin can be repeated at 30-minute intervals if parturition does not progress. Parturition usually occurs within 30 to 60 minutes after the first dose. If parturition does not progress, it could be because of fetal death causing dystocia or uterine inertia due to exhaustion or illness.

The question of when to induce delivery in a mare with a high-risk pregnancy is more difficult to answer than how to induce parturition. The goal of induction is to either remove a pregnancy that is threatening the dam's life with no thought of fetal survival, or to remove a fetus from a perilous environment, in an attempt to improve the likelihood of fetal survival. In the first instance, the decision to induce parturition is easy. In the second, the decision of when to induce is more difficult. Serious limitations on our ability to manage premature foals make preterm induction unwise and expensive. An additional complication is determining the extent of fetal compromise. The essential question the perinatologist must answer is when extrauterine life is superior to intrauterine life. For the foal known to be immature, the answer is probably never. Determination of prematurity is based on breeding dates and mammary secretion electrolyte levels. However, foals that are chronically stressed in utero can have an acceleration of maturity, and thus breeding dates provide only a guideline. Additionally, placental insults can elevate calcium levels in mammary secretions in the absence of fetal maturity.

A few examples may be useful: (1) If a foal is exposed to an acute insult such as maternal colic but the mare's mammary secretion electrolyte levels indicate prematurity, parturition should be induced only if the mare is being euthanized and the owners understand the poor prognosis and probable expense for neonatal care. (2) If the foal is exposed to an acute insult and the mare's mammary secretion electrolyte levels are mature, parturition can be induced if it is thought to be necessary. A large perinatal expense still accrues, but the odds of survival are better than those of the immature foal. (3) If a foal is exposed to a chronic insult such as placentitis, if its heart rate is erratic, or if the mare's progestogen levels are declining but her mammary electrolyte levels are mature, parturition should probably be induced. (4) If a foal is exposed to a chronic insult but the mare's mammary secretion electrolyte levels indicate immaturity, treatment of the primary condition should be instituted and parturition induced either when the electrolytes indicate maturity or if rapid deterioration of fetal heart rate and maternal progestogen concentrations occurs. To induce parturition in mares with high-risk pregnancies remains more of an art than a science. The overriding rule about inducing high-risk mares is to be cautious.

Supplemental Readings

Ousey JC, Dudan F, Rossdale PD: Preliminary studies of mammary secretions in the mare to assess foetal readiness for birth. Equine Vet J 16(4):259–263, 1984.

Santschi EM, LeBlanc MM: Fetal and placental conditions that cause high-risk pregnancy in mares. Comp Cont Ed Pract Vet 17(5)710–720, 1995.

Santschi EM, LeBlanc MM, Matthews PM, Slone DE: Evaluation of equine high-risk pregnancy. Comp Cont Ed Pract Vet 16(1):80–87, 1994.

Santschi EM, Slone DE: Maternal conditions that cause high-risk pregnancy in mares. Comp Cont Ed Pract Vet 16(11):1481–1488, 1994.

Vaala WE, Sertich PL: Management strategies for mares at risk for periparturient complications. Vet Clin North Am Equine Pract 10(1):237–265, 1994.

Parturition and Postpartum Complications

SALLY VIVRETTE
Raleigh, North Carolina

Gestation in horse mares lasts a little more than 11 months, approximately 340 days, with a range of 320 to 360 days. Gestation length does not vary significantly between breeds of horses and is not influenced significantly by the nutritional status of the mare, with the exception of marked undernutrition, which may prolong gestation. The length of gestation is typically longer for mares bred in the winter and spring than for mares bred in the summer and fall.

PREFOALING MANAGEMENT

During the last month of gestation, the mare's serum can be screened for antierythrocyte antibodies. If the antierythrocyte antibody titer is high, the foal may be at risk for developing neonatal isoerythrolysis and should be prevented from ingesting that mare's colostrum. Colostrum with sufficient immunoglobulin concentration from a different mare, also screened for antierythrocyte antibodies, can be administered to the foal to provide passive immunity.

The pregnant mare should be stabled for at least 4 weeks before parturition in the environment in which she will foal. The mare should be vaccinated every 2 months during pregnancy against rhinopneumonitis and, 1 month before anticipated foaling, she should receive a tetanus toxoid-encephalomyelitis-influenza booster vaccine. Pregnant mares should receive exercise daily, either through turn out in large pastures or through light riding, lunging, or hand walking. A regular hoof care program should be followed.

PREDICTION OF PARTURITION

It is not possible to accurately predict the delivery date of a foal based on gestation length alone. Instead, gestation length is considered along with observation of physical signs of impending parturition including udder development and relaxation of the sacrosciatic ligaments and vulva. About 1 month before foaling, the mare's udder increases in size, and in the final week of gestation the teats begin to enlarge and may develop a small bead of wax ("waxing up") at the teat openings. A small amount of milk can be expressed from the teats before foaling and evaluated for color and viscosity. About 1 week before foaling, the milk changes from watery serum-colored to thick honey-like. The physical signs of impending delivery may be subtle in maiden mares.

The mammary secretions before foaling can be evaluated for changes in electrolyte concentrations, which may indicate when the mare will foal (Fig. 1). During the week before parturition, there is usually a marked decrease in sodium and marked increase in potassium concentrations in the mammary secretions. In the 24 to 28 hours preceding parturition, the mammary secretion potassium concentrations are usually higher than the sodium concentrations. Calcium concentrations typically increase during the 24 hours preceding delivery of the foal. Commercial kits are available to evaluate changes in calcium concentrations as a predictor of parturition. These kits have variable accuracy, and test results should be interpreted in conjunction with changes in physical signs of impending parturition in the mare.

PARTURITION

The endocrine changes that initiate parturition are not as well understood in the mare as in other domestic animal species. For example, in domestic ruminants, there is a marked surge of fetal cortisol in the days preceding parturition. This increase in fetal cortisol induces an increase in estrogen and a decrease in progesterone production by the placenta that facilitates the initiation of parturition. An increase in fetal cortisol also occurs before parturition, but its role in equine parturition is unclear. In addition, the decrease in progesterone and increase in estrogen concentrations observed in ruminants is not observed in the horse.

Parturition usually occurs at night and is typically divided into three stages of labor. In stage 1 labor, the mare may appear uneasy, look at her flank, sweat, and pace. Mares in stage-1 labor may progress immediately into stage-2 labor, or may postpone delivery of the foal for hours or days. The beginning of stage-2 labor is marked by the "breaking of the water," which is rupture of the chorioallantois and release of allantoic fluid. The "breaking of the water" may occur with the mare standing or lying down. The abnormality of placenta previa is demonstrated by the velvety-red chorioallantois appearing at the vulvar lips without rupturing (Fig. 2). If this occurs, the membrane should be immediately opened and the foal delivered to decrease potential hypoxia. The majority of mares deliver their foals while recumbent, using both uterine and abdominal muscle contractions. The mare may rise to her feet and walk in a circle a few times during stage-2 labor, presumably in an effort to properly position the fetus. The majority of mares deliver their foals without assistance; therefore, people observing a mare foaling should remain quietly outside of the stall.

Stage-2 labor in the horse always proceeds in a progressive fashion after breaking of the water with the appearance

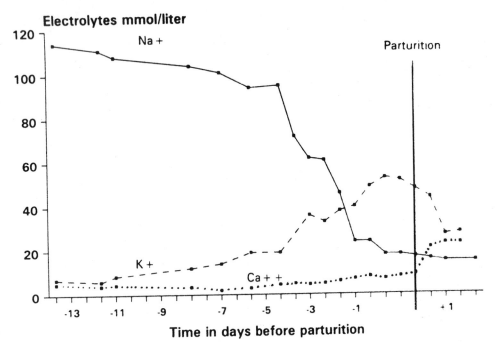

Figure 1. Electrolyte changes in prepartum mammary secretions. Sodium and potassium concentrations are expressed in mmol/L and calcium concentrations are expressed in mEq/L. (From LeBlanc MM: Induction of parturition. *In*: McKinnon AO, Voss JL (eds): Equine Reproduction. Philadelphia, Lea & Febiger, 1992, p 575. Adapted from Ousey JC, Dudan F, Rossdale PD: Preliminary studies of mammary secretions in the mare to assess foetal readiness for birth. Equine Vet J 16:259, 1984.)

of the shiny-white amnion, through which one, and then both of the foal's forelimbs can be seen, and then the foal's muzzle and head. Once the foal's shoulders are visible, the rest of the body is delivered quickly. Stage 2 labor usually lasts less than 20 minutes in most mares, but it may take up to 60 minutes.

The position, presentation, and posture of the fetus before and during parturition have been documented using radiography. The results of this study are represented diagrammatically in Figure 3. The near-term fetus lies in a ventral or ventral lateral position with the head oriented toward the mare's pelvis. Before stage-1 labor, the fetal movements are confined to the head, upper neck, and distal forelimbs. During stage-1 labor, the head and forelimbs extend and rotate into a dorsal position for delivery. In stage-2 labor, the fetal head, forelimbs, and shoulders enter the birth canal, while the hindquarters remain in a ventral position.

After the foal is delivered, the amnion should be gently removed from the foal's head if it is blocking the nostrils. The mare usually remains recumbent for 10 to 15 minutes after delivery of the foal, during which time the umbilical cord remains unbroken. It was previously believed that a substantial quantity of placental blood was passed to the foal during the immediate postpartum period. Later research has determined that blood flow in the intact umbilical vessels is bidirectional and, therefore, does not significantly change the foal's blood volume. In most cases, the umbilical cord is broken as the mare rises to her feet or through efforts of the foal struggling to stand.

In stage 3 labor, the placenta is expelled, usually within 1 hour after foaling. During this time, the mare may lie down and appears colicky. The placenta is typically expelled with the allantoic side of the chorioallantois outermost. The placenta should be examined for abnormalities and completeness during the postpartum evaluation of the mare and foal.

PROLONGED GESTATION

Gestation may be prolonged (>360 days) in association with both normal and pathologic conditions. Mares carrying twin fetuses may experience shortened, normal-length, or prolonged gestation. One of the most common causes of prolonged gestation in the United States is consumption of endophyte-infected fescue pasture during late gestation (see page 571).

INDUCTION OF PARTURITION

Indications for induction of parturition in the mare include the presence of a physical problem such as rupture

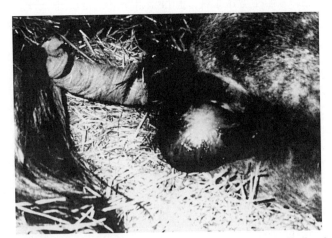

Figure 2. Placental previa in a mare during labor. The dark-colored chorioallantois and pale cervical star are visualized unruptured at the vulvar lips.

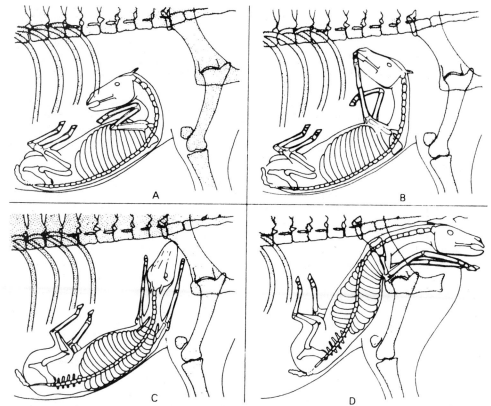

Figure 3. Diagrammatic representation of fetal movements during parturition in the mare. Maternal bones are lightly stippled. *(A)* Near-term fetus is lying in ventral or ventrolateral position with head and forelimbs flexed. *(B)* Before stage 1 labor fetal movements are chiefly confined to head, upper neck, and distal forelimbs. *(C)* During stage 1 labor the head and forelimbs extend and rotate into dorsal position for delivery. *(D)* At stage 2 labor the fetus engages in the birth canal although the distal vertebral column, and hindlimbs are still in ventral position. (From Jeffcott LB, Rossdale PD: A radiographic study of the foetus in late pregnancy and during foaling. J Reprod Fert 27[Suppl]:563, 1979.)

of the prepubic tendon, severe laminitis, and fractured pelvis or other orthopedic problems that limit the mare's ability to position and deliver the foal. It is not advisable to induce a mare to foal because she is undergoing a prolonged gestation that appears otherwise normal. It is not possible to accurately predict fetal maturity based on gestation length alone, and induction of parturition may result in delivery of a dysmature foal. If time and circumstances permit, changes in mammary secretion electrolyte concentrations may be monitored to allow for induction of parturition as close to spontaneous parturition as possible. Specifically, when mammary secretion potassium concentrations are higher than sodium concentrations, and calcium concentrations are above 40 mmol/dl, the likelihood of delivery of a mature foal after induced parturition is enhanced.

Parturition in horses is most effectively induced with the administration of oxytocin. The route of administration, intravenously or intramuscularly, and dose used may vary in reference texts. The horse is extremely sensitive to oxytocin around the time of parturition, and administration of an excessive dose of oxytocin may cause hyperstimulation and spasm of the uterus. Therefore, current recommendations are to use small doses of oxytocin (0.5–10 IU/500 kg IV) given as a bolus or diluted in isotonic fluids and administered through an indwelling intravenous catheter.

This dosage may be repeated at approximately 15-minute intervals. Alternately, a low dose of oxytocin (10–20 IU IM) may be administered to induce parturition. This dose may be repeated at approximately 30-minute intervals.

POSTPARTUM COMPLICATIONS

Prolapsed Uterus

Uterine prolapse is rare in the mare and can occur immediately following, or may occasionally occur days after, parturition. Complications of uterine prolapse include shock, hemorrhage, uterine lacerations, and ischemia of the uterus or abdominal viscera trapped in the uterus. Treatment includes control of straining through administration of sedatives and caudal epidural anesthesia, or by inducing general anesthesia (see page 713). If the intestines are incarcerated in the uterine prolapse, an exploratory celiotomy may be necessary to assess bowel viability and facilitate resection of devitalized bowel. Before replacement of the uterus, the mare's tail should be wrapped and the perineal area cleaned thoroughly. Placement of a catheter in the jugular vein facilitates administration of medications and institution of fluid therapy. The uterus should be supported in a clean sheet or on a tray held at the level of the pelvis to facilitate restoration of circulation to the uterus and viscera trapped in the prolapse. The uterus is cleaned with water and a nondetergent soap, and endometrial lacerations, if present, are sutured with absorbable suture. Complete uterine tears should be sutured using an absorbable suture in an inverting pattern. The uterus should then be gently returned to its normal position, taking special care to prevent perforation or tearing. Administration of oxytocin (10–20 IU IV or IM or preferably divided into multiple sites in the uterine wall), results in uterine contractions and reduction of uterine size, which facilitates repositioning. The uterus is retropulsed, beginning with the uterine body and working gradually, replacing the tip of the horns last. Correct positioning of the uterus and ovaries is important to prevent the prolapse from recurring. This can be achieved by gently inserting a bottle into the uterus and stretching the horns to fully evert them. Following replacement of the uterus, treatment with intravenous isotonic fluids as needed for dehydration and shock should be continued. Flunixin meglumine (0.25 mg/kg IV q.i.d. to 1.1 mg/kg IV b.i.d.) should be administered along with broad-spectrum antibiotics. Oxytocin (10–20 IU IV or IM) can be given to facilitate uterine contraction and involution. Adequacy of tetanus immunization should be ensured. The mare should be closely monitored for secondary complications such as metritis and laminitis.

Invagination of the Uterine Horn

Following parturition, a uterine horn may invaginate, resulting in signs of colic after foaling. The presence of a uterine horn invagination can be determined by palpation per rectum where a short, blunted uterine horn and tense mesovarium is identified. Invagination of a uterine horn may be associated with placental retention. Care should be exercised to avoid traction on the placenta because traction may worsen the uterine invagination. When possible, the placenta should be gently separated from the uterus (see page 560). The invaginated uterine horn can then be replaced in its normal position. This is facilitated by the infusion of 4 to 8 L of warm isotonic sodium chloride solution. Medical treatment for uterine horn invagination is similar to that previously described for uterine prolapse.

Uterine Hemorrhage

During pregnancy and parturition, the utero-ovarian, middle uterine, or external iliac arteries may rupture, resulting in moderate to severe blood loss. Following vessel rupture, the mare may exhibit signs of colic and clinical signs attributable to blood loss including tachycardia, sweating, and pale mucous membranes. When the utero-ovarian or middle uterine artery ruptures, hemorrhage may occur directly into the abdominal cavity or may be contained within the broad ligament. Hemorrhage of a uterine artery into the abdominal cavity or broad ligament may result in death of the mare immediately after foaling. A hematoma within the broad ligament may subsequently rupture into the abdominal cavity, resulting in clinical signs of hemorrhage and possibly death days to weeks following foaling. Fatal uterine artery rupture associated with hemorrhage into the abdominal cavity is seen most often in mares older than 18.5 years. Nonfatal hemorrhage into the broad ligament is more common in younger mares, those with an

average age of 11.5 years. Vessel rupture is most common on the right side, possibly related to the presence of the cecum causing displacement of the uterus to the left, thus putting increased tension on the right uterine artery. An association between serum copper levels, which is important for vessel elasticity, and uterine vessel rupture has also been identified. Mares with fatal uterine artery rupture have reduced serum copper levels compared with younger mares or unaffected older mares. Age-related degeneration of the uterine arteries has also been proposed as a predisposing cause of rupture.

Uterine artery rupture can be diagnosed based on clinical signs of blood loss and mild to severe colic, palpation and ultrasonographic presence of a hyperechoic mass in the broad ligament per rectum, or identification of free blood in the abdomen upon abdominocentesis. A significant decrease in the peripheral blood packed cell volume (PCV) may not be observed for several hours following vessel rupture. Treatment of severe hemorrhage following uterine vessel rupture is often ineffective. Circulating blood volume expansion, through blood transfusion or isotonic intravenous fluid administration, may be instituted following identification of a uterine vessel rupture. In some cases, treatment may include the administration of tranquilizers to keep the mare quiet and analgesics, such as butorphanol (0.01–0.04 mg/kg IM). The effectiveness of less conventional therapy, including the intravenous use of hypertonic saline or naloxone, has not been evaluated.

Uterine Rupture

Uterine rupture may occur following dystocia, fetal malpresentation, or uterine torsion, or after iatrogenic damage following fetotomy or postpartum uterine lavage. Uterine rupture may also occur following an apparently normal uncomplicated delivery. Complications of uterine rupture include herniation of abdominal contents through the uterine rent, peritonitis, and hemorrhage. Physical examination findings include colic, hemorrhage from the vulva, and presence of blood or purulent material on abdominocentesis. Lacerations located in the uterine body or base of the horns can be palpated per vagina. Treatment for uterine rupture includes repair during celiotomy or following prolapse of the uterus. The uterus is repaired with absorbable suture. Care should be taken to avoid incorporation of the placenta into the uterine closure. Postoperatively, oxytocin should be administered to enhance involution of the uterus. Uterine rupture may also be managed conservatively in cases when the tear does not gape and the abdominal contents do not herniate. Management of these mares includes cross-tying and the administration of oxytocin (10 IU q.i.d.), broad-spectrum systemic antibiotics, and nonsteroidal anti-inflammatory drugs. Peritoneal lavage may be employed if necessary. Uterine lavage should be avoided in cases of uterine rupture.

Perineal Laceration and Rectovaginal Lacerations

Lacerations of the vagina, rectum, and perineum occur most commonly in primiparous mares. First-degree perineal lacerations, which involve only the skin and perineal mucosa at the dorsal commissure of the vulva, occur during parturition as a result of stretching as the foal's poll and shoulders pass through the vulva. These lacerations can be repaired at the time of occurrence by simple suturing or performing a Caslick vulvoplasty. Second-degree lacerations occur when the foal's feet pass through the vestibulovaginal junction and lacerate the dorsal vestibular mucosa and the perineal body. During parturition, the foal's forelimb may penetrate through the dorsal vaginal wall and ventral rectal wall. If the foal retracts the limb into the birth canal before delivery progresses, a rectovaginal fistula remains. If the limb of the foal is not retracted and delivery progresses, a third-degree perineal laceration ensues, which includes laceration of all the tissues of the ventral rectum, dorsal vagina, perineal body, and anal sphincter. Second- and third-degree perineal lacerations and rectovaginal fistulas are usually repaired by elective surgery 4 to 8 weeks following injury (see *Current Therapy in Equine Medicine 2*, page 550).

COLIC

Differential diagnosis for colic in the postpartum mare includes a wide variety of causes that result from gastrointestinal or uterine sources. Colic may also be seen in mares during stage-3 labor during expulsion of the placenta. The differential diagnosis for colic in the postpartum mare is shown in Table 1.

Cecal and Large Colon Rupture, and Colon Volvulus

Increased intra-abdominal pressure during parturition may predispose mares to cecal rupture. Extension of the fetal forelimbs during stage-1 labor and possible kicking by the fetal hindlimbs may allow the hind hooves of the fetus to exert sufficient focal pressure against the walls of the large bowel to cause rupture. Pre-existing impaction or large amounts of ingesta may be involved with cecal rupture at the time of parturition, but rupture without evidence of distension has also been observed. Crepitus and gritty peritoneal or serosal surfaces may be felt per rectum in affected horses. Abdominocentesis is useful in obtaining a diagnosis of bowel rupture.

Mares in the first 100 postpartum days appear to have a higher incidence of colon volvulus. The cause of this has not been determined, and management practices to minimize colon volvulus occurrence have not been identified.

Bowel Prolapse

Mares may prolapse bowel through a uterine tear during or immediately following delivery of the foal. In cases in which there is marked contamination of the bowel, treatment options are very limited. In most cases, these mares are euthanized.

Tearing of the Mesocolon

Contusions of the small intestine or small colon, or the attaching mesentery of these structures, can occur without compromising the blood supply. Clinical signs of intestinal

TABLE 1. DIFFERENTIAL DIAGNOSIS FOR COLIC IN THE POSTPARTUM MARE

Placental expulsion and uterine involution	Rupture of the mesocolon—small colon necrosis
Cecal or colonic rupture	Diaphragmatic rupture
Colon torsion	Uterine horn necrosis
Internal hemorrhage	Uterine rupture
Ruptured urinary bladder	Retained placenta

contusion include mild colic. More severe trauma to the mesentery may result in mesenteric rupture. If the blood supply to the adjacent bowel is not disrupted, the mesenteric defect may close or heal, leaving an opening through which intestinal incarceration or strangulation may occur.

Mesenteric tears involving the vascular arcade of the small colon result in segmental ischemic necrosis of the bowel. Peritonitis and bowel rupture may occur if the condition remains untreated. Ischemic necrosis may also occur in cases of rectal prolapse when more than 30 cm of the rectum and small colon are affected.

Clinical signs of small colon necrosis are usually observed within 24 hours after foaling. Initially it may be difficult to differentiate pain of intestinal disease from pain associated with uterine contracture. Signs of small colon problems become more apparent with the development of small colon impaction and onset of intestinal tympany. An important sign in this problem is failure to pass feces after foaling. Findings on palpation per rectum range from no palpable abnormalities to impaction of the small colon. Abdominocentesis is useful in obtaining a diagnosis of small colon necrosis. Exploratory surgery may be indicated; the outcome depends on the time from onset of signs to surgery.

Supplemental Readings

Asbury AC: Care of the mare after foaling. *In* McKinnon AO, Voss JL (eds): Equine Reproduction. Philadelphia, Lea & Febiger, 1992, pp 976–980.

Fisher AT, Phillips TN: Surgical repair of a ruptured uterus in five mares. Equine Vet J 18:153–155, 1986.

Hooper RN, Blanchard TD, Taylor TS, Schumacher J, Varner DD: Identifying and treating uterine prolapse and invagination of the uterine horn. Vet Med 88(1):60–65, 1993.

Jeffcott LB, Rossdale PD: A radiographic study of the fetus in late pregnancy and during foaling. J Reprod Fertil 27[Suppl]:563–569, 1979.

LeBlanc MM: Induction of parturition. *In* McKinnon AO, Voss JL (eds): Equine Reproduction. Philadelphia, Lea & Febiger, 1992, pp 574–577.

Lofstedt RM: Miscellaneous diseases of pregnancy and parturition. *In* McKinnon AO, Voss JL (eds): Equine Reproduction. Philadelphia, Lea & Febiger, 1992, pp 596–603.

Ousey JC, Dudan F, Rossdale PD: Preliminary studies of mammary secretions in the mare to assess foetal readiness for birth. Equine Vet J 16:259–263, 1984.

Rossdale PD, Ricketts SW: Equine Stud Farm Medicine, ed 2. Philadelphia, Lea & Febiger, 1980.

Vivrette SL: The endocrinology of parturition in the mare. Vet Clin North Am Equine Pract 10(1):1–17, 1994.

Zent WW: Postpartum complications. *In* Robinson NE (ed): Current Therapy in Equine Medicine, ed 2. Philadelphia, WB Saunders, 1987, p 544.

Dystocia*

MELVYN L. FAHNING
St. Paul, Minnesota

MICHAEL S. SPENSLEY
Mendota Heights, Minnesota

MATS H. T. TROEDSSON
St. Paul, Minnesota

Dystocia is defined as difficult parturition, and it may be a sign of either maternal or fetal conditions that impede fetal passage through the birth canal. Dystocia in mares is more likely attributable to fetal causes such as malpresentation, malposition, and malposture than to maternal conditions. Considering the adverse effect that dystocia can have on the dam and the neonate, Rice (1994) defined dystocia as any birth that reduces neonatal viability, causes maternal injury, or requires assistance. The incidence of dystocia overall and incidence of different types of dystocia vary among the breeds. The incidence of dystocia among Thoroughbred mares is 4% but is higher in most draft horse breeds and in some pony breeds. Dystocia represents an emergency situation that commands prompt resolution to afford the optimal prognosis for mare and fetus. Manipulation, traction, fetotomy, and cesarean section are the obstetric procedures available for management of dystocia. The economics of practice often play a significant role in determining which course to pursue in resolving dystocia. The lives of the mare and the fetus may be at risk. Although the objective should be the survival of both, unless otherwise advised by the owner and conditions are not prohibitive, the well-being of the mare and her reproductive potential should have priority over the fetus.

Although parturition has been divided into three distinct stages for descriptive purposes, the stages overlap clinically, and normal parturition is observed as a continuous process. During the first stage of parturition the fetus plays an active role, along with myometrial contractions, in assuming correct extremity posture as it positions itself for delivery through the birth canal. The second stage of parturition commences with rupture of the allantochorion and culminates in delivery of the fetus. Myometrial contractions continue during third-stage parturition, which ends with the expulsion of the placenta. In the mare, parturition is a forceful explosive act. Time between rupture of the allantochorionic membrane and delivery of the fetus is normally about 20 minutes. Separation of the fetal membranes from the endometrium may occur within 1 to 2 hours after the second stage of parturition commences; therefore, the retained fetus must be delivered quickly or it will asphyxiate. Primiparous dams generally require longer to expel the fetus than do multiparous dams. Regardless, if the first stage of parturition is prolonged or

delivery of the fetus does not occur within 20 to 30 minutes of allantochorionic membrane rupture, dystocia is possible. The mare should be examined and preparations made to assist the delivery.

APPROACH TO DIAGNOSIS

Pertinent reproductive history should be obtained, including the mare's age, her previous breeding history, and the outcomes of previous pregnancies (i.e., abortion, normal parturition, dystocia). Her present gestational status should be determined; has parturition commenced at term or is hers a preterm or post-term delivery? Her udder should be examined to determine stage of development. Information regarding the progress of the current parturition should be obtained. Time since rupture of the allantochorionic membrane, the duration and intensity of labor, whether any fetal membranes or parts have appeared at the vulva, and previous attempts to assist in delivery should be noted. If the mare is recumbent, one should determine if she has attempted to or been able to rise. Although a complete examination of the mare is optimal, such an examination may best be postponed until after the delivery of the fetus. However, in obtaining the mare's reproductive history, questions regarding her current physical condition should be included. Such predisposing factors as recent weight loss, systemic disease, and trauma should be considered. She should be assessed for signs of hemorrhage, dehydration, and shock.

The basic obstetric equipment required to aid in mare dystocia is similar to that used in other large animals. It is important to have the equipment organized so that it is readily accessible when the obstetric case is presented. Instruments that are easy to handle and convenient to sterilize are best. The basic equipment is shown and identified in Figure 1. Obstetric chains and handles are essential instruments. Chains or ropes can be used as snares on the extremities and can serve as an extension of the obstetrician's second arm outside the mare. Alternatively, an assistant can provide traction while the arm in the vagina/uterus can repel and mutate the affected extremity. One should never overlook the importance of the clean, gentle hands and arms of the clinician in obstetric procedures.

*Portions of this chapter are adapted from Spensley MS: Dystocia. In Smith BP (ed): Large Animal Internal Medicine, ed 2. St. Louis, C.V. Mosby, (with permission).

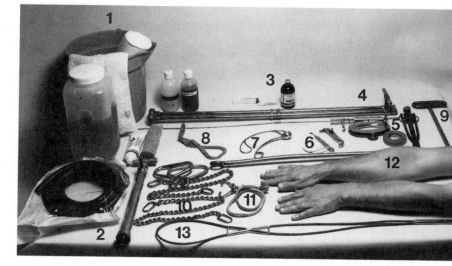

Figure 1. Obstetric supplies and equipment. (1) Supplies for cleansing perineal area of mare and gauze for tail wrap; (2) nasogastric tube and pump for delivery of lubricant into the uterus; (3) lidocaine and syringes to administer epidural analgesia; (4) Thygesen's model fetotome; (5) obstetric saw wire, wire cutter, and wire handles; (6) fetotomy knives; (7) obstetric wire handles; (8) Krey hook; (9) leverage bar for detorsion rod; (10) obstetric chains; (11) obstetric rope with blunt eye hooks attached; (12) clean, gentle hands and arms of the obstetrician; (13) head snare.

PHYSICAL AND CHEMICAL RESTRAINTS

Dystocia may be accompanied by colic and forceful straining. The mare may attempt to lie down and stand repeatedly. This is a characteristic of mares with dystocia that is caused by fetopelvic disproportion, malposture, or fetal impaction. Alternatively, the dam may stand quietly with minimal or no straining, as in cases of uterine inertia, uterine rupture, or exhaustion associated with prolonged dystocia of any cause. Whatever the presentation of the mare, the attending veterinarian must be prepared for unexpected behavior when attempting to perform obstetric examination and procedures. The mare, fetus, attendants, and veterinarians must be protected from injury. The mare should be placed in open-ended stocks with movable sides or in a straw-bedded box stall. During obstetric examination and manipulation, mares may attempt to get up and lie down or they may suddenly collapse. Such sudden movements may cause injury to the mare and veterinarian if rigid, closed-end stocks are used. Minimal physical restraint should be used; however, restraint should be sufficient to permit completion of obstetric examination and procedures with efficiency and safety. Adequate physical restraint may be achieved with a twitch or lip chain. Sidelines and hobbles must be used with care. Chemical sedation should be used with discretion to prevent cardiovascular and respiratory compromise of the mare and fetus. Little is known about the pharmacokinetics of drugs for the gravid mare, her uterus, or fetus. Accordingly, it must be assumed that sedative and anesthetic drugs will depress neonatal and fetal functions at least as much as those of the mare. The effects on myometrial activity of drugs administered to mares experiencing dystocia also must be considered.

While equine practitioners are familiar with the sedative properties of acepromazine,° detomidine,† and xylazine,‡ none of these is approved for use in the pregnant mare.

°*Promaz, Fort Dodge Laboratories, Fort Dodge, IA*
†*Dormosedan, Pfizer Animal Health Group, West Chester, PA*
‡*Rompun Injectable, Bayer, Animal Health Products, Shawnee Mission, KS*

Accordingly, they must be used with caution in the management of dystocia. Acepromazine has little effect on the fetus and is generally considered safe for use in the pregnant mare; however, myometrial activity was reported to decrease following administration of acepromazine to normally cycling mares. Detomidine causes significant fetal cardiovascular compromise and likely diminished placental perfusion. The fetal depressant effects of xylazine are of shorter duration than are those of detomidine. Detomidine and xylazine cause some mares to become hypersensitive over their hindquarters despite appearing to be well sedated. Myometrial activity increases after administration of detomidine or xylazine to mares. Sedative dosages are presented in Table 1.

Practitioners and researchers have determined that several drugs administered concomitantly are safe and effective for use in management of dystocia in the mare. The opioid analgesics morphine° and butorphanol† have been

°*Morphine sulfate injection USP, Elkins-Sinn, Philadelphia, PA*
†*Torbugesic Veterinary Injection, Fort Dodge Laboratories, Fort Dodge, IA*

TABLE 1.   SEDATIVES USED IN THE MANAGEMENT OF DYSTOCIA

DRUG	INTRAVENOUS DOSE	COMMENTS
Acepromazine	0.04–0.06 mg/kg (4–6 mg/100 kg)	Minimal effect on foal
Xylazine	0.3–0.6 mg/kg 0.0625 mg/kg for miniature horses	Beware of hypersensitivity over hindquarters Decreased fetal heart rate (0.5 mg/kg)
Detomidine HCl	0.01–0.02 mg/kg	Beware of hypersensitivity over hindquarters Decreased fetal heart rate Decreased aortic peak velocity flow Placental perfusion probably diminished

From LeBlanc MM, Norman WM: Sedatives and anesthesia of the mare during obstetric manipulation. Proc 38th Annu Conv Am Assoc Equine Pract, 1992, p 619

TABLE 2. SEDATIVES AND ANALGESICS CONCOMITANTLY USED IN THE MANAGEMENT OF DYSTOCIA

DRUG	INTRAVENOUS DOSE (mg/kg)	COMMENTS
Acepromazine	0.02–0.04	
Xylazine	0.2–0.4	
Xylazine	0.25–0.5	Hindlimb weakness, ataxia may
Butorphanol	0.01–0.02	occur; mares may "walk" unless restrained
Xylazine	0.25–0.5	Mares "plant" feet and
Morphine	0.25–0.75	abdominal press is obliterated
Acepromazine	0.04	Acepromazine enhances sedative
Xylazine	0.25	properties of xylazine
Butorphanol	0.01–0.02	
Acepromazine	0.04	Acepromazine enhances sedative
Xylazine	0.25	properties of xylazine
Morphine	0.25–0.75	

Data from LeBlanc MM, Norman WM: Sedatives and anesthesia of the mare during obstetric manipulation. Proc 38th Annu Conv Am Assoc Equine Pract, 1992, p 619

TABLE 3. EPIDURAL ANESTHESIA USED IN THE MANAGEMENT OF DYSTOCIA

DRUG	DOSE	COMMENTS
Lidocaine 2%	1.0–1.25 ml/100 kg	May cause hindlimb weakness and ataxia
Xylazine 10%	0.17 mg/kg; 100 mg/450 kg	Dilute to 10 ml in physiologic saline Preferred for shipment of mare
Xylazine 10%	0.17 mg/kg; 1 ml/454 kg	Rapid onset and
Lidocaine 2%	0.22 mg/kg; 5 ml/454 kg	prolonged duration of analgesia

In part data from LeBlanc MM, Norman WM: Sedatives and anesthesia of the mare during obstetric manipulation. Proc 38th Annu Conv Am Assoc Equine Pract, 1992, p 619

reliably used in conjunction with sedatives. Dosages for concomitantly used drugs are presented in Table 2. Potential complications associated with the use of opioids in horses include excitement, gastrointestinal stasis, and constipation. Simultaneous administration of a sedative reduces the incidence of excitement. Mineral oil should be administered, after resolution of the dystocia, whenever morphine or another opioid is used.

Caudal epidural anesthesia is often an excellent means of facilitating examination and resolution of dystocia and at the same time minimizing trauma to the mare, fetus, and operator. Epidural administration of lidocaine* has been reliably used for perineal anesthesia. After epidural administration of lidocaine, onset of analgesia occurs in several minutes and persists for approximately 2.5 hours. Lidocaine epidural anesthesia may cause hindlimb weakness and ataxia. Safe and effective analgesia has also been induced by epidural administration of xylazine. Although onset of analgesia occurs about 0.5 hours after epidural administration of xylazine, perineal analgesia persists for 3 to 5 hours. Perineal analgesia was recently evaluated after epidural administration of a combination of lidocaine and xylazine. Onset of analgesia occurred, similar to lidocaine alone, in minutes; however, duration of caudal epidural analgesia, approximately 5.5 hours, was significantly longer than after either lidocaine or xylazine alone. Although vaginal sensitivity and the Ferguson's reflex both are reduced by epidural anesthesia, myometrial contractions and abdominal press are not totally eliminated. Time to onset, duration of analgesia, and potential side effects should be considered when deciding whether to manage dystocia on site or transport the mare to a referral hospital. Dosages of epidural anesthetics are presented in Table 3.

Examination of the mare and manipulation of the fetus can be greatly facilitated by anesthetizing the mare and elevating her hindquarters, enabling the fetus and viscera

*Lidocaine injection, Vedco, St. Joseph, MO

to recede cranially into the mare's abdominal cavity, thereby allowing more room for the operator. Intravenous xylazine, followed approximately 5 minutes later with intravenous ketamine,* provides 10 to 15 minutes of general anesthesia (see page 713). Anesthesia can be prolonged by 10 to 20 minutes by the administration of guaifenesin† after xylazine-ketamine induction. Neither xylazine-ketamine nor the addition of guaifenesin to the regimen appears to compromise mare or fetal respiration. Minimal concentrations of inhalation anesthetics, halothane‡ or isoflurane,§ can be added to the regimen to maintain anesthesia for prolonged procedures (e.g., mutation and traction, cesarean section, fetotomy) in the hospital setting when appropriate assistance is available to monitor the mare and foal. The recumbent mare must be carefully monitored to prevent cardiovascular and respiratory compromise when intravenous and/or inhalation anesthesia is employed. Dosages for general anesthetic agents are presented in Table 4.

*Ketaset, Fort Dodge Laboratories, Fort Dodge, IA
†Guilaxin, Fort Dodge Laboratories, Fort Dodge, IA
‡Halothane USP, Fort Dodge Laboratories, Fort Dodge, IA
§Isoflo, Solvay Animal Health, Inc., Mendota Heights, MN

TABLE 4. GENERAL ANESTHESIA USED IN THE MANAGEMENT OF DYSTOCIA

DRUG	DOSE	COMMENTS
Xylazine	1.1 mg/kg	Premedication
Ketamine	2.2 mg/kg	Induction; administration after maximal effect of xylazine is observed
Guaifenesin	1 L of a solution of 5% guaifenesin and 5% dextrose 100 mg/kg when administered with thiamylal sodium	To extend xylazine and ketamine combination 10–20 minutes
Halothane and isoflurane		Profound skeletal muscle and myometrial relaxation

In part data from LeBlanc MM, Norman WM: Sedatives and anesthesia of the mare during manipulation. Proc 38th Annu Conv Am Assoc Equine Pract, 1992, p 619

Tocolysis, the inhibition of labor, has been induced by the β-adrenergic compounds isoxsuprine* (200–300 mg IM) and clenbuterol† (200–300 μg IM or IV). Isoxsuprine and clenbuterol have been used for the treatment of premature labor in human obstetrics and to delay parturition and as an aid in the management of dystocia in veterinary obstetrics. The drugs are available in many countries; however, they are not licensed for veterinary use in the United States.

OBSTETRIC EXAMINATION AND MANIPULATIONS

After the tail has been wrapped, the perineal area should be thoroughly and gently washed and rinsed. Great care must be taken during the examination of the mare's genitalia and the fetus. In addition to the viability of fetus and mare, the mare's future reproductive potential is at risk and must be preserved. The vulva, vestibule, vagina, and cervix should be carefully examined. Vaginal examination should reveal the presentation, position, and posture of the foal and allow the clinician to assess the relative size of the foal's and the mare's pelvis. Fetal oversize is relatively rare in the mare compared with other species. Because of the length of the extremities in the foal, mutation is more difficult than in the cow and requires extensive repulsion to provide adequate room for manipulation. Generous application of lubricants is required in all cases of equine obstetrics. Several liters of lubricants should be infused into the uterus by the use of a nasogastric tube. Lubricating preparations consisting of methylcellulose are superior to mineral oil or soaps. Handling of some of the more common postural abnormalities will be discussed.

Anterior Presentation

Carpal Flexion

One or both limbs may be involved in this condition. With unilateral involvement, one foot may be protruding from the vulva while the flexed carpus is found at the pelvic inlet. If the case is of short duration, the first step is repulsion of the fetus cranially to provide room for extension of the limb. The foot of the affected limb is grasped and while the carpus is pushed dorsally, the foot is moved caudally and up over the brim of the pelvis to the extended position. Care should always be taken to cup the hand over the hoof to protect the uterine wall from trauma. Rotating the carpus laterally facilitates repositioning of the limb. A chain snare may be positioned around the affected limb below the fetlock so that an assistant can apply traction while the obstetrician guides the foot up over the brim of the pelvis. If the carpus is impacted into the pelvis and repulsion is not successful, depending on the viability of the fetus, a fetotomy or cesarean section is the best alternative.

Shoulder Flexion

As with carpal flexion, this condition may be unilateral or bilateral. Externally the clinician observes either one limb and the head protruding or only the head being

presented. Some repulsion is necessary to provide room to allow passage of the obstetrician's arm into the birth canal. Total repulsion of the fetus is necessary to proceed with manipulation. If one can grasp the humerus and bring the distal end caudally, the shoulder flexion is converted to a carpal flexion and one proceeds to correct that as previously described. An obstetric chain can be used as a snare around the distal end of the humerus with traction applied by an assistant to facilitate conversion of the shoulder flexion to carpal flexion. The chain snare is then moved below the fetlock to provide traction to bring the limb into extended position with previously described precautions to protect the uterus. In the event of bilateral shoulder flexion in which the swollen head of a dead foal is protruding through the vulva, it may be impossible to repel the head back into the birth canal. A single fetotomy cut removing the head and as much of the neck as possible should allow mutation of the shoulder flexion into extended position. In cases when extension of the limb in shoulder flexion is not possible and the foal is dead, the limb can be removed at the shoulder by means of a single fetotomy cut. A better option may be to remove the shoulder, head, and neck with a single fetotomy cut.

Lateral Deviation of the Head and Neck

This can be one of the more difficult malpostures to correct because of the length of the foal's neck and head, which makes it very difficult to reach the muzzle of the foal for manipulation. A chain snare positioned around the neck just caudal to the head may provide a point of traction to bring the head sufficiently caudal to grasp it for mutation. A rope snare around the lower mandible is often helpful to achieve this mutation, but caution must be used putting traction on the mandible because of its susceptibility to fracture. If this fails, a cesarean section or a fetotomy cut to remove the head and neck are the next options, depending on the viability of the foal. Those fetuses with a wry or ankylosed neck require fetotomy. Manipulations associated with lateral deviation of the head and neck are illustrated in Fig. 2A to D.

Ventral Deviation of the Head

This malposture is not uncommon in the mare and occurs in varying degrees of severity ranging from only the nose below the brim of the pelvis to a complete nape posture. In mild cases a loop of obstetric chain or rope may be placed over the lower mandible with gentle traction applied to the chain while the foal's forehead is repelled, allowing the muzzle to come up over the brim of the pelvis. Extreme caution must be used in applying traction to the mandible to avoid causing a fracture. With more complete displacement of the head ventrally between the forelimbs, repulsion of the entire fetus should be attempted to reposition the head and neck. The duration of the dystocia and degree of contraction of the uterus around the fetus determine the success of this manipulation. Cesarean section or fetotomy are the alternatives, depending on the viability of the foal.

Foot-nape Posture

This malposture is characterized by one or both forelimbs being displaced so they lie above the extended head.

---

*Duphaspasmin, Solvay Duphar B.V., Weesp, The Netherlands
†Ventipulmin, Boehringer Ingelheim Animal Health, St. Joseph, MO

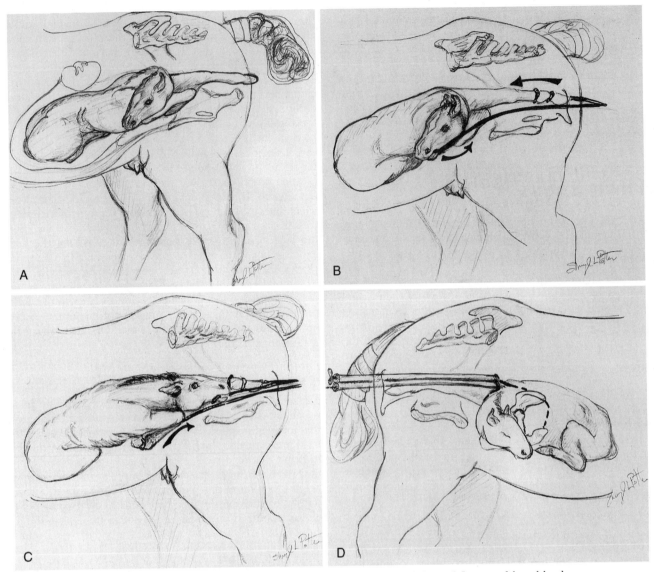

Figure 2. (A) Anterior presentation, dorsal sacral position with unilateral carpal flexion and lateral head deviation. (B) Diagnosis as in A. Correction of lateral head deviation with a snare placed around the lower mandible and repulsion of the fetus anteriorly. (C) Diagnosis as in A. Correction of carpal flexion with the aid of a chain or rope snare around the fetlock. (D) Anterior presentation, dorsal sacral position, bilateral carpal flexion and lateral head deviation. Placement of fetotome and obstetric wire to remove one forelimb and the head and neck.

The slender head of the foal and long forelimbs make this unique posture possible. The muzzle of the foal should be repelled cranially and dorsally while the foot is pushed ventrally and laterally. If bilateral, the other forelimb should be repositioned similarly so the head rests on the forelimbs. The dorsal vaginal wall should be carefully examined for trauma, which can occur from one or both of the feet of the foal.

Dog-sitting Position

This position is easily diagnosed by vaginal examination and is characterized by the head and all four limbs being presented in the pelvic inlet. Traction applied to the forelimbs in this position results in greater impaction. An attempt can be made to repel the hindlimbs out of the pelvic inlet to deliver the foal in anterior presentation. Frequently

this fails, and it is necessary to place traction on the rear limbs while repelling the head and forelimbs to convert the foal to a posterior presentation. The foal then is in a ventral-sacral position and needs to be rotated to a dorsal-sacral position for delivery. Generous amounts of lubricant are necessary for these manipulations. A cesarean section should also be considered if manipulation is difficult.

Transverse Ventral Presentation

This condition is characterized by the fetus lying on its side with the head and two to four limbs extending into the pelvic canal. This presentation is frequently complicated by wry neck. Mutation of these foals is often difficult unless the foal is small and the birth canal and uterus are large and relaxed. If mutation is attempted one should convert the foal's position to a posterior presentation by traction

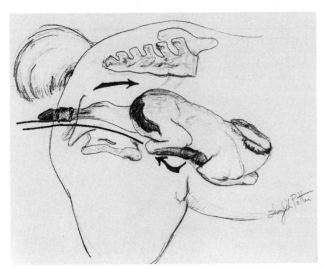

Figure 3. Posterior presentation, dorsal sacral position with unilateral hock flexion. Correction with the aid of a snare around the fetlock and repulsion of the fetus anteriorly.

on the rear limbs and repelling the forelimbs. Adequate lubrication is essential for these manipulations. A cesarean section may be the method of choice to avoid trauma to the mare.

Posterior Presentation

The incidence of posterior presentation in the mare is relatively low, but the incidence of foal mortality is high. Foals in posterior presentation require prompt attention and delivery to prevent asphyxiation from pressure on or premature breaking of the umbilical cord.

Hock Flexion

Hock flexion can occur unilaterally or bilaterally. To bring the limbs into extension, repulsion and traction are

employed. Manual mutation should be attempted by grasping the foot and bringing it medially and dorsally while repelling the hock dorsally and laterally to provide room to bring the hoof over the brim of the pelvis. A snare made with an obstetric chain can be placed around the affected leg below the fetlock, and an assistant can apply traction while the obstetrician guides the foot into extension (Fig. 3).

Hip Flexion

If the foal has bilateral hip flexion, the condition is described as a "breech presentation." Because of the length of the foal's extremities and the forceful contraction of the mare, this can be an extremely difficult malposture to correct. One must consider the possibility of dorsal rupture of the uterus during manipulation. The goal of treatment is to initially convert the hip flexion to a hock flexion and then to full extension of the hindlimbs. It is necessary to repel the foal's perineum cranially and dorsally to bring the flexed limbs within reach to grasp the leg near the hock and, applying traction, to bring the leg into hock flexion. A chain snare around the affected limb at the level of the hock may be helpful to allow an assistant to apply traction while the obstetrician repels the posterior end of the foal. Once the limb is in hock flexion, procedures previously described are applied to convert the limb to full extension.

In some cases it may be impossible to extend the flexed limb. If the foal is dead, removal of one of the flexed limbs by fetotomy may facilitate delivery (Fig. 4A). The obstetric wire is passed from above around one of the flexed limbs and the wire introducer picked up below the limb and brought to the outside, and the fetotome is then threaded. The head of the fetotome should be placed firmly in the perineum. This should ensure that the femur is sectioned through the articular head. This cut maximizes reduction of the foal and minimizes leaving a sharp bony projection that could traumatize the birth canal. Once the detached limb is removed, it may be possible to extend the remaining

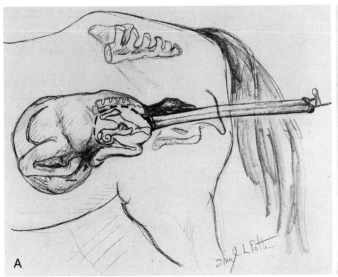

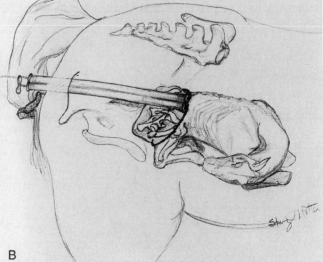

Figure 4. (A) Posterior presentation, dorsal sacral position with bilateral hip flexion (breech position). Illustrates placement of fetotome and obstetric wire for removal of one flexed rear limb. (B) Diagnosis as in A. Illustrates placement of fetotome and obstetric wire to remove entire rump, as described in the text.

TABLE 5. COMPLICATIONS ASSOCIATED WITH DYSTOCIA

COMPLICATION	PREVENTION	TREATMENT	COMMENTS
Retained placenta	When retained placenta is known or suspected, twice-daily uterine lavages; nonsteroidal anti-inflammatory drugs, antimicrobials	See Retained Fetal Membranes, page 560	Probability increases after dystocia
Invagination of uterine horn		Replace tip of uterine horn; lavage uterus	Probability increases after dystocia, retained placenta
Acute metritis	Resolve dystocia under aseptic conditions	Treat retained placenta	
	Examine the placenta for integrity	Uterine lavages twice daily; eventual removal of retained placenta or piece thereof	
		Systemic and uterine antibiotics	
		Nonsteroidal anti-inflammatory drugs	
		Mineral oil p.o.	
		Supportive care of feet	
Endotoxemia	As above, prevention is achieved through removal of retained placenta and uterine lavages	In addition to therapies for retained placenta and metritis, consider fluids, antiendotoxin antiserum, glucocorticoids, anticoagulants and reactive oxygen scavengers	
Laminitis	Correct retained placenta, metritis, and/or endotoxemia	Retained placenta, metritis, and endometritis therapies as indicated	
		Vasodilators	
		DMSO	
		Protective bedding; pad feet	
		See Laminitis, page 737	
Chronic endometritis	Uterine lavages for several days after dystocia	Uterine lavages; intrauterine and systemic antimicrobial therapy	
	Systemic antibiotics and oxytocin following dystocia		
Uterine prolapse	Examine and correct invagination of a uterine horn following dystocia	Sedate, administer epidural anesthesia, remove placenta if easily accomplished and replace uterus	
		Lavage uterus	
		Systemic antibiotics and nonsteroidal anti-inflammatory drugs	
		Observe for metritis, toxemia, laminitis	
Uterine artery rupture	Cautious use of fluid distension of chorioallantoic space (Burn's technique) in predisposed mares (i.e., multiparous mares >11 years old)	If necessary, administer mild sedation, analgesia	Survival chances diminish when broad ligament ruptures, allowing hemorrhage into peritoneal cavity
		Maintain quiet environment (i.e., darkened stall)	Transport of mare, surgery, and heroic strategies usually contraindicated
		Single dose of naloxone 80 mg IV	
Delayed uterine involution	Vigorous uterine and systemic therapies for retained placenta	Uterine lavages during postparturient period and subsequent estrus periods	Probability of occurrence increases after retained placenta
	Repeated oxytocin treatment in predisposed mares	"Short cycle" by administration of prostaglandin $F_{2\alpha}$	
		Repeated oxytocin treatments during postparturient period	
Cervical laceration	Slow traction accompanied by continuous palpation of cervix	Determine tetanus vaccination status and treat accordingly	
	Cautious use of obstetric instruments	Prevent cervical adhesions	
	Generous application of lubricants	Surgery	
Vaginal laceration	Vigilant periparturient observation and prompt intervention when dystocia becomes apparent	Third-degree lacerations require one- or two-step surgical repair	
		Determine tetanus vaccination status and treat accordingly	
		Prevent vestibular adhesions	
Uterine laceration	Vigilant periparturient observation and prompt intervention when dystocia becomes apparent	Surgery	
		Ergonovine maleate to contract uterus, arteries	
		Systemic therapies may be indicated for shock, peritonitis, endotoxemia, and laminitis	
		Prevent endometrial adhesions	
Rectovestibular fistula	Vigilant periparturient observation and prompt intervention when dystocia becomes apparent	Surgical reconstruction	
		Determine tetanus vaccination status and treat accordingly	
Vulvar laceration	First-degree perineal lacerations are common in eutocia and dystocia; however, second- and third-degree lacerations and rectovestibular fistulae may be prevented by keen observation and timely intervention	First- and second-degree laceration may require reconstructive surgery, Caslick procedure, or no surgical treatment	
		Prevent vestibular adhesions	

TABLE 5.   COMPLICATIONS ASSOCIATED WITH DYSTOCIA *Continued*

COMPLICATION	PREVENTION	TREATMENT	COMMENTS
Vaginal/vulvar hematoma		Laxative diet may be indicated until hematoma, inflammation resolve	
Postparturient vaginal necrosis		Debride, disinfect, and prevent vestibular adhesions	
		Laxative diet may be indicated until necrosis, inflammation resolve	
Rectal prolapse		Mild prolapses: epidural anesthetic, manual reposition of the prolapsed tissue, and a purse string suture	Treat immediately to prevent progression of the condition
		Mineral oil p.o., laxative diet	
		Severe prolapses: Surgical resection, guarded to poor prognosis	
Indigestion, constipation	Mineral oil p.o. Bran mash	Mineral oil p.o. Bran mash, laxative diet Nonsteroidal anti-inflammatory drugs to control perineal inflammation	Postpartum perineal inflammation, pain result in reluctance to defecate
Entrapment/ compression/ rupture of intestinal segments	Reduction of roughage ingested late in gestation	Monitor closely; serial abdominocentesis Appropriate supportive treatments (fluids, nonsteroidal anti-inflammatory drugs, antibiotics) Peritoneal lavage Surgery	

limb and accomplish delivery of the foal. In the case of a breech presentation, one should consider placing a loop around the entire rump of the foal as shown in Figure 4*B*, with the head of the fetotome placed dorsal to the sacrum. This results in a reduction of fetal size and, because the distal ends or rear limbs are still attached by skin to the body, facilitates their removal.

Traction

As previously mentioned, relative fetal oversize is uncommon in the mare. Most traction is applied to assist delivery of a foal following correction of a malposture or malposition. Traction should proceed only after maximal dilation of the caudal reproductive tract so as to minimize the potential for injuries to the dam during delivery (Table 5). Mares are especially susceptible to cervical lacerations, which may have detrimental consequences on the dam's future reproductive performance. Traction may be applied by attaching loops of obstetric ropes or chains above the fetlock and a half hitch below the joint. This distributes the traction over a larger area and decreases the possibility of causing a fracture. Slow traction with continuous palpation of cervical stretching by the attending obstetrician is, therefore, recommended in management of equine dystocias. The use of traction should be coordinated with the mare's uterine contractions and abdominal press. The use of two or three persons should be the maximal force applied. Mechanical fetal extractors should definitely not be employed.

The integrity of the birth canal, fluids, and fetal membranes serve as indicators of fetal viability and length of time the dystocia has persisted. Lubrication should be applied continuously during the management of dystocia to prevent damage to the dam's birth canal.

In equine dystocia, if the foal is still alive and dystocia cannot be relieved quickly (20 minutes) or if it is determined that extensive manipulation will be required, general anesthesia may be induced. Examination and manipulation can be greatly facilitated by anesthetizing the mare and elevating her hindquarters, enabling the fetus and viscera to recede cranially into the mare's abdominal cavity, thereby allowing more room for manipulation by the obstetrician.

Supplemental Readings

Arthur GH, Noakes DE, Pearson H: Veterinary Reproduction and Obstetrics, 5th ed. London, Bailliere Tindall, 1982.

Bierschwal CJ, deBois CHW: The technique of fetotomy in large animals. Bonner Springs, KS, VM Publishing Inc., 1972.

Blanchard TL, Varner DD, Elmore RG, Martin MT, Scrutchfield WL, Taylor TS: Management of dystocia in mares: Examination, obstetrical equipment and vaginal delivery. Comp Contin Ed Pract Vet 11:745–753, 776, 1989.

Grubb TL, Riebold TW, Huber MJ: Comparison of lidocaine, xylazine and xylazine/lidocaine for caudal epidural analgesia in horses. J Am Vet Med Assoc 201:1187–1190, 1992.

LeBlanc MM, Norman WM: Sedation and anesthesia of the mare during obstetric manipulation. Proc 38th Annu Meet Am Assoc Equine Pract, 1992, pp 619–622.

Menard L: Tocolytic drugs for use in veterinary obstetrics. Can Vet J 25:389–393, 1984.

Rice LE: Dystocia-related risk factors. Vet Clin North Am Food Anim Pract 10(1):53–68, 1994.

Taylor TS, Varner DD, Martin MT, Blanchard TL, Scrutchfield WL, Elmore RG: Management of dystocia in mares: Uterine torsion and cesarean section. Comp Cont Ed Pract Vet 11:1265–1273, 1989.

Vandeplassche M: Dystocia. In McKinnon AO, Voss JL (eds): Equine Reproduction. Philadelphia, Lea & Febiger, 1993, pp 578–587.

Zent WW: Postpartum complications. In Robinson NE (ed): Current Therapy in Equine Medicine, ed 2. Philadelphia, WB Saunders, 1987, pp 544–547.

Retained Fetal Membranes

MATS H.T. TROEDSSON
St. Paul, Minnesota

MICHAEL S. SPENSLEY
Mendota Heights, Minnesota

MELVYN L. FAHNING
St. Paul, Minnesota

The anatomic structure of the equine placenta is described as diffuse, epitheliochorial, and microcotyledonary. It is composed of the allantochorion, the allantoamnion, and the umbilical cord. Although the actual physical separation and expulsion of the fetal membranes from the uterus occurs during the third stage of labor, important cellular events that involve the microcotyledonary maturation and separation of chorionic villi from the endometrial crypts begin before parturition. Rupture of the umbilical cord in association with parturition is believed to cause collapse of the fetal placental vessels, with subsequent shrinkage of the chorionic villi. The final separation of the interdigitating components of the microcotyledons is most likely the result of myometrial contractions, induced by oxytocin and possibly prostaglandin. Myometrial contractions reduce the uterine size and the amount of circulating blood in the endometrium, resulting in relaxation of the endometrial crypts, which allows the villi to be released.

Retained fetal membranes are defined as the failure of the entire or partial fetal membranes to be expelled for a duration of time that is considered to be longer than normal. During most normal foalings, the separation of the fetal membranes from the endometrium and their subsequent expulsion occurs within 0.5 to 3 hours after the delivery of the foal. However, in 2 to 10% of equine parturitions, the fetal membranes are retained beyond 3 hours after foaling. In most cases, it is the area of the allantochorion near the tip of the nonpregnant horn that fails to separate. The principal cause of retained placenta after term delivery of the equine fetus is believed to be an endocrine imbalance or disturbance in normal uterine contractions, but any swelling at the site of the microcotyledons can cause retention of fetal membranes.

DIAGNOSIS

Retained fetal membranes often follow episodes of dystocia, cesarean section, and fetotomy. Reports of a higher incidence of retained fetal membranes in association with abortion, stillbirth, and twinning may be explained by the high incidence of dystocia in these cases. The incidence of retained fetal membranes is higher in draft horses than in lighter horse breeds.

Diagnosis of retained fetal membranes in the mare may be very straightforward if it is based on the observation of placental membranes hanging from the vulva 3 or more hours after foaling. However, the fetal membranes may fall forward over the pelvis and remain within the uterus without being visible. In such cases, diagnosis of complete or partial retention of fetal membranes may also be made 1 to 2 days after foaling, after observation of signs indicative of metritis such as fever, depression, colic, and laminitis. Following their expulsion, fetal membranes should be kept intact until they can be examined to determine their entirety and integrity. Tears, missing areas of tissue, and areas of chorionic surface devoid of microvilli should be considered evidence of partially retained fetal membranes. Immediate action should be taken to enhance expulsion of retained tissue and minimize complications. Evidence that a portion of the placenta was retained in the uterus or that an area of microvilli was sheared off and retained in the endometrial crypts is indication for transvaginal digital endometrial examination and institution of appropriate therapy.

Vital signs are often normal early in cases of retained fetal membranes. Systemic signs of dehydration, septicemia, toxemia, and laminitis may accompany fetal membranes retained for 24 to 36 hours. Rectal examination and ultrasonography should be performed to determine the degree of uterine involution. Vaginal examination should be performed to determine the area and extent of retention.

TREATMENT

If the retained fetal membranes are protruding from the vulva, they should be "knotted" below the vulva and above the hocks. This prevents the mare from standing and possibly tearing the membranes and reduces contamination of the membranes. The time allowed to lapse between parturition and intervention varies significantly among veterinarians, as do the methods of treatment that have been used in the management of retained placenta. The least invasive method that results in expulsion of the fetal membranes should be employed (Table 1). It is important to institute systemic anti-inflammatory and antimicrobial therapies in cases of retained placenta that are refractory to removal of retained tissue. Oxytocin is the drug most commonly used in mares with retained fetal membranes. Oxytocin (20–120 IU IM) can be administered at 2-hour intervals for up to 8 hours postpartum, until the fetal membranes have been expelled. Slow intravenous infusion of oxytocin (60–100 IU in 0.5 to 2 L of a 0.9% saline solution), over 30 to 60 minutes, often results in the expulsion of the membranes. The authors' experience has been that, if administered

TABLE 1. RECOMMENDED TREATMENTS AND MANAGEMENT OF RETAINED FETAL MEMBRANES (RFM) IN THE MARE

Clinical Presentation	Treatment	Comments
Complete retention of fetal membranes	**RFM 3–8 hours postpartum** Repeated treatments with oxytocin (20 IU IM) every 1–2 hours **RFM >8 hours postpartum** Slow infusion of oxytocin (100 IU in 1 L 0.9% saline) over 30 minutes, followed by 5–10 minutes of walking as needed **Above treatments fail to expel RFM** Infusion of large amounts of fluid into the allantoic cavity (Burns' technique)	The treatment will result in expulsion of RFM in >75% Allantochorion needs to be intact Important to identify the allantochorion from the allantoamnion, and to infuse the fluids strictly into the allantoic cavity (See Fig. 1)
Partial retention of fetal membranes	**RFM are reachable in the nonpregnant horn** Oxytocin (10 IU IV), followed by careful traction of the retained membranes, in utero **RFM cannot be reached, or manual traction fails to expel the membranes** Daily intrauterine infusions with 0.9% saline, lactated Ringer's solution, or a dilute (<2%) povidone-iodine solution	Clinical judgment and care needed to prevent damage to the uterus Intrauterine lavage should be combined with systemic treatments
Additional treatments	**Systemic treatments** *Antibiotics* Penicillin-G proc. (20,000–50,000 IU/kg b.i.d.) Penicillin K (10,000–50,000 IU/kg q.i.d.) Gentamicin (2–4 mg/kg b.i.d. to q.i.d.) Ceftiofur (2.5–5 mg/kg b.i.d.) Amikacin (3.5–7.5 mg/kg b.i.d.) Ticarcillin (40–80 mg/kg t.i.d.) Trimethoprim/sulfa (15–30 mg/kg p.o. b.i.d.) *Anti-inflammatory drugs* Flunixin meglumine (0.25 mg/kg t.i.d.) Phenylbutazone (2–4 mg/kg b.i.d.) Dimethyl sulfoxide (1 g/kg; 10% solution in 5% dextrose) *Vasodilators* Isoxsuprine hydrochloride (1.2 mg/kg b.i.d.) Acetylpromazine (0.02 mg/kg t.i.d.) *Aids in uterine involution* Oxytocin (20–40 IU q.i.d.) Uterine lavage with 3–5 L of lactated Ringer's solution	**Indications** When attempts to expel the entire fetal membrane have failed >12 hours have passed between parturition and expulsion of the fetal membranes Clinical signs of systemic illness **Prevention of endotoxemia** Broad-spectrum antibiotics, effective against gram-negative microorganisms Flunixin meglumine **Prevention of laminitis** Phenylbutazone Isoxsuprine DMSO Support shoeing or padding of the hoof The effect of NSAIDs on myometrial contractility is not clear. The potential benefit of treatment may outweigh the risk Repeated lavages until the effluent is pink or tea-colored Treatment may be indicated in mares with delayed uterine involution, and mares that are scheduled to be bred on foal heat

within 12 hours of parturition, oxytocin (100 IU in 1 L of a 0.9% saline solution) infused over 30 minutes, followed by 5 to 10 minutes of walking as needed, rarely fails to expel the fetal membranes.

Distension of the allantoic cavity by the infusion and trapping of large amounts of a weak (<2%) povidone-iodine solution in water (or 0.9% saline solution) into the allantoic space was reported by Burns and coworkers (1977). This technique is recommended if oxytocin treatment fails to expel the retained membranes. The treatment is most successful if the allantochorion is intact, and it is essential that it is performed correctly.

Following thorough cleansing of the perineal region, the allantochorion needs to be identified and a stomach tube inserted through the opening of the torn end of the cervical star into the collapsed allantoic space (Fig. 1). The membranes should be closed over the tube by the use of the operator's hand or umbilical tape. It is important to not advance the tube too far into the uterus, because of potential damage to the fragile postpartum uterine wall. Up to 12 L of solution of 2% povidone-iodine may be infused into the allantoic cavity using this technique. Note that this method does not allow contact between the infused fluid and the uterine lining. The procedure results in endogenous release of oxytocin and endometrial stretching, which facilitate the release of microvilli from endometrial crypts. The forceful myometrial contractions cause expulsion of the fluid-filled fetal membranes. Good results can be expected even beyond 12 hours after parturition in the presence of inflammatory edema of the microcotyledons. Repeated infusions of the allantoic cavity may, however, be necessary if separation of the retained membranes is incomplete. Flushing and siphoning of fluid from the uterus has been suggested but may not be as successful as infusion of the allantoic cavity.

Manual removal of the retained fetal membranes used

to be common practice, and several different techniques have been reported. However, manual removal may lead to many undesirable complications, including severe hemorrhage and retention of broken microvilli in the endometrial crypts resulting in prolonged inflammation, delayed involution, and possible permanent endometrial damage with lower fertility as a consequence. Accordingly, manual removal of retained fetal membranes should generally be discouraged. An exception may be cases of partially retained fetal membranes, in which a small piece of allantochorion can be reached by a transvaginal approach in the nonpregnant horn. A combination of administration of oxytocin (10 IU IV) and careful traction of the membranes, in utero over a period of 10 to 20 minutes, often results in successful removal of the retained pieces of membranes without complications.

Collagenase injections in the placental umbilical arteries have been suggested to have therapeutic potential in mares with retained fetal membranes. The approach is interesting and needs to be further investigated.

COMPLICATIONS

Complications of retained fetal membranes in the mare include acute metritis, endotoxemia, laminitis, and chronic endometritis. Treatment and prevention of these complications are presented on page 558. If treated properly, retained fetal membranes do not affect the rates of pregnancy after first breeding, pregnancy per season, pregnancy loss, or foaling rates.

Supplemental Readings

Asbury AC, LeBlanc MM: The placenta. *In* McKinnon AO, Voss JL (eds): Equine Reproduction. Philadelphia, Lea & Febiger, 1993, pp 509–516.

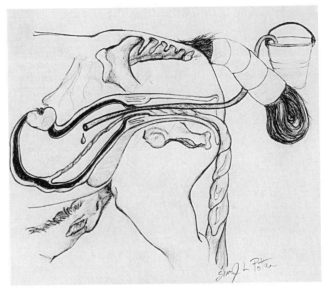

Figure 1. Infusion of large amounts of fluids into the allantoic cavity (Burns' technique). A stomach tube is inserted through the torn end of the allantochorion. Once in the allantoic space, the allantochorion is closed over the tube by the use of the operator's hand or umbilical tape. Up to 12 L of a weak povidone-iodine solution is infused into the allantoic cavity. The procedure induces forceful myometrial contraction, resulting in expulsion of the fluid-filled membranes. (Illustration by Sheryl Potter.)

Blanchard TL, Scrutchfield WL, Taylor TS, Elmore RG, Varner DD, Bretzlaff KN, Martin MT: Management of dystocia in mares: Retained placenta, metritis, and laminitis. Comp Cont Ed Pract Vet 12:563–571, 1990.

Burns SJ, Judge NG, Martin JE, Adams LG: Management of retained placenta in mares. Proc Annu Meet Am Assoc Equine Pract, 1977, pp 381–390.

Threlfall WR: Retained placenta. *In* McKinnon AO, Voss JL (eds): Equine Reproduction. Philadelphia, Lea & Febiger, 1993, pp 614–621.

Perinatal Behavior of the Mare and Foal

J A N E A. B A R B E R
St. Paul, Minnesota

Although play between juvenile horses prepares them for most adult behavior such as sexual activity and dominance hierarchal interactions, the primiparous mare has no behavioral "dress rehearsal" for the act of parturition. Successful periparturient formation of the mare-foal bond and establishment of maternal behavior provide the foal with a source of nutrients, shelter, security, and guidance, and thus are essential for foal survival.

At birth, the foal leaves the sanctuary of the intrauterine environment and receives a rude awakening into the world. The first few hours after birth represent a critical period in the foal's life. The termination of the fetal existence and the transition through the act of birth into the harsh extrauterine environment impose new challenges: respiration, thermoregulation, locomotion, location and ingestion of nutrients, elimination of wastes, and others, each of which must be overcome if the foal is to survive. Within seconds to hours of birth, the foal undergoes both dramatic physiologic change and rapid behavioral development.

When either the mare fails to maternally bond or the foal fails to achieve the necessary adaptations, early detection is of paramount importance to successful resolution of the problem. Timely and accurate identification of the abnormal neonatal or abnormal maternal behavior requires knowledge of the normal foaling process, maternal bond formation, perinatal development, and ontogeny of behavior. A discussion of the parturition process appears in another part of this section (see page 547).

THE MARE-FOAL BOND

Mares form strong maternal bonds with their foals. Formation of the mare-to-foal bond is believed to begin before birth, following rupture of the chorioallantoic membrane and the concomitant discharge of allantoic fluid. The mare sniffs the fluid, often exhibits the flehmen response, and investigates bedding on which fluid has fallen. Shortly after birth, the mare licks the fetal membranes and her foal extensively. After doing this, the mare is able to discriminate between her foal and other foals and rejects attempts to nurse by other foals. Within minutes of parturition, removal of foals elicits distress responses in mares. Olfaction and taste are more important to foal recognition by mares than are vision and hearing. Excessive human intervention in the periparturient period, as a result of either extensive medical treatment or an overzealous owner, may alter the foal's odor and interfere with the development of normal bonding. Without the presence of their foals as a continual reinforcer, mares lose the mothering instinct within 3 or 4 days.

In contrast to the mare's rapid bonding, foals are not strongly bonded to their mothers for the first few days or even the first week of life and will follow any large moving object such as other horses, people, and trucks. Orphan foals will bond to a foster mother until they are several months old. Up to 2 months of age they appear to have little discrimination. During this time, foals are strongly motivated by hunger and are discouraged only by repeated aggressions from antagonistic mares.

ONTOGENY OF BEHAVIOR IN THE FOAL

During their first few hours of life, foals effect rapid and substantial changes in their behavior. The following time line of normal behavioral development may aid the clinician in identifying the abnormal or high-risk foal.

At birth—eyes open, sucking reflex present in response to oral stimulation

At 10–60 seconds—respiratory rhythm established

At 5 minutes—limb movement

At 10 minutes—pupillary responses present

At 30 minutes—binocular orientation, spontaneous sucking reflex present, foal makes attempts to stand

At 45 minutes—auditory orientation with unilateral pinna control

At 60 minutes—ability to stand, walking soon follows standing

At 90 minutes—foal nurses successfully

At 2 hours—defecation (some straining is normally associated with meconium passage)

At 9 hours—urination

SPATIAL RELATIONSHIPS

The bond between mare and foal is most apparent in the close association of the two. During the perinatal period, spatial relationships are characterized by extremely close proximity. On the first day of life, mares and foals spend 100% of the time less than 5 meters apart. Throughout the first week of foal life, mares and foals spend about 95% of the time within 5 meters of each other. Spatial separation gradually increases as foals mature.

This close association is primarily a direct effect of the foal's behavior. During the first few weeks of foal life, mares repeatedly leave their foals, and the foals maintain close proximity by repeatedly approaching their mothers. Mares more frequently terminate nursing bouts during the perinatal period and do so by simply walking away from their foals. This behavior, in combination with isolation from other herdmates, appears to assist with the foal's imprinting on its own mother. Thus, although the foal's following response is innate, selective following of its mother is probably learned. Interference with this learning process may disrupt normal mare-foal bond development.

PROTECTION AND THE RECUMBENCY RESPONSE

The innate following tendency observed in neonatal foals puts the horse into the "follower" category of survival strategies. Follower species usually inhabit open environments such as plains, and follower young typically remain close to their mothers during periods of activity. In contrast, young of hider species (bovidae and most cervidae species) lie still, sequestered for long periods in vegetative cover, while their mothers graze a significant distance away. Follower young do not hide when resting recumbently. Foals are especially vulnerable to predation during periods of deep and rapid eye movement (REM) sleep when they become relatively unresponsive to external stimuli. Neonatal foals are subject to added peril; they spend nearly 40% of the time resting recumbently, and they must often make several attempts before successfully rising, thereby precluding a quick escape from potential predators.

As a result, mares exhibit a protective response to their sleeping foals, which is termed the *recumbency response*. When a mare's foal lies down, she interrupts her normal wandering pattern of grazing to either stand beside or graze in a small circle around her foal. The recumbency response begins to wane gradually when foals are 6 to 8 weeks old.

Mares may protect their foals from other adult conspecifics, as well as humans and potential predators. Maternal protection may entail a simple positioning of the mare between her foal and another approaching horse, or it may involve overt aggression directed against the approaching horse. Some mares may exhibit a greater frequency and intensity of aggression when their sleeping foals are approached by either humans or other horses. In the horse's wild ancestors, evolutionary selection pressure probably favored foal survival of mares that were most alert and aggressive when their foals were sleeping.

MATERNAL AGGRESSION

Maternal aggression is defined as any antagonistic behavior on the part of the mare that is directed toward her foal. Maternal aggression, although infrequently observed, is a normal phenomenon of the mare-foal relationship. In assessing a potential case of foal rejection, the clinician is aided by a knowledge of the contexts in which maternal aggression normally occurs, in addition to the normal frequency and type of aggression.

Mares rarely act aggressively against their foals, especially during the periparturient period. However, when they do so, almost all aggression is associated with the nursing process. A majority (85%) of maternal aggressions occur as foals initiate nursing bouts, specifically during the pre-suck nuzzle portion of the nursing bout. Nuzzling, when accompanied by vigorous head bunting behavior, is likely to be painful and may serve as an aversive stimulus to the mare. Later in the bout, foals begin to suck, which does not appear to be aversive to the mare.

The foal's most common response to maternal aggression is no response at all. When nursing, the foal's head is placed both medial to the mare's hindlimb and ventral to her abdomen, thereby preventing visualization of its mother's head and neck. When maternal aggression takes the form of either laying back the ears or a threat to bite, for example, the foal is probably oblivious to the aggression. A pause in nuzzling is the second most common response to maternal aggression. Maternal aggression almost never results in nursing bout termination.

FOAL REJECTION

A failure in formation of the mare-to-foal bond results in rejection of the foal by the mare. The vast majority of maternal aggression consists of relatively mild encounters of short duration that do not result in dissolution of the maternal bond. Foal rejection, the final outcome of severe prolonged maternal aggression, occurs in less than 1% of all mares. Early warning signs of foal rejection include failure of a mare to protect, exhibit the recumbency response, or maintain close proximity to her neonatal foal. Rejection should definitely be suspected when maternal aggression occurs outside of the context of nursing, occurs at higher frequencies than normal, or consists of greater intensity aggression types.

Several forms of foal rejection are observed. Although foal rejection occurs at widely varying levels of intensity, severe forms are a rare event. The majority of foal rejections are mild and are believed to involve inexperi-

enced primiparous mares. In mild cases of foal rejection, the mare simply avoids her foal. Her ear and tail posture indicates a fear response, and she may actually be rejecting the nursing process and not her foal. Apparently, experience teaches a mare that sucking relieves the pressure and pain caused by a turgid mammary gland. Conversely, the problem of nursing rejection can be aggravated by anything that increases udder or teat sensitivity. This form of foal rejection, although not conducive to nursing, usually does not involve injury to the foal except in cases of stall confinement in which the mare, intent on avoidance, inadvertently tramples on her foal.

Pain-associated foal rejection also occurs. In this form of rejection, mares act aggressively against their foals only when they are experiencing pain, as is the case in some mares with retained placenta. Usually the rejection problem resolves spontaneously after the pain is relieved; acceptance of the foal and maternal bond formation then proceed normally.

Foal rejection can be a displacement behavior. Postparturient mares normally act aggressively against other adult conspecifics. In a typical barn environment, the mare can see, hear, and smell other horses but is prevented from reaching them. The agitated mare then redirects her aggression against her own foal. Displacement rejection can be prevented if the periparturient mare and her foal are separated from the rest of the herd, as well as people, for a few days. Then other horses and people can gradually be reintroduced into the mare's environment in such a way so as not to evoke an aggressive response by the mare.

Iatrogenic foal rejection also occurs. As mentioned previously, maternal behavior is largely dependent upon the mare's receiving appropriate olfactory cues from her foal. Although early handling and socialization of foals is recommended, human intervention beyond that deemed absolutely essential is best delayed until after maternal bond formation has occurred. In this way, significant alterations in the foal's taste and smell can be avoided.

Other forms of foal rejection are more severe. Some mares allow their foals to nurse but attack them under other circumstances. The attack usually consists of bites to the foal's neck and withers. This most serious form of foal rejection may be genetic in origin because it is primarily seen in certain lines of Arabian mares. Unfortunately, this form of foal rejection can be chronic, with the mare repeatedly rejecting her foal year after year.

Treatment and Management

Once it has been determined that a mare is in the process of rejecting her foal, treatment must be instituted immediately. The critical period for maternal bond formation in the mare is believed to be less than 6 hours. Normally, less than 1 hour is required for the mare to be able to discriminate the olfactory characteristics of her foal. Before maternal bond formation, separation of foals from their mothers for even a single day makes the chance for maternal bond formation very low.

Aggressive mares should be restrained in a manner that allows the foal to nurse without risk of injury. One useful method of restraint uses a beam or pole attached parallel to the wall of the stall. The pole is mounted at a height approximately level with the stifle. The pole should be at a distance from the wall that just allows containment of the mare but prevents her forward and lateral movement. The mare should not be able to chase the foal, neither should she be able to kick back caudally or out laterally. Mares should be restrained but should not be left unattended. In one case, a mare was restrained in this manner for 3 weeks before finally accepting her foal.

Protocols for the use of drug therapy in the treatment of foal rejection are not well established. Although both drugs are useful, phenothiazine° (0.6 mg/kg) tranquilization empirically has been more beneficial than xylazine†(1 mg/kg), a sedative analgesic, in promoting the mare's acceptance of her foal. Diazepam‡ (10–20 mg/horse), an anxietiolytic drug, is also helpful in treating mares exhibiting fear responses. Progestogen therapy using altrenogest§ (0.044 mg/kg) raises the threshold for aggression and is the drug of choice in more severe cases of foal rejection in which mares attack their foals.

Behavioral methods can also be useful in stimulating maternal behavior. Maternal behavioral responses are induced by separating the foal from its mother or by orchestrating threats to the foal. Both actions normally elicit strong responses from mares, separation anxiety in the former case and protective behavior in the latter case. These behavioral methods work best when mares are fearful or when the mare is only mildly aggressive toward her foal. One simple means of threatening the foal involves turning both the mare and her foal out into a paddock with other horses. Protective maternal behavior such as maintaining close proximity to her foal, positioning herself between her foal and other horses, or attempting to keep other horses away from her foal may be induced.

°*Promace, Fort Dodge Laboratories, Fort Dodge, IA*
†*Rompun, Haver, Lockhart, Shawnee, KS*
‡*Valium, Hoffman-LaRoche, Nutley, NJ*
§*Regu-mate, American Hoechst Corp., Somerville, NJ*

Punishment is often employed in the routine training of horses and can be used in a behavioral modification program to treat foal rejection. However, administration of an aversive stimulus is not necessarily the same thing as punishment. To be effective, punishment must absolutely meet each of three criteria. First, the punishment must be administered immediately following the occurrence of the inappropriate behavior. Even a 2- or 3-second delay renders the punishment useless. Second, the punishment must be administered in every instance of the misbehavior. Otherwise, the mare receives mixed signals. Third, the appropriate intensity of punishment must be consistently used. When applied to cases of foal rejection, punishment should be administered at the same instant that the mare bites or kicks her foal. Other secondary behavioral problems, such as displaced aggression or association of the presence of the foal or trainer with the punishment, can develop from inappropriate use of punishment. Punishment is definitely contraindicated in cases of foal rejection due to fear and only results in escalating the mare's fear. Given the logistic difficulties of adhering to the three criteria, behavioral modification using punishment should be considered only after the type of foal rejection has been determined and the client has been carefully educated and is capable of complete compliance with the behavioral modification program.

Supplemental Readings

Barber JA, Crowell-Davis SL: Maternal behavior of Belgian (*Equus caballus*) mares. Appl Anim Behav Sci 41:161–189, 1994.
Crowell-Davis SL, Houpt KA: Maternal behavior. Vet Clin North Am Equine Pract 2(3):557–571, 1986.
Houpt KA: Foal rejection and other behavioral problems in the post partum period. Comp Cont Ed 6(3):S144–S148, 1984.
Rossdale PD: Abnormal perinatal behaviour in the Thoroughbred horse. Br Vet J 124:540–553, 1968.
Waring GH: Onset of behavioral patterns in the newborn foal. Equine Pract 4(5):28–34, 1982.

Assisted Reproductive Techniques in the Mare

KATRIN HINRICHS
North Grafton, Massachusetts

Assisted reproduction refers to any method to produce young that goes beyond simply breeding one animal to another. Embryo transfer is a well-established assisted reproductive technique in the horse, and methods for embryo transfer were presented previously (see *Current Therapy in Equine Medicine 3*, page 637). Although freezing and micromanipulating embryos is still problematic in the horse, transporting embryos has become a viable clinical procedure, and techniques for doing so are presented here.

Unfortunately, the success rate of embryo transfer is low in subfertile mares, and some mares are unable to provide an embryo for transfer because of uterine or cervical problems such as chronic endometritis, cervical lacerations, or adhesions. These mares should, however, be able to provide oocytes for fertilization. Techniques for obtaining foals from donor mare oocytes, including oocyte transfer and in vitro fertilization, are currently being developed in the horse.

The appropriate in vitro environments in which to mature horse oocytes and enhance sperm penetration into the egg are currently unclear, as is the best environment for subsequent cleavage and development. As a result, the techniques most likely to succeed clinically are those that involve in vivo fertilization, that is, transfer of an oocyte to a recipient mare with fertilization within the recipient mare's tract. Although techniques for oocyte transfer have been variably successful in producing embryos and foals in research laboratories, they have yet to be used to obtain foals in a clinical situation. The methods described for oocyte transfer here, then, are those that are the most likely to work based on current research reports.

Although these techniques for assisted reproduction in the horse are in their infancy, breakthroughs in equine oocyte transfer and in vitro fertilization have occurred in just the last year. Oocyte transfer has the potential to replace embryo transfer for infertile mares, and could be a viable "treatment" for nonresponsive postbreeding endometritis and other causes of infertility. Progress in in vitro oocyte maturation and fertilization suggests that in 5 years these techniques may also be clinically viable, allowing embryos to be produced and cultured in the laboratory to transferrable size. This would eliminate the need for the exacting synchronization and surgical oviduct cannulation that is necessary for oocyte transfer. In vitro fertilization may also provide some hope of fertility in stallions with conditions affecting sperm quality or ability to ejaculate, because it drastically decreases the number of normal sperm necessary for fertilization. These techniques are already being used clinically in humans and cattle.

EMBRYO TRANSFER

Transporting Embryos

One of the major factors in success of embryo transfer is synchronization of the donor and recipient mares (see *Current Therapy in Equine Medicine 3*, page 638). When transfers are being done in only a few mares, as may happen in clinical practice, two recipient mares are usually synchronized with each donor mare. This is often done by giving daily injections to all mares for 10 days (progesterone/estrogen synchronization), with expected ovulation 9 to 11 days after the end of treatment, a 20-day delay of ovulation from the time the procedure is initiated. Even with this regimen, synchronization of ovulation between donor and recipient cannot be guaranteed. Alternatively, ovariectomized recipient mares may be used, which guarantees synchronization but necessitates surgery on the recipients. These problems may be avoided if a large herd of recipients is available, because a recipient mare ovulating within the desired time in relation to the donor (from about 1 day before to 3 days after the donor) should be available at any time. Obviously, only large facilities are able to keep and monitor a recipient mare herd.

Recently, methods have been developed that allow embryos to be shipped in a commercial semen cooling device* and be transferred after shipment, with pregnancy rates equal to that for directly transferred embryos. Using this method, an embryo can be collected from the donor mare at her home 7 days after ovulation and then shipped to a large facility for transfer into an appropriate recipient mare. For the donor mare's veterinarian, this eliminates the need

for synchronization of the donor and recipient mares and allows concentration on breeding the donor mare and obtaining the embryo.

The methods for evaluating and breeding the donor mare and collecting the embryo are those used for typical embryo transfer (see *Current Therapy in Equine Medicine 3*, page 637). The medium used for embryo collection and for holding the recovered embryo is a modified Dulbecco's phosphate buffered saline (PBS). However, this medium is not optimal for cooling and storing embryos, and thus the embryo must be transferred to a different medium for transport. Although only a few media have been examined for use in storing equine embryos, Ham's F-10 with a bicarbonate buffer provides better embryo viability than does PBS or Hepes-buffered Ham's F-10. Unfortunately, this medium requires special handling, because the bicarbonate buffer system maintains pH based on a 5% carbon dioxide (CO_2) atmosphere.

Ham's F-10, and all other culture reagents mentioned in this chapter, are available from major suppliers.* The Ham's F-10 contains phenol red as a pH indicator; this indicator turns yellow when acid and purple-red when alkaline. At the appropriate pH (about 7.4) the medium is an orange-red or tan. The medium can be gassed by infusing it with medical-grade gas containing 5% CO_2, 5% oxygen (O_2), and 90% nitrogen (N) (obtained in canister form from a medical supplier), or by placing it in a loosely capped container in a 5% CO_2 incubator. For the convenience of the practitioner, some transfer centers supply gassed medium immediately before the embryo recovery is to be performed. This necessitates overnight delivery of the medium, a labor and expense that is wasted if no embryo is recovered. Obviously, the extra time involved in using a CO_2-based medium is a major nuisance in transporting embryos. Workers in Colorado are currently examining cooled storage in other media that contain adequate amounts of bicarbonate but do not require gassing. At this time, however, the recommendation would be to use bicarbonate-buffered Ham's F-10 for cooled, transported embryos.

Once the medium is gassed, it should be capped to prevent CO_2 from escaping. The final medium used to store the embryo should contain 10% newborn calf serum and 100 IU penicillin-100 μg streptomycin per ml. The antibiotics can be obtained by adding 1 ml of penicillin/streptomycin mixture (supplied at 10,000 IU penicillin and 10,000 μg streptomycin per ml as diluted) to 100 ml of medium.

To package the embryo for shipment, a 5-ml clear plastic tube should be half-filled with the transport medium (prepared Ham's F-10). The embryo is transferred from the holding dish into the tube with a minimum of holding medium, using a 1-ml, fire-polished glass pipette or a 25-μl capillary pipette and 1-ml syringe. The embryo should be observed leaving the pipette and entering the fluid in the tube. The tube is then filled with transport medium and capped immediately to prevent gas loss. Paraffin film is wrapped around the top of the tube to ensure a tight seal. The 5-ml tube is placed in a 50-ml centrifuge tube containing 40 ml of transport medium. The centrifuge tube

---

*Equitainer, Hamilton Equine Systems, Danvers, MA

*Gibco Labs, Grand Island, NY; and Sigma Chemical, St. Louis, MO

is then completely filled, capped, and sealed with film. The centrifuge tube is wrapped with 70 to 120 ml of ballast (two ballast bags from the Equitainer or sealed bags containing the appropriate volume of water) and placed in a plastic cup in the isothermalizer of the Equitainer. The remainder of the packaging is as for semen shipment.

Although most transported embryo centers have been shipping embryos by counter-to-counter air services, so that the embryo arrives the same day that it is collected, original research in this area used embryos cooled for 24 hours, achieving pregnancy rates equal to those for fresh embryos. Therefore, shipment of embryos by overnight courier should allow good pregnancy rates.

When the embryo is received, the recipient mare is prepared for transfer. Most research with cooled embryos has used surgical transfer, but there is no evidence that cooled embryos benefit more from surgical transfer than do fresh embryos. When transfer is performed at the same time as collection, pregnancy rates for transcervical transfer are equivalent to those for surgical transfer. The 5-ml tube is removed from the centrifuge tube, and if possible (if the embryo is large enough) the embryo is visualized at the bottom of the tube. The embryo is transferred to a petri dish containing modified Dulbecco's PBS holding medium, which is prepared as for a typical embryo transfer. The embryo may be removed from the transport tube by either pipetting the contents of the tube from the bottom or by pouring the contents of the tube into the petri dish and rinsing the tube. Care should be taken to transfer the embryo out of the transport medium as soon as possible, because the pH of the transport medium starts to rise as soon as it contacts room atmosphere. The embryo is washed by transferring through three to ten 35-mm petri dishes containing holding medium, and then transferred as for a typical embryo transfer.

OOCYTE TRANSFER

Collection of Oocytes From Donor Mares

All follicles present on the mare ovary contain oocytes, but only the dominant preovulatory follicle contains an oocyte that will mature in vivo. This oocyte resumes meiosis in response to luteinizing hormone (LH) (or exogenous human chorionic gonadotropin [hCG]) stimulation, whereas the remainder of oocytes stay in meiotic arrest. Theoretically, all follicles visible on the mare ovary could be aspirated, providing a large number of immature oocytes, and the oocytes could be matured to metaphase II in vitro for transfer. This is currently being done clinically in cattle. Unfortunately, in the horse, the best method for in vitro oocyte maturation has not been determined, and the viability of in vitro matured oocytes is unclear. In addition, the oocyte recovery rate on aspiration of immature follicles has been poor (around 35%) in the horse. At this time, therefore, clinical techniques for oocyte transfer may best concentrate on collection of mature oocytes from the dominant preovulatory follicle of the donor mare, after stimulation of ovulation with hCG. Oocyte recovery rates on aspiration of dominant follicles after hCG stimulation are around 75%.

Oocytes may be collected from mares by puncturing the

follicle with a needle placed through the flank while the ovary is held per rectum or directly via colpotomy, or by transvaginal ultrasound-guided needle placement. To facilitate these procedures, the mare receives acepromazine (10–30 mg IV) and butorphanol (10–15 mg IV) for tranquilization and analgesia, and ampicillin (6 g IV). The mare is restrained in stocks.

Follicle Aspiration With the Ovary Grasped per Rectum

Two people are needed for the procedure: One operator performs the needle puncture and another handles the syringes or vacuum for aspiration and flushing, if done. While flushing of the follicle after aspiration is performed at many laboratories, equivalent oocyte recovery rates may be obtained by aspiration alone in dominant preovulatory follicles 24 to 36 hours after administration of hCG. A 10-by-10-cm area of the flank ipsilateral to the dominant follicle is shaved and disinfected as for surgery. The operator palpates the mare per rectum, clearing intestine away from the inner body wall and estimating the point at which the trochar should be introduced through the flank to be adjacent to the ovary. Lidocaine (20 to 50 ml of a 2% solution) can be instilled into the rectum to aid in relaxation of the rectal wall. A lidocaine bleb is made in the prepared skin at the area adjacent to the ovary, and a stab incision is made into the skin. A 1 cm or smaller diameter trochar-cannula is inserted through the body wall, and the trochar removed. The operator should palpate the end of the cannula on the inside of the body wall to assure that it has passed through the peritoneum. At 8 inches, a 12- to 18-gauge needle is introduced into the abdomen through the trochar cannula. This needle should be attached to a 50-ml syringe via a short extension tube, because this allows the needle to be freely manipulated. The syringes used should be all-plastic° to ensure that they are not toxic to the oocyte.

The ovary with the dominant follicle is grasped per rectum with one hand. The author has found that a rectal sleeve with the fingers cut off over which to place a surgical glove improves the sensitivity of palpation. With the other hand, the operator holds the needle and cannula, with the needle retracted into the cannula. The ovary and cannula are manipulated to place the end of the cannula immediately on the surface of the preovulatory follicle. The needle is then extruded to puncture the follicle. The contents of the follicle are aspirated, fairly slowly, into the empty syringe. As the follicle empties, it is gently massaged by hand per rectum. When the follicle is empty (no further fluid is obtained), the needle is withdrawn, still under a slight vacuum. If flushing is desired, a syringe filled with flush solution (see below) may be attached, with the aspiration syringe, to the extension tubing via a three-way stopcock. When the follicle is almost empty, the stopcock is turned and the flushing solution is instilled into the follicle. It is important to do this before the follicle is completely empty, because it will bleed at that point, and without the heparin in the flushing solution a clot will form and no further aspiration can be performed. An empty syringe is attached to the stopcock, and the follicle contents are aspirated,

---

°Air-tite syringes, Air-tite of Virginia, Virginia Beach, VA

flushed again *with fresh medium*, and aspirated. The number of flushes performed depends upon the time the needle remains in the follicular antrum before the mare's movement causes it to dislodge, but some workers flush follicles up to 10 to 20 times to assure that the oocyte is collected. The oocyte may be obtained in the very last fluid recovered, and thus it is important to continue to aspirate the contents of the extension tube into the syringe while the needle is being withdrawn from the follicle.

An alternative method to the aspiration-flush-aspiration technique is the use of a double-bore needle* that allows flush fluid to enter the follicle during aspiration, for a continuous flushing action. Some workers have reported increased oocyte recovery rates using this method. Use of a vacuum system instead of syringes simplifies the aspiration procedure. If a vacuum system is used, the vacuum should pull the follicle contents into a 100- to 500-ml flask, because the follicular fluid alone from one preovulatory follicle may be as much as 50 ml. The strength of the vacuum depends on the length and diameter of the needle and tubing, but a good guideline is to use the vacuum that allows the flush to enter the collection bottle in a stream, rather than in drops.

Follicle Aspiration With the Ovary Grasped via Colpotomy

This procedure is essentially that described above, with the exception that the hand does not grasp the ovary per rectum, but directly through an incision in the vagina (i.e., via a colpotomy incision). Grasping the ovary directly eliminates the possibility of creating a rectal tear or puncturing the rectum with the cannula or needle, eliminates the need to cope with the tautness of the rectal wall and peristalsis during handling of the ovary, and greatly increases sensitivity, especially the ability to place the cannula and needle on the appropriate area of the ovary and to hold the ovary steady during the procedure. Colpotomy incisions are commonly used to perform ovariectomies, and have a low complication rate. However, the complications can be life-threatening. These include incising the gut, aorta or internal iliac artery during the initial opening of the vagina; evisceration through the vaginal incision after the procedure; and peritonitis.

The mare is tranquilized for the procedure as described earlier and restrained in stocks. The tail is wrapped and tied out of the way, and the perineum is scrubbed and dried. The operator dons a sterile rectal sleeve and gloves. Using sterile lubricant,† the hand is inserted into the vagina. The operator lifts the perineal body at the vestibular-vaginal ring to let air into the vagina. A scalpel blade or bistury is carried into the vagina and an incision is made in the cranial vagina at about 2 o'clock or 10 o'clock to the cervix, according to the side of the preovulatory follicle. The incision is then enlarged manually until the hand may be passed through the vagina and peritoneum into the abdominal cavity. The ovary is grasped and the placement of the cannula, aspiration, and flushing of the follicle are performed as described earlier. After the procedure the mare is held in the stocks for as long as she is tranquil,

and then is stall rested at least overnight to reduce the possibility that gut will be pushed through the incision when the mare exerts herself. The vaginal incision heals rapidly without suturing, and mares appear to have little pain from the procedure.

Transvaginal Ultrasound-guided Follicle Aspiration

The mare is tranquilized and given antibiotics as described earlier and restrained in stocks. The tail is wrapped and tied out of the way, and the perineum is scrubbed and dried. An ultrasound unit with a specialized transvaginal probe is used. Probe adapters are available for some machines, which incorporate the transrectal probe in a rigid extension with a needle guide;* alternatively, a probe produced especially for transvaginal use may be purchased for some machines.† The probe, lubricated with sterile lubricant, is inserted into the vagina, and the ovary is grasped per rectum and drawn caudally to be visualized transvaginally. Specialized probes have a line visible on the screen to indicate the path of the needle; this should be lined up to the center of the follicle if possible. A 60-cm needle (Cook Veterinary Products) is placed through the guide in the probe and is directed into the follicle as visualized ultrasonographically. The follicle is drained and flushed as described earlier.

Sterilization of the transvaginal probe is important to ensure that a minimum of organisms are introduced into the mare's vagina. The needle must remain sterile to reduce the chance of introduction of organisms into the peritoneum or follicle antrum, and to maintain sterility of the recovered fluid. However, the transvaginal probes or adapters are not autoclavable. Sterility can be assured by soaking the probe in a cold sterilant (use only those recommended by the manufacturer); however, even a minute amount of most sterilants can be toxic if they come in contact with the oocyte. Voluminous rinsing with sterile saline should remove most traces of cold sterilant but cannot be guaranteed to do so. Alternatively, the probe and handle can be cleaned and then sheathed in a sterile latex probe cover.‡ Some workers use isopropyl alcohol to clean the probe, although manufacturers state that this may damage the probe. Sterile lubricant is used inside and outside of the probe cover to ensure good contact of the probe with the vaginal mucosa. The needle is passed through the cover at the time of aspiration; the covers are used only once and discarded.

Follicle Rinsing Medium

Excellent results, up to 80% oocyte recovery with subsequent fertilization of recovered oocytes, have been obtained using Dulbecco's PBS with 1% neonatal calf serum and 2 IU heparin/ml for flushing of the follicle. When adding heparin to the flushing medium it is important to use an embryo culture-quality heparin§ and not that used for medical treatment, because the latter has preservatives in it that could be toxic to the oocyte.

---

*Cook Veterinary Products USA, Spencer, IN
†HR Sterile Lube, A.J. Buck, Cockeysville, MD

*Products Group International, Boulder, CO
†Corometrics, Wallingford, CT
‡Cone Instruments, Solon, OH
§Gibco Life Technologies, Grand Island, NY, or Sigma Chemical, St. Louis, MO

Transfer of Oocytes to Recipient Mares

Surgical Transfer to the Oviduct of a Recipient Mare

Because oocytes may be retrieved from follicles immediately before ovulation, it is logical that transfer of these oocytes directly to the oviducts of recipient mares would provide good pregnancy rates. Unfortunately, this has not proved to be the case because studies using this method report pregnancy rates of only 3 to 8%. The most successful results from oocyte transfer to date, 92% embryo development of oocytes transferred from fertile mares, were recently reported by Carnevale and Ginther. The author is currently using a modification of this technique for oocyte transfer and has achieved four pregnancies from four transfers. Their technique necessitates very close synchronization of donor and recipient mare cycles, which would be best obtained by using a progesterone/estrogen/prostaglandin regimen (see *Current Therapy in Equine Medicine 3*, page 637) or by having a large number of recipient mares available from which to choose. Follicular growth in donor and recipient mares should be monitored until the preovulatory follicle in both mares is greater than 30 mm in diameter; hCG (2000 IU IV) is administered at that time. Twenty-four hours after hCG administration, the dominant preovulatory follicles of both donor and recipient mares are aspirated, and the oocytes identified in the aspirate. Oocytes collected 24 hours after hCG stimulation are enclosed in a large expanded cumulus, visible to the naked eye; the oocyte itself is seen under the dissection microscope as a dark circle within the amorphous cloud of cumulus cells (Fig. 1). The recipient mare's oocyte should be identified to ensure that it was recovered so that it is not available for fertilization. The donor mare's oocyte will be matured in vitro in a CO_2 incubator at 39°C; if this is not available, an air-tight container* gassed with medical

---

*Modular incubator chamber, Billups-Rothenberg, Del Mar, CA

grade 5% CO_2 and air and placed in a 39° incubator or water bath will work. The oocyte is transferred into a 35-mm petri dish containing Medium 199 with Earle's salts, with 10% fetal calf serum, 0.2 mM pyruvate, and 50 μg/ml gentamycin, and is incubated for 12 to 20 hours before transfer.

The oocyte transfer is performed after the recipient mare is tranquilized and has received antibiotics as for oocyte recovery, and is restrained in stocks. A flank laparotomy is performed using a line block of 2% lidocaine, entering the peritoneum through a grid or straight incision. The transfer can be performed on the oviduct ipsilateral or contralateral to the ovary containing the preovulatory follicle without influencing results. The ovary is located and exteriorized, and the infundibulum of the oviduct identified. The infundibulum, a thin piece of tissue about 3 cm in diameter, is attached to the ovary at the ventral-lateral border of the ovulation fossa. The dish containing the oocyte is removed from the incubator, and the oocyte is transferred to a petri dish containing a Hepes-buffered medium such as Hepes-buffered Medium 199 with Hank's salts, also at 39°. The cumulus of the oocyte is reduced in size by cutting off the excess with two needles. The oocyte is loaded into a fire-polished glass pipette or a tomcat catheter with a minimum (<1 ml quantity) of medium. To do this, a small amount of medium is loaded, then an air bubble, then medium containing the oocyte. The recipient mare's infundibulum is grasped gently and pulled away from the ovary, and the opening of the ampulla of the oviduct is identified and cannulated with a hemostat or mosquito forcep. The pipette or catheter is inserted approximately 3 cm into the oviductal ampulla and the contents gently expressed. The flank incision is then closed routinely. Flunixin meglumine (1 mg/kg IM) can be given for pain relief.

The recipient should be bred 12 hours before the transfer and again immediately after transfer. Because aspiration and flushing of the recipient mare's follicle may impair luteal function, it is necessary to ensure that progesterone levels are adequate. The recipient mare may therefore be given progesterone in oil (100 mg on the first day and 200 mg each day thereafter for a light-horse mare) until the pregnancy examination is performed. Once the mare is found to be pregnant, progesterone treatment or altrenogest (0.044 mg/kg p.o., s.i.d.) may be continued until secondary corpora lutea have formed (around 50 days).

INTRAFOLLICULAR OOCYTE TRANSFER

Although intrafollicular transfer of oocytes has been successful, yielding up to 40% embryo development (seven embryos from 15 oocytes in one mare), it has not been repeatably successful, because only four of 16 mares produced embryos from transferred oocytes. Intrafollicular transfer is a technique that does not require incubation of recovered oocytes and thus may be more practical for the veterinarian who does not have in vitro culture capabilities in the laboratory. However, because the recipient mare's follicle and oocyte must be left intact, both donor and recipient oocytes may be fertilized. This necessitates recov-

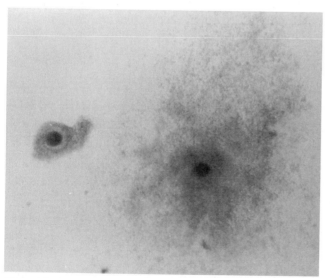

Figure 1. Equine oocytes with compact (*left*) and expanded (*right*) cumuli. The cumulus cells of the expanded oocyte appear darker in the photomicrograph than they do under the microscope.

ering the embryos from the recipient's uterus 7 days after transfer, and performing embryo transfer to secondary recipients. The foals can be identified by blood typing at birth. Methods to mark the donor mare's oocyte before transfer so that the resulting embryo may be identified at recovery are being explored.

The work on this technique was done in the author's laboratory, using oocytes collected from slaughterhouse specimens. These were immature at the time of collection, and were then matured within the recipient mare's follicle. The most repeatable results were obtained when oocytes from large preovulatory follicles were transferred. The following protocol is that which would be used to transfer an oocyte from the preovulatory follicle of a donor mare to the preovulatory follicle of a recipient mare.

Donor and recipient cycles must be synchronized closely, as for oviductal transfer (see above). When the donor and recipient follicles are larger than 30 mm in diameter, the transfer is performed. The donor and recipient mares are prepared for the procedure as described for follicle aspiration. The donor mare's follicle is aspirated to obtain the oocyte, which should be kept at 39° while being held. Because no hCG is given, the oocyte should have a compact cumulus at this time (see Fig. 1). If transvaginal ultrasound-guided needle puncture is used, other follicles visible on the ovary may also be aspirated to increase the number of oocytes obtained. All oocytes recovered should be transferred, regardless of cumulus morphology. The oocytes are loaded into a length of extension tubing by aspiration with a 10-ml Air-tite syringe, then a three-way stopcock is attached to the other end of the tubing. A 10-ml Air-tite syringe is attached to the second port of the stopcock, and the stopcock is then attached by a length of extension tubing to the follicular puncture needle (Fig. 2).

After the donor mare's oocyte has been recovered, the preovulatory follicle of the recipient mare is punctured with the needle/tubing setup containing the oocyte. The puncture is performed as for follicle aspiration, either by flank or by transvaginal ultrasonography. Ten milliliters of follicular fluid are aspirated into the syringe attached to the stopcock, then the fluid in the tubing containing the oocyte is injected into the follicle. Five milliliters of

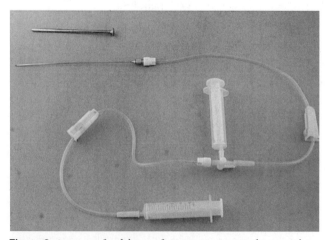

Figure 2. Apparatus for delivery of equine oocytes into the preovulatory follicle in vivo (see text for methods).

the aspirated follicular fluid are injected to ensure that the oocyte is flushed from the tubing into the follicle. The needle is removed from the follicle. Some leakage and decrease in size is apparent in the follicle on ultrasonographic examination after the procedure; echogenic specks within the follicle represent air introduced during transfer. The recipient mare is given hCG as soon as the transfer is complete and is inseminated the following day. A small proportion of these follicles bleed after transfer and fail to ovulate; however, in our study, 16 of 19 mares ovulated normally after transfer (approximately 36 hours after hCG administration).

Because oocyte recovery from the donor mare is done without hCG stimulation, the recovery rate may be less than that for stimulated follicles. However, workers aspirating follicles from pregnant mares have had an 80% recovery rate from unstimulated follicles, using multiple (10–20) flushes of the follicle during aspiration. An alternative method would be to give both donor and recipient mares hCG and aspirate the donor follicle 24 hours later, after the cumulus has started to expand and becomes free from the follicle wall. This procedure successfully produced twins (i.e., an embryo developed from the transferred oocyte) in 2 of 7 transfers.

FUTURE TECHNIQUES: IN VITRO FERTILIZATION

In vitro fertilization (IVF) is still not repeatably successful in the horse, despite almost a decade of work in numerous laboratories. Only two IVF foals have been produced, both from the laboratory of E. Palmer in France. To produce these foals, oocytes were recovered from the preovulatory follicles of mares around 34 hours after hCG administration, or from the oviducts immediately after ovulation, and the oocytes were incubated for another 6 hours before fertilization was attempted.

Other laboratories have reported IVF of in vitro matured oocytes; however, until recently the fertilization rate was very low, with no embryonic development. Successful IVF with embryonic development was reported in 1994. The fertilization rate of horse oocytes appears to be greatly increased by partially dissecting the zona pellucida, or drilling a hole in it chemically, to create a defect through which sperm can enter. Japanese workers reported that zona-free oocytes had a sperm penetration rate of 86%, and partially zona-dissected oocytes had a sperm penetration rate of 52%. Workers in Louisiana achieved a fertilization rate of up to 79% with zona-drilled oocytes, with a morula/blastocyst development rate of up to 36%.

A major problem with IVF after zona drilling or dissection appears to be polyspermy. Deposition of one sperm inside the oocyte by micromanipulation (intracytoplasmic sperm injection, or ICSI) is currently being explored by some laboratories; workers in Louisiana and Colorado achieved fertilization and embryo development using ICSI in 1995, and one foal has been born as a result of this procedure. These techniques show great promise for the development of effective fertilization protocols in the horse. Once a repeatable method for IVF is achieved, the resulting embryos could be cultured in vitro to the blastocyst stage for transfer to the uterus of a recipient mare. Culture to a transferrable stage has already been done successfully with one-celled embryos collected from oviducts after fertilization in vivo.

Supplemental Readings

Carnevale EM, Ginther OJ: Defective oocytes as a cause of subfertility in old mares. Biol Reprod Monograph 1:209–214, 1995.
Cook VM, Squires EL, McKinnon AO, Bailey J, Long PL: Pregnancy rates of cooled, transported equine embryos. Equine Vet J 8[Suppl]:80–81, 1989.
Hinrichs K, DiGiorgio LM: Embryonic development after intra-follicular transfer of horse oocytes. J Reprod Fertil 44[Suppl]:369–374, 1991.
Hinrichs K, Kenney DF, Kenney RM: Aspiration of oocytes from mature and immature preovulatory follicles in the mare. Theriogenology 34:107–112, 1990.
Meintjes M, Bellow MS, Paul JB, Broussard JR, Li LY, Paccamonti D, Eilts BE, Godke RA: Transvaginal ultrasound-guided oocyte retrieval in cyclic and pregnant horse and pony mares for in vitro fertilization. Biol Reprod Monograph 1:281–292, 1995.

Reproductive Aspects of Fescue Toxicosis

JAMES P. BRENDEMUEHL
Auburn University, Alabama

Tall fescue (*Festuca arundinaceae* Schreb.) is a cool-season, seed-propagated, perennial grass that is the most widely grown pasture grass in the humid areas of the southeastern and northwestern United States. It is estimated that over 35 million acres of tall fescue are currently grazed by livestock, including approximately 700,000 horses. Tall fescue is popular as a pasture grass because of its wide range of adaptation, ease of establishment, persistence, disease and drought resistance, long growing season, and good winter growth. An endophytic fungus, *Acremonium coenophialum*, has been shown to be widely spread wherever tall fescue is grown. The endophyte is difficult to control or eliminate from established pastures. Since the early 1980s, surveys from horsemen and practitioners have confirmed reports that pregnant mares grazing fescue incurred myriad reproductive problems that include agalactia, prolonged gestation, thickened placentas, abortion, dystocia, dead or weak foals, and breeding problems.

Infection of tall fescue with the endophyte *Acremonium coenophialum* is associated with the presence of pyrolizidine and ergopeptine alkaloids. The signs of fescue toxicoses may be partially the result of the vasoconstrictive and dopaminergic actions of the alkaloids found in the forage and seed. The ergopeptine alkaloids have been demonstrated in vitro to have a significant effect on peripheral vasoconstriction in the horse. This peripheral vasoconstriction is associated with an increased incidence of laminitis in horses grazing endophyte-infected pastures. Thus, even low concentrations of ergopeptines found in endophyte-infected forage have biologic potency.

CLINICAL MANIFESTATIONS OF FESCUE TOXICITY

Agalactia

Agalactia or hypogalactia is the most commonly reported clinical sign in mares grazing endophyte-infected fescue (Table 1). Mares grazing endophyte-infected fescue exhibit lower prolactin concentrations than mares grazing endophyte-free forage. Hypoprolactinemia associated with endophyte ingestion inhibits normal mammary development in the prepartum period. Prolactin concentrations increase in the immediate prepartum period in the mare and return to baseline levels several weeks postpartum. Episodic increases in prolactin associated with nursing by the foal suggest the requirement of prolactin to maintain lactogenesis.

Prolonged Gestation

Gestation lengths of 13 to 14 months are frequently reported in association with grazing infected fescue. A physiologic lack of readiness for parturition, evidenced by failure of relaxation of pelvic ligaments and musculature, is commonly demonstrated. The combination of prolonged gestation, resulting in abnormally large foals, in conjunction with minimal relaxation of pelvic ligaments, musculature, and cervix leads to a high incidence of dystocia. Parturition-induced injury is common and ranges from vaginal and

TABLE 1.   CLINICAL MANIFESTATIONS OF FESCUE TOXICITY IN THE MARE

Agalactia/hypogalactia	Decreased total progestogens prepartum
Prolonged gestation	Poor neonatal viability
Delayed vernal cyclicity	Reduced colostral IgG absorption
Reduced pregnancy rates	Neonatal hypoadrenalism
Early embryonic death	Neonatal hypopituitarism
Cyclic irregularity	Neonatal hypothyroidism
Corpora luteal persistence	Fetal oversize
Dystocia	Hirsutism
Premature allantochorion separation	Hyperhidrosis
Allantochorion edema	
Increased placental weight	
Retained placenta	

cervical bruising and laceration to death. Malpositioning of the foals contributes to the high incidence of dystocia.

Placenta Alterations

Placental changes in mares consuming endophyte-infected fescue include premature separation of the allantochorion, evidenced by presentation of the cervical star at the onset of stage two of parturition, increased allantochorion weight and thickness, and retained placenta. Biochemical analysis of placentas from mares fed endophyte-infected seed is suggestive of increased cellularity and connective tissue. Transabdominal ultrasonography performed on pregnant mares grazing endophyte-infected fescue indicates an abrupt increase in placental thickness an average of 8 hours before the onset of labor. The increase in thickness is due to edema of the splanchnic mesoderm. Premature separation of the allantochorion occurs in conjunction with the increase in placental thickness.

Foal Viability

Foals born to mares grazing endophyte-infected tall fescue are typically weak at birth with characteristic signs of dysmaturity, including overgrown hooves, irregular dental eruption, fine hair coat, and flexor laxity. Thirty to 70% of foals die at birth or in the peripartum period. Foal weights are greater in endophyte-exposed mares, despite poor muscle mass, which is probably attributable to the increased gestation length. Histologic examination of organs from foals exposed in utero to endophyte-infected fescue demonstrated enlarged, colloid-distended thyroid follicles. At birth, concentrations of tri-iodothyronine, progestogens, adrenocorticotropic hormone (ACTH), and cortisol are lower in foals from mares grazing endophyte-infected fescue.

The high incidence of perinatal morbidity and mortality can also be attributed to failure of passive transfer and neonatal sepsis. Not only do the mares fail to produce adequate colostrum, but there also is decreased absorption of immunoglobulins by the foals. When foals from mares grazing infected fescue are administered high-quality colostrum by nasogastric tube, concentrations of IgG at 24 hours of age are significantly lower than in foals whose dams have not grazed on infected fescue or are removed at 300 days of gestation.

REPRODUCTIVE EFFICIENCY

Mares grazing endophyte-infected tall fescue during winter anestrus and the vernal transition experience their first ovulation 4 to 5 weeks later than mares grazing noninfected grass. This delay in the initiation of ovulation represents a potential 25% loss, 5 of 20 weeks, in the effective length of the breeding season. Mares maintained on infected fescue may be supplemented with artificial light to provide 16 hours of light per day to minimize the delay in ovulation.

Continuous grazing of endophyte-infected fescue during breeding results in a 45% pregnancy rate at 14 days compared with 75% in mares grazing endophyte-free grass. At the end of a 60-day breeding period, the same percentage of mares is pregnant in both groups. A greater incidence

of prolonged luteal activity is observed in nonpregnant mares grazing infected fescue.

Early embryonic death is observed in 30% of mares grazing endophyte-infected fescue compared with approximately 10% of mares grazing endophyte-free pasture. Embryonic development based on vesicle height at day 14 after ovulation is not different between groups for embryos that maintain viability. Embryos that undergo early embryonic loss are smaller at day 14 or irregular in shape. Plasma progesterone concentrations are greater at 21 days after ovulation in endophyte-affected mares in which the embryo remains viable than in endophyte-affected mares that experience early embryonic death or that demonstrate prolonged luteal activity. The progesterone concentrations in all mares experiencing embryonic loss are greater than 6 ng/ml, suggesting a direct effect on the embryo rather than an effect on luteal function. Although abortion has been anecdotally attributed to grazing infected fescue, only two abortions occurred in over 100 pregnancies after 30 days of gestation in a multiyear study.

Thus, grazing endophyte-infected fescue can have a detrimental effect on reproductive efficiency owing to a delay in initiation of ovulation, an increase in cycles bred per pregnancy, prolongation of luteal function, and increased early embryonic loss. When mares must be maintained on endophyte-infected pastures during breeding, repeated examinations to diagnose and monitor pregnancy maintenance are necessary. Weekly or biweekly examination between days 14 and 40 are required to identify mares that have undergone embryonic loss or prolonged luteal function and to maximize reproductive performance.

APPROACH TO DIAGNOSIS

Definitive diagnosis of fescue toxicosis involves the identification of the causative endophytic fungus in forage or seed samples by microscopic examination. In addition, ergopeptine concentrations may be determined by HPLC analysis or specific enzyme-linked immunosorbent assay (ELISA) assays. Hypoprolactinemia is supportive of the diagnosis, but the assay is not commercially available.

Presumptive diagnosis of fescue toxicity in the pregnant mare is based on the failure of normal mammary development in the prepartum period and prolonged gestation in association with consuming tall fescue pasture or hay. Determination of maternal immunoreactive progestogen concentrations using a commercially available progesterone assay° is a very sensitive indicator of endophyte exposure. Mares grazing endophyte-infected fescue after day 300 of gestation fail to demonstrate the typically observed prepartum increase in progestogen concentrations (Fig. 1).

PREVENTION, MANAGEMENT, AND TREATMENT

With the vast acreage covered by fescue, the high percentage of endophyte infection, and the difficulty of eradication, much research has been directed toward minimiz-

---

°*Coat-A-Count Progesterone, Diagnostic Products, Los Angeles, CA*

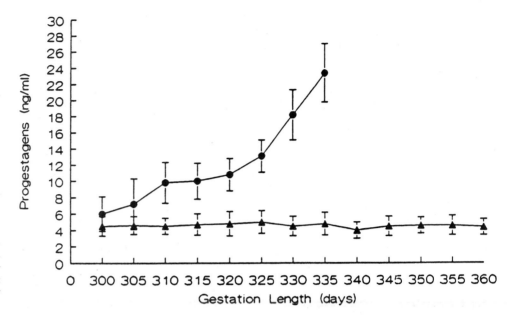

Figure 1. Progestogen concentrations in pregnant mares grazing endophyte-infected fescue from day 300 to parturition ● and mares not consuming infected fescue after day 300 ▲.

ing the toxic effects on pregnant mares. Supplementation of the pregnant mare's diet with selenium and energy, in the form of cracked corn, has failed to demonstrate any beneficial effects on the incidence of reproductive abnormalities in mares grazing infected fescue.

Removal of pregnant mares from endophyte-infected pastures during the last 30 days of gestation to either endophyte-free pastures or to dry lots with feeding of endophyte-free hay has been shown to be effective in eliminating signs of toxicity. If it is impossible to remove the mares, a high-quality legume hay should be fed ad libitum. Mammary gland development of mares that graze fescue should be monitored during the last 30 days of gestation.

In mares failing to demonstrate adequate mammary development, treatment with agents known to stimulate prolactin secretion should be considered to treat or preferentially prevent agalactia. Perphenazine (0.3–0.5 mg/kg p.o. b.i.d.) and reserpine (2.5–5.0 mg per horse p.o. s.i.d.) have been reported to initiate lactation in 1 to 5 days in agalactic mares. Domperidone (1.0 mg/kg p.o., s.i.d.), a dopamine antagonist, has been administered to late-term pregnant mares grazing infected fescue with a reversal of the signs of clinical toxicosis. Domperidone is currently available only on a research basis. Acepromazine (20 mg/horse IM q.i.d.) has been empirically used in agalactic mares. It should be noted that only acepromazine is approved for use in the horse. Adverse reactions to perphenazine have been reported and include excessive muscle tone, incomplete voluntary movements, and apparent excitability.

Attending parturition is recommended because of the risk of dystocia, premature placental separation, and neonatal asphyxia. An alternative source of immunoglobulins must be available to ensure adequate passive transfer of humoral immunity of the foal. Because of poor absorption of orally administered colostrum to postdate foals, it is essential to monitor IgG concentrations and administer plasma or hyperimmune serum in the event of failure of passive transfer. A supplemental nutritional source in the form of commercial mare-milk replacers, goat's milk, or the adoption of the foal by a nurse mare may be employed.

Supplemental Readings

Boosinger TR, Brendemuehl JP, Bransby DL, Wright JC, Kemppainen RJ, Kee DD: Prolonged gestation, decreased triiodothyronine concentration, and thyroid gland histomorphologic features in newborn foals of mares grazing *Acremonion coenophialum*-infected fescue. Am J Vet Res 56:66–69, 1995.

Brendemuehl JP, Boosinger TR, Bransby DI, Shelby RA: The effect of short term exposure to and removal from the fescue endophyte *Acremonium coenophialum* on pregnant mares and foal viability. Biol Reproduction Monograph Series No., 1, 61–67, 1995.

Brendemuehl JP, Boosinger TR, Pugh DG, Shelby RA: Influence of endophyte-infected tall fescue on cyclicity, pregnancy rate and early embryonic loss in the mare. Theriogenology 42:489–500, 1994.

Brendemuehl JP, Williams MA, Boosinger TR, Ruffin DG: Plasma progestogen, tri-iodothyronine, and cortisol concentrations in postdate gestation foals exposed in utero to the tall fescue endophyte *Acremonium coenophialum*. Biol Reproduction Monograph Series No., 1, 53–59, 1995.

Green EM, Loch WE, Messer NT: Maternal and fetal effects of endophyte fungus-infected fescue. Proc 37th Annu Conv Am Assoc Equine Pract, 1991, pp 29–44.

Putnam MR, Bransby DI, Schumacher J, Boosinger TR, Bush L, Shelby RA, Vaughn JT, Ball D, Brendemuehl JP: Effects of the fungal endophyte *Acremonium coenophialum* in fescue on pregnant mares and foal viability. Am J Vet Res 52:2071–2074, 1991.

Redmond LM, Cross DL, Strickland JR, Kennedy SW: Efficacy of domperidone and sulpiride as treatment for fescue toxicoses in horses. Am J Vet Res 55:722–729, 1995.

Care of Stallion Semen

DICKSON D. VARNER
College Station, Texas

The stallion delivers semen to the protective confines of the mare reproductive tract at the time of coitus. For semen evaluation or artificial insemination, humans intercept ejaculated spermatozoa normally en route to the mare. It therefore becomes mandatory that semen be appropriately handled in this "artificial" environment so that: (1) fertilizing capacity of the spermatozoa is retained, and (2) semen quality, as measured during a fertility examination, is an accurate reflection of that produced by the stallion.

COLLECTION OF SEMEN

Ejaculated semen is collected from stallions for artificial insemination of mares, or for assessment of semen quality, as part of a fertility examination. In either case, it is important that the spermatozoa be protected against injury, beginning with the semen-collection process. Numerous factors can result in destruction of spermatozoa, including temperature extremes, excessive light, toxic chemicals, or physical trauma from improper handling. To ensure utmost protection to spermatozoa, semen should be collected using an artificial vagina that has been properly prepared. Most stallions can be readily trained to serve an artificial vagina. Quality of semen collected in a condom is generally quite inferior to that obtained with an artificial vagina, because spermatozoa can be adversely affected by debris from the penis or toxicants within the condom.

Artificial Vaginas

Several models of artificial vaginas are available commercially (Table 1). Each has distinct attributes and limited disadvantages, but all serve their purpose well. Initial cost, maintenance costs, types of accessories, durability, weight,

TABLE 1. SOME MODELS AND SOURCES OF EQUINE ARTIFICIAL VAGINAS

MODEL	SOURCE
Missouri	901 Janesville Ave. Fort Atkinson, WS 53538–0901 (414) 563–2446
C.S.U.	Animal Reproduction Systems 14395 Ramona Ave. Chino, CA 91710 (909) 597–4889
Lane	Lane Manufacturing Co. 2075 S. Valentia Denver, CO 80231 (303) 745–2603
Roanoke	Roanoke A.I. Labs Route 7, Box 230 Roanoke, VA 24018 (703) 774–0676

temperature maintenance, and spermatozoal losses incurred during semen collection should be considered when contemplating purchase of an artificial vagina. Homemade artificial vaginas may also be constructed to meet specific needs.

It is imperative that all components of an artificial vagina coming into contact with semen are nontoxic to spermatozoa. Therefore, reusable items, including semen receptacles and rubber liners, should be properly cleaned and dried before use. Use of soaps and disinfectants to clean these parts is discouraged. Thorough rinsing with deionized water is advised. For disinfection, rubber liners can be submerged in 70% isopropyl or ethyl alcohol for 20 minutes, then air-dried before use. Rubber liners of some artificial vaginas can be toxic to spermatozoa. If possible, sterile, nontoxic disposable artificial-vagina liners or semen receptacles should be used to avoid contamination of semen with toxic chemicals and to minimize transmission of venereal diseases. Some stallions may not ejaculate when the penis enters an artificial vagina fitted with a plastic liner.

A filter should be installed in the artificial vagina before collection of semen. This filter allows the sperm-rich portion of an ejaculate to pass into the semen receptacle, but retains the gel fraction. The result is a higher usable sperm harvest because fewer spermatozoa become entrapped in the gel during collection. Newly developed nylon micromesh filters are preferable to conventional polyester matte filters.

Internal temperature of the artificial vagina normally should not exceed 45 to 48°C at the time of semen collection, because irreversible damage to spermatozoa can result from even short-term exposure to temperatures above this level. If the glans penis is beyond the water jacket of the artificial vagina at the time of ejaculation, as typically occurs when using the Missouri-model artificial vagina, the temperature of the water jacket can be adjusted to 50 to 60°C without temperature-related injury incurred by ejaculated spermatozoa. Only lubricants that are nonspermicidal should be used to lubricate the interior of the artificial vagina.

Other Considerations

Before collecting semen, the stallion's penis, particularly the distal portion, should be cleansed with water, then thoroughly dried. Soaps should be avoided because their use may lead to surface overgrowth with potentially pathogenic bacteria. Bactericidal soaps should be used only when it is necessary to rid the penile surface of bacteria before obtaining urethral culture swabs for bacterial analysis. Semen is generally collected after allowing the stallion to mount a breeding dummy or a receptive and properly restrained mare. Stallions can also be trained to ejaculate while standing.

Ejaculated semen is promptly transported to the laboratory for evaluation and further processing. During transit, semen should be maintained near body temperature (35–40°C) and protected from sunlight. If a filter was incorporated into the artificial vagina during semen collection, it is removed promptly to prevent seepage of gel into the gel-free portion of the ejaculate. Upon arrival in the laboratory, the semen should be promptly placed in an incubator adjusted to 37 to 38°C, then mixed with an appropriate semen extender.

EVALUATION OF SEMEN

Spermatozoal quality and quantity are assessed soon after collection. Color and consistency of the ejaculate are noted, paying particular attention to contamination of the sample with blood, urine, debris, or purulent material. Volume of the gel-free semen is determined by using a graduated cylinder to ensure accurate measurement. Spermatozoal concentration is determined using a hemacytometer counting chamber, or a spectrophotometer (550-nm wavelength) or densimeter properly calibrated using hemacytometer counts.

Evaluation of spermatozoal motility is considered to be a fundamental laboratory test for assessing the fertilizing capacity of an ejaculate. Because spermatozoal motility is extremely susceptible to environmental conditions, it is necessary to protect the semen from injurious agents or conditions before analysis. Taking such precautionary steps helps ensure that the motility estimate is representative of that intrinsic to the stallion and not depressed because of artifactual changes. The following basic steps should be observed to minimize environmental damage to spermatozoa before analysis:

- Collect semen using a properly prepared artificial vagina
- Promptly transport gel-free semen to the laboratory in a warm, light-shielded container, then place semen in an incubator maintained at 37 to 38°C
- Mix gel-free semen with an appropriate prewarmed (37 to 38°C) semen extender within 2 minutes after its collection
- Microscopically examine spermatozoal motility within 10 minutes after the semen is mixed with a semen extender
- Ensure that all equipment and glassware that come in contact with the semen are clean, nontoxic, and prewarmed to 37 to 38°C

To further enhance the reliability of motility estimation, the procedure should be done by an experienced person using a properly equipped microscope. A microscope with a built-in stage warmer and phase-contrast optics is preferred.

Several different techniques and instruments have been developed for objective, unbiased evaluation of spermatozoal motility; however, these methods, such as time-lapse photomicrography, frame-by-frame playback videomicrography, spectrophotometry, and computerized analysis, are too tedious or expensive for routine use. Subjective assessment of motility by visual estimation is more practical. This method is generally quite acceptable, provided that the criteria outlined earlier are met. Dilution of semen to a spermatozoal concentration of approximately 25×10^6/ml is recommended before analysis of motility because variation in spermatozoal concentration can affect subjective measurement of spermatozoal motility. Parameters of measurement generally include (1) percentage of spermatozoa that are motile; (2) percentage of spermatozoa that are progressively motile; and (3) spermatozoal velocity based on an arbitrary scale of 0 to 4. Longevity of spermatozoal motility may also be evaluated, both with raw semen at room temperature (20–25°C) and extended semen at room temperature or refrigerated temperature (4–6°C).

Morphology of spermatozoa is typically examined at $1000\times$ magnification. Major morphologic defects such as abnormal heads, abnormal midpieces, or proximal cytoplasmic droplets are known to interfere with fertility of stallions. A standard bright-field microscope can be used to examine air-dried and stained semen smears. Visualization of structural detail can be enhanced by viewing unstained spermatozoa as a wet-mount, using a microscope with phase-contrast or differential-interference optics. Clinicians who are inexperienced in assessment of spermatozoal morphology are encouraged to submit specimens to a reference laboratory for analysis.

SEMEN EXTENDERS

Semen collected for artificial insemination should always be placed in a semen extender, whether the semen is to be inseminated immediately or preserved. The semen extender enhances spermatozoal survival outside the stallion's genital tract by: (1) providing spermatozoa with metabolizable substrates; (2) accommodating spermatozoal pH and osmotic pressure requirements; (3) protecting spermatozoa against cold shock; and (4) eliminating or reducing bacterial growth in the semen through incorporation of antibiotics. Semen extenders may be purchased commercially or prepared in the laboratory (Table 2). If semen is to be used for insemination soon after collection, it should be mixed with semen extender at a 1:1 to 1:3 ratio (semen:extender). More extensive dilution is recommended if semen is to be stored for a prolonged period of time before insemination.

Milk-based or cream-gel extenders are considered to be optimal for maintaining viability of ejaculated spermatozoa. Egg yolk-based extenders or addition of egg yolk to milk-based extenders can have a depressing effect on spermatozoal function.

Addition of antibiotics to milk-based extender can affect spermatozoal motility following storage. Polymyxin B sulfate should be avoided as an antibiotic for semen extenders if semen is to be stored for prolonged periods because of its suppressing effect on spermatozoal motility. In a recent study, potassium penicillin G appeared to yield better motility results than sodium penicillin G or ticarcillin when added at 1000 IU or 1000 μg/ml. Amikacin sulfate tended to yield better motility results than gentamicin sulfate or streptomycin sulfate. In another study, ticarcillin yielded better results than amikacin sulfate or gentamicin sulfate following semen storage for 24 hours when antibiotics were added at 1000 μg/ml. Following semen storage for 48 hours, ticarcillin and amikacin sulfate yielded the most

TABLE 2.   COMMONLY USED EQUINE SEMEN EXTENDERS

NAME	FORMULA*
Kenney extender	1. Mix nonfat dry milk solids (2.4 g) and glucose (4.9 g) with 92 ml deionized water. 2. Add (a) crystalline penicillin G (150,000 IU) and crystalline streptomycin sulfate (150,000 μg), or (b) gentamicin sulfate (100 mg) mixed with 2 ml of 7.5% sodium bicarbonate.
Modified Kenney extender (Texas A&M University formula)	1. Mix nonfat dry milk solids (24 g), glucose (27 g), and sucrose (40 g) with 907 ml deionized water. 2. Add potassium penicillin G (1,000,000 IU) and amikacin sulfate (1 g).
Skim milk extender	1. Heat 100 ml nonfortified skim milk to 92–95°C for 10 minutes in a double boiler. Cool. 2. Add polymyxin B sulfate (100,00 IU).
Cream-gel extender	1. Dissolve 1.3 g unflavored Knox gelatin in 10 ml sterile deionized water. Sterilize. 2. Heat Half & Half cream to 92–95°C for 2–4 minutes in a double boiler. Remove scum from surface. 3. Mix gelatin solution with 90 ml of heated Half & Half cream (100 ml total volume). Cool. 4. Add crystalline penicillin G (100,000 IU), streptomycin sulfate (100,000 μg), and polymyxin B sulfate (20,000 IU).
Modified cream-gel extender (Neely formula)	1. Heat Half & Half cream (1 pint) to 85–92°C in a glass flask in a double boiler for 10 minutes. Remove scum from surface. 2. Dissolve 6 g unflavored Knox gelatin in 40 ml 5% dextrose and heat to 65°C in a water bath. 3. Add hot gelatin solution to cream and allow to cool covered to 35–40°C. 4. Add potassium penicillin G (1,000,000 IU), or potassium penicillin G (1,000,000 IU) and amikacin sulfate (0.5 g).

*Many different antibiotics and antibiotic dosages have been used with these basic extenders, including: potassium penicillin G (1000–2000 IU/ml), streptomycin sulfate (1000-1500 μg/ml), polymyxin B sulfate (200–1000 IU/ml), gentamicin sulfate (100–1000 μg/ml), amikacin sulfate (100–1000 μg/ml), or ticarcillin (100–1000 μg/ml). Use of gentamicin sulfate or amikacin sulfate may require the addition of sodium bicarbonate to adjust the pH of the extender to 6.8–7.0. The extenders can be stored in small packages at −20°C and thawed immediately prior to use.

favorable results, followed by gentamicin sulfate. Bacterial growth in extended semen may not be adequately controlled through use of any antibiotics used singly. In a recent study, a combination of potassium penicillin G (1000 IU/ml) and amikacin sulfate (1000 μg/ml) improved spermatozoal motility, as compared with either antibiotic used singly, and bacteria were more effectively controlled.

ARTIFICIAL INSEMINATION

Artificial insemination is permitted by the vast majority of United States breed associations. Only sterile, nontoxic disposable equipment should be used for the procedure. All-plastic syringes° are recommended for artificial insemination because the rubber plunger seals of some syringes contain toxic materials that may leach into the semen. All inseminations should be performed using a minimum contamination technique. With the mare adequately restrained, and the tail wrapped and elevated, the area between the base of the tail and ventral commissure of the vulva is thoroughly scrubbed, rinsed, and dried. Particular attention is given to removal of debris from the caudal vestibule and clitoral fossa. Semen contained within a syringe is deposited into the anterior uterine body through an 18- to 22-inch sterile insemination pipette. A sterile or clean plastic shoulder-length sleeve should be worn when passing the pipette through the cervix to the uterine body where the semen is to be deposited.

°Air-Tite, Vineland, NJ

Mares are generally inseminated with 250 to 500 × 10⁶ progressively motile spermatozoa, which is contained in a semen extender. Volume of the inseminate typically ranges from 5 to 20 ml; however, insemination volume can be as high as 50 to 120 ml without a corresponding reduction in fertility, provided that spermatozoal concentration is at least 25 to 50 × 10⁶ sperm/ml. For maximal pregnancy rates, it is best to inseminate mares within 12 to 48 hours before ovulation, although pregnancies have been achieved at a similar rate when mares are inseminated within 12 hours following ovulation. Pregnancy rate following post-ovulation breeding may be increased if semen is placed in a milk-based extender containing heparin (final heparin concentration of 10–40 μg/ml) before insemination. Using semen from fertile stallions, mares may sometimes be inseminated 48 to 72 hours before ovulation with no depression in pregnancy rate.

PRESERVATION OF SEMEN

The number of breed registries in the United States that permit the use of stored (i.e., cooled or frozen) or transported semen is continually increasing. Semen from fertile stallions can often be stored in the liquid state for 24 to 48 hours or longer without a corresponding reduction in fertility. To maximize longevity of spermatozoal viability when stored in this manner, semen should first be mixed with a good-quality semen extender at a high dilution ratio. Best results are obtained when semen is diluted to 25 to 50 × 10⁶/ml before storage, or seminal plasma volume is reduced to only 5 to 20% by dilution with extender or centrifugation and resuspension in extender (i.e., a dilution ratio of 1:4 to 1:19 [semen:extender]). Centrifugation time and g-force must be critically evaluated to determine the appropriate centrifugation technique required to maximize spermatozoal harvest without undue injury to spermatozoa created by the centrifugation process. Supplementation of milk-based extenders with electrolytes, buffers, and energy sources has improved motility of spermatozoa following storage, especially if ejaculated semen is first centrifuged to remove most of the seminal plasma. The safety of these supplements with regard to fertility awaits confirmation.

Both cooling rate and storage temperature have an effect on spermatozoal survival following storage. A storage temperature of 4 to 6°C is considered preferable as long as a relatively slow cooling rate is permitted, especially at temperatures below 20°C. Recent studies have shown that the area of the cooling phase at which spermatozoa are most sensitive to rapid cooling is between 20°C and 5°C. Spermatozoa can be rapidly cooled from 37°C to 20°C, but they require a linear cooling rate of −0.05 to −0.1°C/minute from 20°C to 5°C to maximize spermatozoal motility. Passive cooling systems that permit slow cooling of semen to refrigerated temperature are available commercially. These systems also protect the semen if it is to be shipped to another location. Development of these products has made breeding with "mail order" semen a relatively easy and successful venture for mare owners. Active cooling systems are not yet sold commercially.

Freezing of horse semen has not been as successful as with semen from dairy bulls, probably owing to biophysical and biochemical differences in the spermatozoa of these two species. Pregnancy rate per cycle in mares bred with frozen and thawed semen is reported to range from 70 to 10% or less. Although the upper level of this range would lead one to suspect that it might be commercially feasible, the pregnancy rate is in the 30 to 40% range for many stallions.

A wide variety of extender types have been used to process semen for freezing. No single extender has been identified as superior for this purpose. Most extenders contain a source of lipoproteins. The lipoproteins are adsorbed to the plasma membrane of spermatozoa and aid in stabilizing membranes during the freeze/thaw cycles. Monosaccharides (e.g., glucose or fructose), disaccharides (e.g., sucrose or lactose), and trisaccharides (e.g., raffinose) are also commonly incorporated in semen extenders. Disaccharides and trisaccharides are nonpermeable sugars and are used primarily because of their osmotic effects. Monosaccharides also have osmotic properties. In addition, they can be utilized by spermatozoa as a source of energy. Glycerol is used universally as a cryoprotectant. This molecule is incorporated into the interior of spermatozoa and exerts its effect both intracellularly and extracellularly. Assorted electrolytes, and sometimes detergents, are typical components of freezing extenders as well.

Various packaging systems are available for semen freezing. Most commonly, semen is packaged in polyvinylchloride straws with volume capacity ranging from 0.5 ml to 5 ml. Occasionally, polypropylene bags or flattened aluminum tubes are used as semen packages. These containers accommodate volumes of 10 to 25 ml. Semen is generally thawed in a water bath. Temperature of the water bath and thawing time are dependent on the type of packaging system used when freezing the semen.

Sperm number per package is also subject to considerable variation. Semen processing personnel usually place 100 to 1000 × 10⁶ sperm per package. The number of package units required as an insemination dose varies from one to 10 or more. The veterinarian who is responsible for thawing semen and inseminating mares must obtain written information from the processing facility regarding the number of packages, contents required per insemination dose, and thawing and insemination protocols.

Information available to date suggests that frozen and thawed semen is not dramatically affected by extender type, packaging system, or freezing method (i.e., freezing semen in static nitrogen vapor versus a computerized nitrogen vapor freezer with specific preprogrammed freeze rates). Fertility can be affected by insemination dose. An insemination dose should probably contain a minimum of 200×10^6 progressively motile spermatozoa.

Freezability of semen varies greatly among individual stallions. Ejaculates from a particular stallion can also respond differently to the freezing and thawing processes. Mare owners and their attending veterinarians should contact stallion owners and agents for semen processing facilities to obtain accurate information regarding fertility results with frozen and thawed semen from stallions of interest before contracting for shipment of frozen semen. Pregnancy rate per cycle is the measurement that yields the most information about fertility of semen. A veterinarian should also encourage owners to use only mares that are considered fertile. This policy greatly increases the likelihood of a successful outcome.

Laboratory-based tests are commonly used to evaluate viability of frozen and thawed spermatozoa. The percentage of progressively motile spermatozoa in samples is the most widely employed parameter of measurement. Although post-thaw motility of spermatozoa provides useful information regarding sperm viability, it is not an exact measure of fertilizing potential. Some semen samples express a high percentage of progressively motile sperm yet yield low pregnancy rates. Likewise, some samples contain a lowered percentage of progressively motile spermatozoa but possess acceptable fertility. Investigators have attempted to develop additional tests that would improve the predictive power of laboratory testing. The tests developed to date have not satisfied this need.

Post-thawed spermatozoa are considered to have lowered longevity in comparison with freshly ejaculated spermatozoa. Therefore, insemination of mares with frozen and thawed semen should be reserved for the periovulatory period. The ovaries of mares can be evaluated daily while in estrus until a dominant follicle 35 mm in diameter or larger is detected. As ovulation approaches, the ovaries should probably be examined two to four times daily to more closely predict the exact time of ovulation. Transrectal ultrasonography aides the clinician in detecting ovarian changes consistent with imminent ovulation. Ideally, mares should be inseminated within 6 to 12 hours before ovulation or within 6 hours after ovulation. Some practitioners regularly breed mares both before and after ovulation. The usefulness of this breeding policy has not been critically examined. Administration of human chorionic gonadotrophin (hCG; 2000–2500 IU) to mares with a dominant follicle of specific size (35 mm in diameter) provides additional predictive power regarding timing of ovulation because most of these mares ovulate 36 to 40 hours following injection of hCG.

Supplemental Readings

Amann RP, Pickett BW: Principles of cryopreservation and a review of cryopreservation of stallion spermatozoa. J Equine Vet Sci 7:145–173, 1987.

Bedford SJ, Hinrichs K: The effect of insemination volume on pregnancy rates of pony mares. Theriogenology 42:571–578, 1994.

Fleet TL, Varner DD, Blanchard TL, Vogelsang MM, Thompson JA: Use of heparin to accelerate capacitation of equine spermatozoa *in vivo.* Biol Reprod Monograph Series 1, 1995, pp. 713–718.

Hoyumpa AH, McIntosh AL, Varner DD, Scanlan CM: Normal bacterial flora of equine semen: Antibacterial effects of amikacin, penicillin, and an amikacin-penicillin combination in a seminal extender. Proc 12th Int Cong Anim Reprod, 1992, pp 1427–1429.

Jasko DJ, Bedford SJ, Cook NL, Mumford EL, Squires EL, Pickett BW: Effect of antibiotics on motion characteristics of cooled stallion spermatozoa. Theriogenology 40:885–893, 1993.

Jasko DJ, Lein DH, Foote RH: Determination of the relationship between sperm morphologic classifications and fertility in stallions: 66 cases (1987–1988). J Am Vet Med Assoc 197:389–394, 1990.

Jasko DJ, Martin JM, Squires EL: Effect of insemination volume and concentration of spermatozoa on embryo recovery in mares. Theriogenology 37:1233–1239, 1992.

Kayser JP, Amann RP, Shideler RK, Squires EL, Jasko DJ, Pickett BW: Effects of linear cooling rate on motion characteristics of stallion spermatozoa. Theriogenology 38:601–614, 1992.

Kenney RM, Bergman RV, Cooper WL, Morse GW: Minimal contamination techniques for breeding mares: Technique and preliminary findings. Proc Annu Meet Am Assoc Equine Pract, 1975, pp 327–336.

Kenney RM, Hurtgen JP, Pierson R, Witherspoon D, Simons J: Manual for Clinical Fertility Evaluation of the Stallions. Hastings, NE, Society for Theriogenology, 1983, 100 pp.

McDonnell SM, Love CC: Manual stimulation collection of semen from stallions: Training time, sexual behavior and semen. Theriogenology 33:1201–1210, 1990.

Metcalf L: Maximizing reproductive efficiency in private practice: The management of mares and the use of cryopreserved semen. Proc Soc Therio, 1995, pp 155–159.

Padilla AW, Foote RH: Extender and centrifugation effects on the motility patterns of slow-cooled stallion spermatozoa. J Anim Sci 69:3308–3313, 1991.

Pickett BW, Amann RP: Extension and storage of stallion spermatozoa: A review. J Equine Vet Sci 7:289–308, 1987.

Samper JC: Stallion semen cryopreservation: Male factors affecting pregnancy rates. Proc Soc Therio, 1995, pp 160–165.

Varner DD, Blanchard TL: Current perspectives on handling and storage of equine semen. Proc Annu Meet Am Assoc Equine Pract, 1994, pp 39–40.

Varner DD, McIntosh AL, Forrest DW, Blanchard TL, Johnson L: Potassium penicillin G, amikacin sulfate, or a combination in seminal extender for stallions: Effects on spermatozoal motility. Proc 12th Int Cong Anim Reprod, 1992, pp 1496–1498.

Webb GW, Arns MJ: Influence of modified Tyrode's media on motility of cold-stored stallion spermatozoa. Proc 14th Equine Nutr Physiol Symp, 1995, pp 160–161.

Reproductive Diseases in the Stallion

CHARLES C. LOVE
St. Louis, Missouri

This chapter is an addition to previous editions describing reproductive conditions of the stallion. It is not intended to be complete, but rather to update the clinician on certain facts that may not have been presented in previous editions.

ANEJACULATION

When the clinician is presented with a stallion that will not ejaculate, there are several potential causes of the anejaculatory condition. These range from factors that may be termed psychological to those that are physical in origin. Often the psychological presentation is incorrectly diagnosed when the inability to ejaculate is actually a result of an iatrogenic cause, such as rough handling of the stallion during the breeding process or improper preparation and handling of the artificial vagina during the collection process. It is critical that these more likely potential causes are eliminated before the diagnosis of a psychological problem is accepted.

One way of evaluating the possible contributions of these iatrogenic influences is to eliminate as many of them as possible. This can be accomplished by changing the stallion handler. The most extreme possibility is to turn the stallion out with a mare in estrus. In most instances this cannot be effected because of the risk of injury. An alternative is to allow the stallion, handled in-hand, to breed a mare in estrus, naturally. This method determines whether the artificial vagina is the source of the problem.

Pain can also be the source of ejaculatory dysfunction, and this can also be a very difficult cause to diagnose. Many stallions in which pain is a primary or contributing cause may not exhibit overt signs of discomfort when standing on all four legs, but rather may only demonstrate signs when they are mounted on the mare. This may result from the posture of the stallion during the breeding process, in which the neck is flexed and the hind legs bear more weight than normal, and it may result in a different degree of stress exerted in those areas at the time of breeding. Therefore, because a stallion is sound when exercised or bearing weight on all four legs does not mean that pain is not a primary or a contributing cause of the discomfort. A stallion may pin his ears back when mounted on the mare, may fail to couple well when mounted on the mare because that particular posture is too painful, and may therefore hang back off the mare and have a difficult time achieving intromission.

Diagnostically there are several approaches to take. Initially, a complete lameness evaluation should be performed, concentrating on the neck, back, and hind legs. Evaluation of the neck and back can be difficult because of the limited use of radiography in these two areas. Therefore, careful observation of how the stallion handles himself can be the most important diagnostic sign.

One condition that is an infrequent cause of anejaculation is aortoiliac thrombosis (see page 267). A thrombus is formed in the terminal aorta and can involve the internal and external iliac arteries. A stallion may readily mount the mare and may be able to attain as well as maintain an erection, but the hind legs become fatigued and the stallion discontinues thrusting and is unable to dismount; he may even fall off the mare suddenly. This condition can be easily diagnosed by ultrasonographic and manual per rectum evaluation of the terminal aorta.

Treatment

Phenylbutazone (2.0 g b.i.d. for 3 days, then 1.0 g b.i.d. for 3–5 days) can be administered to determine if musculoskeletal pain is a source of the problem. A diagnosis based on a single administration should be avoided because blood levels of the drug may not have had adequate opportunity to stabilize. The horse's breeding behavior should be re-evaluated following at least 6 to 7 days of therapy.

It is the author's opinion that stallions that are identified as anejaculatory can be treated effectively using a combination of medical and behavioral therapy. This may be because before the onset of clinical signs many of these stallions were behaviorally normal, but as a result of the pain they manifested an abnormal behavior that became the presenting sign. Therefore, to resolve the presenting sign, the root of the problem must be identified.

BACTERIAL COLONIZATION OF THE EXTERNAL GENITALIA

Cultures of swabbings of the stallion external genitalia have become a routine aspect of the breeding soundness evaluation. The intent of these cultures is the isolation and identification of potential bacterial pathogens, such as *Klebsiella pneumoniae* and *Pseudomonas aeruginosa*, from the penis and prepuce. Some of the sites cultured include the preputial folds, the shaft, and the fossa glandis. These sites are usually swabbed before cleansing of the penis. The urethra is also cultured following cleansing of the penis and then immediately following ejaculation. The intent of the latter two swabs is to evaluate potential infections of the internal accessory glands, recognizing that the accessory glands are the most common sites for these types of infections.

Colonization of the external genitalia by bacterial pathogens is more frequent than overt infection of the accessory glands and does not present a risk to the stallion's health.

The major risk is the transmittal of the pathogens to mares during the breeding process.

Adequate acquisition and interpretation of swab culture results are heavily dependent on clinician expertise and familiarity with the process. *Klebsiella* and *Pseudomonas* species are environmental commensals that may be inadvertently isolated and incorrectly implicated as a cause of the infertile condition. However, only select serotypes are associated with infertility in the mare and should be considered pathogenic. The stallion is the source of infection only if the serotype isolated from his external genitalia is the same as the one isolated in the mare. Despite the latter fact, there still may be significant pressure to rid the stallion of this historically significant pathogen.

Treatment

Treatment for colonization of the penis involves topical application of an antibiotic ointment to which the organism is sensitive. Ointment can be applied daily following cleansing of the penis with warm water. Because *Pseudomonas* species are intolerant of acidic conditions, an acidic solution (10 ml concentrated HCl in 1 gallon of water) can be applied to the erect penis daily. In the case of *Klebsiella,* which is intolerant of alkaline conditions, 45 ml of 5.25% sodium hypochlorite can be added to a gallon of water and applied in a similar fashion. This approach has the advantage that both are cheap to make and can be easily applied daily to the affected stallion. In addition, it is unnecessary to use expensive antimicrobials when a bacterial resistance has developed.

SEMINAL VESICULITIS

Infection of the seminal vesicles should be suspected when small to moderate amounts of blood and purulent material are present in the final portions of the ejaculate. This can be ascertained by collecting the ejaculate with an open-ended artificial vagina such that the jets of the ejaculate can be collected and analyzed separately for the presence of blood and leukocytes. The amount of blood and leukocytes can vary from trace to overt amounts, depending on the extent of the condition.

Treatment

Several approaches can be considered for treatment. Systemic therapy can be instituted using antimicrobials to which the organism is sensitive. This can be very expensive and time-consuming, requiring the use of costly antibiotics coupled with administration three to four times per day. In addition, the inflamed accessory gland may limit effective antimicrobial penetration to achieve the required antibiotic level.

Antibiotics may also be applied directly to the lumen of the accessory gland. An endoscope is passed into the urethra to the level of the seminal colliculus, where both the ampullar and seminal vesicular openings are located. A catheter can then be passed through the accessory channel of the endoscope and inserted into the seminal vesicular opening of the affected seminal vesicle.

Despite vigorous therapy, this condition may remain refractory to treatment, requiring a decision on the clinician's part regarding if and how the stallion is to breed. Seminal vesiculitis does not affect the actual quality of the spermatozoa produced by the testes and because it does not cause any systemic signs such as pyrexia, there is no threat to the stallion's health. Although the presence of blood and purulent material may reduce the fertility of a stallion, this condition can be managed to optimize and maintain the stallion's fertility.

Semen extenders (see page 575) can be used to dilute the potential toxic effects of the blood and purulent material. In addition, an antimicrobial to which the bacteria are sensitive can be added to eliminate bacterial growth. When natural cover is required, the extender can be infused into the uterus immediately before the cover so that the semen immediately contacts extender following ejaculation.

OCCLUDED AMPULLAE

The ampullae, the widened terminal portion of the ductus deferens, are not true accessory glands but are considered as such when performing the breeding soundness evaluation. The bulk of the ampulla is composed of the glandular portion that is surrounded by the two layers of smooth muscle. This glandular portion is a relatively large potential space in which sperm can accumulate if they are not normally voided in the urine.

Either one or both ampullae can become occluded with sperm and completely or partially limit the passage of sperm at the time of ejaculation. If blockage is complete in both ampullae, the stallion may be azoospermic; if partial, the stallion may have varying numbers of immotile sperm that may or may not have detached heads. The number of detached heads is probably related to the duration of the condition because the longer the sperm have remained in the ampullae, the greater the effect of the heat stress on the integrity of the neck of the sperm. The condition may also be subclinical if one ampulla is patent and the other is blocked. In the latter case, sperm quality may be unaffected but daily sperm output will be half that expected based on the size of the stallion's testes. Although the condition is fertility limiting, it is not irreversible, but the prognosis is usually excellent, assuming that the testes are able to produce normal sperm.

Diagnosis is usually based on presenting signs and may be confirmed using ultrasonography of the distended ampullar lumen. Enlargement of the lumen as well as the oversize of the ampulla is an infrequent finding in most cases, but may occur in long-standing conditions. A more frequent ultrasonographic presentation is an increase in the luminal diameter without an increase in the outside diameter. This may be accompanied by a hyperechoic line in the lumen, representing the retained spermatozoa.

Treatment

Treatment is directed at "loosening" the accumulated sperm by manual massage of the ampullae per rectum. Massage can be relatively vigorous using the flexed middle finger to knead the ampulla in a longitudinal fashion for about 5 minutes, if the stallion tolerates it. A semen sample should then be collected to see if the blockage is released. Administration of oxytocin (20 IU IV) immediately before semen collection may enhance smooth muscle contraction around the lumen of the ampullae. Oxytocin administration and semen collection should be repeated until the sperm quality has stabilized. This may take 1 to 2 weeks of twice-daily ejaculations, depending on the severity of the condition.

Recurrence is possible after an extended period of sexual abstinence, and therefore the clinician should be particularly aware of stallions presented at the beginning of the breeding season with infertility and semen-related problems.

Supplemental Readings

Kenney RM, Hurtgen JP, Pierson R: Breeding Soundness Evaluation of the Stallion. Hastings, NE, Society for Theriogenology, 1993.
Love CC: Ultrasonographic evaluation of the testis, epididymis, and spermatic cord of the stallion. Vet Clin North Am Equine Pract 8(1)167–182, 1992.
Love CC, Garcia ML, Riera FL, Kenney RM: Evaluation of measures taken by ultrasonography and calipers to estimate testicular volume and daily sperm output in the stallion. J Reprod Fertil 44:99–105, 1991.
Varner DD, Schumacher J, Blanchard TL, Johnson L: Diseases and Management of Breeding Stallions. Goleta, CA, American Veterinary Publications, 1991.

13

THE FOAL

Edited by Guy D. Lester

Immunodeficiencies of Foals

MELISSA TROGDON HINES
Pullman, Washington

Foals at birth are immunologically naive and, although immunocompetent, some aspects of their immune function are diminished when compared with adults. The increased susceptibility of neonates to infection is a well-recognized phenomenon in all species. In foals, bacterial infection, particularly gram-negative septicemia, constitutes a major cause of morbidity and mortality. Although the reasons for the enhanced susceptibility of neonates to infection are not fully understood, inherent deficits in the neonatal immune system may play a role. In addition, several specific immunodeficiencies have been recognized in foals, which are of significance in individual cases.

IMMUNITY IN NEONATES

Most interest has been focused on development of the specific immune system in foals. However, particularly in naive foals, nonspecific immune mechanisms undoubtedly play an important role in resistance to infection. Based on limited studies in foals and on findings in other species, it appears that many components of the nonspecific immune system, such as complement, neutrophils, and macrophages, may be compromised in neonates. For example, there is evidence that foal neutrophils are deficient in phagocytic ability and hydrogen peroxide release, which may predispose to early infection. In addition, once gram-negative infection is established in foals, there is generally a significant decrease in the neutrophil count. Failure of the neutrophil count to subsequently recover has been associated with a grave prognosis. Therefore, future adjunct treatments may include granulocyte transfusions or administration of granulocyte colony-stimulating factor, in an effort to increase neutrophil production and upregulate function.

It is well documented that the specific immune system of foals is competent at birth. Functional T lymphocytes are present in the fetus by 100 days of gestational age, although in vitro assessment of the responsiveness of lymphocytes to phytolectins suggests that cell-mediated immune function may still be immature at birth. Functional B cells are present by 200 days of gestational age, and equine fetuses are capable of producing specific antibody in response to antigen exposure at this age. Detectable quantities of IgM are generally found in the fetal circulation by day 200, and are consistently found in the presuckle sera of normal foals at birth. Wide variation exists in the time of onset of IgG synthesis in utero, which may reflect differences in the antigenic stimulation of fetuses. In general, most foals are born with little or no circulating IgG. In immunologically naive foals, the primary immune response results in detectable serum concentrations of autogenous IgG at approximately 2 weeks of age, with concentrations approaching adult values by 4 months of age. The numbers of circulating B cells may not reach adult values until 3 weeks of age.

COLOSTRAL IMMUNITY

The diffuse epitheliochorial placentation of the mare does not provide for transplacental transfer of immunoglobulins, and therefore the newborn foal depends on the passive transfer of immunity through the ingestion and absorption of colostrum. A specialized secretion of the mammary gland, colostrum is normally produced under hormonal influences during the last 2 to 4 weeks of gestation. Secretion of colostrum by the equine mammary gland occurs only once during each pregnancy and is short-lived, with colostrum usually being replaced by milk within 12

581

hours from the time the mammary gland is first suckled by the foal.

Immunoglobulin is the best characterized component of colostral immunity. The equine mammary gland concentrates immunoglobulins from the circulation. Colostrum contains predominantly IgG and IgG(T), with lower concentrations of IgA and IgM. Specialized epithelial cells in the small intestine are responsible for the nonselective uptake of colostral immunoglobulins by pinocytosis, the efficiency of which is increased by low-molecular-weight enhancement factors present in the colostrum. The uptake of immunoglobulin from the gastrointestinal tract declines over time, with the greatest absorption occurring within the first 6 to 8 hours following birth. Absorption decreases significantly thereafter in most foals, regardless of oral intake. By 24 to 36 hours of age, the specialized enterocytes are replaced by more mature cells unable to take up immunoglobulin. The half life of maternally derived immunoglobulin is 20 to 23 days, and serum concentrations are minimal to absent by 5 to 6 months of age. Because normal foals are producing significant quantities of autogenous immunoglobulin at this age, overall serum immunoglobulin concentrations tend to be lowest in foals at 1 to 2 months of age.

A number of colostral components other than immunoglobulin contribute to protective immunity in neonates. For example, colostrum is a source of complement and lactoferrin, which enhance host defenses. In addition, colostrum activates granulocytes, regulates cell-mediated immunity, and provides a local protective effect in the gastrointestinal tract. Some of these effects may be mediated by cytokines present in the colostrum, such as tumor necrosis factor-alpha, interleukin-1, interleukin-2, interleukin-6 and interferon-gamma. These cytokines may influence maturation of the neonatal immune system through their immunomodulatory effects.

FAILURE OF PASSIVE TRANSFER

Failure of passive transfer (FPT), which is the inadequate transfer of colostral immunoglobulin, is the most common immune disorder of foals, with an estimated incidence of between 2.9 and 25%. Although long recognized as a risk factor for sepsis, the actual significance of FPT remains controversial. Although several studies have demonstrated a positive correlation between FPT and the incidence of equine neonatal sepsis, others have failed to confirm such a relationship, and factors other than the amount of immunoglobulin clearly influence the development of infection. These factors include the type of management, environmental conditions, virulence of pathogens, concurrent stress or disease, and specificity of the antibody. Despite the varying association between FPT and infection, low concentrations of serum immunoglobulin are a predisposing factor for infection, which in many cases can be minimized by management practices. Because of the number of factors contributing to the occurrence of sepsis, the minimal concentration of immunoglobulin necessary for protection varies with the farm and individual situation. Most normal foals nurse by 2 hours of age and obtain an immunoglobulin concentration of more than 800

mg/dl. Currently, complete FPT is most often defined by serum IgG concentrations of less than 200 mg/dl; partial FPT is defined by serum concentrations of 200 to 800 mg/dl, and concentrations higher than 800 mg/dl are considered optimal.

Causes of FPT

Failure of passive transfer can occur as a result of both maternal and neonatal factors. The major causes are listed in the following sections.

Loss of Colostrum via Premature Lactation

Mares that drip milk before parturition have been shown to have lower colostral concentrations of IgG than mares that do not. Although the factors predisposing to this problem are not well understood, premature lactation has been associated with twinning, placentitis, and premature placental separation.

Inadequate Immunoglobulin Content in the Colostrum

This may occur as a result either of a failure to produce an adequate volume of colostrum or a failure of the mammary gland to concentrate an adequate amount of IgG. Although variable, the volume of colostrum normally ingested by healthy light-breed foals is approximately 2 to 4 L during the first 12 hours of life. Agalactia or delayed onset of milk production may occur in association with ingestion of endophyte-infected fescue or with serious illness in the mare. In addition, mares that foal prematurely or in which parturition is induced may not produce enough colostrum of sufficient quality as a result of disruption of the normal sequence of hormonal changes that occur in the final stages of gestation. Generally, subnormal colostral IgG content (<3000 mg/dl) is uncommon in mares that foal at term and do not lactate prior to parturition, but there is wide individual variation in colostral immunoglobulin content, which is partially the result of genetic factors.

Failure to Ingest an Adequate Volume of Colostrum in the Early Postpartum Period

Neonatal weakness or rejection of the foal by the mare are common reasons for inadequate ingestion of colostrum.

Failure to Absorb Colostrum

Malabsorption is incriminated as a cause of FPT when foals that are known to have ingested an adequate volume of high-quality colostrum have a low serum concentration of immunoglobulin. Although the specialized enterocytes responsible for absorption normally appear early in fetal development, many premature foals have low serum IgG concentrations despite ingestion of colostrum. Because many of these foals have concurrent illnesses, it is unclear if the low immunoglobulin concentration is the result of malabsorption or differences in the distribution and catabolism of IgG in sick foals. In addition, it has been suggested that elevated concentrations of endogenous or exogenous glucocorticoids may hasten the maturation of the enterocytes and may decrease the efficiency of absorption.

Assessment of Passive Transfer of Immunoglobulins

Bacteremia in neonatal foals can develop by 24 hours of age or earlier, making the early recognition of FPT important. In foals that nurse within 2 hours of birth, serum concentrations of IgG are detectable by 6 hours of age and generally peak by 18 hours. Thus, routine evaluation of the IgG concentration in foals should generally be performed at 18 to 24 hours of age when absorption from the intestinal tract is essentially complete. Foals that are considered at high risk for FPT or for infection may be evaluated at 6 to 12 hours of age, allowing the oral supplementation of colostrum if the concentration of IgG is very low. It is advisable to assess the immunoglobulin status of all sick neonates.

Several tests are currently available for assessing passive transfer. It is important to remember that total protein determination is generally not useful in the foal for evaluating the passive transfer status, because the total protein is influenced by too many factors to accurately estimate the IgG concentration. The most accurate test to determine serum IgG concentration has been single radial immunodiffusion (RID), although there is still up to 20% variability in results.° The major disadvantage of this test is that results are not available for 5 to 24 hours. Because rapid therapeutic intervention is important in FPT, numerous field screening tests for FPT have been developed. The zinc sulfate turbidity test, which measures total immunoglobulin based on the formation of a precipitate when immunoglobulin combines with zinc ions, has been widely used in multiple species. A commercial test kit is available, or the reagent may be made.† The test requires approximately 1 hour, and under some conditions, the concentration of IgG may be overestimated. The enzyme-linked immunosorbent assay (ELISA), which is designed for the semi-quantitative measurement of IgG in equine serum, plasma or whole blood, utilizes a color spot with calibration standards corresponding to concentrations of 200, 400, and 800 mg/dl of IgG.‡ The assay is rapid, requiring approximately 10 to 15 minutes, and results have correlated well with RID. Other available rapid screening tests include (1) the latex agglutination test, which estimates IgG concentration from the degree of agglutination between IgG in serum or blood and latex beads coated with antibody to equine IgG, and (2) the glutaraldehyde clot test, which is based on the ability of glutaraldehyde to react with gammaglobulin, forming a solid clot.§

Treatment

Although many foals with FPT remain healthy, others rapidly develop sepsis. In addition, there is evidence that once sepsis is established it is more difficult to raise serum concentrations of IgG. Therefore, prevention of FPT by ensuring adequate consumption of colostrum is optimal. When situations do result in diminished passive transfer,

there are no universally accepted recommendations for determining which foals require treatment. It is generally recommended that all foals with serum concentrations of IgG lower than 400 mg/dl receive treatment, whereas treatment of those with concentrations between 400 and 800 mg/dl is dependent on evaluation of other risk factors, such as environmental conditions and concomitant problems.

Oral Supplementation

Foals that do not nurse or in which FPT is identified at less than 12 hours of age can usually be managed by oral immunoglobulin supplementation. Ideally, equine colostrum should be given, with the quantity required depending on the size of the foal, the degree of FPT, the quality of the colostrum, and the efficiency of absorption from the intestinal tract, which is usually unknown. Although good-quality colostrum is typically sticky, thick, and yellow, appearance can be misleading. A more accurate assessment of colostral immunoglobulin content can be made by RID, by the glutaraldehyde clot test, or by the measurement of specific gravity using a colostrometer.° The specific gravity of colostrum is directly correlated with the IgG concentration. Acceptable colostrum should have a minimum specific gravity of 1.060 and an IgG concentration higher than 3000 mg/dl. If colostrum from the mare is not available, frozen colostrum can be given. A colostrum bank can be established by collecting colostrum from mares that die during parturition or that lose their foals. Small volumes can be collected from mares that have high-quality colostrum and healthy foals without adverse effects on the foal. Approximately 200 to 250 ml of colostrum should be collected 1 to 2 hours after parturition, after the foal has suckled several times, and preferably from the teat opposite that from which the foal first nurses. Ideally, banked colostrum should have a high concentration of IgG (>7000 mg/ dl, specific gravity >1.090), and should be free of anti-red blood cell antibodies to avoid neonatal isoerythrolysis. Colostrum can be stored frozen for 18 months without significant loss of IgG, although other components such as complement may be lost. Before administration, colostrum should be thawed at room temperature or in warm water. If a microwave is used, it should be set on low power only, because use of high settings can result in denaturation of immunoglobulin. It is recommended that for a 40- to 50-kg foal, 1 to 2 L be administered in 500-ml increments during the first 8 hours of life, with 1 hour between feedings; preferably administration is begun by 1 to 2 hours of age. This should provide at least 1 g/kg of immunoglobulin if the colostrum is of sufficient quality. Colostrum can be administered via nasogastric tube or bottle.

There are alternative sources of immunoglobulin for oral supplementation if equine colostrum is not available, although most have not been widely used. Bovine colostrum may be safely given to foals and may be of some benefit; however, bovine immunoglobulins appear to have a short half life in foals and are not specifically directed against equine pathogens. Equine plasma or serum may also be substituted for colostrum and administered orally, but because of their low concentration of immunoglobulin

°*Equine RID Kits, VMRD, Pullman, WA; and Equine-RID, Veterinary Dynamics, San Luis Obispo, CA*
†*EQUI-Z, VMRD, Inc., Pullman, WA*
‡*CITE Foal IgG Test Kit, IDEXX Laboratories, Westbrook, ME*
§*Foalchek, Centaur, Overland Park, KS; and Gamma-Check-E, Veterinary Dynamics, San Luis Obispo, CA*

°*Gamma-Check-C, Veterinary Dynamics, San Luis Obispo, CA; and Equine Colostrometer, Jorgensen Laboratories, Loveland, CO*

as compared with colostrum, much larger volumes must be given. A number of concentrated equine serum products and lyophilized or concentrated IgG products have been available.° Although such products may provide adequate immunoglobulin, it is important to remember that for oral administration, most foals deprived of colostrum require 1 g/kg of IgG, or approximately 40 g for a foal of average size, to consistently raise the IgG concentration from 0 to more than 400 mg/dl. All foals receiving any type of oral supplementation should be tested by 24 hours of age to ensure that absorption of immunoglobulin has been adequate. This is especially important if foals are older than 6 hours of age at the time of oral supplementation, because absorption of immunoglobulin may be significantly decreased.

Parenteral Supplementation

Parenteral treatment is required to correct low immunoglobulin concentrations in foals 12 to 24 hours of age or older, because it is unlikely that sufficient amounts of immunoglobulin will be absorbed from the gastrointestinal tract. There are several equine plasma and serum products commercially available for the treatment of FPT.† These products are convenient, free of alloantibodies and infectious agents, and should provide a known quantity of IgG. Some products originate from horses immunized with endotoxin or with specific pathogens and may provide increased amounts of specific antibodies, although the degree of additional protection afforded by these products has not been well documented. One disadvantage of commercial products is that they may actually be lacking in antibodies specific for pathogens in the foal's environment. Plasma harvested from a local donor may provide such antibody. Donors should be negative for equine infectious anemia, and should be screened by a blood-typing laboratory to establish that they are free of antibodies to equine red blood cells. Because plasma separated by sedimentation is commonly contaminated with red blood cells that could sensitize recipients, donors should ideally be negative for the antigens Aa and Qa that are frequently associated with neonatal isoerythrolysis. Because there is considerable individual variation in plasma concentrations of IgG, the IgG concentration in the donor plasma should be measured and should be higher than 1200 mg/dl.

The volume of plasma necessary to bring the concentration of IgG into an acceptable range cannot be accurately predicted, because it depends on a number of factors including the severity of the deficiency, the IgG content of the plasma, and the body weight of the foal. Importantly, the presence of existing sepsis can dramatically alter the distribution and catabolism of antibody, generally increasing the volume of plasma required to raise the serum concentration of IgG in the foal. Even in healthy foals in which the amount of plasma administered is carefully calculated, serum IgG concentrations often fail to reach target values. One general guideline for the parenteral

administration of immunoglobulin is 200 to 400 mg of IgG per kg of body weight; for plasma of average quality, this is equivalent to approximately 20 to 40 ml/kg. The highest serum concentrations of IgG are attained 1 to 3 hours after transfusion. To accurately assess the effects of plasma administration and allow for redistribution to extravascular sites, serum IgG concentrations should be measured approximately 24 hours after transfusion. In a healthy foal of average size, the administration of 20 ml/kg of plasma, or approximately 1 L, typically raises the serum concentration of IgG by a mean of about 200 mg/dl. Therefore, in foals that are severely deficient, more than 1 L is usually required. Generally 30% of the IgG concentration attained at 24 hours is lost by 7 days. In foals with established infection, repeated plasma transfusion may be necessary to maintain high levels of circulating IgG, although the benefit of such therapy has not been determined. It is important to remember that establishing high concentrations of immunoglobulin does not preclude the development of infection, particularly with virulent organisms.

Plasma should be administered intravenously, preferably through an in-line filter. Frozen plasma should be thawed in a water bath at 39 to 45°C (102–113°F), and should be warmed to at least room temperature before administration. Recommendations for the rate of plasma administration are largely empirical. The first 50 ml should be given slowly, and the foal should be closely observed for changes in heart rate, respiratory rate, or general behavior. Subsequently, plasma can be administered at 20 ml/kg per hour, or approximately 1 L/h for a 50-kg foal. Administration should be slower if the foal is oliguric or markedly compromised to avoid overloading the vascular system. If additional plasma is required, the rate of administration is usually decreased, with a second liter given over 2 to 3 hours. Compromised foals may become hypoglycemic if administration of plasma is prolonged, and blood glucose concentrations should be monitored in these foals.

Little information is available on the incidence of adverse reactions to plasma transfusions. Tachycardia, tachypnea, restlessness, and muscle fasciculations or shivering occur with some frequency, and most often resolve after decreasing the rate of administration. In more severe reactions, marked muscle fasciculations, defecation, hypotension, and collapse may be observed. If signs are severe or do not diminish after slowing the rate of administration, the transfusion should be discontinued. Administration of crystalloid fluids may be initiated to maintain the circulatory status. In cases of shock, epinephrine can be given intravenously or subcutaneously at a dose of 0.01 mg/kg in a 1:10,000 dilution (0.1 mg/ml).

OTHER IMMUNOGLOBULIN DEFICIENCIES

Several immunoglobulin deficiencies have been defined in foals in addition to FPT, including transient hypogammaglobulinemia, agammaglobulinemia, and selective IgM deficiency. In these conditions, low serum concentrations of immunoglobulin are typically not recognized until at least 2 months of age if ingestion and absorption of colostrum has occurred. Total lymphocyte counts are generally

°ZooQuest Equine Lyphomune, Diagnon Corporation, Rockville, MD; and Seramune, Sera, Shawnee Mission, KS
†Seramune, Sera, Shawnee Mission, KS; Lake Immunogenics, Ontario, NY; Veterinary Dynamics, San Luis Obispo, CA; and Endoserum, Immvac, Columbia, MO

normal. Although the age of onset and the extent of clinical disease are highly variable, these syndromes are often associated with chronic or recurrent infections beginning at approximately 2 to 6 months of age.

Transient hypogammaglobulinemia is a rare disorder in which the onset of immunoglobulin production, which normally occurs before birth, is delayed until approximately 3 months of age. Therefore, between 2 and 4 months of age, serum concentrations of IgG and IgG(T) are low, and concentrations of IgM and IgA are low to normal. Only rarely reported, the condition may be underdiagnosed owing to its transient nature. Although some cases require support in the form of antimicrobial therapy or plasma transfusions, the prognosis for recovery is excellent.

Agammaglobulinemia is a rare primary immunodeficiency characterized by the absence of circulating B cells and failure to produce immunoglobulin. Cell-mediated immune function is normal. Actually, the disorder is a hypoglobulinemia, characterized by low concentrations of IgG and IgG(T), whereas IgM and IgA are generally absent. Recognized in males of several breeds, there may be a mode of inheritance similar to X-linked hypoglobulinemia of humans. Although plasma transfusions and appropriate antimicrobial therapy are beneficial in the short term, there is no treatment for the condition.

Serum concentrations of IgM are significantly decreased or absent in selective IgM deficiency, whereas concentrations of other immunoglobulin classes are normal or increased. Although several breeds are affected, the condition has been reported most frequently in Arabians and Quarterhorses, and a genetic basis has been suspected, but not proved. Plasma transfusion provides only temporary benefit, because the plasma concentration of IgM is relatively low and the half life of transfused IgM is short. The prognosis is generally unfavorable, with most cases succumbing by 2 years of age; however, recovery has been reported.

It is important to remember that secondary or acquired immunodeficiencies also occur, particularly in seriously ill foals, and in many cases the immunosuppression may be transient. Therefore, a diagnosis of a primary immunodeficiency should not be made without repeated assessment of the immune system. Perinatal infection with equine herpesvirus 1 (EHV-1) has been associated with lymphopenia, necrosis and atrophy of lymphoid tissues, and increased susceptibility to infection. Various immunologic deficits have been recognized in foals between 2 weeks and 4 months of age with oral candidiasis and bacterial septicemia. These immunodeficiencies have been poorly characterized, and their prognosis is grave.

COMBINED IMMUNODEFICIENCY

Combined immunodeficiency (CID) is a lethal primary immunodeficiency characterized by a failure to produce functional B and T lymphocytes. The majority of affected horses are Arabian or part-Arabian, although the disorder has been identified in an Appaloosa. In foals of Arabian breeding, the condition is inherited as an autosomal recessive trait, with an incidence of at least 2 to 3%. This is consistent with a carrier prevalence of approximately 25%.

It appears that Arabian foals with CID have a defect of lymphoid stem cells. The thymic hormones necessary for differentiation of stem cells are produced, but specific maturation pathways are blocked. In human patients with CID, several specific enzyme deficiencies have been identified, and in some affected foals, there is evidence of altered purine metabolism. As a result of the maturation defect, there is a lack of functional T and B cells. Components of the innate immune system, including natural killer cells, neutrophils, macrophages, and complement, appear to be uninvolved.

Foals with CID are highly vulnerable to infection as a result of their inability to mount specific humoral or cell-mediated immune responses. Typically normal at birth, affected foals tend to develop signs of infection beginning at 1 to 2 months of age, as concentrations of maternal antibody wane. The onset of clinical disease varies depending on the adequacy of passive transfer and the degree of environmental challenge. A variety of systemic and localized infections have been recognized, including infections by some agents that are rarely seen in normal foals. Recurrent respiratory infections are especially common, and infections caused by adenovirus or *Pneumocystis carinii* are particularly suggestive of CID. Currently, there is no specific therapy recommended for CID. Supportive treatment, such as antibiotics, plasma, and isolation, can prolong the course of disease, but the foal's condition generally deteriorates and they die by 5 to 6 months of age. Although immunologic reconstitution by bone marrow transplantation from a histocompatible donor is possible, it is not practical.

An accurate diagnosis of CID is essential both because of the grave prognosis and because both parents are identified as carriers. An ante mortem diagnosis of CID is supported by appropriate clinical signs in a foal of Arabian breeding with: (1) persistent lymphopenia, as evidenced by lymphocyte counts less than 1000/μl, and often less than 500/μl; (2) absence of IgM in serum collected either presuckle or after 30 days of age, when colostral IgM is depleted owing to its low concentration and short half life. All suspected cases should be confirmed by necropsy, which reveals gross and histologic evidence of lymphoid hypoplasia in the thymus, spleen, and lymph nodes. It should be remembered that septicemic or other compromised foals, as well as some clinically normal foals, may have low lymphocyte counts, and therefore persistent lymphopenia should be established for a diagnosis of CID. In addition, foals affected with CID do not respond to intradermal injection of phytohemagglutinin, nor do their lymphocytes respond to stimulation by mitogens in vitro.

The prevention of CID relies on the identification of carriers and their removal from the breeding population. Unfortunately, there is currently no reliable method of detection of carriers other than the production of an affected offspring, although a genetic test may be available in the future. Heterozygotes are clinically asymptomatic and have normal lymphocyte numbers and function. For an autosomal recessive trait such as CID, mating of two carriers results in one of four foals being affected, one of four being genotypically normal, and two of four being carriers. Although mating of a carrier and a normal horse does not produce affected foals, half of the offspring may be carriers. Thus, breeders should be advised to avoid use of confirmed carriers for breeding.

Supplemental Readings

LeBlanc MM: Immunologic considerations. *In* Koterba AM, Drummond WN, Kosch PC (eds): Equine Clinical Neonatology. Philadelphia, Lea & Febiger, 1990.

LeBlanc MM, Tran T, Baldwin JL, Pritchard EL: Factors that influence passive transfer of immunoglobulins in foals. J Am Vet Med Assoc 200:179–183, 1992.

Morris DD: Immunologic diseases of foals. Comp Cont Ed Pract Vet 8:S139–S150, 1986.

Perryman LE, McGuire TC: Evaluation for immune system failures in horses and ponies. J Am Vet Med Assoc 176:1374–1377, 1980.

Perryman LE, McGuire TC, Torbeck RL: Ontogeny of lymphocyte function in the equine fetus. Am J Vet Res 41:1197–1200, 1980.

Riggs MW: Evaluation of foals for immune deficiency disorders. Vet Clin North Am Equine Pract 3(3):515–528, 1987.

Robinson JA, Allen GK, Green EM, Fales WH, Loch WE, Wilkerson CG: A prospective study of septicaemia in colostrum-deprived foals. Equine Vet J 25:214–219, 1993.

Prematurity

GUY D. LESTER

ANNE M. KOTERBA
Gainesville, Florida

The premature foal frequently represents a management challenge to even the most experienced equine clinician. The clinical course is typically interrupted by various complications including dysfunction of the musculoskeletal, respiratory, and gastrointestinal systems. Before beginning treatment it is important to provide the owner with an accurate estimation of short- and long-term survival, expected costs, and possible complications. Formulation of an accurate prognosis can itself be a difficult task.

DEFINITIONS

Various terms have been used to describe foals that have the physical characteristics of immaturity. Terms previously cited in the literature include prematurity, immaturity, dysmaturity, ready or unready for birth, intrauterine growth retarded, viable or nonviable, and small for gestational age. Gestational length is variable in Thoroughbreds, ranging from 320 to 365 days with a mean of 341 days. Some have defined prematurity as foals with a gestational age of 320 days or less but, although this definition may hold true for many foals, it is inadequate for others. For example, a 340-day-old fetus may possess many characteristics of immaturity if its normal or expected gestational length is 360 days. The terms *viable* and *nonviable* are also inadequate because they fail to take into consideration the availability of facilities for intensive care. A foal that would die in the field without intervention could be very viable if expertise and facilities were available for treatment. The term *readiness for birth* was formulated on the basis of endocrinologic findings in surviving and nonsurviving premature foals. The terminology is useful but must be considered again in conjunction with other factors, such as skeletal maturity or the presence of peripartum asphyxia to fully formulate an accurate prognosis.

PHYSICAL CHARACTERISTICS

The physical characteristics of prematurity include a low birth weight, weakness, a short and silky hair coat, an increased range of joint motion, rear limb flexural laxity, and incomplete skeletal ossification as assessed radiographically. Premature foals often take longer than normal to stand (>60 min) and nurse from the mare (>120 min). The suckle reflex may lack vigor. A prominent or domed forehead is commonly seen in foals such as twins that have undergone intrauterine growth retardation. In addition to these abnormalities, premature foals that fail to survive often demonstrate flexural laxity of the forelimbs, "floppy" ears, and a progressive deterioration in neurologic function.

FORMULATING A PROGNOSIS

To establish a prognosis for survival, several important factors must be considered. These include the reason for premature delivery, assessment of gestational age and the degree of physical immaturity, factors in the perinatal period, laboratory data, and resources available for care. Although all premature foals are at risk for development of complications, particularly of their pulmonary and skeletal systems, the exposure to chronic in utero stress appears to be the most important determinant of survival during the neonatal period. For example, a foal born early to a mare with chronic placentitis and premature lactation stands a much better chance of survival in the extrauterine environment than a foal that is taken by Cesarean section or induced labor before complete maturation.

The fetal pituitary-adrenal axis controls the final maturation of various organ systems, especially the respiratory tract. The fetal adrenal gland is poorly responsive to adrenocorticotropic hormone (ACTH) until the final 3 to 5 days of gestation when its sensitivity changes, so that there is a large increase in cortisol during the final 24 to 48 hours before parturition. This cortisol surge coincides with maturation of the hematopoietic system, and the healthy newborn foal should have a total white blood cell (WBC) count of more than 5000 cells/μl. Tri-iodothyronine (T₃) also increases late in gestation, such that the normal neonate has circulating levels of T₃ that are 10 to 20 times higher than those seen in the adult animal. These values begin to decline by 24 hours of postnatal life. Thyroid hormones regulate a number of important physiologic functions, including thermogenesis and skeletal development, and may act synergistically with endogenous glucocorticoids to hasten production of surfactant.

Foals suddenly removed from their in utero environment before endocrine maturation is complete have low serum levels of thyroid hormone and cortisol, and when challenged with exogenous ACTH, they fail to adequately increase cortisol. Maturation of body systems that takes place during the final days of gestation has not occurred, and these foals are poorly prepared for survival in the extrauterine environment. In contrast, maturation is hastened when the fetus is exposed to chronic in utero stress, resulting in a foal that despite physical immaturity often has adequate pulmonary and hematologic function. It is possible for foals born as early as 280 days' gestation to survive if they have been exposed to a stressful in utero environment. These foals often require some degree of intensive support during the early neonatal period and are susceptible to potential complications of immaturity, especially developmental disease of the skeletal system. Some of these foals are born with infections and the remainder are at risk to develop bacterial infection.

The premature foal is particularly vulnerable to added stresses during the perinatal period. An episode of asphyxia may severely complicate the clinical course. Likewise, meconium aspiration adds an additional stress on an immature cardiopulmonary system. The successful management of such complications usually requires access to appropriate physical and labor resources. In addition, the owner must undertake a substantial financial commitment because intensive care of the premature foal is likely to be expensive.

Laboratory Assessment

Premature foals that have a low total WBC count (<5000 cells/μl) and a low-to-normal fibrinogen level (100–300 mg/dl) are likely to experience difficulties in the neonatal period. These foals typically have a low neutrophil:lymphocyte ratio, low blood cortisol, and failure to produce an adequate rise in cortisol when challenged with ACTH (0.125 mg ACTH IM) during the first 24 hours after birth. Failure of WBC count or fibrinogen level to increase by day 2 is an additional poor prognostic sign. It is important to determine if sepsis is present because neutropenia is a common hematologic finding associated with infection. A shift toward immature cell types and toxic neutrophils should point the clinician toward a diagnosis of primary sepsis or prematurity complicated by sepsis. Premature foals without septicemia frequently have a positive sepsis score because they share clinical and laboratory features of

septicemic neonates, including neutropenia, hypoglycemia, and systemic weakness (see Neonatal Septicemia, page 595).

Clinical Progression

The clinical progression usually reflects the degree of endocrine maturity; additional perinatal stresses such as asphyxia, sepsis, or meconium aspiration; and the degree of physical maturity. Typically foals born prematurely, but exposed to chronic in utero stress, initially appear weak and depressed. Some require resuscitation after birth. After a longer than normal period of postural adaptation, they usually manage to stand but often need assistance. Suckle reflex and appetite are often reduced or absent, and many need to be fed colostrum and milk via nasogastric tube. They frequently have trouble maintaining their body temperature and blood glucose levels. After the initial 24-hour period, many of these foals improve both in physical strength and mentation. Their appetite for milk often exceeds that of a healthy "term" foal.

The hormonally immature foal commonly requires immediate resuscitation. The condition of these foals often mimics the clinical progression of the hormonally mature or "stressed" premature foals up until 12 to 18 hours of age, after which a range of progressive abnormalities may develop. These include systemic weakness, depression, seizures, respiratory acidosis, and an intolerance to enteral feeding. Cardiovascular collapse may ensue, the first sign of which is a reduction in the intensity of peripheral pulses, followed by oliguria, subcutaneous edema, and worsening neurologic function. Poor tissue perfusion leads to lactate production and a mixed metabolic and respiratory acidosis. Death is certain without aggressive support, and even with high-level intensive care, mortality rates are high.

SPECIFIC PROBLEMS OF THE PREMATURE FOAL

Maintenance of Body Temperature and Blood Glucose

Premature animals appear to be more susceptible to hypothermia than full-term neonates because thermogenic mechanisms likely develop late in gestation. The mature foal can generate body heat through shivering and by metabolizing brown fat, but the premature foal may lack these mechanisms. Low levels of thyroid hormone have also been associated with hypothermia in foals. Body temperature needs careful management because rapid warming may result in peripheral vasodilatation and possibly cardiovascular collapse. Initially, the foal should be covered by blankets and removed from drafts. Intravenous and oral fluids should be warmed before use. Once the foal becomes more vigorous, heat lamps and circulating warm-water blankets can be used. The inadequate glycogen stores of the premature foal put it at risk for hypoglycemia. This is managed acutely by rapid infusion of 10% dextrose solution (10 ml/kg IV) over several minutes, followed by a constant infusion of about 6 mg/kg per minute, approximately 200 ml/hour of a 5% dextrose solution to a 30-kg foal.

Cardiopulmonary System

Premature foals are likely to experience some degree of respiratory insufficiency. The low arterial oxygen concentration in healthy newborn foals is further accentuated in the dysmature or premature foal. Extrapulmonary right-to-left shunts can account for more than 30% of cardiac output in contrast with less than 10% in normal full-term foals. In addition, ventilation/perfusion inequalities may occur as a result of alveolar collapse or atelectasis, the severity of which is influenced by maturation of the surfactant system. Lung surfactant, a mixture of phospholipids (including dipalmitoyl phosphatidylcholine and phosphatidylglycerol), inert lipids, and protein produced from type II alveolar epithelial cells, prevents alveolar collapse by reducing alveolar surface tension. Although surfactant activity can be detected in the fetus by 100 days' gestation, development is not complete until 300 days, or even after birth. Deficiency of surfactant is the major contributing factor in respiratory distress syndrome (RDS) or hyaline membrane disease in premature human infants. Infants with RDS develop a severe respiratory acidosis with secondary hypoxia-induced pulmonary arterial hypertension, reduced cardiac output, and tissue hypoxia. A highly proteinaceous fluid leaks into the interstitium and alveoli. This results in the radiographic finding of air bronchograms. Fibrinogen in the edema fluid is converted into fibrin, the so-called hyaline membranes observed histologically in RDS. Dramatically improved survival rates have been achieved in human infants with RDS since the incorporation of bovine° or synthetic surfactant† into therapeutic regimens. An equivalent syndrome probably occurs rarely in premature foals. In contrast, a clinically less severe form of this syndrome may occur commonly. Lung dysfunction in premature foals often is characterized clinically by reduced ventilation capacity, tachypnea, hypoxemia, and progressive hypercapnia. Radiographically, there is a diffuse increase in interstitial density without alveolar changes (i.e., there are no air bronchograms). Atelectasis, with or without inflammatory cell infiltrates, is observed histologically, but hyaline membrane formation is rare. The administration of bovine surfactant to premature foals at risk for respiratory failure has been purported to be successful, but objective controlled studies are lacking. Unfortunately, the cost of commercial bovine or synthetic surfactant almost always precludes its use in foals at this time. The clinical management of respiratory failure is discussed elsewhere in this text (see page 606).

Management of the failing cardiovascular system is challenging. Successful treatment is reliant upon early detection of falling systemic blood pressure. Maintenance of mean blood pressure higher than 65 mm Hg is critical in the prevention of a fatal downward spiral of cardiopulmonary collapse with secondary renal failure. The initial approach to treatment involves intravenous plasma followed, if necessary, by dopamine infusion at 3 to 5 μg/kg per minute. If this is ineffective, dobutamine infusion (5–20 μg/kg per minute) is added. Preservation of renal function is critical, and the subcutaneous tissues should be monitored for edema. Overadministration of sodium-containing fluids can often result in hypernatremia.

Musculoskeletal System

Skeletal maturity is easily assessed by radiography of both the carpus and tarsus for evidence of incomplete ossification. Management of incomplete skeletal ossification is controversial. Most clinicians believe that exercise should be restricted to minimize collapse of developing carpal or tarsal bones, but forced recumbency may predispose the foal to or exacerbate pulmonary disease. Restricted stall exercise with splinting is commonly recommended. Assessment of joint and tendon laxity is also important. The excessive joint laxity of premature foals predisposes them to acquired angular limb deformities (see page 624).

Immune System

The premature foal is at increased risk for developing secondary bacterial disease. Chronic placental disease is often associated with premature lactation, resulting in an inadequate quality and quantity of colostrum, predisposing to failure of passive transfer. The dams of prematurely induced foals or foals taken by Cesarean section may have failed to produce colostrum. The ability of the premature foal to absorb colostral antibody is assumed to be similar to that of mature foals, but data are lacking to substantiate this fact. Susceptible animals require prophylactic antibiotic therapy.

Ophthalmic Complications

Premature foals are more likely than full-term neonates to develop temporary entropion that commonly causes corneal abrasion and ulceration, which often produce few clinical signs. Therefore, regular fluorescein staining of the cornea is recommended in sick premature foals. The management of entropion and corneal ulceration is described on page 636.

Corticosteroid Therapy

Corticosteroids are important prepartum medications administered to women who are in danger of delivering prematurely. Betamethasone administered systemically crosses the human placenta and hastens maturation of the fetal lung. Unfortunately, the equine placenta appears to be relatively impermeable to exogenous corticosteroids. Betamethasone injected intramuscularly into the foal fetus using ultrasound guidance hastens maturation. Considering the apparent synergism between thyroid hormone and cortisol, it has been suggested in women to combine thyrotropin-releasing hormone (TRH) with betamethasone.

The administration of corticosteroids to premature human infants has not been widely adapted because of the potential for adrenal suppression and sepsis. The use of corticosteroids in newborn foals is likewise controversial. Short-acting prednisolone preparations have been used in our clinic with inconsistent results. It is unlikely that ACTH has therapeutic benefit, but its use coupled with measurement of plasma cortisol concentration may have diagnostic or prognostic value.

°*Survanta, Abbott Laboratories, Abbott Park, IL*
†*Exosurf Neonatal, Burroughs Wellcome, Research Triangle Park, NC*

LONG-TERM SURVIVAL

The short-term survival or hospital discharge rate of foals with a gestational age of 325 days or less is 50% for foals admitted to the University of Florida. These foals were not further categorized according to "readiness for birth" criteria, but survival appeared to be poorly correlated with actual gestational age. Although many surviving premature or twin foals grow into healthy adults, certain problems of prematurity, especially carpal or tarsal bone collapse and angular limb deformities, may linger into adult life. The ability of premature foals to survive and compete at a level equivalent to that of their siblings requires further study, but in a preliminary survey of 23 surviving premature Thoroughbred foals from the University of Florida, premature foals appeared to be less likely to race and earned less prize money than their siblings.

Supplemental Readings

Cottrill CM: Maturation of the cardiopulmonary system. Equine Vet J 14[Suppl]:26–30, 1993.
Koterba AM: Prematurity. *In* Koterba AM, Drummond WH, Kosch PC (eds): Equine Clinical Neonatology. Philadelphia, Lea & Febiger, 1990, pp 55–70.
Thorburn GD: A speculative review of parturition in the mare. Equine Vet J 14[Suppl]:41–49, 1993.

Hypoxic Ischemic Encephalopathy

WILLIAM V. BERNARD
Lexington, Kentucky

The term *neonatal maladjustment syndrome* has been used to describe newborn foals that are exhibiting behavioral or neurologic abnormalities that are not related to infectious or toxic conditions, congenital or developmental abnormalities, or metabolic disorders. These foals have previously been classified as barkers, wanderers, dummies, or convulsants. The syndrome has been divided into four stages, which are preconvulsant, coma or semicoma, and wanderer. Numerous theories are given as the cause of the syndrome. These include central nervous system (CNS) trauma and hemorrhage and CNS anoxia. It appears that the majority of neonates exhibiting CNS signs within the first few days of life have suffered a lack of cerebral oxygen delivery either resulting from a lack of blood flow (ischemia) or decreased arterial oxygen tension (hypoxemia). Therefore, the descriptive term *hypoxic ischemic encephalopathy* (HIE), which has been adapted from human medicine, will be used in the remainder of this discussion.

ETIOLOGY AND PATHOGENESIS

Intracranial hemorrhage as a result of increased CNS pressures during birth or subsequent to trauma has been proposed as a cause of CNS disease in the neonate. Vascular pressure changes and hemorrhage also may occur as a result of asphyxia. Many newborn foals with CNS disturbances have a history suggestive of decreased oxygen delivery during the perinatal period. This, coupled with histopathologic findings similar to those described in other species with experimentally induced asphyxia, suggests that hypoxia and ischemia are important components of this syndrome in foals.

Interference with blood flow and oxygen delivery before birth can result from placental insufficiency or interference with uterine blood flow. A wide variety of conditions can result in interference with blood flow and oxygen delivery during parturition, such as obstruction of umbilical blood flow, premature placental separation, decreased uterine blood flow, and prolonged parturition (dystocia). During normal foaling, the fetus experiences a transient period of anoxia. The normal healthy foal is not affected by this period of oxygen deprivation. However, the compromised foal may not be able to compensate, and a cycle of events leading to exacerbation of the anoxia may result.

Events subsequent to birth can also lead to hypoxia and ischemia. Inadequate cardiac ouput can result in insufficient pulmonary or cerebral blood flow. The transition from fetal to adult circulation is critical to adequate oxygen delivery and can result in periods of inadequate delivery if delayed or if there is a reversion to fetal circulation.

It is likely that responses to hypoxia at the cellular level are the same in all species. Mitochondrial swelling is followed by cytoplasmic vacuolization within minutes of the onset of hypoxia. Events subsequent to the intracellular "edema" include increased cerebral tissue pressure, focally decreased cerebral blood flow, generalized brain swelling, increased intracranial pressure, generalized decreased cerebral blood flow, and cerebral necrosis.

HISTORY

The history of a foal with HIE may include a report of gestational problems in the mare. Examples include vaginal discharge suggesting uterine or placental infection, colic, or other medical problems during gestation, premature lactation, and prolonged or shortened gestational length. Some mares have histories of repeatedly delivering foals that develop CNS signs. It is possible that these mares may have repeated problems during parturition or an inability to form an adequate placental unit. Premature placental separation is also commonly reported in the history of neonates with HIE. Previous reports suggest that delivery of affected neonates may be fast and uncomplicated. However, more recent reports suggest that dystocia is not uncommon in neonates with HIE. Delivery via emergency cesarean section is another risk factor for the development of hypoxic insults before or shortly after delivery.

A very important point to consider is that these neonates may be normal at birth and show no evidence of CNS disease for hours to days after delivery. Alternatively, these foals may exhibit evidence of violent CNS activity immediately or shortly after birth. This variation in onset of clinical signs is likely to be related to the degree of cell damage occurring as a result of the hypoxia-ischemia and possibly to the degree of edema that occurs as a result of cell death.

CLINICAL SIGNS

Clinical signs of HIE in neonatal foals are highly variable. The original descriptions of these foals as "barkers," "wanderers," or "convulsants" indicate the variation in clinical signs. Signs can be mild, such as a loss of affinity for the mare, an inappropriate suckle reflex, wandering, intermittent depression, and star-gazing. Facial spasms, lip curling and chomping, or abnormal respiratory patterns may occur. The abnormal vocalizations (barking) are rarely identified. These foals may sleep deeply and may be difficult to arouse. These "mild" signs may be all that is seen, and the patient may recover without complication. On the other hand, signs may progress to more prominent and severe indications of CNS disease. Foals may become totally unaware of the environment and appear to have blindness of central origin. Seizures may follow and are usually very sudden in onset but are often preceded by one of more of the earlier-mentioned signs. One of the more frequent premonitory signs of seizure is a "stretching" activity that actually may be a mild seizure. While lying down, the foal extends the front legs outward and lifts the head before again relaxing into a sternal sleeping position. Seizures can be of short duration with no subsequent evidence of obvious CNS disease. In more severe cases, seizures are severe and generalized with tonic-clonic convulsions, opisthotonus, and extensor rigidity. Some patients may paddle violently. If seizures are repetitive or continuous, foals are generally stuporous or comatose in the interictal period. Not all HIE patients develop seizures before progressing into a state of stupor.

The onset of clinical signs is extremely variable, and many foals may appear completely normal for hours to days. The onset of seizures has been reported to be as late as 4 to 5 days. Neonates also can be seen with CNS signs immediately after birth. The duration of clinical signs can also vary. These signs can be very brief with single or no seizures to persistent stupor for several days. Usually foals recover in the reverse order in which the CNS signs developed, that is, stupor to awareness of the environment, standing, walking, and suckling. Typically, when foals recover from prolonged CNS derangement, relapses do not occur. However, recurrence of seizures subsequent to prolonged stupor has been seen.

DIAGNOSIS

The diagnosis of the disease is based upon typical clinical signs, historical information, and elimination of other possible causes of CNS disease in the newborn foal. As mentioned, the history often includes such factors as prepartum problems in the mare, problems during delivery, and placental separation or delivery via emergency cesarean section. When parturition includes any of these factors, close observation should ensue, with special attention for early or mild evidence of CNS disease. The signs of CNS disease are not pathognomonic for HIE. Conditions that may also result in seizures include hyponatremia, hypocalcemia, hypoglycemia, hypomagnesemia, metabolic acidosis, generalized sepsis, parasite migration, Tyzzer's disease, viral encephalitis, drug-induced toxicities, hydranencephaly, liver failure, idiopathic epilepsy, and heat stroke. These conditions must be considered in the differential diagnosis but rarely cause seizures in the newborn foal. Those conditions that more frequently cause CNS derangement in the neonate are cerebral contusion or hemorrhage possibly related to episodes of anoxia, hydrocephalus, and bacterial meningitis.

The differentiation of the foal with hydrocephalus from one with HIE can be difficult. Central nervous system abnormalities are not always present at birth in either case. The seizures in foals with hydrocephalus can be very severe, violent, and difficult to control. Foals with meningitis may have fevers. The CNS signs may first appear as period of agitation with pawing, grinding of teeth, or sweating. The CNS signs in foals with meningitis may appear more like those in the adult horse with encephalopathy. These may include continuous and persistent wandering and circling, maniacal behavior, and head pressing.

Results of laboratory data of the equine neonate with HIE are neither specific nor diagnostic. However, an elevated creatinine and elevated muscle enzyme levels are not uncommonly present in foals with HIE. The elevation in creatinine that is seen at birth has been suggested to be related to placental insufficiency, which may be related to a lack of adequate oxygen delivery in utero. The elevation in the muscle enzymes creatine kinase and aspartate aminotransferase may correlate with muscle hypoxia-ischemia or trauma at birth. The leukogram in a foal with meningitis may suggest infection; however, it is not diagnostic. Clinical chemistry levels can be useful in excluding some of the less likely causes of CNS disease, such as metabolic or hepatic disease. Cerebrospinal fluid analysis is not diagnostic in the foal with HIE or hydrocephalus. However, increased cerebrospinal fluid cell counts can be diagnostic of meningitis.

Radiographs of the skull may be useful in cases of severe trauma. Computerized axial tomography or magnetic resonance imaging can be used to diagnose hydrocephalus and is used in human medicine to differentiate hemorrhage from edema.

TREATMENT

The treatment of HIE is symptomatic. Supportive and nursing care are critical to the outcome of the case. The treatment of seizures varies depending on their severity. A seizure that is mild and brief may not need to be controlled. However, if seizures are recurrent or severe, treatment becomes necessary. The control of seizure activity can prevent trauma, reduce the energy consumption of seizures, and allow for better nursing care. A variety of anticonvulsants can be used. Diazepam is the drug of choice for the immediate short-term suppression of seizures; 5 mg can be administered IV to the 50-kg foal (0.1 mg/kg). If this is not effective, repeated doses can be given. Diazepam is safe and fast-acting, but its duration of action is short. If seizures persist, alternate choices of drugs include phenobarbital, phenytoin, or sodium pentobarbital used to effect. Phenobarbital can provide prolonged seizure control and is safe if given slowly and used to effect. The dosage is 10–20 mg/kg as a loading dose (10 mg/kg is often sufficient), diluted in saline and given over a 20–30 minute period. Administration should stop if desired effects are achieved before the full dose is administered. Phenobarbital can be repeated as needed. Once seizures are controlled, oral administration (12 mg/kg b.i.d.) can be used for maintenance. Phenytoin, given initially at 5 to 10 mg/kg IV and subsequently at 1 to 5 mg/kg IV, IM, or p.o. every 2 to 4 hours, may also be used. Disadvantages are the frequency of administration and cost. Intravenous sodium pentobarbital to effect, approximately 2 to 4 mg/kg, may be used in foals with uncontrollable seizures. Marked sedation or anesthesia may occur at higher or more frequent doses.

Broad-spectrum antimicrobial therapy should be considered for the prevention of secondary infection in the compromised patient. Nutritional therapy is of utmost importance and varies with the severity of the condition. If the foal can stand but not suckle, an indwelling nasogastric tube may be used to provide adequate caloric support. The foal requires a minimum of 10% of its body weight in milk over a 24-hour period. Feeding every 1 to 2 hours is preferred. If the patient is recumbent but is able to maintain sternal recumbency, cautious enteral feeding is still possible, but care must be taken not to overfeed the recumbent foal. Enteral feeding must be provided sparingly in the stuporous foal. In these cases, caloric supplementation should be provided with continuous intravenous dextrose administration or more complete parenteral nutrition (see page 600 and *Current Therapy in Equine Medicine 3*, page 747).

Intravenous fluids should be used judiciously in foals with HIE because overhydration may worsen cerebral edema. It is wise to restrict fluid administration unless a secondary complication requires additional fluid therapy. When determining maintenance fluid requirements (4 ml/kg per hour), oral fluid intake must be taken into account. A foal that is receiving 10% of its body weight in milk may not need additional intravenous fluids.

Medications to reduce cerebral edema may be helpful. Intravenous dimethyl sulfoxide or mannitol can be useful in the acute stages of cerebral edema. Dimethyl sulfoxide (0.5–1.0 g/kg as a 10% solution IV) also has been recommended. Hypertonic solutions such as mannitol should be used only if it can be definitively shown that cerebral hemorrhage is not present. In the presence of cerebral hemorrhage, hypertonic solutions can exacerbate edema. The use of corticosteroids is controversial because they can result in immune suppression and can increase cerebral blood flow, which may worsen cerebral edema.

PROGNOSIS

The prognosis for survival is dependent upon the severity of the initial insult and progression of edema and cellular damage. Overwhelming hypoxia can result in a rapid onset of respiratory arrest. If cerebral damage results in fixed, dilated, nonresponsive pupils, the prognosis is grave. The CNS signs in many affected foals may not progress beyond a minimal loss of recognition of the environment, with gradual recovery over a 1- to 2-day period. The prognosis for foals that have seizures is worse than for those that do not. However, if seizures can be controlled, adequate nursing care provided, and secondary complications avoided, the prognosis for these foals is good. Persistence of residual neurologic signs is unusual. When recovery does occur, there does not appear to be a long-term effect on growth or development.

Supplemental Readings

Green SL, Mayhew IG: Neurologic disorders. *In* Koterba AM, Drummond WH, Kosch PC (eds): Equine Clinical Neonatology. Philadelphia, Lea & Febiger, 1990, pp 496–530.

Volpe JJ: Hypoxic ischemic encephalopathy. *In* Neurology of the Newborn. Philadelphia, WB Saunders, 1990, pp 211–369.

Neonatal Isoerythrolysis

JILL JOHNSON McCLURE
Baton Rouge, Louisiana

Neonatal isoerythrolysis (NI) is an immunogenetic disease that affects foals within the first week of life. The principle behind NI is very simple. A mare generates an antibody response against a foreign antigen. In this case, the target antigen is a red blood cell surface molecule, which she lacks on her own cells. These antibodies gain access to the circulation of her foal through ingestion of colostrum. If the foal has on its red cells the target antigen inherited from the sire, the antibodies attach to the red cells and cause their destruction or removal from the circulation. Mares become sensitized or immunized as a result of exposure to blood containing the foreign antigens from transfusion or exposure to blood of a fetus with incompatible blood type as a result of placentitis or at parturition.

For NI to develop, a sequence of events must occur. (1) The mare must be exposed to a red cell factor, the antigen, which she lacks on her own cells, and she must produce antibody to it. (2) She must be bred to a stallion that has this factor on its cells, and (3) the sire must pass the gene for that factor to the fetus, which then makes the factor on its cells. (4) The mare must make colostrum, which contains these antibodies. (5) The foal must ingest and absorb sufficient quantities of these antibodies. (6) The antibodies must combine with the factor on the red cells, which results in their rapid destruction or removal from the circulation leading to anemia.

The two red cell factors or antigens that appear to be most immunogenic and are most commonly associated with problems in horses are Aa and Qa. Only mares that lack these factors can produce antibody to them and are thus at risk. Mares that lack these factors can be identified by blood typing. When examining the blood typing report (Fig. 1), clinicians must look at the list of factors detected for the A system and Q system. The list amounts to a series of lower-case letters from "a" to "g" for the A system and "a" to "c" for the Q system and minus sign. If "a" is not listed under the system, the mare does not have that factor and is considered a higher risk for production of antibodies to that factor and subsequently an NI foal. This assumes that the factor actually occurs in the breed and thus stallions to which the mare may be bred have the factor. For example, factor Qa does not occur in Standardbreds at all, and thus although all mares appear to be at risk, that is they lack Qa, no "incompatible" Standardbred stallions exist to which they may be bred.

NI has occasionally been associated with other red cell factors in horses. Theoretically, any factor lacked by the mare and present in the foal and stallion can be a problem, but the prevalence is so low that it does not warrant taking preventive measures for incompatibilities in these other factors. Virtually all mule pregnancies are incompatible for a red cell factor called *donkey factor*, which has been associated with NI. Not all mares at risk actually become sensitized and produce foals that develop NI.

Horses that lack factor Ca frequently produce anti-Ca antibody. This antibody does not appear to produce NI, and in fact it may confer some degree of protection against sensitization by other factors by rapidly eliminating foreign cells from circulation.

If a mare is known to be at risk either based on knowledge of her blood type or because of previous production of an affected foal, her sera can be tested for the presence of anti-red cell antibodies during the last month of gestation or her colostrum can be tested against the foal's or stallion's red cells before allowing the foal to nurse. If antibody is detected before ingestion of colostrum, the foal can be prevented from ingesting the "tainted" colostrum and an alternate source can be provided.

CLINICAL SIGNS

Typically, signs of disease occur in the first 2 to 24 hours but may occur as late as 7 or 8 days of age. Clinical signs are referable to destruction of red blood cells and resulting anemia and other complications of red cell destruction. Peracute cases may die within several hours and show only pallor, hemoglobinemia, and hemoglobinuria. Clinically these are often weak, depressed, "floppy" foals. Foals that survive for several days or that have a slower and later onset are generally icteric. Tachycardia, tachypnea, and pallor may also be noticeable. Secondary signs resulting from anoxia may include those of central nervous system injury such as depression or seizures. Nephropathy associated with organ failure may result from renal vascular changes and excretion of hemoglobin. Mules suffering from NI frequently manifest thrombocytopenia as well as anemia, presumably because of the presence of anti-platelet antibody as well as anti-red cell antibody.

Delayed onset, after more than 6 days, of acute hemolysis is uncommon and may be due to continued presence of antibody of some class other than IgG. In these cases, the milk gives a positive result on the jaundiced foal agglutination (JFA) test (Table 1), suggesting the continued presence of agglutinins. In these cases it may be necessary to remove the foal from mare's milk.

DIAGNOSIS

Diagnosis may be suspected based on signs of pallor or icterus and concurrent anemia, hemoglobinemia, or hemoglobinuria. Septicemic foals may clinically share many of the features including depression and icterus, but infected foals are not usually anemic.

Diagnosis is confirmed by demonstrating antibody on the surface of red cells using a direct antiglobulin test

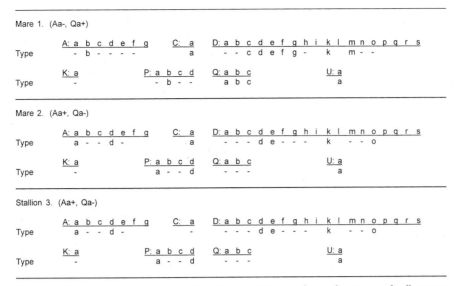

Figure 1. Example of blood typing reports and how to interpret the results. Seven red cell systems are routinely tested. Upper case letters denote the system (gene locus). Lower case letters that follow denote factors associated with the system for which the laboratory tests. Minus signs and lower case letters listed below the system denote those factors that were detected and those that were not in a particular individual.

Mare 1 does not have factor Aa, as indicated by the minus sign under that factor.

Mare 2 does not have factor Qa, as indicated by the minus sign under that factor. A blank under the factor indicated that the factor was not tested for in the laboratory. (e.g., Di, Dp, Dq, Dr, Ds). Mare 1 would be considered at risk because she lacks factor Aa. Mare 2 would be considered at risk because she lacks factor Qa. Stallion 3 would be incompatible with Mare 1 for factor Aa because he has the factor and she does not. The fact that he lacks Qa and Mare 1 has Qa is irrelevant. Stallion 3 would be compatible with Mare 2 because they both have Aa and lack Qa.

(Coombs' test). This test is run on ethylenediaminetetra-acetic acid (EDTA) anticoagulated samples and requires species-specific reagents. Human Coombs' test reagents do not work. Diagnosis is supported by demonstrating anti-red cell antibodies in the colostrum or serum of the mare using agglutination or hemolytic assays.

TREATMENT

Treatment after the ingestion of colostrum and the onset of signs depends on the severity of clinical changes and the speed with which red cells are destroyed. In mild cases when the hematocrit (PCV) remains above 15% and is not decreasing rapidly, little except restriction of exercise may be indicated. In more severe cases, minimizing exertion is imperative because these foals may die while being manipulated or attempting to follow their dams. When the PCV is less than 15%, replacement red blood cells that are resistant to the circulating maternal antibody may be required. Although transfusion may not be necessary if the PCV remains above 12%, if it is at 15% and decreasing, preparation should begin to have the blood ready if the PCV drops to 12% as collecting and processing blood for transfusion takes time.

Selection of a Donor

The key to donor selection is to provide a red blood cell that will not react with the maternal antibodies that the foal absorbed through the colostrum. At this age, the foal has only maternal antibody and no autologous antibody about which the clinician needs to be concerned. From a standpoint of speed and ease, the best donor lacks the factor against which the antibodies are directed (e.g., has the same blood type as the mare with regard to that factor, and has no anti-red cell antibodies in its serum). Whole blood can be used from these horses without additional processing. Depending upon the breed, however, the number of individuals that lack the offending factor and are thus suitable donors varies. For example, in Thoroughbreds, only about one in 50 horses lack factor Aa. This means that only one in 50 Thoroughbreds is a suitable red cell donor to treat a foal affected with NI due to anti-Aa antibody. The odds of randomly selecting a suitable donor are obviously slim.

With advance screening, horses that are Aa and Qa negative and free of antibody can be identified for donors (Table 2). Among the more common breeds in the United States, a suitable Aa and Qa negative donor would most likely be found among Quarterhorses. Because pregnancy is often associated with sensitization against red cells, the use of geldings as blood donors has been suggested. This is a consideration relating to the presence of antibodies in the transfused blood, but has no effect on which red cell factors are present.

If colostrum from the mare is available, a potential donor can be screened in the field by performing the JFA test (see Table 1) using the mare's colostrum and blood from potential donors. The mare's own blood is run as a control and the donors' blood cells should not react at any higher dilutions than the mare's own blood cells.

TABLE 1. JAUNDICED FOAL AGGLUTINATION TEST (JFA)

Materials:
1. Centrifuge capable of centrifuging blood types at moderate speeds (300 to 600 × g)
2. Test tubes, either 13- × 100-mm disposable tubes or blood collection tubes
3. Test tube rack
4. Pasteur pipettes and rubber bulbs or other pipette system to deliver 1.0-ml volumes
5. Room-temperature 0.9% NaCl
6. Colostrum from mare
7. Presuckle blood from the foal, preferably in EDTA anticoagulant
8. Blood from the mare, preferably in EDTA anticoagulant, can be used for a control

Methods:
1. Add approximately 1 ml of 0.9% NaCl to each of 8 tubes
2. Label the first tube SALINE CONTROL
3. In the remaining 7 tubes, prepare serial dilutions (1:2, 1:4, 1:8, 1:16, 1:32, 1:64, 1:128) of the colostrum by adding 1 ml of colostrum to the tube labeled 1:2, then transferring 1 ml of the mixture to the second tube labeled 1:4, and so on until reaching the tube labeled 1:128. Discard 1 ml from the tube labeled 1:128 so that the total volume in each tube is approximately 1 ml.
4. Add one drop of the foal's whole blood to each tube and mix the samples
5. Centrifuge the tubes for 2 to 3 minutes at medium speed (300–500 × g)
6. Invert each tube, one at a time, pouring out the liquid contents; observe the status of the button of the red cells at the bottom of the tube.

Complete agglutination causes the cells to remain tightly packed in the button; strong agglutination causes the cells to remain in large clumps. For weaker agglutination, the cells are in smaller clumps as they run down the side of the tube. When no agglutination exists, the cells easily flow down the side of the tube. The titer is defined as the highest dilution that gives strong agglutination.

If the blood agglutinates in the SALINE CONTROL tube, this may indicate that the foal has already absorbed antibodies and the cells are already coated at the time of collection. Colostrum can be tested on the dam's own cells to be certain that it is not the conditions of the test or viscosity of the colostrum that are causing the agglutination.

Positive reactions at 1:16 or greater in horses and 1:64 or greater in mules are considered significant.

One reliable source of red cells that is not affected by maternal antibody is the dam. The dam's red cells will not be affected by her antibody, but the problem with using the dam's red cells is that they must be washed free of antibody to prevent administration of more offending antibody to the foal. The process of washing allows the red cells to sediment from anticoagulated blood and removes as much of the plasma as possible, followed by addition of several volumes of isotonic saline. The red cells are allowed to sediment again, after which time as much of the saline-diluted plasma as possible is removed. The red cells are then resuspended in isotonic saline at about a 50% suspension. This procedure takes several hours.

The sire of the foal is absolutely not a suitable red cell donor because his red cells share the same red cell antigen as the foal. Administration of more red cells that share the same antigens as the foal will only add to the load of damaged red cells that must be cleared by the reticuloendothelial system and hemoglobin that must be cleared by the kidneys.

In the case of mules with NI, virtually any horse can provide suitable red cells because the factor involved ap-

pears to be a uniquely donkey antigen (i.e., a xenoantigen), and thus it is necessary only to exclude horses with anti-donkey antibody in their serum as donors.

Administration of Erythrocytes

The red cells or whole blood must be administered through a blood administration set with a filter. Failure to do so may result in acute fatal reactions, probably anaphylactoid in nature. The volume of washed red cells or whole blood that can be given is somewhat limited by the size of the patient. In general, as much as possible is given without overloading the blood volume of the patient. The estimated blood volume of a 50-kg foal is 3.5 L, which is 7.5% of body weight. Usually 1 to 2 L of washed cells or whole blood is given initially, with an additional 1 to 2 L per day given over the next day or two if needed. This volume can be expected to increase the PCV about 10 percentage points. The PCV tends to gradually decrease again over the following several days. This is most likely attributable to the continued destruction and removal of the foal's cells, not the transfused cells, if they were compatible with the maternal antibody. If the decline in PCV is gradual, additional transfusions may be unnecessary, even if the levels decrease to around 15%. It may take several weeks for the PCV to return to levels expected for age, keeping in mind that the PCV level of normal foals tends to decrease, often into the 20s, over the first several weeks of life.

PREVENTION

Two general methods exist for prevention of NI. One is to prevent incompatible matings and the other is to prevent

TABLE 2. LABORATORIES PROVIDING EQUINE BLOOD TYPING SERVICES*

Serology Laboratory
University of California
Davis, CA 95616
Telephone: (916) 752–2211

Stormont Laboratory, Inc.
1237 East Beamer St., Suite D
Woodland, CA 95776
Telephone: (916) 661–3078

Dr. Melba Ketchum
Shelterwood Equine Laboratories
Box 215
Carthage, TX 75633
Telephone: (903) 693–6424

Dr. Gus Cothran
Equine Blood Typing Research Laboratory
University of Kentucky
Department of Veterinary Science
Lexington, KY 40546
Telephone: (606) 257–3022

Dr. David Colling
Mann Equitest, Inc.
335 Laird Road
Unit 4
Guelph, Ontario N1H 6J3
Canada
Telephone: (519) 836–2400

*Serum and/or colostrum from the suspect mare are needed to screen for the presence of anti-red cell antibody. ACD anticoagulated blood is generally preferred for screening for red cell antigens.

the offending antibodies from entering the foal. A compatible breeding is to mate a mare and stallion lacking the same factors, therefore precluding the inheritance of those factors by the foal. Compatibility can be determined by routine blood typing of the mare and stallion. When examining the blood typing reports for the mare and stallion (Fig. 1), the list of factors detected for the A system and Q system should be examined. As described earlier, the list amounts to a series of lower-case letters from "a" to "g" for the A system and "a" to "c" for the Q system. If "a" is not listed under the A system for the mare, a compatible stallion would also lack the "a" factor under the A system. If "a" is not listed under the Q system for the mare, a compatible stallion would also lack the "a" factor under the Q system. It is the lack of a factor in the mare that creates the "at risk" situation, not the converse, and thus the presence of the factor in the mare and the absence in the stallion is of no consequence.

The presence of anti-red cell antibodies in the serum of mares late in gestation is presumptive evidence of an impending problem, although because the blood type of the fetus is not known, this does not predict absolutely that a problem will occur with the current pregnancy. Postpartum tests for antibody can be done using either the sire's blood or blood from several horses that are known to possess a spectrum of red cell antigens, known as a panel. Thus, blood from the sire is not necessary to detect problematic antibodies. If antibodies are detected, provisions should be made to either check colostrum for specific reactions with the foal's cells at birth by means of the JFA test (see Table 1), or to arbitrarily withhold the dam's colostrum and provide an alternate source.

The presence of colostral antibodies against red cells can be detected using the JFA test. Mare colostrum is reacted with foal's blood collected before the foal is suckled and a titer determined (see Table 1). Titers of 1:16 or greater are considered significant in horses. Titers of 1:64 or greater of anti-donkey factor are significant in mules. The JFA does not differentiate antibodies against one factor from another; it simply detects the presence of some anti-red cell antibody. If the foal has already nursed and has anti-red cell antibody on its cells, the cells may agglutinate in the JFA test saline control and at all dilutions even in the absence of colostrum; thus, it is important to use presuckle blood to accurately assess the test or the tendency will be to overestimate the titer.

Colostral titers as determined by JFA test generally decrease quite rapidly. It is safe to allow the foal to nurse once the titers decrease below 1:16. This may occur in as little as 4 hours. Recommendations to withhold milk for 24 to 72 hours are probably overly conservative. If colostral antibodies are ingested in the first few hours, the antibody levels may continue to increase in the blood for 24 hours, but probably not because new absorption is occurring but rather because the antibody already in the pipeline continues to reach the blood stream. By milking out the mare and repeatedly testing the milk using the JFA test with the foal's presuckle blood, the foal can safely be returned to the mare as soon as the titer drops, thus saving considerable time and effort required to feed a foal every several hours if it is being withheld from the mare for periods of 1 to 3 days.

Supplemental Readings

Bailey E: Prevalence of anti-red blood cell antibodies in the serum and colostrum of mares and its relationship to neonatal isoerythrolysis. Am J Vet Res 43:1917–1921, 1982.

Bailey E, Albright DG: Equine neonatal isoerythrolysis: Evidence for prevention by maternal antibodies to the Ca blood group antigen. Am J Vet Res 49:1218–1222, 1988.

Bailey E, Conboy HS, McCarthy PF: Neonatal isoerythrolysis of foals; an update on testing. Proc 33rd Annu Conv Am Assoc Equine Pract, 1987, pp 341–353.

Bowling AT, Clark RS: Blood group and protein polymorphism gene frequencies for seven breeds of horses in the United States. Anim Blood Groups Biochem Genet 16:93–108, 1985.

McClure JJ, Koch C, Traub-Dargatz J: Characterization of a red blood cell antigen in donkeys and mules associated with neonatal isoerythrolysis. Anim Genet 25:119–120, 1994.

Scott AM, Jeffcott LB: Haemolytic disease of the newborn foal. Vet Rec 103:71–74, 1978.

Stormont C: Neonatal isoerythrolysis in domestic animals: A comparative review. Adv Vet Sci Comp Med 19:23–45, 1975.

Traub-Dargatz JL, McClure JJ, Koch C, Schlipf JW: Neonatal isoerythrolysis in mule foals. J Am Vet Med Assoc 206:67–70, 1995.

Neonatal Septicemia

MARY ROSE PARADIS
North Grafton, Massachusetts

Septicemia in the neonatal foal is the most common cause of death in the first 7 days of life. It accounts for 33% of foal mortality. The challenges to the equine practitioner are early recognition of the risk factors that may predispose a foal to bacterial infection, early identification of the disease process, and early generation of a strategic intervention plan so that therapy can be initiated before the animal's condition spirals down into irreversible shock. To meet these challenges, the veterinarian must be aware of the normal physiologic events that occur during the perinatal period. Deviations from these events can result and have devastating consequences to the foal.

EARLY RECOGNITION OF RISK FACTORS

The time period before, during, and after birth of an animal is generally considered the perinatal time. Maternal health during the perinatal period can directly influence the health of the foal. This is especially important during the prenatal period. Prenatal infections in the mare, such as pneumonia or enteritis/colitis, have the potential of entering the bloodstream and developing into septicemia. Hematogenous spread of the infection to the foal may occur.

The health of the placenta plays an important role in protecting the foal from possible infection. During the last month of gestation in the mare, the foal gains much of its birth weight and size. The placenta is a unique organ that exerts regulatory control over the nutrients, such as glucose and amino acids, that are delivered to the foal. Disruptions in placental function can have an adverse effect on the fetus or foal. In a recent study, abnormal placentae diagnosed by ultrasound prepartum or visualization at parturition were associated with approximately 79% abnormal foals. The abnormalities included septicemia, prematurity, hypoxia, neonatal maladjustment, limb deformities, twins, and death.

Conditions of the placenta that should be considered high risk for predisposing the foal to septicemia include placentitis and placental separation. Placentitis presents clinically as premature lactation and vaginal discharge. The presumed route of infection is via the cervix. The most commonly encountered infectious agents include fungi and bacteria. *Aspergillus* is the most likely fungus cultured, while *Escherichia coli* and β-hemolytic streptococci are the predominant bacteria recovered. The risk of septicemia in the fetus of the mare with bacterial placentitis is high. Infection can occur in utero as a direct extension of the placentitis. One study reported that 80% of aborted fetuses from mares with acute placental lesions were septicemic. Bacteria could be isolated from the fetal blood, lung, and stomach in these cases.

The clinical signs of placentitis should alert the clinician to the other consequences of this disease. The contaminated vaginal discharge may serve as a source of infection to the newborn foal as it passes through the birth canal during parturition. Premature lactation results in poor-quality colostrum for the foal at birth. Inadequate colostral antibody transfer, otherwise known as partial or complete failure of passive transfer (FPT) is the most common cause of septicemia that occurs after parturition.

The mare's placentation inhibits any in utero transfer of antibodies from the maternal to fetal circulation. Because the foal is born with no IgG and very little IgM, it is susceptible to infection. Colostrum is the first mammary secretion that the mare produces, and it is a distillation of IgG, IgGt, IgM, and IgA. The mare begins colostrum production approximately 3 weeks before parturition and it is only made once. Good-quality mare colostrum contains IgG levels ranging from 4000 to 6100 mg/dl. Extensive premature lactation has the effect of diluting the colostral antibodies to that of normal milk secretion, less than 2000 mg/dl IgG.

Premature placental separation can indirectly increase the risk of the foal's developing septicemia. If the placenta separates during parturition, the foal may experience a period of asphyxia. This lack of oxygen may produce a foal that is neurologically compromised and thus unable to stand and nurse after parturition. Ingestion of good-quality

colostrum must occur within the first 8 to 10 hours after birth. This is the period when the gastrointestinal tract is most receptive to the absorption of the large molecular weight immunoglobulins.

Acceptable levels of antibody transfer in foals range from 500 to 800 mg/dl. The age of the mare also plays a part in determining the amount of colostral transfer that occurs in the newborn foal. Foals born to older mares have an increased risk of not achieving immunoglobulin levels of more than 800 mg/dl. Low environmental temperatures and the amount of solar radiation may also affect colostral and foal serum IgG levels.

Not all foals with low immunoglobulins become septic. Management and environmental factors also play a role in the susceptibility of the foal to infection. Foals that are born into or raised under unsanitary conditions are at higher risk than foals that are born on well-managed farms.

EARLY RECOGNITION OF SEPSIS

Early recognition of sepsis is imperative to the successful outcome of the foal. It is not hard to make a diagnosis of septicemia in the foal that is presented in septic shock. These animals are recumbent and often unaware of their surroundings. Hemodynamically, they have decreased cardiac output and hypotension. On physical examination, this manifests as cold extremities, cyanotic mucous membranes, prolonged capillary refill time, and weak to absent peripheral pulses. The degree of hypotension can roughly be determined by the sequence of loss of peripheral pulses. The more peripheral pulses are the first to be lost. For example, a septic foal would lose the greater metatarsal artery pulse first, followed by the femoral pulse as shock progresses.

The greater challenge comes in recognizing the early signs of sepsis to prevent irreversible shock. These signs can be subtle and variable in each foal. The importance of a thorough perinatal history and physical examination cannot be overstressed. Clues in the history that may be predictive of sepsis include premature lactation, vulva discharge, prenatal illness in the dam, dystocia, a delay in time of standing and nursing in the foal, and foal rejection by the dam. All of these factors should raise the clinician's level of suspicion that this foal may develop a problem.

The practitioner's examination of the foal should begin with observation of the foal's behavior. The normal neonate should be vigorous and active soon after birth. Soon after the foal is expelled from the birth canal, it should become sternal. Within the first hour of life the foal should be scrambling around the stall and making attempts to stand. At this time the foal should also be making suckling motions with its tongue. The normal foal should be standing and nursing by 3 hours of life. Any deviation from this pattern may indicate the possibility of an in utero infection. If infection is not already present, this foal may be predisposed to postnatal infection due to delayed colostral ingestion.

One of the consistent first signs of developing sepsis in the newborn foal is depression and lethargy. Owners may report that their foals are quiet, easy to handle, and appear to sleep most of the time. Normal foals nurse approximately seven times an hour in short 30- to 90-second bursts. The sick foal often has decreased or absent suckle reflex. A distended and leaking mare's udder may indicate that the foal is not nursing as frequently as it should.

Dehydration or hypovolemic shock may be difficult to determine in the sick equine neonate. Tenting of the skin is unreliable because even in the normal foal it remains tented when pinched. The packed cell volume (PCV) and total protein levels (TP) in foals are normally lower than in the adult; therefore, significant increases for a particular foal may be underinterpreted when compared with adult values. The best indicator of dehydration in foals appears to be the observation of sunken eyes. Septic foals quickly lose fluid and fatty tissue behind their eyes. As the globe of the eye retracts in the socket, the foal often develops entropion of the lower lid. This can develop rapidly and is often seen in sick foals less than 24 hours of age.

Other clinical signs of sepsis are variable. The presence of a fever or hypothermia would certainly be cause for concern, but an equal number of septic foals present with a normal temperature. Mucous membranes may be pale, congested, or gray with or without petechiation in the septic newborn. Because of the systemic nature of the disease, many different organs may be involved, presenting their own set of clinical signs.

The lungs are the most commonly affected organ system in the septic foal. Early clinical signs may include an increased respiratory rate and effort. Auscultation of the lungs of a newborn foal is not always helpful in determining the presence of disease. If the examiner hears crackles or wheezes on auscultation, it is certain that the lungs are involved, but quiet lung sounds do not ensure a normal respiratory system. Consolidation of the lungs may be present despite normal findings on auscultation. Thoracic radiographs and arterial blood gas analysis should be considered as important diagnostic adjuncts in the examination of the foal that one suspects is septic. Hypoxemia is often present in foals with respiratory compromise. Eighty-three percent of septic foals in one study experienced mild to severe hypoxemia. Unfortunately, the observation of cyanotic mucous membranes does not occur before the Pao_2 is less than 40 mm Hg.

The second most common system failure presented in septic foals involves the gastrointestinal tract. Enteritis or colitis may occur as a result of ingestion of an infectious agent or through hematogenous spread of bacteria. Clinically this may present as ileus, abdominal distension, colic, and/or diarrhea. Radiography, ultrasonography, and abdominocentesis may be helpful in ruling out other causes for these clinical signs, such as intussusception, volvulus, and bladder rupture.

Other less frequent but equally devastating manifestations of sepsis in the foal include meningitis and septic arthritis. Foals presenting with septic meningitis have a severely depressed mentation that may be accompanied by seizure activity. The affected animals may hold the head and neck in a rigid position and exhibit extensor rigidity of the forelimbs. Focal signs may include strabismus, head tilt, and nystagmus. One of the difficulties in diagnosing septic meningitis is that it mimics many of the clinical signs that are common to neonatal maladjustment syndrome.

The diagnosis is dependent on a cerebrospinal fluid (CSF) analysis. An increased number of white blood cells with the presence of any neutrophils in the CSF should point toward a diagnosis of septic meningitis.

Lameness or joint effusion present in an equine neonate should be diagnosed as septic arthritis or osteomyelitis until proved otherwise. Septic arthritis was a clinical feature of 28% of the septic foals in one study. Osteomyelitis may be present without overt signs of joint swelling. The first clinical observation may be that the foal appears to spend most of its time recumbent. This would be an indication of bone or joint pain. Careful palpation of the joints and the bone proximal to the physeal regions of the long bone should be part of the physical examination.

Foals with septic arthritis or osteomyelitis are prone to develop decubital ulcers over the bony prominences of the shoulder, elbow, hock, stifle, and hip. The first sign of the decubiti is a change in the skin texture from soft and pliable to stiff and leathery. This devitalized skin eventually sloughs, leaving raw, open wounds.

Umbilical remnant infections have been incriminated as a source of the widespread infection that constitutes septicemia. In one study, 25% of the total number of foals that were classified as septic had umbilical infections. Interestingly, if the foal had septic arthritis or osteomyelitis, its chances of having an umbilical infection increased to 50%. External examination of the umbilicus of a foal is important, but it does not completely rule out the possible presence of internal infection. Ultrasonography of the internal structures of the umbilical remnant is important in determining the source of the infection. Structures that should be examined and measured include the umbilical stalk and vein, the two arteries, and the urachus. Enlargement of any of these structures over normal values is indicative of infection.

Laboratory Investigation

Some basic clinical laboratory tests are also very useful in confirming the diagnosis of sepsis. A complete blood count (CBC), blood glucose level, and immunoglobulin determination constitute a good minimal data base. A leukopenia represented by a neutropenia is the most common white blood cell abnormality seen in the septic foal. Toxic changes in the neutrophil may also be noted by the clinical pathologist. Leukocytosis may be seen in foals that have a persistent infection, such as a septic joint.

Septic foals younger than 24 hours of age often have hypoglycemia from their failure to nurse and their lack of glycogen storage. Hepatic gluconeogenesis is depressed by endotoxemia as well.

Because neonatal sepsis has a close association with failure of passive transfer of colostral antibodies, serum IgG levels should be determined in all questionably sick equine neonates. Several field tests are available to evaluate serum immunoglobulins. Two of the more common kits used are the zinc sulfate turbidity test° and an enzyme-linked immunosorbent assay (ELISA) test.† The latter test takes only 15 minutes to perform and can be used on whole blood, plasma, or serum.

°Equine-2, VMRD, Pullman, WA
†Foal IgG Test Kit, CITE, Portland, ME

TABLE 1.   MODIFIED SEPSIS SCORE

Foal's Name _____ Date _____ Total Score _____

Case # _____ Check One:

_____ At admission?
_____ Day subsequent to admission?

Indicate day #: _____

Information Collected:	4	3	2	1	0	This Case
CBC Neutrophil count		<2000/mm³	2000–4000 or >12,000	8000–12,000	Normal	
Band neutrophil count		>200/mm³	50–200		<50	
Doehle bodies, toxic, granulation or vacuolization in neutrophils	Marked	Moderate	Slight		None	
Fibrinogen			>600	500–600	≤400	
Other Laboratory Data Hypoglycemia			<50 mg/dl	50–80	>80	
Immunoglobulin	<200	200–400	401–800		>800	
Clinical Examination Petechiation or scleral injection not secondary to eye disease or trauma		Marked	Moderate	Mild	None	
Fever			>102°F	<100°F	Normal	
Hypotonia, coma, depression, convulsions			Marked	Mild	Normal	
Anterior uveitis, diarrhea, respiratory distress, swollen joints, open wounds		yes			no	
Historical Data Placentitis, vulvar discharge prior to delivery, dystocia		yes			no	
Prematurity (days)		<300	300–310	310–330	>330	
					Total Points	

A score of 11 is used as the cut-off point in determining non-septic (<11) or septic (≥11).
From Brewer BD, Koterba AM: Development of a scoring system for the early diagnosis of equine neonatal sepsis. Equine Vet J 20(1):18–22, 1988.

The taking of blood cultures is advocated in cases of neonatal septicemia because about 80% of confirmed septic foals have a positive blood culture. The problem of relying on blood cultures to confirm a diagnosis of sepsis is that it may take 72 hours or more before the results are available. The need to determine the presence of sepsis is immediate. Because of this need, a sepsis scoring system has been designed. A sepsis score is determined by entering particular historical, physical examination, and clinical pathologic parameters into the system (Table 1). Specific points are assigned to these parameters and a score is calculated. Foals with scores of greater than 11 are considered to be septic. Foals with scores of less than 11 are generally not septic. The sepsis score has proved to be a useful clinical tool, but because it is not 100% reliable, a strong clinical suspicion of sepsis should lead one to treat the foal despite a low score.

EARLY INTERVENTION STRATEGY

The key to a successful outcome when confronted with the possibility of a septic foal is prevention or early inter-

vention. The treatment of prepartum mares with clinical signs of infectious placentitis includes the use of appropriate systemic antibiotics and anti-inflammatory agents. Stall rest may also be important for prolonging gestation. The antimicrobial agents should be chosen on the basis of results of cultures done on the uterine discharge. Late pregnancy in women lowers the plasma concentrations of some drugs by 10 to 50%, but it is not known how antimicrobial distribution is altered in the pregnant mare. Studies on the transfer of antimicrobials across the normal equine placenta have compared trimethoprim/sulfa, penicillin, and gentamicin. Trimethoprim/sulfa was the only one of these three drugs that could be detected in fetal fluids. Placentitis may alter these dynamics.

If significant premature lactation has occurred during the prepartum period, the mare's mammary secretion should be analyzed for immunoglobulin content at the time of parturition. This can be done stall-side with a specific instrument that is calibrated to measure specific gravity of mare's colostrum.° The specific gravity of the secretion is correlated to IgG concentration. A high specific gravity

———————————————————

°Colostrometer, Blue Grass Equine Products, Lexington, KY

indicates a high concentration of IgG. Specific gravities of less than 1.060 are indicative of poor-quality colostrum. If the colostrum is of low quality, the foal should be given colostrum of a known quality from another mare or it should receive a plasma transfusion soon after birth. When the risk of sepsis is high, prophylactic antibiotics should be considered.

In foals that are already showing signs of septicemia, the general goals are to rid the animals of the offending organism through immunologic and antimicrobial support and to prevent the endotoxin released from the bacteria from starting the cascade of irreversible shock.

Immune Therapy

Virtually all septicemic foals have FPT (IgG <800 mg/dl). Exceptions may be those foals that were infected in utero but received adequate colostrum at birth. Plasma transfusions are routine in an attempt to provide immunologic support for these animals. Immunoglobulins opsonize bacteria, which facilitates phagocytosis by neutrophils. Although transfused plasma does not provide the same level of protection as good-quality colostrum, its contribution in the sick foal is important.

In general, the aim of the plasma transfusion is to raise the foal's IgG level up to 800 mg/dl. IgG levels in the normal foal increase at a rate of 20% of the concentration of the transfused plasma for each liter transfused. For example, if 1 L of plasma contains 1000 mg/dl of IgG, the expected rise in immunoglobulin in the foal is 200 mg/dl. The percentage rise in immunoglobulin decreases in the sick foal to approximately 11% of the transfused immunoglobulins. It is postulated that this decreased rise in the sick foal is due to rapid consumption of the immunoglobulins by the infection or sequestration in the extravascular space or areas of inflammation.

Other forms of immunotherapy have been used or are currently being investigated. Hyperimmune serum with antibodies against the rough mutant of *Salmonella* or *E. coli* is used clinically in some neonatal intensive care units as an anti-endotoxin therapy. Various forms of lyophilized or monoclonal antibodies can be used as an oral supplement to colostrum of questionable quality. Because equine colostrum is not readily available, the use of oral bovine colostrum has been investigated. Bovine IgG has a significantly shorter half life than does equine IgG in the foal, and its protective value against specific equine pathogens is unknown.

Antibiotic Therapy

Appropriate antibiotic therapy is important in the elimination of the bacterial infection of the septic foal. Antibiotics should be administered immediately when the foal is suspected of being infected. This means that the practitioner is often asked to make a choice of antibiotic without culture results. Septic foals should be placed on broad-spectrum bactericidal antibiotics that are effective against gram-positive and gram-negative organisms.

In a study involving 53 septic foals, 50% of the foals had a mixed gram-positive/gram-negative infection, and 50% of the foals were infected with a single organism. The most common gram-negative organism cultured was *E. coli*, followed by *Klebsiella, Enterobacter, Actinobacillus, Pseudo-* *monas, Citrobacter, Actinobacter,* and *Salmonella* species. The most common gram-positive organism cultured was *Streptococcus* species. Eighty-nine percent of all the gram-positive organisms were cultured in a mixed infection along with a gram-negative organism.

The sensitivity patterns for these organisms have changed over the past 10 years, probably because of increased resistance developed by the organisms to some of the more commonly used antibiotics. Studies suggest that amikacin and cefotaxime are the most effective in killing the gram-negative organisms found in neonatal sepsis. Two commonly used antibiotics, gentamicin and trimethoprim/sulfa, have lower sensitivity patterns. Ampicillin and penicillin are still effective in killing *Streptococcus* species. Therefore, an appropriate choice to initiate antibiotic coverage may include amikacin and ampicillin. Alternative antibiotic combinations should be considered when culture results are available or if the animal does not appear to be responding (Table 2).

Fluid Therapy

The gram-negative bacteria that are found in neonatal septicemia contain endotoxin in their cell walls. When endotoxin is released in the animal, it initiates a cascade of cytokines that are responsible for many of the behavioral, hematologic, and hemodynamic changes that are seen in septic shock. The most important treatment strategy for diverting the lethal effects of endotoxin involves intravascular fluid expansion. Physiologically balanced crystalloid fluids, such as Ringer's, Ringer's lactate, or acetate, remain in the intravascular space three times longer than dextrose and water solutions; therefore, these types of fluid would be favored in the treatment of septicemia. If the foal is hypoglycemic, dextrose may be added to the crystalloid solution; 100 ml of a 50% dextrose solution may be added to a liter of lactated Ringer's solution. This will make the solution approximately a 5% dextrose concentration.

Because foals have a larger volume of distribution, their normal maintenance fluid requirements are higher than those of an adult horse. Normal healthy foals require approximately 80 to 120 ml/kg per day or 3 to 5 ml/kg per hour. In the 45-kg foal this translates to 3.6 to 5.4 L/day. If the foal is experiencing endotoxemia, these requirements may increase as high as 30 to 40 ml/hour until volume expansion has occurred.

Urinary output should be monitored during fluid admin-

TABLE 2. ANTIMICROBIAL DRUGS USED IN THE TREATMENT OF EQUINE NEONATAL SEPTICEMIA

Drug	Route	Dose (mg/kg)	Interval
Amikacin sulfate	IV, IM	7.5	b.i.d., t.i.d.
Gentocin sulfate	IV, IM	3.3	b.i.d.
Cefotaxime sodium	IV, IM	15–25	b.i.d., t.i.d.
Ceftiofur	IV, IM	2.2	b.i.d.
Penicillin G sodium	IV	20,000–40,000 IU/kg	q.i.d.
Ampicillin sodium	IV, IM	10–15	q.i.d.
Ticarcillin sodium	IV, IM	40–60	t.i.d.
Ticarcillin-clavulanate	IV	50	t.i.d., q.i.d.
Trimethoprim-sulfonamide	p.o.	15–30	b.i.d.

istration. Most foals urinate after approximately 3 L. If this does not occur, one should be suspicious of renal shutdown or a ruptured bladder. In cases of anuric renal failure, dopamine HCl (2–10 μg/kg per minute) increases the sympathetic tone to the splanchnic venous system. Blood flow to the kidneys and the small intestine is increased, increasing urine formation. The use of pressor drugs may also be beneficial in the hypotensive foal. Dobutamine (2–15 μg/kg per minute) is a positive inotrope that increases cardiac contractility without increasing heart rate.

Specific System Therapy

Different manifestations of the septic process have specific therapy that is necessary for a successful outcome. Umbilical remnant infections require surgical removal. Once that foal's condition is stable enough to undergo general anesthesia, the umbilical structures are carefully dissected. Structures that are enlarged or discolored should be removed. Culture of these tissues is often rewarding in determining the causative organism of the septicemia.

Specific intra-articular therapy for septic arthritis is an emergency. Infection in or around a joint results in a rapid influx of inflammatory cells into the synovia. Cell counts can range from 10,000 to greater than 150,000 with protein levels increased above 2.5 mg/dl. The cells and their inflammatory byproducts are very damaging to cartilage cells. Multiple joint lavages with sterile lactated Ringer's solution are very effective in establishing a more normal synovial fluid. Joint flushes should continue on alternate days until joint fluid analysis approaches normal values. In treatment of human septic arthritis, it has been found that a delay of treatment by more than 48 hours causes a significant decrease in prognosis.

Septic foals that present with bacterial pneumonia may progress into respiratory failure with PaO_2 less than 60 mm Hg and $PaCO_2$ higher than 55 mm Hg. These foals require intensive respiratory physiotherapy consisting of oxygen administration and mechanical positive pressure ventilation until the antibiotics and immunologic supports can have a chance to work. This is extremely labor-intensive work and is best performed at an intensive care facility. Hypoxia without hypercapnia often responds to oxygen supplementation. Oxygen can be administered through a face mask or an indwelling nasal oxygen tube.

Corneal ulceration is often a secondary problem associated with the septic foal. As stated before, the eyes of the septic foal often become sunken as the result of dehydration and loss of the infraorbital fat. The common consequence of this retraction of the globe is entropion of the lower lid. The entropion produces irritation and ulceration of the cornea. Aggressive therapy of these ulcers is important. Topical ophthalmic antibiotics should be placed in the eye four to five times a day. The entropion is easily corrected by placing a temporary mattress suture in the lower lid, rolling the eyelashes away from the cornea.

Nutritional Support

The increased survival rates resulting from treatment of the septic foal have coincided with the growing recognition that these foals have special nutritional needs. Although it has been suggested that the metabolic rate of the premature or maladjusted foal decreases to 75% of the healthy recumbent foal, sepsis increases caloric demand of a patient. In the septic human it is estimated that the caloric needs increase from 40 to 50%. The septic patient is in a catabolic state. This is magnified in the foal, which has very few fat reserves and has the needs of growth. In the absence of enteral feeding, the normal foal has only enough glycogen reserves to support metabolism for 2 hours postpartum. If nutrition is not a prominent component of the strategic therapeutic plan for the septic foal, the patient "melts" before the clinician's eyes. Malnutrition compromises the healing process of the foal. There is a decrease in chemotaxis of white cells, complement levels, T-cell activity, and wound healing.

The normal, healthy 45-kg foal ingests approximately 12 to 13 L/day of mare's milk. This provides about 130 to 150 kcal/kg per day (5850–6750 kcal/day). For the first week of life a normal foal feeds on the average of seven times per hour for short periods. If the foal has a good suck reflex, it should be encouraged to suck from the mare. This is the least labor-intensive method of providing nutrition. An indwelling nasogastric tube may be placed in foals that are anorectic. Generally, small amounts (200–500 ml) of mare's milk or milk substitute should be administered every 1 to 2 hours.

As the caloric demand increases with sepsis, it becomes difficult to provide adequate nutrition through enteral means only. The presence of diarrhea or milk intolerance may further complicate the nutritional support of the sick foal. It is important for the health of the gastrointestinal tract to maintain some form of enteral nutrition, but partial or total parenteral nutrition (PPN or TPN) may need to be introduced to the patient. Glucose, amino acids, and lipids are the major components of parenteral nutrition. Vitamins, electrolytes, and trace minerals can also be added.

When considering the use of parenteral nutrition in the critically ill foal, one needs to weigh the advantages and disadvantages. The advantages are obvious in that one can provide the foal with a higher level of nutrition than through enteral formulations alone. Mortality rates in humans with multiple organ failure are significantly higher in those patients with a negative nitrogen balance. The disadvantages of TPN are numerous. They include catheter-related problems, labor intensity, hyperglycemia, and expense. Ideally, the foal should have a sterilely placed central venous catheter that is dedicated to the TPN solution only. Technically a constant infusion pump is needed to deliver the solutions at a constant rate. A veterinarian should be available to monitor the patient and its blood work at frequent intervals. The cost per day of TPN varies with the formulations but the range is from $75 to $150/day.

Calories for energy can be provided by the dextrose and lipid solutions. One g of dextrose contributes 4 kcals of energy whereas 1 g of lipid provides approximately 9 kcals of energy. It is important to use these components to make up the entire energy requirement of approximately 100 to 150 kcal/kg per day in the foal. This allows the amino acid solution to be utilized for protein building rather than as an expensive source of energy calories. This can be accomplished by keeping 100 to 200 non-nitrogen calories/g of nitrogen from amino acids.

Although 50% dextrose has been the traditional source

of energy in TPN solutions, the addition of exogenous lipid has been helpful in many ways. It is an isotonic solution; therefore, it lowers the hypertonicity of the TPN solution, which in turn decreases the incidence of phlebitis. One guideline states that the lipids should not exceed 60% of the nonprotein calories.

To begin TPN or to provide PPN in addition to enteral feeding, it may be advisable to start by providing half the energy needs. As the animal adjusts to the high glucose levels, the energy and protein levels can be increased to the animal's full needs. A simple starting formula includes the following: 10 g/kg per 24 hours of glucose, 2 g/kg per 24 hours of amino acids, and 1g/kg per 24 hours of lipid. The foal would receive approximately 53 kcal/kg and 140 non-protein calories per g of nitrogen. Practically, for the 50-kg foal, this translates to 1 L of 50% dextrose, 1 L of 8.5% amino acids with electrolytes, and 0.5 L of 10% lipid with an approximate cost of $70.

Blood and urine glucose should be measured two to three times a day for foals that are receiving parenteral nutrition. Most foals adjust to the glucose load within the first 24 hours if they are begun on a lower dose at a slow rate. Blood glucose levels that are consistently higher than 250 mg/dl may indicate glucose intolerance. If a further lowering of the glucose concentration does not alleviate the problem, insulin can be started along with the parenteral nutrition.

CONCLUSIONS

The treatment strategies for working with the critically ill foal have become more successful over the last 15 years. Identification of the high-risk mare and foal has enabled practitioners to anticipate problems before they happen and to work toward their prevention. By developing a team approach with the owner, practitioner, and intensive care facility, the prognosis for the septic foal becomes more hopeful.

Supplemental Readings

Baggot JD: Drug therapy in the neonatal foal. Vet Clin North Am Equine Pract 10(1):87–107, 1994.

Brewer BD, Koterba AM: Development of a scoring system for the early diagnosis of equine neonatal sepsis. Equine Vet J 20(1):18–22, 1988.

Hansen TO: Parenteral nutrition in foals and calves. Proc. The application of intensive care therapies and parenteral nutrition in large animal medicine. Aug, 1986, pp 36–38. Sponsored by the University of Pennsylvania School of Veterinary Medicine through a grant from Travenol Laboratories.

Koterba AM, Brewer BD, Tarplee FA: Clinical and clinicopathological characteristics of the septicaemic neonatal foal: Review of 38 cases. Equine Vet J 16:376–383, 1984.

Paradis MR: Update on neonatal septicemia. Vet Clin North Am Equine Pract 10(1):109–135, 1994.

Wilson WD, Madigan JE: Comparison of bacteriologic culture of blood and necropsy specimens for determining the cause of foal septicemia: 47 cases (1978–1987). J Am Vet Med Assoc 195:1759–1763, 1989.

Umbilical Disorders

LUCY M. EDENS
Gainesville, Florida

The umbilicus serves as the portal through which vascular channels travel into and out of the fetus. The umbilicus also provides a route for the elimination of nitrogenous wastes produced by the growing fetus. The proper development and function of the umbilicus is critical for the delivery of a viable foal. In the postpartum period, a number of different abnormalities may affect this structure.

The umbilicus is composed of one umbilical vein, two umbilical arteries, a urachus, and a ring of smooth muscle encompassing the umbilical structures at the abdominal body wall. Immediately after rupture of the umbilical cord, the umbilical arteries and urachus retract caudally into the abdomen toward the urinary bladder. The musculature within the abdominal wall surrounding the umbilicus contracts, narrowing the diameter of the remaining opening; however, this leaves remnants of the umbilical vein and amniotic sac exposed to the outside environment. Under normal conditions, this exposed umbilical stalk dries out and involutes over a 3- to 7-day period, being completely eliminated within 3 to 4 weeks. After delivery, the umbilical vessels no longer are required for the transfer of blood, so they undergo constriction and fibrosis. The umbilical vein

becomes the falciform ligament of the liver and the umbilical arteries develop into the round ligaments of the urinary bladder. The urachus persists as a remnant structure on the apex of the bladder.

Umbilical problems arise during the immediate postpartum period as a consequence of either abnormal involution or bacterial infection. Failure of the smooth musculature within the abdominal body wall surrounding the umbilical vessels and urachus to contract and close the umbilical opening within a few days provides a site for herniation of abdominal contents. Failure of proper urachal closure can result in patency of this structure. Blood clots form and stay within the umbilical vessels after delivery, providing an excellent medium for bacterial growth in an environment that becomes, for all practical purposes, avascular. Thus, the three most commonly encountered umbilical problems are umbilical herniation, persistent or acquired patent urachus, and umbilical abscessation.

UMBILICAL HERNIATION

Failure of the abdominal musculature to properly close around the umbilical structures results in an umbilical hernia. The reason for this failure is unknown, although it has been postulated that the herniation is due to umbilical cord inflammation or an inherited predisposition. The intra-abdominal structures contained within the hernia vary with the size of the defect. Small-diameter (<2 cm) openings almost always resolve spontaneously and are unlikely to cause problems because the omentum is typically the only structure able to fit through this small ring. Larger hernial rings may contain omentum, small intestine, or a combination of these within the sac. The diagnosis of umbilical herniation can often be made by external palpation alone. Ultrasonography of the affected area can be useful in determining the contents and in differentiating other causes of umbilical enlargement such as umbilical abscessation (see *Current Therapy in Equine Medicine* 3, page 417). One important fact to recall when examining umbilical swellings is that nonstrangulating umbilical hernias are not painful; however, umbilical abscesses or strangulating hernias are painful when examined by palpation.

Treatment

Congenital umbilical hernias smaller than 5 cm in diameter that can be manually reduced typically heal spontaneously during the first 6 to 9 months of life. The hernia should be monitored frequently by confirming that manual reduction is still possible. If the hernia persists beyond 6 to 9 months of age or enlarges during the period of observation, more aggressive intervention is indicated. In addition to surgical reduction, either a supportive abdominal wrap or hernial clamps may used to stimulate abdominal wall closure. If clamps are used, they should be placed with the foal in dorsal recumbency to help ensure that no intestinal contents are trapped within the clamp. One potential complication from the use of clamps is the subsequent development of intestinal adhesions because of the inflammatory response that accompanies the necrosis and fibrosis of the abdominal body wall induced by clamping.

Large umbilical hernias, those that are larger than 10 cm in diameter, are unlikely to close without surgical intervention and present a potentially serious problem for the foal. Foals with large hernias should undergo surgical correction within the first 3 months of life.

PATENT URACHUS

Almost immediately after birth and rupture of the umbilical cord, the urachus should retract and the abdominal musculature surrounding the umbilicus contracts, resulting in a cessation of urine flow out of the urinary bladder via the urachus. Failure for this to occur in the immediate postpartum period results in a persistent or congenital patent urachus, whereas re-establishment of urine flow after a normal closure at birth is termed acquired patent urachus. The pathophysiologic mechanisms allowing a congenital patent urachus to develop are unknown. Acquired patent urachus can occur as a consequence of a variety of insults, all of which place tension on the ventral abdominal body wall or are associated with umbilical inflammation. Prolonged recumbency, tenesmus, abdominal distension, umbilical abscessation, and septicemia have all been associated with the occurrence of acquired patent urachus.

Diagnosis

The diagnosis in most cases can be made by observing urine flowing or dribbling from the umbilical remnant. Dermatitis from exposure to urine may be present on the ventral abdominal wall or rear limbs. In cases in which urine has not been noted from the umbilical remnant but a patent urachus is suspected, confirmation can be made on contrast cystography by instilling 100 ml of a 10-part water to one-part iodinated radiographic contrast medium into the urinary bladder after catheterization. Foals with a patent urachus should receive a complete physical examination, complete blood count, fibrinogen estimation, and immunoglobulin quantification to rule out concurrent problems. If a fever, leukocytosis, high fibrinogen, IgG deficiency, or clinical evidence of septicemia is noted, bacterial infection of the umbilicus should be suspected. It is also prudent when evaluating these cases, particularly those foals with an acquired patent urachus, to perform an ultrasound examination of the internal umbilical structures (see *Current Therapy in Equine Medicine* 3, page 417).

Treatment

Foals with an uncomplicated patent urachus often are best managed conservatively with local therapy and elimination of accompanying problems, such as tenesmus. Cauterization of the urachus with silver nitrate sticks, 2% iodine solutions, or local injection of procaine penicillin into the external umbilical remnant is usually curative. External treatments should not be applied proximal to the abdominal body wall because of the risk of enhancing internal urachal abscessation or cystitis. If the problem persists for more than 5 days after resolution of predisposing factors such as prolonged recumbency, surgical removal of the umbilicus should be considered to prevent urachal abscessation, local ascending infection, and possibly septicemia.

In foals with acquired patent urachus coincident with umbilical abscessation or if evidence of umbilical infection develops during the course of treatment, parenteral antimicrobial therapy with broad-spectrum antibiotics should be implemented. Surgical resection of the umbilicus should also be considered to minimize the incidence of septicemia.

UMBILICAL ABSCESSATION

Bacterial infection of the structures within the internal or external umbilical cord is one of the most commonly encountered problems in neonatal foals. These infections originate from contamination of the external umbilical remnant after delivery or from seeding from other sites, particularly the umbilical vessels, during septicemia.

Previously, it was suspected that the umbilicus served as the primary portal of entry for bacteria, but recent evidence suggests that most neonatal septicemias may occur from bacterial translocation across the gastrointestinal wall. Whatever the role umbilical contamination may play in neonatal septicemia, proper care of the umbilical remnant should be a part of any good preventive health program. Solutions recommended for routine use include 2% iodine, 1% povidone-iodine, and 0.5% chlorhexidine. In one study, foals treated with 0.5% chlorhexidine had the lowest number of bacteria cultured from their umbilical cords after treatment, when compared with foals treated with 2% iodine, 1% povidone-iodine, or 7% iodine. In addition, chlorhexidine's reported residual activity, by binding to the stratum corneum, provides a longer duration of antimicrobial activity than any of the other solutions. Strong iodine (7%) solutions should be avoided because of their irritating and locally damaging effects on tissues. In a study comparing local umbilical treatments, four of 10 foals treated with 7% iodine developed a patent urachus within 3 to 5 days of treatment. The tissue damage and necrosis that occur in association with the use of 7% iodine solutions have led to speculation that the incidence of bacterial infections may actually be enhanced because the necrotic tissue provides favorable conditions for bacterial growth.

Diagnosis

Clinical signs of umbilical abscessation may include external umbilical swelling, heat, pain on palpation, patent urachus, or purulent umbilical discharge. When only the internal or intra-abdominal portions of the umbilical cord are affected, the clinical signs are often subtle and therefore difficult to appreciate on physical examination alone. As with many neonatal infections, the first and sometimes only clinical signs observed may be depression and inappetence. Other abnormalities include fever, dysuria, pollakuria, and tenesmus. In a retrospective study of 38 foals with umbilical abscessation, 91% of the foals had external evidence of either umbilical infection or infection at some other visible sight. This finding suggests that the diagnosis can commonly be made during physical examination. A more recent prospective study involving approximately 150 foals indicated that umbilical infections can often be detected with ultrasound before the appearance of external abnormalities. Even in the cases in which the diagnosis is readily apparent on physical examination, it is important to determine the extent of involvement of internal umbilical structures, so that proper treatment recommendations and prognosis can be made. Transabdominal ultrasonography is the best method by which to evaluate internal umbilical structures to determine the severity and extent of infection. For a complete description of this technique, the reader is referred to *Current Therapy in Equine Medicine 3,* page 417.

Clinicopathologic aberrations that may be associated with umbilical abscessation include neutrophilia, toxic changes within the white blood cells, and hyperfibrinogenemia. Because of the association of umbilical infection with septicemia, blood cultures should be obtained, particularly in foals with fever or multiple sites of infection. It is important to note that umbilical remnant infections have been reported in horses up to 16 months of age.

Treatment

Treatment options include surgical resection or medical management. Indications for surgery include evidence of multisystem infection, umbilical vein involvement, uroperitoneum resulting from urachal rupture, or failure to respond to medical therapy. Medical management of umbilical abscessation carries some risk owing to the potential for septic arthritis, pneumonia, peritonitis, uroperitoneum because of urachal rupture, and other life-threatening problems. However, in situations in which economic constraints preclude surgical intervention, medical therapy has been used successfully. Medical therapy consists of prolonged administration of broad-spectrum antimicrobials and encouragement of drainage from the external umbilical remnant if swelling is present. In one study, medical treatment was successful in almost 50% of affected foals. The foals in this study underwent frequent ultrasound examinations and, if the internal umbilical structures continued to enlarge during the course of treatment, or if the foals developed persistent fevers, surgical resection was recommended. Ultrasonographic changes consistent with resolution of the infection were seen in most foals in this study within 3 to 7 days from the onset of treatment.

Bacteria involved in umbilical infections include gram-negative enterics, *Streptococcus* species, *Staphylococcus* species, and occasionally anaerobes. Antimicrobial therapy with intravenous potassium penicillin and an aminoglycoside is preferred, although other treatments including cephalosporins, trimethoprim/sulfa combinations, or metronidazole have all been used with success in some instances. Because of the wide variety of bacteria that may be involved, bacterial culture is indicated in foals undergoing surgical resection. When surgical resection is selected, antimicrobials should be used preoperatively and for at least 5 days postoperatively. Flunixin meglumine (0.25 to 1.1 mg/kg IV or IM b.i.d.) for 3 to 5 days postoperatively minimizes local reaction and incisional pain and may reduce the incidence of postoperative intestinal adhesions to the abdominal incision.

Supplemental Readings

Lavan RP, Madigan J, Walker R, Muller N: Effects of disinfectant treatments on the bacterial flora of the umbilicus of neonatal foals. Proc 40th Annu Meet Am Assoc Equine Pract, 1994, pp 37–38.
Reimer JM: Ultrasonography of umbilical remnant infections in foals. Proc 39th Annu Meet Am Assoc Equine Pract, 1993, pp 247–248.

Neonatal Pulmonary Disease

GUY D. LESTER
Gainesville, Florida

A number of factors clearly separate respiratory diseases in newborn animals from those in older foals and adults. The neonatal foal is susceptible to a range of noninfectious diseases associated with the perinatal period and the transition from fetal to extrauterine environments. In addition, a different spectrum of bacterial and viral agents is responsible for infectious pulmonary disease in this age group. Identification and management of respiratory diseases in newborn animals can be particularly challenging. In contrast to adults, respiratory disease may develop rapidly in neonates, but may also improve at an equally rapid rate.

PULMONARY ADAPTATION

Adaption of the respiratory system to the extrauterine environment involves a complex sequence of events that is easily disturbed by factors that include inadequate lung development, surfactant deficiency, viral or bacterial infection, or meconium aspiration. In the normal newborn animal there is a rapid and smooth transition from a fluid-filled fetal lung to an air-filled structure responsible for whole body gas exchange. This process involves opening of collapsed alveoli and absorption of fluid, a process primarily mediated by a net change in sodium ion transport from secretion to absorption. A highly compliant chest wall, although essential for smooth passage through the pelvis during birth, can contribute to respiratory failure in compromised foals. A flexible chest wall is drawn inward during inspiration, and consequently the diaphragm must contract with greater force to offset this effect. The immune system of the newborn foal is also inefficient relative to that of an older foal or adult. Complement factors, immunoglobulin-secreting plasma cells, and alveolar macrophages are important components of the immune system that are probably deficient at the time of birth. In addition, failure to derive adequate antibody from colostrum (i.e., partial or total failure of passive transfer) can expose the neonatal foal to diseases from common environmental pathogens.

ASSESSMENT OF THE RESPIRATORY SYSTEM

History

To thoroughly assess the respiratory system it is important to consider the history, physical examination findings, and often a number of diagnostic tests. Historical information should include an estimation of gestational age and physical maturity; presence or absence of meconium staining; assessment of colostral quality and quantity; and recognition of maternal problems such as fever, dystocia, placentitis, or vaginal discharge.

Clinical Examination

Although physical examination of the newborn foal can often reveal clear evidence of pulmonary disease, it can also be very misleading. In contrast to older foals and adult horses, newborn animals with pulmonary disease rarely demonstrate cough or nasal discharge. Fever can also be an inconsistent finding, even in foals with severe bronchopneumonia.

During the first 60 minutes of postnatal life, the respiratory rate may be as high as 80 breaths per minute in the healthy foal. The rate should slowly decline to 30 to 40 breaths per minute over the following few hours. Tachypnea, an elevation in respiratory rate, is not only seen with lung disease but is also associated with a variety of extrapulmonary conditions including excitement, pain, fever, anemia, and as a consequence to some metabolic derangements such as acidemia. Unfortunately, it can sometimes be very difficult to distinguish between lung disease and extra-pulmonary causes of tachypnea without pursuing some further diagnostic tests. The depth of breathing is another important observation that should be made. Foals in respiratory distress may demonstrate paradoxical chest wall motion, that is, the chest may move inward during inspiration, a warning sign of impending respiratory failure. In an attempt to maintain adequate lung volumes, the foal with respiratory disease may have a prolonged expiratory phase against a partially closed glottis. This may coincide with an audible expiratory "grunt."

A reduction in respiratory rate can be seen in foals that have been asphyxiated. Periodic breathing patterns can be occasionally observed, especially in premature or dysmature foals and in animals with hypoxic ischemic encephalomyelopathy (HIE). The patterns observed in foals are variable and may include Cheyne-Stokes respiration, in which lengthy periods of apnea are interspersed with short breaths that wax and wane in amplitude, "cluster breathing" in which the duration of apnea is shorter than the breathing phase, or "Biots breathing" in which the breath clusters and apneic periods occur without obvious periodicity. The mechanism responsible for the change in the pattern of ventilation is unknown but may be related to reduced chemoreceptor sensitivity in the brain.

In utero, the foal is exposed to a hypoxic environment, the partial pressure of oxygen being around 30 mm Hg. As an adaptive response to this environment, fetal hemoglobin has a high affinity for oxygen. Because high-affinity hemoglobin persists in the neonate, mucous membrane color usually fails to reflect mild to moderate pulmonary disease, and some foals with mild to moderate hypoxemia can appear bright. In contrast to adult horses, obvious cyanosis

604

does not occur in newborn foals until the arterial partial pressure of oxygen (PaO_2) is very low (<40 mm Hg).

Auscultation of the thorax can also be deceptive. During the first few hours after birth, fluid sounds can normally be auscultated throughout both lung fields and in the trachea. End-inspiratory crackles are also commonly heard over the dependent lung during and shortly after lateral recumbency. This is presumably due to simple atelectasis. Foals with respiratory disease often have obvious abnormal sounds, such as crackles and wheezes, but it is also not uncommon for foals with even severe pulmonary disease to demonstrate little abnormality during auscultation.

Radiography and Ultrasound

Thoracic radiography is an extremely useful diagnostic tool in the work-up of the newborn foal with suspected respiratory disease. Many newer portable machines have sufficient power (100 kVp and 30 mA) to produce good-quality films. By minimizing exposure time, efficient high-speed screens and machines with higher mA capacities can reduce some of the blurring that is a result of the rapid respiratory rate of newborns. The requirement for relatively large screens is probably the biggest limitation for the practitioner. Films are routinely taken with the animal either standing or in lateral recumbency. Radiography is also helpful in following the progression of disease in response to treatment, but it is not uncommon for radiographic changes to lag behind clinical changes. Radiographic differentiation of atelectasis from pneumonia is sometimes difficult, if not impossible. Diffuse pulmonary infiltrates initially clear caudodorsally and with time "settle" caudoventrally in foals that are ambulatory.

Thoracic ultrasound examination is rarely needed in the work-up of respiratory disease in neonates, probably due to the low incidence of pleural disease at this age. It can, however, be of some use in localizing pulmonary abscesses, collapsed or pneumonic lung, or pneumothorax. Ultrasound is of critical importance in the evaluation of cardiac anomalies and the differentiation of cardiac and respiratory causes of hypoxemia.

Measurements of Gas Exchange

Arterial blood gas analysis is probably the most sensitive clinical measurement of lung function. Although collection of the sample is relatively simple, the equipment to process the sample has been limited to institutional or large referral practices. The introduction of cheaper portable units* now allows the field veterinarian to use blood gas analysis. The most common site for sampling arterial blood is the dorsal metatarsal artery. This artery is not usually accompanied by a vein and can be easily palpated in most foals on the lateral aspect of the hind cannon bone. The sample is obtained using either a 1- or 3-ml syringe with the hub filled with heparin and a narrow-gauge needle (25 gauge, 5/8 inch). In some foals a small bleb of 2% lidocaine may facilitate collection. Placement of an indwelling arterial catheter is relatively easy, but it is very difficult to maintain patency for any length of time. The brachial artery is located at the level of the medial collateral ligament of the elbow joint. The artery is covered by the pectoralis

*StatPal II, Unifet, La Jolla, CA

transversus, which is relatively thin at this level, allowing easy palpation of a pulse. The brachial vein runs adjacent to the artery making venous blood contamination of the sample possible. The carotid artery offers yet another site, but hematoma formation is a common sequel to aspiration from this site.

Interpretation of the Blood Gas Data

It is important to note the amount of struggling and position of the foal during sample collection. Lateral recumbency can reduce the PaO_2 by as much as 30 mm Hg. In most foals this reduction is likely to be around 15 mm Hg (PaO_2 of 95 versus 80 mm Hg in standing and recumbent foals, respectively). The PO_2 in venous blood is slightly higher in recumbent than upright foals during the first 5 days of life. Venous samples are usually reserved for investigation of metabolic conditions. The blood gas sample needs to be handled appropriately, paying strict attention to avoidance of air contamination. Such contamination artificially increases the PaO_2 and decreases the $PaCO_2$. If analysis is delayed, the capped sample may be kept for up to 6 hours before processing.

During the first 15 minutes of life, the normal foal, by increasing minute ventilation (the product of respiratory frequency and tidal volume), converts a severe hypoxemia (<40 mm Hg) and hypercapnia (>60 mm Hg) into mild hypoxemia (60 mm Hg) and hypercapnia (50 mm Hg). These values further improve over the following 4 to 6 hours to 75 and 54 mm Hg for PaO_2 and $PaCO_2$, respectively. The PaO_2 is similar to that of an adult animal ($\geq$ 85 mm Hg) by 7 days of age. The lower PaO_2 in newborn foals is most likely due to right-to-left shunting of blood, presumably through the ductus arteriosus. This probably represents about 10% of the cardiac output in healthy newborns. The newborn foal therefore fails to reach the same PaO_2 of adult horses when challenged with 100% O_2 (230–370 mm Hg in foals <4 days of age compared with >475 mm Hg in older foals and adults).

The two most common blood gas derangements of respiratory origin include hypoxemia with normo- or hypocapnia, and hypoxemia with hypercapnia ($PaCO_2$ >50 mm Hg). The first derangement is often treated with oxygen therapy, whereas the management of hypoxemia with hypercapnia can be more complex. If possible, acute hypercapnia needs to be distinguished from chronic hypercapnia. Sudden rises in $PaCO_2$ are usually associated with a more dramatic decrease in blood pH (0.008 units for every 1 mm Hg rise in CO_2) and may lead to circulatory collapse and coma, particularly if accompanied by moderate to severe hypoxemia. Chronic exposure to elevated CO_2 permits adaptation and more subtle clinical effects. The change in pH is less dramatic (0.003 units for every 1 mm Hg rise in CO_2) primarily because of enhanced bicarbonate reabsorption in the proximal tubules of the kidney. This effect probably begins within 6 to 12 hours of exposure to increased concentrations of CO_2 and is maximal by 3 to 4 days. Hypercapnia is further accentuated by a number of factors, including fever and exogenous administration of carbohydrates or bicarbonate. The latter is often clinically relevant and highlights the danger of giving sodium bicarbonate to foals with pulmonary disease. A moderate metabolic acidosis with mild hypercapnia is easily converted into a mild metabolic acidosis and severe respiratory acidosis with exogenous bicarbonate therapy, the net effect being a lower blood pH and a worsening of the clinical condition.

Pulse Oximetry

Pulse oximetry remains largely restricted to institutional practices, although newer devices are now marketed for the private practitioner. Oximetry measures the concentration of oxyhemoglobin in blood by light absorbency. The value is falsely lowered in icteric animals. The technique is useful in monitoring of the anesthetized patient but its value in the conscious foal requires further definition.

Expired CO_2 Concentration

Expired CO_2 concentration, which offers an approximation of $PaCO_2$, can be measured by use of either a mass spectrometer or infrared analyzer.° The values are falsely lowered when the expired gas is aspirated from a circuit that has a high humidity, such as when a heated water humidifier is used in a ventilator circuit. This effect can be reduced by using heat and moisture exchange filters. This equipment is useful in an intensive-care facility, but it is unlikely to be of value to the field practitioner.

THERAPEUTIC STRATEGIES

Resuscitation of the Neonate

The equine veterinarian occasionally must attempt to resuscitate the newborn foal, particularly if it is born after dystocia. The decision to attempt resuscitation must be based on an estimation of the foal's gestational age and physical maturity, probable length and severity of ischemic or hypoxic insult, and assessment of the foal's initial vital signs. Some owners or attendants expect that all reasonable attempts at resuscitation be performed, but successful resuscitation does not necessarily translate into long-term survival. Many foals that have undergone prolonged periods of tissue ischemia or hypoxia often become very challenging and expensive intensive-care patients. Items that may be required for resuscitation should be available before every spontaneous or induced delivery.

Apnea or inadequate ventilation occurs relatively commonly in the foal during the immediate postpartum period. Simple stimulation and postural drainage often induce effective breathing. Stimulation can be accomplished by vigorous rubbing of the skin, stimulation of the nasal mucosa, or manipulation of limbs. Mouth-to-nose resuscitation can be an effective ventilatory stimulant and provide time while other items such as nasotracheal tubes and resuscitation bag are gathered. The mouth, lips, and one nostril are occluded and a sufficient volume of expired air is blown into the open nostril to cause effective chest excursions. Hanging foals by their rear limbs should be discouraged because the intestinal contents further increase intrathoracic pressure and impair diaphragmatic contraction. A gentle incline is usually effective for postural drainage. If an adequate ventilatory response is not obtained within 60 seconds, more aggressive support is indicated.

Examination of the nasal openings and auscultation of the trachea and thorax may confirm the presence of excessive residual fluid or meconium aspiration, which is indicated by a brown nasal discharge. These foals may require more vigorous airway suctioning either by use of a soft catheter and a 60-ml syringe or a portable suction unit. Care must be taken to avoid excessive or prolonged negative pressure. Nasotracheal intubation usually is necessary for effective suctioning of the lower airway. Consequently, the practitioner should have ready access to a variety of cuffed endotracheal tubes (6 mm–12 mm).

If spontaneous ventilation is weak or absent, assisted ventilation may be required. Adult human resuscitation bags are effective in providing temporary intermittent positive airway pressure. Newer devices are now available with adjustable positive end-expiratory pressure (PEEP) valves and can be used with room air or can be attached to an oxygen source. An oxygen demand valve° can be used to assist spontaneous breathing in intubated foals. It is critical to be familiar with this demand valve before using it on an animal. Negative airway pressure created by the foal during spontaneous ventilation causes the valve to open and supplement the breath with oxygen-enriched gas at an increased tidal volume. Oxygen can also be forced into the airway under pressure when a button is depressed. Barotrauma is easily induced through overinflation. If suddenly discontinued, excessive assisted ventilation of newborn foals sometimes is followed by apnea. For this reason, foals should be weaned from assisted ventilation. Doxapram hydrochloride (400 mg total dose infused at a rate of 0.05 mg/kg per min) is a respiratory stimulant that is potentially useful in improving uncomplicated or primary apnea of newborn foals.

The pulse rate and rhythm need to be evaluated in flaccid, unresponsive newborn foals. If bradycardia is present, atropine should be administered (1–2 mg/45 kg IV or intratracheally). It should be appreciated that the pulse rate of normal newborns can vary between 40 and 80 bpm during the immediate postpartum period. Ventricular standstill or asystole can be managed by administration of epinephrine (1:10000, 9 ml/45 kg IV, intratracheally or directly into the ventricle) combined with external cardiac compression (60/min) and assisted ventilation (20/min). In a hospital setting, an electrocardiogram (ECG) should be monitored for response to treatment. It is probably unreasonable to continue external cardiac massage if a spontaneous palpable pulse cannot be achieved after 10 minutes. Significant central nervous system (CNS) damage is reflected by pupils that are unresponsive to light, absent ocular reflexes, and loss of muscle tone.

Basic Respiratory Support

Good airway hygiene is essential. Sick foals tend to lie in lateral recumbency, and this can lead to significant pressure atelectasis and worsening of gas exchange in foals with pre-existing disease. Maintenance of sternal recumbency can be achieved using sandbags or pads, but foals need frequent manual repositioning. Care must be taken not to place focal direct pressure on the thorax, especially in foals

---

°*Multinex, Datascope, Paramus, NJ*

°*Hudson, Temecula, CA*

with fractured ribs. Adjustable V-pads° are very effective for most foals and decrease the labor requirement.

Oxygen Therapy

Intranasal oxygen is usually administered to foals that are hypoxemic (PaO_2 ≤70 mm Hg). If blood gas analysis is not available, the decision to administer oxygen revolves around the presence of one or more of the following clinical signs: membrane cyanosis; restlessness and agitation; tachypnea or hyperpnea; or overt respiratory distress. The most common method involves insertion of a nasal insufflation tube. The oxygen must be humidified by bubbling through sterile water. The translation of oxygen flow rates to an inspired oxygen concentration (FiO_2) is not clear, but a good starting point for most foals is to deliver oxygen at 5 L/minute. Rates of up to 10 L/minute may be required and probably translate into an FiO_2 of around 1.0. The response to therapy needs to be carefully evaluated.

Ideally, an arterial blood gas analysis is obtained to confirm an appropriate rise in PaO_2. The aim should be to maintain PaO_2 at around 70 to 105 mm Hg. If blood gas analysis is not available, clinical improvement can be confirmed, for example, by noting a reduction in rate and/or depth of ventilation, improvement in mucous membrane color, and reduced agitation. It is possible to maintain oxygen therapy in ambulatory foals by attaching the gas line to a flexible coil that is usually used for administration of intravenous fluids. The insufflation tube should be cleaned twice daily and the tubing replaced every 1 to 2 days. An alternative approach involves the placement of an indwelling 8.5 French transtracheal catheter.† Administration of oxygen via this method should allow lower flow rates to be used.

Neonatal foals with moderate to severe respiratory disease often have arterial blood gases consistent with hypercapnic respiratory failure. During prolonged respiratory acidosis, the respiratory stimulation of CO_2 is often lost and respiratory drive is controlled by peripheral chemoreceptors in response to hypoxemia. Consequently, in certain individuals, oxygen therapy, particularly if excessive, may result in an acute elevation in $PaCO_2$ and a reduction in pH due to a loss of hypoxic drive and hypoventilation.

Assisted Ventilation

Mechanical or assisted ventilation is usually indicated during resuscitation (see earlier) or if $PaCO_2$ exceeds 70 mm Hg. The resultant acidemia is potentially life-threatening, particularly if accompanied by moderate or severe hypoxemia. Prolonged high levels of CO_2 can result in generalized CNS depression (CO_2 narcosis) and circulatory failure.

The simplest forms of assisted ventilation, the resuscitator bag and oxygen demand valve, were discussed earlier. Mechanical ventilation has improved considerably over the past decade. Several good references on this subject are cited in Supplemental Readings. Older volume cycle ventilators were unforgiving, resulting in a foal that thrashed and "fought" the ventilator. This necessitated the use of chemically induced paralysis or heavy sedation. Newer ventilators recognize and assist spontaneous breaths and pro-

vide continuous pressure support. Foals with severe respiratory disease often relax or sleep when ventilated appropriately and rarely require sedation. A well-ventilated foal often has a normal PaO_2 and $PaCO_2$, even in the face of severe bronchopneumonia. The guiding principle in the management of bacterial pneumonia should be to ventilate the foal until antibiotics can have time to resolve the active pathology.

Stimulation of central and peripheral chemoreceptors with an infusion of doxapram hydrochloride (400 mg total dose infused at a rate of 0.05 mg/kg per min) frequently resolves the periodic breathing and hypoventilation seen in foals with neurologic depression (HIE). Repeated treatments may be required. Oral caffeine (10 mg loading dose then 2.5 mg/kg s.i.d.) may also be an effective respiratory stimulant.

DISEASES AND SYNDROMES

Congenital Abnormalities

Congenital abnormalities of the respiratory tract include choanal atresia, stenotic nares, abnormalities of the soft palate resulting in dorsal displacement, cervical tracheal bronchus, accessory or ectopic lung lobes, pulmonary lobe hypertrophy, and adenomatoid hamartoma. Foals with dorsal displacement of the soft palate may have clinical signs that include stridor, dyspnea, and dysphagia. Endoscopy reveals a swollen, flaccid soft palate with redundant tissue. Treatment includes anti-inflammatory drugs, enteral feeding, and management of secondary aspiration pneumonia with antibiotics, and, if necessary, oxygen. If no improvement has occurred after 4 days of medical therapy, recommended procedure is a staphylectomy (according to J Am Vet Med Assoc 195(1):1395–1398, 1989).

Infectious Pulmonary Diseases

Bacterial Diseases

The common bacterial organisms associated with pulmonary disease in foals are those that commonly cause septicemia. These include *Escherichia coli*, *Klebsiella pneumoniae*, *Salmonella* species, *Pasteurella* species, *Actinobacillus equuli*, or *Streptococcus* species. Infection most commonly occurs either during or shortly after birth, but also can occur before birth through aspiration of contaminated amniotic fluid in mares with placental infection. Identification of the causative agent should be an important component of the diagnosis. This can be achieved by isolation of bacteria from blood culture or by placental or uterine culture from the mare if in utero infection is suspected. Culture of the airway can be difficult. A transtracheal wash can be potentially dangerous in a severely compromised neonate. An alternative method involves passage of a guarded swab through an endotracheal tube into the lower airway. The tip of the endotracheal tube can also be cultured. Systemic infections can originate from or localize elsewhere in the foal, including the umbilicus, gastrointestinal tract, musculoskeletal system, CNS, skin, and kidneys. The author routinely performs an ultrasound examination of the umbilical structures in foals with probable bacterial pneumonia.

°*Midwest Fabric Products, DeWitt, MI*
†*Scoop Transtracheal Systems, Englewood, CO*

The treatment of bacterial lung disease involves a combination of respiratory support and antibiotic therapy. Oxygen therapy and ventilatory support are dictated by the severity of the lung disease as reflected by clinical signs, radiographic changes, and blood gas analysis. Broad-spectrum antibiotic therapy should begin as soon as lung disease is suspected clinically. A good choice appears to be either penicillin (22,000 IU/kg IV q.i.d. or IM b.i.d.) or ampicillin combined with an aminoglycoside. Gentamicin (6.6 mg/kg IV or IM s.i.d.) is commonly used as a first choice aminoglycoside, but amikacin (20 mg/kg IV or IM s.i.d.) may be more efficacious in suspected nosocomial infections. Adjustment of dose rate and/or frequency may be required based on measurement of peak and trough levels of these drugs. The third-generation cephalosporins, such as ceftazidime, ceftriaxone, or cefotaxime, have advantages over the aminoglycosides in the treatment of confirmed bacterial pneumonia. They have superior penetration into the lung, and effective tissue concentrations are easily achieved by intravenous or intramuscular routes. This class of antibiotic should be reserved for moderate to severe cases of pneumonia to avoid developing drug resistance and because of their cost. Ceftiofur° is a third-generation cephalosporin marketed to treat *Streptococcus equi* subsp. *zooepidemicus* infections and may be an affordable alternative to other similar-class drugs. The drug appears to have good activity against gram-negative bacteria based on in vitro sensitivities. The dosage and efficacy of this drug in the management of neonatal bacterial pneumonia require further definition, but a dose of 5 mg/kg (IM b.i.d.) has been used in our hospital. Prolonged courses (3–4 weeks) of antibiotics are often needed and should be continued until a complete blood count and fibrinogen are normal.

If treated aggressively, neonatal foal pneumonia has little if any detrimental effect on long-term growth and performance. In contrast, if not identified early or if treated inappropriately, neonatal foals with pneumonia can develop persistent lung disease and poor growth.

Viral Diseases

Viruses incriminated as causes of neonatal pneumonia include equine herpesvirus type 1 (EHV-1) and type 4 (EHV-4), equine influenza, and equine viral arteritis (EVA). Of these, EHV-1 appears to be the most important. Adenovirus can be a potential problem in Arabian foals with combined immunodeficiency (CID) syndrome. Herpesvirus or EVA pneumonia is almost always fatal. It is difficult to establish a diagnosis of viral pneumonia ante mortem in neonates. Several factors appear common to EHV-1-infected foals, but at this point in time none should be considered pathognomonic. Infected foals may be icteric with mucosal petechial hemorrhages and may have nonspecific signs of pulmonary disease. Hematologic changes include leukopenia with neutropenia and lymphopenia. Toxicity and depletion of the myeloid cell lines are seen on examination of bone marrow aspirates. Dilation of retinal vessels and a red discoloration to the optic disc have also been reported in EHV-1-infected foals. The antiviral drug acyclovir (5–10 mg/kg p.o. t.i.d.) has been used in suspected cases, but efficacy data are lacking.

°Naxcel, The Upjohn Company, Kalamazoo, MI

Noninfectious Pulmonary Disease

Rib Fractures

In a radiographic survey, 7 of 243 (3%) neonatal foals admitted to the University of Florida with evidence of respiratory dysfunction had rib fractures. It was perceived to be a clinical problem in two foals, one of which developed a fatal puncture to the myocardium and the other a nonfatal hemothorax. Direct pressure to the thorax should be avoided in foals with rib fractures. Treatment is unnecessary.

Pneumothorax

Pneumothorax can occur spontaneously from trauma during birth or as an iatrogenic consequence of excessive positive pressure ventilation. Ruptured alveoli can coalesce to form bullae, and air may dissect through the lung interstitium to form blebs on the pleural surface, which subsequently burst into the pleural space resulting in pneumothorax. The condition should be suspected if the ventilated foal suddenly develops respiratory distress and hypoxemia. Diagnosis is aided by radiography and ultrasound examination, or needle aspiration of air from the pleural space. If signs are mild and nonprogressive, no additional therapy is indicated, but if clinical signs are moderate to severe or progressive, closed suction drainage is required. Massive spontaneous subcutaneous emphysema has been seen in foals in which air has migrated from the pleural space to the mediastinum and subcutaneous tissues.

Meconium Aspiration

Meconium is the sterile concretion of intestinal cells and mucus that forms in the developing digestive tract. Staining of amniotic fluid and the foal with meconium usually reflects pre- or intrapartum asphyxia. Aspirated meconium may obstruct airways, interfere with gas exchange, and act as a nidus for bacterial infection. It is important to clear the nasal passages and ideally suction the trachea. If tachypnea or distress occur, thoracic radiographs and arterial blood gas analysis are warranted. Antibiotics are indicated in these foals.

Milk Aspiration

Aspiration of milk occurs commonly in foals with dysphagia and in sleepy foals that are force-fed. Management of these foals includes cessation of oral feeding until the cause of the dysphagia has been determined and resolved. The resultant lower respiratory disease should be managed as for cases of primary bacterial pneumonia.

Respiratory Distress Syndrome (RDS)/Hyaline Membrane Disease

This syndrome, reported in the premature human infant, lamb, calf, pig, and foal, is caused by a deficiency of surfactant superimposed on a structurally immature lung. An equivalent syndrome is rare in premature foals, but a clinically less severe form may occur commonly. Lung dysfunction in premature foals is characterized by reduced ventilation capacity, tachypnea, hypoxemia, and progressive hypercapnia. Radiographically, there is a diffuse increase in interstitial density without alveolar changes. Atelectasis, with or without inflammatory cell infiltrates, is observed histologically, but hyaline membrane formation is rare. The administration of bovine surfactant to premature foals at risk for respiratory failure has been purported to be successful, but objective controlled studies are lacking. If available, the product should be administered by long catheter through a nasotracheal tube while the foal is in each of four positions: left lateral, right lateral, sternal, and dorsal recumbency. After each administration the foal should be ventilated with a resuscitation bag for 5 to 10 minutes to distribute surfactant into the distal airways. A total dose of 100 mg/kg of bovine surfactant has been suggested. Unfortunately, cost usually precludes the use of surfactant in foal practice. Mechanical ventilation and oxygen are important components of treatment.

Persistent Fetal Circulation

This occurs rarely, but when present can be difficult to differentiate from congenital cardiac anomalies such as critical pulmonic valve stenosis. Both conditions result in respiratory distress, hypoxemia that is not responsive to oxygen therapy, and a loud systolic murmur. Thoracic radiography may be helpful in differentiating the conditions.

Idiopathic or Transient Tachypnea

This syndrome occurs most frequently in Clydesdale foals, but also in other breeds, including Thoroughbreds and Arabians. The syndrome is most commonly seen in association with warm, humid conditions and is thought to be related to either immaturity or dysfunction of thermoregulatory mechanisms. Clinically affected animals have an elevated respiratory rate and rectal temperature. The signs typically develop within a few days of birth and spontaneously resolve within days to weeks. Results of complete blood count, fibrinogen estimation, auscultation of the thorax, arterial blood gas analysis, and thoracic radiography should be within normal limits. Treatment with antipyretics such as dipyrone or flunixin are usually of little help, but dramatic improvement can occur following body clipping, alcohol baths, and placement into a cooler environment. Considering the difficulty in differentiating idiopathic tachypnea from infectious causes, it is usually recommended to place these foals on a course of broad-spectrum antibiotics.

Supplemental Readings

Coons TJ, Kosch PC, Cudd TA: Respiratory care. *In* Koterba AM, Drummond WH, Kosch PC (eds): Equine Clinical Neonatology. Philadelphia, Lea & Febiger, 1990, pp 200–239.

Koterba AM: Respiratory disease: Approach to diagnosis. *In* Koterba AM, Drummond WH, Kosch PC (eds): Equine Clinical Neonatology. Philadelphia, Lea & Febiger, 1990, pp 153–176.

Koterba AM, Paradis MR: Specific respiratory conditions. *In* Koterba AM, Drummond WH, Kosch PC (eds): Equine Clinical Neonatology. Philadelphia, Lea & Febiger, 1990, pp 177–199.

Palmer JE: Ventilatory support of the neonatal foal. Vet Clin North Am Equine Pract 10(1):167–185, 1994.

Bronchointerstitial Pneumonia and Acute Respiratory Distress

W. DAVID WILSON

JEFFREY LAKRITZ
Davis, California

A sporadic, rapidly progressive, high-mortality, acute respiratory distress syndrome (ARDS) has been described in foals aged between 1 week and 8 months. The syndrome appears to be distinct from the acute respiratory distress syndrome seen in neonatal foals and has been encountered in Canada, the northeastern United States, Florida, Kentucky, Oklahoma, California, and Britain, and probably also occurs elsewhere.

ETIOPATHOGENESIS

It is likely that this syndrome does not have a single etiology but rather represents the common reaction of the lung to a number of different insults, the precise nature of which remains to be determined. A viral etiology has been proposed based on the sporadic nature of the disease, the age incidence, and the histologic lesions, which include multinucleate syncytial cells similar to those seen with bovine respiratory syncytial virus (BRSV) infection in cattle. Although viruses such as influenza virus and equine adenovirus are capable of causing diffuse alveolar damage, and certain strains of equine influenza A-equine-2 virus have been reported to induce severe fatal pneumonitis and respiratory distress in foals, viral agents do not appear to be involved in the majority of cases of ARDS.

Pneumocystis carinii has recently been implicated as a potential cause of ARDS in foals, based on the identification of this organism in the lungs of a number of fatally affected foals in Britain, the northeastern US, Canada, Florida, and Japan. This parasite, a unicellular eukaryote of uncertain etiology but possibly a fungus, is generally thought to be an opportunist pathogen of patients with immune deficiency disorders and is well recognized to commonly infect Arabian foals with severe combined immunodeficiency. The identification of *P. carinii* in the lungs of affected foals, many of which are also infected with *Rhodococcus equi*, an organism now recognized to be a common pathogen of human patients with acquired immunodeficiency syndrome (AIDS), has led to the suggestion that these foals may be suffering from an as yet undefined immune deficiency state that may involve defective production of gamma interferon by CD4+ lymphocytes. This concept is further supported by the finding that gram-negative enteric organisms such as *Escherichia coli* are also commonly isolated from the lungs of foals with ARDS. In addition, it is noteworthy that many affected foals were being treated with erythromycin, rifampin, or other antibiotics for a pre-existing respiratory infection, often *R. equi* pneumonia, before the onset of signs of ARDS. Recent studies have documented that erythromycin, administered orally as erythromycin base, causes a profound inhibition of neutrophil migration into pulmonary airways in response to an inflammatory stimulus. It is likely that this effect may inhibit phagocytic clearance from the lower airways and may allow proliferation of opportunist pathogens such as *P. carinii* or gram-negative enteric bacteria, which may then contribute to the development of the alveolar, bronchiolar, and interstitial lesions typically found in affected foals. *R. equi* alone can cause apparent acute-onset respiratory distress because the clinical signs associated with the insidious development of pulmonary consolidation and multiple pyogranulomas may go unobserved by owners or because of acute fulminant infection resulting from massive airborne challenge.

The similarity of the pulmonary lesions seen in affected foals to those seen in cattle with atypical interstitial pneumonia (fog fever) has prompted the suggestion that this syndrome may be caused by ingestion of pneumotoxins such as perilla mint ketone, pyrrolizidine alkaloid, paraquat, or 3-methyl indole. However, the lesions produced by the administration of these compounds to horses do not duplicate all the lesions seen in naturally affected foals. The majority of affected foals seen in the authors' clinic have presented during hot weather (usually in excess of 90°F) or after transportation on hot days, suggesting that heat stress may play a role. A number of foals were being treated with antibiotics before the onset of signs of severe respiratory distress. Bacterial toxins or mediators produced during the pulmonary response to infection may play a role in the pathogenesis of this condition, although direct side-effects of the antibiotic treatment should also be considered. For example, horses occasionally develop hyperthermia during courses of treatment with erythromycin. The ability of the foal to dissipate heat during periods of high ambient temperature may be further compromised by underlying bacterial or viral lung disease, resulting in a progressive cycle of thermal injury to the lung.

PATHOLOGIC FINDINGS

The lungs of affected foals that die are diffusely red, wet, heavy, firm, and fail to collapse when the chest is opened. In many instances the lungs have a mottled lobulated appearance with dark reddened areas interspersed between areas of more normal-appearing lung tissue. Airway lumens usually contain various amounts of pink foamy fluid, and the cut surface exudes fluid and has edematous separation of lobules. A substantial number of foals also have other lung lesions such as *R. equi* pyogranulomas, which represent pre-existing pulmonary disease, and many also show hypoxemia-induced lesions in other organs.

Histopathologic pulmonary lesions include severe, diffuse necrotizing bronchiolitis, alveolar septal necrosis, and filling of alveolar spaces with large numbers of neutrophils and lesser numbers of macrophages, lymphocytes, desquamated pneumocytes, and epithelioid-like cells enmeshed in an eosinophilic proteinaceous to fibrinoid material suggestive of hyaline membranes. Other prominent lesions include congestion and edema of the interstitium, hyperplasia of type II pneumocytes and, in more chronic cases, interstitial fibrosis. Intracellular viral inclusion bodies are not evident. The relative predominance of lesions differs to some extent between foals and probably reflects the severity and chronicity of the condition, pre-existing lung disease, and perhaps the initiating etiologic agent. For instance, diffuse alveolar damage is a prominent early lesion that appears to precede development of necrotizing bronchiolitis, proliferation of type II pneumocytes, and interstitial fibrosis. Multinucleate syncytial cells are present in the exudate, accumulating in bronchioles and alveoli of some, but not all, affected foals, but they appear to be a consistent finding in foals in which *P. carinii* is present.

CLINICAL SIGNS AND DIAGNOSIS

The clinical presentation of affected foals includes an acute or peracute onset of respiratory distress manifested by marked tachypnea, nostril flaring, extended head and neck position, increased intercostal and abdominal effort, and, in many instances, a notable double expiratory lift and "heave line." The majority of affected foals are cyanotic at rest, or become so with minimal exertion, and are febrile, depressed, and reluctant to move or eat. Nasal discharge and cough are frequent but inconsistent findings. Although cough is often part of the history because affected foals often have underlying bacterial pneumonia, the onset of respiratory distress may diminish the frequency of efforts to cough. Thoracic auscultation reveals tachycardia, loud bronchial sounds over central airways, and reduced bronchovesicular sounds in peripheral areas of the lung, suggesting reduced ventilation of small airways. Crackles and polyphonic wheezes are heard in the caudodorsal lung fields of those foals that retain sufficient air movement in the lung periphery, and the sounds tend to become more prominent as ventilation improves in response to treatment. This change in auscultation findings appears to have prognostic value because lung sounds in those foals that die tend to remain bronchial and do not show the increase in adventitious sounds heard in recovering foals. The clinical course in foals that do not survive ranges from less than 24 hours, in which case the presentation may be one of apparent sudden death, to several weeks, although the clinical course is generally less than 7 days.

Laboratory findings include neutrophilic leukocytosis, hyperfibrinogenemia, and hypoxemia with a hypercapnic respiratory acidosis. Other laboratory abnormalities reflecting dehydration, diffuse intravascular coagulation, and hypoxic injury to other organs are seen in some foals. Radiographic findings are variable and frequently include evidence of an underlying disease process such as consolidating anteroventral pneumonia or diffusely distributed pyogranulomas in foals with concomitant *R. equi* infection. However, thoracic radiographs typically show prominent interstitial patterns of increased density with superimposed mixed bronchial and alveolar patterns of varying severity distributed diffusely throughout the lung fields. Foals seen early in the course of the disease may show a diffuse alveolar pattern of increased density reflecting alveolar flooding induced by diffuse alveolar damage. In foals that respond well to treatment, this alveolar pattern resolves over a period of days, but resolution of the prominent bronchointerstitial pattern may be incomplete even after many months. A prominent miliary reticulonodular pattern is found in the majority of foals with *P. carinii* infection but has also been identified in foals with respiratory distress in which *P. carinii* was not identified.

If not precluded by the severity of clinical signs, tracheobronchial aspirates should be collected in an attempt to identify the etiologic agent and guide treatment and, in selected cases, bronchoalveolar lavage (BAL) may also prove helpful, particularly for the identification of *P. carinii*. In addition to routine cytologic examination and bacterial culture, efforts should be made to isolate or identify viruses and *P. carinii* in tracheobronchial aspirates or BAL samples (and in pulmonary tissues of foals that die). *P. carinii*, in its trophozoite, sporozoite, and cyst forms, can be identified by Wright's-Giemsa, toluidine blue O, Gomori's methanamine silver or, optimally, by immunofluorescence staining methods or electron microscopy.

TREATMENT AND PROGNOSIS

This syndrome constitutes a respiratory emergency necessitating aggressive and intensive therapy. A variety of treatments have been used, including oxygen by nasal insufflation or transtracheal percutaneous oxygenation, nebulization, antihistamines, bronchodilators, antibiotics, corticosteroids, nonsteroidal anti-inflammatory agents, and external thermoregulation. The high mortality rate in the face of multiple treatments most likely indicates that no one treatment is highly effective, although the administration of corticosteroids and oxygen, and management of hyperthermia appear to be important. The use of glucocorticoids is further supported by the finding that the risk of respiratory failure and death in human immunodeficiency virus (HIV)-positive human patients with moderate to severe *P. carinii* pneumonia is reduced by early inclusion of these drugs in the therapeutic regimen. Recognition that *P. carinii* may be involved in some foals suggests that specific treatment with antimicrobials, such as trimethoprim-sulfonamide combinations (10–15 mg of trimethoprim/kg of body weight per day), which inhibit folate synthesis, is indicated. The pulmonary interstitial fibrosis seen

in chronic cases and radiographic evidence of a persistent increase in pulmonary interstitial density several months after recovery in a limited number of surviving foals suggest that survival may be accompanied by permanent pulmonary pathology, which can impair future performance.

PREVENTION

Until the etiology of this syndrome is better understood, definitive therapeutic and prophylactic recommendations cannot be made. However, the apparent association with heat stress in some cases suggests that particular care should be taken to control ambient temperature and to protect foals, especially those being treated for respiratory disease, against direct exposure to the sun on hot days. Transporting foals during hot weather should be avoided. Necessary transportation should be performed early in the morning when it is cool, and appropriate ventilation of the trailer should be provided. The recognition that erythromycin may interfere with thermoregulation suggests that foals requiring treatment with erythromycin during hot weather should be carefully monitored and kept in the shade during the hottest portion of the day, preferably by confining them in a cool, well-ventilated area with fans or air-conditioning. Foals that develop hyperthermia should be recognized early and managed aggressively to reduce their core body temperature before severe systemic and pulmonary complications develop. The use of large fans, the application of ice water and alcohol baths and cold water enemas in a shaded or air-conditioned area can be lifesaving under these circumstances. Administration of corticosteroids, flunixin meglumine, or other nonsteroidal anti-inflammatory drugs to hyperthermic foals may help prevent cell death and secondary effects but does not reverse the hyperthermia unless other measures are instituted.

Supplemental Readings

Ainsworth DM, Weldon AD, Beck KA, Rowland PH: Recognition of *Pneumocystis carinii* in foals with respiratory distress. Equine Vet J 25:103–108, 1993.

Buergelt CD, Hines SA, Cantor G, Stirk A, Wilson JH: A retrospective study of proliferative interstitial lung disease of horses in Florida. Vet Pathol 23:750–756, 1986.

Ewing PJ, Cowell RL, Tyler RD, MacAllister CG, Meinkoth JH: *Pneumocystis carinii* pneumonia in foals. J Am Vet Med Assoc 204:929–933, 1994.

Lakritz J, Watson J, Wilson WD, Bryant J, Kann M, Mihalyi J: Pulmonary lavage cell populations in foals treated with erythromycin. In Proc 11th Vet Med Forum Am Coll Vet Intern Med, 1993, p 958.

Lakritz J, Wilson WD, Berry CR, Schrenzel MD, Carlson GP, Madigan JE: Bronchointerstitial pneumonia and respiratory distress in young horses: Clinical, clinicopathologic, radiographic, and pathological findings in 23 cases (1984–1989). J Vet Intern Med 7:277–288, 1993.

Prescott JF: Immunodeficiency and serious pneumonia in foals: The plot thickens. Equine Vet J 25(2):88–89, 1993.

Prescott JF, Wilcock BP, Carman PS, Hoffman AM: Sporadic, severe bronchointerstitial pneumonia of foals. Can Vet J 32:421–425, 1991.

Whitwell K: Pneumocystis carinii infection in foals in the UK. Vet Rec 27:19, 1992.

Foal Pneumonia

W. DAVID WILSON
Davis, California

Pneumonia is the leading cause of morbidity and mortality in foals aged between 1 and 6 months and constitutes a major cause of economic loss to the equine industry. A crude incident morbidity of 6.1% was reported in a large prospective study of foal pneumonia on 167 farms in Texas, although the true incidence of infection of the lower airways of foals is most likely much higher, and many cases of infection undoubtedly go unrecognized and resolve spontaneously. Indeed, careful weekly examination of Thoroughbred foals on farms in Ontario, Canada, demonstrated an average morbidity from bacterial infection of the distal respiratory tract of 82%. The impact of foal pneumonia on individual farms can be devastating. Mortality rates of 5 to 15% are common, although up to 80% of affected foals have died in some outbreaks, especially when *Rhodococcus equi* was the pathogen involved. The spectrum of clinical signs shown by affected foals is broad, reflecting the severity and chronicity of the disease process, the degree of systemic sepsis, complicating environmental influences, and the pathogens involved. Most affected foals show tachypnea, abnormal respiratory character, nasal discharge, fever, and cough, although the latter three signs are not consistent findings, even in severely affected foals.

During outbreaks, the disease process is often well advanced in the first foals to present, but additional foals are almost always infected but not yet showing prominent clinical signs. Identification of these foals, early recognition of new infections, and identification of patterns of spread and predisposing factors are very important if therapeutic and preventive measures are to be cost-effective and successful.

ETIOLOGY

The etiology of foal pneumonia is complex and involves the interaction of a number of predisposing factors with various microorganisms. The majority have bacterial involvement at the time of presentation and in most cases bacterial agents, particularly *Streptococcus equi* subspecies *zooepidemicus* (*S. zooepidemicus*) and *R. equi*, are primary pathogens. In other instances, viral agents such as influenza, equine herpesvirus-1 (EHV-1), EHV-4, EHV-2, rhinoviruses, adenoviruses, and possibly others may be important predisposing factors, although it is usually not possible to isolate the viral agent by the time the foal presents with signs of bacterial pneumonia. Viral agents compromise pulmonary defense by inducing ulceration of the respiratory epithelium, reduced mucociliary clearance, and impaired pulmonary alveolar macrophage function. Primary viral pneumonia due to influenza is recognized occasionally in young foals and can prove fatal in severe

cases. Foals born with congenital EHV-1 infection frequently have severe pneumonic lesions with or without pleural effusion, which is a condition that has a high mortality rate. Outbreaks of EHV-4 are common in sucklings and weanlings, with more severely affected foals showing pneumonic signs during the primary disease and after secondary bacterial infection.

Parasites may predispose to bacterial pneumonia by causing unthriftiness and, in the case of ascarid larvae, may cause pulmonary damage and a mild pneumonia directly during migration through the lung. This may induce eosinophilic bronchitis and pneumonitis, which is a condition also associated with *Dictyocaulus arnfieldi* infection in foals grazed with donkeys, asses, or mules. Most molds and fungi isolated from tracheobronchial aspirates of foals are thought to be environmental contaminants not contributing to the disease process, although *Aspergillus* species, other fungal agents, and the fungus-like organism *Pneumocystis carinii* have been isolated from foals with pneumonia on rare occasions, generally in association with immune deficiency states or prolonged antibiotic treatment. However, it has recently been suggested that *P. carinii* may play an etiologic role in acute respiratory distress syndrome in foals (see Bronchointerstitial Pneumonia, and Acute Respiratory Distress, page 609).

Bacterial pneumonia is generally caused by opportunistic pathogens that are normal inhabitants of the equine upper respiratory tract or the gastrointestinal tract or are environmental contaminants. The frequency of isolation of each bacterial species varies between different geographical locations and polymicrobic infections are common. However, β-hemolytic *Streptococcus* species, especially *S. zooepidemicus*, are the most frequent isolates in all geographical locations, and *S. zooepidemicus* may spread between individuals as a transmissible pathogen. *Streptococcus equi* subspecies *equi* is not commonly isolated from the lungs of foals with pneumonia. *Rhodococcus equi*, a gram-positive pleomorphic rod (coccobacillus), occurs sporadically but is enzootic on some breeding farms. Gram-negative nonenteric bacteria, including *Actinobacillus suis* species, other *Actinobacillus* species, *Pasteurella* species, and *Bordetella bronchiseptica* are also frequently isolated, either alone or in combination with *S. zooepidemicus* or other organisms. *Pseudomonas aeruginosa* and gram-negative enteric bacteria such as *Klebsiella pneumoniae*, *Escherichia coli*, and *Salmonella* species are involved in some cases, particularly in younger foals in which infection was acquired during the neonatal period, and is often associated with generalized sepsis. Other aerobic bacteria, such as *Staphylococcus* species, and anaerobic bacteria, are the etiologic agents in a small percentage of cases. However, anaerobic bacteria are isolated much less frequently from foals with bacterial pneumonia than from adult horses with pneumonia.

EPIDEMIOLOGY

The majority of foals with pneumonia are aged between 4 weeks and 6 months. The particularly high frequency of distal respiratory tract infection in foals between 3 and 5 months of age has led some authors to suggest that this reflects a transient age-related immune deficiency. However, with the exception of a trough in the level of maternal antibody that occurs at this time, standard procedures have failed to demonstrate immunologic defects in the vast majority of affected foals.

Of the interactive environmental and management factors that may predispose foals to the development of pneumonia, high ambient temperature appears to be important, especially when dry dusty conditions prevail. The demands for heat dissipation in hot climates may stress the respiratory system of foals, which appear to be less able than adults to tolerate extremes of temperature. In colder climates, chilling and overprotection from the cold, for instance by reducing ventilation in a barn or excessive application of blankets, also appear to be detrimental. Overcrowding may stress foals and increases the concentration and transmission of pathogens both indoors and at pasture. Grass dies on overcrowded pastures, which then become dusty during dry weather if not irrigated. Dust irritates the respiratory tract and can compromise respiratory defense as well as acting as a fomite for potential pathogens, including *R. equi*. Indoors, warmth and humidity promote survival of pathogens and the stabilization and transmission of infective aerosols. Bedding may act as a source of dust and allergens and as a culture medium for certain bacteria and fungi. Poor stall drainage and sanitation, high temperature, and poor ventilation contribute to the build-up of noxious gases such as ammonia that compromise pulmonary defense. Many handling procedures, transportation, showing, and weaning can be stressful to foals. Weaning also results in the concentration of young susceptible animals and thus promotes disease spread. The common practice of transporting mares and foals to other farms for breeding and the mixing of visiting mares and foals or show horses with the resident foal crop also increases the likelihood of acquiring infections.

The epidemiology of *R. equi* infection has special features that contribute to the development of disease. The organism is a coprophilic soil inhabitant that is resistant to many disinfectants and tolerates desiccation and a wide range of soil pH, surviving in soil containing equine fecal material for at least 12 months. Replication increases with increasing temperature, the optimal temperature for growth being 30°C. *R. equi* has been isolated from the gastrointestinal tract of horses and most other grazing herbivores and appears to multiply in the gastrointestinal tract of foals up to 12 weeks of age. After passage in feces, *R. equi* proliferates rapidly in the aerobic environment of the fecal pat, resulting in 10,000-fold increases in numbers in a period of 2 weeks under optimal conditions of temperature, pH, and moisture. Citrate and propionate, the simple organic acid fermentation products of the large intestine, appear to be important growth factors. On farms on which infection is endemic, the organism has been found in highest numbers in soil in paddocks where horses have grazed and in dust in stables, holding pens, exercise areas, and aisleways where infected foals have been kept. These areas appear to pose the greatest risk to young susceptible foals.

Mare feces and contaminated soil or dirt appear to be important sources of *R. equi* for colonization of the foal intestinal tract during the first few weeks of life. The coprophagic behavior of foals may be important in this regard. This colonization likely does not result in infection of the foal but rather subsequent fecal shedding by foals and their dams, which, along with reduced moisture and increased environmental temperature, promotes multiplication of *R. equi* in fecal pats. Dry windy conditions during the summer months promote dispersion of an increased number of organisms in the air, resulting in an increased aerosol challenge dose at a time when a large number of susceptible foals are present.

PATHOGENESIS

Most infections causing foal pneumonia are thought to be acquired by inhalation of aerosolized or dust-borne pathogens, but hematogenous seeding of the lung as a consequence of septicemia also occurs, especially in neonates. Aspiration pneumonia is encountered occasionally. Infectious agents suspended in aerosols or on dust particles tend to be deposited on the mucosa of the respiratory tract at the bronchiolar-alveolar junction. Colonization of the bronchiolar epithelium by opportunist bacteria occurs when pulmonary defense mechanisms are overwhelmed by massive challenge and when defenses are compromised by predisposing factors such as viral infection, transport stress, dust, or noxious gases. The resulting inflammatory response is characterized by the influx of neutrophils and other inflammatory cells into the airways and pulmonary parenchyma. Degranulation of neutrophils and other inflammatory cells causes damage to the airway epithelium and capillary endothelium, resulting in flooding of the terminal airways and alveoli with inflammatory cells, serum, cellular debris, and fibrin. This bronchopneumonic process is most prominent in the cranioventral portions of the lung, particularly the right lung, and causes reddish purple discoloration as involved areas become consolidated, heavy, and wet. These lesions interfere with gas exchange in affected areas and, if severe enough, the resulting ventilation/perfusion mismatch leads to hypoxemia and clinical manifestations of respiratory disease.

The basis for the pathogenicity of *R. equi*, a facultative intracellular parasite, is its ability to multiply within and destroy alveolar macrophages by inhibiting normal phagosome-lysosome fusion and perhaps by causing nonspecific degranulation of lysosomes. Destruction of macrophages and release of lysosomal products induces tissue damage and provides both a constant source of infection and a stimulus for continued influx of macrophages and neutrophils. The result is persistence of an acute inflammatory response, even in chronic cases, with destruction of pulmonary parenchyma and formation of chronic pyogranulomatous mass lesions in the caudodorsal portion of the lung as well as in cranioventral areas, superimposed upon a prominent consolidating bronchopneumonia. This process appears to progress relatively slowly, and thus signs may not become apparent until several weeks after infection. Incubation periods ranging from 10 days to more than 3 weeks have been noted in natural and experimental infections. Ingestion of large doses of the organism may lead to gastrointestinal lesions, particularly ulcerative enterocolitis and associated lymphadenitis, although the gastrointestinal tract is not thought to be a major portal of entry for pulmonary *R. equi* infections. Significant pyogranulomatous lesions may develop in the hilar, mediastinal, or mesenteric lymph nodes and secondary bacteremia occurs occasionally, resulting in serious sequelae.

The polysaccharide capsule of *R. equi* appears to facilitate infection by helping the organism adhere to cells and may, along with mycolic acid–containing glycolipids, inhibit phagocytosis and killing by phagocytes. Other candidate virulence factors include cholesterol oxidase and choline phosphohydrolase exoenzymes (*equi* factors). Ingestion, phagosome-lysosome fusion and killing of *R. equi* by macrophages and neutrophils is greatly enhanced by the presence of specific opsonic antibody and products of sensitized lymphocytes.

Expression of plasmid-mediated 15- to 17-kilodalton antigens by *R. equi* appears to be essential for virulence, a finding that may prove helpful in developing approaches to immunoprophylaxis and may help explain why infection is endemic on some farms, sporadic on others, and not recognized on most despite the presence of a large number of horses that are shedding *R. equi* in their feces. Survey cultures of feces and tracheal wash samples in endemic herds indicates that the intestinal tract of the majority of foals becomes colonized with *R. equi* and that a substantial number of foals acquire subclinical pulmonary *R. equi* infection. These exposures appear to effectively immunize most foals. Anti-*R. equi* antibodies are common in the horse population and are passively transferred to foals in the colostrum. The decline in levels of passively acquired antibody results in an "antibody trough" at 8 to 10 weeks of age, or earlier if passive transfer is suboptimal, after which levels rise to those seen in adult horses by 6 months of age. It is thought that those foals that develop *R. equi* pneumonia may do so because they receive an overwhelming challenge at a time when passive humoral protection is waning and before the foal has mounted a specific immune response.

CLINICAL PRESENTATION

The history and clinical presentation of foals with infection of the distal respiratory tract varies considerably. The spectrum ranges from an otherwise normal-appearing foal with intermittent coughing and mild mucopurulent nasal discharge to one with a high fever, severe depression, anorexia, profuse purulent nasal discharge, severe respiratory distress, and cyanosis. Tachypnea and altered respiratory character are typical features, even in mildly affected foals, and are best assessed at rest with minimal restraint during the cool part of the day. Respiratory rates greater than 40 per minute in an older foal or weanling at rest are considered abnormal under most circumstances, and resting rates greater than 30 per minute during the cool early morning hours are cause for concern, warranting further evaluation of the foal. Increased intercostal effort, often characterized by asynchronous rib excursion (rippling of the rib cage) is a subtle, but frequent, early sign. More severely affected foals also show nostril flaring, increased abdominal effort, or frank abdominal breathing with minimal costal excursion. These foals are exercise-intolerant; show an anxious expression; are reluctant to lie down, nurse, or move; and may develop signs of severe respiratory distress, cyanosis, and disorientation if stressed or forced to exercise.

Coughing is an important clinical sign, although it is not invariably present, particularly in foals with *R. equi* pneumonia. In early cases, coughing is generally most obvious in the morning when the foal is disturbed or restrained after lying down, or after brief exercise. The nature of the cough varies from intermittent, moist, and shallow to paroxysmal, deep, and hacking. Almost all affected foals cough when a rebreathing bag is applied, whereas normal foals rarely do so. A bilateral mucopurulent nasal discharge is a frequent finding, which varies in amount from profuse to scant and intermittent. In some foals the only evidence of a nasal discharge is dry crusting at the external nares or dried exudate on the dorsal aspect of the front cannon area deposited when the foal wipes its nose. Exudate from the lower airways may be swallowed and not appear as a nasal discharge. Some foals, including a substantial proportion of those with *R. equi* pneumonia, do not have a nasal discharge. Fever, usually in the range of 38.8° to 40.0°C (102°–104°F) but sometimes in excess of 40.5°C (105°F), is a common finding in foals with pneumonia. However, the rectal temperature is frequently normal in foals with infection of the distal respiratory tract but lacking significant parenchymal lesions. Demeanor and appetite are highly variable and do not necessarily reflect the severity of underlying pulmonary pathology. Most affected foals are well grown and in good flesh, but weight loss and stunting may become apparent with chronicity.

Most clinical cases of *R. equi* pneumonia represent the chronic form of the disease with a smaller percentage experiencing a more fulminant subacute form. However, respiratory signs are frequently of acute onset, reflecting the insidious progression of the disease process until sufficient lung is damaged to cause respiratory failure. In addition, the subtle early signs of disease are frequently missed or ignored by horsemen, allowing the condition to progress to a more advanced stage before veterinary help is sought. Although it is not possible to recognize the etiologic cause of foal pneumonia based on clinical signs alone, the clinical presentation and clinical pathology findings in foals with *R. equi* infection present some features that increase the index of suspicion. These include lack of nasal discharge, presence of fever, markedly delayed recovery from application of a rebreathing bag, peripheral neutrophilia and marked hyperfibrinogenemia, and a relatively lower percentage of neutrophils in bronchial lavage fluid than is usually encountered with other bacterial agents.

Auscultation, both at rest and after application of a rebreathing bag, if not precluded by severe respiratory distress, is very helpful in defining the presence, extent, and nature of lung involvement when findings are interpreted in the context of other signs, such as respiratory rate and character. The lung sounds in foals with distal respiratory tract infection vary considerably, and sounds referred from the upper airway can confuse auscultation findings. Foals with a large amount of tenacious exudate in the trachea often have an audible and palpable tracheal rattle. Mildly affected foals have increased audibility and harshness of expiratory and inspiratory bronchovesicular sounds and increased tracheal sounds reflecting the presence of exudate. Occasional inspiratory and expiratory wheezes and crackles are usually audible over involved areas, which are most often located cranioventrally. In many early cases, adventitious sounds are audible only when a rebreathing bag is used. In more severely affected foals, increased tracheal and bronchovesicular sounds are accompanied by fine and course crackles and widespread polyphonic wheezes. In some cases wheezes are audible at the nostrils, with the inciting turbulence also palpable on the chest wall. Lung sounds are diminished over areas of severe consolidation, extensive abscess formation, or pleural effusion. These areas may also show reduced resonance on chest percussion, although pleural effusion is not commonly present in foals with pneumonia.

DIAGNOSIS

Diagnostic evaluation should be directed at the entire herd as well as at further assessment of sick foals. Evaluation of individual foals should establish whether infection of the distal respiratory tract is present and determine the etiology and severity of pulmonary involvement so that appropriate therapeutic measures can be instituted and an accurate prognosis rendered. Important features of the history in affected foals include age; duration and progression of signs; response to treatment; previous cases in the herd including agents isolated, antimicrobial susceptibility, and response to treatment; herd history of viral respiratory disease and vaccination; season; general herd management; parasite control; movement of horses on and off the farm; and the presence of other clinical signs such as diarrhea or lymphadenopathy in the affected foal or herdmates. In addition to examination of the respiratory system, a general physical examination should be performed, paying particular attention to hydration status, mucous membrane color and capillary refill, the umbilicus, joints, and the lymph nodes of the head and neck. *R. equi* infections occasionally cause diarrhea, and up to 30% of foals with *R. equi* pneumonia also show a chronic, active, nonseptic (likely immune-mediated) synovitis characterized by neutrophilia in synovial fluid and joint distension with minimal or absent lameness. Panophthalmitis, septic arthritis, physitis, and osteomyelitis, including vertebral body osteomyelitis, have also been encountered in foals with *R. equi* infection.

The need for ancillary diagnostic procedures is determined by the herd history, the number and value of foals affected and at risk, the time of year relative to the foaling season, management practices, available facilities, severity and duration of clinical signs, treatments used, and response. In foals with pneumonia, measurement of complete blood count (CBC), plasma protein, and fibrinogen concentration commonly shows evidence of a moderate to marked inflammatory response characterized by leukocytosis with neutrophilia, with or without a left shift, and an elevated

fibrinogen concentration. However, there does not seem to be a high degree of correlation between the severity of clinical signs and the magnitude of CBC changes. Indeed, many foals with infection of the distal respiratory tract have a normal leukocyte count. Sequential measurement of plasma fibrinogen concentration often provides a useful means of monitoring response to treatment and helps guide the decision to discontinue treatment. In general, antibiotic treatment should not be discontinued until plasma fibrinogen concentration has returned to the normal range (≤ 400 mg/dl). A CBC test result also allows evaluation of hydration and preliminary screening of the immune system. If the lymphocyte count is consistently low ($<1000/\mu l$), immune function should be evaluated more thoroughly, particularly in Arabian foals. Similarly, the adequacy of colostral antibody transfer should be determined in foals younger than 1 month of age. The thrombocytosis noted consistently in *R. equi* cases by workers in Ireland has not been reported by workers elsewhere. This most likely reflects differences between laboratories in the method used to quantify equine platelets rather than being a unique feature of *R. equi* infections in Ireland.

Tracheobronchial aspiration, with cytologic examination and aerobic and anaerobic bacteriologic culture and susceptibility testing of aspirated material, is the most definitive diagnostic procedure available. The results of bacteriologic culture should be interpreted in the context of the results of cytologic evaluation. Because the number as well as species of bacteria may be important, quantification of growth should be attempted. In the field setting it is not always practical or desirable to perform transtracheal washes on all foals with pneumonia. On breeding farms where multiple cases are likely to occur, especially if *R. equi* has been a problem in previous years, a reasonable approach is to perform tracheal washes on the first few affected foals in an outbreak to establish which organisms are involved and their antibiotic susceptibility patterns. Thereafter, washes should be performed on any foal that is not responding to the chosen treatment, foals with atypical signs, and foals with other evidence such as radiographic changes of *R. equi* pneumonia. Depending on the chronicity of the condition, a period of at least 3 days is generally needed to assess the response to initial treatment. Whenever possible, antibiotic treatment should be discontinued at least 24 hours before performing tracheal washes on foals that are nonresponsive to initial treatment. The recent introduction of aspiration catheters that can be passed through the biopsy port of an endoscope has facilitated collection of appropriate diagnostic samples and provides an alternative to the transtracheal technique. Similarly, the use of a guarded bronchoscope fitted with a clear sterile cellulose acetate sheath provides an excellent method for collection of uncontaminated samples from the lower airways. In addition, endoscopic examination is helpful in ruling out concurrent or predisposing upper airway abnormalities such as guttural pouch empyema, and in documenting bronchial erythema, exudate, and edema, all of which are evidence of inflammation of the distal respiratory tract. Nasopharyngeal swabbing is useful for diagnosing acute viral respiratory tract infections but not bacterial infection of the lower airways.

On cytologic evaluation of smears of the cell pellet from

tracheobronchial aspirates, particular attention should be given to the types and numbers of cells, their state of degeneration, and the presence, number, location (intra- or extracellular), morphology, and staining characteristics of bacteria. *S. zooepidemicus* is frequently recognizable on direct smears by the presence of a prominent halo, representing its nonstaining capsule. Accurate cytologic evaluation aids diagnosis and assists in selection of initial antibacterial treatment before final culture results are available. In foals that have already been treated with antibiotics, bacteria, particularly gram-negatives, are often seen on a direct smear but fail to grow in culture. In *R. equi* infections, false-negative culture results have been noted, but in at least 60% of cases, cytologic examination of tracheobronchial aspirates demonstrates the characteristic pleomorphic gram-positive coccobacilli located intra- and extracellularly. Special staining techniques may be necessary to identify unusual pathogens such as *Pneumocystis carinii.*

Radiography is a useful diagnostic technique, especially in more severe cases in which consolidation or abscessation is suspected or when *R. equi* is the suspected or confirmed pathogen. The procedure is also helpful in evaluating the response to treatment. The presence of air bronchograms in the cranioventral lung field, increase in interstitial density, variously sized "cotton-ball" or cavitary densities in the lung field, and hilar lymphadenopathy are typical radiographic features of *R. equi* pneumonia. Thoracic radiography is particularly useful in the evaluation of pneumonia in neonatal foals because clinical and auscultation findings in this age group frequently do not correlate well with the degree of pulmonary consolidation present. The use of rare-earth screens and air-gap techniques makes it possible to take chest radiographs on smaller foals using some portable radiograph machines (see Table 1 in *Current Therapy in Equine Medicine 3*, p 470). Ultrasound examination is useful, either alone or as adjunct to radiography, when consolidation of the peripheral lung or the presence of pleural fluid is suspected, although the procedure does not detect deep pulmonary lesions surrounded by normally aerated lung.

Currently, no serologic tests reliably detect early infection with the bacterial species commonly associated with foal pneumonia. Sensitive enzyme-linked immunosorbent assay (ELISA) tests, which detect antibodies directed against cell wall components of *R. equi*, are useful for epidemiologic investigation and herd monitoring but are not useful adjuncts to diagnosis. The agar gel diffusion test, synergistic hemolysin inhibition test, and immunodiffusion test, which detect antibodies directed against the cholesterol oxidase coenzyme ("*equi* factor") produced by actively replicating *R. equi* organisms, have been advocated as being useful for the early diagnosis of *R. equi* infections. However, both false-negative and false-positive results have been observed, and there is generally a lag period of several weeks between infection and detection of antibodies using these tests. In addition, an ELISA test has been shown experimentally to be useful in the diagnosis of infection, but the antigens used for the test remain to be defined.

Blood gas analysis is very useful for monitoring the oxygenation and acid-base status during therapy of affected foals showing signs of marked respiratory distress or cyanosis. Culture of blood frequently yields bacterial growth in neonatal foals with pneumonia, and *R. equi* may be isolated from blood of affected foals showing signs of systemic infection. A bronchodilator response test, using atropine or β₂-adrenergic drugs such as clenbuterol or albuterol, may help in the evaluation of those foals that continue to show signs of obstructive lung disease after resolution of the bacterial pneumonia. Other diagnostic procedures that are useful in selected situations include bronchoalveolar lavage, virus isolation, serology for respiratory viruses, fecal flotation, immune function tests, and thoracocentesis. A thorough necropsy examination, including culture and susceptibility testing of pneumonic lesions, abscesses, and exudates, should be performed on any foal that dies.

After completing the diagnostic evaluation and initiating treatment on the first foal(s) presented for examination, herdmates should be screened for evidence of infection and a protocol should be established to facilitate early detection of new infections. On farms on which foals are halter-trained and handled regularly, the best approach is to perform physical examinations on all foals at risk and to perform appropriate diagnostic procedures on those with signs suggestive of infection. Thereafter, careful daily observation, daily or twice-daily recording of rectal temperature, and regular weighing facilitate early detection of new infections. In addition, performance of complete physical examinations, including pulmonary auscultation twice weekly has proven to be successful in promoting early diagnosis of *R. equi* infection and in preventing mortality. If economics permit, routine screening for complete blood count, fibrinogen concentration, and serology for viral infections and *R. equi* may further improve diagnostic sensitivity for early bacterial infection and the identification of predisposing viral agents.

On farms on which foals are unaccustomed to being handled, assembly and restraint for examination may prove unnecessarily stressful to the foals, may distort the findings of clinical and laboratory examinations, and may actually facilitate transmission of infectious agents. A useful approach under these circumstances is to observe all foals at rest in their paddocks during the cool early morning hours before they are disturbed by feeding and other management activities. Foals showing evidence of tachypnea, altered respiratory character, nasal discharge, depression, poor body condition, excessively rough hair coat, repeated coughing when disturbed, or other signs of disease are selected for a more complete physical examination and appropriate further diagnostic evaluation.

TREATMENT

An integrated approach is required that not only destroys the causal organisms with specific antimicrobial therapy, but also improves respiratory function, minimizes stress, and maximizes patient comfort and environmental quality. Restricting exercise is important initially in more severe cases to reduce ventilatory demands. In milder cases and in those that are improving with treatment, limited exercise may be helpful in promoting expectoration. Confinement in a cool, clean, dust- and odor-free, well-ventilated enclosure is indicated to minimize activity and exposure to the elements. Screened doors and wall panels promote ventilation at foal level. Sprinklers can be used to control dust in paddocks and pastures, and feeders should be moved to a grassy area if possible. Other dusty areas such as aisles and stalls in barns should be cleaned and watered down regularly during hot dry periods. Barns with poorly insulated roofs can be cooled with roof-mounted water sprinklers on hot days. Confinement in an air-conditioned stall may be necessary for foals with marked respiratory distress.

Antibacterial Treatment

Systemic antibacterial treatment should be based on the nature and severity of clinical signs, results of culture and susceptibility testing of tracheobronchial aspirates, experience within the herd and locale, and the properties of the chosen drugs that determine their distribution to inflamed lung tissue in therapeutic concentrations (see Table 2 in *Current Therapy 3*, p 471). In addition, the required route and frequency of drug administration, side effects, toxicity, and relative cost of therapy are important considerations. It is generally necessary to initiate antibacterial treatment before the results of culture and susceptibility testing are known, and in many instances treatment proceeds without samples for culture being obtained. Because β-hemolytic *Streptococcus* species are the most common bacteria isolated from pneumonic foals older than 30 days of age, penicillin G is a logical choice for initial treatment in circumstances when *R. equi* has not previously been a problem. This drug also shows activity against many isolates of gram-negative nonenteric organisms such as *Actinobacillus suis* and *Pasteurella* species. When involvement of penicillin-resistant gram-negative organisms is suspected or confirmed, an effective antibiotic that is compatible with penicillin should be included in the regimen. Aminoglycoside antibiotics such as gentamicin or amikacin are logical choices, but these agents should not be used alone because of their poor activity against β-hemolytic *Streptococcus* species. Trimethoprim/sulfonamide combinations (TMS) have a broad spectrum of activity, which includes many of the causal agents of foal pneumonia, and can be administered by the oral route (15–30 mg/kg of combination b.i.d.) to initiate treatment. Trimethoprim/sulfonamide can be used alone or with penicillin G when TMS-susceptible, penicillin-resistant bacteria are present in mixed infections with gram-positive organisms. Ceftiofur, a third-generation cephalosporin antibiotic recently approved for use in horses, has a broad spectrum of activity that includes most of the etiologic agents of foal pneumonia, except *R. equi*. Doses of 2.2 to 5.0 mg/kg IM b.i.d. exceed manufacturers' recommendations but appear appropriate. Antibiotic treatment should be continued for 5 to 7 days after the foal is clinically normal, otherwise a high rate of relapse is encountered. If the foal does not show clinical improvement within 3 to 5 days following initiation of treatment, the therapeutic regimen should be re-evaluated, including a repeated tracheal wash. Chronic cases generally respond more slowly than do acute cases.

The treatment of *R. equi* pneumonia requires special consideration. *R. equi* is susceptible in vitro to a wide range of antibiotics including amikacin, gentamicin, neomycin, chloramphenicol, trimethoprim/sulfonamide, erythromycin, and rifampin. However, the dramatic increase in recovery

rates since the introduction of oral treatment with erythromycin/rifampin makes this the therapeutic approach of choice. These lipid-soluble agents show synergistic activity in vitro; both effectively penetrate cell membranes to achieve therapeutic concentrations in the lung, bronchial secretions, and within phagocytes where the organism multiplies; and both appear to be active in the environment of pyogranulomas, thus sterilizing them. In addition, both drugs show excellent activity against *Streptococcus* species and moderate activity against *Actinobacillus* species, organisms that are frequently isolated along with *R. equi*. Because resistance to rifampin can develop rapidly during therapy, it should not be used alone. Although the vast majority of *R. equi* isolates are susceptible to erythromycin and rifampin, resistant strains have been encountered.

It is recommended that erythromycin (25 mg/kg p.o. t.i.d. to q.i.d.), as the acid-stable estolate or ethylsuccinate esters or as erythromycin base or phosphate, be used with rifampin (5–10 mg/kg p.o. b.i.d.) to initiate therapy. Use of a lower dose of rifampin (2.5–5 mg/kg p.o. b.i.d.) after a positive response has been achieved with the higher dose has proven effective and reduces treatment costs. Rifampin causes reddish discoloration of urine, and the erythromycin/rifampin combination frequently causes the fecal consistency to soften. The occurrence of the latter side effect does not necessitate discontinuing treatment, but these foals should be monitored carefully because a small, but significant, number develop depression, severe diarrhea, dehydration, and electrolyte loss necessitating intensive fluid and electrolyte therapy and cessation of treatment with rifampin and erythromycin. Similar side effects have been noted on occasion when rifampin is used in combination with penicillin G or TMS. Erythromycin and rifampin may give rise to transient signs of partial anorexia, mild colic, and bruxism, which resolve on temporary cessation (one to two doses) of treatment.

Oral erythromycin alone has been used successfully to treat *R. equi* pneumonia, but comparison of efficacy with the erythromycin/rifampin regimen awaits confirmation. In addition, idiosyncratic reactions characterized by hyperthermia, tachypnea, or overt respiratory distress have been seen in foals being treated with erythromycin during hot weather. Diarrhea has been observed occasionally in the dams of nursing foals while the foals are being treated with oral erythromycin, presumably because coprophagic behavior leads to ingestion of sufficient active erythromycin to disrupt the normal gastrointestinal flora of the mare.

The severe consolidating pulmonary lesions that characterize *R. equi* infection necessitate early recognition and prolonged treatment to achieve a satisfactory outcome. Resolution of clinical signs, normalization of plasma fibrinogen concentration, white blood cell (WBC) count and thrombocyte count, and radiographic resolution of lesions are used to guide the duration of therapy, which generally ranges between 4 and 12 weeks. Relapses may occur if treatment is prematurely discontinued. A positive clinical response within 7 days suggests a favorable prognosis. Recovery rates exceeding 80% have been reported for referred, presumably serious, *R. equi* cases.

Although erythromycin and rifampin are the drugs of choice for treating *R. equi* infection, it may be necessary to use other drugs for individual foals. Trimethoprim/sulfonamide (15–30 mg/kg of the combination p.o. b.i.d. or t.i.d.) has proved successful in some foals with mild or early *R. equi* pneumonia but without marked evidence of pulmonary abscessation, and for continued therapy in foals that have responded well to other drugs. Parenteral treatment with gentamicin (2.2 mg/kg to 3.0 mg/kg t.i.d. or b.i.d.) in combination with penicillin G or ampicillin has also proved to be therapeutically effective in some cases.

Clearing Secretions

Maintenance of adequate hydration is important to promote mucociliary clearance and expectoration by reducing the viscosity of tenacious bronchial secretions. This can usually be accomplished by the provision of clean water but parenteral therapy with polyionic electrolyte solutions may be indicated in some cases. Intravenous fluid therapy should be monitored closely because pneumonia predisposes foals to the development of pulmonary edema. Expectorants such as iodides, guaifenesin, volatile oils, and sulfonamides are often beneficial by helping mobilize respiratory secretions. Mucolytics, such as bromhexine hydrochloride or a newer derivative,* can also be beneficial in cases with large amounts of mucopus in the airways. The use of cough suppressants is generally contraindicated but may be needed in the occasional foal that becomes exhausted by paroxysmal coughing.

Nebulization is often helpful in foals with tenacious secretions or a nonproductive cough but is contraindicated in foals with voluminous moist secretions, and the procedure may prove too stressful to some foals. The major functions of nebulization are to humidify, liquefy secretions, relieve bronchospasm, decrease mucosal edema, and kill bacteria. Ultrasonic nebulizers that disperse droplets less than 5 μm in diameter should be used. Saline alone is useful for liquefying tenacious secretions, and saline is also the usual choice as a carrier solution for other agents such as bronchodilators, mucolytics, and antibiotics. The aerosol is delivered through a loose-fitting mask, such as a gallon or half-gallon plastic jug, with 15- to 30-minute exposures at 6- to 12-hour intervals. The following has been reported to be a useful nebulizing formula for foals with pneumonia caused by *R. equi* or gram-negative organisms:

1. Carrier solution: half-strength saline (180 ml)
2. Mucolytic: N-acetylcysteine 20% (5 to 10 ml)
3. Bronchodilator: isoproterenol (2 ml) or isoetharine HCl inhalation, 1% (1 ml)
4. Antibiotic: gentamicin sulfate (150 mg) or kanamycin sulfate (400 mg).

Another nebulizing formula reported to be successful is 10 ml N-acetylcysteine (20%), 10 ml isoetharine HCl inhalation, 1%, 10 ml gentamicin sulfate (50 mg/ml), and 50 ml normal saline.

Maintaining Gas Exchange

Oxygen therapy, using humidified oxygen (6–10 L/minute) delivered by nasal insufflation, via a loose-fitting mask or, in severely hypoxemic foals, via percutaneous transtracheal administration, is indicated in those foals showing severe respiratory distress and persistent hypoxemia or cyanosis. Nonsteroidal anti-inflammatory drugs (NSAIDs) such as phenylbutazone, flunixin meglumine, or dipyrone may be of value in limiting the pulmonary inflammatory reaction, as well as in reducing fever and improving attitude and appetite in febrile, depressed, anorectic foals. However, these drugs may negate the value of temperature in monitoring the effectiveness of therapy, may predispose to gastric ulceration, and can be nephrotoxic in hypovolemic foals. These cases should be monitored carefully and NSAID therapy should be discontinued when the foal's attitude and appetite improve.

The use of bronchodilator drugs in treating foal pneumonia is controversial but it is the experience of the author that some foals judged to have widespread bronchoconstriction on the basis of clinical findings or the results of bronchodilator response tests may benefit considerably from bronchodilator therapy. Aminophylline (5–10 mg/kg p.o. b.i.d.), terbutaline (0.02–0.06 mg/kg p.o. b.i.d.), or clenbuterol (0.8 μg/kg p.o. or IV b.i.d.) have proved beneficial in selected patients, particularly those that have an abnormal respiratory character (increased expiratory effort) and adventitial lung sounds after the bacterial component has been eliminated with antibiotic therapy. Culture-negative cases of this type appear to be suffering from hyperreactive small airway disease with excess mucus secretion similar to that seen in adult horses with chronic obstructive pulmonary disease. Aminophylline treatment should be short term and should be monitored carefully because clinical signs may deteriorate in some foals owing to cardiotoxicity and increased ventilation/perfusion mismatch. In addition, the elimination of aminophylline may be delayed by erythromycin; thus, blood levels may be increased and toxicity potentiated. If the response to environmental improvement (minimum-dust management) and bronchodilator treatment is poor, short-term low-dose treatment with corticosteroids, such as dexamethasone (0.02–0.05 mg/kg s.i.d. for 4–7 days), may be necessary to break the inflammatory, mucus-secreting cycle and promote resolution in foals with hyperreactive airway disease.

Immunotherapy

Supplementation or augmentation of the immune response may be beneficial in selected patients. Plasma transfusion is indicated in young foals with pneumonia and partial or complete failure of passive transfer of colostral antibody and may benefit foals that are hypoproteinemic for other reasons. Specific hyperimmune *R. equi* plasma has been shown to effectively prevent *R. equi* pneumonia following natural and experimental challenge, but the value of hyperimmune plasma in treating established *R. equi* infections appears to be more limited. Immunomodulatory drugs such as mycobacterial cell wall extract and extracts of *Propionibacterium acnes* are nonspecific stimulators of the immune response and have gained widespread use in recent years as adjuncts to conventional treatment of respiratory tract infections, particularly chronic foal pneumonia. Levamisole, a modulator of T cell function, has also been recommended for use in foals with chronic nonresponsive pneumonia. The use of immunomodulatory drugs may increase as the rationale for their inclusion in therapeutic regimens becomes supported by controlled indepen-

---

*Sputolysin, Boehringer Ingelheim, Bracknell, England

dent studies to document their efficacy. The majority of foals with bacterial pneumonia, including those with serious *R. equi* infection, survive and appear to maintain the potential to become successful performance horses.

PREVENTION

The cornerstone of prevention is good herd management. This involves good hygiene and sanitation, maximizing environmental quality, avoiding overgrazing and overcrowding, reducing dust, employing strict parasite control, vaccinating to prevent viral respiratory infections, enforcing rest if viral respiratory infections do occur, maintaining fixed herd groups, separating resident horses from visiting horses, and isolating new arrivals and clinically ill horses. Farms and feeding and watering arrangements should be designed so that foals are dispersed rather than concentrated, and the size of mare-foal bands should be restricted to 10 pairs or less. Foaling management is also very important, in particular the booster vaccination of mares against respiratory pathogens before foaling, ensuring adequate early colostral intake by foals, attention to the foal's umbilicus at foaling, and avoiding transportation and mixing of young foals from different sources. Provision of adequate shade is important for horses pastured in hot sunny climates. Extreme care must also be taken when transporting foals, especially those with respiratory disease, during the summer months, because the interior of horse trailers can become extremely hot, particularly when the trailer is parked. As noted previously, foals should be observed closely for signs of respiratory disease because early diagnosis of pneumonia is important if treatment is to be cost-effective and successful.

Routine preventive measures outlined for the control of foal pneumonia, although helpful, have not prevented serious outbreaks of *R. equi* pneumonia on individual breeding farms. Bearing in mind the coprophilic nature of *R. equi* and the progressive amplification of *R. equi* numbers during the summer months in paddocks, holding pens, barn aisles, and walkways, strict attention to removal of feces from these areas, the use of clean paddocks for foals, promotion of grass growth in paddocks, and reduction of dusty or sandy conditions in the environment of foals are indicated to reduce the level of challenge. Despite the poor results achieved by vaccinating foals or their dams (prefoaling) with *R. equi* bacterins, recent evidence indicates that some factors, which may or may not be specific antibody, present in hyperimmune plasma may be important in conferring resistance to infection. A program whereby hyperimmune plasma (500–1000 ml) is administered to foals during the first month of life and, if necessary, repeated later in the season has greatly reduced the incidence of *R. equi* pneumonia on problem farms. Such hyperimmune plasma is now commercially available* for administration to individual foals or to the entire foal crop on premises with endemic *R. equi* when the expense of this approach outweighs the costs associated with treatment and mortality.

Supplemental Readings

Cohen ND: Causes of and farm management factors associated with disease and death in foals. J Am Vet Med Assoc 204:1644–1651, 1994.

Hillidge CJ: Use of erythromycin-rifampin combination in treatment of *Rhodococcus equi* pneumonia. Vet Microbiol 14:337–342, 1987.

Hoffman AM, Viel L, Juniper E, Prescott JF: Clinical and endoscopic study to estimate the incidence of distal respiratory tract infection in Thoroughbred foals on Ontario breeding farms. Am J Vet Res 54:1603–1607, 1993.

Hoffman AM, Viel L, Prescott JF, Rosendal S, Thorsen J: Association of microbiologic flora with clinical, endoscopic, and pulmonary cytologic findings in foals with distal respiratory tract infection. Am J Vet Res 54:1615–1622, 1993.

Madigan JE, Hietala S, Muller N: Protection against naturally acquired *Rhodococcus equi* pneumonia in foals by administration of hyperimmune plasma. J Reprod Fert 44[Suppl]:571–578, 1991.

Martens RJ, Ruoff WW, Renshaw HW: Foal pneumonia: A practical approach to diagnosis and therapy. Comp Cont Ed Pract Vet 9:S361–S375, 1982.

Prescott JF, Hoffman AM: *Rhodococcus equi.* Vet Clin North Am Equine Pract 9:375–384, 1993.

Sweeney CR, Sweeney RW, Divers TJ: *Rhodococcus equi* pneumonia in 48 foals: Response to antimicrobial therapy. Vet Microbiol 14:329–336, 1987.

Polymune R, Veterinary Dynamics, Chino, CA

Infectious Orthopedic Disease in Foals

JOHN B. MADISON
Gainesville, Florida

Bone and joint infections occur commonly in young foals and may be life-threatening even with early identification and aggressive treatment. These conditions occur most commonly in foals younger than 4 months of age. The infecting organisms typically gain access to the bone or joints via hematogenous spread, although direct inocula-tion and extension of local infections can also occur. Hematogenous spread of organisms from infected umbilical remnants, gastrointestinal tract, or infections localized in the thoracic cavity are most common, although the primary source of infection may reside anywhere.

It is therefore important, when presented with a foal

with infectious orthopedic disease, to make a concerted effort to localize a primary source for the infection. This requires careful and thorough examination of the foal and an ultrasonographic evaluation of the umbilical remnants. Serum should be evaluated for IgG content to ensure adequate passive transfer of colostral immunoglobulin in foals younger than 14 days of age. Thoracic radiographs, transtracheal aspirates, cerebrospinal fluid (CSF) taps, and other diagnostic tests are useful in localizing and identifying the primary source of infection when body systems other than the musculoskeletal system are suspected to be involved. In general, blood culture should be performed before starting antibiotic therapy in an attempt to isolate the etiologic agent. Specific attempts to isolate the offending organism from the sites of bone or joint infections are also essential and are discussed in detail later. It is important to recognize that often organisms cultured from the blood or a primary site of infection such as an umbilical remnant do not match the organisms cultured from the bone or joint infection. In all cases, broad-spectrum antibiotic coverage should be initiated pending the results of the cultures. A parenterally administered combination of an aminoglycoside (either gentamicin or amikacin) with penicillin or ampicillin are commonly used. Antibiotic therapy should be changed to more specific coverage when and if an etiologic agent is identified. Common organisms isolated from foals with infectious orthopedic disease include *Salmonella* species, *Actinobacillus equuli*, *Eschericia coli*, β-hemolytic *Streptococci*, and occasionally *Rhodococcus equi*.

INFECTIOUS OSTEITIS AND OSTEOMYELITIS

In foals, hematogenously spread bone infections nearly always occur at a bone-cartilage interface. The common sites of occurrence are the epiphysis of the long bones, metaphyseal side of the growth plates, costochondral junctions, and articular facets and growth plates of the vertebral bodies. Diaphyseal lesions rarely occur as a result of hematogenous dissemination. The propensity for infections to localize at these sites is thought to be due to sluggish blood flow and vascular stasis as the nutrient vessels approach a cartilage interface, turn back on themselves, and empty into large venous sinusoids.

Diagnosis

The most consistent presenting sign in foals with bone infections is diffuse swelling over the infected region that may range from barely noticeable to quite marked. Usually a pain response is elicited on deep palpation of the area. The degree of lameness observed varies from none to a non-weightbearing lameness. Changes in the hemogram and elevations in plasma fibrinogen are not always present and are unreliable aids in establishing the diagnosis. Radiographic evaluation of suspected sites of bone infection is essential in evaluating the location and extent of the condition. The proximity of the infection to adjacent joints may also be evaluated using radiography. Radiographic changes are often subtle and difficult to interpret early in the course of bone infections. Comparisons with radiographs of the opposite limb are often helpful in determining the signifi-

cance of subtle radiographic changes. Detection of radiographic evidence of bone lysis requires 30 to 50% of the bone mineral content to be removed. As always, subtle changes must be correlated with the clinical examination to assess their significance. As the condition progresses, however, the presence of bone lysis becomes more obvious. Nuclear scintigraphy may be useful in selected cases in localizing sites of infection; however, the intense uptake of technetium-99m methylene diphosphonate typical of infected bone may be obscured by the normally intense uptake at osteochondral junctions in young foals. Indium labeling of white blood cells, although more specific in localizing areas of infected bone, is impractical because of the extended period of isolation required for adequate clearance of the radiopharmaceutical.

Joint effusions commonly occur in joints adjacent to areas of bone infection. It is important to assess whether these effusions are septic as a result of extension of the infection into the joint or whether they are merely nonseptic sympathetic effusions occurring in response to local inflammation. Arthrocentesis and cytologic evaluation of the synovial fluid differentiate septic from nonseptic effusions.

Culture

In addition to blood culture and culture of suspected primary sites of infection, specific culture and Gram's stain of infected bone is often helpful in elucidating the etiologic agent and guiding the selection of appropriate antibiotic therapy. If the bony lesion can be localized radiographically, culture of the infected bone may be obtained in many instances under sedation and local anesthesia. A Michele trephine or curet may be inserted through a small stab incision and samples of bone obtained. Alternatively, a 4.0- or 4.5-mm drill bit may be inserted in the infected bone and the drillings harvested from the flutes of the bit for culture and Gram's stain. Bone specimens are easily obtained from many sites, particularly the distal limbs. Unfortunately, not all sites are easily accessible for culture, and the clinician must weigh the risks of obtaining a specimen, for example, damage to adjacent soft tissue structures or seeding previously sterile joints with bacteria, against the benefit of isolating the etiologic agent.

Treatment

The cornerstone of therapy for bone infections is long-term antimicrobial treatment. Although surgical debridement of infected bone as an adjunct to medical therapy is, in theory, desirable, the extent and location of bone infections in foals often makes surgical treatment impractical. Surgical debridement of infected bone as a rule should be reserved for those cases not responsive to medical management. There are three notable exceptions, however, when surgical intervention is indicated. These are (1) joint infections that occur as a result of extension of epiphyseal bone infections into the joint; (2) bone infections accompanied by draining sinuses and sequestra; and (3) focal and easily accessible bone infections that can be debrided without risking the integrity of the bone or damage to surrounding soft tissue structures.

As mentioned previously, broad-spectrum antibiotic therapy should be initiated pending identification of the etiologic agent. Once the etiologic agent has been identified, the treatment may be changed to an appropriate oral antibiotic, if possible. Antibiotic therapy should continue for weeks to months to achieve resolution of the problem. The difficult dilemma facing the clinician is when to change to oral antibiotic coverage and which antimicrobial to choose in cases when an etiologic agent has not been identified. Prolonged parenteral broad-spectrum therapy is expensive and requires either long-term maintenance of intravenous catheters or repeated painful intramuscular injections. In the absence of culture and sensitivity results to guide the selection of oral antibiotics, enrofloxacin (2.5 mg/kg p.o., b.i.d.) may be a reasonable choice. Other oral antimicrobials such as trimethoprim/sulfa, rifampin, chloramphenicol, and erythromycin have been used successfully, either alone or in combination, to treat susceptible organisms. There has been some reluctance to use enrofloxacin in the foal because of the concern that the severe destruction of articular cartilage observed in young dogs would also be seen in the foal. The author is not aware of any documentation of this side effect in foals at this dose and has used enrofloxacin in foals without causing lameness. Until further studies of the safety of this antimicrobial have been conducted, owners should be warned of the potential but unknown risk of serious joint damage with use of enrofloxacin.

Other strategies for delivering antimicrobials to the site of bone infections such as the use of antibiotic-impregnated polymethylmethacrylate beads or regional vascular or intraosseous perfusion of antibiotics are under investigation and show promise in the management of difficult infections; however, these techniques are not yet widely used.

SEPTIC ARTHRITIS

The majority of cases of septic arthritis in foals can be divided into two categories: (1) hematogenously spread septic arthritis, and (2) infection caused by direct penetration of the joint either iatrogenically or via a wound or by extension of an inflammatory process from tissues adjacent to the joint.

Diagnosis

The presenting clinical signs for foals with septic arthritis are the acute onset of severe lameness coupled with a marked effusion in the affected joint. Fever and hemogram changes may or may not be associated. Aspiration of synovial fluid for cytology and culture are essential diagnostic aids. Normal synovial fluid has a nucleated cell count of less than 500 cells/μL and a total protein level of less than 2.0 g/dl. The majority of cells in normal synovial fluid are monocytes, lymphocytes, and synovial lining cells. The predominant cell type in inflamed synovial effusions, regardless of cause, is the neutrophil. As a general rule the neutrophils tend to be well preserved in nonseptic suppurative effusions and tend to be degenerating and karyolytic in septic effusions. Nucleated cell counts higher than 20,000 cells/μl in foals with hematogenously acquired septic arthritis are essentially diagnostic. Inflamed painful joints with nucleated cell counts higher than 10,000 cells/ml must be presumed to be infected until proved other-

wise. Other synovial fluid components that change with sepsis are an elevation in the total protein (>2 g/dl), and a decrease in mucin clot formation and viscosity. These changes support the diagnosis of septic arthritis but are not pathognomonic.

Culture

Definitive diagnosis of joint sepsis can be made when positive culture results are obtained. It is important to recognize, however, that cultures of infected joints yield bacteria only 50 to 60% of the time. This is due to the low concentration of bacteria in the fluid and bacteriostatic properties of synovial fluid itself. Culture of synovial membrane does not, in most instances, enhance the ability to recover organisms from septic joints. This is probably due to the fact that the bacteria do not tend to colonize the synovial membrane but instead live in fibrin clots coating the synovial lining and floating free in the joint. Although it is probably warranted to obtain synovial biopsies at the time of surgery for culture, specific efforts to obtain synovial membrane for culture are not warranted. Highest yield of positive culture results is achieved by one of two methods. The method the author prefers is to obtain as large a volume of synovial fluid as possible, centrifuge the fluid, and culture the pellet. The fluid may be stored in a sterile container such as a capped syringe under refrigeration until presentation to the laboratory. Alternatively, a large volume of synovial fluid may be inoculated into blood culture media. The media should be incubated for 24 hours under aerobic and anaerobic conditions then subcultured on blood agar. This method has the disadvantage of adding 24 hours to the time before initial culture results can be obtained. Regardless of the method chosen, greater numbers of positive culture results are obtained if large volumes of synovial fluid are submitted. The use of antibiotic removal devices or sodium polyanetholsulfonate tubes should be considered for submission of synovial fluid samples obtained after the administration of antibiotics. All positive culture results from aseptically obtained joint fluid should be considered significant. Organisms that are not typical equine pathogens such as *Staphylococcus epidermidis*, *Aspergillus*, and *Candida* species can cause septic arthritis if inoculated into joints.

Histopathology

Histopathologic evaluation of synovial membrane biopsy specimens as an aid in distinguishing infectious arthritis from other causes of joint inflammation in horses is of little or no value. The organisms are rarely identified in the synovium of biopsy specimens from infected joints even with the use of special stains. Furthermore, the response of the synovium to inflammation is characteristic, varying only in degree and not varying in response to the insult. In addition, widely varying degrees of synovial membrane histologic response can be seen in synovial membrane biopsy samples taken from different areas of the same joint.

Treatment

Treatment of septic arthritis should be initiated as soon as the condition is encountered. The author considers these patients to be medical-surgical emergencies. The earlier one intervenes, the less likely that chronic drainage systems will be necessary to obtain joint sterility. Several important principles should be kept in mind when treating cases of infectious arthritis.

1. Some form of joint drainage should be employed in all cases.

2. Broad-spectrum parenteral antibiotics at appropriate dosages and frequency should be administered pending culture results.

3. Nonsteroidal anti-inflammatory drugs (NSAIDs) should be administered for their analgesic and anti-inflammatory effects.

4. Radiographs should be obtained at the onset of treatment.

5. Adequate rest must be allowed following resolution of the problem.

Antibiotic therapy should begin as soon as septic arthritis is suspected, but preferably after obtaining synovial fluid for culture and cytology tests. This necessitates choosing antibiotics before specific culture and sensitivity results are obtained. In foals *Salmonella* species, *Actinobacillus*, *Escherichia coli*, and *Streptococci* are the most common organisms encountered. Based on the wide variety of organisms encountered, broad-spectrum antibiotic coverage is essential until specific culture and sensitivity results can be obtained. The parenteral route of administration is preferred initially to ensure that adequate levels of antimicrobials are being achieved. Penicillin G (22,000 IU/kg IV, q.i.d.) in combination with either gentamicin (6.6 mg/kg IV, s.i.d.) or amikacin (20 mg/kg IV, s.i.d.) are good choices.

Once culture and sensitivity results are obtained, antibiotics should be changed to effective specific therapy for the organisms cultured. Antibiotic treatment should continue *at least* 3 weeks after the resolution of lameness or removal of a closed suction drain. In the absence of positive bacterial culture results, despite repeated attempts, the author often changes to enrofloxacin (2.5 mg/kg p.o., b.i.d.) or oral trimethoprim/sulfa (20 mg/kg of combination p.o. b.i.d.) in combination with rifampin (5 mg/kg b.i.d.) following drain removal.

The decision on what type of drainage to employ depends on the duration of the infection, economic considerations, and in foals, the number of joints involved. Infections present for less than 48 hours may be adequately managed with through-and-through lavage. This is best accomplished using the arthroscope; however, it can be easily performed in the sedated foal by using a soft catheter for fluid ingress and a stab incision for fluid egress. Use of a small stab incision allows removal of fibrin clots not removed with needle lavage. The skin of the stab incision should be closed using one or two sutures, much like an arthroscopy portal. Lavage should be performed using a balanced pH-adjusted polyionic solution such as Plasmalyte A which is pH 7.4.* Adding antibiotics or antiseptics to the lavage fluid is probably of limited value, and these substances can cause chemical irritation of the already inflamed synovial lining. Essentially all antibiotics used routinely in equine practice achieve good levels in the synovial fluid when administered systemically.

Infected joints that have not responded to through-and-

through lavage or in which disease is more chronic should have some type of chronic drainage established. Two options are leaving a small arthrotomy open to drain or the use of closed suction drainage systems. The latter, although requiring careful management, are in the author's opinion superior to open arthrotomies for several reasons. Problems with the formation of synovial fistulae, drying of articular cartilage, and joint capsule fibrosis at the site of the arthrotomy are avoided by using the closed suction drains. Horses with closed suction drains in place walk nearly sound because their joint is being continually decompressed. When properly maintained, these drains do not tend to plug and maintain continuous joint decompression for as long as they are left in place. We have used these drains in foals for as long as 3 to 4 weeks without encountering problems with superinfection.

Treatment recommendations for the chronically infected joint are to perform an initial arthroscopic evaluation of the joint with thorough lavage and removal of as much fibrin as possible. The author does not advocate extensive synovectomy because of the hemarthrosis that results and because the bacteria probably do not colonize the synovium itself, but live in the layer of fibrin deposited on the synovium. Following arthroscopic examination, a flat latex fenestrated drain is placed in the joint, and the drain exit tubing is tunneled subcutaneously for 5 to 15 cm before exiting the skin. The drain is attached to a 60-ml syringe and a pin is inserted through the syringe plunger. The pin holds the plunger in place, thus maintaining continuous suction. Continuous suction must be maintained to keep the drain functioning properly. Great care is taken to ensure that nothing returns to the joint through the drain system. The drain is kept in place until the character of the synovial fluid retrieved is normal, the volume of synovial fluid decreases, and the synovial fluid aspirated is sterile. This can take anywhere from several days to several weeks to achieve. This drainage system has been used in nearly every joint in the appendicular skeleton, including the shoulder and stifle.

In the absence of associated osteomyelitis, the prognosis for rendering an infected joint sterile using this system is good to excellent. If the joint infection occurs as a result of extension of a bone infection into the joint or if the bone has become infected as a consequence of the septic arthritis, the prognosis for achieving joint sterility is substantially worsened. In these cases, arthroscopic exploration and debridement of the infected bone are strongly recommended. In either case, the ultimate prognosis for return to athletic function depends on the amount of cartilage matrix damage done before joint sterility is achieved. This depends on, among other factors, the organism cultured, its virulence and antibiotic susceptibility, and the duration of the infection prior to establishment of joint drainage.

Aftercare

Enzymes released from neutrophils and chondrocytes are in large part responsible for the degradation of cartilage matrix and collagen that occurs in septic arthritis. Destruction of cartilage matrix results in mechanically inferior cartilage that is not able to withstand excessive forces. For this reason a period of rest of 1 to 2 months after resolution of the septic arthritis is recommended before the mare

*Normosol R, Baxter Healthcare, Deerfield, IL

and foal are allowed full pasture exercise. As previously mentioned, antibiotic therapy should continue for at least 3 weeks past the resolution of clinical signs. Intra-articular injection of hyaluronic acid is beneficial in helping to resolve the synovitis. Intra-muscular polysulfated glycosaminoglycan° (1 mg/kg IM q5days) is recommended because of its ability to inhibit chondrodestructive enzymes. Physical therapy including hand walking and passive range of motion is important in minimizing scarring and fibrosis, which can limit range of motion. Physical therapy also probably enhances cartilage nutrition.

IMMUNE-MEDIATED SYNOVITIS

An important consideration for polyarthritis in foals is immune-mediated joint disease. These foals can be distinguished from foals with septic polyarthritis primarily on the degree of lameness and on synovial fluid cytology test results. Foals with immune-mediated joint disease tend to be stiff rather than overtly lame. Usually at least four or more synovial sheaths are involved. These can be joints, tendon sheaths, or bursae. Cytologic evaluation of synovial

°*Adequan, Luitpold Pharmaceuticals Inc., Shirley, NY*

fluid reveals nucleated cell counts below 20,000 cells/ml with well-preserved neutrophils and large mononuclear cells. This syndrome results from the deposition of immune complexes in the synovial lining with subsequent complement fixation and synovitis. There is usually an inflammatory focus elsewhere, for example, pneumonia, umbilical remnant infection, or diarrhea, that should be investigated. About one third of foals with *Rhodococcus equi* pneumonia exhibit immune-mediated polysynovitis. The diagnosis can be confirmed by immunofluorescent staining of synovial membrane biopsy specimens. These joints do not need to be lavaged.

Supplemental Readings

Madison JB, Scarratt WK: Immune-mediated polysynovitis in four foals. J Am Vet Med Assoc 192:1581–1584, 1988.
Madison JB, Sommer M, Spencer PA: Relations among synovial membrane histopathologic findings, synovial fluid cytologic findings, and bacterial culture results in horses with suspected infectious arthritis: 64 cases (1979–1987). J Am Vet Med Assoc 198:1655–1661, 1991.
Montgomery RD, Long IR, Milton JC, DiPinto MN, Hunt J: Comparisons of aerobic culturette, synovial membrane biopsy, and blood culture medium in detection of canine bacterial arthritis. Vet Surg 18:300–303, 1989.
Schmid FR: Principles of diagnosis and treatment of bone and joint infections. *In* McCarty DJ (ed): Arthritis and Allied Conditions: A Textbook of Rheumatology, ed 10. Philadelphia, Lea & Febiger, 1985, pp 1627–1650.

Noninfectious Musculoskeletal Disorders of Foals

ROBERT J. HUNT
Lexington, Kentucky

Foals are susceptible to an array of developmental abnormalities involving the musculoskeletal system. Some conditions are evident at birth, whereas others evolve with development of the foal. Many have a genetic component influencing the onset of problems, and almost all are influenced by environmental or management factors. It is important for the veterinarian to recognize which problems may be influenced in a positive fashion by intervention, which problems should be left alone, and which foals should be euthanized because of a faulty gene pool or for humane purposes. The following is a review of the common musculoskeletal conditions of the foal that have a significant impact on the equine industry.

FLEXURAL LIMB DEFORMITIES

Flexural deformities refer to hyperflexion and failure to fully extend a given area. They may occur during development of the fetus in utero, shortly after birth, or later as the foal is developing. In utero flexural deformities, most commonly involving the carpus or a combination of carpus

and fetlock, are responsible for a substantial portion of the dystocias in mares. Other variations of in utero deformities involve the hindlimbs and spine.

The etiology is rarely determined but causes include in utero malposition of the fetus, exposure of the mare to influenza, and ingestion of Sudan grass or loco weed. Although a genetic link has not been proved, there are instances of mares and sires producing contracted foals over consecutive years.

Treatment for foals with flexural deformities that develop in utero varies with the severity of the deformity. If the foal can extend the limb adequately to allow support and ambulation, most deformities resolve spontaneously or respond to heavy bandages or splinting. Moderate deformities that necessitate assisting the foal to stand and nurse require application of splints or casts as well as administration of oxytetracycline (2–3 g slowly IV). This may be repeated daily or every other day for several treatments unless complications arise. Treatment of foals with severe flexural deformities should be discouraged, and the use of splinting or cast application is generally futile. Aggressive surgery should be discouraged because of a poor outcome.

Even after physically straightening the limbs by aggressive physiotherapy, some foals with severe deformities are unable to advance the limbs properly and have a spastic, hyperreflexive action of the limb when splinted. Without splints the limbs collapse forward, suggesting neurogenic involvement of the extensor muscle group. The extensor tendons are intact in these foals. Although foals with this disorder may be salvaged, it is unlikely that they will ever attain athletic ability. It is generally more practical to euthanize foals with severe flexural deformities.

Foals that acquire carpal or fetlock flexural deformities several weeks to months after birth are managed by dietary restriction and limiting exercise initially by stall confinement followed by gradual turn out in a dry lot. Grain or other sources of high energy and protein for the mare should be limited, and a modified nutritional program based on recommended nutritional guidelines should be followed. In extreme cases, limiting the foal's access to milk from high-producing mares by muzzling the foal and stripping the mare may be attempted. Alternatively, the owner may choose to wean the foal to control the foal's dietary intake. Carpal flexural deformities that develop when the foal is older than several weeks of age may require weeks to months to correct.

Splints and tetracycline may be of benefit. Pressure sores often develop with protracted use of splints, and the benefit is temporary if other management changes are not employed. Oxytetracycline likewise results in temporary improvement of the carpus but may result in hyperextension of the fetlocks. These effects are generally temporary and the long-term effects are neither deleterious nor beneficial without other treatments, such as dietary changes and exercise control.

Rupture of the Common Digital Extensor Tendon

Rupture of the common digital extensor tendon is often mistaken for flexural deformity of the fetlock or carpus because of the knuckling forward when the foal attempts to walk. The disorder may be recognized shortly after birth or generally by 3 to 4 days of life, although it may occur in foals up to 3 weeks of age. Diagnosis of common digital extensor tendon rupture is based on the clinician's ability to extend the limb to a normal position, the presence of a fluctuant swelling over the dorsolateral surface of the carpus, and palpable laxity or defect in the extensor tendon over the dorsal surface of the third metacarpal bone. Ruptured extensor tendons may occur concurrently with flexural deformities, especially in premature contracted foals. Treatment consists of heavily padding the lower limb and application of a splint over the dorsal or palmar surface of the limb. Dorsally placed splints are most effective if the bandage does not slip or rotate; this may be accomplished by first taping the bandage to the leg. Casting is occasionally used but is not generally necessary. Foals typically begin advancing the limb properly after several days to several weeks of age and should be restricted to a stall until the knuckling forward ceases.

Coronopedal Deformity

Coronopedal deformity (club foot) is occasionally seen at birth or within the first few days of life but most commonly develops between 2 and 6 months of age. The early clinical signs consist of a prominent bulge at the coronary band, increase in length of the heel relative to the toe of the hoof, and failure of the heels to adequately contact the ground after trimming. Eventually the foot develops a boxy, tubular shape with a dish along the dorsal surface. Many foals with coronopedal deformity also develop a "back in the knee" conformation. The etiology of the deformity is multifactorial, with genetics, diet, and exercise being the most commonly incriminated factors. Development of the condition may also occur as a consequence of a protracted lameness originating elsewhere in the limb. If lameness accompanies the deformity it is important to rule out other sources of lameness through physical evaluation, local anesthesia, radiographs, or other diagnostic aids.

If the newborn foal is able to ambulate without knuckling forward, the syndrome spontaneously corrects within a few days or responds to oxytetracycline. If the foot is flexed beyond an angle of 90°, splinting or casting is necessary. Toe extensions along with splinting are helpful but alone are generally ineffective.

Initial treatment of coronopedal deformity in the older foal consists of limiting the exercise, lowering the heels by trimming, and reducing the dietary intake to mare and foal. If the toe becomes worn excessively, toe extensions constructed from composite materials may aid in protection of the toe temporarily and serve as a lever arm for the toe. Elevating the heels has also been used to reduce tension on the deep digital flexor tendon and promote weightbearing on the foot. Although this appears to make the foal more comfortable initially, it is difficult to lower the heels at a later date and establish a normal hoof conformation. In addition, glue-on shoes are frequently used. These shoes tend to promote a boxy or tubular conformation of the hoof over time and their use in foals should be discouraged.

If no improvement is achieved after 1 to 2 months of conservative treatment, surgical intervention by use of a distal check ligament desmotomy may be indicated. When combined with a long-term trimming program, this improves the conformation of the hoof and hoof angle, and generally improves the "back at the knee" conformation. Owners should be made aware of the potential for a blemish at the surgery site.

Foals that have a hoof angle greater than 90° are candidates for salvage by performing a deep digital flexor tenotomy. Generally, if allowed to progress to this severity, relative shortening of the joint capsule or surrounding soft tissues precludes successful management by conservative means or distal check desmotomy. These animals may be useful as pets or for light riding, but it is unlikely that they will be successful athletes.

ANGULAR LIMB DEFORMITIES

Angular limb deformity refers to a deviation of the limb in the frontal plane and may be congenital or acquired in origin. Valgus deformities are those in which the limb deviates laterally distal to a reference point, whereas varus deformities deviate medially. Rotational deformities often occur concurrently with angular deformities either as a result of actual rotation of the bony column or from uneven loading of the hoof wall owing to the angular deformity. Typically, foals with valgus deformities rotate outwardly (supinate), whereas those with varus deformities rotate inwardly (pronate). Rotational deformities associated with rotation of the bony column improve little if any with correction of the angular deformity, and those associated with a nonbalanced foot generally resolve with trimming of the foot and correction of the valgus or varus deviation.

A mild to moderate degree of carpal valgus deviation is present at birth in many foals. The vast majority of these foals spontaneously undergo correction during the first few weeks to months of life. Varus deformity of one hind fetlock is common in Thoroughbred foals, which almost always spontaneously corrects if the sesamoids and flexor tendons are in proper alignment with the third metatarsal bone and fetlock joint when viewed from the plantar aspect of the limb.

The causes of angular limb deformities are unknown but are probably multifactorial. Premature or dysmature neonates that have incomplete ossification of the cuboidal bones and excessive laxity of periarticular supporting structures are often born with or develop angular limb deformities. Incomplete ossification occurs in foals of inadequate gestational age and in foals that were growth-retarded due to maternal disease, placental insufficiency, or twinning. Other causes of congenital angular deformities include inappropriate intrauterine positioning, loco weed ingestion, nutritional imbalances, and hypothyroidism.

Development of angular limb deformities in the postnatal foal is the result of a discrepancy in growth and development between the medial and lateral sides of the limb. This discrepancy may occur anywhere along the bony column but most commonly involves the physis, epiphysis, or metaphysis. Diaphyseal curvature or rotation and articular deformities occur less commonly. The etiology and pathogenesis are largely unknown but may include focal overloading and physeal trauma, physeal inflammation, factors associated with developmental orthopedic disease such as mineral imbalances or other dietary or environmental factors, and possibly genetic causes.

Treatment

Treatment of angular limb deformities varies depending on the severity of the deformity, age of the foal, and the presence of accompanying problems. Premature foals with incomplete ossification or periarticular laxity are at high risk of sustaining permanent deformation, fracturing, or crushing the cuboidal bones. It is important to minimize the amount of exercise for these foals to reduce the amount of loading on the immature bones. Splinting or casting until ossification occurs is recommended to reduce the chance of bony injury. This is, however, not without complications such as worsening the degree of laxity or development of decubitus sores. Providing ample padding, changing the splints two to three times daily, inspection of the limbs, and aggressive physiotherapy may reduce these complications. Foals that undergo crushing or fracture of the cuboidal bones of the carpus seldom develop into sound athletes, although they may occasionally be sound enough for light riding or raising as pets. Most with malformed tarsal bones withstand breaking and training but have soundness problems racing.

Management practices used in the treatment of angular limb deformities include exercise restriction and modification of the turn-out schedules of the mare and foal. Manipulation of hoof balance of the foal is also used commonly. This should be done with caution; excessive misbalancing of the foot should be avoided because of the possibility of creating a deformed foot or a deformity elsewhere in the limb. Simple balancing and leveling of the foot on a 2-week basis generally suffices.

External coaptation in the form of tube casts, splints, and articulating braces have been used with success. Cost of materials, time involved with application and removal, and the complications of pressure sores make the use of these devices less favorable options.

Surgical intervention for correction of angular limb deformities is indicated if there is worsening in the deformity during the first several months of age or failure to improve a moderate to severe deformity within 3 to 4 weeks of age. The vast majority of foals with angular limb deformities have corrected spontaneously; surgery is often performed as an attempt to take advantage of the rapid growth potential of the foal and ensure correction of the deformity before losing this growth potential. The surgical procedures in common usage for correction of angular limb deformities are hemicircumferential periosteal transection with periosteal elevation (HCPT/PE) and transphyseal bridging. HCPT/PE is performed on the relatively slowly developing (concave) side of the limb, whereas transphyseal bridging is used to retard the faster-developing side of the limb. Transphyseal bridging may be performed with screws and wires or with staples constructed of titanium or stainless steel. Because of their speed of placement and removal as well as the cosmetic appearance, staples are preferable.

Carpal valgus deformities of less than 10° in foals younger than 4 to 5 months of age benefit from HCPT/PE. Carpal varus deformities respond less favorably and may require transphyseal bridging at a later date. Transphyseal bridging of carpal angular limb deformities may be performed until 14 to 16 months of age but is more appropriately performed by 9 months of age. Angular deformities of the fetlocks require intervention by 1 to 2 months to achieve correction with HCPT/PE and by 4 months with transphyseal bridging. Tarsal deformities should be corrected on a similar timeframe as carpal deformities.

PHYSEAL DEFORMITIES

Physeal dysplasia is one of the most common manifestations of the developmental orthopedic disease complex recognized in foals. It is believed to be similar in pathogenesis to osteochondrosis and, therefore, involves a defect in endochondral ossification at the metaphyseal physis. There is also a mechanical influence of compression-induced ischemia of the affected area, which eventually results in cartilage necrosis, collapse of the physis, and premature closure of the epiphysis.

Physeal dysplasia is commonly referred to as *epiphysitis* or *physitis*; these terms may be inaccurate because it is not the epiphysis that is primarily involved and there is not necessarily an active inflammatory process. It has been associated with rapid growth, genetic predisposition, and the dietary associations of the developmental orthopedic disease complex.

Clinically the disease is recognized as a firm enlargement, most commonly involving the medial aspect of the distal metacarpal/metatarsal physis or the distal radial physis. The swelling may be warm and is usually sensitive to palpation. Lameness may be present in the early stages.

Physeal dysplasia of the distal metacarpus/metatarsus is recognized between 3 and 6 months of age, whereas the distal radius is affected between 6 and 20 months. Although both sexes are affected, rapidly growing fillies are generally the most severely involved and are especially prone to developing varus deformities as a sequela. Other clinical signs include development of an upright conformation to the point of knuckling and trembling at the fetlock.

The diagnosis of physeal dysplasia is based on the clinical signs. Radiographic changes include widened and irregular physes, lysis and sclerosis, bony flaring of the metaphysis, and periosteal proliferation.

Treatment

Treatment of physeal dysplasia is usually conservative and begins with assessment and modification of the nutritional program of the foal to correct errors. If the foal is still sucking the mare, grain intake to the mare should be kept to a minimum or the foal should be weaned so that diet may be controlled.

Exercise in the form of pasture turn out is generally reduced but not eliminated unless lameness is evident or the foal develops a rapid onset varus deformity associated with the physeal dysplasia. Phenylbutazone may be used at a low dosage rate (2.2 mg/kg s.i.d.) if lameness and pain are associated with the disease. Agents to facilitate cartilage repair such as polysulfated glycosaminoglycans are employed anecdotally, although their efficacy has not been documented.

Physeal dysplasia is generally self-limiting and has a good prognosis for complete recovery. Exceptions to this are foals that collapse the medial side of the growth plate and develop varus limb deformity or flexural limb deformities.

OSTEOCHONDROSIS

Osteochondrosis is one of the most common orthopedic diseases encountered in equine practice, and it is included as a part of the developmental orthopedic disease complex. It is probably far more common than clinically recognized, with many cases resolving uneventfully. Osteochondrosis is an arrest or delay of endochondral ossification in areas where cartilage is destined to become bone. The disease is manifested as focal areas of detached cartilage or as cartilage retention and cyst formation in subchondral bone.

The etiology of osteochondrosis is multifactorial, and in most instances the precise cause or group of factors involved is not determined. Heredity; exercise; trauma; corticosteroids; and dietary influences of vitamins A, D, and E, the trace minerals copper, zinc, molybdenum, calcium, and phosphorus, excess energy, and protein have been incriminated as potential factors involved with the onset of the disease.

Clinical Signs

Clinical signs vary depending on the joint involved, age of the animal, and extent of the lesion. Joint distension and pain on palpation of the involved region may be evident, and lameness varies from imperceptible to severe. Lesions may go undetected until the foals develop into yearlings or begin the early stages of training. Conceivably, all joints or areas of cartilage destined to become bone may be involved, but those most commonly affected include the stifles, hocks, and fetlocks. Less commonly involved areas are the shoulder, elbow, knee, coxofemoral joint, and cervical spine.

The Stifle

The most commonly affected regions of the stifle are the lateral trochlear ridge and the medial condyle of the distal femur. Other sites include the lateral femoral condyle, medial trochlear ridge, intertrochlear groove, the patella, and the proximal tibial plateau. Clinical signs of osteochondrosis of the stifle are typically noticed in late weanlings to yearlings. Lesions involving the femoropatella joint (trochlea or intertrochlear groove) generally present with effusion and varying grades of lameness. A defect may be detected in the cartilage upon careful palpation of the joint. Cyst-like lesions of the medial femoral condyle do not typically have increased joint distension, but the animal may be sensitive to palpation of the condyle with the limb flexed. Intra-articular anesthesia of the involved joint generally results in a marked improvement in the degree of lameness.

The diagnosis of osteochondrosis of the stifle is confirmed radiographically. During the acute stage of lameness and joint distension of the femoropatellar joint, radiographs may be normal. It may require 3 to 4 weeks from the onset of disease for lesions to become detectable radiographically. Cyst-like lesions of the medial femoral condyle are usually radiographically evident with the onset of clinical signs.

The Tarsus

Osteochondrosis of the tarsus most frequently involves the distal intermediate ridge of the tibia. Other sites are the lateral trochlear ridge of the talus, medial trochlear ridge, medial and lateral malleolus of the tibia, and cuboidal bones of the distal tarsal joints. Affected foals do not typically demonstrate an overt lameness unless severe joint distension is present, an osteochondral fragment is dislodged, or the bony lesion is excessively large. The lesion may be an incidental finding detected on radiographs, or there may be joint distension.

Metacarpophalangeal Joint

Osteochondrosis of the metacarpophalangeal joint may be seen as early as a few months to several years of age. In foals, lesions may be recognized as incidental findings on radiographs or may be associated with joint distension and varying degrees of lameness. The most commonly involved areas are the distal sagittal ridge of the third metacarpal bone, the palmar/plantar proximal aspect of the first phalanx, cyst-like lesions of the distal condyle of the condyles of the third metacarpus and first phalanx, and the dorsomedial and dorsolateral rim of the proximal first phalanx.

Other Areas

Other less commonly affected areas involved include the coffin joint, pastern joint, carpal joints, elbow, shoulder, and cervical vertebra. As with other more commonly affected joints, the lesions may be incidental findings or may be associated with mild to pronounced lameness.

Treatment

Treatment of osteochondrosis depends on the type and location of the lesion; clinical signs; and age, intended use, and value of the animal. The majority of osteochondrosis lesions detected as foals are self-limiting. Conservative treatments include exercise restriction, nonsteroidal anti-inflammatory drugs, and articular medications such as polysulfated glycosaminoglycans or hyaluronic acid. Consideration should be given to the fact that the immature cartilage and bone of foals are softer than those of skeletally mature animals and, if possible, surgery should be delayed until the foal is a yearling if excessive curettage is anticipated.

As a general rule, detached osteochondral flaps or fragments warrant surgical removal, although many of these eventually resolve. Scalloped-appearing lesions with a sclerotic margin seen radiographically do not necessarily benefit from surgery unless there is detached cartilage present.

Cyst-like lesions vary in their clinical presentation as well as in their response to surgery; controversy exists as to the benefits of surgical intervention. Surgical procedures for specific sites are thoroughly discussed in surgical texts.

Supplemental Readings

Auer J, Martens R, Morris E: Angular limb deformities in foals. Part 1: Congenital factors. Comp Cont Ed Pract Vet 4:S330–S339, 1982.
Auer JA, Martens RJ, Morris E.: Angular limb deformities in foals. Part II: Developmental factors. Comp Cont Ed Pract Vet 5:S27–S35, 1983.
Bohanon TC: Developmental musculoskeletal disease. In Kobluk CN, Ames TR, Geor RJ (eds): The Horse: Diseases and Clinical Management, vol 2. Philadelphia, WB Saunders, 1995, pp 815–858.
Douglas J: The pathogenesis and clinical manifestations of equine osteochondrosis. Vet Med 87:826–833, 1992.
Gabel AA, Knight DA, Reed SM, Pultz JA, Powers JD, Bramlage LR, Tyznik WJ: Comparison of incidence and severity of developmental orthopedic disease on 17 farms before and after adjustment of ration. Proc Am Assoc Equine Pract, 1987, pp 163–170.
Pool R: Developmental orthopedic diseases in the horse: Normal and abnormal bone formation. Proc Am Assoc Equine Pract 1987, pp 43–49.
Rose JA, Sande RD, Rose EM: Results of conservative management of osteochondrosis in the horse. Proc Am Assoc Equine Pract 1985, pp 617–626.
Wagner PC, Watrous BJ: Equine pediatric orthopedics: Part 4—physitis (epiphysitis). Equine Pract 12(7):11–14, 1990.
Watson DE, Selcer BA: Radiographic signs of osteochondrosis in horses. Comp Cont Ed Pract Vet 14:809–815, 1992.

Evaluation of Colic in the Neonatal Foal

MARTIN FURR
Leesburg, Virginia

The clinical presentation of foals with colic, with or without abdominal distension, is fairly common in equine practice (Table 1). Accurate diagnosis is critical for successful management of these conditions, because there is little room for error in treatment of problems of the neonatal foal. Particularly challenging is the determination of the need for exploratory surgery. No specific clinical examination findings unequivocally indicate that surgical or medical treatment is indicated, and thus synthesis of the results of diagnostic procedures is important in determining correct treatment. Many of the diagnostic methods applicable to the adult with abdominal pain are not useful in the neonate, and conversely, many techniques valuable in the neonate are not employed in the adult.

PHYSICAL EXAMINATION

A complete physical examination is imperative because many conditions such as sepsis or congenital abnormalities can lead to ileus, abdominal distension, and colic. The initial examination should be directed toward determining the nature and extent of all the foal's physiologic abnormalities, assessing gastrointestinal patency, ruling out sepsis, and determining the adequacy of passive transfer of immunoglobulins. Particular attention also should be directed toward assessment of abdominal circumference, presence of ascites, function of the cardiovascular and respiratory

TABLE 1.   CAUSES OF COLIC IN THE FOAL

Obstructive	Congenital
Meconium	Ileocolonic aganglionosis
Ingested foreign material	Atresia coli
(hair, bedding, string, rope)	Atresia ani
Torsion/volvulus	Uroperitoneum
Intussusception	Urachal leakage
Physiologic (ileus)	Urinary tract disruption
Gastric ulcer disease	Peritonitis
Infectious	Hernias
Rotavirus	Inguinal
Enteritis	Diaphragmatic
Sepsis	Scrotal

systems, presence of congenital defects, passage of stool, and urinary tract integrity.

Abdominal circumference can be measured with a cloth tape measure. Subsequent measurements to determine if distension is progressing need to be made in the same region and therefore the site of the initial measurement should be marked by shaving a small area. If abdominal distension exists, determining if it is the result of peritoneal or gastrointestinal accumulation of fluid or gas is key to the evaluation. Ascites can readily be confirmed by ultrasonography.

The cardiovascular system should be examined by evaluating mucous membrane color and moisture, capillary refill time, and pulse quality. Knowledge of the foal's hydration status does not aid in determining the cause of the colic, but does assist in development of a treatment plan.

The presence of dyspnea should prompt thoracic radiography and an arterial blood gas evaluation. Dyspnea could be associated with primary respiratory disease or sepsis, diaphragmatic hernia, fluid in the pleural cavity (an effusion, blood, chyle, or serum), fractured ribs, or diaphragmatic compression from bowel distension.

A digital rectal examination should be performed to determine if a meconium impaction exists. This can cause signs ranging from mild colic to complete obstruction. The absence of fecal material on the hindquarters or the presence of clear, clean mucus on the finger after a digital examination may suggest bowel atresia. Foals that are all white, are the offspring of overo-overo breedings, and show signs of abdominal pain should be suspected of having colonic aganglionosis, so-called lethal white foals. Such foals have varying degrees of colic and progressive abdominal distension. The presence of diarrhea makes a diagnosis of enteritis fairly straightforward, but foals can have fairly severe discomfort, ileus, and abdominal distension before passing abnormal stool. Thirty percent of foals eventually determined to have neonatal sepsis are presented with diarrhea.

The neonate with colic should also be evaluated thoroughly for metabolic derangements such as hypoglycemia, failure of passive transfer, and electrolyte disorders. Typically, the foal with a ruptured bladder is hyponatremic and hyperkalemic if it has continued to nurse the mare. If the foal has received intravenous fluids, however, these characteristic changes may be obscured or delayed. Similar electrolyte changes can be seen in cases of septicemia, renal failure, and enteritis, necessitating the need for additional diagnostic tests before surgical intervention. Typically these tests include abdominal ultrasound and abdominal fluid collection and evaluation.

Because the neonatal foal has little energy reserve upon which to draw, foals with colic and abdominal distension are likely to develop hypoglycemia. If the foal is not fed, as is often necessary in cases of colic, it is even more imperative that supplemental glucose be provided as 5 or 10% dextrose via intravenous drip. Although this will not provide adequate nutritional support, it can be used to maintain serum glucose for up to 24 hours, during which time a more definitive nutritional plan can be implemented.

Serum IgG levels should always be determined in the neonate with colic or abdominal distension to detect failure of passive transfer. Correction of this condition is critical to the overall management of such cases. Levels higher than 800 mg/dl are suggested, and several different methods, many of them stall-side, are available to determine serum IgG levels (see page 582).

Abdominal Radiography

Abdominal radiography is often very helpful in evaluating abdominal distension and colic in the neonate. Evaluating such radiographs is often not straightforward, however, and some degree of experience is necessary. Serial radiographs may be helpful in determining the significance of specific questionable lesions. A lateral view of the abdomen is routinely performed with the foal standing, although views of recumbent foals are often of benefit. Usually, the abdomen can be imaged on one 14 × 17 inch cassette and the approximate technique for the typical neonatal Thoroughbred foal is 85 kVp and 20 mAs, using a 10:1 focused grid and a focal film distance of 180 cm. These are guidelines only, and the technique may need to be modified based upon the specific equipment in use. The stomach is usually noted in the cranial central abdomen and usually is gas- and fluid-filled. Small intestinal distension with multiple erect and inverted U-shaped loops of bowel is consistent with obstructive disease (Fig. 1). Ileus produces diffuse small intestinal distension only (Fig. 2). Gas shadows are seen in the bowel wall in cases of pneumatosis intestinalis, and they suggest necrotizing enterocolitis. Large colon distension is often noted in cases of ileus, and displacements can occasionally be noted radiographically as a severely distended and distorted colon. Ascites is indicated by the presence of a fluid line on the films taken with the foal standing. Radiography is less valuable than ultrasound in characterizing peritoneal fluid, because it is sometimes difficult to determine if the fluid is intra-abdominal or within the large bowel. Pneumoperitoneum, which can be the result of gastrointestinal perforation or can follow abdominocentesis, is detected by an increased lucency of the film, with enhanced visualization of serosal surfaces.

Contrast studies that can be performed to further assess the bowel include barium enemas and an upper gastrointestinal series. These should be performed after routine

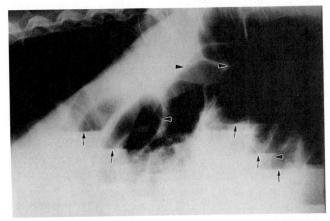

Figure 1. Abdominal radiograph of a foal with a strangulating obstruction of the intestine. Note the multiple fluid lines (*arrows*) and inverted loops of distended bowel (*arrowheads*). Surgery is indicated in such cases.

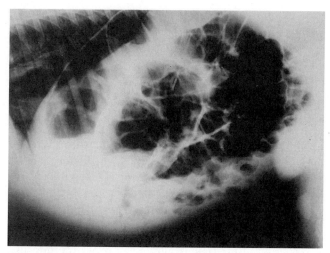

Figure 2. Abdominal radiograph of a foal with diffuse small intestinal ileus and distension. In contrast to the foal in Figure 1, there are no fluid lines or distended loops of bowel seen. This foal responded well to medical treatment.

films have been taken to establish a technique. The technique should then be increased by 10% to compensate for the radiodense contrast material. To perform an upper gastrointestinal series, 5 ml/kg of barium sulfate suspension is administered by nasogastric tube after a 4-hour fast. Serial radiographs are performed immediately after administration, at 5, 15, and 30 minutes, then at 2-hour intervals until the contrast medium has reached the small colon. In a normal foal, the stomach should empty within 2 hours. Duodenal strictures, as well as diffuse ileus, delay gastric emptying markedly. Mucosal erosion and ulceration can sometimes be seen, and filling defects of the stomach suggest gastric abscesses, foreign bodies, or masses. Filling defects of the proximal duodenum confirm duodenal stricture. An upper gastrointestinal series is contraindicated in the presence of severe small intestinal distension. The greatest value of this procedure lies in evaluating gastric emptying and the proximal duodenum for the presence of strictures. More distal lesions are difficult to interpret.

Barium enemas are useful to confirm an obstruction of the rectum or small colon. A well-lubricated enema tube should be gently passed into the rectum after evacuation of fecal material. Barium sulfate suspension (180 ml) is slowly infused while the anus is occluded around the tube. A radiograph of the caudal abdomen is performed immediately after instillation of the barium. Filling defects, obstructions such as meconium impactions, and atresia can be diagnosed with this method.

Ultrasonography

A 7.5- or 5-MHz scan head, preferably with a built-in standoff, is most useful for the evaluation of colic and abdominal distension in the neonate. The abdomen should be prepared by clipping the hair and applying ultrasound couplant gel. The examination is most productive if the foal is standing, because this allows the small intestine to drop to the ventral body wall. In a routine examination, the urachus, umbilical vein, umbilical arteries, bladder, peritoneum, and segments of small intestine can be easily

visualized via a ventral portal. Small intestinal segments can be examined and the thickness of the wall and the presence of distension determined. Normal bowel wall should be about 2 to 3 mm in thickness, and bowel greater than 4 mm in thickness is abnormal, suggesting inflammation, cellular infiltration, or edema. Suspicious areas can be compared with other segments of the bowel to determine the presence of focal thickening. Fluid filling, as is noted with diarrhea and enteritis, appears as round areas of bowel filled with composite fluid. Gas-distended bowel has a hyperechoic (echogenic) line at the surface of the bowel with little visualization beyond that surface. Small focal areas of gas may sometimes be seen within the wall of the bowel in cases of necrotizing enterocolitis. Intussusceptions have a characteristic "bull's eye" appearance with several concentric rings. This observation may be coupled with bowel distension in other small intestinal segments. Bowel motility can also be assessed using ultrasound and a lack of contractions of small intestine confirms ileus, which can be of physiologic or obstructive origin.

Abdominocentesis

Abdominocentesis should be performed with caution, because enterocentesis is more likely to occur and to have serious consequences in the neonate than the adult. Enterocentesis is particularly risky in the foal with gas- or fluid-distended bowel. Information gained by radiography and ultrasound examination should aid the clinician in deciding if abdominocentesis is warranted. The ultrasound examination can determine if large volumes of intraperitoneal fluid or localized pockets of fluid that can be tapped are present, thus increasing the diagnostic yield and decreasing the risk of bowel penetration. Use of a short teat cannula also reduces the risk of bowel penetration. If a needle is used, the thin bowel can easily be lacerated when the foal moves, resulting in abdominal contamination.

To perform an abdominocentesis with a teat cannula, place a subcutaneous bleb of 2% lidocaine or carbocaine, followed by a stab incision with a number 15 blade through the skin at the most dependent part of the abdomen. The teat cannula can then easily be advanced through the body wall. Analysis of abdominal fluid should include assessment of color and clarity, white blood cell count, total protein, and cytologic assessment of fluid. Fluid that is serosanguinous uniformly throughout the collection suggests devitalized bowel, with transudation of leukocytes, erythrocytes, and protein. An increased intra-abdominal protein and leukocyte count suggests intra-abdominal sepsis, which could be due to an abscess, umbilical remnant infection or abscessation, generalized sepsis, or other causes. Foals with severe enteritis may have only slight changes in the composition of the peritoneal fluid. A ratio of peritoneal fluid to serum creatinine greater than 2:1 confirms uroperitoneum, which can arise from a ruptured bladder or torn urachus. Blood can be recovered in cases of intra-abdominal hemorrhage or when the teat cannula punctures the spleen. A splenic sample has a higher hematocrit than peripheral blood, whereas in cases of hemorrhage the hematocrit and total protein equal or are less than peripheral blood. In the case of bowel perforation or enterocentesis, cytologic evaluation of peritoneal fluid reveals feed material and a mixed population of bacteria, whereas intra-abdominal sepsis may result in the presence of bacteria and degenerative neutrophils.

If enterocentesis is performed during the abdominocentesis, the foal should be placed on broad-spectrum antibiotics, preferably including metronidazole (10–15 mg/kg p.o. or IV q.i.d.). Nonsteroidal anti-inflammatory drugs and heparin (40–50 IU/kg SC or IV) should be used also, to help minimize the risk of intra-abdominal adhesions.

CASE SYNTHESIS AND MANAGEMENT

If physical obstruction is confirmed or suspected, immediate surgical exploration is indicated. If ileus, rather than physical obstruction, is considered to be the cause, medical treatment is indicated. The foal's condition should be closely monitored during diagnosis and initial medical treatment. If improvement in the clinical condition is not noted within 1 to 2 hours after initiating treatment, surgical exploration should again be considered. If pain or abdominal distension persists or worsens during this period, surgical exploration is indicated. Persistent pain or progressive distension are probably the most common and reliable indications for surgery in the foal. The decision for surgery should not be delayed, because the neonatal foal's condition deteriorates rapidly, and persistent distension of the bowel can lead to further metabolic compromise and bowel adhesions.

Medical management of the foal with colic or abdominal distension should have the following goals: (1) correction of the primary problem, (2) correction of metabolic or electrolyte abnormalities, (3) decompression of the bowel, (4) relief of pain, and (5) resting the bowel if intestinal distension exists.

If the ileus is the result of a specific medical condition, it is necessary to address the primary problem directly. Perinatal asphyxia and sepsis are multisystemic disorders that require aggressive supportive care for survival (see pages 604 and 595). Meconium impaction is the most common cause of colic in the neonate, and it may lead to complete obstruction if it is not passed normally. Foals should be administered an enema, using either warm, soapy water or a commercial Fleet enema. Fleet enemas work well and are convenient, and the short insertion tube is safe. If a warm water enema is to be performed, a lubricated soft red rubber stallion catheter can be gently passed to the approximate level of the pelvic inlet and the solution gently administered by gravity flow. The operator should be careful not to tear the rectum, which is very delicate in the neonate. If the meconium is not passed, the enema can be repeated in 2 to 4 hours. In this author's experience, additional treatments are rarely successful if two enemas have not led to significant improvement. If after two enemas the impaction is still present, or there is continued pain and distension, surgical removal is indicated. Use of irritant cathartic compounds such as castor oil is not recommended. These compounds may also produce diarrhea if used injudiciously. Acetylcysteine enemas are of little value. Manual removal of meconium using forceps is not recommended because of the risk of rectal trauma or penetration.

Correction of electrolyte abnormalities, metabolic derangements, or dehydration is vital because any of these conditions can lead to ileus and colic. Specific electrolyte abnormalities should be corrected using the appropriate replacement solution. Hyponatremia can be corrected using 0.9% sodium chloride (NaCl) solution or hypertonic (5%) NaCl. Hypertonic saline should not be administered as a bolus because there is potential for neurologic sequelae. Hyperkalemia can be treated with the administration of fluids that lack potassium combined with intravenous 5% dextrose infusion. Simple dehydration can be readily corrected with standard commercial polyionic replacement solutions. These solutions can be administered at 1.5 times maintenance rates (1.5 × 100–120 ml/kg per day) until the hydration status is normalized. Hypoglycemia, which often accompanies disease of the neonate, is corrected with intravenous infusion of 5 or 10% dextrose at a rate of 2 to 4 mg/kg per minute of dextrose. It is important to give this as a constant infusion rather than a bolus. Bolus dosing may lead to a rebound hypoglycemia that is more severe than the original problem.

Decompression of the bowel decreases pain and ameliorates distension-induced ileus. A nasogastric tube can be passed routinely, and gastric decompression can be achieved. The nature or amount of reflux obtained has little bearing upon the decision for or against surgery, however, because it is often difficult to retrieve reflux fluid even when it is present. The tube should be left in place and capped to prevent aspiration of air. It is usually very difficult to achieve significant decompression of the small and large intestine via a nasogastric tube; however, gastric decompression followed by treatment with analgesics may alleviate pain sufficiently to diminish ileus. Trocharization of the neonate is almost never justified and should be performed in only the most extreme circumstances, because severe peritonitis is ensured. In some circumstances, if distension and pain continue or progress, surgical decompression may be necessary, often leading to dramatic improvement.

Although decompression of the bowel is important in controlling pain, pharmacologic pain control is also needed. Conservative doses of flunixin meglumine (0.25 mg/kg) are often adequate for the neonate. Other nonsteroidal anti-inflammatory drugs can be used, but flunixin is probably safest in the foal. Xylazine should be used with caution because of the potential for cardiovascular compromise. Intravenous cimetidine (6.6 mg/kg q.i.d.) or ranitidine (1.5 mg/kg IV t.i.d.) should be administered to the foal with colic owing to the risk of gastric ulceration.

Enteral feeding of foals with colic or abdominal distension is contraindicated. Nursing from the mare can be limited by use of a muzzle, or by separating the pair with a partition. The foal should be supported with intravenous fluids and dextrose during this period to prevent hypoglycemia and dehydration. If the duration of enteral rest is longer than 48 hours, intravenous nutritional supplementation is highly desirable. The duration of enteral rest necessarily varies with the specific inciting cause, but 24 hours is probably the minimal duration. In cases of enteritis, 3 to 5 days is sometimes necessary before the foal can tolerate enteral feeding. Findings at surgery dictate the duration of enteral rest in foals that had a surgical procedure performed. When oral feeding is to be reintroduced, 4 ounces of water, or a water and dextrose solution, should be given every 2 hours. If no intolerance is noted, the volume can be increased with subsequent feedings until a volume of 12 to 16 ounces of water or glucose solution is tolerated. Once this is achieved, diluted (50:50) water and milk or milk substitute can be given. If no intolerance is noted after several feedings, the strength of the solution can be increased to normal. Obviously, this process requires some patience, but reintroducing enteral feeding too rapidly often results in recrudescence.

Supplemental Readings

Cohen ND, Chaffin MK: Intestinal obstruction and other causes of abdominal pain in foals. Comp Cont Ed Pract Vet 16(6):780–790.
Cudd TA: Gastrointestinal system dysfunction. *In* Koterba AM, Drummond WH, Kosch PC (eds): Equine Clinical Neonatology. Philadelphia, Lea & Febiger, 1990, pp 367–442.
Reef VB: Ultrasonographic evaluation and diagnosis of foal diseases. *In* Robinson NE (ed): Current Therapy in Equine Medicine, ed 3. Philadelphia, WB Saunders, 1992, pp 417–422.

Diarrheal Diseases of Foals

NOAH D. COHEN
College Station, Texas

Diarrhea is one of the more prevalent problems of foals. Because diarrheal diseases of foals are often infectious, veterinarians must consider not only needs of affected foals but also those of in-contact foals and horses. Identifying the cause of diarrhea in foals can be challenging because the list of differential diagnoses is large and because the diagnostic methods have limitations.

ETIOLOGY

Infectious Causes

Viruses

Rotavirus is a common cause of diarrhea in foals up to 3 months of age. Clinically affected foals become depressed, have decreased appetite, and are usually febrile. These signs are generally followed within 24 hours by diarrhea that typically resolves in 3 to 5 days but may persist longer. Younger foals are usually more severely affected. Infected foals older than 1 month may not develop diarrhea. Foals that recover may have diminished rate of growth.

Rotaviral diarrhea can occur as an outbreak or as sporadic cases. The organism may be shed by adults that are carriers, asymptomatic carrier foals, infected foals that have not yet developed diarrhea, foals with diarrhea, and those that are recovering. Shedding has been detected from 2 days before the onset of signs until 6 days after resolution, but intermittent shedding has been described up to 8 months after resolution of diarrhea. The organism may persist in the environment for up to 9 months.

Diarrhea due to adenovirus may precede obvious signs of the usual respiratory infection. Immunodeficiency is often an important factor in adenoviral infection. Coronavirus and parvovirus have been associated with diarrhea, but their role in pathogenesis remains unknown. Coronavirus also has been isolated from apparently healthy foals.

Bacteria

Salmonellosis is considered the most common cause of bacterial diarrhea and enteritis in foals. Infected foals may become septicemic, and bacteria may disseminate to other organ systems, such as joints. *Salmonella* septicemia often occurs without diarrhea.

Clostridium perfringens types A, B, and C have been associated with enteritis, colic, and death in foals. The disease appears to be sporadic, rapidly progressive, and generally fatal. Affected foals are usually younger than 7 days old, and signs are often seen in 1-day-old foals. Diarrhea is often hemorrhagic. Viral gastroenteritis may predispose to enteric infection with *C. perfringens*. In the United States, *Clostridium difficile* was initially associated with fatal, hemorrhagic necrotizing enterocolitis in foals younger than 3 days old. Subsequently, this agent has been associated with mild to moderate diarrhea among foals of various ages.

Escherichia coli has rarely been associated with diarrhea in foals. Enterotoxigenic *E. coli*, common among calves and other animals, has only been reported once in a foal in the United States. Current evidence indicates that *E. coli* is an uncommon cause of foal diarrhea.

Foals infected with *Rhodococcus equi* infection are usually examined for respiratory disease, but occasionally infected foals 1 to 4 months of age may have acute or, more often, chronic diarrhea. These foals often have pyogranulomas in the lungs, colon, and mesenteric lymph nodes, or ulceration of lymphoid tissue in the colon.

Enterotoxigenic *Bacteroides fragilis, Leptospira interrogans,* and *Campylobacter jejuni* have been isolated from foals with diarrhea, but the clinical importance of these agents remains unclear. *Campylobacter jejuni* also has been isolated from foals without diarrhea.

Helminths and Protozoa

The prevalence of diarrhea associated with *S. westeri* infestation is unknown, but it appears rare in the absence of infection with an extremely large number (i.e., millions) of larvae. Mild enteritis may develop in infected foals, and it has been speculated that this predisposes foals to infection with other enteric pathogens. The most common route of infection is ingestion of milk that contains larvae, but larvae may directly penetrate the skin.

Foals may develop diarrhea, fever, and colic when infected at a young age with a heavy load of larvae of *Strongylus vulgaris*. Clinical signs may be observed as early as 7 days after ingestion of third-stage larvae, when they migrate through the arteries supplying the intestine. The importance of large strongyles as a cause of diarrhea in foals has been questioned. Cyathostomes can cause diarrhea in adult horses and weanlings, but their role in foal diarrhea is unknown. Infection with *Parascaris equorum* has been more commonly associated with intestinal obstruction than diarrhea.

Although reports of equine cryptosporidiosis are rare, cryptosporidial infection may be an underrecognized cause of diarrhea in foals. Clinical signs in foals appear to vary with age and immune status. Cryptosporidial diarrhea appears to be more prevalent during the first 4 weeks of life, but older foals, weanlings, and yearlings can be affected. Among foals with combined or other immunodeficiency, signs are often severe and rapidly progressive. Among immunocompetent foals, clinical signs associated with cryptosporidial infection can vary from inapparent to those of fatal enterocolitis. Inapparent infections may represent a source of infection for other foals. Cryptosporidial diarrhea is usually mild or self-limiting among immunocompetent foals. In foals 3 to 6 months of age, the diarrhea may be more chronic and can persist until foals are 9 to 12 months of age.

Although the oocysts of *Eimeria leukarti* have been reported in the feces of 40 to 80% of foals, the significance of this agent as a cause of intestinal disease is unknown. Experimental infection has not caused diarrhea, and natural infection does not appear to be associated with diarrhea.

Noninfectious Causes

Noninfectious diarrheas are frequently recognized and are associated with foal heat, nutritional causes, gastric ulceration, and antibiotic administration. Diarrhea associated with foal heat is considered the most common diarrhea in younger foals, and usually develops between 7 and 12 days of age. Proposed causes include changes in milk composition, maternal estrus, ingestion of foreign material, carbohydrate malabsorption, parasitic infections, and overeating. The pathogenesis remains unknown, but the problem does not appear to be exclusively attributable to changes in milk composition, maternal estrus, or *Strongyloides westeri*. Evidence exists that hypersecretion of fluid into the small intestine overwhelms the colon and thereby causes loss of fluid and electrolytes. Feces are soft to watery in consistency, but rarely profuse. The diarrhea is generally self-limiting. Occasionally, replacement of fluid and electrolytes is required.

Overfeeding can result from inappropriate feeding of an orphan foal or excessive sucking of the mare. In the case of the orphan, the required amount of milk replacer may be overestimated or it may be prepared too concentrated or too dilute. Even commonly used commercial milk replacers may not be tolerated by some foals. Although generally self-limiting once overfeeding is terminated, this cause of diarrhea can be problematic if unrecognized.

Some foals consume excessive roughage, sand, or dirt, which can cause irritation of the gastrointestinal tract resulting in enteritis. Coprophagy, which is common among foals, may also introduce fiber that osmotically changes fecal consistency, or bacteria that alter the flora of the intestinal tract, resulting in diarrhea.

Deficiency of lactase with subsequent lactose intolerance has been described in foals, and lactase deficiency should be suspected when diarrhea is associated with ingestion of milk, and resolution of diarrhea occurs when milk is withheld. Lactase deficiency may be a congenital problem or may be acquired as a result of enteric diseases that result in loss of lactase-producing intestinal cells.

Clinically important gastric ulceration frequently can develop concurrent with other medical problems. Several syndromes are thought to exist based on age of the foal and location of the lesions. Lesions in the stratified squamous mucosa adjacent to the margo plicatus are observed among foals older than 60 days. The lesions occur along the lesser curvature of the stomach and may extend to the cardia. Diarrhea is the most common clinical sign, but inappetence, weight loss, depression, and colic also may be observed. Gastroparesis and gastroesophageal reflux may result from these ulcerations or from lesions in the glandular mucosa of the stomach or in the duodenum.

Various antimicrobial agents such as trimethoprim-sulfonamide combinations and tetracyclines have been associated with induction of diarrhea in horses. Prophylactic administration of antimicrobials to newborn foals increases the risk of diarrhea. Diarrhea may result from alteration of the normal flora of the gastrointestinal tract, direct toxic effects to the intestine, and alterations of bile acids or pancreatic enzymes. Although orally administered antimicrobials have been chiefly implicated, agents administered parenterally that undergo enterohepatic circulation can also alter the normal gastrointestinal flora.

ASSESSMENT AND INITIAL MANAGEMENT

Assessment and initial management must be based upon consideration of both the affected animal and the group or herd from which it was derived. Diagnostic efforts to identify causal agents often are more important in reference to the herd than to the individual. The diagnostic plan should include an accurate medical history, thorough physical examination, blood samples for hematologic and biochemical analyses, and fecal samples or intestinal contents for detection of enteropathogens.

The history helps to formulate the list of differential diagnoses. A farm history of current or past diarrheal disease of foals could help to indicate the cause. The age of the foal, peripartum events, duration and progression of clinical signs, and dietary history also may provide important diagnostic clues. For example, onset of hemorrhagic diarrhea shortly after birth is more consistent with clostridial diarrhea than with cryptosporidiosis or rotaviral diarrhea.

The examination of foals with abdominal disease is described on page 627. Foals with diarrhea should undergo a similar evaluation because diarrhea can develop concurrent with other gastrointestinal disorders, including causes of colic that require surgical intervention. Many causes of diarrhea result in signs of abdominal pain before abnormal feces are observed.

Clinicopathologic data may provide useful diagnostic and prognostic information. A complete blood count should be evaluated for evidence of anemia, hypoproteinemia, inflammatory response, and sepsis (see page 595). Sepsis, indicated by leukopenia, left shift, toxic neutrophils, and lymphopenia, is commonly seen in neonatal foals as a primary entity or as a result of acute bacterial enteritis or severe viral enteritis. An older foal may have a focus of sepsis such as an intra-abdominal abscess caused by *R. equi* that is associated with diarrhea. Such a focus may be characterized hematologically by neutrophilia, hyperfibrinogenemia, and possibly a degenerative shift and toxic changes of neutrophils.

Foals with diarrhea are frequently dehydrated, have abnormal serum concentrations of electrolytes, and are in a state of metabolic acidosis. Healthy foals younger than 2 months of age often have lower concentrations of sodium and higher concentrations of phosphorus than adult horses. Hyponatremia and hypochloremia are common among foals with enteritis and diarrhea. Hyponatremia can result in weakness or neurologic signs that are the result of cerebral edema. Although the plasma concentration of potassium is variable, depending on the degree of metabolic acidosis and renal compromise, the majority of foals with diarrhea are hypokalemic. Foals also are often hypoglycemic because of decreased sucking.

Radiography and ultrasonography are important diagnostic aids for evaluating foals with abdominal distension. Presence of erectile distended loops of small intestine is most consistent with a diagnosis of obstructive disease and may help to differentiate obstruction from enteritis. Foals with diarrhea or enteritis often have an increased amount of gas accumulation throughout the gastrointestinal tract without discrete distension of loops of small intestine. Mechanical and nonmechanical obstructions often cannot be definitively distinguished using radiography. Intraperitoneal accumulation of fluid may be imaged radiographically and differentiated from intraintestinal accumulation of fluid. Contrast radiography using barium sulfate (5 ml/kg of barium sulfate as a solution of 30% weight/vol) administered by nasogastric tube can identify gastric filling defects or duodenal strictures, but sensitivity is poor.

Ultrasonographic evaluation of the abdomen is often beneficial in the diagnosis of various conditions causing colic, including strangulating obstruction, intussusception, ascarid impaction, and colonic impaction. Foci of infection may be detected, such as abscesses of the mesentery, that may be associated with diarrhea. The small intestine can be readily imaged and assessed for wall thickness, luminal content, and peristaltic activity. Strangulated sections of small intestine usually have a thickened, hypoechoic wall, a fluid-distended lumen, and decreased peristaltic activity; however, similar sonographic findings may be apparent in foals with severe enteritis.

Endoscopy can be of value in foals with diarrhea caused by gastric ulceration. Diagnosis by clinical signs alone is

not recommended because signs of gastric ulceration can accompany other gastrointestinal disorders. In the absence of equipment to perform gastroscopy, however, diagnosis may be based on exclusion of other disorders and response to antiulcer therapy.

Identifying the Cause of Diarrhea

Specific strategies can be used to identify the cause of diarrhea. Lactase deficiency can be diagnosed by comparing lactose and glucose absorption curves during a lactose tolerance test. In the identification of enteropathogens (Table 1), diagnostic sensitivity is improved by collecting and promptly submitting fresh fecal samples to the laboratory.

Viruses and Bacteria

Diagnosis of rotavirus infection is based on history, clinical signs, and detection of rotavirus in feces by electron microscopy or an enzyme-linked immunosorbent assay (ELISA). Diagnostic efforts should not end with detection of rotavirus because healthy foals may shed rotavirus in feces, and concurrent infection with another enteric pathogen is possible.

Diagnosis of infection with *Salmonella* is based on microbiologic culture of feces. Because false-negative results occur, at least five negative results should be obtained to be confident that a foal is not shedding salmonellae. As with rotavirus, concurrent infection with other enteropathogens is possible.

Diagnosis of diarrhea caused by *C. perfringens* is based on isolation of the organism and demonstration of toxins in

TABLE 1. DIAGNOSTIC TESTS USED ON FECAL SAMPLES

Procedure	Comments
Microbiologic Culture	
Salmonella	Repeated samples are necessary
Campylobacter	Agent is of questionable importance
Clostridium difficile	Quantitative culture helpful
Clostridium perfringens	Must also identify toxin concurrently
Rhodococcus equi	Limited value, quantitative culture may help
Escherichia coli	Questionable importance
Immunoassays	
C. difficile toxin IFA	Availability may be limited
Cryptosporidium IFA	Highly sensitive and specific
Rotavirus ELISA	Results correlate well with electron microscopy
Fecal Flotation	
Cryptosporidium	Sheather's sugar solution; prompt processing required
Strongyles	Limited value because of false positives and false negatives
Strongyloides westeri	Eggs one half size of strongyle-type eggs
Acid-Fast Staining	
Cryptosporidium	Fast, simple, inexpensive, experience beneficial
Electron Microscopy	
Rotavirus	Can examine feces for many viruses; availability

feces or intestinal contents. Unlike *C. perfringens*, demonstration of *C. difficile* in feces appears sufficient to attribute diarrhea to the organism because shedding by asymptomatic horses and foals is negligible. An immunofluorescence assay to detect toxin produced by *C. difficile* is available at some veterinary diagnostic laboratories.

Isolation of *R. equi* from feces is not diagnostic because it can be isolated from the gastrointestinal tract of healthy foals. Quantitative culture may be more reliable as an indication of enteric infection. Diagnosis is based on exclusion of other causes of enteritis; concurrent pulmonary infection with *R. equi* should raise suspicion.

Nematodes

Fecal examination for *Strongyloides westeri* and strongyles can be unrewarding. Patent infections with *Strongyloides westeri* can be diagnosed by fecal flotation with salt or sugar solutions. Typical embryonated eggs are approximately one half the size of a *Strongylus* egg. For strongyles, correlation between fecal egg count and diarrhea is poor. Foals affected during the prepatent period may not shed eggs in feces, and high egg counts may be observed in foals without signs of disease. Strongyle eggs observed in the feces of foals younger than 6 months of age are likely to be a result of coprophagy rather than patent intestinal infection.

Cryptosporidia

Various methods are available for detection of cryptosporidial oocysts. Currently, three techniques are used commonly at veterinary diagnostic laboratories: flotation, acid-fast staining, and detection by an immunofluorescence assay (IFA).

After flotation in Sheather's sugar solution, oocysts appear spherical, 4 to 6 μm in diameter and pink-tinged by bright-field microscopy under high-power (oil-immersion) microscopy. Samples should be processed and examined within 30 minutes because oocysts collapse and lose their spherical shape when left in Sheather's sugar solution.

Acid-fast staining of fecal specimens is widely used for detection of *Cryptosporidium*. The technique is simple and staining kits are commercially available.* The oocysts appear as red spheres against a dark background. Although limitations of the sensitivity and the specificity have been described for acid-fast staining, the author often uses this technique because it is simple, rapid, and cheap.

High sensitivity and specificity have been described for IFA tests. A commercial IF assay† simultaneously detects cryptosporidial and giardial organisms. Although several ELISA tests have been developed for detection of *Cryptosporidium* in samples from human beings, to date, no ELISA has been validated for use in foals.

The pattern of oocyst shedding by foals appears to be of variable duration (1–19 weeks) and can be intermittent. Shedding may be antecedent, concurrent, or subsequent to onset of diarrhea. Because of the variable duration and the intermittent pattern of shedding, at least three multiple samples should be submitted to detect *Cryptosporidium* in feces from foals. In people, identification of oocysts is more likely in watery stool. Concurrent infection with other enteropathogens may be observed. Cryptosporidial organisms can be detected in fresh postmortem tissue samples fixed routinely and stained appropriately.

TREATMENT

Because the clinical condition of foals, particularly neonates, can deteriorate rapidly, initial assessment often entails concurrent therapeutic intervention to stabilize the patient's condition before determining a cause of diarrhea. Many therapeutic interventions, including intravenous or enteral administration of fluid and electrolytes, provision of caloric needs, prevention or treatment of hypogammaglobulinemia, prevention of infection, and alleviation of pain, are similar regardless of the cause of diarrhea.

Fluid and Electrolyte Balance

Restoring circulatory volume and correcting electrolyte and metabolic imbalances by administration of oral or parenteral fluids or both are priorities for successful management of diarrhea in foals. If metabolic acidosis is not severe, intravenous administration of a balanced polyionic electrolyte solution such as acetated Ringer's solution or lactated Ringer's solution is adequate. Acidosis and hyponatremia may be treated with isotonic sodium bicarbonate (1.3%, 12.5 g of sodium bicarbonate per liter of distilled water). Potassium (not to exceed 0.5 mEq/kg per hr) may be added to intravenous fluids of a hypokalemic foal. Dextrose solutions (2.5–5.0%) may promote movement of potassium into cells, and provide a small proportion of a foal's caloric needs. For neonatal foals with hypoglycemia and unknown electrolyte and acid-base status, a solution of 2.5% dextrose and 0.45% saline can be used.

Foals with less severe derangements of fluid and electrolyte balance can be treated with commercially available oral electrolyte solutions. Many foals do not consume these solutions voluntarily, but they can be fed with a bottle or a nasogastric tube. At any time, no more than 1% of body weight (i.e., 1 pint per 100 lb) should be administered. Oral electrolyte solutions that contain glucose are preferred because of glucose-ionic cotransport. Glucose and electrolyte solutions provide 25% or less of the foal's caloric needs, and therefore should not be used as a means of total nutritional support for more than 24 hours.

Caloric intake may be decreased in diarrheic foals because of decreased ingestion or decreased absorption of nutrients. In addition, illness often increases caloric requirements of foals. Caloric needs of the foal with diarrhea must be maintained by nursing, enteral supplementation via bottle or nasogastric tube, or parenteral alimentation. Some conditions, like lactase deficiency, are exacerbated by enteral feeding. Foals with lactose intolerance can be fed yogurt, which contains lactase, or mare's milk pretreated with a commercially available lactase.* Milk should be withheld if clostridial enteritis is suspected.

Failure of passive transfer of immunoglobulins (FPT) may be a predisposing factor for diarrhea, a result of diarrhea because the foal fails to ingest colostrum because

---

*Kinyoun AF Stain, BBL Microbiology Systems, Cockeysville, MD
†Meridian Diagnostics, Cincinnati, OH

---

*LactAid, LactAid Inc., Pleasantville, NJ

of pain, or an unrelated, concurrent finding. Hypoproteinemia accompanies FPT and is common with enteric infections caused by invasive organisms such as *Salmonella*. If FPT or marked hypoproteinemia (<4 g/dl) is identified, administration of plasma (1–3 L IV) may be of benefit. Generally, 1 L of plasma containing 1.5 to 2.5 g/dl of protein can be expected to raise the total protein concentration of a 50-kg foal by about 200 mg/dl for approximately 10 to 12 hours. The rate of decline may be accelerated by increased catabolism or gastrointestinal loss. Alternatively, administration of *Salmonella typhimurium* antiserum° to hypoproteinemic endotoxemic foals not only helps to restore normal concentration of protein, but can also increase IgG concentration and may help to neutralize circulating endotoxin. The rise in total protein concentration following 500 ml of *S. typhimurium* antiserum intravenously is similar to that seen after 1 L of a commercially available plasma product.† The *S. typhimurium* antiserum should be diluted before use.

Antimicrobial Therapy

Broad-spectrum antimicrobial therapy may be indicated in foals with suspected primary or secondary bacterial enteritis, peritonitis, or bacteremia. Microbiologic culture of blood and feces should be obtained before initiation of antimicrobial treatment. Parenteral antimicrobials that do not undergo significant enterohepatic circulation are generally preferred to diminish the potential for induction or exacerbation of diarrhea. Trimethoprim-sulfonamide combinations undergo enterohepatic circulation but are frequently selected because of their broad antimicrobial spectrum and ease of administration by the oral route. Fecal consistency should be monitored among foals receiving trimethoprim-sulfonamide combinations.

If clostridial enteritis is suspected, administration of Na or K penicillin (≥22,000 IU/kg IV q.i.d.) is indicated. When enteritis caused by *B. fragilis* is suspected, metronidazole (10–20 mg/kg p.o. or IV b.i.d. or q.i.d.) should be added to the treatment regimen. Erythromycin with or without rifampin is considered the drug of choice for *R. equi* infection (see page 617). Erythromycin can cause diarrhea in horses, but this side effect is generally manageable. The prognosis for enteritis caused by *R. equi* is guarded and treatment must be prolonged. Paromomycin (100 mg/kg, p.o. s.i.d.), an aminoglycoside, has been used with varying success to treat calves and lambs with cryptosporidial diarrhea.

Anti-inflammatory and Anti-diarrheal Agents

Nonsteroidal anti-inflammatory drugs have been advocated for use in diarrheal diseases because of their anti-inflammatory, analgesic, and possibly antisecretory effects. These agents must be used cautiously in dehydrated, diarrheic foals because they can cause gastrointestinal ulceration and nephrotoxicity. Low doses of flunixin meglumine (0.25 mg/kg IV t.i.d.) are less toxic and combat endotoxemia.

Intestinal protectants often exert a beneficial effect in foals with diarrhea, especially when the foal is otherwise clinically normal. Preparations containing bismuth subsalicylate seem superior to those containing kaolin, pectin, or activated charcoal. Bismuth subsalicylate neutralizes bacterial toxins, has some antibacterial activity, and may exert an antisecretory effect by its antiprostaglandin action. It can be administered at a dosage of 2 to 6 ounces every 6 to 8 hours; the drug results in darkened feces. Constipation can result from overuse of these products, and may cause abdominal pain. If the intestinal protectant does not exert a beneficial effect within 48 hours, continued administration probably is not warranted. Because of bulk-forming and potential salutary effects on colonic mucosa, 1 to 2 ounces of psyllium mucilloid may be added to the bismuth protectant twice daily. The author has used the antidiarrheal agent loperamide° (2–4 mg p.o. b.i.d. to t.i.d.) in foals and found it to be effective. Caution must be used when administering antidiarrheal agents to foals with clinical or clinicopathologic evidence of toxemia. Delay or cessation of fecal passage in toxemic animals may lead to increased time for absorption of endotoxin and other toxins from the gut. Because of the autoinfective stage of the life cycle of *Cryptosporidium*, it may be inadvisable to administer any agent that will prolong transit time in foals with cryptosporidial diarrhea. Management of foals with cryptosporidiosis is supportive; currently, effective specific treatment is not available.

Other Supportive Therapy

Gastric ulcers may be a cause of diarrhea or may develop as a secondary problem. In the author's clinic, drugs used commonly to treat gastric ulcers in foals include ranitidine (4.4–8.8 mg/kg p.o. b.i.d. or t.i.d.; 2–4 mg/kg IV b.i.d. or t.i.d.) and sucralfate (1–4 g p.o. b.i.d. to q.i.d.).

In managing foals with colic and diarrhea, general nursing care and close monitoring of physical condition are necessary. Maintaining a clean environment is helpful to decrease the prevalence of concomitant infectious diseases.

CONTROL AND PREVENTION

Because many of the causes of diarrhea in foals are infectious, efforts at control and prevention are essential and must be well planned. The veterinarian must be prepared not only to treat individual foals that are ill, but to consider the entire farm population and farm management program to control and prevent diarrheal disease. The initial approach to control of diarrhea among foals must be to provide care for sick foals and implement diagnostic testing, as described earlier. Consideration must then be given to methods for isolation, hygiene, disinfection, and prevention.

Isolation

Diarrheic foals should be isolated from other foals and horses because they can amplify and transmit infection. Special effort should be made to isolate foals younger than 2 weeks of age because of their apparently increased susceptibility to infection. Isolation in a separate facility is

°*Endoserum, Immvac, Columbia, MO*
†*HiGamm-Equi, Lake Immunogenics, Ontario, NY*

°*Imodium A-D, McNeil-PPc, Fort Washington, PA*

preferred, but often isolation must occur within a stall or small paddock. When entering the isolated area, personnel should wear plastic boot covers or dedicated rubber boots that do not have deep treads and that can be scrubbed and disinfected; disposable latex gloves; disposable surgical masks; and protective clothing such as disposable gowns or coveralls. Separate instruments such as stomach tubes and buckets should be maintained for each isolation stall or area. Foot baths equipped with a brush to scrub boots should be available for use when entering and leaving the stall; these should contain phenolic compounds and be deep enough to immerse soles. The duration of isolation should be based upon the particular infectious agent involved, but must extend well beyond initial resolution of clinical signs.

Disinfection and Hygiene

For many infectious causes of diarrhea such as rotavirus or *Salmonella* species, carriers and environmental contamination are the principal sources of infection. Removing organic materials and using appropriate disinfectants to decrease contamination in the environment is essential. Removal of fecal material is probably most important. Phenolics are recommended over sodium hypochlorite (bleach) or quarternary ammonium compounds as disinfectants because the latter disinfectants are inactivated in the presence of organic material and they do not kill rotavirus. Cryptosporidial oocysts can remain viable in the environment for months. Formalin (10%), ammonia (5%), steam, and sodium hypochlorite (undiluted bleach) have some efficacy against the oocysts, but each requires at least several minutes of direct contact. Disinfecting foaling areas between use is important; foaling in pasture or in areas that can be more easily disinfected such as stalls with cement rather than dirt floors may decrease the risk of transmission of infectious agents. People handling sick foals should wash their hands thoroughly and for at least 30 seconds with a disinfecting soap between contact, and should take precautions to avoid wearing contaminated clothing from stall to stall. Immunosuppressed people should not provide care

to diarrheic foals, because many causal agents such as *Salmonella* species and cryptosporidia are zoonotic.

Prevention

Vaccines for prevention of rotavirus in other species probably do not afford protection to foals. A continuing problem with diarrhea caused by *C. perfringens* was alleviated after type C and D toxoid manufactured for ruminants was administered to pregnant mares. However, types A and B also have been reported to cause diarrhea among foals. No evidence exists that administering *C. perfringens* antitoxin manufactured for sheep is beneficial to foals.

Anthelmintic treatment of the dam shortly after foaling helps to decrease the incidence of *S. westeri* infections in foals. Anthelmintics that are reportedly effective include ivermectin, benzimidazoles, and febantel. These agents may also be administered to diarrheic foals shedding *S. westeri* eggs in feces.

The most important principle in control and prevention of diarrheal disease among foals is use of good management. Overcrowding should be avoided. Efforts to control or prevent exposure to extremes in environmental temperature by provision of adequate shade must be made. The importance of sanitation and cleanliness must be emphasized to caretakers. Some evidence indicates that foaling outdoors decreases the prevalence of diarrhea in regions where the weather is clement during foaling season. Separating foals by age group may decrease the prevalence of disease.

Supplemental Readings

Cohen ND, Chaffin MK: Causes of diarrhea and enteritis in foals. Comp Cont Ed Pract Vet 17:568–574, 1995.

Semrad SD, Shaftoe S: Gastrointestinal diseases of the neonatal foal. *In* Robinson NE (ed): Current Therapy in Equine Medicine, ed 3. Philadelphia, WB Saunders, 1992, pp 445–455.

Smith BP: Another view of approaching a herd problem of foal diarrhea. Proc 38th Annu Meet Am Assoc Equine Pract, 1992, pp 183–189.

Traub-Dargatz JL, Gay CC, Evermann JF, Ward ACS, Zeglen ME, Gallina AM, Salman MD: Epidemiologic survey of diarrhea in foals. J Am Vet Med Assoc 192:1553–1556, 1988.

Xiao L, Herd RP: Review of equine *Cryptosporidium* infection. Equine Vet J 26:9–13, 1994.

Ocular Problems in the Foal

D E N N I S E. B R O O K S
C A R O L K. C L A R K
Gainesville, Florida

Normal embryogenesis of the foal eye results in a fully developed globe and adnexa at birth. Reduced tear secretion, a round pupil, reduced corneal sensitivity, lack of menace reflex during the first 2 weeks after birth, and lagophthalmos may be found in neonates. The hyaloid artery remnants may contain blood for several hours after birth and generally disappear by 3 to 4 months of age. Lens Y sutures are often prominent and should not be mistaken for a cataract. Young horses have a round optic disc with smooth margins that is located in the nontapetal retina. Tapetal color is related to coat color, with most horses having a blue-green tapetum, although combinations of red, orange, and blue can be found. Color-dilute foals may have no tapetum and have exposure of the choroidal vasculature, giving a red fundic reflection.

CONGENITAL AND INHERITED DISORDERS (see also page 355)

Microphthalmia

Microphthalmia, a congenitally small globe, is common in foals and may be unilateral or bilateral. A small palpebral fissure and prominence of the nictitans is noted in affected foals. Microphthalmia is generally associated with other ocular abnormalities, such as cataracts, and the eyes are usually blind. The bony orbit may also become malformed as the foal ages. Entropion may also occur because of lack of support from the small globe and may be associated with mild to severe ulcerative keratitis. Corneal ulceration due to entropion and microphthalmia may necessitate entropion repair or enucleation of nonvisual globes.

Dermoids

Dermoids of the eyelids, cornea, and conjunctiva are reported in foals. Corneal and conjunctival dermoids may look like aberrant pigmentation, with lack of hair follicle development. Depending on the location, superficial to deep keratectomy or blepharoplasty is indicated to remove the dermoid before the hairs grow enough to cause ocular irritation.

Nasolacrimal System Atresia

Eyelid or nasal lacrimal puncta atresia must be differentiated from acquired obstruction of the nasolacrimal drainage system. The clinical signs are unilateral or bilateral, chronic mucoid, and eventually mucopurulent discharge (often copious) in a young horse. Some horses may not present until clinical signs become severe at 1 to 2 years of age. If the nasal opening is present, it may be possible to flush the nasolacrimal system from the nares and cause a dilation over the site of the eyelid punctum. Once the site is identified, a cutdown through the conjunctiva establishes patency. A stent may be needed in the nasolacrimal system for several weeks to prevent healing over of the puncta. The presumptive diagnosis of nasal puncta atresia may be made by noting the lack of a distal opening of the nasolacrimal duct at the mucocutaneous junction within the nares. Nasolacrimal duct agenesis may also accompany the nasal puncta atresia. Contrast dacryocystorhinography should confirm the diagnosis. Referral for creation of a new distal opening and duct is indicated in many cases.

Persistent Pupillary Membranes

Remnants of the anterior tunica vasculosa lentis, or persistent pupillary membranes, can leave strands of iridal tissue arising from the midiris collarette and passing to the lens, iris, or to the cornea. Nonprogressive corneal opacity results if the persistent pupillary membrane is adherent to the cornea, or a cataract can result from lens involvement. Persistent pupillary membranes generally regress over the first 6 to 12 months of life.

Congenital Lens Luxation

Because of defective zonule formation, the lens may luxate to an anterior or posterior position. Posterior luxation does not necessitate surgical intervention; however, anterior movement usually requires lens removal to prevent secondary glaucoma.

Cataracts

Congenital cataracts are the most frequent congenital ocular defect in foals. Most are bilateral. Heritable, traumatic, nutritional, and postinflammatory etiologies have been proposed. A dominant mode of inheritance has been reported in Belgian and Thoroughbred horses. Morgan horses have nonprogressive, nuclear, bilateral, symmetrical cataracts that do not seriously interfere with vision.

Healthy foals with cataracts, no uveitis, visual impairment, and the personality to tolerate the administration of topical therapy are candidates for cataract surgery. Brisk pupillary light reflexes and a blink response to bright light usually indicate a functional retina. If the retina is not visible preoperatively, ocular ultrasound examination is indicated to ensure that a retinal detachment is not present. Because of hereditary congenital stationary night blindness in the Appaloosa, preoperative electroretinography should be considered in this breed.

The most common technique for removal of congenital cataracts in foals is phacoemulsification. Recent advances in the surgical technique have increased the success to nearly 75% in foals. Surgical success is highest in foals operated on when they are younger than 6 months of age, although the risk of ocular complications is always present. The visual outcome of cataract surgery can be difficult to evaluate in young horses. Most reports of successful cataract surgery in adult horses indicate vision is functionally normal. The horse with no lens is quite far-sighted postoperatively, but this optical effect does not appear to be important to their vision.

ENTROPION

Inversion of the lower or upper eyelids may occur in foals as a primary condition or may be a consequence of microphthalmia, dehydration, malnutrition, prematurity/dysmaturity, eyelid trauma, or cicatricial formation after trauma. The treatment in foals with secondary entropion is to evert the eyelid with temporary nonabsorbable sutures in a vertical mattress pattern or with surgical staples until the causative mechanism is resolved. Alternatively, a subcutaneous bleb of procaine penicillin can be injected to cause eversion of the eyelid. Blepharoplastic procedures may be necessary in primary entropion cases or in those due to trauma.

CONJUNCTIVITIS AND SUBCONJUNCTIVAL HEMORRHAGE

Primary conjunctivitis caused by environmental irritants such as hay, sand, dirt, and ammonia is more common than secondary conjunctivitis in neonates with recumbent foals especially at risk. Secondary conjunctivitis associated with pneumonia is usually found in older foals (1–6 months of age). Etiologic agents include adenovirus, equine herpesvirus-1 (EHV-1), equine viral arteritis (EVA), influenza virus, *Streptococcus equi* subspecies *equi* infection (strangles), and *Rhodococcus* and *Actinobacillus* species infections. Clinical signs are ephiphora, chemosis, and hyperemia. If a bacterial component is present, the ocular discharge becomes mucopurulent. Conjunctival cytology and culture methods can be useful in the diagnosis of infectious conjunctivitis. Intranuclear inclusion bodies may be found in viral etiologies. Therapy begins with copious flushing of the conjunctival sacs to remove an underlying irritant. Patency of the nasolacrimal duct should be established because obstructions can exacerbate the condition. Broad-spectrum antibiotic ophthalmic ointments or eye lubricants are used as indicated. Corticosteroid ophthalmic preparations are also useful if no corneal ulcer is present.

Subconjunctival or episcleral hemorrhages can result from birth trauma and generally do not require treatment. These hemorrhages can be separated from conjunctival hyperemia by topical administration of phenylephrine, which greatly relieves superficial conjunctival congestion. Traumatic hemorrhages are generally quite large and must be differentiated from petechial or ecchymotic hemorrhages suggestive of a coagulation disorder.

CORNEAL ULCERS

Corneal ulcers are defects in the corneal epithelium that may also involve the stroma, Descemet's membrane, and the endothelium. Every ulcer in a horse is potentially serious and sight-threatening because the equine cornea appears prone to develop infection and heals slowly with extensive scarring. Corneal ulceration in foals requires early clinical diagnosis, laboratory confirmation, and appropriate medical and surgical therapy. Both bacterial and fungal keratitis may present with a mild, early clinical course, but the conditions require prompt therapy if serious ocular complications are to be avoided.

The environment of the horse is such that the conjunctiva and cornea are constantly exposed to bacteria and fungi. The conjunctival microbial flora of the horse varies, depending on the season and geographic area. Many bacterial and fungal organisms normally found in the horse conjunctival flora are potential ocular pathogens. *Fusarium* species and *Aspergillus* species are both common causes of equine fungal keratitis in the United States. Gram-negative bacteria known to be associated with equine corneal ulcers include *Pseudomonas* species and assorted coliform bacteria. *Staphylococcus* and *Streptococcus* species are gram-positive bacteria found in infectious equine keratitis. Mixed bacterial and fungal infections can be present.

Clinical History and Appearance

Neonatal foals, especially those under intensive care, should be monitored daily for corneal ulcers. In general, clinical signs in foals are not as obvious as in the adult horse. Foals with corneal ulcerations generally have only mildly painful lesions and exhibit slight photophobia, blepharospasm, and increased tearing. The eyelashes are pointed downward, rather than perpendicular to the corneal surface. The corneal surface of superficial ulcers appears dull, cloudy, and roughened. The corneal stroma may appear to be melting in rapidly progressive infected ulcers. In acute cases, signs of anterior uveitis and corneal vascularization may not be clinically evident, but they become prominent as the corneal disease progresses.

Infection should be considered in almost any ocular inflammation and in every corneal ulcer in the foal. Fungal involvement should be suspected if there is a history of corneal injury with vegetative material or if a corneal ulcer has received prolonged antibiotic and/or corticosteroid therapy with poor or no improvement. Infection is suggested by rough margins, stromal opacity, or exudate.

Diagnostic Techniques

The diagnosis of a corneal ulcer is made by the application and retention of fluorescein dye on the cornea. It is strongly recommended that corneal swab cultures and corneal scrapings for cytology testing be obtained to initiate appropriate medical therapy. Samples for aerobic and fungal culture are best taken before fluorescein stain and topical anesthetic have been administered. Vigorous corneal scrapings, at the edge and base of the lesion, to detect bacteria and hyphae can be obtained with topical anesthesia and the blunt handle end of a sterile scalpel blade. Superficial swabbing cannot be expected to yield the organisms in a high percentage of cases. Multiple scrapings and the use of several stains and culture growth media increase the chance of isolating a fungus. Immediate cytologic evaluation and Gram's stain can direct therapy by identifying etiologic agents present. A superficial corneal ulcer that does not show rapid improvement in 24 to 48 hours suggests that an underlying cause of the ulcer has not been detected (e.g., infection, lagophthalmos).

Medical Therapy

Medical therapy almost always comprises the major thrust in ulcer control in foals, albeit tempered by judicious use of adjunctive surgical procedures. First, bacterial and fungal growth must be halted and the microbes rendered nonviable. Secondary anterior uveitis must then be controlled to prevent blinding sequelae. Corneal perforation caused by direct microbial extension or indirect stromal proteolysis (melting) must be averted. Treatment frequently needs to be sustained for weeks or, occasionally, months.

Therapeutic Methods

Horses with ocular disease are often in pain, and topical treatment is usually difficult. Techniques that are particularly useful in treating severe eye disease in the horse include subconjunctival injections of medication and subpalpebral lavage systems. Soft contact lenses* are available to fit the foal cornea. They are used to enhance epithelial adhesion in recurrent corneal erosions. Tinted lenses are used to cover corneal scarring. The lenses may have a use as slow-release drug delivery systems.

---

*Contact lenses to fit foals and horses may be ordered from The Cutting Edge, NNQ Inc., 870 N. Circle Dr., Diamond Springs, CA 95619 USA; Tel 916/621-2275

Topical Antimicrobial Therapy

Superficial ulcers can be treated with broad-spectrum antibiotics such as polymyxin, bacitracin, and neomycin or with chloramphenicol. Deeper ulcers involving the corneal stroma often require more specific antibiotics in fortified concentrations (Table 1). Gentamicin, tobramycin, and amikacin are usually effective against bacterial ulcer pathogens. Miconazole° (10 mg/ml) and natamycin† have been used successfully topically to treat fungal ulcers in horses. Some clinicians also suggest topical treatment with 1 to 6% tincture of iodine in the routine management of fungal ulcers.

Uveitis Control

In foals, as in adult horses, iridocyclitis (anterior uveitis) is the usual and expected sequel to ulcerative keratitis. Anterior uveitis in horses with corneal ulcers should be treated by both topical and systemic routes. (For specific therapy see Iridocyclitis.) Foals on topical atropine should be watched closely for symptoms of colic.

Collagenolysis or Melting Prevention

Severe corneal inflammation resulting from bacterial (especially, *Pseudomonas* species) or fungal infection may result in sudden, rapid corneal liquefaction and perforation. Activation and/or production of proteolytic enzymes by corneal epithelial cells, leukocytes, and microbial organisms are responsible for stromal collagenolysis (melting). The appearance of a gray, mucoid corneal exudate should herald immediate action. Five to 10% acetylcysteine‡ or sodium ethylenediaminetetraacetic acid (EDTA)§ should be instilled hourly, in addition to the other indicated drugs, until stromal liquefaction ceases. Autogenous serum from the foal or its mare may also be effective in arresting corneal melting when used topically (q1h).

Adjunctive Surgical Therapy

Keratectomy may prove useful (1) in the early stages of ulcerative keratomycosis, while the infection is confined to the corneal epithelium and anterior half of the corneal stroma, and (2) in the later stages of stromal mycosis if the epithelium has healed over the ulcer to cause a stromal abscess.

To augment lost corneal thickness and strength, deep corneal ulcers threatening perforation may require conjunctival flap placement. If the apposed conjunctiva adheres to the denuded stroma, drug penetration may be impeded, but ocular perforation will be averted.

Panophthalmitis following perforation through a stromal ulcer has a poor prognosis for the foal eye. Medical therapy must include injection of antimicrobial drugs into the anterior chamber and/or the vitreous, as well as systemic antibiotics. Whether or not treatment is applied, phthisis bulbi is likely to result after a chronically painful course. Enucleation may be necessary in some cases.

°*Monistat IV, Janssen Pharmaceuticals, Piscataway, NJ*
†*Natacyn, Alcon, Ft. Worth, TX*
‡*Mucomyst, Mead Johnson, Evansville, IN*
§*Sodium Versenate, 3M Co, St Paul, MN*

Inappropriate Therapy

Corticosteroid therapy by all routes is contraindicated in the management of equine corneal infections. Even topical corticosteroid instillation, to reduce the size of a postmycotic corneal scar or blood vessels, may be disastrous if fungi remain indolent in the corneal stroma. Topical corticosteroids may encourage growth of bacterial and fungal opportunists by interfering with nonspecific inflammatory reactions and cellular immunity. Fungi have been shown, clinically and experimentally, to behave more aggressively and penetrate deeper into the cornea in the presence of corticosteroids.

NONINFECTIOUS PERSISTENT CORNEAL EROSIONS

Etiology

Very slow-healing superficial corneal ulcers are commonly encountered in recumbent neonatal or premature foals. The ulcers prove to be frustrating for both the owner and veterinarian because they are resistant to normal ulcer treatments, often without apparent reason. The lesions are only mildly painful if painful at all, the corneas fail to vascularize, and the ulcer exhibits no or slow evidence of healing. All of these ulcers retain fluorescein dye and are noninfectious initially, with some having a noticeable lip of epithelium at the edge of the ulcer. One theory as to the cause of this condition in equine neonates is the diminished level of corneal sensitivity that is found in these foals. Corneal insensitivity is associated with delayed corneal healing and ulceration in other species. Inadequate or poor nutrition in the sick neonate can also lead to delayed healing.

The most important diagnostic consideration for ulcers in equine neonates is to determine whether the corneal ulcer is not healing owing to a primary corneal defect or is a consequence of some other ocular condition. Bacterial and fungal infections cause slow healing but generally deteriorate quickly. Noninfected ulcers can remain relatively static for quite some time. Fungal ulcers in neonates may also progress slowly. The authors recommend corneal cytology and culture studies for all slow-healing ulcers in foals.

Distichia or ectopic cilia are infrequently found in foals but are capable of causing persistent ulcers. A thorough ocular examination may be necessary to detect them. If abnormal eyelashes are indeed causing delayed corneal healing, they are adjacent to the corneal defect. The conjunctival sacs should be checked for foreign objects such as dirt or sand, which can also cause chronic ulcers. If the foals are blinking poorly or entropion is present, corneal ulcers will heal slowly.

Treatment

Therapy is directed at treating the underlying cause, if it can be identified, removing abnormal epithelium, and promoting adhesion of the epithelium to the stroma. If all indications are that the ulcer is primary, the cornea should be topically anesthetized and the epithelium gently debrided with a dry, soft cotton swab. All of the loose, abnormal epithelium should be removed to let the healing pro-

TABLE 1. COMMON THERAPEUTIC AGENTS USED IN OCULAR DISEASES OF FOALS

Category/Drug	Indications/Comments	Dosage
Topical		
Antibiotics		
Bacitracin, neomycin, polymxyin	Superficial corneal ulcer, broad-spectrum	Ointment q4–8h
Chloramphenicol	Superficial corneal ulcer, broad-spectrum	1% ointment q4–8h
	Good corneal penetration	0.5% solution q2–4h
Amikacin (250 mg/ml)	Deep, stromal corneal ulcer	Dilute with saline or artificial tears
	Broad-spectrum	6.7 mg/ml q2–4h
	Good for *Pseudomonas*	Fortified = 50 mg/ml
Gentamicin	Deep, stromal corneal ulcer	0.3% solution
	Gram-negatives including *Proteus, Pseudomonas, Staphylococcus*	Fortified = 8–11 mg/ml
Tobramycin	Deep, stromal corneal ulcer	0.3% solution
	Drug of choice for *Pseudomonas*	0.3% ointment
		Fortified = 8 mg/ml
Antifungals		
Miconazole 1% (10 mg/ml)	Broad-spectrum	Use 1% IV solution topically q2–6h
	Good corneal penetration	Intracameral injection: 0.1 ml of 1 mg/ml solution
Natamycin 5% suspension	Broad-spectrum, poor corneal penetration	Topically q1–2h for 3 days, then reduce frequency
Silver sulfadiazine 1%	Inexpensive, also antibacterial	Topically t.i.d.
Antivirals		
Trifluridine 1%	Good corneal penetration	q2–6h
Idoxuridine	Epithelial disease only	0.1% solution q2–6h
		0.5% ointment q4h
Mydriatics/Cycloplegics		
Atropine 1%	Mydriasis and cycloplegia	Solution: can use 1% to 3% prn
		Ointment: prn to achieve dilation
Tropicamide 1%	Short-acting, diagnostic use	
Phenylephrine 10%	Not cycloplegic, can use with atropine	Use alone or combine 2.5% phenylephrine and 1% atropine
	Conjunctival hyperemia	
NSAIDs		
Suprofen 1%	Anterior uveitis, can use with corneal ulcer	b.i.d. to t.i.d.
Flurbiprofen 0.03%	Anterior uveitis, can use with corneal ulcer	b.i.d. to t.i.d.
Corticosteroids		
Prednisolone acetate 1% suspension	Anterior uveitis, without corneal ulcer	b.i.d. to q.i.d.
	Most potent available	
Dexamethasone 0.1% ointment	Anterior uveitis, without corneal ulcer	b.i.d. to q.i.d.
Anticollagenases		
Acetylcysteine 20%	Can be irritating, refrigerate	Dilute to 5–10% with saline q1h until liquefication stops (48–72 h)
Serum or plasma	Also promotes epithelial adherence in indolent ulcers	Use q2–4h, refrigerate, replace after 3 days
Miscellaneous		
Tissue plasminogen activator (TPA) Activase 20 mg/ml	Fibrinolytic, not for recent hemorrhage	Dilute with balanced salt soln. to 500 μg/ml Intracameral injection 50 μg (0.1 ml) topically, b.i.d. to q.i.d.
NaCl 5% ointment	Reduces corneal edema	Dilute with saline to 50 IU/ml,
Regular insulin (100 IU)	Stimulates corneal healing	Refrigerate, replace after 3 days Topically, q4h
Hyaluronic acid 0.2%	Provides matrix for corneal adhesion	Topically, q2h
Adequan 100 mg/ml		Topical use: dilute with artificial tears 5 mg/ml t.i.d.
Systemic		
NSAIDs		
Flunixin meglumine	Intraocular, extraocular inflammation	0.5 mg/kg p.o. IV, or IM q12–24h
	Can cause GI ulceration	
Phenylbutazone	Intraocular, extraocular inflammation	2 mg/kg p.o. IV q12–24h
	Can cause GI ulceration	
Corticosteroids		
Prednisone	Anterior uveitis, nonseptic	0.5 mg/kg s.i.d. p.o.
Dexamethasone	Initial therapy of nonseptic anterior uveitis, not for maintainance	0.02 mg/kg s.i.d. p.o., IV, or IM
Glaucoma Drugs		
Demacarium bromide 0.25%	Increases outflow by causing miosis	Topically b.i.d.
Timolol maleate 0.5%	β-Adrenergic blocker, decreases aqueous production	Topically b.i.d.
Acetazolamide 250 mg tablets	Carbonic anhydrase inhibitor	1 to 3 mg/kg s.i.d. p.o.

cess begin again. Debridement may need to be repeated every 3 to 4 days.

Antibiotic solutions are indicated to prevent infection. Ointments or solutions containing gentamicin should be avoided because they are known to retard corneal healing. Five percent sodium chloride ophthalmic ointments or solutions* are beneficial in removing the superficial corneal edema associated with persistent ulcers. The serum or plasma of the affected foal or its mare can be used topically to help the epithelium adhere and prevent stromal melting from collagenase enzymes in the tears. Insulin has been used topically as a corneal epithelial growth promotant, and topical hyaluronic acid can provide a matrix for epithelial migration, adhesion, and proliferation (see Table 1).

Contact lenses serve as bandages and are helpful in healing superficial ulcers. Contact lenses in sizes for horses are available. Temporary tarsorrhaphies can also accomplish the same function.

Superficial punctate or grid keratotomy may also be necessary in refractory ulcers in foals. In this procedure, a series of shallow punctures into the anterior stroma of the ulcer bed and 1 to 2 mm of the adjacent epithelium are made with a sterile 25-gauge needle. Alternatively, the needle may be dragged in lines across the ulcer bed to form a grid pattern to speed healing. Topical anesthesia and sedation are necessary, and care should be exercised during the procedure so that the cornea is not penetrated.

IRIDOCYCLITIS

Systemic disease can cause iridocyclitis because of two mechanisms: (1) the anterior uvea can act like a lymphoid organ to create an immune-mediated inflammation with a subsequent sterile uveitis and hypopyon; and (2) direct invasion of an organism, although less common, can occur to create an infectious uveitis. Both mechanisms can result in blindness, and attempts to diagnose the cause early and treat aggressively are imperative. Organisms associated with equine uveitis are *Salmonella*, *Rhodococcus*, *Escherichia coli*, *Streptococcus equi* subspecies *equi*, *Actinobacillus equuli*, adenovirus, and EVA.

Clinical Signs and Diagnosis

Lacrimation, blepharospasm, photophobia, and lethargy can be seen in eyes with iridocyclitis or anterior uveitis. These signs are often less apparent in foals than adults. Corneal edema, conjunctival hyperemia, and ciliary injection often alert the owner or veterinarian to the problem. Aqueous flare, hyphema, fibrin, and hypopyon can be observed with a bright external focused light or with a slit beam of light. Miosis is usually a prominent sign in cases of anterior uveitis and can result in a misshapen pupil, posterior synechiae, fibrin and pigment deposition on the anterior lens capsule, and cataract formation.

It is imperative to immediately employ a fluorescein dye test to differentiate a painful eye with anterior uveitis caused by ulcerative keratitis from an eye with anterior uveitis and no corneal ulcer or abscess. Although corticosteroids are the treatment of choice for anterior uveitis,

they can lead to the rapid demise of an eye with a corneal ulcer.

Severe anterior segment inflammation often prevents an adequate fundic examination of the acutely affected eye. However, as the pupil dilates and the ocular media clear with successful treatment, the clinician should evaluate the fundus for evidence of active or inactive chorioretinitis. If the anterior uveitis cannot be controlled, blindness will result subsequent to cataract formation or severe chorioretinitis.

Treatment

The major goals of treatment of foals with anterior uveitis are to preserve vision and decrease pain. Anti-inflammatory medications, specifically corticosteroids and nonsteroidal anti-inflammatory drugs (NSAIDs), are used to control the intense intraocular inflammation that can lead to blindness. A complete ophthalmic examination reveals the signs of uveitis and determines if a corneal ulcer is present. The presence of an ulcer precludes the use of topical corticosteroids but not topical NSAIDs. Medication can be administered topically, subconjunctivally, orally, and parenterally. The requirement for frequent application of topical medications is most easily accomplished with the aid of a subpalpebral lavage system. The medications are administered every 1 to 6 hours, depending on the severity of the disease, and tapered as the problem resolves.

Prednisolone acetate* (1%) is the most potent and penetrable corticosteroid available for topical administration. Dexamethasone† (0.1%) preparations are also a very good choice of topical corticosteroid. Preparations of hydrocortisone, as commonly found in "triple" antibiotic/steroid combinations, penetrate the cornea poorly and are usually not potent enough at the onset of the disease to suppress the intraocular inflammation.

When frequent application of topical steroids is not practical, the use of subconjunctival steroids provides adequate levels of steroids. Again, the clinician must be absolutely sure that the cornea is not ulcerated or at risk of ulceration before injecting the steroids. As in intravenous injections, once a subconjunctival injection is made, there is no stopping the effects until the drug has totally dissipated from the subconjunctival space. Most commonly, methylprednisolone acetate‡ (20 mg q1–3 weeks), or triamcinolone acetonide§ (20 mg q1–3 weeks) is used.

The NSAIDs inhibit the enzyme cyclooxygenase, which is responsible for prostaglandin synthesis. Only a few topical antiprostaglandins are currently available, and their efficacy in the treatment of neonatal iridocyclitis has not yet been thoroughly investigated. The authors have had positive experience with topical 1% suprofen‖ (q.i.d.) in horses. It can help to reduce intraocular inflammation when an ulcer is present.

Flunixin meglumine¶ (0.5mg/kg b.i.d.) used orally or parenterally is especially effective in reducing uveal exudation and relieving ocular discomfort. Alternatively, phenyl-

---

*Muro 128, Bausch and Lomb, Tampa, FL

*Pred Forte, Allergan Pharmaceuticals, Irvine, CA
†Dexair, Pharmafair, Hauppauge, NY
‡Depo-Medrol, The Upjohn Company, Kalamazoo, MI
§Kenalog, Westwood-Squibb, Buffalo, NY
‖Profenol, Alcon, Ft. Worth, TX
¶Banamine, Schering-Plough, Kenilworth, NJ

butazone (2 mg/kg s.i.d. or b.i.d.) orally or intravenously can be used. Oral corticosteroids (prednisone 0.5 mg/kg s.i.d.) can also be of benefit in controlling the inflammatory response as long as concurrent systemic disease or the presence of corneal ulcers do not preclude their use. These drugs can cause gastroduodenal ulceration and should be used judiciously. Ranitidine (1 mg/kg IV, b.i.d.) and sucralfate (20 mg/kg p.o. t.i.d. to q.i.d.) may be indicated for gastric ulcer prophylaxis when using systemic NSAIDs in foals.

Mydriatics/cycloplegics are effective in stabilizing the blood-aqueous barrier. Relaxation of the ciliary muscles also eliminates ciliary spasm, a major factor in ocular discomfort. Pupillary dilation protects the visual axis from occlusion and may minimize synechiae development. The two most common drugs used to allow pupillary dilation and reduction of pain are atropine and tropicamide,° both parasympatholytic drugs. Although atropine can last several days in the normal eye, its effect is only a few hours in duration in the inflamed foal eye. Gut motility should be monitored when using ocular atropine. If gut motility decreases during treatment with atropine, the clinician can either discontinue the drug or change to the shorter acting tropicamide before development of a hypomotile colic. Phenylephrine can also be used as a direct mydriatic, but it is not cycloplegic. The authors often use a combination of phenylephrine 2.5% and atropine 1% to obtain maximal dilation in the inflamed foal eye. Injectable atropine can be administered subconjunctivally for a repository effect (5 mg/injection).

Broad-spectrum antibiotics with good corneal penetration such as chloramphenicol are advised as prophylaxis and treatment of infections in the anterior chamber.

Tissue plasminogen activator (TPA) has been used to speed up fibrinolysis and clear hypopyon. With the foal under heavy sedation or general anesthesia, an intracameral injection of 50 mg can be made at the limbus with a 27-gauge needle. TPA should be avoided if hemorrhage has been present for less than 48 hours.

Depending on the cause, the overall prognosis for anterior uveitis is usually guarded. The owner should be educated immediately about the potentially severe nature of this disease and the possibility of loss of sight. Treatment of the disease can be both time-consuming and expensive.

GLAUCOMA

Glaucoma is an elevation in intraocular pressure that is detrimental to normal ocular function. The abnormal rise in intraocular pressure is caused by an obstruction to the outflow of aqueous humor. The condition eventually results in optic nerve damage and blindness. Glaucoma can be a sequela to anterior uveitis. Congenital glaucoma is reported in foals and associated with developmental anomalies of the iridocorneal angle (i.e., goniodysgenesis). No particular breed predisposition is reported for glaucoma in equine neonates.

The clinical signs of early glaucoma include generalized corneal edema, deep linear corneal band opacities, lens

luxations, and a fixed dilated pupil. The linear corneal band opacities are a consistent feature of equine glaucoma, and histologically they represent thin areas of Descemet's membrane. Buphthalmia occurs if the intraocular pressure remains elevated.

Therapy for equine neonatal glaucoma is aimed at preserving vision and minimizing discomfort. It is a difficult disease to manage in the foal, with little to no chance of preserving vision unless the condition is detected and treated early. Glaucoma may be treated medically or surgically, but surgical therapy may be best for goniodysgenic foals. Therapy is directed at decreasing the intraocular pressure by reducing production or, more importantly, increasing outflow of aqueous humor.

Outflow should be increased with topically applied miotics, and aqueous production should be reduced with a β-adrenergic blocker, 0.5% timolol maleate.° Systemically administered carbonic anhydrase inhibitors, such as acetazolamide† (1–3 mg/kg p.o.) and NSAIDs, such as phenylbutazone or flunixin meglumine, may be beneficial in foals with glaucoma (see Table 1).

Surgical therapy for glaucoma in the horse is directed toward reducing production of aqueous humor by damaging the ciliary body with nitrous oxide (cyclocryotherapy) or laser energy (cyclophotocoagulation). Surgery has the best potential for preserving vision in glaucomatous eyes if the glaucoma is detected early. High-flow gonioimplants should be considered to increase aqueous outflow in foals. Modified canine gonioimplants or dual-tube gonioimplants have been used in glaucomatous horses. Chronically painful and blind buphthalmic globes should be enucleated or have an intrascleral prosthesis implanted.

DISEASES OF THE RETINA AND OPTIC NERVE

Variations of the normal equine fundus are numerous and primarily related to coat color. The retinal vasculature is classified as "paurangiotic" because the retinal vessels are small and extend only a short distance from the optic disc. The tapetal fundus is usually yellow to blue-green with small dots (stars of Winslow) distributed in a uniform pattern throughout the tapetal fundus. These represent end-on views of choroidal capillaries. The optic disc is oval to round, pink-orange in color, and located slightly temporal in the inferior quadrant of the nontapetal fundus.

Neonatal maladjustment syndrome (NMS or hypoxic-ischemic encephalopathy) is commonly associated with ocular abnormalities. Lesions described include small, round retinal hemorrhages; hemorrhages on the optic disk; pupil asymmetry; corneal edema; and ulcerative keratitis. Hemorrhages found associated with NMS disappear in several days if the foal survives.

Congenital alterations in the equine neonatal ocular fundus are uncommon. Blind foals often display a searching nystagmus. Colobomas of the optic nerve head are excavations of the optic disc containing retinal vessels, glial tissue, and a paucity of neural tissue. They are generally incidental

°Mydral, Optopics, Fairton, NY

°Timoptic, Merck Sharp & Dohme, West Point, PA
†Acetazolamide, Schein Pharmaceuticals, Port Washington, NY

findings but can be bilateral and, if large, can be associated with blindness. Retinal dysplasia is a developmental or postinflammatory problem of the retina that develops in utero in which the sensory retina is "folded" to form rosettes of neural tissue. Retinal dysplasia in foals is generally bilateral, not heritable, but often associated with other congenital ocular problems. Retinal detachments may be unilateral or bilateral and can be associated with other ocular abnormalities. The detached retina can be observed through the dilated pupil as a floating veil of opaque tissue in the vitreous. If bilateral, the foal will have been blind since birth and may have nystagmus. Chorioretinitis may be noticed in foals born to mares suffering from respiratory and other systemic diseases in late gestation. Peripapillary small circular lesions with a hyperpigmented center and a depigmented peripheral ring characterize these chorioretinal scars. Optic nerve hypoplasia and optic nerve atrophy are diagnosed by direct ophthalmoscopy in foals and may be the result of developmental or inflammatory processes. Foals with optic nerve hypoplasia display smaller-than-normal discs and may retain some vision depending on the degree of hypoplasia. Foals with optic nerve atrophy have pale discs with no retinal vessels and are blind with fixed and dilated pupils.

Supplemental Readings

Latimer CA, Wyman M: Neonatal ophthalmology. Vet Clin North Am Equine Pract 1:235–259, 1985.
Lavach JD: Large Animal Ophthalmology. St. Louis, C.V. Mosby, 1990.
Roberts SM (ed): Congenital ocular anomalies. Equine ophthalmology. Vet Clin North Am Equine Pract 8(3):459–478, 1992.

Sedation and Anesthesia in Foals

JEFF C.H. KO

LUISITO S. PABLO
Gainesville, Florida

This article presents sedation and general anesthesia of the foal in a problem-oriented style to suit the practitioner's need as a quick reference. The authors arbitrarily consider neonatal foals to be younger than 2 weeks old, young foals to be 2 weeks to 3 months of age, and juvenile foals to be older than 3 months.

INDICATIONS FOR SEDATION AND ANESTHESIA

Noninvasive and minimally invasive procedures such as radiography, catheter placement, cast application, abdominocentesis, arthrocentesis, respiratory support via mechanical ventilation, and minor laceration repair require sedation with or without concurrent use of local anesthesia. Major procedures such as surgical repair of a ruptured bladder, musculoskeletal and ocular trauma, fracture repair, umbilical remnant resection or hernia, and gastrointestinal impaction or intussusception require general anesthesia to provide immobilization, muscle relaxation, and analgesia during the surgery.

CARDIOPULMONARY AND ANESTHETIC CONCERNS REQUIRING SPECIAL ATTENTION

The resting heart rate (80–120 bpm) of the neonatal foal is higher than that of the adult horse and is necessary to maintain the high cardiac output that supports the greater metabolic rate of the neonatal foal. The large surface area-to-body mass ratio in the neonatal foal results in significant heat loss and partially contributes to the high metabolic requirement. The neonatal foal heart has a relatively fixed stroke volume and poorly developed sympathetic innervation, resulting in limited cardiac reserve for situations such as hypovolemia, hemorrhage, and dehydration, in which there is a decrease in preload, or for situations such as systemic vasoconstriction, which increases afterload. Because cardiac output in the neonatal foal is heart-rate-dependent, decreases in heart rate reduce cardiac output. Sedatives may have a more profound impact upon cardiac output and tissue perfusion in the neonatal foal than in the adult. Xylazine and detomidine increase afterload while causing bradycardia, whereas acepromazine decreases preload via vasodilation. In contrast, inotropic agents increase heart rate and cardiac output. Infusion of dopamine and dobutamine (3–5 μg/kg per minute IV) increases heart rate and blood pressure.

A low lung functional residual capacity coupled with high blood flow to the brain makes induction with inhalational anesthetics relatively fast in foals. Hypoxia, hypercapnia, and respiratory acidosis develop more easily in neonates compared with juvenile foals as a result of the immature respiratory control mechanisms, heightened sensitivity to sedatives and anesthetics, hypoventilation, airway closure, and atelectasis. Reversion to the fetal circulatory pattern with anatomic shunting, and reopening of the ductus arteriosus and foramen ovale may occur if hypoxia-induced elevation of pulmonary vascular resistance persists in the neo-

TABLE 1.   DRUGS USED FOR CHEMICAL RESTRAINT AND SEDATION IN STANDING FOALS

Age	Drugs	Dosages	Route
Younger than 3 months Older than 2 weeks	Diazepam or midazolam	0.05–0.2 mg/kg	IV, IM
	Acepromazine	0.02–0.04 mg/kg	IV, IM, SQ
	Promazine	0.25–0.5 mg/kg	IV, IM, SQ
	Xylazine	0.2–1.1 mg/kg	IV, IM, SQ
	Detomidine	10–40 μg/kg	IV, IM, SQ

nate. The small functional residual capacity and presence of shunts contribute to the rapid onset of hypoxia during periods of apnea and atelectasis under anesthesia. Oxygen insufflation and assisted or controlled ventilation may be required during profound sedation and general anesthesia. Close monitoring of cardiopulmonary parameters during sedation and general anesthesia is required for safe anesthesia.

ADVANTAGES OF FOAL SEDATION IN THE PRESENCE OF THE DAM

Although the foal is the patient that deserves all the attention, one must not forget about the mare. The dam's presence during sedative injection or anesthesia induction usually provides a calming effect on the foal, reducing the stress of handling. Once the foal is sedated or general anesthesia is induced, the mare can be taken away. Care must be taken with protective mares, which may strike, bite, or kick when the foal is being handled and taken. It is a good idea to sedate the mare as soon as the mare and the foal are brought up to the induction area. The mare can be sedated with xylazine (0.2–0.4 mg/kg IV) or detomidine (5–10 μg/kg IV). To prevent agitation during separation, additional sedation with acepromazine (0.04–0.06 mg/kg IM) may be administered to the mare to provide a longer sedative duration (2–3 hours) when she returns to her stall.

SEDATIVE AGENTS FOR USE IN THE FOAL

Neonatal foals can usually be physically restrained for diagnostic procedures. However, physical restraint becomes progressively more difficult with increasing age. Several sedative agents are available for chemical restraint in the young and juvenile foal (Table 1). Phenothiazines such as acepromazine (0.02–0.04 mg/kg IV, IM, SQ) or promazine (0.25–0.5 mg/kg IV, IM, SQ) may be used. These drugs reduce anxiety and fear and cause minimal respiratory depression. The disadvantages of these drugs are slow onset, long duration of action, poor analgesia and muscle relaxation, and production of hypotension at moderate sedative doses.

Benzodiazepines such as diazepam (0.05–0.2 mg/kg, IV, IM) and midazolam (0.05–0.2 mg/kg IV, IM) are useful sedatives. Midazolam is water-soluble and has a shorter duration of action than diazepam. Diazepam is a propylene glycol-based drug. The absorption of diazepam following intramuscular or subcutaneous injection is slow and unreliable, especially with subcutaneous administration. Cardiac depression or arrest following rapid intravenous injection of diazepam can occur because of arrhythmogenic activity of propylene glycol. The advantages of benzodiazepines include good sedation, relative safety, minimal cardiopulmonary depression, and good muscle relaxation. Furthermore, a specific reversal antagonist, fulmazenil,* is available. The latter agent is administered at a dose of 0.75 to 0.1 mg/kg IV. The disadvantages of benzodiazepines are poor analgesia and required recordkeeping for controlled substances.

Thiazine agents such as xylazine and detomidine are very potent sedatives. These agents produce rapid onset of profound sedation, muscle relaxation, and analgesia. Severe ataxia or lateral recumbency commonly follows administration in the foal. Antagonists such as yohimbine (0.125 mg/kg IV), tolazoline (0.5 mg/kg IV) and atipamezole (0.05–0.1 mg/kg IV) may be used for reversing anesthetic effects of xylazine and detomidine. Disadvantages of thiazine agents include profound cardiovascular depression with bradycardia, reduced cardiac output, and hypotension. One study of xylazine (1.1 mg/kg, IV) in healthy 10- and 28-day-old foals concluded that the heart rate decreased between 20 and 30% without observed second-degree heart block. Blood pressure initially increased and then decreased, with mean arterial blood pressure maintained above 60 mm Hg. Respiratory rhythm was profoundly disrupted, and partial upper airway obstruction occurred for up to 20 minutes. $PaCO_2$, PaO_2 and pH were not affected during the 2-hour period following xylazine administration. The authors caution the use of xylazine in sick foals with hypovolemia or respiratory disease, because foals may not be able to compensate for xylazine-induced hypotension, bradycardia, and upper airway obstruction. The use of detomidine (10–40 μg/kg IV) is considered to be less desirable than xylazine because of a higher incidence of cardiac arrhythmia. In the authors' hospital, midazolam and diazepam are preferred sedatives in younger foals. In foals younger than 2 months old, low doses of xylazine (0.2–0.5 mg/kg IV) or acepromazine (0.015–0.03 mg/kg IV) can be used for sedation.

INTRAVENOUS ANESTHETIC COMBINATIONS FOR SHORT-DURATION CHEMICAL RESTRAINT

Several combinations of drugs are capable of inducing chemical restraint accompanied by lateral recumbency in

---

*Mazicon, Hoffman-LaRoche, Nutley, NJ

the foal (Table 2). In the neonate, short-term chemical restraint can be induced with intravenous diazepam or midazolam (0.1–0.2 mg/kg) followed within 5 minutes by ketamine (0.5–1 mg/kg). This combination produces lateral recumbency that lasts approximately 15 to 30 minutes. The authors consider this combination relatively safe and effective. In a seriously compromised foal, midazolam or diazepam alone may produce satisfactory chemical restraint. The benzodiazepine/ketamine combination produces minimal analgesia, and thus a local anesthetic may be needed for invasive procedures.

A xylazine/propofol combination may be a viable option when immobilization or short-term anesthesia is required and rapid recovery is desired. Neonatal foals can be premedicated with xylazine (0.5 mg/kg IV) induced with a propofol bolus (2.4 mg/kg IV), and maintained with propofol infusion (0.3 mg/kg per minute) for up to 2 hours. Muscle relaxation is good and recovery is smooth and rapid, approximately 30 minutes. Blood pressure is maintained as well as when foals are anesthetized with inhalants, and only a mild respiratory acidosis occurs. However, the cost of propofol may preclude its routine use in foals.

In young foals, intravenous injection of xylazine (0.3–1.0 mg/kg) followed 2 minutes later by butorphanol (0.1–0.2 mg/kg) induces profound sedation and lateral recumbency for approximately 15 to 40 minutes. Bradycardia and second-degree heart block may occur with this combination. It may be necessary to treat the bradycardia with atropine (20–40 μg/kg, IV). In the juvenile foal, xylazine (0.5–1.0 mg/kg), followed in 1 to 2 minutes by ketamine (1–2 mg/kg) induces a lateral recumbency of 15 to 30 minutes. Other methods of inducing short-duration chemical restraint in the juvenile foal include slow intravenous infusion of 1 L 5% guaifenesin mixed with either 2 to 3 g thiopental or thiamylal or 1 g ketamine and administered to effect. When compared with other bolus injection techniques, the infusion of this combination provides more precise control of the depth of anesthesia. If the foal appears to be too deeply anesthetized once it attains lateral recumbency, the infusion can be stopped. If the foal is in a light plane of anesthesia, the infusion rate may be increased until the desired anesthetic plane is reached. The guaifenesin-ketamine infusion method is suitable in the minimally compromised neonatal and young foal. However, one should remember that the cardiopulmonary depression and recovery duration with this infusion combination is dose-dependent. The infusion duration should be limited to 30 minutes.

PREPARING THE FOAL FOR INHALATION ANESTHESIA

The cardiopulmonary function of the foal, including heart rate, heart rhythm, ventilation pattern, oxygenation, and body temperature, should be closely evaluated. If a foal tolerates handling, preclipping the surgical site decreases the total general anesthesia time. The foal's mouth and oral cavity should be washed to remove foreign material. Nasogastric feeding tubes should be removed to ensure adequate breathing. Preplacement of a venous catheter helps in administration of fluids or emergency drugs. The hydration of the foal should be assessed, and blood glucose, serum electrolyte concentration, and acid-base status determined before beginning general anesthesia. A water-circulating blanket and heat lamps are needed if the foal has a low body temperature. An ophthalmic ointment should be applied to the eyes once the foal is anesthetized.

A small-animal anesthesia machine equipped with 22-mm breathing hose and 5-L rebreathing bag and a double CO_2 absorption canister can be used for foals weighing up to 100 kg. Juvenile foals may require a large-animal anesthesia machine with 52-mm internal diameter breathing hose, 15- or 30-L rebreathing bag, and a 6500- to 8000-ml CO_2 absorber canister. The surgery table may need to be modified to accommodate the long legs of the foal and provide proper support when the foal is placed in either lateral or dorsal recumbency.

INDUCTION OF ANESTHESIA BY USE OF INHALED AGENTS

Anesthesia in the neonatal foal may be induced with either isoflurane or halothane in oxygen. The mare is sedated and the foal is physically restrained in the induction area. A nasotracheal tube, measuring 7 to 9 mm internal diameter and approximately 55 cm in length, lubricated with 2% lidocaine gel, is passed into the ventral meatus of the nose. The foal's head and neck are extended to facilitate nasotracheal intubation. The foal may swallow as the naso-

TABLE 2. INTRAVENOUS DRUGS USED FOR SHORT-TERM CHEMICAL RESTRAINT AND INDUCTION OF LATERAL RECUMBENCY IN FOALS

Age	Premedication	Induction	Duration
3–10 days°	Xylazine 0.5 mg/kg	Propofol 2.4 mg/kg bolus followed by 0.3 mg/kg infusion	60–122 minutes
Younger than 3 months	Diazepam or midazolam 0.1–0.2 mg/kg	Ketamine 0.5–1 mg/kg	15–30 minutes
2 weeks to 3 months	Xylazine 0.3–1.0 mg/kg followed by butorphanol 0.1–0.2 mg/kg in 5 minutes	None	15–40 minutes
Older than 3 months	Xylazine 0.5–1 mg/kg or detomidine 10–20 μg/kg	Ketamine 1–2 mg/kg	15–30 minutes
	Xylazine 0.5–1 mg/kg or detomidine 10–20 μg/kg	1 L of 5% guaifenesin containing 2–3 g of thiopental or thiamylal or 1–2 g of ketamine	The infusion should be limited to 30 minutes

°See text for details.

tracheal tube approaches the laryngeal opening. The nasotracheal tube may then be moved back and forth inside the pharynx to accomplish the intubation. Upon successful entrance into the trachea, air flows freely out of the nasotracheal tube and condensation forms within the tube during each expiration. The tube cuff is inflated, and the nasotracheal tube is securely taped on the foal's jaw and connected to the anesthetic breathing circuit. The foal is preoxygenated with oxygen, 3 to 5 L/min for 2 to 3 minutes, and anesthesia is induced with either isoflurane or halothane. The vaporizer is turned on while oxygen flow is maintained at the same rate. If the foal is relatively healthy, "crash induction" may be used with the vaporizer setting turned immediately to 4 to 5%. Once the foal attains lateral recumbency, the vaporizer setting is reduced to 2%. For compromised foals, a "gradual induction" is preferred. The vaporizer is initially set at the lowest setting, gradually turned up in 0.5 to 1% increments up to 4 to 5% with every 3 to 4 breaths, and the foal is immediately positioned for surgery upon the loss of consciousness. If the surgical procedure lasts longer than 30 minutes, the nasotracheal tube should be replaced with a larger internal diameter oral tracheal tube to reduce the work of breathing. In addition to nasotracheal intubation, foals may be premedicated with the aforementioned sedatives and anesthesia induced with isoflurane or halothane via face mask. Alternatively, induction may be accomplished with intravenous anesthetics (guaifenesin-ketamine or xylazine-ketamine) followed by oral tracheal intubation and inhalant anesthetic maintenance.

MONITORING DURING THE INTRAOPERATIVE AND POSTOPERATIVE PERIODS

Cardiopulmonary function, depth of anesthesia, body temperature, and blood glucose level of the foal should be monitored during intraoperative and postoperative periods. Maintaining adequate tissue perfusion with oxygenated blood is essential for safe anesthesia. Heart rate and rhythm can be monitored by use of electrocardiography. Bradycardia and other arrhythmias should be treated accordingly (see page 606). Monitoring arterial blood pressure provides quantifiable information regarding cardiovascular function. The pulse pressure and capillary refill time may give crude indications of the blood pressure, but are not quantitative. Direct invasive arterial blood pressure measurement via facial, auricular, or dorsal metatarsal arterial cannula provides an accurate, beat-to-beat continuous blood pressure reading. Furthermore, it also provides an access for arterial blood gas sampling. This technique is, however, technically difficult, expensive, and invasive. Indirect noninvasive measurement can be accomplished using an occlusive pneumatic cuff over a peripheral artery coupled with an ultrasonic Doppler flow detector and a sphygmomanometer. This method measures systolic pressure only. A second noninvasive method uses an automated oscillometric device,° which measures systolic, diastolic, and mean pressure. Indirect measurement of blood pressure is not reli-

able during periods of hypotension and does not provide continuous monitoring. The mean arterial pressure needs to be maintained above 60 to 70 mm Hg for adequate tissue perfusion. Blood pressure may be improved by lightening the plane of general anesthesia, rapid intravenous fluid administration (10 ml/kg lactated Ringer's solution), and inotropic agent infusion such as dopamine and dobutamine (2–5 μg/kg per minute). The presence or absence of ocular reflexes and level of blood pressure can be used to monitor the depth of anesthesia. Loss of palpebral and corneal reflexes, accompanied with low blood pressure, is indicative of deep anesthesia. The presence of palpebral reflex and high blood pressure indicates a light anesthetic plane. Other information such as heart rate and respiratory rate assists the determination of the depth of anesthesia.

The oxygenation of the blood may be assessed by mucous membrane color or pulse oximeter or arterial blood gas analysis. Mucous membrane color provides qualitative information but is unreliable in the presence of anemia and peripheral vasoconstriction. Pulse oximetry° is a noninvasive method for monitoring arterial oxygen hemoglobin saturation (SpO_2). Pulse oximeter values of 70%, 80%, and 90% approximately correspond to PO_2 values of 40, 50, and 60 mm Hg. Arterial hemoglobin saturation should be maintained above 90% (normoxia) or PaO_2 above 60 mm Hg in the anesthetized foal. In case of hypoxia (SpO_2 <90%), tissue oxygenation can be improved by increasing inspired oxygen concentration (100% O_2 supplementation) and increasing oxygen delivery to the tissue by increasing blood pressure. In anemic foals, increasing hemoglobin concentration by means of a blood transfusion increases oxygen-carrying capacity of the foal and therefore improves tissue oxygenation.

Anesthetic agents generally depress respiratory function through direct actions on the central nervous system and peripheral chemoreceptors and by relaxation of respiratory muscles. Hypoventilation either as a result of low respiratory rate or low tidal volume (i.e., shallow chest excursion) may be observed clinically. However, these clinical observations provide only crude information. A foal with apparently normal chest excursion and respiratory rate may have high CO_2 concentrations. Ventilation is best monitored by measurement of $PaCO_2$. Normal $PaCO_2$ should be between 35 and 45 mm Hg. If ventilation is inadequate, the $PaCO_2$ will be high. Conversely, hyperventilation results in low $PaCO_2$, provided that CO_2 production is constant. $PaCO_2$ can be measured invasively using arterial blood gas samples or can be estimated noninvasively by use of capnography.† Capnography, involving a sensor connected between the endotracheal tube connector and the anesthetic breathing circuit Y piece, provides a constant breath-to-breath measurement of end-tidal CO_2 (alveolar tension of CO_2, $PACO_2$). In the absence of ventilation/perfusion mismatch, $PaCO_2$ should equal $PACO_2$. If CO_2 concentration is high, assisted or controlled ventilation is indicated to improve ventilation of the foal. This can be done by increasing either the foal's respiratory rate or tidal volume.

Body temperature should be continuously monitored. If the temperature is below 37°C (101°F), a water-filled heat-

---

°Dinamap, Criticon, Tampa, FL; or Vet/BP 6000, SDI, Waukesha, WI

°Vet/Ox 4402 and Vet/Ox Plus 4700, SDI, Waukesha, WI
†Vet/Cap 7000, SDI, Waukesha, WI

ing blanket and/or heat lamp should be provided. Hypoventilation and hypothermia prolong recovery from general anesthesia. Blood glucose level should be monitored before, during, and after surgery. In cases of hypoglycemia (i.e., glucose concentration is less than 70 mg/dl) 5% dextrose solution should be provided and blood glucose concentration rechecked in 30 minutes.

During the recovery period, oxygen can be administered through the endotracheal tube via anesthetic breathing circuit or E tank of oxygen equipped with flow meter and plastic tubing. Extubation is achieved when the foal exhibits vigorous swallowing and chewing motions. Foal recovery can be facilitated by bringing the mare to the recovery area as soon as the foal is extubated and assumes sternal recumbency.

Supplemental Readings

Dunlop CI: Anesthesia and sedation of foals. Vet Clin North Am Equine Pract 10(1):67–85, 1994.

Klein L: Anesthesia for neonatal foals. Vet Clin North Am Equine Pract 1(1):77–89, 1985.

Matthews NS, Chaffin MK, Erickson SW, Overhulse WA: Propofol anesthesia for non-surgical procedures of neonatal foals. Equine Pract 17(3):15–20, 1995.

Robertson SA: Sedation and general anesthesia of the foal. *In* Robinson NE (ed): Current Therapy in Equine Medicine, ed 3. Philadelphia, WB Saunders, 1992, pp 474–478.

Tranquilli WJ, Thurmon JC: Management of anesthesia in the foal. Vet Clin North Am Equine Pract 6(3):651–663, 1990.

Webb AI: Restraint and anesthesia of the foal. Robinson NE (ed): Current Therapy in Equine Medicine, ed 2. Philadelphia, WB Saunders, 1987, pp 203–205.

TOXICOLOGY

Edited by Francis D. Galey

Toxic Plants

MIKE MURPHY
St. Paul, Minnesota

JOHN REAGOR
College Station, Texas

This chapter on toxic plants differs from the ones in previous editions of this book because it is organized around clinical signs rather than the toxic plants themselves. The major presenting signs induced by toxic plants are oral ulcers and dysphagia, colic, peripheral edema, laminitis, photosensitization, hemoglobinuria or myoglobinuria, failure to thrive, hyperexcitability or seizures, ataxia or stringhalt, and sudden death. Details of treatment of individual plant toxicities can be found in *Current Therapy in Equine Medicine 2,* page 672, and *Current Therapy in Equine Medicine 3,* page 372.

ORAL ULCERS AND DYSPHAGIA

Oral ulcers (see also pages 156 and 386) have been observed in horses following ingestion of various plants such as foxtail and bristlegrasses (*Setaria* species), sandburs (*Cenchros pancufloris* species) and cacti, which induce physical trauma, or those such as buttercups (Ranunculaceae), which contain caustic agents. A diagnosis may be supported by identification of the plants in hay or on pasture with evidence of ingestion or identification of plant fragments in the stomach contents or gastrointestinal reflux from an affected animal. Buttercups are not toxic in hay.

Chewing of food but failure to swallow food boluses (i.e., dysphagia) may follow ingestion of white snakeroot (*Eupatorium rugosum*) or, in central California, yellow star thistle (*Centaurea solstitialis*) or avocado (*Persea americana*).

COLIC

Horses may develop colic following ingestion of some toxic plants or toxic seeds. Plants that cause oral ulcers may also traumatize the gastrointestinal tract and induce signs of colic. The most common weed seeds that contaminate horse feed and induce colic are mustard (*Brassica* species) and corn cockle (*Agrostemma githago*). Seeds can be identified in feed and toxicity prevented by feeding screened grains and avoiding the inclusion of grain screenings in horse feed. Colic may be an initial sign in horses that ingest nightshades (*Solanum* species) in hay or on pasture, or after eating plants like oleander (*Nerium oleander*) that contain cardioactive glycosides or plants such as oak (*Quercus* species) that contain tannins.

Nightshades grow throughout the United States, and all species are considered potentially toxic. However, they are not usually consumed by horses even when they make up most of the available forage. Poisoning usually follows either ingestion of contaminated hay or pastures treated with a phenoxy herbicide, such as 2,4-D. Clinical signs are referable to the central nervous system (CNS) or gastrointestinal (GI) system or both. Gastrointestinal signs include anorexia, colic, and diarrhea. Signs referable to CNS damage include depression, dyspnea, muscle trembling, weakness, paralysis, or convulsions before death. Treatment is symptomatic. Some animals with severe CNS signs have recovered following treatment with dimethyl sulfoxide (DMSO, see page 303).

PERIPHERAL EDEMA AND LAMINITIS

Horses may develop limb edema ("stock up") and occasionally laminitis ("founder") after exposure to hoary alyssum (*Berteroa incana*), on pasture or in hay, or black walnut (*Juglans nigra*) shavings as bedding. Facial edema has been observed in horses after ingestion of avocado (*Persea americana*).

Hoary alyssum (*Berteroa incana*) has recently been associated with dependent limb edema, transient fever, and occasionally laminitis. The plant is commonly found throughout the north central and northeastern United States in waste areas, disturbed soils, and as a contaminant in alfalfa and other hay fields. In the spring or early summer, the plant may be ingested when other forage is not available or it is available at any time of year when baled in hay. The toxin in hoary alyssum and its toxicity are currently unknown, but animals are reported to develop signs within 2 to 3 days of ingesting contaminated hay. Animals with limb edema normally recover 2 to 4 days after removal of the source and routine supportive treatment.

A syndrome similar to hoary alyssum toxicity has been observed in the southwest United States in horses that ingested *Lesquerella*, also a mustard, but a cause-and-effect relationship has yet to be confirmed by experimental feeding trials.

Horses in contact with fresh wood shavings comprised in whole or in part of black walnut have developed laminitis, limb edema, and lethargy. The use of these shavings in bedding is not advised. Aeration of shavings or use of "old" shavings has been suggested as a means of preventing the problem, but is not recommended because these procedures have not been proved to decrease the risk of toxicity. The toxicity of shavings from butternut (*Juglans cinerea*) and English walnut (*Juglans regia*) have not been determined. To be safe, they should be considered potentially toxic. Removal of animals from the bedding and routine management of laminitis (see page 737) generally results in an uneventful recovery.

PHOTOSENSITIZATION

Primary and secondary photosensitization are distinguished clinically by elevated liver enzymes in cases of secondary photosensitization. Plants causing primary photosensitization include buckwheat (*Fagopyrum saggitatum*), St. John's wort (*Hypericum perforatum*), Bishop's weed (*Ammi majus*), Dutchman's breeches (*Thamnosma texana*), and parsley (*Cymopterus watsonii*). Secondary photosensitization requires liver damage, the ingestion of chlorophyll, and, of course, exposure to sunlight. Secondary photosensitization is rarely reported in horses; however, it has occurred in horses ingesting alsike clover (*Trifolium hybridum*), kleingrass (*Panicum* species), or lantana (*Lantana camara*).

Lantana may be found as an escaped ornamental shrub across the southern United States. The clusters of blooms vary from pink and white to orange and yellow to orange and red. The toxicity is highly variable, and plants with darker flowers appear to be more toxic. Lantana causes liver damage, secondary photosensitization, gastroenteritis, and some loss of renal function. Affected animals avoid the sun because of pain that results from the edema, necrosis, and epithelial sloughing of the unpigmented areas of skin. Mild to severe diarrhea may also be noted, and colic may

be observed early in the syndrome. Clinical chemistry profiles demonstrate markedly elevated plasma levels of aspartate aminotransferase (ALT), lactate dehydrogenase (LDH), alkaline phosphatase (AP), and gamma-glutamyl transferase (GGT). Poisoning is prevented by proper pasture management, because the plant is not normally consumed in significant amounts if other forage is available.

HEMOGLOBINURIA AND MYOGLOBINURIA

Discolored urine may be observed in horses following ingestion of dried maple leaves (*Acer* species) or trematone-containing plants such as white snakeroot (*Eupatorium rugosum*) or rayless goldenrod (*Isocoma wrightii*).

Red maple, *Acer rubrum*, is classically associated with toxicity, but all maples (*Acer* species) should be considered potentially toxic. Horses that ingest the wilted leaves may exhibit polypnea, tachycardia, icterus, cyanosis, scleral petechiation, and brownish discoloration of the urine, methemoglobinemia, or acute death. The toxin responsible for the methemoglobinemia and Heinz body formation is not yet identified. Poisoning generally occurs in September or October when the leaves wilt, fall, and cover other available forage in the pasture or paddock. Ingestion of 1.5 and 3 pounds of wilted leaves by a 500-kg horse is reportedly toxic and lethal, respectively. If maple toxicity is suspected and the animal is alive, anemia, hemoglobinemia, Heinz bodies, increased ALT, sorbitol dehydrogenase (SDH), plasma protein, and bilirubin test results may be used to support the diagnosis. Centrilobular hepatic degeneration, pigment-induced renal degeneration and erythrophagocytosis in the spleen, adrenal, and liver with comparable gross lesions are observed histologically. A blood transfusion or intravenous fluids may be indicated in severely affected animals.

White snakeroot (*Eupatorium rugosum*), also referred to as snakeroot or richweed, is found in the eastern half of the United States in wooded pastures, and along lakes and streams. Rayless goldenrod (*Isocoma wrightii*), also called jimmy weed or burrow weed, grows in the southwestern region in open pastures along dry stream beds. Horses ingesting either plant may exhibit signs of sluggishness, gait stiffness, ataxia, base-wide stance, partial throat paralysis, severe sweating, or sudden death without previous signs. Poisoning generally occurs on wooded pastures in October or November when forage is covered with snow and horses graze stalks available above the snow as their only forage source, or at any time of year, when the weed is baled in hay. The toxin, tremetone, remains active in hay. Occasionally, newly introduced animals ingest snakeroot or rayless goldenrod when other forage is available. On a dry matter basis, ingestion of 0.5 to 2% body weight by a horse is lethal. Clinical chemistry results from affected animals commonly demonstrate markedly elevated levels of the muscle enzymes creatine kinase (CK), ALT, and LDH. Skeletal and myocardial degeneration and necrosis are seen histologically.

FAILURE TO THRIVE

Horses may fail to thrive (i.e., be "poor-doers") because of hepatic or renal disease. Pyrrolizidine alkaloid-containing plants are known hepatotoxins and include hound's tongue (*Cynoglossum officinale*), groundsel (*Senecio* species), rattlebox (*Crotalaria species*), heliotrope (*Heliotropium* species), and tarweed (*Amsinckia* species). Numerous common names exist for the *Senecio* species including stinking willie, wooly groundsel, thread-leaf groundsel, Riddell's groundsel, bitterweed, and broom groundsel. *Amsinckia* is also commonly called fiddleneck. Cockleburs (*Zanthium strumarum*) in the two- to four-leaf stage, kleingrass (*Panicum* species), and lantana (*Lantana camara*) may induce hepatic necrosis. Horses have been reported to experience renal damage following ingestion of large numbers of acorns from certain oak trees (*Quercus* species).

Clinically, animals with minimal exposure to these plants and those early in the toxic syndrome present as poordoers. Those receiving greater exposure progress through rough hair coats, depression, and anorexia to icterus, ascites, emaciation, diarrhea or constipation, head pressing, occasionally mania, and eventually death. Clinical chemistry findings early in the syndrome reflect hepatic damage such as elevated SDH, ALT, and GGT. Later in the syndrome elevated bilirubin, lowered albumin, decreased albumin-to-globulin ratios, and perhaps compensatory polyclonal gammopathy are observed. Histologically, lesions vary from hepatic necrosis and hemorrhage to fibrosis. Megalocytosis is said to be diagnostic for pyrrolizidine alkaloid poisoning. A latent period of at least 3 weeks is required following ingestion for the megalocytes to appear. The hepatocyte nucleus increases in size without mitosis.

Kleingrass (*Panicum* species) is a recently introduced perennial grass found in improved pastures in the southwestern United States. It is used for both grazing and hay. Toxicity in horses in usually seen when the animals consume kleingrass hay as their only roughage source. The highest concentrations of hepatotoxic saponins are found during times of rapid growth. Thus, higher quality hay is likely to be more toxic than that containing overmature plants. Affected animals have elevated ALT, LDH, AP, and bilirubin. There is no specific treatment. Poisoning can be prevented by not feeding kleingrass hay or not forcing horses to ingest a large amount of the grass on pasture.

HYPEREXCITABILITY AND SEIZURES

Horses can have seizures for 3 to 4 weeks following ingestion of bracken fern (*Pteritium aquilinum*).

Animals poisoned by loco weeds from *Astragalus* and *Oxytropis* species also exhibit signs of CNS disease varying from hyperexcitability and trembling to ataxia, depression, emaciation, and paralysis. Many species of *Astragalus* and *Oxytropis* are found in the western half of the United States, and they vary greatly in toxicity. Some are not toxic. Horses must consume large amounts of the plant, 30% body weight, over a period of weeks to months to become affected. "Loco" horses are dangerous to ride despite apparent recovery following removal of the plant. Loco weeds are thought to be addictive; however, this has been questioned. These weeds are not highly palatable, but once animals begin consuming them they must be moved to a range that is free of the weed to discontinue ingestion. Animals introduced to ranges containing loco weeds are much more likely to be poisoned than horses raised on ranges containing the plant.

ATAXIA AND STRINGHALT

A small percentage of horses consuming large amounts of sorghum forage or hay develop sorghum cystitis. Most cases are the result of the animals grazing fields planted with a sorghum-Sudan hybrid. Affected animals exhibit varying degrees of hindlimb ataxia. Signs may progress from urine dribbling and scalding to complete paresis of the rear limbs. The syndrome is the result of nerve degeneration, and consequently, affected animals virtually never recover. Prevention of the syndrome centers on restricting access of horses to sorghum pasture or hay.

Singletary pea (*Lathyrus hirsutus*), also known as wild winter pea or caly pea, was at one time planted over a wide area of the southern, far western, and northwestern United States. It has become naturalized in many of these areas where there is adequate rainfall. The plant produces desirable nutritious forage, and poisoning is confined to consumption of the seeds. Horses ingesting hay containing singletary pea pods for weeks to months develop clinical signs. Affected horses are usually noted to stand with their hind legs and feet too far forward. Horses also have partial paralysis of the hind legs, and animals forced to move do so in a stringhalt fashion. Most animals recover when the source of singletary pea seeds is removed. To prevent the problem, hay meadows containing singletary pea should be harvested before the setting of seed pods.

Outbreaks of stringhalt have occurred periodically in the western United States and in Australia and New Zealand. The cause for these outbreaks has not been identified, although ingestion of toxic weeds such as flatweed (*Hypochoeris radicata*) has been implicated.

SUDDEN DEATH

Horses may be found dead following ingestion of plants containing cardioactive compounds or those containing cyanide. Other differential diagnoses should include ingestion of blue-green algae or organophosphates. Plants containing cardioactive compounds include milkweeds (*Ascelpias* species), rhododendrons (*Rhododendron* species) or azaleas (*Rhododendron* species), oleander (*Nerium oleander*), foxglove (*Digitalis* species), and yews (*Taxus* species), including both English and Japanese varieties. Cyanide-containing plants include fruit trees, members of the *Prunus* species such as apple, cherry, and plum, or sorghum-Sudan hays (*Sorghum* species).

Numerous milkweeds are found throughout the United States, and although a large number of common names are used to describe these plants, almost all of them contain the term "milkweed." Azaleas or laurels are not only ornamental plants in the southern United States but also houseplants throughout the country. Foxglove is native in Europe and an ornamental found commonly in flowerbeds throughout the world. Oleander is an ornamental plant found throughout the southern half of this country along roadways and in flowerbeds. The milkweeds are commonly seen in pastures throughout the country, but because they are highly unpalatable, they are ingested only under circumstances of severe overgrazing. The other three plants are ingested when animals are allowed to graze yards or roadways, when trimmings are thrown over a fence to the horses, or when weather causes the leaves to fall and blow into the pasture or paddock. When ingestion of the plants occurs, the animals are often just found dead. Rarely, signs of anorexia, colic, or diarrhea are observed. Each of the plants contains one or more cardiac glycosides, which cause an atrioventricular block that progresses to asystole. The cardiac glycosides are quite toxic; ingestion of 0.05 to 2% body weight of milkweed is fatal. Because of this degree of toxicity and the rapid onset of death, plant parts may be found in the stomach contents on necropsy. Treatment is rarely possible, leaving prevention as the method of controlling toxicosis from these plants.

Yew or ground hemlock is commonly planted as an ornamental shrub around foundations in the northern half of North America. Animals ingesting the plant are found dead. Rarely, trembling, incoordination, collapse, diarrhea, bradycardia, and acute cardiac failure may be observed up to 2 days after ingestion because the toxin depresses myocardial conduction and depolarization. *Taxus* species are readily consumed by livestock, especially in winter months, when other forage is not available, or any time of year when the prunings are thrown over the fence. Yew is quite toxic, 0.1 to 0.5% body weight being lethal, and a diagnosis of poisoning is commonly made by identifying plant parts in the stomach contents.

Supplemental Readings

Beier RC, Norman JO: The Toxic Factor in White Snakeroot: Identity, Analysis & Prevention. Proc. Public Health Significance of Natural Toxicants in Animal Feeds, 1990.

Cheeke PR, Shull LR (eds): Natural Toxicants in Feeds and Poisonous Plants. Westport, CT, AVI Publishing Company, 1985.

Kingsbury JM (ed): Poisonous Plants of the United States and Canada. Englewood Cliffs, NJ, Prentice-Hall, 1964.

Kownacki AA, Tobin T: Plant toxicities. In Robinson NE (ed): Current Therapy in Equine Medicine. Philadelphia, WB Saunders, 1983, pp 595–607.

Murphy M, Reagor J: Toxic plants. In Robinson NE (ed): Current Therapy in Equine Medicine, ed 3. Philadelphia, WB Saunders, 1992, pp 372–377.

Oehme F: Plant toxicities. In Robinson NE (ed): Current Therapy in Equine Medicine, ed 2. Philadelphia, WB Saunders, 1987, pp 672–682.

Diagnostic Toxicology

FRANCIS D. GALEY
Davis, California

Rapid, accurate diagnosis is critical to the treatment and prevention of diseases caused by toxic agents. Treatment of most toxicoses is supportive, and therefore prevention of further cases is usually the primary goal. The practitioner must determine if the horse's clinical signs are the result of a toxic agent, the nature of the agent and its source, and the best way to minimize exposure.

The chapters in this section discuss therapy with an emphasis on understanding, identification, and exclusion of potential etiologies. Dose-response concepts, the amount of a poison needed to cause toxicosis, are included where appropriate. This section discusses correct, timely diagnosis as a means of preventing illness in additional animals. The discussion is not intended to be all-inclusive. Rather, it builds on information presented in earlier editions of *Current Therapy in Equine Medicine*. The topics were selected because of their relevance to the horse, the availability of new information, or their absence from earlier editions of this book. This edition includes expanded information on forensic toxicology. Chapters on poisonous plants, mycotoxins, and feed-associated toxicants have been completely rewritten. In addition to updates throughout, topics that are covered in expanded detail include selenium poisoning and fescue toxicosis.

Poisoning may affect many animals and may stimulate considerable emotion and publicity. Unfortunately, there is no magic test for all possible toxicants. Therefore, this chapter suggests a systematic approach to suspected poisonings. Examples are used when possible.

The approach to a toxicology case involves fitting together several pieces of a puzzle. Often parts of the story are not present. Negative findings may be as important as pathognomonic findings. Frequently no single pathognomonic finding is present, and a composite of several criteria must be evaluated to arrive at a diagnosis. The approach begins with a comprehensive history, followed by clinical examination, diagnostic pathology testing, analytic chemistry tests, and bioassay.

HISTORY

The history must include a description of the clinical syndrome; herd dynamics, including animal movement, location, and new introductions; management practices; the source and type of feed; the source of water; and environmental conditions. Questioning should be systematic, with findings carefully noted and maps drawn of the premises. Recent movements of animals and shipments of feed should be noted and all sources of feed, water, and bedding identified. Dates of most recent shipments should be recorded as appropriate. If the feed is mixed elsewhere, the practitioner should determine whether the mill also mixes feeds for other animal species. Incorporation of cow feed into a horse ration can result in potentially toxic exposure of horses to feed additives such as monensin and other antibiotics. The relationship between the time of initial exposure to a material and the onset of clinical signs can also provide clues to the diagnosis. Recently, nine horses developed head pressing, aimless walking, and convulsions within 4 weeks of being fed corn screenings. Affected horses died within 1 week of onset of clinical signs. The major lesion was leukoencephalomalacia. The corn screenings were found to contain 38 ppm (parts per million) of fumonisin.

The regional environment, especially industry or dumps in the vicinity, must be investigated. Determination must be made whether animals are downstream or downwind from contaminated areas, such as piles of lead-laced mine tailings. The immediate environment should also be examined. Location of farm chemicals should be noted, because feeding accidents have occurred when insecticides are stored near vitamin-mineral mixes. Feed preparations are examined on site and at the mill, because mixing errors are a common source of toxicosis. Recently trimmed hedges or hedge clippings that are accessible to the horse should be looked for. Clippings from some hedges such as yews (*Taxus* species) or oleander (*Nerium oleander*) can cause sudden death if eaten by horses. Fields must be examined for overgrazing or evidence of consumption of toxic plants.

Feeds should be sampled systematically. Samples of concentrates to be screened for toxicants must be obtained from the mixing bin and feed troughs. Feed ingredients should also be sampled. If screening of as-fed materials yields a positive result, the various ingredients can be tested to determine the source of the toxicant.

Hay, forage, and pasture samples should be obtained and examined for potentially poisonous plants and evidence of consumption. Plants for identification should be sampled in their entirety, wrapped in a moist paper, and taken to an herbarium or cooperative greenhouse. Once the plant is identified, the practitioner can judge the potential hazard or consult with a veterinary toxicologist. If local identification is not possible, plants can be pressed, dried, and mailed to a diagnostic laboratory. Hay from several sites in a stack should be examined. Weeds should be sampled with a notation of the relative prevalence in the stack or lot. A diagnosis is rarely found when a flake of hay is selected at random and sent to a laboratory for plant identification. Alternatively, the plant can be pressed onto a high-quality office copier. The resulting copy can then be faxed to the diagnostic laboratory for quick identification.

All samples of feed and forage should be representative of their original lot. Each bin should have several areas cored, or sampled and pooled. Several parts of several bales from each stack of hay should be sampled and pooled. Pooling is appropriate only for samples from the same bin or stack of hay; otherwise, the samples should be kept separate. This is critical because toxicants are not always present uniformly in a bin. For example, some mycotoxins are often localized in certain areas within a bin. Once the management, environmental, and feed records are complete, the clinician can concentrate on the clinical syndrome at hand.

CLINICAL EXAMINATION

Evaluation of clinical signs is the next step in piecing together the toxicology puzzle. The incidence of poisoning; the signalment of affected animals; and the nature, rapidity of onset, severity, and progression of clinical signs should all be observed. Some problems, such as ingestion of some plants and feeds, or improper or inappropriate injection of drugs or other chemicals, may result in sudden death with little evidence of specific intoxication. Other cases with nonspecific signs may be more insidious in onset, such as gradual weight loss from ingestion of loco weed or pyrrolizidine alkaloids. Conversely, a clinical sign may be very specific, such as laminitis from exposure to black walnut shavings or paralysis due to botulism. Some cases may not involve clinical signs. For example, residues from some plants like jimsonweed (*Datura* species), which contains tropane alkaloids like scopolamine, may lead to positive drug test results in samples from equine athletes. Regardless of the type of clinical signs, it is important to rule out nontoxic causes of clinical signs and avoid focusing too rapidly on toxicology.

Clinical laboratory data may also be useful. Complete blood cell counts may suggest a type of anemia or infection, and serum biochemistry assays can help identify affected organ systems. A clinical biochemistry test that is especially useful in toxicology is the assay of acetylcholinesterase activity of whole blood. Depression of the activity of this enzyme suggests exposure to a carbamate or organophosphorous insecticide. Whole blood, serum, gastrointestinal (GI) contents, and urine are all useful for toxicology testing (Table 1).

PATHOLOGY

If animals have died, complete necropsies should be performed, because the toxicologic or forensic necropsy is usually critical to the diagnosis of a toxicology case. In some instances, such as pyrrolizidine alkaloid toxicosis, histologic examination may provide the only concrete diagnostic information. The necropsy (see page 655) should be systematic and samples should be properly obtained for bacteriologic, virologic, histologic, and toxicologic examinations. Specimens that should be obtained for toxicology testing are listed in Table 1. It is often helpful to hold samples frozen until other testing is complete to ensure that the most useful and pertinent battery of chemical analyses is assigned. Not all samples will be needed, but it is easier to save samples and discard them later than to somehow regenerate them after the fact.

The samples should be examined before they are shipped. Parts of poisonous plants and fragments of lead have been found in the GI contents of animals that have died suddenly. Specimens should be properly labeled, sealed, and frozen. Inclusion of a complete written history of the case with the samples helps the toxicologist order the appropriate tests and adequately interpret the results.

TABLE 1.   SAMPLES, AND AMOUNTS OF EACH, THAT ARE NEEDED FOR TOXICOLOGIC ANALYSIS*

Sample	Amount	Condition	Examples
Ante Mortem			
Whole blood	5–10 ml	EDTA anticoagulant	Pb, As, Se, cholinesterase
Urine	100 ml	Plastic screw-capped vial	Drugs, some metals
Serum	10 ml	Remove from clot. Special trace element tubes, especially for Zn	Trace elements, drugs, nitrates, electrolytes
CSF	1 ml	Clot tube	Sodium
GI contents	500 g	Obtain representative sample: both feces and stomach content	Pesticides, plants (e.g., alkaloids, oleander), metals, feed-associated toxicants
Hair	2 g	Rarely useful, call laboratory, wash before sampling	Chronic selenosis, do not use Se shampoo to wash
Postmortem			
Urine	100 ml	Plastic screw-capped vial	Drugs, some metals
Serum	20 ml	Remove from heart clot	Drugs, nitrates, electrolytes
Liver	250 g	Plastic (foil if organics)	Pesticides, metals, organics
Kidney	250 g	Plastic (foil if organics)	Metals
Brain	50%	Split sagittally, send half in formalin to pathologist, half frozen in plastic to analyst	Organochlorines, sodium, cholinesterase
Fat	250 g	Foil inside plastic	Accumulated organochlorines
GI contents	500 g	Obtain representative sample: both cecal and stomach content.	Pesticides, plants (e.g., alkaloids, oleander), metals, feed-associated toxicants
Ocular fluid	0.5 ml	Send entire eye	Nitrate, salts (e.g, magnesium)
Bone	100 g	1 long bone	Fluoride
Miscellaneous		Injection sites, spleen	Some drugs
Environment			
Baits, etc.	200 ml or g	Clean mason jar (liquid), plastic	Unidentified chemicals, feed additives, pesticides, etc.
Concentrates	1 kg plus	Plastic sack, box, representative sample is imperative	Mycotoxins, feed additives, plants, pesticides, metals
Forage	1 kg plus	Plastic sack, box, representative sample is imperative	Plants, pesticides
Plants	Plant	Fresh, or pressed and dried. Send all plant parts	Identification
Water	1 L	Clean mason jar, foil under lid for metals, plastic if organics	Metals, nitrates, pesticides, sulfate, algae

*With the exception of whole blood and very dry samples (e.g., some feeds), all samples should be submitted frozen. Separate tissue samples should be properly fixed in formalin for histologic analysis as well, but fixed tissue is not useful for any of the listed chemistry assays. Do not submit material in syringes.

ANALYTICAL TOXICOLOGY

Analyses are readily available for several classes of toxicants, including heavy metals, pesticides, feed additives, drugs, and some natural toxins (see Table 1). Analytical chemistry involves much more than putting a minute amount of material into a machine. Analyses often require a great deal of preparatory chemistry and significant quantities of material. Thus, analyses for the most likely agents should be based on historical, clinical, and pathologic data. A diagnostic laboratory should be consulted regarding the specimen sizes and times that are required for testing.

Although tissues are useful for many chemistry tests, the best sample for analysis is often the feed source or GI contents. This is because the animal's body, especially the liver, has not yet had a chance to metabolize and dilute the parent compound. Following metabolism, many compounds, especially drugs, are concentrated in the urine during the excretory phase. In addition, many compounds, such as mycotoxins, do not appear in tissue in detectable levels even in poisoned animals. Thus, sampling from the source, GI tract, and urine is often essential in obtaining a diagnosis.

BIOASSAY

There are two types of bioassay. In some situations, the response of affected animals to specific therapy is a legiti-mate diagnostic bioassay. This approach should be used with caution and only when the diagnosis is reasonably certain. Some therapeutic agents, such as atropine, which is used to treat organophosphorous or carbamate insecticide poisoning, are themselves potentially very hazardous to the horse.

The other category of bioassay involves feeding a suspected toxin or source of toxin to laboratory animals. This is done only when other diagnostic avenues have been exhausted.

PREVENTION AND TREATMENT

At the end of the initial toxicology case work-up, the veterinarian will probably have formed some opinion of the source and nature of the intoxication. Exposure of horses to suspected material should be eliminated immediately. This may involve removal of animals from a pasture if plant toxicosis is suspected. If removal from the pasture is impractical, horses may be provided with adequate feed to prevent continued consumption of noxious weed. If hay and grain are suspected sources, the feed remaining in troughs or racks should be completely replaced. Similar measures should be taken if bedding or water is suspected.

Once further exposure to a suspected agent has been prevented, horses must be clinically evaluated for possible treatment. Because many toxicants lack specific antidotes, treatment frequently consists of nonspecific support and alleviation of clinical signs. If appropriate, horses recently exposed to a suspected toxicant should be treated with an oral absorbent such as activated charcoal (2 g/kg body weight as a slurry in water, administered via nasogastric tube). Horses with impaired intestinal motility should receive mineral oil, but mineral oil and activated charcoal inactivate each other and should not be mixed. If a horse showing signs of colic has been treated with mineral oil and a toxicant is still suspected, activated charcoal can be administered 3 or 4 hours later if GI motility is normal.

In the case of specific clinical problems, the practitioner must avoid administering drugs that are metabolized by, excreted by, or have an impact on the organs affected by the toxin. Once test results are complete and the toxicant has been identified, treatment can be modified accordingly.

Supplemental Readings

Blodgett DD: The investigation of outbreaks of toxicologic disease. Vet Clin North Am Food Anim Pract 4:145–158, 1988.

Hancock DD, Blodgett D, Gay CC: The collection and submission of samples for laboratory testing. Vet Clin North Am Food Anim Pract 4:33–60, 1988.

Osweiler GD, Carson TL, Buck WB, Van Gelder GA: Diagnostic toxicology. *In* Clinical and Diagnostic Veterinary Toxicology, ed 3. Dubuque, IA, Kendall/Hunt Publishing, 1985, pp 44–51.

Forensic Necropsy of the Horse

BILL JOHNSON
Davis, California

The practitioner is sometimes called upon to perform a postmortem examination on a horse that is either insured for large sums of money, or because the circumstances of the horse's death are likely to be the subject of a lawsuit. Typical veterinary necropsy training is oriented toward finding diseased conditions or describing traumatic injuries. Minimal attention is given on how to approach cases that may represent malicious or possible litigious acts. These cases must be handled in a manner that will protect the rights of all parties involved. The practitioner must be a neutral observer, making trained, intelligent observations and reporting findings without prejudice. Good planning, thorough necropsy technique, and accurate records are a must since these cases may end up in litigation 5 or 10 years after the original examination.

These cases can be very time consuming. If you do not have the time, tell the client and suggest referral. If you do the necropsy you have accepted the responsibility for the case. Failure to follow accepted procedure in handling such a case may result in professional embarrassment in court or possibly your being named in a later lawsuit. If transportation is possible and postmortem decomposition during shipment is not a factor, it is best to send these cases to a qualified animal disease diagnostic laboratory. If this is not possible, the following is a guideline to help protect the interests of all parties.

PREPARATION

Take the time to obtain a thorough history. Identify the proper owner. If the animal is insured, get the name and address of the insurance company and permission to communicate with them directly. If the animal is insured, there may be specific requirements in the policy that must be executed before the company will settle a death claim. It is best to call the insurer and find out what their requirements are. Be sure to inquire of the owner or attendee about any previous health problems, present ration, any changes in ration, previous medications, any environmental changes, any changes in the daily routine of the horse and a description of the clinical abnormalities, if any, noted prior to death. Accept this information as opinion and not as fact. Let your observations during the necropsy confirm or raise questions about the history.

THE NECROPSY

Identify the horse as well as possible. Ask the owner or the attendant if there are any identifying marks. If possible photograph the animal with pictures of the limbs, head, body, and any tattoos or lack of tattoos. Record, on the report, a description of markings and tattoos. Write what you can clearly see; when a tattoo is illegible, draw what you can see. With Arabians, clip the neck and draw the figures just as you see them. Report only what you can testify to, not what is on the registration papers.

Get rid of your prejudices before starting the necropsy. It is fine to have a most likely diagnosis, but do not focus on that possibility to the point that other possibilities are ignored. Keep your mind strictly on what you are doing. Based on the clinical history, determine what organs or organ systems need particularly close scrutiny. Use a good systematic necropsy technique. A systematic approach will ensure that all organs are examined and that any previously unforeseen problems will be recognized.

Record the nutritional condition of the animal and its state of postmortem decomposition. Remember that the obvious is not always as it seems. Ruptured stomachs and bloody-appearing intestines can be postmortem artifacts. When faced with a possible lesion, remember the processes of inflammation. True lesions should have hemorrhage or fibrin and swelling that may be the result of edema or accumulation of a cellular exudate. Fibrin may be visible as readily apparant adherent white tags or as subtle dull granularity. Any ante-mortem stomach rupture should have areas of hemorrhage or fibrin release at the margins of the tear. Omentum or other organs should be lightly adherent to the edges of the ruptured organ. The serosa next to the tear may be dull and granular due to fibrin release rather than having the normal smooth and shiny appearance. What is often termed hemorrhagic enteritis is often only blood-engorged capillaries and venules in the intestinal villi with postmortem imbibition of hemoglobin. Cases of enteritis should have some combination of necrosis, mural edema, adherent fibrin, or blood. On the other hand, do not be misled by normal-appearing intestines or organs. Inflammatory changes may be so subtle that they can only be seen microscopically in formalin-fixed sections.

Constantly ask yourself questions based on what you are seeing. Do your findings match the owner's ante-mortem observations? Is there marked subcutaneous bruising that suggests a prolonged agonal death? A history of, "just found dead," with no subcutaneous bruising might suggest a malicious poisoning. In such cases, special attention should be paid to the jugular furrows and the intimal surfaces of the jugular veins for any evidence of an injection.

Even though the circumstances seem unusual, the death may be from natural causes affecting a vital organ. The heart should be closely examined. Check for subepicardial edema around the coronary groove as gross evidence of subtle inflammation. You may want to remove the heart and major vessels intact and do a water ejection test. For this, cut the top off of the auricles and remove the postmortem blood clot. Continuously flood the lumen of the auricle and then squeeze the corresponding ventricle, which will force the atrioventricular valve to close. Any serious valvular insufficiencies can be noted then. Loose tags of a ruptured cordia tendinae can be seen floating in the ejected water, adjacent to a segment of valve that does not completely close. Also collect sections of heart in formalin as there may be microscopic areas of inflammation around the bundle of His or around the sinoatrial node or atrioventricular node. You may need to consult an anatomy book for the location of these structures. Record all the organs that you examine, even though they appear normal. In five years' time, on the witness stand, you may not remember if you examined the adrenal glands.

Carefully examine the organ system that makes the animal particularly valuable. If it is a valuable breeding stallion, make a good examination of the testicles and genital tract. Be assured that if the animal is insured for a large sum of money because it is a valuable breeding animal, the insurance company will be asking you for confirmation that the horse's reproductive tract was sound. Failure to do this could cost your client money. The limbs of valuable racing horses should be examined, especially the front limbs. Examine the suspensory apparatus for inflammatory changes, also the carpal and pastern joints, which are particularly susceptible to articular damage. While lesions in these organs would not account for death, the description of healthy organs will help the owner and the insurance company agree on the value of the animal. Inversely, if irreparable damage is noted in the organ, it will increase your degree of suspicion surrounding the circumstances of death of the animal.

SPECIMEN COLLECTION

Collect 1-cm-thick sections in 10% formalin for histopathology of any abnormal organs plus sections of organs that could physiologically account for the reported clinical signs. If the animal was just found dead, collect a wide assortment of tissues. In all cases, routine sections of kidney, spleen, liver, heart, lung, brain, stomach, small and large intestine, and cecum should be collected. When the history or findings dictate, collect proper specimens for microbiologic examination.

If the history in any way suggests intentional or malicious death, collect samples for toxicology. If possible, check with a toxicologist before the necropsy for any special samples or handling instructions. If this is not possible, use the guidelines suggested on page 654 for collection, handling, and shipping of samples.

Be diligent and tenacious with your postmortem examination. These qualities will usually be rewarded. The best example the author can recount was demonstrated in a racehorse that had an ill-defined lameness in a front limb followed by complete inability to use or even bear weight on the limb. A complete scapular or humeral fracture was diagnosed and the horse humanely euthanized. At postmortem, no fractures were found grossly or with radiographs but examination of the spinal cord revealed severe unilateral lesions of equine protozoal myelitis.

Finally, immediately record all findings. To quote an old proverb, "The historical accounts from the dullest pencil are clearer than those from the brightest mind."

Supplemental Readings

Edwards WC, Johnson BJ: A veterinarian's guide: Equine insurance examinations. Equine Pract 8(6):19–22, 1986.

King JM, Dodd DC, Newson ME: Necropsy of the horse, part 1. Mod Vet Pract 59:897–899, 1978.

King JM, Dodd DC, Newson ME: Necropsy of the horse, part 2. Mod Vet Pract 60:29–32, 1979.

King JM, Dodd DC, Newson ME: Necropsy of the horse, part 3. Mod Vet Pract 60:109–112, 1979.

Taylor RJ, Sexton JW: Medical-legal aspects of veterinary medicine. Am Assoc Vet Lab Diagnosticians, 25th Annu Proc, 1982, pp 499–509.

Medicolegal Investigation of the Sudden or Unexpected Equine Death: Toxicologic Implications

JOHN C. HALIBURTON
Amarillo, Texas

WILLIAM C. EDWARDS
Stillwater, Oklahoma

Equine practitioners are occasionally required to use their clinical, anatomic, and pathologic expertise in the practice of postmortem diagnostic medicine. These skills, combined with sound postmortem investigative techniques and an understanding of the unique and detailed requirements of forensic medicine, are essential prerequisites for the equine practitioner in the practice of equine medicolegal postmortem medicine.

When there are no imminent legal questions overshadowing the death of a horse, a thorough gross postmortem examination may be all that is required to satisfactorily conclude the case. Unfortunately, equine deaths occur in which the answers to the questions of cause of death and manner of death may have great legal consequence. It is in this type of case that a comprehensive toxicologic examination may be required.

Equine insurance mortality policies commonly contain exclusions, especially in cases of death due to poisoning. In these cases, the accurate and conclusive determination of the cause and manner of death is crucial to the validity of the claim and ultimately to the liability of the insurance company.

Some veterinarians not experienced in the practice of veterinary postmortem medicine may not understand the difference between the cause of death and the manner of death. The cause of death can be simply defined as any injury or disease condition that results in death. Examples of cited causes of death may be lymphosarcoma, cantharidin poisoning, or electrocution. The manner of death explains how the cause of death came about. Manner of death can be from natural, accidental, intentional, or undetermined causes. The manner of death is an opinion based on the facts associated with the circumstances of the death that are supported by pathologic, toxicologic, and other laboratory findings. A sudden or unexpected equine death should be investigated with the suspicion of a chemical or drug toxicosis at the top of the list of probable cause. Table 1 lists some toxicologic as well as nontoxicologic causes of sudden or unexpected death that may be considered in the investigation of such cases.

This chapter focuses on the logistics and techniques of conducting a postmortem investigation in cases of sudden or unexpected equine death in a manner that will provide the toxicology laboratory with the required information and appropriate specimens. The chapter also addresses the role of the equine practitioner in the testimony phase of the medicolegal case.

POSTMORTEM INVESTIGATION

When first contacted about conducting a postmortem investigation, a record should be made of the date, time of day, method of contact (i.e., telephone, letter) and the identity of the party or parties requesting the services. During the initial conversation, the practitioner should clearly establish who is requesting the services, whether it is the owner or the insurance company, or other party. Additionally, important information that should be obtained includes the name, address, and telephone number of (1) the horse owner and legal representative, and (2) the insurance company and its claim representative. Case information such as the name, age, gender, and breed of the horse and its identification number should be obtained. The time and date of death and the location of the horse should also be recorded at this time.

The veterinarian assigned to conduct the postmortem examination may be owner-appointed or one selected by the insurance company. The party that does not appoint the primary examiner may request that a second veterinarian be present and assist in the procedure. It is strongly recommended that regardless of the situation, the presence of another veterinarian be requested to assist and witness the procedure and validate specimen collection and specimen apportionment.

Once the decision is made to accept the case, the practitioner should obtain a detailed history of medical problems, management, nutrition and training, and related activities associated with the management and health of the horse. It should also be ascertained if there were any unusual circumstances before, during, or after the discovery of the death. Clinical signs are very important presumptive indicators to the toxicologist and should be described in detail when available.

The practitioner should at this stage of the investigation evaluate and discuss with both parties the necessity and the feasibility of transporting the horse to an animal disease diagnostic laboratory that is staffed and equipped to con-

TABLE 1.   SOME CAUSES OF SUDDEN, UNEXPECTED DEATH IN HORSES

Agent	Source	Agent
Toxins		*Infectious/Microbial/Protozoal/Parasitic Agents*
Strychnine	Rodenticides	Botulism
Phosphides		Septicemia
Anticoagulants		Endotoxemia
Organophosphates	Insecticides	Anthrax
Carbamates		Salmonellosis
Nicotine		Tetanus
Mercury	Fungicides	Rabies
Metaldehyde	Molluscicide	Insect-borne viral encephalitides
Arsenic	Herbicides	Herpesvirus
Cyanide	Predator control products	Protozoal myeloencephalitis
Fluoroacetate		Verminous myelitis
Amphetamines	Illicit drugs	Anemia/exsanguination
Cocaine		
Heroin		*Metabolic Agents*
Morphine		Hypomagnesemia
Lead	Environmental/industrial	Hypocalcemia
Insulin	Pharmaceutical	Hypoglycemia
Succinylcholine	Neuromuscular blocking agent	
Electrolytes	Potassium chloride, magnesium sulfate	*Physical Causes*
Selenium	Vitamin/mineral injectables	Trauma
Iron salts		Electrocution
Vitamins A, D, E		Lightning strike
Oleander	Toxic plants	Suffocation
Yew		Gunshot
Hemlock		
Jimsonweed		*Natural/Genetic Causes*
Milkweeds		Hyperkalemic periodic paralysis
Maple		Cardiac conductive disorders
Snakeroot/goldenrod		Cerebral thromboembolism
Ionophores	Feed-related	Aortic aneurysm
Antibiotics		Neoplasia
Mycotoxins		*Iatrogenic Causes*
Cantharidin	Blister beetle	Intracarotid injection

duct comprehensive and specialized postmortem examinations.

Frequently, when the postmortem examination is to be performed in the field (i.e., on site or in a veterinary clinic), the insurance company requests that a specific laboratory or even a specified individual be consulted before starting the postmortem examination. This is not done to question the competency of the practitioner but to ensure that all specimens required by the laboratory are collected, preserved, packaged, and transported in a manner that documents specimen integrity and ensures expedient delivery to the laboratory.

The technique for postmortem examination is described on page 655.

SPECIMEN SELECTION

Collection and preservation of postmortem samples that are suitable for laboratory analysis are the responsibility of the postmortem examiner. The specimens and the amount required to conduct a thorough toxicologic examination vary according to the circumstances of the case and the laboratory conducting the analyses. In some situations, the combined findings of the case investigation and postmortem examination allow the toxicologist to direct the initial analyses toward a specific toxic agent such as a drug, drug group, or chemical, which greatly simplifies the toxicologic examination. In many cases of sudden or unexpected death, the case investigation and pathologic findings do not provide pertinent information as to the identity of a possible toxic agent. In this type of case, the toxicologist has to initiate the analytic investigation from a broad, comprehensive screening approach, commonly referred to as "the general unknown" analysis.

In a comprehensive search for an unknown toxic agent, it may be necessary to analyze a wide variety of postmortem materials. Some of the more universally preferred specimens in "the general unknown" analysis are listed in Table 1 on page 654. The amount of each specimen to be collected is also a critical factor. As a rule of thumb when collecting specimens for submission to the toxicology laboratory, the clinician should collect as much as possible, especially with blood, urine, and stomach content. In addition to the specimens listed in Table 1, it may be necessary to collect representative samples of feeds, feed ingredients, water, plants, chemicals, drugs, bedding materials, or other suspicious substances found in the case investigation.

STANDARD SAMPLES FOR TOXICOLOGY ANALYSIS

Stomach Content

Oral ingestion or oral administration is a common route of exposure in equine poisonings. The high concentration of the toxic agent in the stomach content makes this specimen a preferred sample in "the general unknown" analysis. The total amount (i.e., the weight) of stomach content should be recorded so that total dose calculations can be conducted. A small, portable bathroom scale and a 5-gallon bucket generally work well for this procedure. After determining the weight, the stomach contents should be thoroughly mixed and the required aliquots taken for submission to the laboratory.

Urine

Many chemicals and the majority of drugs are excreted in the urine either unchanged or as a metabolite. This makes urine a valuable specimen in "the general unknown" analysis. Urine does not require extensive preparation for analysis and is ideal for quick, simple, qualitative spot test analyses. There is an old axiom that says, "If the toxic agent is present in drop amounts in the blood, it may be present in bucket amounts in the urine." The major liability of urine as a primary toxicologic specimen is that it is not always available at the time of postmortem examination.

Liver

The liver is the primary site of xenobiotic biotransformation and thus tends to collect many toxic agents in higher concentration than that found in the blood and other body tissues. Because of this fact and the availability of sizable quantities, the liver is a valuable specimen for toxicologic examination.

Blood

Unlike the situation in human forensic medicine, in which the interpretation of toxicologic results is routinely based on blood levels, interpretive toxicokinetic blood levels are not as well defined in equine forensic medicine. However, blood still has its role in the comprehensive toxicologic examination and should be collected when available.

Kidney

When urine is not available, the kidney is a recommended specimen for screening procedures. It is especially useful in the analysis of heavy metal toxicoses.

Brain

The brain is without question the most difficult postmortem specimen to collect but can be the pivotal specimen in the totally unknown case investigation. Brain analysis is particularly useful in the search for toxic agents that are highly lipid-soluble, such as organochlorine and some organophosphate insecticides.

SPECIMEN COLLECTION AND SUBMISSION

The collection of duplicate and sometimes triplicate samples for submission to the toxicology laboratory should be made in clean, secure containers. Whirl-pak bags are ideal for collection, shipment, and storage of nonfluid specimens. Fluid samples are best placed in leak-proof, polypropylene, screw-top containers. If the specimens are hand-delivered

to the laboratory, glass containers are acceptable. If the specimens are courier-delivered, glass containers are not recommended because of potential for breakage and contamination of other specimens.

Proper identification of all specimens is a necessity for the toxicology laboratory and an absolute must in forensic cases. Each container should be identified as to its contents, the name of the horse, and time and date of collection. Each should be initialed by the person who collected the sample.

Specimens should be delivered to the laboratory in a timely manner. If delivery to the laboratory can be made within 6 hours of collection, refrigeration (i.e., ice-cooled) is the only preservation required. If the delivery time is 6 hours or longer (i.e., overnight) the specimens should be frozen and packaged in ice or dry ice for shipment.

Because of the large caseload and limited storage facilities, most toxicology laboratories can only keep submitted specimens for a limited period of time. This situation combined with the fact that it may take 1 to 4 years for a case to reach the courtroom can create problems in the preservation of required evidence. The practitioner should discuss this issue with the laboratory and determine those specimens that can be stored and for how long.

Chain of Custody

Forensic equine death investigation cases require not only sound postmortem investigative and diagnostic skills but also detailed and accurate documentation of collection, possession, and transference of possession of all evidence collected in the case, including postmortem specimens submitted to the laboratory. This is commonly known as the *chain of custody record*. The chain of custody record specifically identifies each specimen, the condition of the specimen, the container in which it is packaged, the time and date of transfer and receipt, and the individuals involved in the transfer and receipt. Failure to maintain a complete chain of custody record can result in the inadmissibility of crucial laboratory results because sample integrity cannot be documented.

PRETRIAL AND TRIAL TESTIMONY

It is equally important for equine practitioners to understand their role in the testimony phase of a forensic case as it was in the medical/scientific investigative phase. By definition, the word *forensic* means belonging to or suitable to the courts of law. Therefore, the practitioner must always remember that all examination findings, observations, conclusions, and other activities performed in the case investigation are discoverable and open to examination in a court of law.

Forensic equine cases fall into one of two categories: civil or criminal. Civil cases are the predominant type encountered and generally involve a tort claim or breach of contract between two or more parties. The classic example of this type of case involves an owner, the plaintiff, who is filing suit against an insurance company, the defendant, for failure to pay the death benefit premium on an insurance policy. The insurance company's basis for denial of payment may be based on the issuance of a poisoning exclusion policy, and their position is that the facts in evidence support poisoning as the cause of death. Criminal cases are those in which state or federal statutes have been violated and criminal charges are filed by the government. This type of case can involve fraud, income tax invasion, or racketeering charges associated with the filing of a fraudulent equine mortality death claim.

As a participant in the trial phase of a forensic case, the practitioner may serve as one of two types of witness: the lay witness or the expert witness. The lay witness (sometimes called *witness of fact*) may only testify to what the person saw, said, smelled, touched, or did; the person cannot testify to what others have said (i.e., hearsay) nor can the person express opinions or conclusions about any aspect of the case. The function of the lay witness is to give factual information and, as such, the person is not required to be qualified by the court. On the other hand, the expert witness is an individual who by virtue of specialized education and training and qualification by the court (i.e., by judge's ruling) is allowed to testify not only on the given facts but is allowed to establish the facts, interpret the facts, and give opinions and conclusions on these facts. Expert witnesses must demonstrate to the court their expertise and defend these qualifications in court before being allowed to testify. It is the practitioner's job as an expert witness to assist the judge and jury in understanding the medical and scientific aspects of the postmortem investigation as they relate to the probable cause and manner of death. The practitioner does not have to be concerned with any aspects of the toxicologic findings. A toxicologist should be brought in to act as the expert in this area.

Regardless of the practitioner's role as a witness, the key to giving competent and accurate testimony is to construct and maintain accurate and detailed records and to thoroughly review and understand those records before giving testimony.

CONCLUSION

The procedures described and recommendations given in this chapter are fundamental to conducting competent and thorough equine forensic death investigations.

Systematic postmortem investigative procedures, proper specimen selection, specimen collection, specimen identification, specimen security, and specimen submission to the toxicology laboratory require foresight and planning on the part of the practitioner as well as good communication with the toxicologist. The equine practitioner can function as a competent and reliable witness in forensic equine cases by keeping accurate and detailed records of all activities associated with the investigation of the case.

Supplemental Readings

Edwards WC, Johnson BJ: A veterinarian's guide: Equine insurance examinations. Equine Pract 8(6):19–22, 1986.

Meads R: Ready or not? Don't be afraid of litigation—Be prepared. Pet Vet 2:12–14, 1990.

Osweiler GD, Carson TL, Buck WB, VanGelder GA: Clinical and Diagnostic Veterinary Toxicology, ed 3. Dubuque, Kendall/Hunt Publishing, 1985.

Poynter DF: The Expert Witness Handbook: Tips and Techniques for the Litigation Consultant. Santa Barbara, Para Publishing, 1987.

Industrial Toxicants

E. MURL BAILEY, JR.
TAM GARLAND
College Station, Texas

Intoxicated horses continually confront veterinary practitioners with therapeutic and prophylactic problems. The widespread necessary use and misuse of pesticides and industrial chemicals in North America causes accidental intoxications in animals. The likelihood of intoxications in horses makes it imperative that veterinarians attempt to educate their clients about the inherent dangers of chemicals and pesticides. Proper handling and storage techniques and appropriate usage of these compounds lessen the number of intoxications. This chapter briefly identifies some common industrial toxicants and describes the therapeutic and management procedures that should be instituted to treat the resulting diseases.

INORGANIC CHEMICALS

Most inorganic chemicals, when ingested in sufficient quantities, induce gastrointestinal signs. Horses acutely intoxicated with these agents exhibit colic, tenesmus, profuse diarrhea, shock, dehydration, coma, and death. Until a correct diagnosis is obtained, fluids, analgesics, and antispasmodics should be used to maintain the life of the affected horse. In most cases, initial maintenance of life is more important than the subsequent application of appropriate antidotal therapy. Inorganic chemicals must be differentiated from other causes of acute abdominal pain such as: blister beetle toxicity; various plants including castor bean (*Ricinus communis*) and sesbania (*Sesbania vesicaria* and *S. drummondii*); acute salmonellosis; colitis; intestinal torsion; and anterior mesenteric artery thrombosis. Unusual instances of chemical spills, drainage through dump sites, or leaching from mining operations may cause hazardous levels of certain heavy metals to appear in water offered to horses. Aluminum, beryllium, boron, chromium, cobalt, copper, iodide, iron, manganese, molybdenum, and zinc are examples of such potential metal contaminants.

Fluorides

Fluorine (F₂) rarely occurs in nature except in the form of fluorides. Fluorides are ubiquitous in varying amounts in soil, water, atmosphere, vegetation, and animal tissues. Inorganic fluorides are the most important sources of fluoride toxicosis, fluorosis, in animals. Organic fluorides occur in nature and in some commercial products, but have not been implicated as inducing problems in horses.

Fluoride concentrations greater than 3 ppm in water can cause mottling of developing teeth. Water containing more than 4 ppm of fluoride is only marginally safe for horses, and water containing more than 8 ppm should be avoided. Phosphorus feeding supplements should be defluorinated and should not contain more than 0.3% (3000 ppm) fluoride. A total daily dietary concentration of 40 ppm (calculated as dry matter) consumed for a prolonged period is considered the maximal tolerable level for horses.

Fluoride intoxication may occur as acute or chronic. The acute syndrome follows accidental ingestion of high levels of fluorides, and the clinical signs are as described in the introduction to this section. The sources of such poisonings in livestock are usually sodium fluorosilicate used as an insecticide, and contaminated water, vegetation, and feeds. The clinical signs associated with the predacide sodium fluoroacetate (Compound 1080) have no relationship to the clinical signs of either acute or chronic fluoride intoxication.

Chronic fluorosis is much more common in horses than the acute form. The variable and extended interval between ingestion and clinical signs complicates the diagnosis. The insidious onset and signs, such as nonspecific lameness and general debilitation, cause fluorosis to be confused with other chronic diseases. Horses with moderate to marked fluorosis appear unthrifty even when ample amounts of quality feed are available. The hair coat becomes rough and dry, and winter coats are shed slowly in the spring. Horses with marked fluorosis are often lame and unable to perform normally.

One of the most sensitive indicators of fluorosis in young horses is dental lesions, which appear before other signs. Ingested fluoride affects enamel and dentine formation during tooth formation. Affected teeth have a characteristic mottling, staining, hypoplasia, and hypocalcification, and are subject to excessive abrasion. There may be evidence of soreness and sensitivity to heat and cold in the teeth, resulting in chewing and then expelling (quidding) of the feed. (See page 149 for the differential diagnosis of quidding.) The central portion of affected cheek teeth may be lost, allowing food particles to be forced into the pulp cavity. Mandibular abscesses may subsequently form, which must be differentiated from actinomycosis or other mandibular diseases. Infected areas are often 4 to 6 cm in diameter and can include a fistulous tract that drains from the ventral aspect of the mandible.

Fluoride is stored in bone, within certain limits, without demonstrable changes in structure and function. However, if excess fluoride is ingested for a prolonged period, structural and functional bone changes appear at sites of greatest metabolic activity and in bones under the greatest stress from weightbearing and locomotion. The first palpable lesions are usually bilateral hyperostotic lesions on the metatarsal and metacarpal bones, mandibles, and ribs. The first and second phalanges may have abnormal periosteal hyperostosis, particularly at tendon insertions. Often the third phalanx is enlarged with a layer of very rough-textured bone. This increases pressure within the hoof, leading to a laminitis syndrome. Lameness problems may improve following removal of the fluoride; however, affected bones and teeth may not improve. Because fluorosis does not primarily affect the intra-articular structures, it must be differentiated from the bony changes in equine osteoarthritis, which are initially intra-articular, with marginal lipping in advanced cases.

When fluorosis is suspected and clinical signs are absent, urinalysis can aid diagnosis. Fluoride concentrations in urine appear to vary with specific gravity and should be standardized. Typically, urine values have been corrected to a specific gravity of 1.040, although other bases have been used. Normal urine fluoride levels are less than 6 ppm. Diagnostic fluoride levels are higher than 15 to 20 ppm.

Bone samples can be obtained by biopsy or at necropsy for analysis of fluoride content and gross and microscopic evaluations. Normal bone fluoride levels are 400 to 1200 ppm, whereas diagnostic levels are more than 3000 ppm. Hair, skin, hooves, and soft tissues have no characteristic changes and only small (less than 2.5 ppm) amounts of fluoride are retained in soft tissues. Correlating clinical findings, biopsy results, and necropsy observations with the fluoride content of the water and forage feed often helps corroborate suspected fluoride toxicosis.

No treatment or prophylactic measures completely prevent the toxic effects of excess fluoride ingestion, but aluminum salts such as aluminum sulfate, aluminum chloride, calcium aluminate, and calcium carbonate partially reduce fluoride effects. Although these measures do not eliminate a fluoride problem, they often ameliorate its severity.

Mercury

Mercury poisoning of horses is rare but has occurred sporadically in the past, usually as a result of feeding seed grains treated with organomercurial fungicides. Mercury for seed dressings was banned in 1970, but other causes have included ingestion of mercurial ointments, batteries, and pharmaceuticals. Mercury has caused concern because it persists in the environment, and some forms have the tendency to accumulate in the food chain. The source and frequency of exposure to mercury determine the morbidity, which is generally high with a guarded prognosis, among affected animals.

Organic mercury is more readily absorbed than the metallic or inorganic forms. Digestive tract irritation and subsequent kidney and central nervous system (CNS) effects may be seen, depending upon its form and concentration in the feed or water consumed. Inorganic and phenylmercury compounds generally cause hyperemic to hemorrhagic and necrotic gastroenteritis and colitis along with pale swollen kidneys. Histologically, there is epithelial necrosis of alimentary mucosa and renal tubules. The severity and course of the toxicosis is reflected in the clinical pathology changes indicating renal damage. Alkyl mercury toxicosis produces mainly neurologic lesions. Microscopically focal malacia of the cerebral cortex, demyelination, astrogliosis, microgliosis, loss of granular cells in the cerebellum, and fibrinoid degeneration of CNS arterioles are evident.

Demonstration of a source of mercury is important in diagnosis because the availability of this toxicant is limited. Inorganic mercury has the highest tissue residues in the kidney, whereas both brain and kidney accumulate high concentrations of alkyl mercury. These tissues may be used for analysis. In acute cases, kidney cortex and liver are expected to contain in excess of 10 ppm mercury on a wet-weight basis. Brain tissue should be collected for chemical analysis and examination for microscopic lesions if alkyl mercury poisoning is suspected. Mercury poisoning has been confused with viral encephalitis, salmonellosis, inorganic or organic arsenic poisoning, and lead poisoning. The maximal tolerable level of organic or inorganic mercury in the diet of horses is considered to be 2 ppm.

Treatment of either inorganic or organic mercury toxicosis in livestock is often unsuccessful. No therapeutic regimens have been established for horses but extrapolation from cattle dosages is recommended. Dosing of a saline cathartic such as sodium sulfate (3 g/kg p.o.), following removal from the source, should be helpful. Sodium thiosulfate has been advocated, because mercurials may be complexed with the sulfhydryl radical. The recommended dosage for adult cattle is 30 g orally in a 10% solution. Dimercaprol,° a 10% oil suspension, is recommended as an antidote for mercury toxicosis. It is given intramuscularly at 2.5 to 5.0 mg/kg body weight every 4 hours for 2 days, three times a day on the third day, and then twice daily for 10 days or until recovery. An alternative therapy suggested for mercury toxicosis has been D-penicillamine,† given orally at dosage levels of 3 to 4 mg/kg every 6 hours for 10 days.

ORGANIC COMPOUNDS

Polyhalogenated Biphenyls

Polyhalogenated biphenyls (PHBs) (polybrominated biphenyls [PBBs] and polychlorinated biphenyls [PCBs]) are extremely stable industrial chemicals sold under the trade names of FireMaster and Arochlor. PHBs' resistance to degradation or metabolic transformation increases with the level of halogenation. Like other halogenated hydrocarbons, PHBs are highly lipophilic and are selectively deposited in body fat.

The toxic syndromes associated with PHBs in horses have not been defined. In cattle, PBBs have produced various disease syndromes encompassing anorexia, decreased milk production, increased frequency of urination

and lacrimation, and some lameness. Subsequent clinical signs included hematomas progressing to abscesses and weight loss even though the ration had been changed and appetites were normal. In addition, abnormal hoof growth, hair that became matted and fell out, and skin on the neck, shoulder, and thorax becoming thickened and wrinkled have been described. Prolonged gestation, lack of udder development, dystocias as a result of large calves that were delivered dead or died soon after birth, and development of postparturient metritis were common. Pathologic lesions were consistent with the various disease syndromes. Disease syndromes and lesions in horses are similar to those in cattle.

There is no specific treatment available for PHB toxicosis. Sources of PBBs should be eliminated, and animals exhibiting clinical signs of illness should be treated symptomatically.

Phenolics

Phenolic chemicals are very useful because of their multiple-use properties consisting of antimicrobial effect, environmental stability, and solubility and mixability with numerous other organic chemicals. Pure phenol is an excellent disinfectant, but is too toxic for routine environmental and animal applications. Phenol derivatives have reduced toxicity while retaining the germicidal properties. Chlorine and other radicals have been added to the benzene ring of phenol to develop myriad useful commercial materials, such as disinfectants and fungicides, and components of multimixture materials that are likely to be disposed of and made available inadvertently to grazing animals.

Exposure to phenolic chemicals is via accidental application or via direct exposure through the carelessness of an uninformed owner. Dietary contamination can occur through sprays applied in feeding areas or through mistaken chemical identity.

Phenolics are rapidly absorbed from the intact skin or from the digestive tract, and these tissues may show evidence of corrosion. Early signs include incoordination, mild muscular fasciculation, depression leading to coma, and deepening coma with terminal respiratory failure. Likewise, an increase in red blood cell and intravascular hemolysis may occur. Icterus is progressive until death. Mild poisoning may result in clinical signs occurring and regressing within 24 hours; more severe poisoning may produce death within 24 to 36 hours.

Necropsy lesions are consistent with the protein-coagulation properties of phenolic chemicals. Congestion of internal organs and generalized icterus are apparent. The skin or digestive tract contents may have a characteristic phenol odor. Microscopically, there is coagulation necrosis of epithelial cells, moderate hepatocyte degeneration, and non-specific nephrotoxic changes.

History and evidence of contact with phenolic-containing materials are invaluable for the diagnosis of phenolic poisoning because clinical signs are not sufficiently specific. The presence of one or more animals with clinical signs should suggest the possibility of phenol toxicity. Urine from suspect animals may be used in a rapid test.

No specific treatment exists for phenolic intoxication; however, preventing further exposure and initiating supportive therapy are advisable. Washing the exposed skin with soap and water and applying sodium bicarbonate bandages reduce the topical effects, whereas administration of activated charcoal is effective in binding unabsorbed phenolic chemicals in the digestive tract. Glyceryl guaiacolate or methocarbamol may be used to control muscle fasciculations. Glucose may have some benefit in reducing liver damage and maintaining renal function. Recovery from phenolic poisoning is still largely determined by the total dose absorbed and the animal's ability to detoxify and excrete the offending chemical.

Coal Tars

Coal tar poisoning, which is most often associated with swine, is an acute, highly fatal disease. It produces characteristic liver lesions that may be undetected until necropsy. Phenol, creosols, and a variety of aromatic hydrocarbons (naphthalene, naphthalene derivatives, anthracene, and anthracene oils) are the toxic agents found in plumbers' pitch, linoleum, and tar paper materials. Young animals are most susceptible, primarily because of their developing eating habits. Death from this toxicosis may occur several decades after the last known pasture contamination with clay pigeons because the toxic compounds are environmentally stable.

The most common syndrome is a rapid clinical course and sudden death, but without diagnostic signs. This sudden death, often associated with exertion, results from increased thoracic and abdominal fluid accumulation. Occasionally, a more chronic illness is observed, with evidence of anorexia, depression, weakness, a rough hair coat, anemia, and icterus. The characteristic lesion is a markedly swollen liver with a mottled appearance. Changes usually involve the entire liver, but in those animals that survive for several days or in those animals with subclinical effects, the lesions may be confined to local or peripheral areas. No good therapeutic regimen for coal tar intoxications exists other than symptomatic treatment with liver-sparing amino acids.

Herbicides and Fungicides

Treatment of most poisoning cases caused by herbicides and fungicides is symptomatic and supportive in nature because of the lack of specific antidotes. Activated charcoal (1–3 g/kg) and a saline cathartic (1–3 g/kg) mixture should be given if exposure has been oral.

Animals intoxicated with sodium chlorate, which forms methemoglobin, should be given a 1% intravenous solution of methylene blue at a rate of 8.8 mg/kg. This must be given slowly, and the animal must be closely observed, because an overdose of methylene blue also causes methemoglobin formation. Because sodium chlorate is not rapidly biotransformed, a poisoned animal may have to be treated for several days to ensure proper recovery. Other supportive measures should be instituted.

Hexachlorobenzene

Hexachlorobenzene (HCB) is a fungicidal agent for treatment of seeds and occurs as a byproduct of a number of industrial processes and a variety of agricultural chemicals. Thus, HCB environmental contamination is extensive. HCB is a stable, persistent chlorinated hydrocarbon that is highly lipophilic and is selectively deposited in the body fat. The liver is the only tissue that tends to accumulate the metabolites, which include pentachlorophenol and pentachlorothiophenol.

Signs of HCB intoxication during and after prolonged exposure are tremors, ataxia, weakness, paralysis, porphyria, possible photosensitization, and weight loss. Pathologic changes reported are blood cell disorders, neurologic abnormalities, and hepatomegaly. No specific treatment is available. Animals showing clinical signs should be treated symptomatically.

Biomagnification of HCB occurs in animals at concentrations 6 to 50 times the dietary level during long-term exposure. Therefore, concentrations in finished feeds should not exceed 0.02 to 0.05 ppm, depending on duration of exposure. The Environmental Protection Agency has set an interim tolerance for HCB in cattle, sheep, goats, and horses of 0.5 ppm.

Pentachlorophenol Poisoning

Lumber treated with wood preservatives, such as pentachlorophenol (PCP), creosote, and related phenolic compounds, is often used to construct animal facilities. Routes of exposure are via skin contact with treated lumber, erroneous topical application of chlorinated compounds, licking or chewing on treated portions of stabling, or consumption of contaminated feeds. In unusual circumstances, respiratory exposure may occur through the housing of animals in poorly ventilated barns that have been heavily treated with pentachlorophenol. PCP is an "uncoupler" of oxidative phosphorylation and induces the development of unusually high body temperatures. Clinical signs associated with PCP include hyperpnea and dyspnea, weakness, intense sweating, and tachycardia, leading to coma and death. Treatment for PCP intoxication is nonspecific, but should include fluid therapy, cold water enemas, and generalized treatment for overheating. Once an animal is exhibiting severe clinical signs, the prognosis becomes poor.

Tetrachlorodibenzodioxin (TCDD)

Dioxins, which are highly toxic to rodents and birds, have a lesser toxicity in horses and humans. Dioxins provide an example of how a chemical can unexpectedly occur in a horse's environment.

Many horses, birds, rodents, cats, and dogs died after being exposed to a horse arena in eastern Missouri. The problem started 4 days after the arena had been sprayed with waste oil for dust control. It was subsequently discovered that the waste oil was a distillate residue from chlorophenol manufacture. This byproduct, among other substances, contained 300 to 356 ppm of 2,4,7,8-tetrachlorodibenzo-p-dioxin, one of the most toxic synthetic substances known.

The clinical signs in horses included polydipsia, anorexia, severe weight loss, colic, alopecia, skin and oral ulcers, dependent edema, conjunctivitis, joint stiffness, and laminitis. Of 85 horses ridden in the arena, 58 became ill and 43 died.

There is no known treatment for TCDD intoxication. Prevention is the only help.

Petroleum Products

Horses generally avoid feed, forage, or water-containing petroleum products, and cases of petroleum product toxicity in horses are rare and most are minimally toxic. However, horses exhibiting pica or those confined to areas containing petroleum products may ingest these materials. Various petroleum or petroleum-based products may be applied by owners to control insects or to treat skin conditions with "home remedies." Petroleum products include kerosene, gasoline, and other fuel oils, waste crankcase oil, and crude oil or partially refined petroleum materials. Petroleum distillates may be used as vehicles for pesticides. Waste oil materials are used to reduce dust in arenas. Used petroleum materials may contain contaminants, such as lead, PCP, or TCDD.

The clinical signs of petroleum product toxicity depend upon the product being applied, its contaminants, and the route of exposure. Ingested petroleum products may produce salivation, blistering of the muzzle and mouth, colic, diarrhea, and 1 to 3 days of reduced appetite. Petroleum products applied to the skin produce local irritation with some hair loss. The horse may rub the involved area, producing additional inflammation and possible bleeding. Inhalation may occur when stables are sprayed with petroleum products, resulting in mild respiratory tract irritation. Coughing, sneezing, increased respiratory rate, and pulmonary congestion may develop following heavy exposure.

The treatment for petroleum product toxicity varies with the type and extent of exposure. Often, conservative and supportive therapy is sufficient, whereas with conditions such as aspiration pneumonia from petroleum product droplet inhalation, the most vigorous antibiotic and supportive therapy is ineffectual. Generally, the petroleum material should be removed from contact with the animal as soon as possible. Osmotic cathartics should be used to empty the digestive tract, and soap and water should be used on the skin to remove topically applied petroleum materials. Soft feed reduces irritation to the mouth and digestive tract. With severe gastrointestinal irritation, parenteral fluid therapy or nasogastric tube feeding may be necessary. Soothing ointments may be used topically to protect irritated skin, and antibiotics may be employed to reduce the potential for systemic infections.

Chromated Copper Arsenate-Treated Lumber

Intoxications associated with lumber treated with chromated copper arsenate (CCA) have been reported in cattle and suspected in horses. The cases in cattle were associated with ashes from treated lumber or sawdust and shavings used as bedding. A case of severe colic was seen in some cribbing horses. The horses survived but exhibited gastrointestinal distress and diarrhea. The CCA wood preservative consists of varying concentrations of arsenic acid (As_2O_5), chromic acid (CrO_3) and copper oxide (CuO).

The clinical signs in animals ingesting CCA-treated lumber products are similar to, if not identical with, arsenic intoxication. The roles of chromic acid and copper oxide in the development of the disease syndrome associated with CCA-treated lumber ingestion are unknown, but may be additive in nature. Diagnostic levels of arsenic (>10 ppm) have been found in livers and kidneys of animals dying after ingesting these products. Additional clinical signs associated with arsenic intoxication are as described in the section on inorganic chemicals (earlier). Treatment of CCA-intoxicated horses should include oral and/or intravenous sodium thiosulfate. The use of dimercaprol (BAL) should be considered in valuable animals.

Supplemental Readings

Bailey EM: Management and treatment of toxicosis in cattle. In Howard JL (ed): Current Veterinary Therapy: Food Animal Practice 2. Philadelphia, WB Saunders, 1986, pp 341–349.
Bailey EM, Garland T: Class Notes for Veterinary Toxicology, College Station, TX, College of Vet. Med. TAMU, 1995.
Edwards VC, Coppock RW, Zinn LL: Toxicosis related to the petroleum industry. Vet Hum Toxicol 21:328–337, 1979.
National Research Council: Mineral Tolerance of Domestic Animals. Washington, DC, National Academy of Science, 1980.
Oehme FW: Arsenic. In Robinson NE (ed): Current Therapy in Equine Medicine, ed 2. Philadelphia, WB Saunders, 1987, pp 668–670.
Oehme FW: Water quality. In Robinson NE (ed): Current Therapy in Equine Medicine, ed 2. Philadelphia, WB Saunders, 1987, pp 682–685.
Osweiler GD, Carson TL, Buck WB, van Gelder GA (eds): Clinical and Diagnostic Veterinary Toxicology, ed 3. Dubuque, IA, Kendall/Hunt Publishing, 1985.
Roberts MC, Seawright AA: The effects of prolonged daily low level mercuric chloride dosing in a horse. Vet Hum Toxicol 20(6):410–415.
Rowe LD, Dollahite JW, Camp BJ: Toxicity of two crude oils and of kerosene to cattle. J Am Vet Med Assoc 162:61–66, 1973.
Short SB, Edwards WC: Are your patients safe from unnecessary mercury poisoning? Vet Med March:287–293, 1988.
Shupe JL: Fluoride toxicosis. In Mansmann RA, McAllister ES (eds): Equine Medicine and Surgery, ed 3. Santa Barbara, CA, American Veterinary Publications, 1982, pp 199–203.
Teske RH: Polybrominated biphenyls. In Howard JL (ed): Current Veterinary Therapy: Food Animal Practice 2. Philadelphia, WB Saunders, 1986, pp 448–449.
Teske RH: Polychlorinated biphenyls. In Howard JL (ed): Current Veterinary Therapy: Food Animal Practice 2. Philadelphia, WB Saunders, 1986, pp 449–450.
Thatcher CD, Meldrum JB, Wikse SE, Whittier WD: Arsenic toxicosis and suspected chromium toxicosis in a herd of cattle. J Am Vet Med Assoc 187(2):179–182, 1985.
van Gelder GA: Tetrachlorodibenzodioxin (TCDD) toxicosis. In Mansmann RA, McAllister ES (eds): Equine Medicine and Surgery, ed 3. Santa Barbara, CA, American Veterinary Publications, 1982, p 189.

Feed-Associated Poisoning

MERL F. RAISBECK
Laramie, Wyoming

Equine poisoning most frequently results from ingestion. Although there are numerous potential feed contaminants, certain toxicants cause trouble much more frequently as the result of use in other domestic species, extreme potency in horses, or both.

IONOPHORES

The carboxylic ionophores such as monensin are added to the rations of poultry, swine, and cattle as coccidiostats and to enhance feed utilization. Chemically, the class is characterized by the ability to form lipid-soluble complexes with cations such as sodium or potassium. This property facilitates cation diffusion across biologic membranes. Although the ionophores have a good safety margin in target species, they are extremely toxic in equidae, apparently as the result of slower metabolism by these species.

Ionophore toxicity in any species is the result of the ionophore's ability to destroy transmembrane electrochemical gradients. Because many homeostatic mechanisms depend upon such gradients, disruption results in cell death. In equidae, the principal targets are mitochondria of highly energetic tissues such as the myocardium, kidney, diaphragm, and musculature.

Manufacturers and some researchers tout the relatively low toxicity of certain ionophores in horses. However, the relative hazard of products formulated for poultry or cattle under field conditions does not differ greatly between the different ionophores. Although horses may occasionally be poisoned as a result of access to cattle supplements on pasture, poisoning is usually the result of improper incorporation of medicated premixes into horse rations. Horses and other equidae should not be exposed to products containing ionophore feed additives under any circumstances.

Clinical Signs

The clinical signs of acute ionophore intoxication in horses are progressive and vary somewhat with dose and between individual animals. Signs usually include anorexia, abdominal pain, profuse intermittent sweating, and posterior ataxia characterized by a stiff gait and reluctance to move. Tachycardia and hypotension may occur within 8 to 12 hours after exposure, especially in peracute cases. Terminally, some horses may become hypertensive. Polyuria and tenesmus occur soon after intoxication. Later, poisoned animals may become oliguric. Hematuria is evident after 24 hours in some animals. Death may result from hypovolemic shock compounded by electrolyte losses within 24 to 48 hours of intoxication. Individuals that survive sublethal doses may succumb to complications of myocardial necrosis and scarring weeks or even months later.

Diagnosis

No practical method exists for detecting the ionophores in vital samples from acutely poisoned horses. For therapeutic purposes, diagnosis must be based upon clinical signs, clinicopathologic findings, and feed analysis. As signs develop, water loss from renal tubular damage is reflected in increased packed cell volume (PCV) and plasma protein concentration and by increased output of urine with a low specific gravity. Blood urea nitrogen (BUN) and creatinine levels may also become elevated. Later, elevated plasma levels of creatinine phosphokinase (CPK) and lactate dehydrogenase (LDH) coincide with skeletal and myocardial muscle necrosis. Serum calcium and potassium levels become depressed soon after the onset of clinical signs, and some individuals become hyperglycemic. Horses that die acutely may not have any diagnostically useful postmortem lesions. Horses that die later in the course of the disease may show degeneration and necrosis of myocardium, skeletal muscle, and renal cortex.

Therapy

No specific antidote is available for ionophore intoxication. Vitamin E and selenium provide some protection against monensin intoxication in cattle and swine, but the therapeutic utility in the horse is dubious. Calcium channel blockers have been suggested, but they actually potentiate monensin toxicity in rodents.

As with any oral intoxication, the first priority should be blocking absorption of toxicant remaining in the gastrointestinal (GI) tract. Either activated charcoal or mineral oil orally prevents uptake of the compound from the gut. Saline cathartics may also be useful to speed elimination, but autonomic cathartics and cardiac glycosides should be avoided. Supportive therapy includes aggressive parenteral fluid therapy to correct hypovolemia and support cardiovascular and renal function. If clinical laboratory support is readily available, it is desirable to monitor serum potassium levels and to use supplemental potassium to correct hypokalemia. However, supplemental calcium is not indicated unless hypocalcemia become severe.

Therapeutic management of horses that survive acute intoxication is primarily supportive. The author is aware of instances in which an apparently recovered horse or pony died peracutely weeks or months after recovering from acute monensin intoxication. In each instance, exercise or some other stressor appeared to induce arrhythmias, and the animal "dropped dead" in midstride. Thus, nursing care and stress reduction are indicated for several months in convalescing animals. In addition, owners should be warned against riding affected animals for several months after apparent recovery and not until the animals have been exercised hard with no signs of cardiac damage.

ANTIBIOTIC-ASSOCIATED COLITIS

The unique nature of the equine digestive system renders horses especially vulnerable to antibacterial agents. Fatal colitis in horse and ponies has resulted from feeding lincomycin, tylosin, tetracycline, and neomycin. Other antibacterial feed additives may also be capable of causing antibiotic-associated colitis, but this has not yet been documented. The pathogenesis of antibiotic-associated colitis is very poorly understood. Although there is agreement that the primary insult is antibiotic-stimulated overgrowth of toxigenic bacteria, their identity is controversial. In fact, there is no reason to doubt that different microbial genera may be involved in different cases. The variable nature of antibiotic-associated colitis is substantiated by the experimental observation that lincomycin (5 mg/kg p.o.) killed four of four ponies in one experiment, but had no observable effect on four additional ponies 3 months later. It is likely that antibiotic-associated colitis results from synergistic effects between diet, environment, and drug.

Clinical Signs

The onset of antibiotic-associated colitis is usually delayed 24 to 48 hours after oral exposure to contaminated feedstuffs. Initial clinical signs include profuse, watery, nonhemorrhagic diarrhea, anorexia, and lethargy. As the condition progresses, animals exhibit colic, moderate to severe tachycardia, muddy mucous membranes, and fever. Borborygmus may be decreased or absent. Severely affected animals become prostrate and die within 3 to 5 days. Clinicopathologic findings are typical of shock and dehydration. An initial transient neutropenia may be seen, but most cases are not examined until the hemogram has progressed to severe leukophilia and neutrophilia. The PCV and total protein levels are markedly elevated. The principal gross lesions are an edematous colon distended with serosanguinous fluid and a hemorrhagic adrenal medulla. Diffuse ecchymotic hemorrhages may be present on many of the visceral organs and blood may clot poorly. Most horses that survive the acute onslaught later develop laminitis. Although antibiotic residues may occasionally be detected in GI contents, the suspected feedstuff is the optimal sample for analysis.

Therapy

Because the bacterial agents responsible for the condition have not been conclusively identified, there is no specific antidote. Oral exchange resins such as cholestyramine ameliorate antibiotic-associated colitis in hamsters by preventing absorption of bacterial toxins, but these agents have not been evaluated in horses. Activated charcoal and mineral oil may be useful. Intravenous fluids should be tailored to replace fluid and electrolyte losses and should be used aggressively from the onset of clinical signs. Parenteral gentamicin and flunixin appear beneficial in resolving the acute crisis, as is phenylbutazone in ameliorating the subsequent laminitis. Rest and supportive care must be extended throughout convalescence to prevent a relapse.

BLISTER BEETLE (CANTHARIDIN)

Historically, blister beetle (*Epicauta* species) poisoning in horses fed alfalfa was a serious problem primarily in the southern Great Plains of the United States. Changes in alfalfa hay production during the last two to three decades have resulted in cases as far north as Illinois and Minnesota. The toxin, cantharidin, is contained in the hemolymph of adult beetles that feed on alfalfa in mid- to late summer. If the insects are trapped and crushed by crimping-type mowers, the toxin becomes incorporated into the hay and may remain toxic for years. Experimentally, as few as two to five beetles may produce colic in horses.

Clinical Signs

The severity of clinical signs varies with the dose of toxin from mild depression and anorexia to severe shock and death. Initial signs include anorexia, colic, apathy, and behavior that suggests oral irritation. Later, tenesmus and diaphragmatic flutter may be evident. Clinicopathologic findings include decreased serum calcium and magnesium concentrations, hypoproteinemia, low urine specific gravity, hematuria, and azotemia. Chemical analysis of urine and ingesta is essential to confirm a diagnosis of blister beetle intoxication. Considering the very small concentration usually present in urine, several hundred milliliters of urine may be necessary for successful analysis.

Therapy

Treatment is symptomatic. Mineral oil administration and osmotic diuresis speed elimination of the toxin. Gastrointestinal protectants should be given to minimize gastrointestinal damage and associated pain. Intravenous fluid replacement therapy should be tailored to the individual case by frequently monitoring serum electrolyte levels. If this is not possible, supplemental magnesium is indicated early in the disease. In horses that survive more than 24 to 48 hours, measurement of CPK levels may be used as a prognostic indicator of myocardial damage.

Alfalfa growers should inspect their fields before cutting when there is a possibility of insect swarms. Affected areas should either not be cut for hay or should be treated with malathion, and the appropriate withdrawal period observed before cutting. Horse owners should be aware of the potential hazard associated with feeding alfalfa and should buy hay only from reputable, known sources.

DICOUMAROL AND ANTICOAGULANT RODENTICIDES

Dicoumarol is a fungal metabolite of coumarin found in spoiled sweetclover hay. Once produced, the toxin may persist in hay for years. Although poisoning is most commonly reported in cattle, horses are also susceptible. Horses have also been poisoned by accidental incorporation of anticoagulant rodenticide baits in feedstuffs.

Clinical Signs

Clinical signs reflect bleeding and hypovolemia. Affected animals may exhibit pale mucous membranes, weak rapid pulse, and generalized weakness. Bleeding and bruising are common; however, the particular sites affected are more a function of the probability of local injury than of the toxin itself. Hematomas are commonly noted in areas of the neck, trunk, or limbs where there has been pressure or bruising, and in joints. Blood may be present in feces and around other orifices. Epistaxis is frequently one of the first signs in horses. Hematomas in various body cavities may result in blindness, paresis, lameness, or dyspnea.

Citrated blood may be evaluated for prothrombin (PT) and activated partial thromboplastin times (APTT), but the activated clotting time assay (ACT) has the dual advantages of being inexpensive and simple enough to run in the field or veterinary clinic. Definitive diagnosis requires identification of dicoumarol in blood, liver, or feed, but prolonged APTT, PT, or ACT results together with exposure to spoiled sweetclover are sufficient criteria for treatment.

Therapy

Vitamin K_1 is the specific antidote for dicoumarol poisoning and usually returns PT to normal within 12 to 24 hours. Specific dosage regimens are the subject of some controversy. With simple dicoumarol (sweetclover) poisoning, 1 to 2 mg/kg given in divided subcutaneous doses is usually sufficient. If the animal was poisoned by one of the newer anticoagulant rodenticides such as diphacinone or brodifacoum, treatment should be repeated as indicated by monitoring clotting times for 2 to 3 weeks.

Menadione, vitamin K_3, is of little benefit in anticoagulant poisoning and may cause acute renal failure in horses. It is therefore not recommended. Although intravenous vitamin K_1 preparations are available, intravenous administration has been associated with a high incidence of adverse reactions. Phenylbutazone, salicylates, aminoglycosides, and sulfonamides may potentiate the effects of anticoagulants and thus are contraindicated.

Severely anemic patients should be transfused with whole blood. If possible, blood from the donor and recipient should be cross-matched before transfusion, especially if the recipient has been transfused previously. Transfusions of whole blood or plasma reverse bleeding, but the transfused clotting factors are soon exhausted and bleeding resumes. Additional fluids may be indicated for the severely hypovolemic patient. Thoracocentesis may be necessary if there is severe dyspnea due to hemothorax.

SELENIUM

Selenium (Se) was first associated with poisoning of horses and cattle during the 1930s. In some geographic areas, notably the western Great Plains, selenosis may result from naturally seleniferous feedstuffs produced on high-selenium soils. In the rest of North America, selenosis is an iatrogenic disease associated with oversupplementation.

Clinical Signs

Clinical signs of selenosis in horses are determined by the dose and duration of Se exposure. Relatively large doses of Se (on the order of 5 mg/kg) may result in acute poisoning characterized by gastrointestinal, renal, hepatic, and cardiac damage. Lassitude, anorexia, and colic are followed by muscular weakness, frequent urination, dys-

pnea, and recumbency. The pulse and respiration rate are likely to be increased, but systemic blood pressure is decreased, as reflected in prolonged capillary refill time and cold extremities. Terminal signs include cyanotic mucous membranes and coma.

Chronic selenosis, either from Se feedstuffs or from oversupplementation, results in hair loss and damage to epithelial structures of the hoof. Signs first appear 30 to 90 days after introduction to a toxic diet. Affected horses exhibit a slight erythema, swelling, and alopecia of the skin just proximal to the coronary band. These signs are rather subtle and may not be noticed by the owner. Approximately 10 days after the initial swelling, a horizontal crack develops just distal to the coronary band, and affected animals become noticeably lame. At about the same time, hair shafts in the mane and tail become quite friable and prone to breakage, leading to alopecia. As the hoof grows out, the crack deepens, and eventually the entire toe sloughs off the hoof. Lameness becomes so severe that affected animals refuse to rise, even to eat or drink, and the animals become severely debilitated. Contrary to statements in many older texts, horses do not become blind.

Therapy

No specific antidote is available for either acute or chronic selenosis. Although there are substances (notably arsenic and the cyanogenic glycosides) that speed elimination of selenium, they are impractical as therapeutic agents. Supportive therapy for acute poisoning should be aimed at replacing fluid losses, treating shock, and easing gastrointestinal irritation. Glutathione precursors such as N-acetylcysteine should theoretically be helpful, but there are no controlled studies to confirm this. The prognosis of acute selenosis is very grave, with or without treatment.

Chronic selenosis may be treated successfully in horses if owners are willing to commit to a prolonged course of nursing care. Easily available clean water and feedstuffs with a low selenium content are the cornerstones of therapy. Adequate bedding should be provided to prevent or alleviate pressure sores in animals that will spend much time recumbent. Heart bar shoes, a sand floor, and analgesics should be used to minimize pain associated with hoof separation. In the author's experience, it requires 6 to 12 months to return an affected animal to soundness.

Other feed-associated poisonings include aflatoxicosis (see page 669) and botulism (see page 326).

Supplemental Readings

Amend JF, Mallon FM, Wren WB, Ramos AS: Equine monensin toxicosis: Some experimental clinicopathologic observations. Comp Cont Ed Vet 2:S173–S183, 1980.

Amend JF, Nichelson RL, King RS, Mallon FM, Freeland L: Equine monensin toxicosis: Useful ante-mortem and post-mortem clinicopathologic tests. Proc 31st Annu Meet Am Assoc Equine Pract, 1985, pp 361–371.

Casper H, Willard J: Moldy Sweet Clover Poisoning. Extension monograph. Fargo, ND, North Dakota State University, 1986.

Kohn CW: Colitis-X. In Robinson NE (ed): Current Therapy in Equine Medicine. Philadelphia, WB Saunders, 1983, pp 200–207.

Prescott JF, Staempfli HR, Barker K, Bettoni R, Delaney K: A method for reproducing fatal idiopathic colitis in ponies and isolation of a clostridium as a possible agent. Equine Vet J 20:417–420, 1988.

Raisbeck MF, Dahl ER, Sanchez DA, O'Toole D, Belden EL: Naturally occurring selenosis in Wyoming. J Vet Diagn Invest 5:84–87, 1993.

Schmitz DG: Cantharidin toxicosis in horses. J Vet Intern Med 3:208–215, 1989.

Schoeb TR, Panciera RJ: Pathology of blister beetle (*Epicauta*) poisoning in horses. Vet Pathol 16:18–31, 1979.

Smyth JBA, Wang JH, Barlow RM, Humphreys DJ, Robins M, Stodulski JBJ: Experimental acute selenium intoxication in lambs. J Comp Pathol 102:197–209, 1990.

Whitlock RH: Colitis: Differential diagnosis and treatment. Equine Vet J 18(4):278–283, 1986.

Witte ST, Will LA, Olsen CR, Kinker JA, Miller-Graber P: Chronic selenosis in horses fed locally produced alfalfa hay. J Am Vet Med Assoc 202:406–409, 1993.

Mycotoxins

KONSTANZE H. PLUMLEE
Davis, California

This chapter describes six mycotoxins that are reported to cause clinical disease in horses. Fescue toxicosis is also associated with a fungus, but is discussed elsewhere (see page 670).

FUMONISIN B$_1$

Corn can be contaminated with *Fusarium moniliforme* to produce mycotoxins called fumonisins. Fumonisin B$_1$ is the most common fumonisin found. The mold is usually found in corn, such as screenings, that has been damaged by insects or adverse weather conditions. *F. moniliforme* has also been isolated from pelleted feeds. Most strains of this fungus do not produce toxins; therefore, finding moldy feed does not necessarily mean that the feed is toxic. Furthermore, feed that looks normal can contain mycotoxins. Therefore, a diagnosis cannot be based on visual evaluation of the feed.

Fumonisin B$_1$ concentrations in excess of 10 ppm in the feed can cause disease in horses. Contaminated feed is usually ingested over several weeks before clinical signs occur. Disease is usually seen from late fall through early spring when wet weather follows a dry growing season. Morbidity may be low, but mortality may reach 100%.

This mycotoxin can affect the nervous system or the liver of horses. Lower doses over a longer period of time are more commonly associated with neurologic disease, whereas high doses of the mycotoxin may cause hepatosis.

The neurologic disease is known as *leukoencephalomalacia*. Clinical signs usually appear suddenly and include ataxia, blindness, depression, hyperexcitability, and head pressing. Death frequently occurs within 1 to 3 days of the onset of clinical signs. Sudden death, without prior clinical signs, has also been reported. Animals that survive often have persistent neurologic deficits.

The primary lesion of leukoencephalomalacia is liquefactive necrosis of the white matter of one or both cerebral hemispheres. Lesions may also occur in the cerebellum, brain stem, or spinal cord. The gray matter is affected occasionally. The protein concentration and white cell counts in the cerebrospinal fluid (CSF) are elevated. Hemorrhage, malacia, and perivascular cuffing in the brain can be present histologically.

The hepatic form of fumonisin B$_1$ toxicosis may be accompanied by icterus, edema, hemorrhage, and hepatoencephalopathy. Serum bilirubin concentrations and hepatic enzyme activities may be increased. Lesions include centrilobular necrosis, periportal fibrosis, periportal vacuolation, and bile duct proliferation. Recovery from hepatosis is more likely than from the neurologic disease.

The pathophysiology of either form of toxicosis is not completely understood. Treatment consists mostly of supportive care because no antidote exists. Aggressive treatment with anti-inflammatory drugs may aid in survival in some patients. Diagnosis is based on history, clinical signs, lesions, and the presence of toxic levels of fumonisin B$_1$ in the feed. To date, the only successful preventive measure is to test feed for the mycotoxin before feeding it to horses. It is recommended to not feed corn that contains excessive broken kernels or debris, such as corn screenings.

SLAFRAMINE

Red clover and other legumes can be infested with *Rhizoctonia leguminicola* to produce a disease in the forage known as *black patch*. This disease appears on the stems and leaves as dark spots or concentric rings. This fungus is commonly found in soil and is transmitted in the seed. During wet, humid weather, the fungal mycelia grow in the cotyledons. The fungus can produce a toxic metabolite, slaframine.

Slaframine is known as "slobber factor" because the most common clinical sign is excessive salivation. Anorexia, diarrhea, frequent urination, and excessive lacrimation have also been reported. The disease usually occurs after consumption of second-cutting legume hay or forage with black patch. It has been diagnosed in the United States and Canada.

Slaframine may interact with one or more of several muscarinic receptor subtypes. In clinical trials, preadministration of muscarinic antagonists, such as atropine, blocks the production of excessive salivation. However, clinical signs are not alleviated if the atropine is given after the slaframine. Although a successful treatment has not been found, signs disappear within 2 to 4 days after the animal has been removed from the source of the slaframine.

LOLITREM B

Perennial ryegrass staggers occurs when perennial ryegrass is infested with the fungus *Acremonium lolii* to produce a mycotoxin, lolitrem B. The fungus is propagated through the ryegrass seed, and 75% of the fungal mycelia are found in the lowest 2 cm of the plant. Some seed lines of perennial ryegrass are resistant to the fungus; however, these seeds produce poor stands of grass and so are not favored by producers.

Ryegrass staggers has been reported in western North America, New Zealand, and Australia. The disease is seen mostly in the summer and early fall when pastures are drought-stressed and overgrazed. At that time, the animals are more likely to graze the lower part of the plant where most of the fungus is found. Clinical signs usually appear several days after a heavy dew or light rainfall.

Initially, the clinical signs include head tremors and muscle fasciculations of the neck and legs. A head nod develops, and the animals sway while standing as the disease progresses. Dysmetria, collapse, and tetanic spasms occur if the animals are excited or forced to move. After a few minutes, the animal recovers from the tetany and walks with a relatively normal gait. Death can occur if the animal suffers an accident such as drowning during a tetanic episode.

Gross lesions usually are not seen in animals affected with ryegrass staggers. Chronically affected animals may have loss of Purkinje's cells in the cerebellum. The toxic mechanism of lolitrem B is not known.

No reliable treatment is available for ryegrass staggers. Animals with mild clinical signs usually recover in a few weeks after removal from the ryegrass. Management strategies focus on minimizing animal exposure to the infested ryegrass. Strategies include proper management to avoid overgrazing of pastures, offering alternative feed sources, or removal of animals from ryegrass pastures during late summer and fall when the disease is more likely to occur.

PASPALITREMS

Dallis grass (*Paspalum dilatatum*) and bahia grass (*Bahia oppositifolia*) can become infested with the fungus *Claviceps paspali*. This fungus overwinters in the soil, releasing its spores when the grasses flower. The spores germinate in the flowers and invade the ovaries of the plant. A sticky exudate called honeydew is produced. The fungus replaces the ovary, hardens, and forms a sclerotium or ergot. The fungus can produce a group of toxic metabolites known as the paspalitrems.

When these toxins are ingested, they can produce a disease known as paspalum staggers or dallis grass staggers. This disease has been reported in cattle, sheep, and horses in the southern United States and New Zealand. Cattle are more often affected than horses or sheep, probably because they are more likely to graze the seed heads where the toxin is located.

The paspalitrems are tremorgenic, causing clinical signs similar to those seen with perennial ryegrass staggers, but not as severe. No gross or microscopic lesions have been reported in affected animals.

The mechanism of action of the paspalitrems is not well understood. No specific treatment for the disease is available. Therefore, treatment is based on supportive care and removing the animals from the infested pasture. Mowing the field decreases the number of toxic seed heads. Affected animals recover within a few weeks after being removed from the source of the toxins.

MACROCYCLIC TRICHOTHECENES

Stachybotrys atra (S. alternans) is a soil fungus that grows well on cellulose-rich substrates. It appears as a sooty, black accumulation on straw or hay. This fungus produces several mycotoxins, known collectively as the macrocyclic trichothecenes. Stachybotryotoxicosis has been reported in horses, swine, sheep, and cattle. Horses seem particularly susceptible; thousands of horses have reportedly died from this disease in Europe, Africa, and the Soviet Union. As of yet, no cases have been reported in North America.

Stachybotryotoxicosis can occur in horses as either a chronic or peracute disease. The chronic form is the more common manifestation and can occur in three stages. The first stage involves inflammation of the lips and oral mucosa that can proceed to necrosis. The horse may refuse to eat and can have nasal discharge and excessive salivation. The swelling can continue to the subcutaneous tissue, lymph glands, and eyes, resulting in conjunctivitis and excessive lacrimation. This stage may be mild or may last for up to one month.

The second stage of the chronic form can occur if the horse continues to eat contaminated feed. The animal develops leukopenia with a marked decrease in neutrophils. The animal also has decreased thrombocytes and an increased clotting time. The second stage usually lasts 2 to 7 weeks.

The third stage usually lasts for only a few days. It is accompanied by an increased severity of the leukopenia and thrombocytopenia. The animal can also develop an elevated body temperature, colic, and an arrhythmic, weak pulse. The horse will become recumbent and die.

The peracute or atypical form of stachybotryotoxicosis usually occurs after the horse consumes a larger amount of toxin. Reported clinical signs include nervous system irritability, cardiac and circulatory depression, colic, pulmonary edema, and cyanosis. The animal usually dies in 1 to 3 days after exposure.

Postmortem lesions are primarily hemorrhage and necrosis of the serous and mucous membranes of the digestive tract. Diagnosis is based on finding the mycotoxins in the hay or straw being fed to animals with appropriate clinical signs and lesions.

Treatment is limited to supportive care because no antidote is available.

AFLATOXINS

Many cereal grains, especially peanuts, corn, and cottonseed, can be contaminated with *Aspergillus flavus* and

Aspergillus parasiticus. These fungal species can produce aflatoxins, especially under wet, warm conditions. Although aflatoxicosis has been widely reported in many species, reports in horses have been scarce. Horses seem to be more resistant to the disease, although when it does occur, the clinical signs and lesions are similar to those reported in other species.

Clinical signs of aflatoxicosis in horses include depression, anorexia, weight loss, icterus, and subcutaneous hemorrhages. Some horses have increased body temperatures. Death occurs several days after the onset of clinical signs. The liver is the primary organ affected. The most consistent clinical pathology finding is a dramatic increase in plasma levels of sorbitol dehydrogenase (SDH). The levels of gamma-glutamyl transferase (GGT) are often elevated in many horses. A defect in hemostasis is a common sequela to the liver disease, and affected animals often have increased prothrombin time, resulting in subcutaneous hemorrhage.

Microscopically, the liver has centrilobular necrosis with varying degrees of biliary hyperplasia. Lipid accumulation has been noted in the proximal tubules, liver, and myocardium. Cerebral edema and neuronal degeneration have been seen in some cases.

Diagnosis is based on clinical signs, lesions, and finding aflatoxin in the grain being fed. A correlation exists between the presence of aflatoxin B and kojic acid, a chemical found in moldy feed. Kojic acid fluoresces under ultraviolet light, and thus feed can be screened with a black light. However, false-positive and false-negative results have been reported with this screening method, and thus it is not recommended for making a diagnosis. Determining the actual concentration of aflatoxin in the feed is the only definitive method of making a diagnosis. Occasionally, a diagnosis has been made by finding aflatoxins in the liver of affected horses. However, aflatoxins are quickly metabolized and thus usually are not found in the liver.

Treatment is limited to supportive care because aflatoxisis has no antidote. Clinicians must choose medications carefully because the liver and possibly the kidneys are compromised. If subcutaneous hemorrhage is present, treatment with vitamin K_1 may be beneficial.

Supplemental Readings

Aller WW, Edds GT, Asquith RL: Effects of aflatoxins in young ponies. Am J Vet Res 42:2162–2164, 1981.

Angsubhakorn S, Poomvises P, Romruen K, Newberne PM: Aflatoxicosis in horses. J Am Vet Med Assoc 178:274–278, 1981.

Asquith RL, Edds GT: Investigations in equine aflatoxicosis. Proc 26th Annu Conf Am Assoc Equine Pract 26:193–199, 1980.

Burrows GE, Edwards WC, Tyrl RJ: Toxic plants of Oklahoma: Grasses. Okla Vet Med Assoc J 39:25–29, 1987.

Cole RJ: Fungal tremorgens. J Food Protection 44(9):715–722, 1981.

Galey FD, Tracy ML, Craigmill AL, Barr BC, Markegard G, Peterson R, O'Connor M: Staggers induced by consumption of perennial ryegrass in cattle and sheep from northern California. J Am Vet Med Assoc 199:466–470, 1991.

Hagler WM, Behlow RF: Salivary syndrome in horses: Identification of slaframine in red clover hay. Appl Environ Microbiol 42:1067–1073, 1981.

Hintz HF: Molds, mycotoxins, and mycotoxicosis. Vet Clin North Am Equine Pract 6:419–431, 1990.

Latch GCM.: Endophytes and ryegrass staggers. *In* Lacey J (ed): Trichothecenes and Other Mycotoxins. New York, John Wiley & Sons, 1985.

McCue PM: Equine leukoencephalomalacia. Comp Cont Ed Pract Vet 11:646–650, 1989.

Mortimer PH, di Menna ME: Interactions of *Lolium* endophyte on pasture production and perennial ryegrass staggers disease. *In* Lacey J (ed): Trichothecenes and Other Mycotoxins. New York, John Wiley & Sons, 1985.

Nicholson SS: Tremorgenic syndromes in livestock. Vet Clin North Am Food Anim Pract 5:291–292, 1989.

Plumlee KH, Galey FD: Neurotoxic mycotoxins: A review of fungal toxins that cause neurological disease in large animals. J Vet Intern Med 8:49–54, 1994.

Smith JE, Henderson RS: Stachybotryotoxicosis in horses. *In* Mycotoxins and Animal Foods Boca Raton, FL, CRC Press, 1991, pp 682–683.

Sockett DC, Baker JC, Stowe CM: Slaframine (*Rhizoctonia leguminicola*) intoxication in horses. J Am Vet Med Assoc 181:606, 1982.

Tantaoui-Elaraki A, Mekouar SL, Hamidi ME, Senhaji M: Toxigenic strains of *Stachybotrys atra* associated with poisonous straw in Morocco. Vet Human Toxicol 36:93–96, 1994.

Wilkins PA, Vaala WE, Zivotofsky D, Twitchell ED: A herd outbreak of equine leukoencephalomalacia. Cornell Vet 84:53–59, 1994.

Wilson TM, Ross PF, Rice LG, Osweiler GD, Nelson HA, Owens DL, Plattner RD, Reggiardo C, Noon TH, Pickrell JW: Fumonisin B_1 levels associated with an epizootic of equine leukoencephalomalacia. J Vet Diagn Invest 2:213–216, 1990.

Fescue Toxicosis

ELEANOR M. GREEN
Knoxville, Tennessee

MERL F. RAISBECK
Laramie, Wyoming

Tall fescue (*Festuca arundinaceae*) was associated with agalactia, prolonged gestation, and stillborn foals in pregnant mares for many years before documented reports appeared during the early 1980s. Since that time, grazing tall fescue during late pregnancy has been incriminated as causing abortion, dystocia, premature separation of the chorion, and thickened and retained placentas. These, in turn, may result in sterility, death, and high foal mortality. Given the ubiquitous nature of fescue pastures in the southeastern United States, approximately 35 million acres, and its increasing presence nationwide, the potential magnitude of this problem becomes evident.

FESCUE TOXINS

The exact identity of the tall fescue toxins is the subject of some debate. Nonetheless, it is widely accepted that the toxicity of tall fescue in both ruminants and horses is due to one or more vasoactive ergopeptine alkaloids, such as ergovaline. Although these alkaloids are pharmacologically similar to the ergot alkaloids produced on grains by *Claviceps*, they are produced within the fescue stem and leaf by the fungus *Acremonium coenophialum* and remain active in hay.

Because *A. coenophialum* spends its entire life cycle within the vegetative parts of its host plant, tall fescue, it is impossible to recognize an infected plant visually. Determining the extent of endophyte infection in a pasture requires laboratory analysis of a representative sample of plants collected from that pasture. Infection rates greater than 80% are commonly held to pose a severe hazard to pregnant mares, although infection rates as low as 5% are not necessarily safe. Pastures should be evaluated in the fall before the breeding season.

At present, analysis of the fescue endophyte is done either by microscopic examination or by one of several immunoassays. Diagnostic methodologies vary between laboratories, and thus it is best to consult with the laboratory doing the analysis regarding the specific number of samples, requirements for preservation, and shipping methods before sampling. The local county agent should be able to assist with locating a convenient testing laboratory. Currently there are no analytic methodologies sufficiently sensitive or robust for routine use in detecting the toxic alkaloids in affected mares or foals.

PATHOPHYSIOLOGY

The dopaminergic fescue alkaloids inhibit prolactin secretion by the anterior pituitary gland. As the name suggests, prolactin is integrally involved in the process of mammary gland development and lactation. In horses, high circulating levels of prolactin are most critical in the process of lactation during the last 2 weeks of gestation and the first few weeks after foaling. Underlying dopaminergic mechanisms may be common to the seemingly diverse effects of fescue on the pregnant mare and foal, although the exact mechanisms for abnormalities other than agalactia are not clear. Mares grazing endophyte-infected tall fescue pastures during late gestation have decreased serum concentrations of prolactin and progesterone and increased serum concentrations of estrogen. Prolonged gestation may result in oversized foals, which create problems with delivery. Paradoxically, these oversized foals may appear dysmature, with large poorly muscled frames, abnormal eruption of teeth, and overgrown hooves.

Mortality associated with parturition appears to be related not only to foal size, but also to the physiologic unreadiness of the mare and foal for parturition. Inadequate relaxation of the pelvic ligaments and musculature result in dystocia and soft tissue trauma to the reproductive tract. The full-term fetus does not contribute adequately to parturition because it fails to position itself properly during delivery. The placenta begins to thicken several hours before parturition, leading to premature separation of the chorion. The placental abnormalities result in neonatal asphyxia.

There is new evidence that nonpregnant mares grazing endophyte-infected tall fescue have some fertility problems. The estrous cycle is altered owing to prolonged diestrus, more estrous cycles are required for pregnancy, and there is also a higher incidence of early embryonic loss.

PREVENTION, THERAPY, AND MANAGEMENT

Prevention is the most effective and economical approach to fescue toxicity in mares. The most effective method of prevention is to avoid infected fescue pastures before day 21 of gestation and after day 300 of gestation (i.e., avoid the first 21 days and last 30 days of gestation). Endophyte-infected fescue can be: (1) replaced with endophyte-free fescue; (2) replaced or diluted with other forages and feedstuffs during late pregnancy; or (3) managed to prevent flowering.

Because infected fescue seed is the principal means of propagation by the endophyte, relatively clean pastures can be established by planting only endophyte-free seed (Table 1). *A. coenophialum* can be eliminated from infected fescue

TABLE 1. MANAGEMENT OF ENDOPHYTE FUNGUS-INFECTED PASTURE

Determination of Infection	
When to Test:	
Forage	May through December (ideally in fall)
Stored seed	Anytime
Procedure for Sampling:	
Seed from field	Random samples representative of field
	30 sample sites/field
	Total of 2 oz of seeds
Stored seed	Single sample for <2000 lbs
	Seed from several bags; mix subsamples
	Total of 2 oz of seeds
Forage	Random samples representing all areas seeded at different dates
	30 sample sites/field or 5/acre
	3 *stems* per sample site
	Cut large green stems at ground level and at top to fit test tubes
	Fill test tubes $\frac{1}{2}$ full with water.
Methods of analysis	Tissue-staining microscopy
	ELISA (antifungal rabbit antibodies)
	Tissue-print immunoblot
Pasture Management Options	
Complete renovation	Kill with herbicides or tillage
	Replant with certified fungus-free fescue seed or other grass seed
	Infected seed becomes endophyte-free if stored 2 years, heat treated, or fungicide treated
Dilution of infected herbage	Overseed with legume every 2 years
	Maintain legume rate of 20%
	Mow frequently
	Supplement with alfalfa hay ad lib

Extrapolated from Livestock Nutrition Laboratory Services, P.O. Box 1655, Columbia, MO 65205; test tubes can be ordered from this address.

TABLE 2. MANAGEMENT OF BROOD MARES GRAZING ENDOPYHYTE FUNGUS–INFECTED PASTURE

Diet	
Avoid affected herbage	Remove to endophyte fungus-free
During first 21 days of gestation	pasture
During last 30 days of gestation	Dry lot; provide alfalfa or
	endophyte-free hay.
If impossible to avoid infected	Provide high-quality alfalfa hay ad
pasture, dilute endophyte	lib
fungus (cannot depend on this	Pasture management, as described
method)	in Table 1

Lactation	
Monitor mammary gland	Last 30 days of gestation
development	
If milk not observed 1–2 weeks	Some potential drugs for inducing
before due date, remove from	prolactin and subsequent
fescue pasture and/or initiate	lactation:
medication to induce prolactin.	Domperidone (1.1 mg/kg p.o.
These drugs may be	s.i.d.)
administered beginning 10–20	Perphenazine (0.3 to 0.5 mg/kg
days before expected foaling	p.o. b.i.d.)
date (ideal) or upon recognition	Reserpine (2.0 to 2.5 mg/day/
of agalactia after foaling (less	horse p.o. s.i.d.)
desirable)	

Parturition	
Attend parturition	Prepare for dystocia
	Record predicted date of
	parturition
	Could monitor late-term fetus as
	parturition nears
	Veterinarian should be contacted
	in advance of mare's due date
	Ideally veterinarian should attend
	the birth
	Emergency situation if red bag is
	observed, foal is malpositioned,
	or if foal is not delivered within
	30 minutes!
	Manually assisted delivery ideal, if
	successful
	Cesarean section is an option if
	foal still alive
	Fetotomy as last resort

seed by a number of simple methods such as heat, long-term storage, or fungicide treatment, and endophyte-free seed is commercially available. Unfortunately, the relationship between tall fescue and *A. coenophialum* is symbiotic rather than commensal or parasitic. Endophyte-free fescue is considerably less hardy than infected fescue, negating one of the prime virtues of this species as a pasture grass. Thus, endophyte-free pastures require better management than infected pastures and can prove difficult to establish in the more southern states. If the endophyte-infected grass and seed are not completely eliminated before planting endophyte-free fescue or other pasture grasses, endophyte-infected grass eventually dominates the mix. Ammoniation of endophyte-infected hay results in increased serum prolactin concentrations in cattle; however, the safety and efficacy of this process has not been evaluated in horses.

In circumstances where outright replacement of infected fescue is impractical, dietary dilution of the fescue alkaloids

by overseeding pastures with legumes such as red or white clover, or by supplemental feeding with good-quality legume hay may be tried. Optimally, overseeding should be repeated as necessary, usually every 2 years, to result in 20% dietary legumes. It should be noted that dilution with legumes did not alter the incidence of fescue toxicosis in one study of pregnant mares.

Both the endophyte and its associated toxins tend to peak as the fescue flowers and are concentrated near the seedhead of infected plants. Thus, the total dietary alkaloid concentration can be decreased by mowing or grazing infected pastures so as to prevent setting seed. It must be stressed, however, that this procedure does not decrease the overall infection of a pasture and is thus a temporary measure.

The most commonly reported problem in mares that graze tall fescue pastures is agalactia or hypogalactia (Table 2). Even after initiation of lactation, colostrum quality may be poor, resulting in immunocompromised foals. Mammary development should be monitored in mares on fescue during the last month of pregnancy, and if insufficient, measures should be instituted to promote mammary development and milk production. Domperidone, perphenazine, and reserpine are reportedly beneficial in stimulating mammary development and lactation and in preventing the other described reproductive abnormalities when treatment is initiated before parturition. Domperidone is currently available only a field-trial basis, although it is expected to be approved for use in pregnant mares in the very near future. Domperidone is administered orally at a dose of 1.1 mg/kg once daily, starting 10 to 20 days before parturition. Perphenazine, approved only as a human drug, is effective at a dose of 0.3 to 0.5 mg/kg b.i.d. A rare side effect of perphenazine is extrapyramidal signs, including

TABLE 3. MANAGEMENT OF THE FOAL BORN TO A MARE GRAZING ENDOPHYTE FUNGUS–INFECTED PASTURE

Prepare for	Veterinarian should be informed of mare's due date
neonatal	Fetus could be monitored during late gestation
emergency	Ideally veterinarian should attend the birth
and critical	*Emergency* situation if red bag is observed, if foal is
care	malpositioned, or if foal is not delivered within
	30 minutes!
	Foal may require treatment in neonatal intensive
	care unit
Ensure adequate	Colostrum from dam (unlikely)
antibodies	Quality colostrum from colostrum bank
	Quality colostrum from another mare
	Antibodies given intravenously (plasma, serum)
	Measure foal's serum IgG before and after
	treatment
	Monitor closely for signs of sepsis
Nutrition	Daily requirement for average foal is 150 kcal/kg
	Mare's milk
	500 ml/hr
	Cow's milk (2%)
	Supplemented with 20 g dextrose/L
	500 ml/hr
	Commercial milk replacers, as directed
	Nurse mare
	Nurse goat
	Parenteral nutrition, if necessary

excitability and hyperesthesia. These signs have consistently resolved upon cessation of treatment; if signs do not resolve, diphenhydramine (Benadryl) is warranted. Reserpine has been used at a dose of 2.0 to 2.5 mg/kg per horse s.i.d. P.O. Reserpine is a potent drug with prolonged pharmacologic action and potentially severe side effects.

The mare should be closely monitored for problems during foaling because of the high probability of dystocia, neonatal asphyxia, and agalactia. An alternate source of both antibodies, such as colostrum from another mare, and nutrients (see page 582) should be readily available. If there is any question as to whether the foal has nursed adequately, supplemental colostrum should be given (Table 3).

Although the ideal prevention for fescue intoxication in pregnant mares is avoidance of the toxin, the widespread use of this grass as a forage source ensures that veterinarians and livestock owners will be confronting this problem for the foreseeable future. Endophyte-infected fescue can be safely used as a forage for pregnant brood mares if proper management and therapeutic measures are followed.

Supplemental Readings

Boosinger TR, Brendemuehl JP, Bransby DL, Wright JC, Kemppainen RJ, Kee DD: Prolonged gestation, decreased triiodothyronine concentrations, and thyroid gland histomorphologic features in newborn foals of mares grazing *Acremonion coenophialum*-infected fescue. Am J Vet Res 56:66–69, 1995.

Brendemuehl JP, Boosinger TR, Pugh DG, Shelby RA: Influence of endophyte-infected tall fescue on cyclicity, pregnancy rate and early embryonic loss in the mare. Theriogenology 42:489–500, 1994.

Cross DL: Effects and remedial therapy associated with the toxins of fescue in gravid mares. Proc 40th Annu Meet Am Assoc Equine Pract, 1994, pp 33–34.

Cross DL, Redmond LM, Strickland JR: Equine fescue toxicosis: Signs and solutions. J Anim Sci 73:899–908, 1995.

Green EM, Loch WE, Messer NT: Maternal and fetal effects of endophyte fungus-infected fescue. Proc 37th Annu Meet Am Assoc Equine Pract, 1991, pp 29–44.

Redmond LM, Cross DL, Strickland JR, Kennedy SW: Efficacy of domperidone and sulpiride as treatments for fescue toxicosis in horses. Am J Vet Res 55:722–729, 1994.

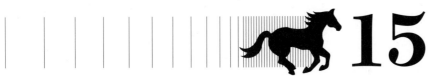

15

NUTRITION

Edited by Laurie Lawrence

Selecting and Utilizing Manufactured Feeds

LESLIE H. BREUER, JR.
East Alton, Illinois

The process of formulating and manufacturing horse feeds has become more sophisticated in the past 20 years as a result of the application of new research results and from the influx into industry of qualified equine nutritionists. Although these changes have resulted in more effective products and programs, there also has been a large increase in the number of horse feed types and forms available to the consumer. This chapter provides information for practitioners to use in evaluating feeding programs on horse farms and in selecting the appropriate feeds to improve the general health and productivity of horses. The practitioner should be able to provide a general evaluation of the nutritional program and determine whether there is a need to obtain assistance from other sources to help solve possible nutritional problems. Characteristics of manufactured feeds are discussed, along with suggestions on evaluating and selecting feeds to meet nutritional needs encountered under typical field conditions.

Advantages accrue to both the client and practitioner from using manufactured feeds. All the required nutrients can be combined in one or two products in the correct quantities in stable available forms, which are uniformly blended into a palatable manufactured feed. By using a manufactured feed, the client is saved the time and inconvenience of locating all the ingredients needed and properly formulating and feeding the resulting home mix. When manufactured feeds are used, the practitioner can be more confident that the nutritional recommendations are being carried out properly. From an economic standpoint, the use of manufactured feeds may be more cost-effective than generally assumed.

Although there are advantages to the use of manufactured feeds, both client and practitioner should be aware that there are no specific regulations or guidelines that must be followed in formulating and manufacturing horse feeds as long as the feeds do not contain drugs regulated by the Food and Drug Administration or Environmental Protection Agency. The labeling of horse feeds is regulated by commercial feed control laws passed and enforced by the individual states. Thus, it is possible for an individual or business entity to begin the manufacture and sale of a nutritional product or feed with no demonstrated nutritional expertise or product performance just by preparing a label that conforms to state feed control laws and paying the appropriate tonnage tax. Thus, there is a need for an informed consumer.

TYPES OF MANUFACTURED FEEDS

The system outlined in Table 1 for classifying manufactured horse feeds is intended to help explain the differences between the wide variety of feed and nutritional products offered to the horse owner. The system arranges feed types in the order of increasing complexity from those containing a limited number of nutrients to those that are complete feeds containing all nutrients and ingredients required by horses. The first group of feed types usually provides nutrients required in small quantities and are used to supplement other feeds. For example, the first type listed is a vitamin supplement containing one or more vitamins. The next is a multivitamin-mineral supplement containing vitamins and trace minerals. Some multivitamin-mineral supplements may contain nutrients such as essential fatty acids and amino acids as well as various "exotic"

TABLE 1. TYPES OF SUPPLEMENTS AND MANUFACTURED HORSE FEEDS

Vitamin supplements
    Single vitamins—vitamin A, vitamin E, vitamin B$_{12}$, etc.
    Combined vitamins—fat-soluble, water-soluble, or both
    Vitamins with additions—yeast, extracts, etc.
Multivitamin/trace mineral supplements
    Combined vitamins and trace minerals
    Vitamins and trace minerals with additions—yeast, extracts, "natural" ingredients, etc.
Mineral supplements
    Salt (NaCl)—with or without trace minerals
    Electrolytes—combinations of NaCl and KCl, with or without the addition of other minerals and sugar
    Calcium/phosphorus mixes—usually a combination of Ca and P but may be one or the other; percentages of each must be shown on feed tag
    Ca/P mixes with trace minerals—iron, copper, manganese, iodine, selenium, and other minerals may be added; vitamin A may also be added
Protein supplements
    Protein ingredients only
    Protein ingredients with other nutrients added—one or more nutrients may be added, including synthetic amino acids, salt, calcium, phosphorus, trace minerals, and vitamins
Energy feeds
    Grain and grain byproduct mixes only
    Energy ingredients with other nutrients added—one or more nutrients may be added including protein, minerals, and vitamins
Roughage feeds
    Roughage or forage ingredients only
    Roughage ingredients with other nutrients added—one or more nutrients may be added, including energy, protein, minerals, and vitamins

ingredients. The vitamin supplement segment of the feed industry often seems to place more emphasis on the length of the ingredient list and the content of various exotic ingredients than on meeting recognized nutritional needs. Generally, horse owners do not consider these supplements as part of the feeding program but rather as "insurance" to correct unrecognized deficiencies present in horse rations. This rationale is often erroneous, because the supplements may actually be providing excessive levels of nutrients such as iodine, vitamin A, and vitamin D, which can have deleterious effects. In addition, the cost may be excessive, especially when several different supplements are combined. The client may be well advised to spend less on supplements and more on good hay and grain feeds.

Mineral supplements may provide the major minerals, trace minerals, or a combination of both. Plain salt (NaCl) and trace mineralized salt are the most common mineral supplements. Trace mineralized salt may contain just enough trace mineral to color the salt, or it may contain enough trace minerals in available forms to make a significant contribution to the trace mineral content of the daily ration. The mineral supplement category also includes mixes of various combinations of calcium, phosphorus, potassium, magnesium, sulfur, and other minerals that may be combined with salt, trace minerals, and one or more vitamins. Sometimes, salt is added to a mineral mixture to encourage consumption, and salt is also used to limit excessive consumption. Mineral supplements should be formu-

lated and selected to compensate for deficiencies in the basic ration of a horse—for example, high phosphorus to balance alfalfa hay or high calcium to balance grain. Mineral supplements are generally fed free-choice but also may be mixed with a grain feed. When fed free-choice, consumption should be estimated by total disappearance to determine whether consumption is adequate. Unfortunately, when fed free-choice to groups of horses, uniform consumption of a mineral supplement by all horses cannot be ensured. Individually feeding supplemental minerals in a grain mix is the most accurate method for controlling mineral intake.

Protein supplements may be simple high-protein ingredients such as soybean meal, linseed meal, or milk protein, or they may be manufactured feeds in which protein ingredients have been fortified with other nutrients such as vitamins, trace minerals, calcium, phosphorus, salt, and the synthetic amino acids, lysine and methionine. Young growing horses, brood mares, and other horses that require protein supplementation of hay and cereal grain rations for optimal production usually also need other supplemental nutrients such as vitamins and minerals. Inclusion of these nutrients with the protein makes it possible to use only one supplement to furnish all the extra nutrients needed when hay and cereal grains such as plain oats and corn are fed to horses, and it simplifies the feeding process. Some manufactured protein supplements fortified with other nutrients are designed to be fed in certain situations—for example, to horses on pasture, or with a particular type of hay.

Energy feeds are added to horse rations when more energy is needed for growth, reproduction, or performance than can be provided by hay or pasture alone. Grains, grain byproducts, and other ingredients containing starch, digestible fiber, and fat may be used. Often, these ingredients are blended with molasses. Protein, vitamin, and mineral supplements can be added directly to the manufactured grain mixes to produce final rations of forage and grain that need no further supplementation. The use of commercial grain mixes that already include the appropriate supplements is a convenient, effective way to provide nutritionally balanced rations for horses fed hay or pasture.

Manufactured high-roughage feeds may be formulated to furnish the forage or fiber requirements of horses. Such feeds are usually based on alfalfa hay but may also contain beet pulp and other sources of fiber. High-roughage feeds are usually manufactured in pellet or cube form but may also be available in a coarse form blended with molasses. These roughage products may be combined with energy, protein, mineral, and vitamin sources to create a "complete" feed, which satisfies all the dietary requirements of the horse, including the need for a fiber source. Complete feeds with roughages are particularly useful in feeding horses with respiratory difficulties, dental problems, or digestive tract limitations.

With information available on the classes of feeds being fed, judgments can be made on whether nutritional deficiencies are likely to be contributing to problems with productive efficiency or health. Recommendations can be made to change feeds or to use supplements to fortify the horse rations.

PHYSICAL FORMS OF MANUFACTURED FEEDS

A list of feed processing methods and feed forms is shown in Table 2. Processing may decrease the need for

TABLE 2. FEED PROCESSING METHODS

Rolling, crimping, or flaking	Mechanical flattening by crushing between rollers, usually with application of water or steam
Cracking	Mechanical reduction by crushing between rollers
Micronizing	Mechanical and chemical alteration by application of dry heat and rolling
Grinding	Mechanical size reduction by impact or rolling
Pelleting	Compaction of feed ingredients by grinding, adding steam, and forcing through a die using mechanical force
Extrusion	Ground ingredients with steam and water are forced through a die under high pressure, which causes the starch in grains to expand and undergo physical and chemical changes

chewing and affect digestive rate and site of digestion of certain feeds but has not been shown to cause large changes in total digestibility of feeds. Much of the crimping and flaking of grains is done for cosmetic reasons. Horses with good teeth and sound mouths are able to chew and extract most of the nutrients from unprocessed forages, oats, and corn. Processing improves utilization of harder, more dense grains such as barley and sorghum grains. Fine grinding and pelleting result in some improvement in feed utilization, especially in horses with poor or no teeth or in those that do not chew for other reasons.

The pelleting process involves the use of a mechanical force to press a feed mix, which has been heated with steam, through a small die. The temperature and pressure involved in pelleting are often high enough to partly sterilize the feed and may also damage some of the vitamins. Extra vitamins may be added to a pelleted feed to compensate for destruction during the pelleting process. Pelleted feeds have some advantages in that the ingredients cannot be sorted by horses, they stay in usable condition longer, and they can be handled and stored in a more economic bulk form. The extrusion process resembles pelleting but uses higher pressures, which results in expansion and other changes in the structure of the feed ingredients. The effects of extrusion can also help improve feed utilization in horses with chewing and digestion problems and can be used to provide a matrix to carry fat in a dry, relatively palatable form. Because they are expanded, extruded feeds weigh less per unit of volume than most other feed types. Extrusion may slow the rate of feed consumption when horses are group-fed and may help reduce the incidence of digestive upsets and colic under some management systems. With the exception of certain horses with chewing, digestive, or respiratory problems, the selection of a feed form is largely a matter of personal preference and the owner's prejudices and feeding management systems.

DETERMINING NUTRIENT CONTENT OF FEEDS

Several sources of information about the nutrient content of feeds are available. State feed control laws require

certain nutrient guarantees to be placed on feed tags or in the copy on feed bags. Protein, fat, and fiber guarantees have been required for many years, but are often shown as minimums or ranges. Recently, some states have increased labeling requirements to include information on calcium, phosphorus, copper, zinc, vitamin A, and selenium, if the ingredient listing on the tag or bag indicates that sources of these nutrients have been added to the feed.

No information is included on feed tags concerning digestible energy or caloric content of the feed. However, reasonably accurate estimates of the energy value of both manufactured feeds and forages must be known to evaluate or develop a feeding program for horses. Fiber levels are sometimes used to estimate energy values in manufactured feed and are based on equations developed for forages. Such estimates do not account for the value of added fat and certain byproduct ingredients, and thus they are accurate to about ±20%. Information on caloric values may be furnished in literature accompanying the feed or may be obtained from the nutritionist responsible for formulating the feed, especially if feeding studies have been done with horses. The nutritionist may also be able to furnish more precise information on other nutrients, if necessary.

If adequate nutritional information cannot be obtained from the tag copy or manufacturer, feed samples can be submitted to a competent independent laboratory, such as the Northeast DHI Forage Testing Lab at Ithaca, NY, which runs assays of protein, minerals, and estimated energy values at a nominal cost. For the analytic information to be useful, it is critical that care be taken to obtain a representative sample of the feed. This normally involves taking samples from several bags, compositing the samples, mixing well, and then taking a subsample for submission to the laboratory. The estimated energy values reported by the laboratory should be specific for horses. The error in estimating energy value discussed earlier still applies.

Once nutrient concentrations in hay and feeds are known, it is necessary to get good quantitative information on hay and feed consumption to calculate daily nutrient intakes and compare with estimated requirements. It is important that all feeds, including all supplements, be included in the calculations. Because most horse owners do not typically weigh feeds for horses, it is usually necessary to assist them in converting the volume of the can or scoop used in feeding grain and the amount of hay fed to a weight basis to obtain useful quantitative information. This is best accomplished by weighing the ration ingredients with a scale.

METHODS USED IN FORMULATING FEEDS AND FEEDING PROGRAMS

The stage of life cycle and activity of horses determine the quantities and ratios of nutrients to calories required in a ration. The amount of a ration to feed is determined by the caloric content of the ration relative to the animal's total requirement for calories. For example, 16 pounds of a ration containing 1 Mcal per pound is required to meet a total caloric requirement of 16 Mcal. Once the energy content has been determined, the concentration of each of the other nutrients can be set to meet the total requirements of the horse. If 1.6 pounds of protein are required by a horse, and 16 pounds of ration will be fed, the ration should contain 10% protein to satisfy the total protein requirement. The nutrient-to-calorie ratios required by horses of different body weights are similar at comparable stages of life cycle and level of activity. For example, the same ration can be used to meet requirements for all the nutrients of mature, idle 300-kg, 500-kg, and 700-kg horses once the quantities fed are adjusted to meet caloric requirements.

Nutrient requirements used to develop feeding programs for horses are usually based on National Research Council (NRC) estimates, with appropriate allowances to compensate for animal variations. Most NRC values are estimated to be average, minimum requirements. Under many circumstances, average or minimum is not satisfactory because of individual variation in nutrient requirements and utilization of feed ingredients. Thus, each nutritionist or nutrition department may develop modifications of NRC nutrient requirements, which are then used to formulate rations. Modifications of the NRC requirements often provide an extra allowance of 5 to 10% for major nutrients such as energy and protein, and up to 100% for other nutrients such as copper.

The formulation of a complete feed with roughage to satisfy nutritional requirements is relatively straightforward because the product makes up the total ration. However, the formulation of most other manufactured feed products is more complicated because the major components of the daily ration, pasture or hay, are not controlled by the nutritionist and can vary greatly in nutrient content. Thus, it is necessary to estimate consumption and nutritional value of pasture or hay and then provide guidelines or feeding directions for the feed products to account for variations in quality and quantity of forages consumed. A typical recommendation is to provide 1 to 1.5% of body weight of hay or pasture daily, assuming that the forage has an average nutritional value, such as that of a good grass or a legume and grass mix. Feeders are advised to fine-tune the rations by adjusting forage quality or quantity or by adjusting the quantity of grain concentrate fed, depending on animal response in body condition or performance. To reduce the risk of digestive disturbances, the quantity of hay fed should not go below a minimum of 1% of body weight. Some horse owners, especially those who are new and inexperienced, need advice and guidance on making such adjustments. The practitioner is often in a position to provide invaluable assistance in this area.

Manufactured feeds should be selected to complement the forage component of the ration. The major nutrient furnished by forages is energy, and to a lesser extent, protein and minerals. However, the available or digestible energy, as well as the protein level and quality in most forages, is too low to support desired levels of performance in young growing horses, lactating brood mares, and many performance horses. In addition, most forages grown in temperate climates are low in phosphorus and trace minerals. Therefore, energy and protein along with added minerals and vitamins must be supplemented in the daily ration of many horses. Generally, horses with lesser requirements can consume rations with supplemental nutrients in moderate excess of their requirements with few or no detrimental effects, other than economic. However, poor performance results if horses with higher nutrient requirements receive rations with inadequate levels of nutrients. Thus, for both performance and economic reasons, feed manufacturers commonly develop a "line" of feeds designed for horses with different nutritional requirements. The basic "line" normally consists of three or four products. Products designed to meet the needs of foals and young horses usually have the highest nutrient density. Such products may contain 15 to 18% protein, supplemental amino acids, and relatively high levels of vitamins and minerals as required by the young horse. Another product in the line may contain 12 to 14% protein and somewhat lower levels of vitamins and minerals to satisfy the needs of yearling horses, performance horses, and breeding horses. An additional product designed for the mature, idle horse may contain 9 to 11% protein and relatively lower levels of vitamins and minerals. A grain feed with little or no fortification may also be included in the line of feeds.

Multiple lines may be offered, based on differences in nutrient density resulting from the addition of fat or fiber ingredients. Lines also may be available in alternate physical forms such as coarse-textured or pelleted or extruded feeds. The practitioner and horse owner should get descriptive literature and other information from the feed manufacturer to enable them to select an appropriate product to satisfy animal needs and owner preferences.

FEED FORMULATION

The technique generally used to formulate feeds is a mathematical process involving the solution of a large number of simultaneous equations by a computerized method called *linear programming*. The use of computers in feed formulation makes it possible to balance rations for large numbers of nutrients and to account for variations in nutrients and physical qualities of ingredients used in formulation. With proper quality control of ingredients, manufacturing process, and final product, it is possible to make products that are highly consistent in nutritional value and physical quality.

In the formulation process, the nutritionist provides a list of ingredients that can be selected and a list of nutrient levels and constraints that must be met in the final solution. The constraints may include maximal and minimal amounts of individual ingredients and nutrients as well as desired physical attributes of the final product. Because more than one solution is usually possible, the program chooses the solution that has the lowest ingredient cost. This is often referred to as the "least cost" formula. However, the list of ingredients offered and requirements and constraints imposed are the factors that actually determine cost and final value of the formula. A reputable feed manufacturer uses a qualified equine nutritionist to supervise formulation of horse feeds. Feeds are not normally interchanged between species without modification. Ideally, feed formulations for horses are evaluated by controlled feeding tests with horses.

SELECTION OF FEEDS FOR SPECIAL PROBLEMS

Developmental Orthopedic Disease (DOD)

Bone development problems in young horses are one of the more frequent and complex problems that practitioners encounter. Overwhelming evidence exists that nutrition is one of a number of factors involved in the expression of this disease. It is sometimes possible for the practitioner to quickly evaluate the possibility of nutrition being a contributing factor by making a qualitative ration evaluation. Most pastures and hays are deficient in phosphorus and trace minerals relative to the needs of young growing horses. Phosphorus deficiency is further complicated when legumes such as alfalfa are fed, because the large quantity of calcium in legumes may decrease utilization of the phosphorus and trace minerals present. Forage-related mineral problems tend to occur when forages are the only or predominant component of the diet of young horses. This situation is most common on horse farms with abundant pastures and in the intermountain and western areas of the United States where alfalfa may be the only hay available for feeding. Some bone problems in young horses can be reduced by supplementing the diet with phosphorus and trace minerals. Because of the lack of uniform consumption when mineral supplements are fed free-choice, the most successful method of supplementing minerals is to feed manufactured feeds with the minerals added. This practice has the added benefit of reducing the amount of hay fed, and it reduces problems from excessive calcium when only alfalfa hay is fed. Substituting alfalfa and grass-mixed hays for purely alfalfa hay or using more mature, lower quality alfalfa hay also reduces excessive calcium intake.

An alternative situation may occur when horses are fed limited pasture and hay and large quantities of unsupplemented grains, such as oats, corn, or barley. Such horse diets contain relatively high levels of phosphorus and energy and may be deficient in calcium and trace minerals. The dietary adjustments are opposite to those described earlier, in that the quantity and quality of hay should be increased and the grain should be reduced and supplemented with calcium, phosphorus, and trace minerals.

Sometimes, custom-made rations are considered as a solution to such problems. However, the formulation and production of custom-made feeds is not always possible or practical because of the costs and inefficiencies involved in customizing small quantities of feed. In addition, custom-made feeds may not be necessary because feed manufacturers may already have a product available that corrects the nutritional deficiencies. For best results, dietary analyses can be carried out using procedures described previously to evaluate feeding programs for young horses and correct nutritional deficiencies or imbalances. It may be desirable to control growth rates of very rapidly growing horses by restricting amounts of hay and grain fed and by modifying rations to furnish more digestible energy from fiber and fat and less from ingredients containing starch and sugar.

Laminitic Horses

Feeding hay and manufactured feeds that contain fiber and fat, rather than starch and sugars, as the predominant sources of digestible energy can help manage this problem.

Horses With Heaves (COPD)

The manufactured feeds most useful for horses with heaves are complete feeds with a high fiber level that eliminate the need for feeding hay. Generally, these feeds contain no alfalfa or oats, rely on beet pulp as a fiber source, and contain molasses to control feed dust.

Geriatric Horses

Using feeds processed by grinding, pelleting, or extrusion to decrease or eliminate the need for chewing and to facilitate digestion helps improve feed utilization by aged horses. Feeds with high palatability and supplemental protein, vitamins, and minerals encourage adequate feed consumption and ensure that the nutrients needed to build and hold body condition in aged horses are available. Choking problems in older horses that do not chew or salivate well can be alleviated by adding water directly to the feed to make a mash.

"Hot" Horses

Anecdotal evidence exists that behavioral problems indicated by hyperactivity, poor concentration, and handling problems can be reduced in certain horses by feeding rations in which digestible fiber and fat are substituted for some of the starch and sugar.

Tying Up

Anecdotal evidence suggests that partly replacing starchy feeds with digestible fiber and fat sources along with adequate supplementation of salt and electrolytes can help control tying up problems.

Supplemental Readings

Cunha TJ: Horse Feeding and Nutrition, ed 2. San Diego, Academic Press, 1991.

Lewis LD: Feeding and Care of the Horse. Baltimore, Williams & Wilkins, 1995.

National Research Council: Nutrient Requirements of Horses, ed 5. Washington DC, National Academy Press, 1989.

Feeds and Feeding in the Northeastern United States

HAROLD F. HINTZ
Ithaca, New York

HEATHER JAQUAY
Liverpool, New York

PAUL SIROIS
Ithaca, New York

COMMON FEEDS AND THEIR COMPOSITION

Most of the horses in the Northeast United States are pleasure horses, and the typical horse owner has two to three horses. Furthermore, this typical pleasure horse owner has limited acreage and does not grow any of the grain fed to horses. The majority of the horses are fed commercial grain mixtures. The Northeast is supplied by several national and regional feed manufacturers as well as many local operations. Thus, there are many sources of commercial grain mixtures. Some owners purchase a commercial supplement containing protein, vitamins, and minerals to mix with grain either in home mixtures or commercial mixtures. The grains most commonly fed to horses in the Northeast are oats and corn, although some barley may also be fed. The Northeast is an oats-deficient area, and the production of oats in New York continues to decline, with an almost 50% decrease in acreage of oats harvested from 1984 to 1994. Only 12,000 acres of barley were harvested in New York in 1993. The amount of corn imported for horse feed varies from year to year depending on the weather and quality of the New York corn crop. Therefore, much of the grain fed to horses in the Northeast may be imported into the area.

The commercial feeds may also contain some coproduct feeds such as dehydrated alfalfa leaf meal, hominy feed, wheat bran, corn gluten meal, beet pulp, molasses, wheat midds, distiller's dried grains, dried brewer's grains, soybean hulls, and soybean meal. Analyses of grains and other ingredients commonly used in commercial horse feeds that have been conducted by the Northeast Dairy Herd Improvement Forage Laboratory (NEDHIA Forage Lab) are summarized in Table 1. The data are classified by customer's address, but as mentioned above, the customer may have purchased grain grown outside the Northeast area.

Horses in the Northeast are fed a variety of legumes and grasses or mixtures of the two. The most common legume harvested as hay in the Northeast is alfalfa. Alfalfa and alfalfa mixtures account for 52% of the tonnage of hay produced in New York. In the New England states, alfalfa and alfalfa mixtures account for only 26% of the tonnage produced. Some red clover and birdsfoot trefoil hay are also produced for horses. These two legumes may tolerate wet, poorly drained soils better than alfalfa, but, in general, neither produces nearly as well as alfalfa.

It has been estimated that at least 75% of the grass hay produced in New York and New England is timothy. Orchardgrass is second in production. However, orchardgrass matures early when the weather is less likely to cooperate at the proper time for harvest. Thus, orchardgrass is likely to be harvested at a maturity that is later than recommended. The later harvest results in a crop with higher fiber content, lower protein and digestible energy, and decreased palatability. Bromegrass is the third most commonly used grass, but its use has been declining because of the difficulty of maintaining a stand. Bromegrass cannot tolerate intensive cutting management. Of course, most of the forage in the Northeast is fed to ruminants. Therefore, the figures cited earlier cannot be used to estimate the

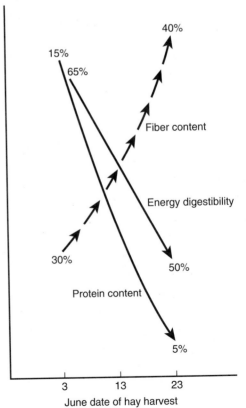

Figure 1. Effect of date of harvest on the composition of timothy hay grown in New York.

TABLE 1. ANALYSES OF GRAINS AND COPRODUCTS
May 1994–April 1995

State	Dry Matter %	Crude Protein %	NDF %	Ca %	P %	Mg %	K %	Cu ppm	Zn ppm	Mn ppm	No. Samples Col 1–7	No. Samples Col 8–10
Barley												
NY	86.8	13.4	25.3	0.13	0.42	0.15	0.65	7	44	25	17	12
	7.4°	2.4	16.0	0.13	0.05	0.03	0.21	5	17	14		
PA	88.1	11.3	21.5	0.11	0.39	0.14	0.65	5	39	24	10	9
	5.1	1.5	4.6	0.10	0.05	0.02	0.65	3	9	8		
Corn												
NY	88.1	9.6	9.9	0.04	0.29	0.13	0.42	3	29	11	98	39
	1.7	2.9	3.9	0.09	0.06	0.02	0.08	2	26	13		
PA	88.4	9.3	10.6	0.03	0.29	0.12	0.41	2	26	12	21	14
	2.0	1.5	2.6	0.05	0.05	0.03	0.07	3	11	10		
Oats												
NY	90.3	12.4	23.3	0.11	0.42	0.16	0.53	4	38	39	6	5
PA	91.1	15.9	20.6	0.09	0.54	0.18	0.51	3	43	45	3	2
Hominy Feeds												
NY	88.2	10.7	17.3	0.04	0.50	0.21	0.01	3	39	12	18	12
	2.4	1.3	—	0	0.11	0.05	0	3	9	4		
Wheat Midds												
NY	89.7	17.8	39.0	0.11	0.96	0.41	1.11	7	84	113	25	23
	1.3	2.0	6.5	0.03	0.27	0.11	0.22	2	18	28		
PA	92.6	25.7	57.0	0.52	0.73	0.25	0.06	11	100	52	18	12
	1.1	3.3	7.7	0.18	0.12	0.03	0	3	14	6		
Corn Gluten Feed												
NY	88.4	21.3	39.6	0.07	0.87	0.38	1.34	5	67	21	13	10
	1.2	1.8	—	0.03	0.18	0.06	0.28	2	9	7		
Distiller's Grains												
NY	89.6	26.5	22.3	0.29	0.83	0.34	1.16	7	57	29	56	35
	1.3	2.6	8.8	0.18	0.06	0.03	0.11	5	7	13		
PA	90.3	28.4	39.2	0.16	0.81	0.34	1.08	5	66	30	9	8
	0.7	1.5	7.2	0.15	0.06	0.03	0.07	3	15	18		

°Standard deviation

relative amounts of legumes and grasses fed to horses. However, it is generally assumed that timothy hay is the most commonly used forage for horses in the Northeast.

The composition of the forage depends on several factors. Species, legumes versus nonlegumes, and stage of maturity at harvest are probably the most important factors. The effect of harvest date on composition of timothy hay grown in New York is shown in Figure 1. If possible, timothy in New York should be harvested by about June 15. The protein content and energy digestibility decrease and crude fiber content increases as the plant matures. Quality would be higher if the hay could be harvested earlier, but yield would be lower. Soil type, fertilization, and climate are also important factors that influence composition.

Grass species usually provide only two cuttings per year. Legumes may provide three cuttings. The first cutting is more likely to be harvested at a later stage of maturity than the second cutting because of the more variable weather early in the season. The first cutting is likely to have more weeds. Preservatives such as propionic salts allow harvesting of hay at higher than usual moisture content

without spoilage and thus help counter weather effects. No adverse effects on the health of the horse have been reported in horses consuming properly preserved hay. Some horses may reduce their intake until they become accustomed to the hay. Of course, if inadequate amounts of the preservative are used, the hay spoils.

The data in Table 2 are classified simply according to legume, mixed mostly legume, and mixed mostly grass, as is the method of operation of the NEDHIA Forage Lab. Although alfalfa cubes and pellets may be imported from Midwestern states, the Northeast area is a forage-exporting area. Therefore, the use of the customer's address to sort the samples submitted to the forage laboratory should be a reasonable method to indicate analyses of forages grown in New York and Pennsylvania. The number of forage samples submitted from the New England states was much smaller than from Pennsylvania and New York, and therefore they were combined. The data were fairly consistent among the states. As expected, legume and mostly legume hays contain a higher concentration of protein, calcium, and potassium and lower fiber concentration than grass or mostly grass hays. Copper and zinc contents were similar

TABLE 2.   ANALYSES OF HAY
May 1994–April 1995

State	Dry Matter %	Crude Protein %	NDF %	Ca %	P %	Mg %	K %	Cu ppm	Zn ppm	Mn ppm	No. Samples Col 1–7	No. Samples Col 8–10
					Legume Hay							
NY	90.6	17.9	46.4	1.29	0.25	0.27	2.40	9	24	32	340	57
	1.3°	2.5	6.2	0.24	0.05	0.05	0.44	2	14	12		
PA	90.4	18.0	47.3	1.25	0.26	0.26	2.50	9	24	36	201	28
	1.0	2.4	6.0	0.21	0.05	0.03	0.43	2	5	12		
NE	91.2	17.6	46.0	1.34	0.26	0.25	2.60	8	22	32	45	16
					Mixed—Mostly Legume							
NY	90.7	15.8	52.5	1.10	0.24	0.26	2.20	9	24	41	1483	133
	1.1	3.0	6.7	0.27	0.05	0.05	0.42	3	6	28		
PA	90.5	16.8	50.5	1.17	0.25	0.26	2.30	9	26	49	520	42
	1.0	2.9	6.8	0.24	0.05	0.03	0.44	4	9	31		
NE	91.2	15.7	53.5	0.97	0.26	0.25	2.35	8	25	40	54	11
					Mixed—Mostly Grass							
NY	91.5	11.8	61.1	0.73	0.22	0.23	1.87	8	25	52	2034	144
	1.1	3.3	6.6	0.27	0.05	0.05	0.52	3	7	35		
PA	91.4	11.8	60.5	0.75	0.23	0.22	1.86	9	27	70	548	88
	1.0	3.3	6.8	0.27	0.06	0.05	0.51	7	10	36		
NE	92.0	11.7	62.4	0.60	0.24	0.22	1.99	8	25	50	258	29
					Grass							
NY	91.8	10.7	63.2	0.62	0.22	0.22	1.79	9	27	63	1283	113
	1.0	3.0	5.9	0.22	0.06	0.05	0.53	3	9	52		
PA	91.9	11.0	63.0	0.57	0.24	0.22	1.90	8	30	76	479	62
	0.9	3.0	5.8	0.19	0.06	0.05	0.57	3	12	44		
NE	92.6	11.6	63.2	0.56	0.25	0.22	1.97	8	26	28	179	32

°Standard deviation

for all classes of hay and provided less than the National Research Council (NRC) recommendation. Manganese content was quite variable. Selenium content of hay in the Northeast is likely to be less than 0.05 ppm.

FEEDING PRACTICES COMMON TO THE AREA

A wide variety of feeding practices are used. As mentioned earlier, many of the horses are pleasure horses maintained on small units. On such units, a "pasture" is more likely to be used for exercise than as a source of nutrients. Many horses are maintained in boarding stables, and, again, pasture is not usually a primary source of nutrients.

Large breeding farms are also present in which pastures can be important sources of nutrients. May and June are usually the months of greatest pasture production (Fig. 2). The pastures are usually a mixture of grasses and legumes. Most pastures in the Northeast consist of cool-season forage species such as orchardgrass, bluegrass, and quackgrass growing in association with white clover or some other legumes. The other legumes may be alsike, birdsfoot trefoil, or red clover. Both alsike and birdsfoot trefoil are hardy legumes but are not particularly preferred by horses. A pasture of exclusively alsike can lead to photosensitiza-

tion. Pure stands of alsike are not common, and horses usually prefer other plants; therefore, photosensitization is rarely encountered. Red clover infested with the fungus *Rhizoctonia leguminicola* may cause slobbers. The fungus is usually considered to be more of a problem when moisture is plentiful. However, the fungus tends to predominate on the lower part of the plant so that, during drought, when the pasture is grazed closer to the ground, animals may develop slobbers. The only treatment for slobbers is

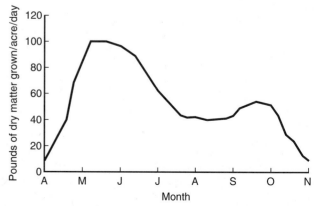

Figure 2. Pasture growth rate (pounds of dry matter per acre per day) over time (adapted from Emmick and Fox).

to remove the animals from the pasture. It may require up to 3 days after removal from the pasture for the horses to cease slobbering.

Grain feeding practices vary greatly. Ready availability and price are probably the two factors that dictate choice of feed and site of purchase. Concern has been expressed about the dangers of mycotoxins in corn, but it is difficult to determine the impact of the concerns on the choice of grains. Of course, the traditional favorite is oats. Most owners buy a commercial grain mixture that usually contains oats and/or corn; a pellet containing vitamins, minerals, and a protein source; and some molasses. This mixture is called "sweet feed" because of the molasses. Texturized feed is the most common form of the grain mixture fed. In this type, the grain mixture may be processed. The oats may be crimped or rolled but may be fed whole. The corn is usually cracked or steam-flaked. The second most commonly used type of commercial grain is pelleted. Pelleted feeds usually contain some wheat midds to increase pellet durability, but the major ingredients are usually the same as those found in texturized feeds. Pelleting prevents the horse from sorting the feed. The third type of feed is extruded. Feed to be extruded is mixed with steam before being expressed through a die. The product is less dense than pelleted feed because of the air holes resulting from the steam. Extruded feed has some advantages such as a slower rate of intake because of its bulky nature. The slower rate of intake has been reported to decrease the incidence of digestive problems. It has also been suggested that the extrusion process increases efficiency of energy utilization because relatively more of the starch is digested in the small intestine and less reaches the large intestine. The end product of starch digestion in the small intestine is glucose, whereas it is volatile fatty acids (VFA) in the large intestine. Glucose is utilized more efficiently than VFA. However, the extrusion process adds considerably to the price of the feed.

The incorporation of fats and oils in commercial feeds has increased in recent years. Some owners also add processed animal fat or pour vegetable oil directly on the grain mixture. Corn oil and soybean oil are probably the oils most commonly used. Animal fat can also be used effectively by the horses and is incorporated in some commercial feeds. Processed animal fat is also available. The fat may be spray-dried or treated to form beads so that it can be added more easily to grain mixture on the farm. The addition of fats and oils increases energy density, does not affect palatability, and has become popular with owners of performance horses.

Some owners add oats or corn, particularly in winter, to a commercial grain. Extensive dilution with oats or corn changes the nutrient balance and is contraindicated. For example, mixing a commercial grain with oats (1:1) decreases the calcium content by half and greatly reduces the trace mineral concentration.

Complete feeds (i.e., feeds that are designed to be used without additional forage) are, under some circumstances, preferred by horse owners. Such feeds can effectively reduce exposure to dust for horses with respiratory problems. They may also reduce "hay belly" on some horses, and thus make the horse more attractive. The most common fiber source is dehydrated alfalfa. Beet pulp also is used successfully. Wood chewing and other stereotypic behaviors may increase without the intake of some long forage. Therefore, some long hay is usually recommended.

FEEDING PROBLEMS COMMON OR UNIQUE TO THE AREA

The following is a list of problems that have been observed in the Northeast related to feeding horses. The list is not intended to rank the problems in order of prevalence but rather to describe situations that the veterinarian may see in practice.

1. Overfeeding of energy to horses at maintenance and to young horses. Results may include obesity and increased risk of colic in the mature horse and increased stress on the developing skeleton in the young horse. Proper monitoring of horses by the use of weight tapes, scales, or body condition scores should be encouraged.

2. Overfeeding of protein to maintenance or performance horses. Elevated protein concentrations are seldom needed for other than growing horses. Horse owners should realize that energy adjustments are usually more important than protein adjustments for mature horses. Excessive protein increases urine output and water intake, may increase feeding costs, and is not environmentally sound.

3. Inadequate management of pasture. Many pastures become exercise yards rather than sources of nutrients because of overgrazing and lack of proper management such as rotational grazing, weed control, and fertilization. Proper management may increase nutrient intake from pasture and perhaps is more economical.

4. Simple nutritional deficiencies have become less common because of the increased use of commercial feeds. Calcium deficiency, nutritional secondary hyperparathyroidism, is still reported sporadically as a result of feeding a ration of grass hay and high amounts of grains such as oats and corn. Grains contain almost no calcium. Selenium deficiency, or white muscle disease in foals, still occurs when only homegrown grains and forages are used. The soils in the Northeast are low in selenium, and thus the forages are low in selenium. As mentioned earlier, forages in the Northeast are also low in copper and zinc. Commercial feeds are usually fortified with copper and zinc.

5. Excessive iodine intake by pregnant mares, either from overzealous supplementation of iodine or mixing mistakes, has been reported. The foal may be born with goiter. For example, one owner was feeding one pound of a supplement containing seaweed to pregnant mares rather than the one ounce that was recommended. Sixty percent of the foals on that farm had goiter at birth.

6. Accidental exposure to ionophores, such as monensin, which may be found in heifer, steer, and poultry rations. Excessive intake of ionophores can cause cardiac problems and death.

7. One of the most common causes of concern is the geriatric horse. The number of geriatric horses over 20 years of age has been increasing, and such horses now constitute 10 to 15% of the equine population. Older horses may have dental problems, hormonal changes, and

decreased digestive efficiency. Old horses do not need special diets unless they begin to lose body condition and the loss in condition cannot be accounted for by another disease process. In such situations, it may be necessary to increase the protein and phosphorus concentration, provide a highly digestible fiber source such as beet pulp, and increase energy density, perhaps by adding fat. Many commercial feeds designed for geriatric horses are now available. Reports from horse owners using such feeds have been favorable.

Supplemental Readings

Agricultural Statistics. USDA. National Agricultural Statistics Service. 1993.

Emmick DL, Fox DG: Prescribed grazing management to improve pasture productivity in New York. USDA Soil Conservation Service, 1993, pp 1–44.

National Research Council: Nutrient requirements of horses, 5th revised ed. Washington, DC, National Academy Press, 1989.

New York Agricultural Statistics. New York Department of Agriculture and Markets. 1993–1994.

Ralston SL: Clinical nutrition of adult horses. Vet Clin North Am Equine Pract 6(2):339–354, 1990.

Feeds and Feeding in the Southern United States

EDGAR A. OTT
Gainesville, Florida

COMMON FEEDS AND THEIR COMPOSITION

Pastures and Hays

The warmer temperatures, higher humidity, and longer growing seasons of the southern United States favor different forages than are commonly used in horse feeding programs of the north. The tropical and subtropical grasses provide the foundation for many horse-feeding programs. However, at certain times of the year, pasture quality or quantity may not be adequate. Under these conditions and for those animals that are stalled or kept in drylot paddocks, hay is necessary. With the exception of the alfalfa producers of the southwest, seasonal factors often affect the ability of southern producers to produce high-quality hay. Therefore, many southern horse owners rely on northern hay for their horses. Discussions on the temperate grasses and legumes are found in other chapters in this section.

Perennial Grasses

Bahiagrass, the Bermudagrasses, and the digitgrasses are the most frequently used pasture forages in the southeast. Bahiagrass and the Bermudagrasses have long growing seasons, often from March through November or until first frost. The digitgrasses, such as Pangolagrass, have shorter seasons and require higher temperatures and more moisture. Tropical and subtropical grasses have lower nutrient content than temperate grasses but are still excellent sources of nutrients for horses. The nutrient content of these forages can be influenced by soil fertility, moisture availability, and plant maturity. Crude protein, neutral detergent fiber (NDF), acid detergent fiber (ADF), calcium, phosphorus, and trace mineral concentrations can vary considerably, even in samples collected on farms in the same general area. Table 1 shows the composition of pasture samples clipped from Bahiagrass pastures on 13 horse farms in July. The nutrient content of this grass can vary

between different pastures on the same farm and with different soil types, fertility, or management programs. Nutrient content of Bahiagrass also varies with the month of the year (Table 2), with the highest nutrient value generally occurring in the spring.

Bahiagrass is one of the best pasture grasses for the southern states because of the durability of the sword. It tolerates traffic well and produces copious amounts of seed, which naturally reseeds areas where the grass may be destroyed by traffic or overgrazing. Bahiagrass matures quickly, and thus pastures must be mowed at regular intervals to keep the forage quality high. In the summer this may be 14- to 21-day intervals, but in the spring and fall the interval may be as long as 56 days. Bahiagrass does not make very good hay because the nutrient value decreases rapidly as the grass matures. Fiber concentrations increase and energy value and protein decrease with maturity.

Numerous varieties and strains of Bermudagrass are found. Coastal Bermudagrass is the most widely grown variety and is well adapted to most of the southern states. It can be utilized as both a pasture forage and as a hay crop. Bermudagrass starts growing when nighttime temperatures exceed 55°F and continues until first frost. Coastal Bermudagrass can produce three to five cuttings of hay per year, depending upon moisture availability and soil fertility. The cutting interval varies with moisture availability. Well-managed coastal Bermudagrass hay fields produce 4 to 6 tons of hay/acre annually.

Digitgrasses such as Pangola grow best when temperatures are high and moisture is readily available. When properly managed, they can be productive pastures. Because it grows best when it is raining frequently, good Pangola hay is difficult to make, but some fall cuttings are successful. The nutrient compositions of Bahiagrass, Bermudagrass, and Pangolagrass are summarized in Table 3.

Fescue is a productive, cool-season forage that is used

TABLE 1. NUTRIENT CONTENT OF BAHIAGRASS PASTURE*

Farm	DM %	DE† Mcal/kg	CP %	NDF %	ADF %	Ca %	P %	Mg %	K %	Na %	Fe mg/kg	Mn mg/kg	Zn mg/kg	Cu mg/kg	Co mg/kg	Se mg/kg
Mean	23.6	2.03	11.1	75.7	36.9	0.29	0.28	0.24	1.92	0.04	85	75	34	9.6	0.09	0.06
SEM	0.84	0.02	0.39	0.76	0.48	0.02	0.01	0.01	0.08	0.001	8	11	2	0.8	0.01	0.01
Range	17.6–30.8	1.75–2.27	8.4–14.4	71.7–80.5	32.5–41.9	0.19–0.4	0.18–0.41	0.17–0.37	1.4–3.2	0.02–0.05	31–182	9–264	19–71	5.2–18.5	0.03–0.23	0.02–0.14

*From Ott EA, Brady J, Mack L: Nutrient composition of bahiagrass pastures in Marion County Florida. Department of Animal Science Research Report AL-1989-1, University of Florida, 1989. Samples collected in July, 1987. Two samples were collected from each farm and labeled A and B.

All values are on a dry matter basis except for dry matter values, which are as collected.

†Estimated using the equation $DE = 4.22 - 0.111\ ADF\% + 0.0332\ CP\% + 0.00112\ (ADF\%)^2$; from National Research Council (Subcommittee on Horse Nutrition): Nutrient Requirements of Horses. Washington, DC, National Academy Press, 1989.

DE = digestible energy; SEM = standard error of mean; DM = dry matter; CP = crude protein; NDF = neutral detergent fiber; ADF = acid detergent fiber.

TABLE 2.   INFLUENCE OF MONTH ON NUTRIENT CONTENT AND IN VITRO ORGANIC MATTER DIGESTIBILITY (IVOMD) OF BAHIAGRASS PASTURES*

	Month													
Element	Jan	Feb	Mar	April	May	June	July	Aug	Sept	Oct	Nov	Dec	Mean	SEM
Crude protein (%)	7.25	7.65	13.00	9.55	10.8	9.65	9.35	8.35	8.95	8.50	7.80	8.30	9.10	0.45
IVOMD %	35.5	38.5	62.0	47.0	52.5	54.5	50.0	47.5	46.5	40.0	40.0	38.0	46.0	2.3
Ca %	0.42	0.40	0.38	0.39	0.42	0.35	0.30	0.33	0.29	0.35	0.36	0.40	0.36	0.007
P %	0.13	0.14	0.20	0.17	0.22	0.18	0.22	0.19	0.20	0.18	0.16	0.17	0.18	0.003
Mg %	0.16	0.16	0.17	0.16	0.22	0.17	0.24	0.26	0.24	0.18	0.24	0.22	0.20	0.005
K %	0.36	0.31	0.86	0.60	1.07	0.85	0.97	0.90	0.87	0.50	0.52	0.65	0.71	0.08
Na %	0.04	0.02	0.03	0.02	0.04	0.04	0.04	0.03	0.03	0.06	0.04	0.04	0.04	0.001
Fe mg/kg	48	42	60	48	46	42	46	39	38	36	42	46	44	1.8
Mn mg/kg	62	73	87	58	50	36	40	29	38	50	61	64	54	4.9
Zn mg/kg	18	18	28	17	22	22	20	14	18	14	12	17	18	1.1
Cu mg/kg	2.4	2.5	3.8	2.2	3.9	3.6	3.4	3.0	2.7	2.4	3.6	3.6	3.2	1.9
Co mg/kg	0.06	0.05	0.18	0.05	0.06	0.04	0.04	0.03	0.06	0.05	0.06	0.08	0.06	0.004
Se mg/kg	0.08	0.08	0.08	0.09	0.06	0.06	0.06	0.04	0.05	0.06	0.08	0.06	0.07	0.001
Mo mg/kg	1.2	1.0	0.08	0.6	0.6	0.6	0.7	0.4	0.5	0.6	2.2	1.5	0.9	0.15

*Means are based on 21 samples each month taken for two consecutive years.
Dry matter basis.
From Espinoza JE, McDowell LR, Wilkinson NS, Conrad JH, Martin FG: Monthly variation of forage and soil minerals in Central Florida. I. Macro-minerals. Commun Soil Sci Plant Anal 22:1123, 1991; and Espinoza JE, McDowell LR, Wilkinson NS, Conrad JH, Martin FG: Monthly variation of forage and soil minerals in Central Florida. II. Trace minerals. Commun Soil Sci Plant Anal 22:1137, 1991.

in horse pastures in the northern portions of the southern states. Tall fescue is commonly infested with an endophyte that causes parturition problems and agalactia in mares. Mares should be removed from fescue pasture at least 28 days before foaling to minimize the problem.

Annual Grasses

These grasses are used to extend the grazing season on many southern horse farms. Ryegrass and the cereal grains (rye, oats, and wheat) are planted in the fall (October or November) to provide winter and early spring grazing. Ryegrass provides the longest grazing season but requires more moisture in the fall to get it established than the cereal grains. Some producers prefer to plant a mixture to ensure success. These forages can be seeded into prepared seedbeds or they can be overseeded on perennial grass sods. On prepared seedbeds, the forage should be at least 6 inches tall before it is grazed. Overseeded pastures can be grazed earlier. Care must be taken when introducing horses to these pastures, because the lush grass can cause laminitis and colic if the animals are allowed to overeat. Horses should be grazed for only one or two hours for the first few days and the grazing time gradually increased until the animals are grazing continuously.

Legumes

Alfalfa, Alyceclover, peanut, and the rhizoma peanut make excellent hay for horses but are generally not used as pasture crops. The exception is the rhizoma peanut, which can be planted with a perennial grass to provide a mixed pasture. Very little alfalfa is grown in the south except for the irrigated areas of the southwest. In other areas, high humidity and high water tables make it difficult to maintain stands and to harvest the crop. Alyceclover and the peanut varieties are well adapted to the climatic conditions of the south, but weather conditions often make it difficult to put up quality hay.

Grains and Byproduct Ingredients

With contemporary transportation and marketing systems, most of the grains and byproduct ingredients that originate in the north are available to feed manufacturers and farm owners of the south. These are discussed elsewhere. Those ingredients that originate in the south include sorghum grain, cottonseed meal, cane molasses, rice bran, cottonseed hulls, and peanut hulls.

Sorghum Grain

Sorghum grain can be used in horse feeds, but only if the grain is adequately processed. For coarse feeds such as

TABLE 3.   NUTRIENT COMPOSITION OF SOUTHERN FORAGES*

Forage	DE Mcal/kg	CP %	Lysine %	Ca %	P %	Na %	Mg %	K %	Fe mg/kg	Mn mg/kg	Zn mg/kg	Cu mg/kg	Co mg/kg	Se mg/kg
Bahiagrass, fresh	2.03	11.1	0.36	0.35	0.20	0.04	0.24	1.92	85	75	34	6.2	0.06	0.06
Bermudagrass coastal, hay	2.00	11.2	0.35	0.36	0.24	0.04	0.20	1.5	74	57	25	6.2	0.05	0.05
Pangolagrass, fresh	1.95	9.1	NA	0.38	0.22	NA	0.18	1.42	NA	NA	NA	NA	NA	NA

*Dry matter basis.
From National Research Council (Subcommittee on Horse Nutrition): Nutrient Requirements of Horses. Washington, DC, National Academy Press, 1989, Table 6–1A.
NA = no value available.

sweet feeds or textured feeds, steam flaking is preferred. For pelleted feeds, grinding or dry rolling is most suitable. Palatability of sorghum grains may not be comparable to that of other feed grains, and thus some restriction on the portion of sorghum in the concentrate may be appropriate.

Cottonseed Meal

This meal can be used as a source of protein in horse feeds if the following limitations are considered. Cottonseed meal is lower in lysine than soybean meal, and thus lysine supplementation may be necessary. Cottonseed meal contains gossypol, which reduces the iron availability in the diet. Only low-gossypol cottonseed meal should be used in horse feeds.

Peanut Meal

Peanut meal also has a lower lysine content than soybean meal, and thus appropriate lysine supplementation may be appropriate if peanut meal is included in horse feeds.

Cane Molasses

This mainstay of horse feeds is used as an economical energy source in the south, but it also serves to bind the concentrate ingredients together so that they do not separate. It is also used to reduce dust and increase the palatability of horse feeds.

Rice Bran

This palatable, high-fat (15%) ingredient is being used extensively in horse feeds. It becomes rancid if the fat is not stabilized, and thus care must be taken to ensure that only stabilized material is included in horse feeds. Rancid products have low palatability.

Cottonseed Hulls and Peanut Hulls

These products have very limited feeding value in horse diets. They may be used as a source of fiber, but their digestibility is very low. They are also occasionally used as carriers for trace mineral or vitamin premixes. When used for this purpose they are usually present at 0.5% of the product or less.

High temperatures and humidity of the summers in the south, especially the southeast, influence the shelf life of processed feeds and feed ingredients. Care must be taken to rotate feed supplies and purchase only amounts that can be fed in 1 to 2 weeks. Feed ingredients should be processed only as required for manufacture of horse feeds. High temperature and high humidity increase the rate at which molds propagate and fats go rancid. Most feed manufacturers add mold inhibitors and additional antioxidants to their products in the summer to help extend shelf life.

FEEDING PRACTICES AND PROGRAMS

Feeding programs can generally be divided into either pasture programs or confinement programs, with some animals experiencing both. In either case it is important to understand that the forage is the foundation of the feeding program. The remainder of the ration is designed to properly supplement the forage to meet the needs of the animal.

When hay is fed, it is fairly easy to determine or estimate the amount the animal is consuming, especially if the animal is being fed in a stall. In group feeding situations, one generally assumes that the animal is receiving about the average for the group. Thus, if one 24-kg bale is fed to three horses each day, one assumes that each animal is consuming about 8 kg of hay daily. This assumption only applies if all hay is being consumed and all horses have equal access to the hay. Thus, it may be necessary to observe the feeding situation. It is often difficult to determine the quantity and quality of the pasture intake. It is generally assumed that the animal will consume a quantity of pasture equivalent to the amount of hay required by the animal. That is, if the animal needs 2.0 kg hay per 100-kg body weight, it will likely consume an equivalent amount of pasture dry matter.

Once the contribution of the forage to the feeding program has been assessed, the remainder of the ration (concentrate and/or supplement) can be formulated or selected to balance the nutrient needs of the animal being fed. For many horses, pasture, water, and a free-choice complete mineral mixture providing salt, calcium, phosphorus, and trace minerals meet the animal's needs. For those with increased nutrient requirements due to growth, reproduction, or work, additional supplementation may be necessary. Table 4 gives the approximate composition of concentrate feeds recommended for various classes of horses when legumes, alfalfa, clovers, peanut, and others make up the forage portion of the ration. Bahiagrass, Bermudagrass, Pangolagrass, and other grasses are typically lower in energy, protein, and calcium than the legumes; Table 5 shows the approximate composition of concentrates that are appropriate when grass forage is fed. Expected forage and concentrate intakes for horses of different classes are shown in Table 6. The variation in intake is the result of individual differences and typical capacity limits imposed by activity requirements.

FEEDING PROBLEMS COMMON TO THE SOUTH

Sand Colic

Light sandy soils, overstocking, poor pasture management, inadequate nutrient supplementation, and drought conditions often lead to horses pulling or digging grass and consuming considerable quantities of sand. If large quantities of sand accumulate in the cecum and large colon, sand colic may occur. The problem is often treated with a mineral oil drench, but may recur at any time. The daily use of high-fiber ingredients such as wheat bran or various psyllium products appears to benefit some animals. Others may require periodic mineral oil drenches or modification of their environment to control the problem.

Anhidrosis

Anhidrosis is primarily a problem in the Gulf Coast states and the Caribbean basin. Its cause is not known. Physiologic, psychologic, and nutritional components ap-

TABLE 4. RECOMMENDED NUTRIENT CONTENT OF CONCENTRATES* TO BE FED WITH LEGUME FORAGES†

	DE Mcal/kg	CP %	Lysine %	Ca %	P %	Na %	Fe mg/kg	Mn mg/kg	Zn mg/kg	Cu mg/kg	Co mg/kg	I mg/kg	Se mg/kg	Vit. A IU/kg
Mature horses														
Maintenance	3.0	10.0	0.35	0.40	0.30	0.40	120	120	120	35	0.2	0.2	0.2	4000
Mare, late gestation	3.0	10.0	0.35	0.40	0.30	0.40	120	120	120	35	0.2	0.2	0.2	4000
Mare, early lactation	3.0	12.0	0.50	0.55	0.45	0.40	120	120	120	35	0.2	0.2	0.2	6000
Mare, late lactation	3.0	12.0	0.50	0.55	0.45	0.40	120	120	120	35	0.2	0.2	0.2	6000
Working														
Light	3.0	10.0	0.35	0.40	0.30	0.40	120	120	120	35	0.2	0.2	0.2	4000
Moderate	3.0	10.0	0.35	0.40	0.30	0.40	120	120	120	35	0.2	0.2	0.2	4000
Intense	3.3	12.0	0.42	0.44	0.33	0.40	120	120	120	35	0.2	0.2		4000
Young horses														
Nursing foal, 4 mo.	3.0	15.0	0.65	0.70	0.60	0.40	150	150	150	35	0.2	6.2	0.2	6000
Weanling, 6 mo.	3.0	15.0	0.65	0.70	0.60	0.40	150	150	150	35	0.2	0.2	0.2	6000
Yearling, 12 mo.	3.0	12.0	0.42	0.55	0.45	0.40	120	120	120	35	0.2	0.2	0.2	6000
Long yearling, 18 mo.	3.0	12.0	0.42	0.55	0.45	0.40	120	120	120	35	0.2	0.2	0.2	6000
Two-yr-old	3.0	12.0	0.50	0.45	0.35	0.40	120	120	120	35	0.2	0.2	0.2	6000

*As fed basis.
†Examples of legume forages: alfalfa, clover, peanut.

TABLE 5. RECOMMENDED NUTRIENT CONTENT OF CONCENTRATES* TO BE FED WITH GRASS FORAGES†

	DE Mcal/kg	CP %	Lysine %	Ca %	P %	Na %	Fe mg/kg	Mn mg/kg	Zn mg/kg	Cu mg/kg	Co mg/kg	I mg/kg	Se mg/kg	Vit. A IU/kg
Mature horses														
Maintenance	3.0	10.0	0.35	0.40	0.30	0.40	120	120	120	35	0.2	0.2	0.2	4000
Mare, late gestation	3.0	13.0	0.45	0.50	0.40	0.40	120	120	120	35	0.2	0.2	0.2	4000
Mare, early lactation	3.0	15.0	0.52	0.65	0.45	0.40	120	120	120	35	0.2	0.2	0.2	6000
Mare, late lactation	3.0	15.0	0.52	0.65	0.45	0.40	120	120	120	35	0.2	0.2	0.2	6000
Working														
Light	3.0	12.0	0.50	0.40	0.30	0.40	120	120	120	35	0.2	0.2	0.2	4000
Moderate	3.0	12.0	0.50	0.40	0.30	0.40	120	120	120	35	0.2	0.2	0.2	4000
Intense	3.0	13.0	0.55	0.44	0.33	0.40	120	120	120	35	0.2	0.2	0.2	4000
Young horses														
Nursing foal, 4 mo.	3.0	18.0	0.80	0.90	0.65	0.40	150	150	150	35	0.2	0.2	0.2	6000
Weanling, 6 mo.	3.0	18.0	0.80	0.90	0.65	0.40	150	150	150	35	0.2	0.2	0.2	6000
Yearling 12 mo.	3.0	15.0	0.65	0.65	0.45	0.40	120	120	120	35	0.2	0.2	0.2	6000
Long yearling, 18 mo.	3.0	13.0	0.60	0.50	0.40	0.40	120	120	120	35	0.2	0.2	0.2	6000
Two-year-old	3.0	12.0	0.50	0.45	0.35	0.40	120	120	120	35	0.2	0.2	0.2	6000

*As fed basis.
†Examples of grass forages: Bahiagrass, Bermudagrass, fescue.

TABLE 6. EXPECTED FEED CONSUMPTION BY HORSES* (% BODY WEIGHT)

	Forage	Concentrate	Total
Mature horses			
Maintenance	1.5–2.0	0.–0.5	1.5–2.0
Mare, late gestation	1.0–1.5	0.5–1.0	1.5–2.0
Mare, early lactation	1.0–2.0	1.0–2.0	2.0–3.0
Mare, late lactation	1.0–2.0	0.5–1.5	2.0–2.5
Working			
Light	1.0–2.0	0.5–1.5	1.5–2.5
Moderate	1.0–2.0	0.75–1.5	2.0–2.5
Intense	0.75–1.5	1.0–2.0	2.0–2.5
Young horses			
Nursing foal, 3 mo.	0	1.0–2.0	2.5–3.5
Weanling, 6 mo.	0.5–1.0	1.5–3.0	2.0–3.5
Yearling, 12 mo.	1.0–1.5	1.0–2.0	2.0–3.0
Long yearling, 18 mo.	1.0–1.5	1.0–1.5	2.0–2.5
Two-yr-old, 24 mo.	1.0–1.5	1.0–1.5	2.0–2.5

*Air dry feed (about 90% DM).

Intake may also be influenced by feeding experience of the animal. An animal restricted to low-quality forage for extended periods may develop increased capacity. An animal restricted to a high-grain, low-forage intake for extended periods may have a reduced capacity.

pear to contribute to the problem, and considerable variation between animals is known to occur. Animals born and raised in the north have been known to develop the condition shortly after arriving in the south. Animals born in the south have been known to develop the condition at age 12 or even older. Severely anhidrotic animals have become normal when shipped north. Some animals perspire normally in the spring and fall but are anhidrotic in the summer. No cure for this condition has been documented; however, a nutritional supplement providing elevated tyrosine has been shown to benefit some animals.

Mineral Deficiencies and Toxicities

Variations in forage mineral concentrations often make balancing the diet a major challenge. The minerals that are most likely to be provided in inadequate amounts or in improper proportion to other minerals include calcium, phosphorus, sodium, zinc, copper, and selenium. Calcium and phosphorus are most frequently a problem when horse owners combine grains, such as oats, and forages without balancing the calcium and phosphorus. A problem may also occur when a commercial product designed to be fed with one type of forage (grass or legume) is fed with another forage. Sodium and sometimes chloride deficiencies can result in inadequate water intake and dehydration; they occur most commonly in animals that perspire heavily and are not provided with adequate salt.

Trace mineral deficiencies occur most frequently in areas where forage mineral concentrations are low and inadequate supplementation is provided to the animals. The addition of trace minerals to the concentrate and the use of free-choice complete mineral mixture or trace mineralized salt is recommended. Examples of acceptable mineral mixtures are shown in Table 7.

Excess intakes of some minerals can cause toxicities. Iodine intakes of 40 mg/day by gestating mares have been shown to result in foals born with goiters. Excessive iodine intake is usually the result of feeding ingredients that are high in iodine (kelp), using high-iodine products designed for other purposes, or formulation errors. Excessive selenium intake can cause hair and hoof problems. This toxicity is usually caused by high natural concentrations in locally grown forage because of high soil selenium or use of multiple supplements containing selenium.

MAKING ON-THE-FARM RECOMMENDATIONS

Veterinarians often encounter disease conditions such as multiple colics, laminitis, developmental orthopedic disease (DOD), poor body condition, and other signs that should stimulate a review of the farm's feeding program. It is not necessary to be a nutritionist to solve basic feeding management problems present on many farms. However, it is important to address the program with a professional and systematic approach.

As a veterinarian, remind yourself that there are about as many ways to feed a horse properly as there are horse owners, and do not assume that the existing program is a problem just because it is different from others with which you are familiar. Assessment of the program may proceed as follows:

1. Is there a general indication of a nutritional or feeding management problem? If the program is not broken, do not try to fix it.

2. If there is a problem, let the signs point you toward a potential solution. For example, a high incidence of impaction colic may suggest inadequate water intake (dehydration), poor-quality forage high in ADF, dental problems, or possibly inadequate exercise. Skeletal problems may suggest inadequate nutrient balance in the diet. Remember, however, that there may also be genetic and conformational causes. Inadequate body condition usually suggests inadequate energy intake.

3. Whenever there is a problem, evaluate the forage program first. If animals are pastured, is adequate forage available? If not, is hay being provided? How much? It may be necessary to observe the animals to determine

TABLE 7. FREE-CHOICE MINERAL MIXTURES FOR HORSES*

Element	Complete Mineral	Trace Mineralized Salt
Calcium, %	12–16	—
Phosphorus, %	6–8	—
Salt, %	20–25	90–95
Iron, mg/kg	5357	5357
Manganese, mg/kg	5357	5357
Zinc, mg/kg	5357	5357
Copper, mg/kg	1000	1000
Cobalt, mg/kg	18	18
Iodine, mg/kg	18	18
Selenium, mg/kg	18	18

*Nutrient concentrations are based on an assumed intake of 2 ounces (56 g) per day. If intake is significantly above 2 ounces for several weeks, a lower concentration of trace minerals would be appropriate.

whether adequate hay is available for the animals and if all of the animals have an adequate opportunity to eat. Is the forage quality acceptable? It may be useful to have an analysis of the forage performed.

4. If the forage program appears to be adequate, the need for supplementation should be assessed. If a concentrate is being fed, how much does each animal receive daily? Is the concentrate fed individually or group-fed? If it is group-fed, do all animals have an equal opportunity to eat? Do they all eat? Does the concentrate match the animal and forage?

5. Evaluate supplements being used. Is a supplement necessary? If free-choice minerals are available to the animals, are they appropriate to the feeding program? Are they being consumed?

Supplemental Reading

National Research Council (Subcommittee on Horse Nutrition): Nutrient Requirements of Horses. Washington, DC, National Academy Press, 1989.

Feeds and Feeding in the Northwestern United States and Western Canada

ROBERT J. COLEMAN
Edmonton, Alberta, Canada

Climate and growing conditions affect the availability and nutritional content of feedstuffs in Western Canada and the Northwestern United States. The challenge for horse owners is to use the available feedstuffs to the best advantage in producing feeding programs that meet the nutrient requirements and maximize performance of the horses being fed.

FORAGE

When selecting a forage for horses, it is important that the forage be free of mold and dust, be palatable, and provide a significant amount of nutrients to meet the horses' requirements. Horses should be fed forage at a minimum intake of 1% of body weight. Intakes of high-quality forage can be 1.5 to 2.5% of body weight or higher.

The average nutrient values for some of the common forages used for feeding horses in Western Canada are listed in Table 1 and Table 2. Alfalfa, a legume, is grown throughout the Northwestern United States and Western Canada. It is a very productive forage and produces a highly nutritious feed that is relatively high in energy, protein, and calcium. Under normal growing conditions, alfalfa can produce from 1 to 4 cuts of hay per year. Typically two cuts of hay are obtained from alfalfa; however, in areas where growing conditions (temperature and moisture) and length of season are favorable, up to four cuttings are possible. In general the later cuts (2nd, 3rd, and 4th) contain higher levels of energy and protein than the first cut because weather conditions allow harvesting of the forage at a more immature stage of growth. As the hay matures the nutritional value decreases. It is recommended that alfalfa be harvested at 10% bloom to obtain

TABLE 1.   NUTRIENT COMPOSITION OF FORAGES FED IN ALBERTA*

Hay Type	Moisture %	DE† Mcal/kg	ADF %	Protein %	Calcium %	Phosphorus %	Magnesium %	Potassium %
Alfalfa	11.1 ± 4.0	2.76	34.4 ± 5.9	17.9 ± 3.2	1.76 ± 0.5	0.22 ± 0.05	0.31 ± 0.09	1.82 ± 0.55
Mixed (alfalfa/grass)	10.3 ± 3.7	2.76	30.7 ± 5.5	14.8 ± 3.9	1.58 ± 0.5	0.18 ± 0.06	0.24 ± 0.17	1.35 ± 0.50
Brome	11.1 ± 4.3	2.66	36.0 ± 4.1	9.6 ± 3.4	0.52 ± 0.24	0.16 ± 0.06	0.18 ± 0.06	1.64 ± 0.56
Timothy	11.6 ± 4.0	2.62	38.0 ± 4.3	8.3 ± 2.9	0.48 ± 0.23	0.14 ± 0.05	0.12 ± 0.05	1.22 ± 0.29
Native grass	10.0 ± 3.8	2.61	38.3 ± 4.3	8.2 ± 2.8	0.46 ± 0.18	0.13 ± 0.06	0.13 ± 0.06	0.98 ± 0.44
Oat hay (greenfeed)	13.4 ± 4.9	2.68	34.8 ± 5.2	9.4 ± 2.7	0.37 ± 0.18	0.21 ± 0.06	0.20 ± 0.08	1.74 ± 0.50

*Values are means and standard deviations and represent feeds analyzed at the Alberta Agriculture Soil and Feed Testing Laboratory, 1967–1994. Data were compiled by Abdul Suleiman, Laboratory Nutritionist.

Except for moisture, all values are on a 100% dry matter basis.

†DE is calculated using % ADF (100% dry matter basis); for alfalfa, DE Mcal/kg = $3.617 - (0.025 \times \%ADF)$; for other forages DE = $3.38 - (.02 \times \%ADF)$. The DE formulae are derived from research at the Ruminant Forage Evaluation Unit at the University of Alberta and overestimate the DE values for horses. To convert to DE for horses, a factor of 0.85 is used.

TABLE 2. TRACE MINERAL COMPOSITION OF COMMON FORAGES FED TO HORSES IN ALBERTA*

Hay Type	Copper mg/kg	Manganese mg/kg	Zinc mg/kg	Selenium mg/kg
Alfalfa	7 ± 2.6	41 ± 34	25 ± 12	0.28 ± 0.28
Mixed (alfalfa/grass)	6 ± 1.8	48 ± 17	23 ± 7	0.35 ± 0.26
Brome	5 ± 2.5	72 ± 36	19 ± 8	0.16 ± 0.15
Timothy	4 ± 3.0	48 ± 32	21 ± 9	0.11 ± 0.12
Native	5 ± 3.6	55 ± 34	20 ± 8	0.13 ± 0.12
Oat hay (greenfeed)	5 ± 2.6	54 ± 26	23 ± 8	0.15 ± 0.17

*Values are averages and standard deviations, and represent feeds analyzed at Alberta Agriculture Soil and Feed Testing Laboratory, 1967–1994. Data were compiled by Abdul Suleiman, Laboratory Nutritionist.

All values are expressed on a 100% dry matter basis.

a high-quality feed. Care must be taken when harvesting and baling alfalfa hay as this forage can become dusty and moldy. Alfalfa hay can be very effective in meeting the energy and protein requirements of young, growing horses and of mares during late gestation and lactation. For many mature horses at maintenance, the intake of good-quality alfalfa must be controlled to avoid excess weight gains.

Timothy and brome are the most commonly grown grass hays for horses. While they are lower in energy and protein than alfalfa hay, they are useful in feeding programs for mature horses at maintenance, performance horses, and broodmares in early gestation. When these feeds are used for the mare in late gestation, the mare in lactation, or young, growing horses, greater amounts of supplemental energy and protein will be required to meet the higher nutrient requirements of these horses. Timothy and brome are commonly found in forage mixtures with alfalfa rather than as pure stands. The mixed forages do not have as high a level of energy and protein as pure alfalfa but are higher than the pure grass hay. Mixed hay gives horse owners more flexibility in feeding and allows one forage to be used for a wide range of horses with minimal supplementation required.

Other legumes such as red clover and sweet clover and grasses such as wheat grass, orchard grass, and creeping red fescue are also grown in the Northwestern United States and Western Canada. These feeds are adapted to different climatic and growing conditions and can provide palatable, nutritious forage. Often horse owners do not use these forage species for horses because they are not considered common or typical horse feeds. As with other forages for horses, it is important that these alternative forages be free of dust and mold. Of particular concern are sweet clover and red clover, which can mold during the hay-making process. Feeding moldy sweet clover can cause sweet clover poisoning, which is the result of the mold-forming dicoumarol, an anticoagulant. Moldy red clover has been associated with excessive salivation or slobbers in the horse.

Native grass hay or wild hay includes a wide range of plant species. Anecdotal information suggests that native or prairie hay has unique nutritional qualities when fed to horses. From a nutrient analysis, native hay is similar to other grass forages in energy, protein, and minerals. A benefit of prairie/native hay is that the hay is generally dust- and mold-free, as are most grass hays.

Oat hay (in some areas called oat greenfeed) is harvested from oats when the grain is in the late milk to dough stage. Oat hay can be used as a feed for horses, particularly mature horses at maintenance. It is an excellent source of energy and protein, but although horses consume it readily, waste can be very high. It is important with oat hay to have a feed analysis done to check the level of nitrate. No scientific information is available regarding nitrate toxicity in the horse, but forages with nitrate (NO_3) levels above 1.0% are not recommended for horses. On average, oat hay in Alberta has had a nitrate (% NO_3) level of 0.26% (dry matter basis), which is considered safe. However, cereal crops that have been damaged by hail, frost, or drought can have nitrate levels that exceed 1.85% (dry matter basis), which is toxic to ruminants. Nitrate levels in the total diet for horses should not exceed 0.50%.

Pasture can be both an area for exercise and a major source of nutrients for horses. In order for the pasture to be a source of nutrients for the entire grazing period, a mixture of early- and late-maturing forage species should be used. Horse owners should consult with their extension service to find information on the most suitable types of plants for pasture in their area. The grazing season in Western Canada runs from May through October, depending on growing conditions.

Stocking rates reflect growing conditions, whether the pasture is improved pasture or native range, and the level of management applied to the pasture (fertilization, weed control, other factors). By using good pasture management practices, a balance between forage availability and use can be established. This balance maintains the productivity of the pasture for many seasons. A rule of thumb for horse owners to follow is not to start grazing a pasture until there is at least 15 to 20 cm (6–8 inches) of new growth, and the pasture should not be grazed below 5 to 10 cm (2–4 inches). Under good conditions on improved pasture, a 500-kg horse requires four to five acres for the summer grazing season.

GRAIN

In Western Canada, many horse owners depend upon locally available grains as a concentrated energy source rather than commercially manufactured feeds. Although most cereal grains can be fed to horses, oats, barley, and wheat are readily available in the Northwestern United States and Western Canada. Tables 3 and 4 give nutrient values for oats, barley, and wheat. Oat grain is the traditional favorite of horse owners. The digestible energy (DE) content of Alberta oats is somewhat higher than reported for oats in the NRC (1989). Alberta oats have less fiber and a higher bushel weight than average oats. As fiber content decreases and bushel weight increases, digestible energy content also increases (see Table 3).

Barley is a dominant feed grain in Western Canada. The DE content of barley is higher than for oats, and barley is often mixed with oats to increase the energy content of the grain mix while maintaining a reasonable level of fiber. Barley can also be readily fed as the only grain, but it is often labeled as a "hot" feed, and some horse owners do not consider it suitable for horses. Care must be taken to

TABLE 3. NUTRIENT COMPOSITION OF WHOLE GRAINS FED IN ALBERTA*

	Moisture %	Bushed Weight lbs/bu	Digestible Energy†Mcal/kg	Protein %	Calcium %	Phosphorus %	Magnesium %	Potassium %
Oats	10.0 ± 1.7	40 ± 3.8	3.53	11.5 ± 1.8	0.09 ± 0.03	0.35 ± 0.05	0.14 ± 0.03	0.47 ± 0.10
Barley	11.6 ± 1.8	47 ± 4.6	3.73	12.3 ± 1.7	0.07 ± 0.03	0.38 ± 0.06	0.15 ± 0.02	0.53 ± 0.10
Wheat	12.0 ± 1.8	60 ± 4.5	3.90	15.8 ± 2.1	0.06 ± 0.04	0.39 ± 0.05	0.17 ± 0.02	0.40 ± 0.09

*Values are means and standard deviations, and represent feeds analyzed at Alberta Agriculture Soil and Feed Testing Laboratory, 1967–1994. Data were compiled by Abdul Suleiman, Laboratory Nutritionist.

Except for moisture, all values are on a 100% dry matter basis.

†Digestible Energy (DE) calculated based on bushel weight.

Oats DE Mcal/kg = [((Bu wt − 40) × .01) + 1.6] × 2.2046

Barley DE Mcal/kg = [((Bu wt − 48) × .01) + 1.7] × 2.2046

Wheat DE Mcal/kg = [((Bu wt − 60) × .01) + 1.77] × 2.2046

ensure that horses are fed an appropriate amount and that they are adapted to the grain gradually, as is the case when any new feed is introduced in the feeding program.

The use of wheat in horse diets is generally not recommended or practiced because of the potential for digestive disturbance owing to the high gluten content. The increased management required when feeding a high-energy, low-fiber feedstuff such as wheat reduces its usefulness as routine feed grain for horses.

Corn is generally not used in horse diets in Western Canada because of limited availability and expense. However it is a good source of energy and is used in the production of some commercial sweet feeds.

PROTEIN SUPPLEMENTS

The protein source typically used in horse diets is soybean meal. However, canola meal is also a good protein source, is readily available in Western Canada, and can be used in diets for horses. Limited research comparing canola meal to soybean meal for horses suggests that canola meal is an effective protein supplement. Canola meal is somewhat lower in protein quantity and quality than soybean meal, but it may be an economical alternative in some feeding situations. The differences between canola and soybean meal are noted in Table 5.

FEEDING PRACTICES

The feeding suggestions that follow are formulated to meet minimum nutrient requirements as suggested by

NRC (1989). These ration suggestions do not take into account environment or individual nature of the horse, and adjustments to the programs are required to account for these factors. The nutrient levels of the feeds used in the examples are listed in Tables 1 to 4.

MAINTENANCE

The foundation of feeding programs for mature idle horses is good-quality forage. Horses can easily consume 1.5 to 2.5% of their body weight of forage on a daily basis. Good-quality forage, when consumed at these levels, provides adequate amounts of energy, protein, and calcium. In certain instances because the level of phosphorus in the forage is below the level that meets the horse's requirement, supplementation is required. The levels of copper and zinc typically found in Western Canadian forages do meet the horse's requirements. Horse owners should offer a suitable mineral supplement to ensure adequate intakes of phosphorus and a fortified trace mineral salt to ensure adequate intakes of copper, zinc, and manganese. Table 6 provides information on the typical types of mineral supplements available in Western Canada. When these products are offered free-choice, horses at maintenance usually consume enough to meet their requirements.

Brood Mares

The mare's production cycle can be divided into the following categories: early to midgestation, late gestation, and lactation (Table 7). By defining the various stages of production, horse owners can easily feed their mares to meet the nutrient requirements for each production stage.

TABLE 4. TRACE MINERAL COMPOSITION OF WHOLE GRAINS FED IN ALBERTA*

	Copper mg/kg	Manganese mg/kg	Zinc mg/kg	Selenium mg/kg
Oats	4 ± 1.7	45 ± 14	33 ± 8	0.10 ± 0.09
Barley	6 ± 2.5	18.5 ± 6	41 ± 10	0.10 ± 0.09
Wheat	4 ± 1.2	36 ± 11	42 ± 8	0.19 ± 0.14

*All values are based on 100% dry matter.

Values are averages and standard deviations, and represent feeds analyzed at Alberta Agriculture Soil and Feed Testing Laboratory, 1967–1994. Data were compiled by Abdul Suleiman, Laboratory Nutritionist.

TABLE 5. COMPARISON OF NUTRIENT CONTENT OF SOYBEAN MEAL AND CANOLA MEAL*

	Canola	Soybean
Crude protein %	40.9	54.0
Digestible Energy Mcal/kg	3.11	3.73
Lysine %	2.29	3.44
Calcium %	0.69	0.29
Phosphorus %	1.30	0.71

*Values are expressed on a 100% dry matter basis.

Values as given by NRC, 1989.

TABLE 6.   RANGE OF TRACE MINERAL LEVELS COMMONLY FOUND IN LIVESTOCK MINERALS AND TRACE MINERALIZED SALTS

	Ca	P	Cu	Zn	Mn	Se*
	%	%	ppm	ppm	ppm	ppm
1:1 Livestock mineral	16	16	2000–3000	4000–10,000	3000–6000	25–100
Trace mineralized salt	0	0	2000–3000	4000–10,000	3000–6000	40–100

*The livestock mineral products and the fortified trace mineral salts can be purchased with or without selenium. If products contain selenium, the range of selenium levels are indicated in the table.

Early to Midgestation

For mares that were not in foal the previous year, this period starts at conception and ends after the eighth month of pregnancy. For mares with foals at side, this stage extends from weaning until the end of the eighth month of gestation. During this stage, growth of the fetus ranges from 0.09 to 0.25 kg/day, and thus the nutrient demands of the fetus on the mare are minimal. As long as the mare is in good body condition, she can be fed similarly to a mature horse at maintenance. Because forages may be low in certain minerals, it is essential that adequate levels of phosphorus, copper, zinc, manganese, and selenium are provided. For example, 8.2 to 9 kg/day of good-quality legume or grass hay provide adequate amounts of energy, protein, and calcium for a 500-kg mare in early gestation. In addition, a 1:1 livestock mineral and trace mineralized salt should be available free-choice.

Late Gestation

This production stage includes months 9, 10, and 11 of pregnancy. At this time, the developing foal is growing at an accelerated rate and gains 60% of its birth weight in the last 90 days of gestation. Although the energy and protein requirements can usually be met by feeding high-quality forage alone, additional minerals are again required. In early gestation, the mare needs about 15 g (0.5 ounces) of mineral intake per day, whereas in late gestation the mineral intake increases to 55 to 60 g (2 ounces) per day to meet phosphorus needs (see Table 7).

Some mare owners may want to include a small amount of grain in the ration of mares in late gestation. Grain is included for two reasons. First, it is easier to meet the mare's nutrient requirements when a combination of hay and concentrates are fed. Some mares do not consume enough forage to meet their energy needs. This is especially true if the forage quality is low and if intake of the forage is low or variable. Total dry matter consumption may also decline in the last month of gestation. Second, with the increased mineral needs at this stage, many mares may not eat 55 to 60 g (2 ounces) of minerals on a free-choice basis, and adding the mineral to some grain increases palatability and ensures adequate mineral intakes.

Lactation

Mares in early lactation have the highest requirements for energy, protein, calcium, and phosphorus. Lactating mares often have an increased capacity for feed consumption and may consume feed at a rate in excess of 2.5% of body weight. Good-quality forage still forms the foundation of the feeding program, but to meet the mare's requirements it is important to feed a balanced ration of hay and grain. The grain portion of the ration should be formulated to provide the nutrients that the forage portion does not provide. For example, when grass hay is the primary forage, the mare requires a protein supplement in addition to oats or another grain (see Table 7).

Body Condition

A great deal of research has been done on the effects of body condition on reproductive performance. Several body condition scoring systems have been developed, but the ones that are used most commonly in the United States and Canada are based on a scoring system (1–9) developed at Texas A&M University, where 1 is equivalent to extremely thin and 9 is equivalent to extremely fat. Table 8 gives a brief summary of a condition scoring system. A more complete description can be found in the NRC publication (1989).

Research has indicated that for most mares, a minimum body condition score of 5 is required for good reproductive performance. Therefore, for most practical situations, maintaining mares in a body condition of 5 to 6 is reasonable, although a somewhat higher condition score does not appear to be detrimental to reproductive efficiency.

TABLE 7.   ACCEPTABLE FEEDING PROGRAMS FOR 520-KG BROOD MARES*

	Ration 1	Ration 2
Early gestation		
Alfalfa/grass hay	8–9 kg	—
Grass hay	—	9–10 kg
1:1 Mineral†	Free choice	Free choice
Trace mineralized salt	Free choice	Free choice
Late gestation		
Alfalfa/grass hay	10 kg	—
Grass hay	—	8.5 kg
Oats	—	1 kg
1:1 Mineral	55 g	55 g
Trace mineralized salt	Free choice	Free choice
Lactation		
Alfalfa/grass hay	9 kg	—
Grass hay	—	9 kg
Oats	4 kg	3.25 kg
Protein supplement (30%)	—	1 kg
1:1 Mineral	55 g	—
Trace mineralized salt	Free choice	Free choice

*The programs assume that the mare is in good body condition at the onset of gestation.

†Free-choice consumption should be 15 g/d for 1:1 mineral and 20–30 g per day for salt.

See Table 6 for typical mineral product analyses.

During lactation, a mare's body condition has little effect on her ability to produce milk. However, mares that are in marginal body condition (below 5) during the rebreeding period may have reduced reproductive efficiency. Because the nutrient demands of lactation are so high, there is little opportunity to adjust the mare's body condition during lactation to enhance her reproductive efficiency. Therefore, the mare must be in optimal body condition at foaling.

If a mare loses body condition during lactation and has a poor or marginal condition score at weaning, the feeding program must be designed to ensure adequate energy intakes for restoration of body fat reserves to a condition score of 6 or better. These feeding program changes can range from increasing the amount of hay available to maximize consumption (9–11 kg/day) or adding 2.25 to 3.0 kg of grain to a base ration of 6.75 to 7.25 kg/day of good grass or legume hay.

Because of the time it takes to increase body condition, changes in the feeding program should start early in the fall (right after weaning), to allow enough time to improve the mare's body condition before the coldest part of winter. Research suggests that the pregnant mare in early to mid-gestation builds up body condition easily on a good feeding program.

Young, Growing Horses

For feeding the young, growing horse (6–12 months of age) it is recommended that owners use a commercial foal ration to supplement good-quality forage (Table 9). When fed in amounts indicated, these feeds provide the nutrients required by the young, growing horse in a balanced form. A typical foal ration that can be fed from weaning to 12 months of age should contain the following minimal nutrient levels: DE 3.00Mcal/kg, protein 17%, lysine 0.85%, calcium 0.85%, phosphorus 0.70%, copper 30 ppm, zinc

TABLE 9. ACCEPTABLE FEEDING PROGRAMS FOR WEANLINGS (6 MONTHS OF AGE) WITH AN EXPECTED MATURE BODY SIZE OF 500 KG*

	Ration 1	Ration 2
Alfalfa/grass hay	4 kg	—
Timothy hay	—	3.65 kg
Foal ration†	2.25 kg	2.70 kg

*Body weight = 215 kg; daily gain 0.55 kg/day
†Approximate composition: DE = 3.0 Mcal/kg; crude protein = 17%; lysine = .85%; calcium = 0.85%; phosphorus = 0.7%; copper = 30 ppm; zinc = 130 ppm; manganese = 90 ppm; selenium = 0.2 ppm; vitamin A = 7000 IU/kg.

130 ppm, manganese 90 ppm, selenium 0.2 ppm, vitamin A 7000 IU/kg.

When selecting a forage for the young horses, owners should select hay that provides a reasonable level of nutrients to meet requirements, is free of dust and mold, and is palatable. The use of an alfalfa/grass mixed hay is a good choice because this hay provides reasonable levels of energy and protein. If a grass hay is selected, more of the foal ration is required to meet the requirements of the young, growing horse.

FEEDING PROBLEMS COMMON OR UNIQUE TO THE AREA

Trace Minerals

Increased emphasis is being placed on trace mineral requirements of the horse. Of particular interest are the trace minerals copper, zinc, manganese, and selenium. The levels of trace minerals found in forages and grains are noted in Tables 2 and 4. Typically, forages in Western Canada are below NRC (1989) requirements for copper and zinc. Grain is generally deficient in copper but adequate in zinc.

Manganese levels in forage are generally adequate, but wide variations can exist owing to growing conditions and the amount of grass in the forage. Grass forages generally contain higher levels of manganese than do legumes. The manganese levels in grain are also quite variable, with levels that are below requirements (in barley) to levels that meet or exceed requirements (in wheat and oats).

Since the early 1970s, when low trace mineral levels were noted in Western Canadian forages, trace mineralized salts and livestock minerals fortified with trace minerals have been available to horse owners. The levels of copper, zinc, and manganese typically found in these products are noted in Table 6. Use of these products to supply copper, zinc, and manganese is recommended.

Selenium levels in forages vary with growing conditions and with the soil type. Forages grown on seleniferous soils tend to have higher levels of selenium. Table 2 gives the average selenium values for a number of Western Canadian forages. On average, these feeds supply an adequate level of selenium. However, the variability is great and levels as high as 30 mg/kg have been reported in some Western Canadian forages.

Feeding forages with 10 to 30 ppm selenium can result in chronic toxicity. Typical signs of chronic selenium toxicity

TABLE 8. EXAMPLE OF A SCORING SYSTEM THAT CAN BE USED FOR EVALUATING BODY CONDITION IN HORSES

Score	Description of Horse
1	Bony structures are easily visible including the ribs, spine, neck, and pelvis. Animal is in very poor condition.
2	Many bony structures are visible, but horse is not as thin as 1.
3	Horse is noticeably thin, but there is some fat present between the ribs and over the spine and pelvis.
4	Ribs are visible and spine protrudes slightly along back, but the neck and shoulder are not noticeably thin.
5	Ribs are not visible but can be felt easily. Other body parts blend together smoothly.
6	Horse is fleshier than 5 and may have a slight crease along spine over the loin area. Ribs are still easy to feel.
7	Fat deposition around the tailhead, neck, and ribs is becoming noticeable. Many horses have a crease along the spine over the loin. Ribs are harder to feel.
8	Neck is thickened and definition between body parts is absent. Ribs are very difficult to feel; horse is obviously fat.
9	Horse has large fat deposits over entire body. Horse is extremely fat.

include loss of vitality, anemia, lameness, poor hair coat, loss of mane and tail hair, and hoof deformities or loss. Forages, pastures, or hay containing such high levels of selenium are not very common but can occur if grown on seleniferous soils.

In addition to finding very high selenium levels in some forages, it is also possible to find forages that are severely deficient in selenium. Selenium concentrations as low as 0.01 ppm have been found in routine forage samples. These levels are well below the requirement of 0.1 mg/kg and require supplementation.

The variability in selenium levels occurs across the area and a feed analysis is recommended to determine the selenium level in the forage being used. Once the selenium content of the feed has been determined, an appropriate supplement can be selected. The salt and mineral mixtures available have a wide range of selenium levels and because of potential toxicity, horse owners should use mineral or salt products that contain selenium at 40 mg/kg or less. Only one product, either the salt or the mineral, should contain selenium.

Winter

Winter weather in the area is characterized by very cold temperatures and snow. Although the variation is great, parts of Western Canada experience winter temperatures as low as −40°C (−40°F). The colder temperatures accompanied by snow and wind can make for very harsh conditions for horses kept outside.

Horses begin to acclimatize to winter conditions in early September as day length shortens. This acclimatization is in the form of increased hair coat and, if adequate feed is available, an increase in body condition because of increased body fat reserves. The increased hair coat and body condition provide insulation against the cold. The fat reserve also can be used as an energy reserve when the temperature drops. Horses that are to be wintered outside should be in a body condition of about 6 before the onset of winter, and should be fed in such a manner as to maintain that level of condition. In most feeding situations, horse owners should react to a decrease in temperature by increasing the feed offered.

Energy is the nutrient most affected by ambient temperatures, and weight loss is the main nutritional problem associated with winter feeding. As the temperature decreases below the horse's lower critical temperature (LCT), more energy is required to maintain body temperature. Researchers at the University of Saskatchewan have suggested that −15°C (5°F) is the LCT for mature horses. This LCT is based on ambient temperature only and does not take into account wind, humidity, or precipitation. Wind and precipitation also increase the horse's maintenance energy requirement.

The DE requirement increases at the rate of 2.5% for every 1°C below −15°C (5°F). To meet a horse's increased energy requirement, horse owners can feed more hay or add grain to the feeding program. In general, horse owners need to provide an additional 0.20 kg of good-quality hay or 0.15 kg of grain for each 1°C below −15°C. For example, horses being fed at −20°C require additional hay in the amount of 1 kg/day to meet their energy requirements. Examples of feeding programs that can meet a horse's

requirements at −10° and −20°C are found in Table 10. Horse owners should use high-quality forage as the basis for all feeding programs, but this is most critical during the winter. Horses eat more high-quality forage than lower quality forage, and the high-quality forage has a higher heat increment (HI), which is the heat produced when the feed is digested. This heat can be used by the horse to keep warm. Continuous feeding distributes the effects of the HI over a 24-hour period. If high-quality forage is in limited supply, grain is required to meet the horse's energy requirement.

Horses have an excellent ability to handle the cold temperatures of winter with little discomfort if provided with adequate feed, water, and shelter. Shelter protects the horse from moisture and wind, which reduce the insulating capacity of the horse's hair coat. A 15-mph wind will make −15°C (−5°F) weather seem like −25°C (−13°F). Cold, wet weather can increase a horse's energy requirement by 50%. Three-sided sheds provide shelter from wind and moisture, but even a 20% porosity wind fence provides some protection from the wind. Winter grazing has a cost that is usually not included when nutrient needs are predicted. As snow cover increases, horses need to work harder to uncover feed. In addition, the winter pasture is generally of a lower quality (lower energy, higher fiber) and of limited supply, making it difficult for the horse to consume enough feed to meet its requirements. The energy cost of grazing can be as high as 35% above maintenance, and thus when the cost of grazing is coupled with a decrease in temperature below the horse's LCT, meeting the horse's energy requirement becomes more challenging. Good-quality hay should be provided whenever forage intake from pasture is limited.

Even when very good-quality forage is provided free-choice, some horses may not consume enough forage to meet their maintenance requirement during winter and require some additional energy supplementation from grain. Horse owners need to routinely check their horses to ensure they are maintaining their weight and staying in good health. This means a routine check in which body

TABLE 10. FEEDING SUGGESTIONS FOR A MATURE HORSE (500 KG) OVER WINTER*

	Temperature		
	−10°C	−20°C	
Rations Based on Mixed Hay		Ration 1	Ration 2
Alfalfa/grass hay	8.6 kg	9.5 kg	8.2 kg
Oats			1.1 kg
1:1 Mineral†	30 g	30 g	30 g
Trace mineral salt†	15 g	15 g	15 g
Rations Based on Grass Hay		Ration 3	Ration 4
Timothy hay	9.0 kg	10.4 kg	8.2 kg
Oats			1.5 kg
1:1 Mineral	30 g	30 g	30 g
Trace mineral salt	15 g	15 g	15 g

*Assumes horse starts the winter in good body condition.
Does not account for effects of wind or moisture on the horse.
†Mineral analyses are found in Table 6.

condition is manually assessed, because a long winter hair coat can hide a thin horse.

Although cold primarily affects the horse's energy requirement, it is important to provide adequate intakes of protein, minerals, and vitamins. The mineral supplement chosen should provide adequate phosphorus because many forages are marginal in phosphorus content, and cold temperatures can reduce phosphorus digestibility.

Water is required when horses are fed hay during the winter. Heated water ($>2°C$) should be available free-choice. Snow is not an adequate source of water. Horses wintered with snow as a water source have an increased incidence of impaction colic.

Alsike Clover

Alsike clover is a short-lived perennial legume that grows well in cool, moist areas. In certain regions of Alberta, alsike clover is the legume of choice for hay and pasture mixes because it is an easily established legume that thrives in areas where other legumes (i.e., alfalfa) do not grow well. However, since the 1930s, alsike clover has been implicated as a cause of alsike clover poisoning in horses.

Alsike clover poisoning in horses is characterized by loss of body condition, hepatic failure, and various degrees of neurologic impairment. These clinical signs have been associated with horses fed alsike clover as either hay or pasture. Although alsike clover is strongly implicated in this disease, a cause-effect relationship has not been identified.

In addition to alsike clover poisoning, photosensitization of horses on alsike clover forage also occurs. Current information suggests that this problem is a form of trefoilosis and is not related to alsike clover poisoning. The photosensitization occurs on the unpigmented parts of the horse. The photosensitization is a reversible condition when the horse is removed from the source of alsike clover and the exposure to sunlight is reduced. It has been noted that if the photosensitization is extensive, there may be some scarring and loss of hair.

It is hypothesized that the problems associated with alsike clover are related to growing conditions: cool, wet weather followed by warm, sunny weather. To prevent problems with alsike clover poisoning or photosensitization, it is recommended that alsike clover not be used in hay or pasture mixtures for horses.

MAKING RECOMMENDATIONS ON THE FARM

When evaluating a current feeding program or setting up a new one, certain information is needed. A feed analysis of all forages is very useful. Pasture analysis is somewhat difficult to determine because one never knows what the horses are actually consuming, unless time is spent observing them. If pasture samples are collected, they should be collected from areas that are being actively grazed or are likely to be grazed by horses (not from areas that are being avoided by the horses). Hay is easier to sample. When taking a hay sample, clinicians must use a forage probe and randomly sample a minimum of 20 bales from each lot of hay. The random core samples are mixed and sent to a laboratory for analysis. Core samplers are available from agricultural representatives or county extension personnel.

The types of analyses required depend on the horses being fed, and whether there is a specific problem on the farm. The suggested analyses include:

1. Recreation horses—moisture, acid detergent fiber (ADF), protein, calcium, phosphorus
2. Performance horses (training stable)—moisture, ADF, protein, calcium, phosphorus, and selenium
3. Breeding farm (brood mares and young growing horses)—moisture, ADF, protein, calcium, phosphorus, copper, zinc, manganese, and selenium. Nitrate should be included whenever greenfeed is being used.

Some laboratories automatically provide a DE or total digestible nutrients (TDN) value. These values are calculated from the chemical analysis. The acid detergent fiber (ADF) value, is often used to predict the DE value. Many equations for predicting DE have been developed for ruminants, but these overestimate the DE value of the forage for horses. The DE values given in Table 1 were calculated using formulae developed by the Ruminant Feed Evaluation Unit at the University of Alberta in Edmonton and should be adjusted for use in horse feeding programs. An adjustment factor of 0.85 is used in Alberta.

Once a forage analysis has been performed, appropriate commercial feeds or supplements (mineral, protein, energy, vitamin) can be selected to complement the forage to the best advantage of the horses. If commercial feeds are being used, a tag provides information regarding the nutrient composition of the feed. In Canada, the feed tag provides information on protein, fat, fiber, calcium, phosphorus, selenium, and vitamins A, D, and E.

To accurately assess a feeding program, it is necessary to have estimates of feed consumption. Horse owners tend to use volume measures and may not know how much feed they are actually providing. It is important to know how much concentrate is being fed especially when grain intakes exceed 3.5 to 4.0 kg/horse per day. A set of scales is useful to find out how much feed is being offered. When possible, it is best to get some estimate of actual consumption, as well as the amount of feed offered. For example, if hay wastage is high because of poor palatability or poor feeding conditions, actual nutrient intake may be much lower than that which would be predicted from the amount of feed offered.

Look at the horses to get an understanding of the horses that are there, their current body condition, and how they are being fed (i.e., large groups or individually, mares and foals, or horses in training). In group feeding situations, some horses may not get adequate feed.

Check the water source. Lack of water quickly reduces feed intake. Horses need clean, fresh water, free-choice all year (except when hot from exercise).

Keep the feeding programs simple. Maximize the use of good-quality forage, and supplement only the nutrients that are required.

Supplemental Readings

Cymbaluk NF, Christison GI: Environmental effects on thermoregulation and nutrition of horses. Vet Clin North Am Equine Pract 6(2):355–372, 1990.

Henneke DR, Potter GD, Kreider LJ: Body condition during pregnancy and lactation and reproductive efficiency of mares. Theriogenology 21:897–909, 1984.

Hintz HF: Horse Nutrition: A Practical Guide. New York, NY, Arco Publishing, 1983.

Lewis LD: Equine Clinical Nutrition: Feeding and Care. A Lea & Febiger Book. Williams & Wilkins, Media, PA, 1995.

Nation PN: Alsike clover poisoning: A review. Can Vet J 30:410, 1989.

National Research Council: Nutrient Requirements of Horses ed 5. Washington, DC, National Academy Press, 1989.

Feeds and Feeding in the United Kingdom

PAT HARRIS

Waltham-on-the-Wolds, England

Over the last few decades the number of horses being used for leisure purposes in the United Kingdom, including domestic riding and various sporting activities, has increased greatly. It has been estimated that there are around 500,000 horses, nearly one million regular riders, and 1.24 million occasional riders. An indication of the number of horses involved in the competitive aspects of the industry is given in Table 1, but many more people also compete at the local unregistered level. The single largest annual cost associated with owning a nonlivery competition horse is the feeding bill, which represents approximately 19% of the total costs (Table 2).

COMMON TYPES OF FEEDSTUFFS

Concentrates

Most of the grains fed to horses in the United Kingdom are processed in some manner, even if this processing is just cracking or grinding. Micronizing and steam cooking of cereals are increasing in popularity, especially with the increasing use of coarse mixes. Micronizing involves the heating of grain with infrared heaters to around 300°F for 25 to 50 seconds, which results in kernel swelling, cell rupture, and reduced moisture content.

Oats are the traditional cereal grain fed to working horses. There is now a variety of oat produced without husks, referred to as "naked" oats, which tend to have higher levels of certain amino acids, digestible energy (DE) content, and oil level, and are less dusty than conventional oats (Table 3). Naked oats are used mainly in the racing industry but seem to be generally increasing in popularity. Because of their nutrient composition, naked oats can be fed at lower rates (25–50% less by weight) than other cereals.

Because oats are considered to be a "heating" feed, oat-free "cool mixes" or "non-heating" products are very popular. Barley is generally fed rolled or cooked to increase digestibility. Maize (corn) is generally micronized or flaked before feeding rather than being fed cracked. The use of more modern cooking processes has increased the utilization of wheat as a high-energy foodstuff in compound coarse mixes and home-mixed cereal rations. Wheat bran is still fed, especially under the more traditional feeding regimens, but there is increasing awareness of bran's nutri-

TABLE 1. APPROXIMATE NUMBER OF HORSES INVOLVED IN THE MAIN COMPETITIVE SEGMENTS OF THE HORSE INDUSTRY IN THE UNITED KINGDOM

Discipline	Approximate Number
Horse trials (registered)	7000
Advanced	700
Dressage (registered)	5500
Advanced	150
Show jumping (registered)	15,500
Endurance (registered)	2500
Horse driving trials (registered)	800
Polo (estimated)	7500
High goal	1500
Race training (estimated)	17,000
Thoroughbred stallions (estimated)	1000
Thoroughbred mares covered/year (estimated, including Ireland)	18,500
Thoroughbred foals/year	13,000

TABLE 2. AVERAGE ANNUAL EXPENDITURES PER HORSE OWNER FOR A NONLIVERY COMPETING HORSE*

Item	Cost as % of Total
Feed	19.4
Transport	15.5
Stabling	15.1
Veterinary fees	10.3
Competition	9.3
Insurance	8.8
Tack	7.2
Equipment	4.6
Shoeing	7.3
Security	2.5

*As reported by a recent survey for *Horse and Hound*. Total annual cost = 6,046 pounds.

TABLE 3. COMPARISON OF TYPICAL NUTRIENT CONTENT OF "NAKED" AND CONVENTIONAL OATS

Nutrient	Naked Oats	Conventional Oats
Protein (% of DM)	14.6	12.5
Fat (% of DM)	10.6	0.5
Crude fiber (% of DM)	2.4	12.5
Ash (% of DM)	2.2	na
DE (MJ/kg)[1]	17.3	12.4
ME (MJ/kg of DM)[2]	15.2	11.5
Calcium (g/kg of DM)	0.8	0.8
Phosphorus (g/kg of DM)	5.0	0.35
Arginine (g/kg)	9.5	8.0
Cystine (g/kg)	4.5	2.0
Histidine (g/kg)	4.0	2.0
Isoleucine (g/kg)	5.5	6.0
Leucine (g/kg)	10.5	10.0
Lysine (g/kg)	5.5	4.0
Methionine (g/kg)	2.5	2.0
Phenylalanine (g/kg)	7.5	7.0
Threonine (g/kg)	5.0	4.0
Tryptophan (g/kg)	na	2.0
Tyrosine (g/kg)	5.5	6.0
Valine (g/kg)	7.5	7.0
Linolenic acid (% in fat)	1.2	na
Palmitic acid (% in fat)	15.1	na
Linoleic acid (% in fat)	38.0	na
Stearic acid (% in fat)	1.35	na
Oleic acid (% in fat)	43.2	na
Other fatty acids[3]		

[1]Digestible energy as estimated for swine; 1 Mcal = 4.18 MJ.
[2]Metabolizable energy as estimated for ruminants.
[3]Concentrations of myristic, palmitoleic, and others <1%.

tional deficiencies, and its use is diminishing. However, wheat bran mash is still fed occasionally following hard work and during convalescence.

Several forms of treated soybeans commonly are added to compound feeds as a source of essential amino acids. Because the expelled meal and full-fat meal are sometimes unpalatable, the full-fat flake, which has usually been micronized, tends to be the form that is used as a top dressing to balance "cereal straights." Sugar beet, a byproduct of sugar beet processing, is usually molassed. It has been estimated that 10 to 12,000 tonnes (1000 kg = 1 tonne) of sugar beet are sold to horse owners directly. For home feeding the sugar beet is usually purchased as dehydrated shreds or compressed pellets, which are soaked before use. Small quantities of extruded unmolassed sugar beet may be included in compound feeds. Oil or fat is an increasingly common supplementary feedstuff given either to improve coat condition or to increase the energy density in the feed. Vegetable oil and fish oil are the common types used as a top dressing. Cod liver oil is a relatively common supplement and is fed in small quantities, primarily to improve coat quality. Although some horses refuse to eat feed containing cod liver oil, the majority do not appear to find small quantities unpalatable.

Roughages

The hay types available often are categorized as meadow, seed, or legume hay. A guide to average United Kingdom hay composition is given in Table 4. Meadow hays are usually made from permanent pastures and can contain a number of plant varieties including several different types of grass. Seed hays are usually made from pastures that have been seeded specially with one or two grass species, most commonly rye or timothy. The amounts of DE and crude protein in seed hays are frequently lower than in meadow hay. The DE content of seed hay on a dry matter (DM) basis tends to be around 8 to 10 MJ/kg DM (1 Mcal = 4.18 MJ) and the protein concentration ranges from 4 to 8% compared with protein levels of around 8 to 12% DM and DE of around 9 to 11 MJ for meadow hay. Alfalfa hay is not commonly fed in the United Kingdom because it tends to be expensive because it usually has to be imported. Thus, its regular use is limited to some racing yards and breeding studs. The alfalfa chaffs, however, are being fed increasingly as part of the forage portion of the diet.

The protein, mineral, and energy levels of hay can be affected by the type of grass species present, the stage of growth when the hay was harvested, and the area where it was grown. The leaf-to-stem ratio, lignin, crude protein, ether-soluble extract, and ash content (on a DM basis) tend to be higher in the grasses cut early in the year. Crude protein levels in grasses, for example, can be as high as 20% (dry matter basis) in April and as low as 2.5% in September. Soluble carbohydrate levels can be affected by plant species, and by cultivars within the species. In a study carried out in Scotland, Italian ryegrasses had a higher average content of soluble carbohydrate than timothy, fescue, and cocksfoot (181 ± 9.6; 110 ± 10.7; 96 ± 14.4; and 79 ± 4.1 g/kg DM, respectively).

The unpredictable weather conditions in the United Kingdom means that hay quality can be very variable, and hay is often dusty with a high fungal spore count. A number of approaches to solve this problem have been used. It is quite common practice to soak hay before feeding, although the optimal soaking time is controversial. It has been suggested that soaking be limited to 10 to 30 minutes because soaking for 12 hours decreases water-soluble carbohydrate and nitrogen content. In addition, the soak liquor may represent a potential hazard to the environment.

TABLE 4. COMPOSITION OF HAYS AND HOMEMADE HAYLAGES (MEAN AND RANGE)[1]

Nutrient[2]	All Hays	Horse Hays	Haylages
DM (%)	84.8 (82–92)	85.6	60.8 (50–75)
pH	na	na	5.7 (5–6)
Ammonia (as % of total nitrogen)	na	na	1.0 (<1–4)
CP (% of DM)	8.4 (4.5–10.5)	7.5	8.8 (7–13.5)
MADF (% of DM)	37.1 (35–40)	43.7	35 (31–39)
DE (MJ/kg)[3]	8.5 (6.5–10)	7.2	8.5 (7.5–11)
Ash (% of DM)	(6–8)		6.1 (6–8)

[1]Data from ADAS Equine Consultancy; values represent mean and range.
[2]DM = Dry matter; CP = crude protein; MADF = modified acid detergent fiber; DE = digestible energy; na = not available.
[3]DE content is estimated; 4.184 MJ = 1 Mcal.

Similar effects are not observed when the hay is soaked for 30 minutes or less. The number of respirable particles still is reduced significantly with short but thorough wettings.

In traditional haymaking, harvesting tends to be delayed until a mature stage of growth with a relatively high dry matter content is reached. When combined with unpredictable weather conditions, this often results in hays of very variable composition and nutritional value. Barn-dried hay is made from grass that is wilted initially in the field when weather conditions are good and then artificially dried in a barn. The wilted grass may be loosely packed into special buildings where warm dry air is blown through it for 8 to 10 days before it is baled. More commonly, the hay is baled and then stacked, and air is blown across the stack for several days.

In Western Europe, the amount of forage preserved as silage now exceeds the amount preserved as hay. Silage accounted for about 40% of preserved forage in 1975, about 57% in 1985, and accounts for an even higher proportion now. The use of alternative forage sources also has increased in the horse industry, particularly the big bale silage products often referred to as haylages. The term *haylage* tends to be used when the dry matter is greater than 40%, whereas the term *silage* is used when dry matter is less than 40%. Both homemade and commercially produced haylages are used for horses. The homemade varieties tend to be very variable in composition. In the commercial production of haylages, plants are wilted to a dry-matter concentration of around 50 to 60% and then placed into semipermeable plastic packages where a mild anaerobic lactic fermentation occurs (stabilizing at around pH 4.5 to 5.5). Suppression of clostridial activity is achieved by the relatively high dry matter and low pH. Haylages tend to have a protein level of 9 to 12% (dry matter basis) and a DE value of around 9 to 11 MJ/kg, although the reported ranges for homemade silages tend to be slightly wider (see Table 4). The modified acid detergent fiber (MADF) level in commercial haylage is around 32 to 36% (dry matter basis). A recent study found better apparent digestibility of organic matter, acid detergent fiber (ADF), crude protein and energy from a commercial haylage (predominantly ryegrass) compared with timothy hay in ponies (15, 10.5, 72, and 28%, respectively).

Poor-quality big bale silage may present particular health problems but, if properly made, can be a useful forage source and may substantially reduce the respiratory challenge to the horse. Larger yards may feed straight silage, although the silage production has to have been carefully controlled so that it is appropriate for horses, especially with respect to the pH, dry matter content, protein level, and the potential risks of bacterial contamination.

Chaff (i.e., forage chopped into short pieces, often around 2–5 cm in length if produced commercially) is commonly added to concentrate feed. The use of manufactured chaff is increasing, especially the alfalfa types, which are considered good sources of calcium. A common inclusion level is around 0.5 kg/feeding. There are four main types of chaff available in the United Kingdom: molassed straw chaffs, which contain around 40 to 60% molasses and straw and may also contain limestone, herbs, seaweed, minerals, and vitamins; high-temperature dried alfalfa chaff with 10 to 20% molasses; a 50:50 straw and alfalfa mix

TABLE 5.   EXAMPLE COMPOSITIONS OF THREE TYPES OF CHAFF FED TO HORSES IN THE UNITED KINGDOM

Nutrient[1]	Alfalfa Chaff With Molasses	Alfalfa Chaff With Naked Oat Straw	Molassed Straw Chaff
CP (%)	15.0	10.5	4.0
DCP (%)	11.25	8.0	3.0
Fiber (%)	32.0	38.0	26.0
Oil (%)	3.0	2.0	0.8
Ca (%)	1.6	1.0	0.5
P (%)	0.3	0.2	0.03
DM (%)	90.0	85.0	
DE MJ/kg[2]	9.0	7.0	9.3

[1]Abbreviations: CP = crude protein; DCP = digestible crude protein; DM = dry matter; DE = digestible energy.
[2]1 Mcal = 4.184 MJ.

chaff; and unmolassed pure hay or straw chaff (Table 5). Homemade chaff is still fed, but mainly in the larger yards. Straw is not highly regarded as a long forage source in the United Kingdom, especially for young animals with an immature hindgut. In addition, straw is believed to increase the risk of impactions and chronic obstructive pulmonary disease (COPD).

Typical nutrient ranges for pasture in the United Kingdom are shown in Tables 6 and 7, but pastures vary in composition from region to region and from season to season. Calcium levels, for example, can decrease significantly during the winter and the calcium-to-phosphorus ratio may become inverted. Certain geographic areas may have pastures that are deficient in trace elements, particularly copper, zinc, manganese, and selenium. It is therefore important to appreciate which areas are likely to be deficient, especially if the pasture is the main source of nutrients. Standard grazing levels vary, but the commonly recommended rule of thumb is 2 acres (1 acre = 0.405 hectares) for the first animal and then 1 acre for each subsequent animal, depending obviously on whether the pasture is the sole source of nutrients. Perhaps the most frequent poisoning that occurs in grazing animals, including the horse, in the United Kingdom results from the eating of common ragwort (*Senico jacobaea*), which contains an alkaloid that can cause permanent liver damage. A wide

TABLE 6.   TYPICAL MINERAL AND TRACE ELEMENT RANGES IN UK GRASSLAND[1]

Calcium (g/kg of DM)	3.0–10.0
Phosphorus (g/kg of DM)	1.5–4.5
Potassium (g/kg of DM)	15.0–28.0
Magnesium (g/kg of DM)	1.0–2.7
Sodium (g/kg of DM)	1.0–3.0
Sulphur (g/kg of DM)	1.5–4.5
Iron (mg/kg of DM)	30–400
Zinc (mg/kg of DM)	12–60
Manganese (mg/kg of DM)	25–250
Copper (mg/kg of DM)	2.0–15
Molybdenum (mg/kg of DM)	0.1–7.0
Iodine (mg/kg of DM)	0.1–0.4
Cobalt (mg/kg of DM)	0.03–2.0
Selenium (mg/kg of DM)	0.02–0.2

[1]Data from Adas Equine Consultancy.

TABLE 7. TYPICAL COMPOSITION OF ESTABLISHED HORSE PASTURES IN THE UNITED KINGDOM[1]

Nutrient[2]	(Range)
DM (%)	14–22
CP (% of DM)	18–24
Sugars (% of DM)	6–20
MADF (% of DM)	18–24
Ash (% of DM)	6–9
DE (MJ/kg DM)[3]	11.5–12

[1]Data from Adas Equine Consultancy.
[2]DM = dry matter; CP = crude protein; MADF = modified acid detergent fiber; DE = digestible energy.
[3]Estimated value; 1 Mcal = 4.184 MJ.

variety of other plants can cause toxicity to a greater or lesser extent.

Supplements

A bewildering array of supplements is available for horses. These supplements range from the broad-spectrum vitamin/mineral supplements to those providing a specific nutrient, as well as those sold as digestive aids such as yeasts and probiotics. Salt is sometimes added to the diets of intensively exercising horses. Salt licks or rock salt tend to be available in many animals' boxes or mangers. There seems to be an ever-expanding range of trace element supplements available, many of which include organic sources of the trace elements including chelates and proteinates. Many supplements are given with little knowledge of their compatibility with the basal diet constituents or with the other supplements in use. The indiscriminate use of supplements can sometimes lead to oversupplementation of certain nutrients or interactions and interferences between nutrients.

FEED PROCESSING AND COMMERCIAL FEEDS

The compound feed market in the United Kingdom is subject to large seasonal variations, but in general, the amount of commercial feed produced in the United Kingdom has increased in the last 5 years (Table 8). The market has become increasingly fragmented with the development of many smaller niche markets, such as the veteran animal and the convalescent animal. The major companies tend to have a wide range of feeds for different life stages and different exercise types, which are available in a number of different forms. This perhaps reflects the feeding trends within the growing leisure section of the horse market, wherein the individual owner wishes to feed a diet specifically targeted to the animal's needs. However, the bulk of the feed sold still tends to be the general maintenance and light work cubes and mixes.

Compound feeds are processed in a number of ways. Nuts/pellets/cubes (2–15 mm diameter) are very popular, especially for horses at maintenance or light work. Extruded feeds are not very popular, although they may be added to coarse mixes. Over the last 15 years, coarse mixes (sweet feed) have increased in popularity. Coarse mixes

contain processed cereals with molasses or glucose syrup and other ingredients such as grass nuts or pellets, sugar beet pellets, and balancing pellets, which usually contain protein, vitamins, and minerals. The mixes for the higher performance animals tend to contain a lower proportion of the grass pellets. Locust beans, a bitter-sweet, fairly aromatic feedstuff, may also be added to coarse feeds to increase palatability. Locust beans are usually imported and tend to vary in quality. A relatively recent development is the inclusion of herbs in some coarse mixes.

Most feed manufacturers guarantee that their products are free from caffeine and theobromine and state that they are therefore suitable for animals competing under Fédération Equestre Internationale or Jockey Club rules.

FEEDING PRACTICES

No uniform feeding program exists for horses, and it is likely that almost any permutation of feeding regimen could be found somewhere in the United Kingdom. Most people feed at least twice a day, and a few of the racing yards feed three to four times a day. Overall intake recommendations tend to be 2 to 2.5% body weight on a DM basis. Most United Kingdom nutritionists recommend that fiber intake should be at least 1% of body weight, and many of the compound diets advertise a high fiber content as a major selling point. Actual fiber intake varies according to the animal, type of performance expectations, and owners' preferences. In addition, seasonal variations in feeding practices occur, often reflecting the usage of the animal and the availability of pasture. Approximately 64% of respondents to a survey* kept their animals on their own land or stables and 76% used grass as part of the animal's diet. In the leisure and breeding industry, many horses are wintered outside with rugs but are often brought in at night and given a small feed, plus forage. Native animals often winter out, usually with the provision of hay.

*IPC Magazines, *Equestrian Group*

TABLE 8. APPROXIMATE AMOUNT OF COMPOUND FEEDS MANUFACTURED FOR HORSES IN THE UNITED KINGDOM FROM JANUARY 1991 THROUGH 1995[1]

Month	1991	1992	1993	1994	1995
January	8.1	16.5	14.4	13	15.5
February	12.6	12.7	11.6	12.2	13.7
March	10.8	14.2	13.4	13.5	16.9
April	11.3	13.6	12.6	12.8	12.5
May	7.6	9.3	10.9	9.1	10.7
June	6.5	7.8	7.6	8.9	9.2
July	6.8	9.2	7.8	8.8	8.1
August	6.6	9.3	8	10	11.4
September	9.2	11.6	11.3	13.8	15.3
October	11.3	14.7	12.5	14.9	13.8
November	11.8	13.2	14.5	15.8	14.9
December	11.9	14.7	13.9	15.2	17.3
TOTAL	114.5	146.8	138.5	148	159.3

[1]Figures in thousand tonnes (1 tonne = 1000 kg). Data supplied by the Ministry of Agriculture Fisheries and Foods (MAFF), statistics (Commodity & Food) Branch A. These figures may change due to notification of amendments or receipt of late survey returns.

The majority of hay being fed, other than in the big, flat racing yards in Newmarket, tends to be rather poor-quality meadow or ryegrass, which sometimes contains a small proportion of timothy. Alfalfa and timothy hays from the United States or Canada are often used in Newmarket and other racing centers. The amount of hay being fed varies greatly between racing yards, with 3.5 kg/day being around the average, which means that these animals may be receiving a far lower fiber intake than recommended. An increasing number of trainers are feeding haylages. The actual moisture level of haylage can range from 25 to 40%. The relatively high and variable moisture level means that if haylages are fed at the same inclusion rate (weight for weight) as hay, problems due to a lowered intake of fiber as well as other nutrients may arise. A low-fiber intake may contribute to behavioral disturbances, among other problems.

Common feeding practices range from feeding the more traditional home mixes to feeding compound manufactured feeds. Very few people feed a diet consisting of roughage and a simple single grain or compound feed. Many people add other feedstuffs and supplements, including soaked sugar beet or straight molasses, primarily as palatability enhancers. Other common additives include cod liver oil or other types of fat, carrots, and one or more vitamin and mineral mixes. Salt is commonly provided as a salt block on the wall or in the feed manger, or salt is added to the feed. Ground limestone is another common additive. Several examples of diets given to race and eventing horses are given in Table 9. In a survey* 50% reported that they used feed supplements regularly and 36% occasionally.

———————————————
*IPC Magazines, *Equestrian Group*

Herbs are currently in vogue with the horse-feeding public, especially the individual owner and rider. Several of the manufactured feeds contain one or more herbs. Conclusive scientific evidence for the validity of their inclusion in horse feeds is still lacking, although anecdotal and historical evidence suggests that they might have a role to play in certain circumstances. Much more work is needed, however, to substantiate their use.

Some of the larger hunting and racing yards still feed the more traditional racing diet of oats, bran, and hay. Canadian oats have been very popular recently. An "oat balancer" may be added to correct the mineral and vitamin deficiencies and the amino acid deficiencies likely to result from such a diet. The flat racing trainers tend to be more traditional than the National Hunt trainers, who tend to feed cubes and mixes only or to use a compound feed as a large percentage of the diet. It has been estimated that up to 90% of yards use one or more supplements. Many of the top yards, across all disciplines, feed some form of vitamin and mineral supplement even if a balanced compound feed is being fed. Many racing yards feed some form of electrolyte mix and various ergogenic aids. There has been increasing interest in creatine and carnitine. L-carnitine plays an important role in energy metabolism. Although several conditions associated with L-carnitine deficiency have been described in humans, none has been identified in the horse to date. Although supplements are available, little or no information exists on their efficacy in the horse. Similarly, little or no information exists on the efficacy of creatine supplements to enhance performance in the horse. Copper may be recommended to help with various conditions from poor performance to developmental orthopedic disease (DOD), although ways of accu-

TABLE 9. EXAMPLES OF TYPICAL DIETS BEING FED TO RACE AND EVENT HORSES IN THE UK

Feedstuff	Racing Stable A	Racing Stable B	Racing Stable C	Racing Stable D (3-yr-olds)	Racing Stable D (2-yr-olds)	Eventing Stable E	Eventing Stable F	Eventing Stable G
Forage	3–5 kg ryegrass or timothy/ ryegrass mix	3–5 kg timothy hay	3–4 kg ryegrass	1.5 kg alfalfa hay and 4.5 kg timothy hay	1.5 kg alfalfa hay and 4.5 kg timothy hay	5–6 kg hay (permanent meadow)	5–7 kg hay (permanent meadow)	5–6 kg hay (permanent meadow)
Chaff	—	0.5 kg hay or alfalfa	0.5 kg hay	—	—	—	—	0.5–1 kg
Oats	—	6–9 kg	3.5–4.5 kg	5 kg	0.5 kg	4–5 kg	—	—
Compound manufactured feed	6–9 kg coarse mix (sweetfeed) or cubes (14–16% CP)	—	3.5–4 kg cubes	—	2.5 kg coarse mix	1.5 kg oat balancer	4–5 kg coarse mix	3–5 kg coarse mix
Bran	—	0.5 kg	0.3 kg	0.5 kg	—	—	—	—
Salt	Salt lick	?	Salt lick	70 g	70 g	—	28–56 g	28–56 g
Soybean	—	0.1 kg full-fat flakes	—	—	—	—	—	—
Others	—	Honey; cod liver oil	Honey; cod liver oil	100 g limestone flour; cod liver oil; general vitamin mix	75 g limestone flour; 25 g dicalcium phosphate; cod liver oil; general vitamin mix	3–5 oz soy/corn oil; electrolyte supplement	Soy oil	Carrots; sugar beet; molasses

As provided by a number of equine nutritionists; thoroughbred horses with a body weight of 430–510 kg; fresh weight/day.

rately evaluating copper status in the horse are not routinely available.

FEEDING RECOMMENDATIONS AND EXAMPLES OF NUTRIENT INTAKES

There are no United Kingdom or European nutritional guidelines equivalent to those of the National Research Council (NRC). Most of the larger feed manufacturers provide free advice, via their associated nutritionists, based on current research and individual personal experiences and opinions. Some manufacturers may be able to design specific feeding regimens and products to address particular problems associated with an area or feedstuffs used. Independent and semi-independent nutritionists are also available, who provide advice, often in collaboration with the attending veterinarian.

A few studies have compared nutrient intakes of horses in the United Kingdom with NRC (1989) recommendations. The results of a survey of the concentrate feeding practices of a number of Thoroughbred studs in Ireland are given in Tables 10 and 11. When the mean nutrient intakes (using estimated pasture intakes) were compared against calculated NRC requirements for a pregnant mare, a 10-month-old foal, and a 17-month-old yearling, nutrient intakes exceeded requirements in all cases except for the

TABLE 11. MONTHLY MEAN CONCENTRATE INTAKES (± SEM) OF BROOD MARES, WEANLINGS, AND YEARLINGS ON THOROUGHBRED STUDS IN IRELAND[1]

	Weaned Foal	Yearlings	Pregnant Mare	Lactating Mare
August	2.5 ± 0.30	—	0 ± 0	—
September	2.1 ± 0.22	—	0.3 ± 0.19	—
October	2.6 ± 0.18	—	0.9 ± 0.28	—
November	3.2 ± 0.17	—	3.5 ± 0.42	—
December	3.7 ± 0.17	—	5.0 ± 0.37	—
January	—	4.0 ± 0.21	5.6 ± 0.32	7.7 ± 0.41
February	—	4.3 ± 0.22	6.0 ± 0.29	7.7 ± 0.4
March	—	4.2 ± 0.25	6.1 ± 0.29	7.5 ± 0.4
April	—	3.4 ± 0.28	—	—
May	—	1.4 ± 0.27	—	—
June	—	1.2 ± 0.22	—	—
July	—	2.4 ± 0.36	—	—
August	—	5.7 ± 0.42	—	—
September	—	7.9 ± 0.46	—	—
October	—	8.5 ± 0.41	—	—

From O'Donohue PD, Smith FH, Strickland KL: Feed intake on Irish Thoroughbred stud farms. Proc 14th Equine Nutr Physiol Soc, Ontario, CA, 1995, p 229.
[1]Estimated amount of air-dried feed (kg/day) as determined from surveys of farms. In August, the values for weanlings are derived from information from only 6 farms; all other values are derived from information from at least 30 farms.

TABLE 10. UTILIZATION OF VARIOUS FEEDSTUFFS BY IRISH THOROUGHBRED STUD FARMS FOR PREGNANT MARES AND YEARLINGS

Type of Concentrate Feedstuff[1]	Pregnant Mares[2]	Short Yearling	Long Yearling
Straights			
Barley	6.5%	6.7%	2.3%
Dried sugar beet pulp	21.7%	20%	11.4%
Maize flaked	4.3%	4.4%	6.8%
Molasses	17.4%	17.8%	20.5%
Oats	84.8%	82.2%	72.7%
Wheat bran	47.8%	42.2%	47.7%
Grass meal	2.2%	2.2%	2.3%
Linseed/flaxseed	2.2%	4.4%	2.3%
Milk	0	0	2.3%
Soybean meal	28.3%	20%	20.5%
Commercially Compounded Feeds			
Complete feeds	0	0	2.3%
Oat replacer feeds	60.1%	60%	78.6%
Balancers/conditioners	21.7%	28.9%	36.4%

Values represent percentage of stud farms on which each feed was routinely used. Number of farms surveyed: pregnant mares, n = 46; short yearlings, n = 45; long yearlings, n = 44.
From O'Donohue DD, Smith FH, Strickland KL: Feed intakes on Irish Thoroughbred stud farms. Proc 14th Equine Nutr Physiol Soc, Ontario, CA, 1995, p 229.
[1]Horses had access to pasture on almost all farms surveyed. In general, animals were housed inside only during the night in the winter. The housing regimen varied with the stud involved, the age of the animal, and the time of the year.
[2]Pregnant mare, last trimester of gestation; short yearling, about 10 months of age, long yearling about 17 months of age.

weaned foal. For the weaned foal, the intakes of protein and lysine were deficient at the lower dry matter intakes and marginal at the higher intakes.

A survey of the feeding programs used in a few of the top horses in several disciplines indicated that many upper level performance horses are being fed less energy than the NRC (1989)-stated requirements.* Advanced dressage horses received slightly more energy and protein than is recommended, whereas novice event horses were being fed slightly more than the stated NRC requirements for protein. All of the performance horses in the survey were being fed levels of calcium, magnesium, phosphorus, potassium, copper, iodine, iron, cobalt, vitamin A, and vitamin D in excess of the NRC (1989) requirements. Intakes of vitamin E, manganese, zinc, and selenium were similar to NRC recommendations in most cases. Sodium intakes tended to be at or slightly lower than NRC. The survey did not account, however, for all sources of minerals and vitamins such as vitamin and mineral supplements.

Supplemental Readings

Harris PA, Frape DL, Jeffcott LB, Lucas DM, Meyer H, Savage CJ: Equine nutrition and metabolic diseases. In Higgins AJ, Wright IM (eds): The Equine Manual. London, WB Saunders, 1995, pp 123–185.
Hollands T: Feeding the three-day event and dressage horse. Recent Advances in Equine Nutrition (Proceedings of the Kentucky Equine Research, Inc., Short Course), Lexington, KY, 1995, pp 163–177.
National Research Council. Nutrient Requirements of Horses. Washington, DC, National Academy Press, 1989.
O'Donohue DD, Smith FH, Strickland KL: Feed intakes on Irish Thoroughbred stud farms. Proc 14th Equine Nutr Physiol Soc, Ontario, CA, 1995, p 229.

*See Hollands T in Supplemental Readings.

MISCELLANEOUS
Edited by N. Edward Robinson

Immunizations

L. MICHAEL SCHMALL
Columbus, Ohio

Vaccinations against infectious diseases are an essential component of any disease control or preventive medicine program. Although no vaccination can claim to be 100% effective in preventing disease, significant reductions in morbidity and mortality are the result of a well-conceived and applied vaccination program. The overall goal of decreasing the incidence of infectious diseases should include proper isolation procedures for new arrivals, adequate ventilation in stalls and barns, adequate feed, access to clean water, and opportunity for horses to receive exercise. Reducing stress and minimizing factors that can cause immunosuppression in the animals should also be considered when attempting to control disease.

Commercial vaccines are currently available for the major equine infectious diseases—eastern, western, and Venezuelan encephalomyelitis; tetanus; influenza; equine herpesviruses 1 and 4; rabies; botulism; equine monocytic ehrlichiosis (Potomac horse fever); equine viral arteritis; strangles; and anthrax. These vaccines come as single entities or as multivalent combinations. The choice as to product varies, depending on practitioner preference; time of year; animal use; potential exposure to the infectious agent; and the age, sex, and other features of the animal to be vaccinated. Any vaccine used should be a United States Department of Agriculture (USDA) licensed product that has been properly handled to ensure safety and efficacy. Unless there are well-established clinical data to indicate otherwise, all vaccines should be used in accordance with manufacturer recommendations. For maximal efficacy, only those horses that are healthy should be vaccinated. Horses that are ill or incubating disease may respond to vaccines in an unpredictable fashion. Adequate records of all vaccinations and associated adverse reactions should be kept for each animal for future reference.

Vaccines can be classified as either modified live or killed product. With the modified live vaccine, an attenuated strain of the organism is used to produce a clinically inapparent form of the disease that results in the animal mounting an immune response that protects against challenge with the wild strain. With the killed products, the viral or bacterial organisms have been inactivated by physiochemical means and are used as the immunizing agent. More commonly, a portion or an extract of the organism is used as the vaccine. Toxoids are inactivated forms of a toxin. These are used as immunogens for tetanus and botulism. Antitoxins are preformed antibodies against a specific agent that provide only short-term passive immunity for the patient.

Vaccination programs are custom-tailored depending on age, sex, use, risk of exposure, and other factors. The following recommendations are general guidelines and should be modified as needed.

ADULTS AND YEARLINGS

The largest group of horses that are exposed to and have the greatest risk of acquiring infectious diseases on a more or less continual basis are the yearling to adult horses. These are the horses that are repeatedly moved to and from stables, tracks, farms, and show rings. They come into contact with numerous potential carriers of infectious disease, particularly respiratory diseases, and are subjected to changes in management.

Tetanus

Tetanus remains a constant threat to the horse population. Clinical disease, which is caused by the neurotoxin of *Clostridium tetani*, is extremely difficult, if not impossible, to treat and usually results in the death of the animal. This organism is present in the gastrointestinal tract and feces of normal horses, and the potential is always present for the contamination of penetrating wounds and injuries. Protection involves the production of antibodies directed against the neurotoxin. This is achieved by use of tetanus toxoid, the inactivated toxin. Animals that have not previously been vaccinated should receive an initial dose of tetanus toxoid, followed by a booster dose 3 to 6 weeks later. Routine immunizations should then be on an annual basis. Administration of tetanus toxoid may be repeated if the horse sustains an injury and more than 6 months has elapsed since the last booster. Horses with an injury in which the vaccination status is unknown should be given tetanus antitoxin along with a dose of tetanus toxoid. The toxoid should be repeated 4 weeks later. Tetanus antitoxin provides immediate protection against the toxin but lasts only 3 to 4 weeks. A serious complication can arise after administration of tetanus antitoxin. The antitoxin is of equine origin and has the potential to produce hepatitis (serum sickness) in a small percentage of horses. Hepatitis usually develops several weeks following the administration of antitoxin. This product should be reserved for use in nonvaccinated horses, nonvaccinated mares, and newborn foals.

Encephalomyelitis

Three strains of viral-induced encephalomyelitis are of clinical concern in the United States—eastern, western, and Venezuelan. The most serious of these three is the eastern variety, which may be associated with mortality rates of up to 90%, followed by the Venezuelan and western strain, which results in the lowest mortality. These diseases are transmitted by blood-sucking insects, most commonly the mosquito, from wild bird and rodent reservoirs. Horse-to-horse transmission does not occur except with Venezuelan equine encephalomyelitis (VEE). The potential for human exposure and disease exists with each of the virus strains. Although Venezuelan encephalitis is not currently found in the United States, it is present in the horse populations in Mexico and other countries of Central and South America. Vaccination for VEE is not currently included in vaccination recommendations unless the animal will be transported to an endemic area. Inactivated vaccines incorporate both the eastern and western strains or all three strains. Unvaccinated horses should receive a two-dose series at a 2- to 3-week interval. Routine vaccinations are then administered on an annual basis before the emergence of the mosquito vector or in the event of an outbreak of the disease. In the warmer climates, where the vector is present year round, boosters should be given on a semi-annual basis.

Influenza

Equine influenza is a highly contagious and rapidly spread disease of the respiratory system. Clinical signs include depression, fever, muscle stiffness and soreness, anorexia, cough, and nasal discharge. Perhaps the greatest concern with this disease is the potential for the development of secondary bacterial infections, which can range from mild bacterial pneumonias to serious pleuropneumonia. The major difficulty with current vaccines is the inability to confer a long-lasting immunity. Even immunity in recovered horses is insufficient to protect for more than several months. Available inactivated vaccines incorporate the common strains of the equine influenza virus, A/equine 1 and A/equine 2. Although influenza viruses are constantly undergoing antigenic shift, there is sufficient cross reaction with the vaccinal strains to provide some degree of immunity. However, this is less than optimal, which means that even vaccinated animals can develop the disease when a newer antigenic strain is encountered. Manufacturers of most products recommend an initial two-dose series followed by semiannual vaccinations. This program is sufficient for most horses without high risk of exposure. Those animals that travel extensively, are shown or raced, or are exposed to a large number of other horses need to be vaccinated more frequently. Current recommendations are that vaccines be given every 2 to 3 months. Even at this frequency, vaccination may not provide full protection against the disease.

Equine Herpesvirus 1 and 4 (Rhinopneumonitis)

Two distinct strains of equine herpesvirus (EHV) that are of clinical significance are identified—EHV-1 and EHV-4. EHV-1 produces three clinical syndromes: respiratory disease, abortion, and encephalomyelitis. EHV-4 has been primarily associated with respiratory disease. The respiratory disease of both EHV-1 and EHV-4 occurs most frequently in younger animals and resembles a mild influenza-like condition. Older horses typically have some acquired immunity and do not develop a serious clinical form of respiratory disease. An acquired immunity to either the abortion or the neurologic forms of the disease does not seem to occur. Both a modified live and a killed vaccine that incorporate both viral strains are available. Vaccination is best done in a manner similar to that for influenza with the same restrictions. Maximal protection is maintained by vaccinating every 2 to 3 months. If horses are not in contact with a large number of outside animals, semiannual vaccinations may be sufficient.

Streptococcus equi (Strangles)

Strangles is a streptococcal bacterial disease that is spread by direct contact with infected horses or carriers. It affects primarily young horses but can afflict animals of any age. Clinical signs include fever, depression, anorexia, profuse mucopurulent nasal discharge, and enlargement of the submandibular and retropharyngeal lymph nodes and lymph nodes of the head and face. Inactivated M-protein extracts of the bacterial organism have largely replaced the whole cell bacterins. Recommended vaccinations are a two- or three-dose series at 2- to 4-week intervals followed by annual boosters. In situations in which animals are at high risk, it has been suggested that boosters be given at 6-month intervals. Unfortunately, the vaccines do not fully protect against the disease. The vaccines do, however, lessen the incidence and severity of the disease and work well in situations in which animals are vaccinated before exposure or at the time the first case is diagnosed. This may be the limiting factor in the overall efficacy in that most horses may not be vaccinated before exposure.

Rabies

Although rabies is not a common clinical condition in horses, its uniformly fatal outcome and its public health significance make this disease of major importance. Horses are frequently kept in environments where infected wildlife pose a potential risk. It is important that the vaccine used for immunization is one that has been approved for use in horses. It is recommended that an initial two-dose series, with doses given 1 month apart, be followed by annual boosters.

Potomac Horse Fever (Equine Monocytic Ehrlichiosis)

Potomac horse fever (PHF) is a seasonal diarrheal disease most frequently seen in late spring through the early fall months. The reservoir and method of transmission of the causative organism, *Ehrlichia risticii*, are not well established. Horse-to-horse transmission does not appear to be a significant factor. Clinical signs include febrile response, anorexia, lethargy, decreased intestinal tract sounds, colic, diarrhea, dehydration, and laminitis. Vaccination recommendations are an initial two-dose series at a 2- to 4-week interval followed by boosters at 6- to 12-month intervals. Vaccinations should be given just before the period of greatest risk. Although the degree of immunity may not be fully protective, it does appear to lessen the clinical severity of the disease.

Anthrax

Anthrax is a fatal septicemic disease produced by *Bacillus anthracis*. It is endemic to certain geographic locations where soil conditions are suitable to maintain the organism. The disease develops following wound contamination or ingestion of the bacterial spores. Because of severe adverse effects of the vaccine, vaccination should be considered only for those animals at significant risk. Two doses of vaccine are administered subcutaneously at a 2- to 3-week interval. Subsequent vaccinations are on an annual basis.

BROOD MARES

Brood mares should receive all annual vaccinations before breeding. This includes tetanus, encephalomyelitis, influenza, EHV-1 and 4, rabies, and PHF vaccinations. Following confirmation of pregnancy, vaccines should not be given, unless necessary, during the first 90 days of pregnancy to minimize the risk of embryonic loss or damage to the developing fetus. Pregnant mares should be routinely immunized against tetanus, influenza, encephalomyelitis, and EHV-1 and 4, 4 to 6 weeks before foaling to provide maximal maternal antibody levels in the colostrum, which can be passed on to the foal. Other diseases that are of specific importance to the brood mare are botulism and equine viral arteritis.

Equine Herpesvirus 1 and 4

A major concern when dealing with pregnant mares is the possibility of infections with EHV-1 and 4. The potential is for these viruses, particularly EHV-1, to induce abortion or produce weak nonviable foals. Infection in mares is usually inapparent, in that the mare shows minimal signs of respiratory disease. The abortions occur several weeks after the infection. Manufacturer recommendations are that mares be vaccinated at 5, 7, and 9 months of pregnancy. Many veterinarians suggest that an additional vaccination be given at 3 months of pregnancy. Both killed and modified live vaccines are available for use. At present, only the killed product is labeled for use in pregnant mares, although many practitioners use the modified live product.

Botulism

The toxicoinfectious form of botulism, caused by the neurotoxin of type B *Clostridium botulinum*, is a clinical condition that affects primarily foals (shaker foals). This disease is considered endemic in several areas of the country. If mares are going to foal in areas where botulism has occurred, vaccination with an approved toxoid is necessary. The protocol is for three doses administered 1 month apart, with the last dose being given 2 to 4 weeks before foaling. Annual boosters should be given 4 weeks before foaling.

Equine Viral Arteritis

Equine viral arteritis (EVA) is an infectious disease that produces abortion; embryonic death; fever; and generalized edematous swelling of the legs, face, and genital areas of affected horses. Seroprevalence data indicate that this virus is widespread in Standardbreds with little clinical disease, whereas the opposite holds true for Thoroughbreds and other breeds. The disease may be transmitted from horse to horse, but a major route of spread is through semen from infected stallions to susceptible mares. This established protocol to control the disease suggests that vaccination be considered only if the mare is going to be bred to a stallion that is a known carrier of the virus. Only under special circumstances is vaccination recommended for nonpregnant mares. Because of the regulatory issues involved with the international movement of seropositive horses, it is recommended that any use of the vaccine be coordinated with state and federal regulatory officials.

STALLIONS

Stallions should receive vaccinations using the schedule for adult horses, including tetanus, encephalomyelitis, rabies, and PHF vaccines, with the following exceptions.

Influenza and EHV-1 and 4

Stallions should be immunized with these products before and every 2 months throughout the breeding season. The febrile response that accompanies infection with these viral organisms can seriously decrease stallion fertility for several weeks.

Equine Viral Arteritis

The clinical presentation of this disorder has already been discussed. Vaccination is most commonly used in mares being bred to an already infected stallion. However, vaccination has also been used to prevent establishment of the disease in noninfected stallions. A significant drawback to routine use is that vaccination can result in virus shedding in the semen. Use of this product should be considered on a individual case basis, because the same concerns and restrictions on the international movement of seropositive mares apply to stallions.

FOALS AND WEANLINGS

Vaccination of foals and weanlings is open to debate. Foals are immunocompetent at birth and do develop active immunity. The difficulty lies in the interference of maternal antibodies absorbed from the colostrum. Ideally, it is best to know when maternal antibody titers have declined to a level that will no longer interfere with the development of active immunity. In most situations that occurs around 12 weeks of age, and many veterinarians begin to vaccinate foals at 3 to 4 months of age in accordance with manufacturer recommendations. However, many choose to start vaccination at an earlier time. This is particularly true if the vaccination status of the mare is unknown or the mare did not receive the proper immunizations before foaling. More recent information indicates that, at least for influenza, it may be advantageous in terms of producing a long-lasting immunity to withhold vaccination of foals for influenza until they reach 6 months of age. This does, however, leave a significant period of time in which they may be at greater risk of acquiring infectious diseases.

Tetanus

Current recommendations are that the foal receive an initial two-dose series of tetanus toxoid, 3 to 6 weeks apart, beginning at 3 to 4 months of age. As mentioned, many practitioners vaccinate at a much earlier age with the toxoid with little or no apparent problem. The major concern is the potential for interference with the vaccine by maternal antibodies. This may not be as much of a problem if the mare was not properly immunized before foaling. A common practice is for newborn foals to be given tetanus antitoxin. This provides significant protection for 2 to 4 weeks. A potential adverse reaction associated with the administration of tetanus antitoxin or biologics of equine origin is Theiler's disease, or acute hepatitis.

Encephalomyelitis

Vaccination against eastern and western encephalomyelitis should begin at 3 to 4 months of age unless the foal was born to a vaccinated mare late in the season. Maternal antibodies provide adequate protection for 5 to 6 months and may be sufficient to protect late-born foals until the next spring. The initial vaccination is a two-dose series at 3- to 4-week intervals followed by annual boosters.

Influenza

Current recommendations for the vaccination of foals for influenza are influenced by various factors. If the foals are born to a well-vaccinated mare and are not exposed to large numbers of other horses, it may be possible to delay vaccination until 6 months of age. If the mare has been vaccinated but the exposure risk is high, it is preferred that vaccination be started at 3 to 4 months of age. Vaccines should be given every 4 to 6 weeks until 7 months of age. If the mare was not vaccinated and the risk of exposure is

high, vaccination can begin as early as 1 to 2 months of age at 4- to 6-week intervals.

Equine Herpesvirus 1 and 4

The recommendations for equine herpesvirus vaccination parallel those for other age groups. An initial two-dose series is followed by boosters at 3-month intervals.

Streptococcus equi

Immunization of foals with any of the strangles vaccines usually begins at 2 to 3 months of age. This is particularly important on premises where there is a high incidence of the disease. Protocols usually suggest a two- or three-dose series at 2- to 4-week intervals. It is frequently necessary to give boosters to foals at 6 months of age to provide proper immunity.

Rabies

Vaccination of foals against rabies should begin at 3 to 4 months, followed by a booster at 1 year of age. Additional boosters are given annually.

Potomac Horse Fever

The recommendations for vaccination of foals for PHF is for an initial two-dose series followed by a booster at 1 year of age.

Vaccines for other infectious diseases, such as leptospirosis, have been reported as being used in horses. Unfortunately, because there is little data supporting their safety or efficacy and because they are not approved for use in horses, they cannot be recommended.

Adverse reactions are not unusual but are for the most part not serious. Because most vaccines are administered intramuscularly, reactions are usually limited to localized swelling and muscle soreness at the site of injection. These reactions usually respond to nonsteroidal anti-inflammatory drugs (i.e., phenylbutazone), application of cold packs to the swollen area, and, if desired, topical application of dimethyl sulfoxide (DMSO) or DMSO and steroid combinations. Occasionally, an abscess may develop at the site of injection. Apart from the costs of treatment and the loss of use, such problems are not a major issue. However, there are rare occasions when animals may experience a severe anaphylactic reaction or develop an acute severe necrotizing myositis as the result of a vaccination. These are life-threatening situations and must be recognized quickly and treated aggressively. Such potential adverse reactions must be recognized when using any product.

Supplemental Readings

Rose RJ, Hodgson DR: Manual of Equine Practice. Philadelphia, WB Saunders, 1993.

Rumbaugh GE: Vaccination programs. *In* Robinson NE (ed): Current Therapy in Equine Medicine. Philadelphia, WB Saunders, 1983, pp 40–43.

Subcommittee on Vaccination Guidelines of the AAEP Biologic and Therapeutic Agents Committee (Wilson DW, Kanara EW, Spensley MS, Powell DG, Files WS, Steckel RR): Guide for vaccination of horses. J Am Vet Med Assoc 207(4):426–431, 1995

Wilson WD, Spensley MS: Preventive medicine programs. *In* Robinson NE (ed): Current Therapy in Equine Medicine, ed 3. Philadelphia, WB Saunders, 1992, pp 35–50.

Parasite Control Programs

THOMAS R. KLEI
Baton Rouge, Louisiana

The principal internal parasites of horses are nematodes. The species of primary importance have changed during the past decade in developed regions of the world because of the advent and use of highly effective anthelmintics. Nonetheless, these organisms remain a serious threat to equine health. Other parasites including tapeworms and botfly larvae, although of arguable significance, are also considered in the formulation of most internal parasite control programs. The focus of most control strategies is the regular use of anthelmintics. The overuse of these drugs has raised concern recently because of the potential for the induction of drug-resistant strains of cyathostomes and the possibility of adverse effects on free-living organisms in the pasture environment. The rational formulation of individual parasite control programs should be based on a knowledge of available anthelmintics, the characteristics of the horses involved and their environment, the potential for the use of nonanthelmintic control methods, and the advantages and disadvantages of currently used strategies.

ANTHELMINTICS

A large number of anthelmintics are currently available for use in the horse (Table 1). These compounds include drugs in six major classes. For purposes of rotational treatment regimens, compounds should be alternated between classes because side resistance generally occurs within drug classes. Anthelmintics are equally effective by all routes of administration as long as the appropriate dosage based on weight is given.

Avermictins/Milbemycins

The avermictins are macrocyclic lactones that interact with gamma-aminobutyric acid (GABA) receptors and invertebrate glutamate-gated chloride channels to disrupt neuromuscular function of nematodes and arthropods. Ivermectin, the avermectin currently available for use in horses, has a broad range of activities at a low dose. Its activity against adult and migrating larval nematodes and all stages of *Gasterophilus* species larvae is unique. Since its introduction, the prevalence of summer sores caused by larvae of *Draschia megastomum* or *Habromena* species, dermatitis associated with *Onchocerca cervicalis* microfilariae, and colic induced by migrating larvae of *Strongylus* species have been markedly reduced. It is likely that ivermectin has played a significant role in these phenomena. Treatment of mares with ivermectin within 24 hours of parturition markedly reduces transmission of *Strongyloides westeri* to foals. This compound is not effective against the tapeworms *Anoplocephala* species or adults of *Onchocerca cervicalis*. Activity against encysted larvae of the cyathostomes is also lacking. Cyathostome eggs normally reappear

TABLE 1. DOSAGE, SAFETY, METHOD OF ADMINISTRATION, AND EFFICACY OF EQUINE ANTHELMINTICS

Drug Class	Anthelmintic	Relative Onset of Action	Dosage (mg/kg)	Safety Index*	Method	Mean Efficacy (%)†				
						Bots	P. equorum	Strongyles Large	Small	O. equi
Avermectin/milbemycin	Ivermectin	Slow	0.2	10	S,O	99	100	100	100	100
Avermectin/milbemycin	Moxidectin	Slow	0.4	5	O	90	100	100	100	100
Benzimidazole	Thiabendazole	Slow	44–88‖	13	S,F,O	0	42	97	95	95
Benzimidazole	Mebendazole	Slow	8.8	45	S,F,O	0	97	80–97	87	97
Benzimidazole	Fenbendazole	Slow	5–10‖	200	S,F,O	0	85	95–97	97	97
Benzimidazole	Oxfendazole	Slow	10	10	S,F,O	0	85	97	97	97
Benzimidazole	Oxibendazole	Slow	10–15	60	S,O	0	85	97	97	97
Probenzimidazole	Febantel	Slow	6	33	S,F,O	0	97	97	97	97
Pyrimidine	Pyrantel pamoate	Slow	6.6	20	S,F,O	0	95	70–77	95	50
Imidazothiazole—simple heterocyclic	Levamisole-piperazine	Fast‡	8/88¶	<3	S	0	100	63–97	97	90
Simple heterocyclic	Piperazine	Fast	88–110§	17	S	0	97	5–50	95	50
Organophosphate	Trichlorfon	Fast	40	1	S,O	95	97	0	0	95
Organophosphate	Dichlorvos resin pellet	Fast	35	3	F	90	97	75–97	90	95

S = stomach tube; F = feed; O = orally as paste or drench
*Safety index (Dose at which clinical signs first appear)/(Minimum therapeutic dose)
†Applies to susceptible parasites only; resistant populations may be encountered, especially small strongyles
‡Due to piperazine
§As piperazine base
‖Higher doses required for *P. equorum*
¶As levamisole/piperazine base

in feces 8 to 10 weeks following ivermectin treatment. This period may be shorter in younger stock that are likely to be more heavily infected. Concern has been raised regarding the potential negative environmental impact of this class of compounds on freeliving arthropods, particularly dung beetles. However, data on this topic regarding the use of the drug in horses are conflicting, and negative effects on the equine pasture environment have not surfaced. Moxidectin is a milbemycin in this group of compounds that has been introduced for use in horses in some parts of the world. It has a range of activity similar to that of ivermectin. Differences between these two compounds and their uses will undoubtedly be determined in the near future.

Benzimidazoles

A number of benzimidazoles in various formulations and mixtures are available as products for use in the horse. The primary mode of action of these drugs is disruption of microtubule formation by binding to the protein tubulin. These compounds are highly effective against most nematodes living within the gastrointestinal tract, although some variation in the spectrum of activity exists (see Table 1). In this regard, fenbendazole is less effective against *Strongyloides westeri* than are other drugs in this class. The reduced efficacy of thiabendazole against *Parascaris equorum* may be helpful in situations where heavy infections are expected, and killing of large numbers of worms may cause intestinal impaction and rupture. The phenylguanidine, febantel, is considered to be a pro-benzimidazole and is metabolized to fenbendazole in vivo. It should be considered to be a benzimidazole for the purposes of drug class rotation. Some benzimidazoles have been demonstrated to be highly effective against migrating large strongyles and encysted cyathostome larvae when used at elevated dosages for prolonged periods. An example of this is the use of fenbendazole at 10 mg/kg for 5 days. As noted later, resistance to benzimidazoles by cyathostomes has become widespread.

Pyrimidines

The pyrimidines approved for use in the horse are the pyrantel salts, pyrantel pamoate and pyrantel tartrate. The mode of action of these compounds seems to be as cholinergic agonists. Pyrantel tartrate, the most recently introduced, is used as a daily food supplement and functions in a prophylactic manner. This formulation and method of delivery have proven to be highly effective in most circumstances. However, its effectiveness in foals that are heavily challenged may be reduced, and special efforts are necessary to ensure compliance in all situations. Use of the prophylactic formulation in young animals also eliminates or delays the development of acquired immunity in these animals. The pyrantel salts are unique as equine anthelmintics in that they are effective against the common tapeworm *Anoplocephala perfoliata*. At the recommended dosage for nematode control, this efficacy is between 80 and 90% when administered as a paste or liquid. This level of efficacy is effective in reducing total tapeworm populations. Efficacy is increased to more than 90% at 2 times this dosage. The low-dose feed-additive formulation of pyrantel

tartrate that is administered daily also appears to have some effect when administered for at least 30 days.

Other Anthelmintic Compounds

A number of other compounds in various formulations and mixtures are available (see Table 1). In general, many of these are less useful than those mentioned earlier in that they have a reduced spectrum of activity and lower safety indexes. Some mixtures, particularly those that include benzimidazoles, have a synergistic activity and are useful in control of benzimidazole-resistant cyathostomes.

FACTORS TO CONSIDER

No single parasite control strategy is ideal for all horses under all management conditions or for use in all regional environments. A number of different but interrelated factors must be considered before the development of programs that suit individual needs.

Cyathostomes as Primary Targets

As indicated earlier, the use of highly effective antiparasitic compounds has reduced the prevalence of *Strongylus* species, the most pathogenic of internal parasites. Effective control of these parasites has focused attention on the cyathostomes. It has been determined that cyathostomes, once considered to be nonpathogenic, promote colic, have a negative impact on development, cause a general loss of condition, and are responsible for larval cyathostomiasis. The latter condition, although difficult to diagnose, is associated with a sudden onset of diarrhea, loss of condition, and in some cases death. This syndrome occurs more commonly in young horses and is associated with the synchronous emergence of large numbers of encysted larvae into the lumen of the large intestine. This phenomenon is seasonal, as is the syndrome, and is most common during the winter or early spring months. Anthelmintic treatment to remove these encysted stages as part of the therapy for this condition is of questionable value and may depend on the degree of damage already done to the mucosa. As noted earlier, elevated dosages of benzimidazoles for prolonged periods have been reported to be efficacious against these larval stages.

Noncyathostome Parasites

In situations in which parasite control is closely monitored and the horses in question have no contact with horses that have not been treated and quarantined, elimination of some parasites such as the large strongyles, *Onchocerca*, and spiruroid stomach worms is possible. However, these parasites have not been eliminated from the general horse population, and caution should be taken to ensure that they do not enter closed herds. Foals and weanlings are susceptible to nematodes not commonly seen in adult animals. Infection with *P. equorum* may be particularly damaging. Control for these parasites should begin before 10 weeks of age, the prepatent period of these worms, which not only eliminates parasites within the horse but also reduces contamination of the environment with the long-lived infective eggs of these worms. Ivermectin is highly effective against the migrating stages of these parasites. The significance of infections with stomach botfly larvae (*Gasterophilus* species) or tapeworms (*A. perfoliata*) has not been demonstrated experimentally and is open to debate. However, until these agents have been shown to be nonpathogenic, their control should also be considered in formulating individual programs.

Level of Control Required

The degree of parasite control necessary to maintain optimal health in a given horse is dependent on a number of factors. These include the animal's age, its use, management conditions and stocking rates, and its potential exposure to heavily infected horses. Thus, mature horses used for recreation, which are maintained at low stocking rates of less than 1 horse per acre, may be able to be maintained in excellent health with only 2 anthelmintic treatments per year. Such a program is unsuitable for athletic horses or mares on a large breeding farm. Variations can even occur within such environments. As an example, nursing mares are affected more by parasite infections than non-nursing mares in the same environment and may require more intense parasite control.

Acquired Immunity

Evidence of acquired resistance to reinfection with *P. equorum* and *S. westeri* is abundant and is presumed to be related to immunity. Control programs that are vigorous and initiated early in the life of the foal, before 6 to 8 weeks of age, may actually delay the acquisition of immunity and increase the duration of infection with these parasites. Acquired resistance to strongyles is not complete, is more difficult to assess, and its level is likely to be controlled by genetic factors. Control programs that exclude or greatly minimize infection are likely to reduce the development of immunity and increase the risk of parasite-associated disease when animals are exposed to heavy parasite challenge. This is an easy concept to express but a difficult one to put into practice. The level and duration of exposure to strongyle infection that are necessary to induce a protective resistance are unknown. Thus, in the ideal situation, young horses should receive the minimal level of treatment sufficient to produce maximal health. As horses mature and acquire resistance, only a small portion of any band remains susceptible. These individuals carry the majority of the strongyle burden in the population and are responsible for pasture contamination. Identification of these horses and their treatment uses acquired immunity in parasite control and minimizes the use of anthelmintics.

Climate

Seasonal variations in climate, primarily temperature and rainfall, affect the development and survival of strongyle larvae on pasture and thus pasture infectivity. In northern temperate regions, severe winters reduce pasture infectivity, and the major period of strongyle transmission is during the summer months. In these regions, control of strongyle infections in mature horses has been accomplished by the strategic treatment to remove luminal parasites during the spring and early summer. This reduces pasture contamination and reinfection. In tropical and semitropical regions, this seasonal cycle is reversed, and the optimal period of transmission is during the cooler

winter months. The hot temperatures during the summer months reduce survival of larvae on pasture and pasture infectivity. In these environments it may be possible to eliminate summer treatments in mature horses.

Drug Resistance

Resistance to anthelmintics in the horse is limited to the cyathostomes. The most widespread resistance documented has been to the benzimidazoles, but incidences of resistance to phenothiazine, piperazine, and pyrantel have been reported. For some time, benzimidazole-resistant cyathostome populations were demonstrated to be susceptible to oxibendazole. However, as might be expected with prolonged widespread use, resistance has developed to this drug as well. Resistance has a genetic basis, and frequent repeated use of the same class of anthelmintic selects for resistant populations. Resistance to ivermectin has not been reported, even though the drug has been used repeatedly and excessively on some farms for long periods. The reasons for this absence of resistance to this compound is not clear. Resistance to ivermectin has been demonstrated against trichostrongyle nematodes of ruminants, and it is unlikely that this apparent refractoriness is due to differences in the biochemistry of cyathostomes. A potential explanation may be related to the large refugum of cyathostomes that escape ivermectin selection pressure. This population includes those hypobiotic and developing larvae encysted in the mucosa, which may be greater than 80% of the total worm burden. Larvae developing on pasture constitute another potentially large refugum population. Thus, the absence of efficacy against mucosal larval stages of the cyathostomes may have prolonged the usefulness of this compound. It has been speculated that the prolonged daily use of pyrantel tartrate in its low-dose formulation would result in an increased incidence of resistance to pyrantel compounds. However, this has not been the case.

CONTROL PROGRAMS

A number of different strategies have been proposed and are used in horse parasite control. These are not all uniformly accepted, and all have some advantages and disadvantages. Each is reviewed below.

Interval Treatment

Interval treatment or fast rotation programs are those that alternate different anthelmintic classes during the year at predetermined periods. Intervals used vary from 1 to 2 months. An advantage of this type of program is that it allows for the elimination of parasites every year that are not uniformly killed by all drugs such as *Gasterophilus* species larvae and *A. perfoliata*. This rotational scheme was designed to increase intervals between treatments with the same drug class and thus slow the development of resistance. However, such rotational methods have induced multiple drug resistance in trichostrongyle nematodes of sheep under experimental conditions, and it is hypothesized that similar results could occur in horses. This has not been demonstrated. Another potential disadvantage of this type of program is that the period following treatment when eggs of cyathostomes reappear; the egg reappearance period (ERP) varies with different drugs and with the infection burden of the horse. Thus, the ERP following ivermectin treatment of mature horses is generally 8 to 10 weeks and that of other drugs is 4 to 6 weeks. Young horses with heavier parasite burdens may also have shorter ERP. Using a standard interval between treatments with different drug classes thus does not always maximally reduce pasture contamination. In some instances, this may be an advantage in that it allows for a minimal exposure to occur and some protective immunity to develop.

Annual Rotation

Annual rotation or slow rotation programs use the same anthelmintic at appropriate intervals throughout the year based on ERP. Drug classes are alternated yearly. The advantage of these programs is that theoretically they minimize the potential development of multiple drug-resistant cyathostome populations. In addition, these programs are easy to implement in that they do not require decision making during the year. This approach may not be appropriate in all circumstances in that these programs do not take into account the variable efficacies of drugs against a broad range of parasites and focus only on the cyathostomes.

No Rotation

The continued regular use of one effective drug until it no longer reduces cyathostome numbers as indicated by fecal egg counts is practiced. This type of control is generally limited to the use of ivermectin or the low-dose feed-additive formulation of pyrantel tartrate. The advantage of this type of vigorous treatment strategy is that it provides for maximal reduction of parasite burdens and is easily implemented. One would predict that this type of program would induce a rapid induction of drug resistance. As noted earlier, however, this has not been the case with ivermectin. Horses raised using such management practices are likely to have a marked delay in the development of an acquired resistance.

Targeted Treatments

It has been suggested for some time that regular treatment of only those horses with significant fecal egg counts would be an effective means of cyathostome control. This type of program has the advantage of minimizing the use of anthelmintics and using naturally acquired resistance as a supplement to control. Implementation of this strategy necessitates the regular use of quantitative fecal examinations. Although these examinations are not difficult and require only minimal equipment, regular decisions on the significance of the results obtained are required. As might be expected, a uniform opinion on the significance of fecal egg count levels in eggs per g of feces (EPG) is not available, and data are limited. However, treatment of individuals when cyathostome counts are higher than 100 to 200 EPG has been effective in minimizing pasture contamination in this system. This type of control program is not useful in young animals because of the absence of acquired immunity, which results in generally higher parasite burdens.

Strategic Treatment

Strategic treatment programs are based on the use of effective anthelmintics to eliminate luminal cyathostome burdens before the season of the year that is optimal for parasite development on pasture. This strategy reduces pasture contamination and thus reinfection. These types of programs have been effective in controlling cyathostomes in yearlings and mature horses in northern temperate regions by using treatments in the spring and early summer and again in the fall. Similar programs have been reported to be effective in southeastern regions of the United States by beginning these treatments in the early fall. A modification of this approach is to treat horses with a larvicidal dose of anthelmintic, such as that described earlier, before exposure to pasture during the optimal transmission season. This approach minimizes the use of anthelmintics, prolonging drug usefulness. A drawback to this method is that it is based on an understanding of the local epidemiology of cyathostome infections that may not be as clear as the examples used. Furthermore, these types of programs may not be as effective in young stock.

MEASUREMENT OF TREATMENT EFFECTIVENESS

Measurements of the efficacies of individual drugs and evaluation of the total control program on an annual basis are essential. Although the exact determination of existing parasite numbers is not possible, adult worm burdens can be estimated by EPG counts. This method is effective for infections of *P. equorum*, *S. westeri*, and cyathosomes. Fecal flotation methods are not reliable for infections of *Anoplocephala* species, spiruroid stomach worms, or *Oxyuris equi*. The modified McMaster method is a quantitative procedure that can be accomplished without a centrifuge and is suitable for clinical work. The special chambered slides required for this procedure or complete kits can be purchased.[*] Determination of individual drug efficacy should be based on results of the fecal egg count reduction tests, which can be accomplished by counting EPG of individual horses at the time of treatment and again 10 to 14 days after treatment. These tests should be conducted at a time when egg counts are expected to be at their highest. Average reductions should be 90% or greater. If values are much less than this, it is likely that drug-resistant cyathostomes are present.

SUPPLEMENTS TO ANTHELMINTIC TREATMENT

A number of supplemental approaches to the use of anthelmintics have been suggested and are aimed at the reduction of pasture contamination with infective larvae. Rotation of stock to clean pastures, particularly at times of the year when larval survival is expected to be minimal, may be an effective supplement to anthelmintic control. However, pasture space is often limited, and the moving

---

[*]*Advanced Equine Products, Issaqua, WA*

of horses to clean pasture following treatment may actually enhance the selection of drug-resistant populations of cyathostomes. Harrowing of pastures to scatter manure with the thought of lowering the survival of strongyle larvae may be effective if done during seasons detrimental to larval survival. Nonetheless, under some circumstances, harrowing has had the opposite effect, and foals maintained on harrowed pastures have had greater parasite burdens. The biweekly mechanical removal of feces has been shown to have a beneficial effect in temperate regions but is labor-intensive, and vacuum equipment for this purpose is expensive. Grazing of pastures alternately with ruminants may also serve to reduce equine parasite burdens. However, this method also has not proved to be uniformly effective and may expose horses to increased numbers of *Trichostrongylus axei*, which in large numbers has been demonstrated to be pathogenic in the horse.

GENERAL RECOMMENDATIONS

Although no single control strategy is optimal in all instances, the principles outlined above should be useful in the construction of individual programs in any instance. In addition, there are some general actions that can be emphasized.

1. Ensure the use of the proper dosage of anthelmintic based on accurate weight
2. Alternate classes of compounds if possible to prolong the effectiveness of anthelmintics
3. Monitor deworming programs and drug efficacies on an annual basis using the fecal egg count reduction test
4. Implement treatment schedules that provide sufficient control to maximize health while minimizing the use of anthelmintics
5. Use nonchemical control strategies when feasible.

Supplemental Readings

DiPietro JA: Internal parasite control programs. *In* Robinson NE (ed): Current Therapy in Equine Medicine, ed 3. Philadelphia, WB Saunders, 1992, pp 51–55.
DiPietro JA, Klei TR, French DD: Contemporary topics in equine parasitology. Comp Cont Ed Pract Vet 12:713–721, 1990.
Herd RP (ed): Parasitology. Vet Clin North Am Equine Pract 2:2, 1986.
Klei TR: Recent observations on the epidemiology, pathogenesis and immunology of equine helminth infections. *In* Plowright W, Rossdale DD, Wade JF (eds): Equine Infectious Disease VI. Proc Sixth Int Conf, Newmarket, England, R&W Publication, 1992, pp 129–136.
Love S: Parasite-associated equine diarrhea. Comp Cont Ed Pract Vet 14:642–649, 1992.
Slocombe JOD: Anthelmintic resistance in strongyles of equids. *In* Plowright W, Rossdale DD, Wade JF (eds): Equine Infectious Disease VI. Proc Sixth Int Conf, Newmarket, England, R&W Publication, 1992, pp 137–143.
Uhlinger CA: Uses of fecal egg count data in equine practice. Comp Cont Ed Pract Vet 15:742–749, 1993.

Anesthesia of Horses in the Field

GEORGE BOHART
East Lansing, Michigan

The equine practitioner is often faced with the task of performing surgery under field conditions. These procedures may be performed on an elective or emergency basis. Castration is the most common equine surgical procedure performed, but cryptorchidectomy, laceration repair, umbilical herniorraphy, fetal extraction, dental procedures, minor upper airway surgeries, and minor orthopedic surgeries may also be performed under field conditions. Although the surgical procedures performed in the field are often the same as those performed in the traditional hospital setting, management of general anesthesia may be quite different.

A wide variety of sedatives, tranquilizers, analgesics, muscle relaxants, and induction agents are available to the equine practitioner. The goal of the equine anesthetist should be to produce a smooth induction with ample anesthesia time followed by an uneventful recovery while maintaining control of the patient at all times. General anesthesia is only as safe as the person administering it: a successful outcome depends as much on the practitioner's anesthesia

skills and judgment as on the anesthetic protocol selected. Familiarity with an anesthetic protocol increases the probability of recognizing an adverse event and intervening with appropriate treatment. Formulation of an anesthetic plan should be based on the practitioner's knowledge of available drugs, type and duration of surgical procedure to be performed, and condition of the patient.

PREANESTHETIC PREPARATION

Preoperative evaluation of the patient is the foundation upon which an anesthetic protocol is formulated. An accurate, detailed medical history should be obtained before general anesthesia. A special effort should be made to determine prior medical problems and previous drug treatments. Known adverse reactions or sensitivities to drugs should be noted and those drugs avoided when formulating the anesthetic plan. Before general anesthesia, a complete physical examination must be performed. Many times, the horse is closely examined exclusively for the presenting surgical problem. It is important to examine the entire horse with particular attention placed on the respiratory and cardiovascular systems. Horses younger than 1 year of age, horses with a recent history of shipping, and horses with reactive airway disease are especially prone to subclinical respiratory disease. Assessment of the cardiovascular system should detect rhythm disturbances and murmurs. A minimal laboratory data base of complete blood count and total plasma solids is recommended. When abnormalities are noted on the physical examination or laboratory tests, appropriate diagnostic procedures should be performed to determine the underlying cause. When laboratory tests are unavailable, or in patients that require emergency surgery and anesthesia, the equine practitioner must rely on clinical judgment. Patients requiring emergency surgery that are not good candidates for general anesthesia should, if possible, be operated on while standing, using local anesthetic and sedation techniques. Owners should always be advised of the potential risks associated with general anesthesia and the surgical procedure being performed on their horse.

Ideally, food but not water is withheld for approximately 12 hours before general anesthesia. In many settings, withholding of food is impractical, especially when the horse is housed outside and individual stall space is not accessible. Horses housed in barns may become extremely agitated when excluded from the normal feeding schedule. To avoid this problem, horses may be fed a small portion of their morning ration and the remainder after surgery. The horse should be groomed and its weight determined by weighing on a scale or estimated with a girth tape. When using anesthetic protocols that require an intravenous catheter, it should be placed in the jugular or cephalic vein before induction. Rinsing the mouth thoroughly with a hose or dose syringe prevents aspiration of food particles during anesthesia.

An additional dilemma of field anesthesia is that the surgeon and anesthetist are often the same person. Every effort should be made to promote efficient use of the anesthetic time by anticipating equipment and drug needs before surgery begins. Preclipping and scrubbing of the surgical site while the horse is standing maximize the anesthetic time available for surgery. Precautions should be taken to prevent the development of anesthesia-related myopathies or neuropathies that can occur in recumbent horses. The down forelimb should be pulled forward to prevent radial nerve paralysis. If required, the head should be padded and strict attention paid to halter buckles that may impinge on the facial nerves. It takes only a few minutes to cause nerve damage in a recumbent horse; therefore, it is imperative that the anesthetist prepare the induction area by removing rocks, ropes, and other items that may injure the patient.

INJECTABLE ANESTHESIA

Many drug combinations have been used successfully for equine field anesthesia. The most common combination consists of using an α_2-adrenoceptor agonist as a preanes-

thetic medication followed by ketamine* a dissociative anesthetic, as the induction agent (Table 1). An advantage of this protocol is that intravenous catheterization is not essential. Xylazine,† detomidine,‡ and romifidine§ are the three most commonly used α_2-agonists in the horse. All produce dose-dependent sedation and muscle relaxation, whereas only xylazine and detomidine possess analgesic properties. In the healthy horse, xylazine (0.8–1.1 mg/ kg IV), detomidine (0.02–0.04 mg/kg IV), and romifidine (0.08–0.1 mg/kg IV) produce sedation characterized by lowering of the head, slight ataxia, and buckling of the knees. In foals younger than 2 weeks of age, α_2-agonists should be used cautiously because of the potential for severe cardiopulmonary complications. A reduced dose of xylazine (0.25–0.5 mg/kg IV) is recommended for preanesthetic sedation of neonatal foals. Peak sedation occurs within 5 minutes after intravenous administration of xylazine. It may take slightly longer for signs of peak sedation to become apparent following intravenous administration of detomidine. In fractious or anxious horses in which intravenous injection is difficult, xylazine or detomidine may be administered intramuscularly at twice the intravenous dose. Peak sedation occurs within 20 minutes following intramuscular administration of xylazine and within 30 minutes following intramuscular administration of detomidine. In horses in which parenteral administration of preanesthetic medication is difficult, detomidine may be administered orally (0.05–0.07 mg/kg) to produce mild to moderate sedation. The degree of sedation achieved is approximately three quarters of that following the same dose administered intramuscularly. The detomidine is "squirted" into the horse's mouth using a small syringe and requires up to 45 minutes for peak sedation to occur. If sedation is inadequate following IV, IM, or p.o. administration of α_2-agonists, small supplemental doses may be administered intravenously until signs of adequate sedation occur. Following satisfactory sedation with an α_2-agonist,

---

*Ketaset, Fort Dodge Laboratories, Fort Dodge, IA
†Rompum, Miles Inc., Agriculture Division, Animal Health Products, Shawnee Mission, KS
‡Dormosedan, Pfizer Animal Health, West Chester, PA
§Sedivet, Boehringer Ingelheim (Canada) Ltd., Animal Health Division, Burlington, Ontario, Canada

TABLE 1.   INTRAVENOUS ANESTHETIC TECHNIQUES

Premedication	Dose (mg/kg) IV	Dose (mg/kg) IM	Induction Agent	Dose (mg/kg) IV
Xylazine	0.8–1.1	2.2	Ketamine	2.2
or			*or*	
Detomidine	0.02–0.04	0.06	Ketamine	2.2
or			+,	0.1
Romifidine	0.08–0.1	—	Diazepam	
Acepromazine	0.04	—	5% Guaifenesin	50–100 or to
+ Butorphanol	0.01–0.04	—	*followed by*	effect
or				
Xylazine	0.5–0.8	1.5	Ketamine	2.2
or			*or*	
Detomidine	0.015–0.025	0.04	Thiopental	4.0–6.0

ketamine is administered (2.2 mg/kg IV). The horse usually becomes recumbent within 2 minutes and may be directed into left or right lateral recumbency by controlling the head during induction. Anesthesia following ketamine induction is characterized by poor muscle relaxation with active ocular and laryngeal reflexes. Duration of surgical anesthesia is about 15 to 20 minutes. The horse usually rolls into sternal recumbency within 25 to 30 minutes, and most stand a few minutes later. Recoveries are usually smooth following xylazine-ketamine, with most horses standing at their first attempt. These horses seldom need assistance during or following recovery. Recoveries following detomidine-ketamine may be slightly uncoordinated, with some horses requiring more than one attempt to stand.

Xylazine, detomidine, and romifidine may induce sinus bradycardia and first- or second-degree atrioventricular block. This effect is especially prominent in the "fit" or athletic horse but may occur in any patient; for these reasons, the pulse rate should always be determined before and after administration of α_2-agonists. Three options are available in the face of severe bradycardia: cancellation of general anesthesia, waiting for the bradycardia to subside, or administration of atropine° (0.01–0.05 mg/kg IV) or glycopyrrolate† (0.005 mg/kg IV) to reverse the bradycardia. Potential complications associated with the administration of anticholinergic agents in the horse include gastrointestinal stasis and occasionally colic. Therefore, except in the case of surgery that cannot be postponed, it is usually best to reschedule general anesthesia until a later date. At that time a protocol should be selected that excludes the use, or reduces the dose of α_2-agonists. The opioid agonist-antagonist butorphanol‡ (0.01–0.04 mg/kg IV) may be combined with xylazine, detomidine, or romifidine to provide additional analgesia and augment sedation. The dose of xylazine and detomodine may be decreased by approximately one quarter when combined with butorphanol. Used alone, opioids may produce central nervous system (CNS) excitement in the horse, especially at higher doses. It is not unusual for butorphanol to cause mild excitement manifested as sweating, slight muscle tremors, and twitching of the lips and face.

A common replacement for α_2-agonists is the phenothiazine tranquilizer, acepromazine§ (0.04–0.06 mg/kg IV or IM). Peak sedation following either route of administration occurs in 20 to 30 minutes. The sedation produced by acepromazine is not as profound or predictable as that of α_2-agonists, and horses are easily aroused in noisy environments. Phenothiazine tranquilizers induce dose-dependent vasodilation by suppression of CNS sympathetic activity and peripheral α-adrenoceptor blockade. This results in decreased arterial blood pressure, packed cell volume, and total protein concentration. Acepromazine should be avoided in hypovolemic, stressed, or very excited horses because of the potential for development of significant hypotension. Although acepromazine is not contraindicated in male horses, it should be used cautiously owing to

the uncommon complication of persistent penile paralysis. Acepromazine is a poor analgesic and lacks good muscle relaxant properties. Butorphanol and α_2-agonists may be combined with acepromazine to provide analgesia and enhance sedation. Anesthetic inductions using acepromazine followed by ketamine are frequently difficult, and many practitioners find this combination unacceptable. The addition of guaifenesin,° a centrally acting muscle relaxant, is highly recommended to improve the quality of induction and anesthesia when using acepromazine as the preanesthetic sedative. Generally, the preanesthetic sedation does not have to be as profound when guaifenesin is included in the anesthetic protocol. When bradycardia or atrioventricular block is an anticipated complication of using α_2-agonists, the addition of guaifenesin to the anesthetic protocol decreases the intravenous and intramuscular dose of xylazine and detomidine by approximately one third to one half. Guaifenesin is administered as a 5% solution (50–100 mg/kg IV) to produce a pronounced head drop, buckling of the knees, and ataxia. To prevent prolonged ataxia and produce a smooth induction, it should be administered rapidly in 2 to 3 minutes using a pressurized delivery system. Once the horse becomes "wobbly," a bolus of ketamine is administered (2.2 mg/kg IV). An intravenous catheter is recommended when administering guaifenesin because of the large volumes required and risk of tissue inflammation resulting from perivascular administration. Concentrations greater than 5% should be avoided owing to increased intravascular hemolysis and risk of thrombosis. The addition of guaifenesin to the anesthetic protocol extends the anesthesia time and may prolong recovery times in horses anesthetized with ketamine.

Guaifenesin and ketamine may be combined and used for induction. The induction dose of ketamine is calculated and combined with 500 ml of 5% guaifenesin or 1 to 2 g ketamine is placed in 1 L of 5% guaifenesin solution. The ketamine-guaifenesin combination is administered to effect following adequate preanesthetic sedation. Combination techniques are not as predictable and require more personnel to assist the horse during induction owing to a longer transition period from standing to lateral recumbency. This limits the usefulness of "mixed bag" inductions to situations where extra personnel are available.

The benzodiazepine diazepam† has minimal cardiopulmonary effects in the horse. In the sick or debilitated neonatal foal, diazepam (0.1–0.2 mg/kg IV) is a safe and effective substitute for xylazine when using ketamine as an induction agent. In the adult horse it is a useful substitute for guaifenesin when additional muscle relaxation is required. Following adequate preanesthetic sedation with an α_2-agonist, diazepam (0.05–0.1 mg/kg) is combined with ketamine in the same syringe and administered intravenously. Horses tend to "dog-sit" following injection of a diazepam-ketamine bolus, allowing the anesthetist to easily guide the horse into lateral recumbency. Incorporation of diazepam into a xylazine-ketamine anesthetic protocol extends the surgical anesthesia time by a few minutes and depresses the brisk ocular and laryngeal reflexes associated with ketamine anesthesia. It is an especially good adjunct

---

°Atropine L.A., The Butler Company, Columbus, OH
†Robinul-V, Fort Dodge Laboratories, Fort Dodge, IA
‡Torbugesic, Fort Dodge Laboratories, Fort Dodge, IA
§PromAce, Fort Dodge Laboratories, Fort Dodge, IA

°Guailaxin, Fort Dodge Laboratories, Fort Dodge, IA
†Diazepam, Elkins-Sinn, Cherry Hill, NJ

to xylazine-ketamine anesthesia to inhibit retraction of the testes into the inguinal canal during castration of young colts. Recoveries following xylazine-diazepam-ketamine anesthesia are usually smooth and coordinated, with the horse standing on the first attempt.

A 1:1 combination of tiletamine, a dissociative anesthetic, and zolazepam, a benzodiazepine, is marketed as Telazol° for use in veterinary medicine. Telazol (1.1 mg/kg IV) administered following α_2-agonist sedation produces swift and smooth inductions similar to those of ketamine-diazepam. Duration of recumbency is 32 ± 7 minutes. Recoveries following Telazol are often difficult, with the horse making several attempts to stand.

The ultrashort-acting thiobarbitutrate thiopental† is another alternative to using ketamine as an induction agent. Thiobarbiturate solutions are alkaline and cause severe tissue damage and skin sloughing following perivascular injection; for these reasons, venous catheterization is recommended. Following adequate preanesthetic sedation, thiopental is administered as a 4 to 10% solution (4–8 mg/kg IV). Thiopental doses are administered at the upper limits of the dose range following premedication with xylazine or detomidine. The addition of diazepam or guaifenesin allows thiopental to be administered at the lower limits of the dose range. Diazepam forms a precipitate if combined with thiopental but may be administered intravenously as a separate bolus immediately before induction. Guaifenesin is administered as a separate infusion followed by thiopental or 1 L of a 5% solution may be combined with 2 g thiopental and administered to effect in adult horses. Thiopental produces anesthesia characterized by quiet ocular and laryngeal reflexes with less swallowing when compared with ketamine. Many surgeons prefer xylazine-guaifenesin-thiopental over xylazine-ketamine for surgeries of the upper airway. Inductions with thiopental are usually swift, with the horse characteristically buckling all four legs at once. Although some horses tend to fall backward following a thiopental bolus, the possibility of a rough induction may be reduced by adequate preanesthetic sedation and inclusion of guaifenesin or diazepam in the anesthetic protocol. Horses often need several attempts to stand following use of thiopental, and assistance is recommended to ensure a safe recovery.

°*Telazol, Aveco Company, Fort Dodge, IA*
†*Pentothal, Abbott Laboratories, North Chicago, IL*

EXTENDING ANESTHESIA

Prolongation of anesthesia is often necessary under field conditions. In the best possible scenario a plan for extending anesthesia should be formulated before it is needed. Extension of anesthesia may be accomplished initially by "topping off" the horse with ketamine using one quarter to one half the original dose. Repeated administration of ketamine without repetition of xylazine increases the likelihood of a difficult recovery. Supplemental doses of xylazine (0.2–0.4 mg/kg IV) are recommended if more than one additional dose of ketamine is required. Diazepam (0.04–0.06 mg/kg IV) may be administered to provide intraoperative muscle relaxation. A combination of 500 mg xylazine and 1000 mg ketamine mixed in 1 L 5% guaifenesin solution may be used to continue anesthesia. The xylazine-guaifenesin-ketamine mixture is infused at a rate of 2.0 to 3.0 ml/kg per hour or to effect. A detomidine-guaifenesin-ketamine combination may be used to continue anesthesia by replacing the xylazine in the above mixture with 10 mg of detomidine. The infusion rate for detomidine-guaifenesin-ketamine is 3.2 ml/kg per hour or to effect. An intravenous catheter is required when using a "mixed bag" technique to extend the anesthesia time. Repeated administration of thiobarbiturates often results in prolonged, rough recoveries; consequently, thiopental is not recommended for extending anesthesia. General anesthesia should not be maintained for more than 40 to 60 minutes with injectable techniques because of the hypoventilation and hypoxemia associated with recumbency in anesthetized horses. Procedures lasting longer than 1 hour should be performed in an equine hospital with a secured airway, inhalant anesthesia, and diligent monitoring of respiratory and cardiovascular variables.

Supplemental Readings

Brock N, Hildebrand SV: A comparison of xylazine-diazepam-ketamine and xylazine-guaifenesin-ketamine in equine anesthesia. Vet Surg 19(6):468–474, 1990.

Diamond MJ, Young LE, Bartram DH, Gregg AS, Clutton RE, Long KJ, Jones RS: Clinical evaluation of romifidine/ketamine/halothane anaesthesia in horses. Vet Rec 132:572–575, 1993.

Hamm D, Turchi P, Jöchle W: Sedative and analgesic effects of detomidine and romifidine in horses. Vet Rec 136:324–327, 1995.

Malone JH, Clarke KW: A comparison of the efficacy of detomidine by sublingual and intramuscular administration in ponies. J Vet Anaes 20:73–77, 1993.

Taylor PM, Luna SPL: Total intravenous anaesthesia in ponies using detomidine, ketamine and guaiphenesin: Pharmacokinetics, cardiopulmonary and endocrine effects. Res Vet Sci 59:17–23, 1995.

Quarantine Considerations and Medical Management of Horses During International Shipment

TIMOTHY CORDES
Riverdale, Maryland

RICHARD MITCHELL
Monroe, Connecticut

The international transport of horses, once reserved for only the most famous equine athletes, has become commonplace in this decade. In the United States the desire to own the European Warmblood; the dramatic growth in the disciplines of dressage, eventing, and show jumping, with the eagerness to compete abroad, have contributed to this development. As horse sports grow throughout the world, there will be an increase in the demand to ship equine athletes to more remote locations under more strenuous conditions. With the tremendous expansion in this segment of the horse industry, it is prudent for equine practitioners to familiarize themselves with the details of preparations for international shipping and the medical management of horses during that transportation.

TRANSPORT AGENT

Reputable horse brokers are familiar with equine import and export prerequisites; many have computer data bases that can rapidly generate updated international health certificates for review. However, veterinarians must be the final authority because it is the certification, with their signature as an accredited veterinarian, that goes before the appropriate United States Department of Agriculture (USDA) officials for endorsement.

In addition, veterinarians must work closely with an experienced transport agent on the details of the trip itinerary beyond the airplane and horse van; these may include scheduling, routing, stabling, and emergency planning. The horse's schedule should allow time for acclimation and recovery from stressful competitions, and the route should take into account temperature and time of day, heavy traffic, and border or ferry crossings. Stables and holding facilities must be suitably ventilated and bedded, and may require vector-proof screening. It is essential to identify emergency phone numbers and locations of equine hospitals along the proposed route.

Veterinarians should seek advice from a knowledgeable broker regarding all contingencies, because they may affect shipping costs to the owner and veterinary fees. Clients should be encouraged to seek competitive bids from several carriers and demand that quotes be in writing. Clients should be informed that problems upon departure and arrival are not uncommon. Equine air transport cost is rated by the pallet, which usually accommodates a three-stall container. On departure, if a horse becomes ill or has test results that are anticomplementary or positive for a restricted disease, the cost of the pallet will be divided among the owners of the remaining horses. On arrival, if a horse becomes ill, all of the other horses must remain in quarantine. Fees for a country's government quarantine may include overtime charges, and extended stays can be costly.

IMPORT CONSIDERATIONS

Horses imported into the United States are held at one of four USDA quarantine facilities, located in Newburgh (New York), Miami (Florida), Honolulu (Hawaii), and Los Angeles (California). At the very least, each horse is tested for equine infectious anemia (EIA), piroplasmosis, dourine, and glanders. Additional testing is based upon the existence, in the country of origin, of endemic diseases foreign to the United States; this also affects the length of quarantine. Horses from most European countries stay less than 3 days; from South American countries with Venezuelan equine encephalomyelitis (VEE), 7 days; and from African and Asian countries with African horsesickness, 60 days. Breeding stock from contagious equine metritis (CEM) countries may be quarantined at state-approved facilities for a testing protocol lasting up to 60 days.

Because of the constant developments in regulations and technology, and the ongoing outbreaks of disease in foreign countries, the authors recommend that questions be directed to the office of the USDA Area Veterinarian In Charge (AVIC) in the veterinarian's state.

The veterinarian should keep all these factors in mind when conducting or consulting in a purchase examination overseas. They should remember to conduct all blood tests required for import well before they plan to conclude the examination and approve shipment. If such timing is not feasible, it must be assured that the final sale is contingent upon the appropriate testing results and health certification. Although veterinarians may use the services of any laboratory they choose, the only official testing is conducted while the horse is in USDA quarantine by the USDA National Veterinary Services Laboratories. It is wise to remind clients to reserve space at the quarantine facility, because the facilities are often booked well in advance.

EXPORT CONSIDERATIONS

Equine practitioners should remember three factors when making preparations to transport horses abroad. First, any American horse that has been outside this country for a period of time is considered to be of foreign origin and must comply with all United States import requirements upon return. Canada is the only exception. Second, it is wise to conduct blood tests before departure, because a delay with one horse affects the entire consignment. Third, each foreign country has very specific, and often variable, temporary and permanent equine import or entry requirements. The authors recommend that each accredited practitioner contact the USDA AVIC in the state, or the state of origin, to make the necessary arrangements well in advance of the departure date. Veterinarians must work closely with the AVIC, because it is this person who will finally endorse the health certification. Preparations normally include testing, vaccinations (or certification of status), and pre-export isolation. The European Union requires a 30-day pre-export quarantine before dispatch for permanent exports; arrangements may be made with the USDA authority to set up private pre-export isolation, rather than using a commercial isolation facility.

MEDICAL MANAGEMENT

Because horses must be transported as quickly and efficiently as possible, this often involves air travel. Several unique aspects to air travel must be taken into consideration when transporting horses. Three major areas of concern in transporting horses over long distances are: (1) behavioral modification; (2) physical safety; and (3) stress management. Although these concerns are not unique to air travel, they take on a different look when compared with land transport. The land travel that horses may face subsequent to arrival at the port of entry must also be considered. Horses that are intolerant of travel-related stress may develop febrile respiratory disease, colic, or laminitis.

Behavioral Modification

The environment of an airport can produce myriad frightening stimuli for the horse. Horses that have traveled frequently and are accustomed to machinery and busy surroundings may not require special restraint or sedation. Fractious horses may require some form of chemical or physical restraint to be loaded and fly safely. The use of chemical restraint should be performed with the regulations of impending competition in mind.

Acepromazine (0.04–0.06 mg/kg IV) effectively quiets a moderately nervous horse 4 to 6 hours and can be repeated if necessary. Because this drug may be detectable for 4

days if an enzyme-linked immunosorbent assay (ELISA) is used for detection, one should carefully consider an alternative if the horse is to compete within a few days of arrival. Detomidine (0.01 mg/kg IM) produces satisfactorily heavy sedation with less ataxia than when administered intravenously. Of course, if rapid sedation is appropriate, intravenous administration can provide profound help in handling the fractious horse during loading. The duration of effect of detomidine administered intramuscularly is about 3 hours, and the dose can be repeated. This drug is unlikely to be detected if it is administered more than 2 days before competition. Butorphanol (0.01–0.02 mg/kg IV) can be used in conjunction with other medications such as detomidine to minimize kicking. The duration of effect is usually about 3 hours. This drug usually has a longer withdrawal time (4 days) than detomidine and should therefore be reserved for special problems.

Physical Safety

The veterinarian should oversee the preparation of the horses for shipment. The individual needs and shipping characteristics of each horse, if known, should be considered. Some horses ship better in "double stalls," whereas others are better transported in closed crates. How a horse has been transported previously may well determine the type of plane in which it should be shipped. Smaller planes (DC-8, 737) transport horses in open stalls placed on standard cargo pallets. Larger aircraft (747) normally use a closed crate that resembles a two-horse trailer without wheels. Special arrangements for placement of various pallets in the aircraft may be necessary when mares and stallions are shipped together.

It may be appropriate to use protective equipment for transport. Leg wraps should be used only on horses that are accustomed to them, because wraps can initiate unnecessary kicking and treading in some horses. The use of helmets, hock boots, and other protective devices may be appropriate in some individuals, and their use should be dictated by previous experience with the horse. The use of kick pads can significantly reduce the incidence of hind leg injuries. Adequate bedding in the crate provides better footing and minimizes slipping.

It is important to restrict excessive movement on the part of the horse while providing enough room to allow the horse to adjust position comfortably, especially during take-off and landing. When horses are transported in open pallets, head restraint is essential. The horse should be provided with enough freedom for comfort but not enough to contact the adjacent horse. Neck straps are normally used in open pallets to prevent rearing and possible escape from the stalls.

Stress Management

A management program for controlling stress-related disease in the horse must include an adequate immunization schedule. This is often dictated by the age of the horse, its level of activity, and the regulations of the destination country. An initial two-dose series of influenza vaccine (no closer than 21 days but no greater than 92 days apart) and annual revaccination are required for all Federation Equestre Internationale competitions, and a vaccination record must be entered in the horse's passport. This vaccination schedule is a bare minimum and probably is inadequate for real protection. Regularly scheduled boosters for various respiratory diseases may be essential to provide an optimal level of protection. The use of other vaccines, such as those against encephalomyelitis (eastern equine [EEE], western equine [WEE], and Venezuelan equine [VEE]) should be used in accordance with the laws of the destination country. The use of immune stimulatory agents is quite controversial at the present time, but it is probably unwise to use these agents just before shipment because they may increase the stress level of the horse.

A thorough pretravel physical examination can aide the veterinarian greatly in evaluating the horse if it becomes ill subsequent to travel. A respiratory examination using a rebreathing bag can help immensely in the early detection of subtle lung disease. A pretravel complete blood count can establish baseline hematologic values. The horse should receive a balanced ration at regular and frequent intervals to promote normal gastrointestinal function. The use of supplemental vitamins (B complex and vitamin C) may be of real value in stressful situations.

Maintaining good hydration is very important during air travel. Extended air travel can be quite dehydrating, and poor hydration may contribute to impaction colic. Good-quality fresh water should be available before and during the flight. Supplemental oral electrolytes may be of benefit in increasing the moisture content within the bowel and preventing impaction. Many practitioners administer intravenous balanced electrolyte solutions immediately before travel to ensure adequate hydration of the horse. Five to ten liters of balanced electrolyte solution° may be used.

°Plasmalyte, Baxter, McGaw Park, IL

Vitamin B complex° and sodium ascorbate (2.5 g) may be added to these solutions. Many horses that are good travelers may not require such measures, and climatic conditions may be a factor in determining the need for this type of therapy. Intravenous fluid therapy can be beneficial for those horses that become febrile following travel, and may reduce the need for antipyretic medications, which may present a problem for later drug testing.

Horses that are known to be stressed by travel and to subsequently develop respiratory disease may benefit from prophylactic antibiotic therapy before, during, and after travel. Treatment with ceftiofur or gentamicin, for example, must be restricted to individuals with a previous history of travel-related respiratory problems. Horses that are very tense or tend to brace themselves constantly while in motion may benefit from nonsteroidal anti-inflammatory medications such as ketoprofen or flunixin meglumine and muscle relaxants such as methocarbamol (5–10 g IV) before and after travel. If the horse is to compete in the near future, it is wise to remember that medications may affect the results of drug testing.

Careful evaluation of each horse following travel can help minimize post-travel illness. A brief general physical examination with measurement of body temperature and pulse and respiratory rate and thorough auscultation of the chest may reveal subtle problems that can be curtailed with appropriate therapy before more serious illness develops.

Supplemental Reading

Code of Federal Regulations, Animal and Animal Products, Title 9, Parts 91 through 94. Office of the Federal Register of the National Archives and Records Administration (Special Edition of the Federal Register), January 1, 1996.

°B-complex fortified (10–20 ml), Phoenix Pharmaceuticals, St. Joseph, MO

New Perspectives on Antimicrobial Chemotherapy

ROBERT D. WALKER
East Lansing, Michigan

Since the publication of the last edition of this book (see *Current Therapy in Equine Medicine 3*, pages 1–13) there have been many new developments in the field of antimicrobial chemotherapy. These include in vitro antimicrobial susceptibility testing results that are specific for veterinary medicine and an increased understanding of pharmacokinetic and pharmacodynamic principles that relate to host-bacterial pathogen-drug interactions. These developments help the equine practitioner to provide the optimal concentration of an active antimicrobial agent at the site of infection for an appropriate length of time. In

addition, the concept of professional flexible labeling is now a reality. This will change how antimicrobial agents are approved and increase their potential for improved clinical efficacy.

To explore these new developments, it is necessary to briefly review some concepts. These include (1) physiologic factors associated with the host that result in the development of infection; (2) methods of identifying the bacterial pathogen or at least gaining a general understanding of the pathogen based on the animal's clinical presentation; (3) methods of determining the pathogen's antimicrobial susceptibility profile (i.e., its antibiogram); and (4) pharmaco-kinetic and pharmacodynamic relationships of the antimicrobial agent, host, and bacterial pathogen.

PHYSIOLOGIC FACTORS CONTRIBUTING TO INFECTION

Most equine bacterial pathogens are part of the horse's normal flora. Beginning at birth, these bacteria develop a win-win relationship with the host. When this relationship is disrupted, the host is at risk of developing an infectious disease. In general, there are two criteria necessary for a bacterium to cause disease. First, it must be able to multiply in or on host tissue. Second, it must be able to resist host defense mechanisms long enough to reach sufficient numbers to cause overt disease. Thus, to cause disease, a bacterium must be able to breach the host's nonspecific defense mechanisms, proliferate to the point where its metabolites disrupt normal host cell function, and avoid the lytic effects of the host's specific immune system. Penetrating wounds, including insect vectors, are a frequent mechanism by which a bacterium may breach the host's nonspecific defense mechanisms. Such injuries introduce bacteria into otherwise sterile tissue where they may proliferate and, if not contained, spread to other body sites. However, the single greatest contributing factor to the development of infectious disease of bacterial etiology is stress.

Stress may be manifested in a variety of ways but the results, to varying degrees, are always the same. When stressed, an animal generally experiences (1) an increase in mucus production on mucous membranes, especially of the upper respiratory tract, resulting in a change of receptor sites on mucosal epithelium; (2) a decrease in the efficacy of nonspecific defense mechanisms (i.e., neutrophils); and (3) a decrease in efficacy of the specific immune system.

A change in receptor sites on mucosal epithelial cells results in a loss of the normal flora for that body site. Those receptor sites may then be colonized by bacteria that have a greater potential to cause disease at that body site. An example would be a change from a gram-positive flora to a gram-negative flora in the upper respiratory tract. To counter the effects of the stress, the clinician needs to minimize or eliminate the cause of the stress and reduce the number of bacteria and their toxic metabolites at the site of the infection. Unfortunately, there are many instances when surgical intervention or lavage cannot be used to reduce the number of bacteria and their toxic metabolites. Under those circumstances, and even with surgical intervention or lavage, the ability of the bacteria to multiply needs to be reduced. This reduces the spread of bacteria and their toxic metabolites to adjacent tissue and allows the host's phagocytes and specific immune system to successfully contain and eliminate the invading bacteria.

IDENTIFYING THE ETIOLOGIC AGENT

Gaining reasonable assurance as to the identity of the infecting organism can be accomplished by using bacterio-logic statistics, Gram staining material taken directly from the site of infection, or through isolation and identification of the pathogen from a properly collected specimen. Bacteriologic statistics involve the use of one's clinical experience, the clinical presentation, and the animal's history to determine the organism most likely to be the etiologic agent. For example, acute nasopharyngeal inflammation that results in abscessation of the regional lymph nodes and a mucopurulent nasal discharge in a 3-year-old horse is most likely to be caused by *Streptococcus equi*. On the other hand, pneumonia in a 6-week-old foal with watery diarrhea may be caused by any one of a number of bacteria and thus requires culturing the lower respiratory tract to determine the etiologic agent.

One of the most important steps in obtaining infected tissue for Gram staining or culture is sample collection. Properly collected specimens frequently provide the identity of the etiologic agent, whereas improperly collected specimens are not useful in distinguishing the etiologic agent from contaminating organisms. For example, there are numerous species of bacteria and fungi in hay. When a transtracheal wash is performed on a horse that has not had access to hay for 4 to 5 hours, the etiologic agent causing respiratory distress will most likely be in pure culture. On the other hand, if the transtracheal wash is performed within a couple of hours after the horse has had access to hay, there will be several different colony types on the resultant culture plate, including fungi. The clinician must then try to determine which of the various species is the etiologic agent.

Once a specimen has been properly collected and transported to the laboratory for analysis, one of the simplest and most useful tests is the Gram stain, for which kits are inexpensive and commercially available. This technique can be used to identify the presence and morphologic features of microorganisms in body fluids that are normally sterile, in draining tracts, and in septic incision sites. Although the visualization of bacteria on a slide using a Gram stain rarely reveals the bacterium's identity, it can provide useful information pertaining to therapy. For example, gram-positive cocci in chains suggests the presence of streptococci. Streptococci isolated from a purulent lesion in a horse are most likely group C streptococci, which are susceptible to penicillin. On the other hand, gram-negative rods, cocco-bacilli, and gram-positive cocci from a postsurgical wound are indicative of a polymicrobial infection that requires bacterial culture to determine the etiologic agents and their antibiogram.

Unfortunately, bacteriologic statistics and Gram staining procedures may not always reveal the identity of the etiologic agent. Under such circumstances, bacteriologic cultures may be necessary. There are several methods available for the rapid identification of pathogenic bacteria isolated from clinical material, most of which are readily available to an equine practitioner. This, in conjunction with the commercial availability of prepared media, makes it possible for the modern equine practitioner to perform basic diagnostic bacteriology. When performed correctly, in-house diagnostic bacteriology testing reduces the cost and the length of time required for microbiologic results. Such results can reduce the time required to verify the accuracy of empirically administered antimicrobial agents.

Culture samples for pathogen identification and susceptibility testing must be collected before beginning antimicrobial therapy. This is particularly true for life-threatening or otherwise serious infections. Once antimicrobial therapy has been started, cultures are usually rendered sterile, even though viable organisms remain in the host.

CHOOSING THE APPROPRIATE ANTIBACTERIAL AGENT

Successful antimicrobial chemotherapy depends on the selection of the appropriate antimicrobial agent and the appropriate dosage regimen. Before choosing an empirical regimen, the equine practitioner needs to consider the site of the infection, whether the infection is mono- or polymicrobial, the potential etiologic agents, the nature of the infectious disease process, and the pharmacokinetic and pharmacodynamic properties of the selected agent.

Choosing an appropriate antimicrobial, like determining the etiologic agent, may be based on clinical experience or laboratory testing. For example, in the horse, most pyogranulomatous infections are caused by β-hemolytic streptococci. These organisms are uniformly susceptible to penicillin and thus do not need susceptibility testing. On the other hand, staphylococci and most of the gram-negative bacterial pathogens in the equine environment vary in their susceptibility to antimicrobial agents. The author's laboratory has isolated 20 *Staphylococcus aureus* from numerous postsurgical wounds that have been resistant to the β-lactams tested (i.e., penicillins and cephalosporins), and to erythromycin, gentamicin, tetracycline and trimethoprim/sulfa. The only active antimicrobial agents were amikacin, vancomycin, clindamycin, and ciprofloxacin. None of these agents is considered a drug of choice in the horse and, in fact, only amikacin and vancomycin and possibly ciprafloxicin can be used safely, but not without a great deal of expense.

Because the susceptibility profile for most staphylococci and gram-negative bacteria is unpredictable, susceptibility testing should be performed. Currently, there are a number of methods for conducting susceptibility testing. The method most commonly used in veterinary medicine is the disk diffusion test, which is inexpensive and flexible in terms of the antimicrobial agents that can be tested. The results have a reasonable correlation with clinical outcome. However, the results are qualitative (i.e., they are reported as susceptible, intermediate, or resistant) and lack the quantitative information the equine practitioner can use to increase efficacy or reduce costs of therapy. Another limitation of this test has been the determination of the interpretive criteria. *Susceptible* implies that blood levels, following recommended doses of the antibacterial agent, should be sufficient to inhibit the growth of the isolated pathogen. *Resistant* suggests that the isolated pathogen would not be inhibited by the achievable systemic concentrations. Unfortunately, these interpretive criteria are based on human serum concentrations of the drug and verified by human clinical trials. The source of these data, at least in the United States, is the National Committee for Clinical Laboratory Standards, Subcommittee on Antimicrobial

Susceptibility Testing (see NCCLS Document M2-A5 in Supplemental Readings).

A susceptibility testing method that is gaining in popularity in both human and veterinary medicine is the microdilution test. Several companies currently produce custom microdilution plates. The antimicrobial concentration may be supplied in a dehydrated form for storage at room temperature for up to 12 months, or frozen for storage at −70°C for up to 6 months. Microdilution plates may also be prepared in-house if appropriate quality control (QC) measures are followed and appropriate QC organisms are tested with each assay (see NCCLS Document M7-A3 in Supplemental Readings). Although microdilution testing gives quantitative information (i.e., minimal inhibitory concentrations), most commercial plates also provide interpretive criteria (i.e., susceptible, intermediate, and resistant). Microdilution testing is, however, less versatile and more expensive than the disk diffusion test. In addition, without knowing the pharmacokinetic parameters of the antimicrobial agent in the target animal, knowledge of the minimal inhibitory concentration (MIC) may be of little value unless it is very low.

When considering the clinical application of the in vitro results, it is important to consider the optimal use of the antimicrobial agents. Penicillin, as with all β-lactam antimicrobial agents (i.e., all penicillins, cephalosporins, carbepenems, and monobactams) exhibits time-dependent killing. In other words, increasing the concentration of the drug four to 16 times the MIC does not dramatically increase the rate of killing (Fig. 1) (see Craig and Ebert, 1991 in Supplemental Readings). Rather, the length of time the bacteria are exposed to the drug dictates the rate of killing. On the other hand, most bactericidal antimicrobial agents that interfere with DNA or RNA synthesis exhibit concentration-dependent killing (see Fig. 1); in other words, the rate of killing increases as the drug concentration increases above the MIC for that bacterial pathogen. Thus, antimicrobial agents may be classified as those that exhibit time-dependent killing such as penicillin and cephalosporins, those that demonstrate concentration-dependent killing such as aminoglycosides or fluoroquinolones, and those that are generally considered to be bacteriostatic, such as tetracyclines and erythromycin. For example, an MIC of 1.0 μg/ml for gentamicin may be less desirable, even though it is lower than an MIC of 2.0 μg/ml for ampicillin, when one considers the pharmacokinetic/pharmacodynamic relationship of these two drugs in the horse. When administered at 2.2 mg/kg q8h, the peak serum concentration (serum C_{max}) of gentamicin is approximately 5 μg/ml and would produce a C_{max}/MIC of 5. Clinical studies in human medicine have demonstrated that a serum C_{max}/MIC ratio of 10 for aminoglycosides predicts a 90% or greater favorable clinical outcome, whereas a ratio of 5:1, as presented in the example earlier, predicts a positive clinical response of 70% or less. By contrast, when sodium ampicillin is administered at 11 mg/kg q12h, the serum concentration would remain above an MIC of 2.0 μg/ml for approximately 10 hours or 83% of the dosing interval. Studies have demonstrated that the serum concentration of β-lactam antimicrobials such as ampicillin should exceed the MIC of gram-negative bacteria for at least 50% of the dosing interval for a successful outcome. In the

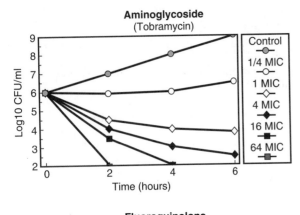

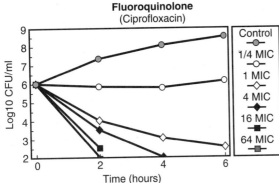

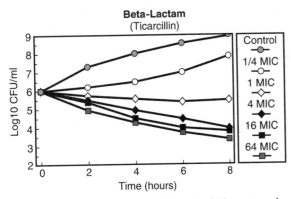

Figure 1. Effect of the concentration of antimicrobial agents on the rate of bacterial killing. In the case of an aminoglycoside (tobramycin) and a fluoroquinolone (ciprafloxacin), the rate of killing is a function of drug concentration, in the case of a beta-lactam (ticarcillin), the rate of killing is independent of drug concentration.

specific but also designed especially for the more common animal species encountered by most veterinary practitioners. In December 1994, this subcommittee, through the NCCLS, published a Proposed Standard for Susceptibility Testing of Bacteria Isolated from Animals (see NCCLS Document M31-P in Supplemental Readings). Although many of the interpretive criteria contained in this proposed standard are still based on human pharmacokinetics and breakpoint values, some are specific to veterinary medicine. As the document moves through the approval process, and as more antimicrobial agents are approved for use in veterinary medicine, the interpretive criteria for determining bacterial susceptibility will be more animal species-specific.

CHOOSING THE APPROPRIATE DOSE AND DOSING REGIMEN BY USE OF PHARMACOKINETIC AND PHARMACODYNAMIC RELATIONSHIPS

The most significant factor determining the efficacy of β-lactam and most bacteriostatic antimicrobial agents (i.e., erythromycin and tetracyclines) is the time that serum levels exceed the MIC of the pathogen. For the aminoglycosides and fluoroquinolones, the most significant factor is how much the concentration of the drug exceeds the MIC. This new information has led to a more complete understanding of the pharmacodynamic parameters associated with drug-bacterial pathogen-host interactions. Historically, the only pharmacodynamic properties that were considered were the interactions between the bacterium and the drug, and these were restricted to MIC and minimal bactericidal concentration (MBC). If the MIC and MBC were the same or very close, the antimicrobial agent was considered to be bactericidal. If there were several dilutions between the MIC and the MBC, the antimicrobial agent was considered to be bacteriostatic. More recent studies have suggested that several other factors need to be taken into consideration when looking at the pharmacodynamic properties of an antimicrobial agent. These include (1) first exposure effect; (2) increased bacterial killing rates with increased concentrations of drug; (3) in vivo postantibiotic effect (PAE); (4) sub-MIC effect; and (5) postantibiotic leukocyte enhancement (PALE).

The first exposure effect and increased bacterial killing rates with increased concentrations of the drug are closely associated pharmacodynamic effects. Although most bactericidal antibacterial agents exhibit some increased killing with increased concentrations of the drug, this effect is far more pronounced for the aminoglycosides and fluoroquinolones than for the β-lactams. In other words, as the concentrations of these agents increase above the MIC of a bacterium, such as *Escherichia coli* or *Pseudomonas aeruginosa*, the rate at which the bacterium is killed increases accordingly. This can be compared with a β-lactam such as ticarcillin, with which the increase in killing is restricted to concentrations two- to four-fold greater than the MIC (see Fig. 1). For the bacteria that survive their first exposure to a drug such as gentamicin, there is a period of time during which there is a down-regulation of

example given earlier, the time above the MIC was greater than 80% of the dosing interval. Thus, although gentamicin has a lower MIC than ampicillin, the drug of choice, based on pharmacokinetic and pharmacodynamic properties of the two drugs, is ampicillin.

In the past, veterinary practitioners have been hampered by not knowing the serum concentrations of common antimicrobial agents used for different animal species. Lacking this information, they have relied on interpretive criteria based on data from human medicine. Recently, the NCCLS formed a subcommittee on Veterinary Antimicrobial Susceptibility Testing (VAST). The objective of this subcommittee was to develop interpretive criteria for antimicrobial susceptibility testing that was not only veterinary medicine-the subsequent uptake of drug by the bacterium. If the second exposure occurs before the bacteria recover from this first exposure, they will be less susceptible to antimicrobial effects. Thus, an initial exposure to a higher concentration of gentamicin results in an increased killing of the bacteria. A longer dosing interval then allows the surviving bacteria to recover before being rechallenged by the drug.

A third pharmacodynamic effect that is closely associated with these two events is the PAE. This term describes the persistent-suppression of bacterial growth that can occur after a limited exposure to an antimicrobial agent. This phenomenon was first discovered shortly after the introduction of the penicillins for clinical use. Initially, it was thought to be an in vitro phenomenon. However, studies with animal models suggest that in vitro PAE, although usually shorter, is a good predictor of in vivo PAE. A notable exception is with the penicillins and streptococci in which substantial PAEs have not been reproduced in various animal models. This may be due to the slow growth rate of streptococci in vivo compared to in vitro.

All antimicrobials appear to produce an in vivo PAE against *Staphylococcus aureus* but vary in their ability to exert an in vivo PAE against streptococci, the Enterobacteriaceae and other gram-negative bacteria such as *P. aeruginosa*. For these organisms, penicillins and cephalosporins produce little or no in vivo PAE. In contrast, antimicrobial agents such as aminoglycosides or fluoroquinolones that inhibit protein or nucleic acid synthesis produce prolonged in vivo PAE. The site of infection may also affect the duration of in vivo PAE, probably due to the duration of time that the concentration of the drug exceeds the MIC of the pathogen in the different tissues.

The clinical importance of an in vivo PAE is obvious. Prolonged in vivo PAE prevents the regrowth of the bacteria when serum and tissue concentrations fall below the MIC of the invading organism and allows for longer dosing intervals. Several studies of gram-negative sepsis have demonstrated that the efficacy of the aminoglycosides and the fluoroquinolones is dependent on the total amount of drug administered at a given time, rather than how frequently it is administered. This is in marked contrast to the β-lactams, whose efficacy is based on the frequency of dosing rather than the concentration of the drug. The only parameter to which one can attribute the differences between the β-lactams and aminoglycosides is the presence or absence of a PAE.

Investigations of the pharmacodynamic properties of gentamicin in humans have demonstrated that once-daily dosing of aminoglycosides provides similar or greater efficacy than more frequent dosing and may reduce oto- and nephrotoxicity. A recent study (see Godber and colleagues in Supplemental Readings) investigated the pharmacokinetic parameters of gentamicin administered as a single versus three-times-daily dosing regimen in horses. Each horse received gentamicin for 10 days with a 30-day washout period between dosing regimens. There was no evidence of nephrotoxicity with either dosing regimen. However, the serum and tissue concentrations of gentamicin administered once daily were significantly higher than those obtained by three-times-a-day administration. When administered at 6.6 mg/kg q24h, C_{max}/MIC for a common equine isolate of *P. aeruginosa* isolate was 98, 11, and 8 for

serum, tissue cage fluid and bronchial secretion concentrations, respectively. When dosed at 2.2 mg/kg q8h, the ratios were 7, 4, and 0.5. These results suggest that once-daily dosing provides peak serum concentrations that may provide an optimal pharmacodynamic relationship for treatment.

As stated earlier, the in vitro PAE are shorter but otherwise may be good predictors of in vivo PAE, with the exception of the streptococci. The longer in vivo PAE may be attributed to higher exposure concentrations, increased length of exposure, slower growth rate of the bacteria in vivo, postantibiotic leucocyte enhancement (PALE), and sub-MIC effect. The PALE is the increased susceptibility of bacteria to the activity of neutrophils, following exposure to an antibiotic. The PALE may be enhanced by the postantibiotic sub-MIC effect (PA SME), which occurs when bacteria are exposed to a high inhibitory concentration of a drug followed by concentrations that are below the MIC. Prolonged PAEs and a pronounced rate of killing promote long PA SME. Clinically, it may not be necessary to distinguish between the effects of the PAE and PA SME, because the combination of the two contributes to prevention of bacterial regrowth between doses. What is important is that these pharmacodynamic properties can influence the frequency of dosing with certain antibacterial agents without adversely affecting the clinical outcome.

Knowledge of how to use MIC with pharmacokinetic and pharmacodynamic parameters will enhance the equine practitioner's ability to use information provided by the new Professional Flexible Labeling (PFL) initiative. With PFL, a practitioner will be able to choose a dose based on the MIC of the bacterial pathogen and the pharmacokinetic and pharmacodynamic properties of the drug. Thus, if the pathogen has a low MIC and the antimicrobial demonstrates time-dependent killing, the practitioner may choose to use a low dose administered more frequently. On the other hand, if the pathogen has a high MIC, the bioavailability curve should provide the clinician with the information needed to select a more appropriate dose. Similar guidelines will also be provided for antimicrobial agents that exhibit concentration-dependent killing.

Supplemental Readings

Cars O, Odenholt-Tornqvist I: The post-antibiotic sub-MIC effect in vitro and in vivo. J Antimicrob Chem [Suppl D]31:159–166, 1993.

Craig W: Pharmacodynamics of antimicrobial agents as a basis for determining dosage regimens. Eur J Clin Microbiol Infect Dis [Suppl 1]12:6–8, 1993.

Craig WA, Ebert SC: Killing and regrowth of bacteria in vitro: A review. Scand J Infect Dis [Suppl]74:63–70, 1990.

Giguère S, Sweeney RW. Bélanger M: Pharmacokinetics of enrofloxaxin in adult horses and concentration of the drug in serum, body fluids, and endometrial tissues after repeated intragastrically administered doses. Am J Vet Res 57:1025–1030, 1996.

Godber LM, Walker RD, Stein GE, Hauptman JG, Derksen FJ: Pharmacokinetics, nephrotoxicosis and in vitro antibacterial activity associated with single versus multiple (three times) daily gentamicin treatments in horses. Am J Vet Res 5:613–618, 1995.

Leggett JE, Ebert S, Fantin B, Craig WA: Comparative dose-effect relations at several dosing intervals for beta-lactam, aminoglycoside and quinolone antibiotics against Gram-negative bacilli in murine thigh-infection and pneumonitis models. Scand J Infect Dis [Suppl]74:179–184, 1990.

National Committee for Clinical Laboratory Standards. Performance

Standards for Antimicrobial Disk Diffusion Susceptibility Tests, Fifth Edition; Approved Standard. NCCLS Document M2-A5. Villanova, PA, 1993.

National Committee for Clinical Laboratory Standards. Methods for Dilution Antimicrobial Susceptibility Tests for Bacteria that Grow Aerobically, Third Edition; Approved Standard. NCCLS Document M7-A3. Villanova, PA, 1993.

National Committee for Clinical Laboratory Standards. Performance Standards for Antimicrobial Disk and Dilution Susceptibility Tests for Bacteria Isolated from Animals; Proposed Standard. NCCLS Document M31-P. Villanova, PA, 1994.

Walker R: Antimicrobial chemotherapy. *In* Robinson NE (ed): Current Therapy in Equine Medicine, ed 3. Philadelphia, WB Saunders, 1992, pp 1–13.

Nonsteroidal Anti-inflammatory Drugs

LAURIE A. MITTEN
Pullman, Washington

KENNETH W. HINCHCLIFF
Columbus, Ohio

Nonsteroidal anti-inflammatory drugs (NSAIDs)—in particular phenylbutazone, flunixin meglumine, dipyrone, ketoprofen, meclofenamic acid, and naproxen—are commonly used medications in horses. Their anti-inflammatory, analgesic, antiendotoxic, antipyretic, and antithrombotic properties make them useful in a variety of clinical situations. Postoperative inflammation and soft tissue injuries are frequently treated with NSAIDs to provide analgesia and to reduce heat, edema, and swelling. Phenylbutazone is used to alleviate lameness caused by degenerative joint and navicular disease, laminitis, and tendinitis. Flunixin meglumine is often administered to horses with abdominal pain. Clinical signs associated with endotoxemia, a common problem in horses with colitis, often improve after NSAID administration. Nonsteroidal anti-inflammatory drugs are the treatment of choice for pyrexia caused by inflammatory and infectious conditions. Aspirin is used to prevent thrombus formation, a frequent problem in endotoxemia, thromboembolic colic, and laminitis, although its efficacy in improving clinical signs is unproven.

CLINICAL PROPERTIES

Anti-inflammatory Properties

The anti-inflammatory properties of NSAIDs are well known and are attributed to their ability to inhibit the production of inflammatory prostaglandins. Tissue damage results in the production of numerous mediators of the inflammatory process, including histamine, bradykinin, 5-hydroxytryptamine, leukotrienes, platelet-activating factor, and prostaglandins. In addition, several of these mediators may act synergistically to increase blood flow to inflamed tissues and increase vascular permeability. Prostaglandin E_2 (PGE_2), with prostacyclin, produces erythema and edema via vasodilation. Phenylbutazone and flunixin meglumine decrease the concentrations of PGE_2 and prostacyclin in inflamed tissue in horses. Plasma concentrations of NSAIDs do not always correlate with their anti-inflammatory effects, possibly because plasma concentrations of the NSAID may be lower than concentrations in inflammatory exudate or concentrations in synovial fluid of inflamed joints. The ability of NSAIDs to concentrate in an inflammatory exudate is attributed to leakage of albumin, to which NSAIDs are highly bound across damaged endothelium.

Analgesic Properties

Prostaglandins produce pain in inflamed tissue and potentiate the pain response to chemical (histamine and bradykinin) and mechanical stimulation by lowering the threshold of polymodal nociceptors of C-fibers. Nonsteroidal anti-inflammatory drugs reduce pain in inflamed tissue by reducing local prostaglandin production. Therefore, an NSAID does not exhibit its analgesic properties until prostaglandins formed before its administration have dissipated. Recent studies provide evidence that prostaglandins in the spinal cord play an important role in processing of pain information. Nonsteroidal anti-inflammatory drugs may have a central action by inhibiting the formation of prostaglandins within the spinal cord. For example, flunixin meglumine may have some central effect that accounts for its superior analgesic property in horses with colic. However, phenylbutazone is usually preferred as an analgesic for musculoskeletal problems, such as degenerative joint disease or laminitis, that result in lameness.

Antiendotoxic Properties

Several studies have documented the beneficial effects of NSAIDs for treatment of endotoxemia in horses. Flunixin meglumine is superior to phenylbutazone and selective thromboxane inhibitors in treatment of experimental endotoxemia. Pretreatment with flunixin meglumine prevents endotoxin-induced increases in blood lactate and plasma prostaglandin concentrations and improves clinical signs of horses given endotoxin. However, there is no difference between treatment with flunixin (1.0 mg/kg IV) or ketoprofen (2.2 mg/kg IV) on plasma prostaglandin, tumor necrosis factor, and leukotriene concentrations in horses given endotoxin. Administration of flunixin meglumine at a low dose (0.25 mg/kg IV) before administration of endotoxin significantly decreases plasma thromboxane concentrations and alleviates abdominal pain in ponies. This low dose of flunixin meglumine is unlikely to mask the clinical parameters necessary for further patient assessment.

Antipyretic Properties

The anti-pyretic effects of NSAIDs are attributable to their ability to prevent PGE_2 formation. Fever is usually the result of infection or inflammation. Subsequent production of interleukin-1 and tumor necrosis factor results in increased production of PGE_2 in the vascular organs in the preoptic hypothalamic areas of the central nervous system. Prostaglandin E_2 acts locally within the hypothalamus to elevate the hypothalamic set point, the temperature about which body temperature is maintained. Nonsteroidal anti-inflammatory drugs prevent the increase in body temperature (fever) by blocking the formation of PGE_2 and promote return of the body temperature set point to normal. The NSAIDs do not influence body temperature when it is elevated by exercise or increased ambient temperature. Phenylbutazone, flunixin meglumine, and dipyrone are frequently used as antipyretic agents, but dipyrone has poor analgesic and anti-inflammatory properties.

Anti-thrombotic Properties

The antithrombotic actions of aspirin are well described in humans and are documented in horses. The antithrombotic action of NSAIDs is due to inhibition of production of thromboxane A_2 (TXA_2), a potent platelet aggregator and vasoconstrictor, by thrombocytes. Thrombocytes do not have the deoxyribonucleic acid (DNA) material necessary to synthesize protein; therefore, irreversible inhibition of thrombocyte cyclo-oxygenase renders thrombocytes incapable of producing TXA_2. Aspirin irreversibly inhibits cyclo-oxygenase, whereas phenylbutazone and other commonly used NSAIDs reversibly inhibit the enzyme (see mechanism of action). The antithrombotic actions of aspirin therefore last the lifespan of the thrombocytes, which ranges between 8 and 10 days. Phenylbutazone, flunixin meglumine, and aspirin decrease platelet aggregation and increase template bleeding times in horses; however, aspirin is the most potent and most long-lasting agent. Aspirin is effective when administered every 48 hours, even though it has a shorter half life than other NSAIDs (Table 1). Aspirin has several advantages over reversible inhibitors of cyclo-oxygenase such as flunixin meglumine and phenylbutazone. Low aspirin doses and a long dosing interval minimize the risk of the toxic effects of NSAID therapy. In addition, low aspirin doses do not affect the synthesis of prostacyclin, the principal prostaglandin synthesized by endothelial cells, a vasodilator and inhibitor of platelet aggregation. Therefore, administration of aspirin on alternate days may be of value in treatment of diseases associated with thrombus formation, including endotoxemia, thromboembolic colic, and thrombophlebitis.

MECHANISM OF ACTION

Prostaglandins and thromboxane are a group of related lipid molecules derived from phospholipid portions of cel-

TABLE 1. PHARMACOKINETICS OF COMMONLY USED NSAID IN HORSES

	Elimination Half Life (h)	Volume of Distribution (L/kg)	Bioavailability (%)
Phenylbutazone	3.5–6.1	0.15	90
Flunixin meglumine	1.6	0.21	80
Ketoprofen	1–2	0.16	NA
Dipyrone	4.7	0.18	NA
Meclofenamic acid	2.5	0.13	65
Naproxen	4–5	0.13	50
Aspirin	0.11	0.08	NA

NA = not available

lular membranes. Arachidonic acid, released by the action of phospholipase A_2 on membrane phospholipids (phosphatidylcholine, phosphatidylethanolamine, and phosphatidylinositol), is metabolized by either 5-lipoxygenase (LOX) to leukotrienes or cyclo-oxygenase (COX) to prostaglandins and thromboxane. All NSAIDs inhibit the formation of prostaglandins and thromboxane through inhibition of COX, but they do not prevent the binding of arachidonic acid metabolites to receptors. Cyclo-oxygenase, also known as prostaglandin G/H synthetase, has both cyclo-oxygenase and peroxidase activities and catalyzes two reactions. The first reaction is the cyclo-oxygenase reaction, by which arachidonic acid is converted to prostaglandin G_2 (PGG_2). The second is a peroxidase reaction, reducing PGG_2 to prostaglandin H_2 (PGH_2). These reactions occur at distinct, but neighboring, catalytic sites of the COX molecule. Nonsteroidal anti-inflammatory drugs only block the cyclo-oxygenase activity without affecting the peroxidase activity. Two COX isoenzymes (COX-1 and COX-2) exist. COX-1 is constitutively expressed in most tissues and is involved in maintaining physiologic cellular functions, such as interaction between vascular endothelium and platelets. COX-2 is expressed only after cellular activation in response to various stimuli, including trauma and presence of various cytokines. Adverse effects of NSAIDs occur with inhibition of COX-1, whereas the beneficial anti-inflammatory effects are observed with inhibition of COX-2. The effect of different NSAIDs on either COX-1 or COX-2 may vary, but this variation is not recognized as being of clinical significance. The exact mode and magnitude of inhibition of COX varies and is complex. Aspirin irreversibly inhibits cyclo-oxygenase by acetylating a serine residue, whereas phenylbutazone, flunixin meglumine, and indomethacin inhibit cyclo-oxygenase reversibly. Flunixin meglumine is the most potent NSAID used in equine medicine, with meclofenamic acid and phenylbutazone being less potent and dipyrone and aspirin being the least potent.

PHARMACOKINETICS

Nonsteroidal anti-inflammatory drugs are weak organic acids that are highly protein bound. Chemically, the NSAIDs are classified as either carboxylic or enolic acids, with subgroups classified by their structural differences. Phenylbutazone, oxyphenbutazone, and dipyrone are enolic acids and are classified in a subgroup as pyrazolones. Carboxylic acid subgroups include the salicylates (sodium salicylate, acetylsalicylic acid); propionic acids (naproxen, ibuprofen); anthranilic acids (meclofenamic acid); aminonicotinic acids (flunixin meglumine); and indolines (indomethacin).

The volume of distribution, elimination half life, and oral bioavailability for the commonly used NSAIDs in equine medicine are presented in Table 1. The volume of distribution is small for NSAIDs, because of the high level of protein-binding of the drugs. The majority of NSAIDs are metabolized to inactive metabolites, with the exception of phenylbutazone and dipyrone. The main metabolites of phenylbutazone are oxyphenbutazone and gamma-hydroxyphenbutazone. Oxyphenbutazone is an active metabolite; however, it has less pharmacologic activity than phenylbutazone. The bioavailability of phenylbutazone after oral administration is variable and is affected by type of feed and by product used (i.e., paste or powder), and it may also be dependent on time of day of administration.

TOXICITY OF NSAIDs

The use of NSAIDs in horses has been generally regarded as safe, even though NSAID-induced gastrointestinal, renal, hematologic, and hepatic disease is recognized in human beings and other species. It is now recognized that gastrointestinal and renal disease may result from excessively high doses and prolonged administration of NSAIDs to horses. Gastrointestinal disease resulting from NSAID use frequently results in a protein-losing enteropathy with gastrointestinal ulcers predominately occurring in the large colon. Nonsteroidal anti-inflammatory drugs may result in renal papillary necrosis in horses, but pre-existing factors such as hypovolemia must usually be present. Gastrointestinal and renal toxicity induced by NSAID use can occur at the same time.

Gastrointestinal Toxicity

The clinical signs of gastrointestinal disease induced by NSAIDs are usually nonspecific but include colic, fever, bruxism, and ventral edema. Diarrhea may or may not be present. Similar clinical signs are often present in horses with colitis accompanying salmonellosis and Potomac horse fever, for which NSAIDs are indicated. Prolonged and excessive use of phenylbutazone occurs during treatment of conditions such as laminitis and degenerative joint disease. Therefore, it is important to obtain a thorough history about previous use of NSAIDs, especially the dose, frequency, and duration of administration.

The first hematologic abnormalities noted in cases of NSAID toxicity are usually hypoproteinemia and hypoalbuminemia. The latter is a very sensitive indicator of NSAID toxicity and can even occur in horses receiving the recommended dose of phenylbutazone. Such horses may have no evidence of colonic ulcers at necropsy. Neutropenia with a left shift and electrolyte abnormalities, hyponatremia, and hypochloremia, presumably associated with gastrointestinal loss of sodium and chloride, are common. Although dehydration may be present, its severity cannot be assessed from the plasma protein concentration because of the concurrent hypoproteinemia. Hydration, therefore, must be evaluated from clinical signs, serum creatinine concentration, and packed cell volume.

The pathogenesis of NSAID-induced gastrointestinal disease is related to inhibition of synthesis of prostaglandins, which have a physiologic role in protection and growth of the gastrointestinal tract. These prostaglandins, in particular PGE_2, increase mucosal blood flow and mucus secretion, decrease gastric acid and pepsin secretion, accelerate cell proliferation, and stabilize cell membranes. Inhibition of production of these important prostaglandins results in gastrointestinal ulcers in the large colon, especially the right dorsal colon, and in the cecum, small intestines, and oral mucosa. Phenylbutazone absorption onto the fibrous and cellulose components of the diet and its release during fermentation may account for the presence of lower gastrointestinal tract ulcers. Ulcers range from shallow to deep and perforating, with bacterial invasion common. The large ulcers are associated with vasculitis and thrombosis of submucosal vessels. In foals, gastric ulcers are more common than colonic ulcers.

Although the breed and age of the horse, the specific NSAID, the formulation, and the route of administration influence the gastrointestinal toxicity of NSAIDs, the most important factors are the dose and duration of administration. Most reports of gastrointestinal toxicity involve phenylbutazone administered at 8 to 14 mg/kg p.o. q24h for 7 to 14 days, although toxicity may occur at lower dose rates. Flunixin meglumine is reportedly less toxic than phenylbutazone, and ketoprofen is the least toxic. Although both oral and systemic administration of NSAIDs may result in toxicity, phenylbutazone paste is reported to be more toxic than the powder formulation.

The prognosis for resolution of NSAID toxicity is poor. Sucralfate, a protectant that may also increase local prostaglandin production, and histamine H_2 antagonists such as ranitidine and cimetidine, which decrease acid secretion, are effective in treatment of gastric ulcers. Sucralfate has also been recommended for treatment of right dorsal colitis, but its effectiveness in treatment of colonic ulcers is unknown. Misoprostol (a synthetic analogue of PGE_2) decreases gastric acid secretion and may provide gastric mucosal protection, but its effectiveness in providing colonic mucosal protection in horses is unknown. Diarrhea and colic may result from its use. Misoprostol is an abortifacient in human beings; pregnant women should not handle the drug, and it should be used with caution in pregnant mares, if at all. Providing dietary linoleic acid (n-6 or the omega-6 polyunsaturated fatty acids) by feeding safflower or coconut oil may increase arachidonic acid availability and formation of protective prostaglandins. Feeding a low-bulk, low-roughage diet and administration of psyllium mucilloid is reported to be successful in treatment of horses with right dorsal colitis.

Renal Toxicity

The clinical signs of renal disease associated with NSAID use are nonspecific but include polyuria, polydipsia, weight loss, and depression. Blood chemistry abnormalities include, but are not limited to, azotemia, hyponatremia, and hypochloremia. Urinalysis reveals isosthenuric urine in the face of an elevated serum creatine concentration. Proteinuria and granular casts may also be detected on urinalysis.

Renal disease induced by NSAIDs is the result of loss of renal prostaglandins. Prostaglandin E_2 is a local vasodilator that helps to maintain renal blood flow and glomerular filtration rate in the face of adverse circumstances such as dehydration and hypotension. Prostaglandins may accentuate renin release in response to the adrenergic activation of β-adrenoceptors that occurs in hemorrhage or dehydration. Prostaglandins also play a role in regulation of sodium and chloride, and they influence water metabolism by antagonizing the effects of antidiuretic hormone.

Renal papillary necrosis, acute renal insufficiency, nephrotic syndrome and interstitial nephritis, sodium and fluid retention, and hyperkalemia occur in human beings receiving NSAIDs. However, the only form of NSAID-induced nephrotoxicity recognized in horses is renal papillary necrosis, which occurs when NSAID administration is coupled with dehydration. Papillary necrosis is thought to be the result of medullary ischemia.

Treatment of renal papillary necrosis includes withdrawal of NSAIDs and nephrotoxic antibiotics, administration of intravenous fluids for correction of dehydration, and replacement of fluids lost in diuresis. Prevention of renal toxicity is achieved by minimizing the use of NSAIDs in hypovolemic horses and prevention of dehydration, especially when administration of NSAIDs is coupled with a nephrotoxic antibiotic such as an aminoglycoside.

Cellulitis

Cellulitis and thrombophlebitis are reported to occur following intramuscular, intravenous, or perivascular injections of various NSAIDs. The reactions are the result of the acidic nature of the drug and its concentration in solution. Flunixin meglumine is recommended for both intravenous and intramuscular administration, but the latter route has been associated with rare cases of clostridial myositis and cellulitis, including botulism, which is usually fatal. Phenylbutazone is recommended only for intravenous or oral administration. Perivascular injections result in inflammation, sloughing of surrounding tissues, and thrombophlebitis.

Other Adverse Effects

Blood dyscrasias have been described in horses receiving phenylbutazone, but the syndrome is not well documented. Transient elevations in liver enzymes occur in horses given toxic doses of phenylbutazone, but values return to normal when the phenylbutazone dose is decreased. Premature closure of the ductus arteriosus and fetal pulmonary hypertension can occur when pregnant women receive NSAIDs. This has not been reported in foals, even with frequent administration of NSAIDs to pregnant mares and even though phenylbutazone crosses the equine placenta. Aspirin can potentiate bronchoconstriction in asthmatic human patients, but administration of NSAIDs to horses with chronic obstructive pulmonary disease does not cause airway obstruction.

Supplemental Readings

Cohen ND, Carter GK, Mealy RH, Taylor TS: Medical management of right dorsal colitis in 5 horses: A retrospective study (1987–1993). J Vet Intern Med 9:272–276, 1995.

Cunningham FM, Lees P: Advances in anti-inflammatory therapy. Br Vet J 150:115–133, 1994.

Higgins AJ, Lees P: The acute inflammatory process, arachidonic acid metabolism and the mode of action of anti-inflammatory drugs. Equine Vet J 16:163–175, 1984.

Kallings P: Nonsteroidal anti-inflammatory drugs. Vet Clin North Am Equine Pract 9(3):523–541, 1993.

Fluid and Electrolyte Therapy

L. MICHAEL SCHMALL
Columbus, Ohio

Clinical conditions that require appropriate fluid therapy are commonplace in equine medicine and may represent the most critical and perhaps the least addressed component of many diseases. Frequently, intravenous fluids are required if treatment is to be successful and the animal is to have maximal chance of survival. Fluid administration is necessary to maintain vascular volume, cardiovascular performance, tissue perfusion, and oxygenation, and to correct for specific electrolyte and acid-base imbalances. Intravenous fluids may be necessary for a short-term replacement therapy or for extended periods, in which case maintenance and replacement requirements must be taken into account. Occasionally, the oral route of administration may be used if the gastrointestinal system has not been damaged and absorptive mechanisms are intact.

Appropriate fluid therapy includes assessment of fluid and electrolyte deficits, selection of the proper solution, evaluation of therapeutic efficacy, and consideration of adverse reactions. This chapter addresses these areas, along with a brief discussion of general principles of water and electrolyte compartmental distribution, types of fluids available for use, and routes of administration. Fluid requirements for specific diseases, which are addressed in detail elsewhere, are not included.

WATER AND ELECTROLYTE DISTRIBUTION

Approximately 60% of the adult and up to 80% of neonatal body weight is water that distributes freely along osmotic gradients between the intracellular (ICF) and extracellular (ECF) fluid compartments. The ICF accounts for approximately two thirds and ECF one third of total body water. ECF may be further subdivided into plasma volume and transcellular fluid (interstitial fluid and lymph), which account for approximately 8 to 12% and 15% of total body weight, respectively. ECF osmolality is maintained principally by sodium and chloride, whereas potassium and phosphates account for the majority of the osmotic forces in the ICF. Decreased water volume in either ECF or ICF results in a distribution imbalance and subsequent changes in osmotic forces that will redistribute water between the two compartments until a balance is re-established. For instance, an acute loss of fluid from the extracellular compartment effectively increases the osmotic forces. Fluid moves from the intracellular compartment until equilibrium is re-established.

The ionic compositions of the extracellular and intracellular compartments are significantly different. Sodium is the major extracellular cation and is responsible for the maintenance of the compartmental osmotic forces and extracellular fluid volume. Serum sodium concentrations are used clinically to estimate changes in total body sodium stores but are not totally reliable. Serum sodium is dependent on the exchangeable sodium content of the ECF, the exchangeable potassium content of the ICF, and total body water (TBW), and can be defined by the following relationship:

$$\text{Serum Na}^+ = \frac{\text{exchangeable Na}^+ + \text{exchangeable K}^+}{\text{TBW}}$$

Consequently, hypernatremia, or relative water deficit, may be the result of increases in exchangeable Na^+, K^+, losses in TBW, or a combination of these factors. Conversely, hyponatremia, or relative water excess, may be the result of increases in TBW or decreases in exchangeable Na^+ or K^+. Clinically, hypernatremia occurs when Na^+ concentration exceeds 146 mEq/L, and hyponatremia when Na^+ concentration is less than 132 mEq/L. Hyponatremia is most frequently seen with diarrheal diseases, in which large volumes of sodium are lost with only partial replacement of losses concurrent with water intake. Hypernatremia is rarely seen but may occur with overzealous or inappropriate fluid replacement.

Potassium is the major intracellular cation, with only 2% of the total body potassium being found in the ECF. Potassium functions in the ICF in a manner analogous to sodium in the ECF. Plasma concentrations of potassium are tightly regulated and, as such, extracellular fluid concentrations of potassium are unreliable estimates of total body potassium balance. Hyperkalemia is rarely seen in the horse with the exception of cases of impaired renal function or severe acidosis. In contrast, hypokalemia is frequently seen, particularly in anorectic animals, those with severe diarrheal disease, or those that are recovering from gastrointestinal surgery and are on restricted diets. Large-scale electrolyte imbalances are frequently associated with severe potassium losses and may be accompanied by alterations in neuromuscular or myocardial function. Potassium deficits are quickly corrected once the animal resumes eating hay.

Chloride and bicarbonate are the major anions in the ECF and exhibit a reciprocal relationship. Hypochloremia is usually the result of increased loss from the upper gastro-

intestinal tract, as with duodenitis-proximal jejunitis, or losses from sweating. Bicarbonate is the major buffering system and, as such, reflects alterations in acid-base status; marked decreases are frequently observed in mild to severe cases of acidosis. However, intravenous bicarbonate solutions should be used cautiously because excessive administration may result in the development of metabolic alkalosis, hypernatremia, hypokalemia, and hyperosmolality.

ASSESSMENT OF FLUID LOSSES

Initial assessment of fluid and electrolyte losses requires a thorough history and physical examination. Dehydration is assessed clinically on the basis of dry mucous membranes, decreased skin turgor, reduced urine production, and muscular weakness. Unfortunately, using these criteria, recognizable changes in hydration status are not apparent until deficits approach 5% of body weight. As such, an adult horse may have a fluid deficit close to 20 L before dehydration becomes clinically apparent. On the basis of clinical assessment, dehydration is graded as mild (5 to 7%), moderate (7 to 10%), or severe (greater than 10% of total body weight). When there are significant fluid losses, clinical signs of hypotension may develop; these signs include decreased jugular distensibility, increased heart rate, increased capillary refill time, decreased peripheral pulse, and cold extremities. Packed cell volume (PCV) and total protein concentration (TPP) are the most commonly used laboratory indicators of dehydration. However, these parameters can be affected by other factors. PCV can be significantly increased by splenic contraction and release of marginated erythrocytes. Protein loss from the gastrointestinal or urinary tract or reduced hepatic production reduces the validity of TPP as an estimator of hydration status. Blood urea nitrogen (BUN) and serum creatinine concentrations are increased in horses with acute fluid losses and are used diagnostically. All laboratory data are of limited use unless they are evaluated in the context of the animal's clinical condition.

Acid-base imbalances often are present in situations in which fluid therapy is indicated. Metabolic acidosis is more frequently encountered, particularly with gastrointestinal disease, diarrhea, or renal failure. Decreased peripheral perfusion, increased lactic acid production, and increased base loss all contribute to the development of acidosis. A compensatory respiratory alkalosis with a reduction in P_{CO_2} may be seen in these animals. Polyionic solutions or solutions containing high concentrations of bicarbonate (up to 5% $NaHCO_3$) are used to correct this condition. It is best to assess the degree of acidosis before administration of large quantities of bicarbonate. Hypochloremic metabolic alkalosis is most commonly seen after strenuous exercise in endurance horses and with early intestinal obstruction. Treatment to replace chloride deficits should be with sodium and potassium salts.

Samples for blood gas analysis should be collected anaerobically in heparinized syringes and may be stored for up to 4 hours before analysis. A laboratory equipped with a blood gas machine or a portable blood gas analyzer is preferable. If not available, a measurement of total carbon dioxide content provides an alternative. Approximately 95%

for the administration of large volumes of fluids are commercially available. Several types of catheters are available, with the choice dependent on cost, duration of fluid administration, potential for the development of complications, and clinician preference. Most common choices include 14- and 16-gauge Teflon, polyurethane, and silicone elastomer. The latter two are associated with a lower incidence of complications and thrombosis and are preferred for those situations in which long-term fluid therapy is required. The jugular vein is readily accessible and is used for most fluid administration. However, thrombosis of the jugular veins and compromise of venous return can lead to severe swelling of the head. For this reason, the lateral thoracic vein is often selected in those horses at high risk for the development of thrombosis. The cephalic and saphenous veins may also be used when necessary. Strict adherence to aseptic technique cannot be overemphasized and is essential for maintenance of catheter patency and to minimize complications. Catheters should be checked frequently and flushed with an appropriate anticoagulant such as heparinized saline. The catheter should be removed if any evidence of thrombosis, infection, or reaction at the catheter site is observed.

The volume of fluids necessary to effectively resuscitate horses in severe states of hypovolemia is frequently on the order of 20 to 40 L and can be as great as 80 to 100 L during the first 2 to 3 days of hospitalization. Fluid amounts of 60 to 90 ml/kg are frequently administered during the first hour to small animals and humans in shock. Such volumes are difficult to achieve in the horse but can be attained by using two intravenous catheters and fluid pumps. A volume of 10 to 20 L of fluid is given rapidly over a 1-hour period followed by maintenance at slower rates.

Supplemental Readings

Carlson GP: Fluid therapy. *In* Robinson NE (ed): Current Therapy in Equine Medicine. Philadelphia, WB Saunders, 1983, pp 311–318.

Carlson GP: Fluid therapy in horses with acute diarrhea. Vet Clin North Am 1(2):313–330, 1979.

Rose RJ: A physiological approach to fluid and electrolyte therapy in the horse. Equine Vet J 13:7, 1981.

Rose RJ: Electrolytes: Clinical applications. Vet Clin North Am 6(2):281–294, 1990.

Spier SJ, Snyder JR, Murray MJ: Fluid and electrolyte therapy for gastrointestinal disorders. *In* Smith BP (ed): Large Animal Internal Medicine. St. Louis, CV Mosby, 1990, pp 708–714.

Medical Management of Eventing Horses

LISA WILLIAMSON
Athens, Georgia

This chapter focuses on the role of the treatment veterinarian in combined-training competitions. Management of medical problems that commonly arise in combined-training horses are reviewed. Veterinarians interested in providing services at combined-training events should learn about the sport and its rules, particularly those governing the use of medications during competition.

BRIEF OVERVIEW OF COMBINED TRAINING

Combined training is a demanding triathletic sport that originated from military training exercises. The two most common types of combined-training events are horse trials and 3-day events. Horses competing in a horse trial perform consecutively a dressage test, a cross-country test, and a stadium jumping test over 1 to 2 days. The 3-day event is similar to a horse trial in that the horse is tested first in dressage and last in stadium jumping. The greatest difference between the two competitions arises in the second test: horse trial horses perform a cross-country test, whereas the 3-day event horse performs four distinct exercises (phases A–D) that are collectively referred to as the

speed and endurance test. Phases A and C, also called "roads and tracks," are endurance phases performed primarily at a trot (220 m/minute). Phase B is a steeplechase phase performed at recommended speeds of 640 to 690 m/minute (depending on the level of competition) that lasts approximately 3.5 to 5 minutes. Phase D, the final phase, is a cross-country test performed at a gallop over solid obstacles and variable terrain. The 3-day event is a more demanding and formal competition than the horse trial, and involves greater veterinary supervision.

Formal inspections are conducted during the 3-day event by the veterinary delegate (veterinary judge) and the ground jury (layperson judges) to determine the suitability of the horse to continue in competition. In addition, veterinary examinations are performed when the horse arrives at the event, and after phase D. The veterinary delegate, the associate veterinarian, and, in international competition, the foreign veterinary delegate, compose the Veterinary Commission. These veterinarians serve in a judicial and regulatory capacity, and therefore have different responsibilities than the treatment veterinarians. Although they supervise veterinary services and emergency care, the veterinary delegate and associate veterinarian should avoid providing medical attention to horses in competition because it could create a conflict-of-interest situation.

TREATMENT VETERINARIANS

Treatment veterinarians are responsible for providing medical care to horses during competition. Emergency veterinary services must be available on the grounds to treat horses on course during the cross-country or speed and endurance test, and during the stadium jumping test. Managers of large 3-day events commonly employ multiple emergency treatment veterinarians on speed and endurance day to provide rapid assistance to horses on course. Veterinarians in well-equipped emergency vehicles are stationed on the cross-country course, beside the steeplechase course, at the end of phases C and D, and in the stable area. The treatment veterinarians, veterinary delegate, associate veterinarian, and event management should all be in communication by radio during the speed and endurance test. Emergency protocols should be thoroughly discussed and understood by all emergency care providers before the speed and endurance test so that emergencies that arise can be handled smoothly and efficiently.

Veterinarians stationed out on course during the speed and endurance phase provide the initial care and stabilization of the sick or injured horse. As soon as the horse's condition is stabilized, the horse should be transported off the course in a designated horse ambulance to the stable area for further assessment and treatment. Because spectators are allowed on the course in roped-off walkways, a horse requiring emergency assistance can quickly draw a large crowd. Screens should be available to separate the public from treatment areas on course, because well-intentioned spectators can encumber medical efforts.

Treatment veterinarians on course must be prepared to perform euthanasia if necessary. However, if the horse is not suffering excessively, it should be transported to the stable area for further assessment, and the veterinary delegate, owner or agent, and (if applicable) the insurance company representative, should be consulted before a final decision is made. Written permission for euthanasia should be obtained from the owner or agent whenever possible. A horse that dies on the grounds during the event should have a postmortem examination performed by a pathologist at a diagnostic laboratory or veterinary college. This measure helps dispel rumors as to the cause of the horse's death, and is particularly important if the animal is insured.

In some situations, such as in the case of a fracture, referral to a surgical facility may be the best course of action after the injury is stabilized. Clearly printed directions to the designated veterinary treatment hospital should be prepared ahead of time to expedite the referral process.

The treatment veterinarian needs to be well equipped to handle various emergency situations. Table 1 lists suggested equipment and supplies but is not necessarily all-inclusive. In addition to being well prepared to handle horse emergencies, the veterinarian needs to pack personal provisions and clothing that accommodate variable weather conditions.

MEDICATION RULES

The treatment veterinarian needs to be familiar with the rules regarding medications and drug testing. In the United States, most combined-training competitions are run under American Horse Show Association (AHSA) rules. A few major 3-day competitions are run under the Federation Equestre Internationale (FEI) rules, however. The distinction is important because the AHSA rules for medications differ from FEI rules. Copies of the AHSA and FEI rules are available on request.* Failure to understand and comply with the medication rules can result in serious repercussions for the horse owner, trainer, and veterinarian.

The AHSA forbids the use of any substance that can affect performance, such as stimulants, depressants, tranquilizers, and local anesthetics. In addition, furosemide and other diuretics are forbidden because they interfere with detection of forbidden substances. The AHSA restricts the use of nonsteroidal anti-inflammatory drugs. To comply with the rules, the maximal dose for phenylbutazone per day is 4.4 mg/kg, and for flunixin meglumine is 1.1 mg/kg per day. The two anti-inflammatory agents should not be used concomitantly, and should not be given for more than 5 consecutive days. Furthermore, neither drug should be given within 12 hours of competition, or unacceptably high plasma levels can result. These recommendations should not be considered absolute for every horse and every situation, however, because many factors can affect drug clearance from the body. The permissible level for phenylbutazone is 1.0 μg/ml, and for flunixin meglumine is 0.2 μg/ml. If both phenylbutazone and flunixin meglumine are found in the same sample, neither can be present at more than a trace level. The use of methocarbamol is also restricted; plasma levels cannot exceed 4.0 μg/ml. To comply with this ruling, veterinarians must not exceed a dose of 11 mg/kg per 12 hours, and may not administer the drug within 6 hours of competition. Trace levels of theobromine, salicylic acid, arsenic, nandrolone, dimethyl sulfoxide (DMSO), and hydrocortisone are allowed, because low levels can arise from endogenous and dietary sources.

A horse or pony that receives any medication containing a forbidden substance is not eligible for AHSA Competition unless (1) the medication is necessary for treatment of an illness or injury; (2) the animal is withdrawn from competition for 24 hours after receiving the medication; (3) the drug is administered by a licensed veterinarian (or in his or her absence, the trainer); and (4) an AHSA Drugs and Medications Report is properly filled out, signed, and filed with the show steward or technical delegate within 1 hour of treatment, or within 1 hour of returning to duty.

The FEI currently has a "no foreign substance" rule. Before January 1994, phenylbutazone use was restricted but allowed. However, under the new regulations, a detectable plasma level of phenylbutazone or any other forbidden medication is considered to be in violation of the rules. Traces of theobromine, salicylic acid, arsenic, nandrolone, DMSO, and hydrocortisone are permissible, because small levels of these substances could arise endogenously or from ingesting normal foodstuffs. If a veterinarian treats a horse before or during an event, treatment must be declared on an Authorization Form for Medication, which is obtained

---

*Copies of the AHSA drug and medication pamphlets can be obtained through the AHSA Drugs and Medication Office (telephone 800–MED–AHSA). The FEI rules are available through the AHSA New York office; telephone 212–972–2472, by request for the International Department.

TABLE 1. SUGGESTED EQUIPMENT FOR THE TREATMENT VETERINARIAN

Personal items	DMSO for intravenous and topical use
Clipboard	Bandage materials (sheet cotton, roll cotton, gauze sponges,
Pen	Kling wrap, Vetwrap or nondisposible wraps)
Name tag	Casting material
Rain gear	Splints
Waterproof shoes/boots	Euthanasia solution
Sun hat	Sedatives (xylazine, detomidine)
Drinking water	Analgesics (butorphanol)
Snacks	Injectable anesthetics (ketamine hydrochloride, glycerol
Written materials	guiacolate)
Billing sheets	Local anesthetics
Current drug rules (AHSA or FEI)	Ophthalmic equipment and treatments (atropine and antibiotic
Medication report forms	ointments, eye wash, fluorescein dye strips, ophthalmoscope)
Copies of printed directions to designated referral hospital	Suture material
Euthanasia permission forms	Surgical instruments
Drugs/supplies	Sterile gloves
Thermometer(s), stethoscope	Rectal sleeves, rectal lubricant
100 L (or more) of balanced electrolyte solution (for IV use)	Syringes, needles (various sizes)
Intravenous administration sets and catheters	Methylprednisolone sodium succinate (four 500-mg vials)
Fluid stand	Calcium gluconate solution
Electrolytes for oral rehydration (table salt, Morton Lite salt)	Radiograph machine, cassettes, protective aprons, gloves
Tape (Elastikon, white, duct)	Electrocardiograph machine
Bucket	Surgical preparation set
Twitch	Lavage solution (normal saline)
Lead rope, halter	Clippers
Hoof equipment (testers, knives, nail pullers, rasp)	Extension cord
Assorted nasogastric tubes	Wire cutters
Stomach pump, dose syringe	Oscillating saw (to cut PVC splints)
Laxatives (mineral oil, psyllium, magnesium sulfate)	Refractometer
Antibiotics (injectable, oral)	Centrifuge
Topical antiseptic preparations	Capillary tubes, clay, reference chart for reading hematocrit
Nonsteroidal anti-inflammatory agents	Flashlight, lantern
Muscle relaxants	

from the veterinary delegate. The veterinary delegate and ground jury review the information and decide whether to allow the horse to start or continue in competition. The FEI rules allow for the use of oxygen insufflation and administration of intravenous balanced electrolyte solutions and glucose-containing solutions for up to 3 hours after the last horse has completed the speed and endurance test. Horses receiving either or both of these therapies must be examined by the veterinary delegate before the third inspection to ensure that the horse is physiologically fit to continue in competition.

MANAGEMENT OF SPECIFIC MEDICAL PROBLEMS

Problems requiring veterinary attention can be divided into several categories: infectious, metabolic, and traumatic. Because horses in competition are subjected to transport stress and exposed to different populations of horses, the necessity for managing acute infectious respiratory and digestive diseases can arise at the competition. Every effort is made at the time of arrival at a 3-day event to identify and isolate horses suspected of having infectious diseases to prevent spread of the disease. The majority of conditions requiring veterinary attention at combined-training competitions are either metabolic or traumatic problems, and most arise during the cross-country or speed and endurance tests.

Fluid Therapy

The physiologic basis for fluid therapy in eventing horse is discussed briefly in this section. Many metabolic problems discussed later in this chapter are treated with fluids. The reader can refer back to this section as needed.

Fluid and electrolyte losses in sweat contribute to the development of many metabolic problems. Under temperate ambient conditions, 3-day event horses typically lose, on average, 4% of their body water during the speed and endurance test without showing obvious signs of compromise. Hot and humid conditions; rough terrain; and prolonged, difficult exercise efforts intensify these losses and increase the likelihood that physiologic changes will become pathologic. Because horse sweat is somewhat hypertonic relative to plasma, hypotonic to isotonic dehydration develops with prolonged sweat losses. A state of voluntary dehydration can ensue because the stimulus to drink is triggered by increased plasma osmolality. Horses do not voluntarily replace their entire fluid deficit until electrolytes are also replenished. Sodium is particularly important because it is the main determinant of the extracellular fluid volume.

Eventing horses lose large quantities of sodium, chloride, calcium, and potassium in sweat. Metabolic acidosis with partial respiratory compensation is the most common acid-base profile immediately after the speed and endurance test. As ventilatory efforts normalize and lactic acid is dissipated during recovery, mild hypochloremic metabolic alkalosis is the predominant pattern.

The horse should be assessed to estimate the degree of dehydration and the severity of the disease state. The route and rate of administration can then be determined, based on these findings. Intravenous fluid therapy is indicated for horses that need rapid correction of moderate-to-large fluid and electrolyte deficits, and in horses for which diuresis is indicated, for example in horses with severe exertional rhabdomyolysis. Intravenous fluids should be sterile and isotonic and should have electrolyte composition similar to that of plasma. Lactated or acetated Ringer's solution and plain Ringer's solution are all reasonable choices for fluid therapy. Isotonic sodium chloride can be used initially, but should not be used for the long term without monitoring the electrolyte and acid-base status, because acidosis, hyperchloremia, hypernatremia, and hypokalemia can result. The treatment veterinarian must be prepared to administer large volumes of fluids, and the person responsible for having the fluids on hand should be decided well ahead of the event. Managers of some large 3-day events actually purchase 100 to 200 L of fluids to have on hand, but in most cases it is the responsibility of the treatment veterinarian to secure the fluids. Five-liter bags are more convenient than 1-L bags, and plastic bags are easier to store and have fewer breakage problems than glass bottles. An administration set with a Y connector makes fluid therapy more convenient by facilitating the administration of two 5-L bags of fluids simultaneously.

The rate of administration varies with the situation. Horses in hypovolemic shock can be started on fluids at an initial rate of 20 to 40 ml/kg per hour until their condition is stabilized, and then a slower rate of administration is used (5–10 ml/kg per hour). As a rule of thumb, 10 L can be delivered through a 14-gauge catheter placed in the jugular vein in approximately 1 to 1.4 hours by gravity flow (20 ml/kg in a 500-kg horse). If faster flow rates are required, a larger gauge catheter or a catheter placed in both jugular veins, and possibly a fluid administration pump are needed. The packed cell volume (PCV), total protein concentration (TP), and the pulmonary status of the patient should be assessed frequently to avoid hyperhydration. Because the lung is a shock organ in the horse, it is possible to create pulmonary compromise in severely ill horses and horses with pre-existing lung disease at extremely high flow rates. Once fluid and electrolyte balance is restored, fluid therapy can continue at a maintenance rate (2–4 ml/kg), or therapy can be discontinued if the horse is voluntarily consuming food and water.

Hypertonic saline has been used successfully to temporarily restore intravascular volume in horses with hypovolemic shock caused by rapid blood loss and endotoxemia. However, it is less appropriate to treat hypovolemic shock caused by exercise-induced dehydration with hypertonic saline, particularly if the plasma electrolyte status is unknown. Rapid replacement with isotonic fluids is preferred as the initial therapeutic choice for hypovolemic shock associated with exhaustive exercise. If hypertonic saline is used, it must be followed with large volumes of balanced isotonic electrolyte solution because its effects on intravascular volume are transient.

Oral fluid therapy via a nasogastric tube is a safe, economic, and effective alternative route, and can be used as an adjunct to intravenous fluid therapy. Oral fluid therapy is appropriate for horses with mild-to-moderate fluid and electrolyte deficits that have adequate gastrointestinal motility and are not exhibiting reflux when a nasogastric tube is introduced into the stomach. The temperament of the horse also is a factor in the decision whether to use this route of fluid therapy; some horses violently resist nasogastric intubation and can endanger themselves and the people attending them in their struggles.

The most beneficial oral rehydration fluids are isotonic to slightly hypotonic relative to plasma and contain sodium and chloride as their principal ions. Most 400- to 550-kg horses can handle 4 to 8 L of fluids via a nasogastric tube every 30 to 60 minutes (David Hodgson, University of Sydney, Australia, personal communication). Gastric emptying occurs in 15 to 20 minutes, and absorption occurs in 60 to 90 minutes. Absorption is slowed by hypertonicity, whereas glucose concentration and temperature of the rehydration solution have little impact on absorption rate.

An isotonic rehydration fluid that yields approximately 150 mEq/L of chloride, 136 mEq/L of sodium, and 14 mEq/L potassium can be prepared by dissolving 20 g Morton's Lite salt (1/2 NaCl and 1/2 KCl) and 70 g table salt (NaCl) in 10 L water. The salt can be weighed out and stored in packages before use for the sake of convenience.

Heat-Related Illnesses (Heat Stroke and Heat Exhaustion)

Heat stroke and heat exhaustion can occur in any environmental conditions, but are more likely to occur in a hot, humid environment when thermoregulatory mechanisms are compromised. Unacclimatized unfit horses are more prone to heat-related problems, as are horses with thermoregulatory abnormalities such as anhidrosis. A distinction can be made between heat stroke and heat exhaustion, but both conditions share some common features and therapeutic approaches.

Heat stroke occurs when heat gain from metabolic and environmental factors exceeds heat loss to the magnitude that tissue damage can occur. The degree of damage is related to the degree as well as the duration of the hyperthermia. Heat stroke can occur during exercise and during confinement in an excessively hot, poorly ventilated trailer or stall. Heat stroke can lead to neurologic, renal, cardiovascular, and gastrointestinal dysfunction, and ultimately the demise of the patient. Clinical signs include neurologic dysfunction ranging from weakness, depression, and ataxia, to collapse, convulsions, and death; rectal temperature of 106 to 110°F; prolonged capillary refill; tachycardia; tachypnea; and reduced sweat production to the point that the skin is actually hot and dry. Early recognition of clinical signs and appropriate treatment improve the overall prognosis.

Therapy is aimed at cessation of further heat generation; external cooling; and correction of fluid, electrolyte, and acid-base abnormalities. If it can walk, the affected horse should be moved to a shaded area and cooled with high-output fans. Unnecessary tack should be immediately removed and the horse left unblanketed. Ultimately the prognosis can depend in part on how rapidly the body temperature is brought into a safer range. Studies have shown that, in hot humid conditions, application of cool-to-cold water over the entire body surface safely and rapidly decreases body temperature in healthy horses with exercise-induced hyperthermia. Horses with extreme elevations of body temperature in hot environments should be cooled by spraying or sponging cool water on the horse's entire body surface. Particular attention should be given to cooling the head, if the horse will tolerate it, to augment selective brain cooling. The warmed water should be scraped off the body surface and cool water reapplied and removed until the body temperature is sufficiently reduced. The rectal temperature should be monitored during cooling and cooling methods adjusted according to response. Intravenous fluid therapy should be started to improve movement of heat from the core to the skin via the circulation, and to correct pre-existing fluid and electrolyte deficits. The use of corticosteroids is controversial, but short-acting corticosteroids such as methylprednisolone sodium succinate (2–4 mg/kg IV) can be considered for patients showing neurologic signs and to reduce tissue inflammation. Nonsteroidal anti-inflammatory drugs are ineffective in reducing hyperthermia originating from exertion or environment, but they can be used to reduce inflammation once the animal has been sufficiently rehydrated.

Exercise-associated heat exhaustion occurs as a result of protracted fluid and electrolyte losses during exercise. Depletion of energy reserves during exhaustive exercise can contribute to exhaustion. Dehydration and electrolyte abnormalities contribute to thermoregulatory compromise and abnormalities in the cardiovascular, nervous, muscular, gastrointestinal, and renal systems. Clinical signs include depression, disinterest in food and water, elevated rectal temperature, tachycardia, tachypnea, flaccid anus, dry oral membranes with capillary refill time longer than 2 seconds, and reduced sweat production. Synchronous diaphragmatic flutter (thumps) can develop as a result of increased irritability of the phrenic nerve as a consequence of acid-base and electrolyte abnormalities. The phrenic nerve contracts as the atria beat, creating a "twitch" in the flank with every heartbeat. Myopathy and colic may be additional complaints. Treatment consists of fluid therapy to correct fluid and electrolyte deficits, and body cooling, as detailed under the heat stroke section. If body temperature is over 104°F, particularly if ambient conditions are hot or humid, application of cool water over the entire body surface should be used to cool the horse. Specific problems, such as colic and myopathy, need further evaluation and treatment. Synchronous diaphragmatic flutter resolves once the horse's metabolic alkalosis and hypocalcemia are corrected. The importance of treating horses with vigorous fluid therapy cannot be overstressed, particularly if nonsteroidal anti-inflammatory therapy is used. The postexhaustion syndrome is best known in endurance horses, but it can be a serious complication of any strenuous horse sport when protracted sweat losses have occurred. The postexhaustion syndrome is characterized by myonecrosis, renal failure, laminitis, and a high mortality rate.

Rhabdomyolysis (see also page 115)

Exertional myopathies are the most common metabolic problems encountered in eventing horses during competition. Contributing factors include but are not limited to fluid and electrolyte imbalances, increased exercise intensity, and adverse environmental conditions. In the 3-day

event, most cases are recognized during the 10-minute mandatory hold between phase C and cross-country. The most common presentation is progressive stiffening of one or more legs. The large muscle masses of the hind legs and back are most commonly affected. Other signs include tachycardia, tachypnea, anxiety or depression, anorexia, and increased sweating over involved muscle masses or the entire body. Some horses demonstrate vague signs of abdominal pain, and gastrointestinal motility can be reduced or absent. Severely affected horses can become recumbent. Other signs of moderate-to-severe involvement include swollen, tense muscles that are painful to palpation, and the presence of dark blackish-to-brownish-red urine that tests positive for blood on urine reagent strips. Severely affected and improperly treated horses can die because of involvement of the diaphragm and from multiple organ failure.

The main therapeutic goals when treating exertional rhabdomyolysis (ER) are prevention of further muscle damage, restoration of fluid and electrolyte balance, and control of pain and anxiety. The severity of the clinical signs can be used to determine the extent of the treatment. In mild cases, cessation of exercise, oral fluid therapy, and anti-inflammatory agents usually achieve satisfactory results. If the condition worsens or does not rapidly respond to initial therapy, more vigorous therapy is indicated. Moderate-to-severe cases require aggressive intravenous fluid therapy. Oral fluid therapy can be used in addition to intravenous therapy to augment rehydration. When in doubt about how aggressively to treat a case of ER, the horse is given intravenous fluid therapy until a urine sample can be evaluated for presence of myoglobin. It is far better to treat this condition aggressively rather than inadequately, because long-term damage to the kidneys and other organs can result from inadequate restoration of fluids. In particular, horses with myoglobinuria need intravenous fluid therapy to reduce the likelihood of myoglobin-induced nephrotoxicity. Fluid therapy not only should correct pre-existing deficits, but also should be continued until adequate diuresis is achieved. In the absence of laboratory support, urine color is a useful field indicator of therapeutic effectiveness. Diuresis should continue until voluminous quantities of clear, dilute urine are being produced. The veterinarian must be prepared to use 30 to 80 L (or more) to achieve this goal.

Nonsteroidal anti-inflammatory drugs (NSAIDs) such as flunixin meglumine (0.5 mg/kg IV), phenylbutazone (2.2 mg/kg IV or orally), or ketoprofen (1–2 mg/kg IV) are commonly used to relieve inflammation and pain. If NSAIDs are used, the veterinarian must ensure that the horse is well hydrated. The NSAIDs block the local prostaglandin-mediated vasodilatory mechanism that protects the kidney in low blood flow states, and can therefore cause ischemic damage to the kidneys if given to hypohydrated horses, particularly if high doses are used. Once the horse is rehydrated, DMSO can be given for its anti-inflammatory and diuretic properties and its protective effect on the renal tubules, at a dose of 10 mg/kg given slowly intravenously diluted in a 10% solution.

Low doses of xylazine (0.2–0.3 mg/kg) and butorphanol (0.01 mg/kg) work very well in combination to calm affected horses and provide analgesia. Use of acetylpromazine is contraindicated in hypovolemic, anxious, painful, or combative horses. Acetylpromazine's hypotensive properties cause many horses with these pre-existing problems to lose consciousness (faint), and should therefore be avoided when treating this condition.

Muscle relaxants can be used to alleviate some of the muscle tension and pain. Methocarbamol is a centrally acting muscle relaxant that can be administered intravenously at a dosage range of 4 to 25 mg/kg to achieve rapid results. If given IV, methocarbamol should be administered slowly to avoid central nervous system side effects arising from the effects of the polyethylene glycol base, and given only after the horse's hydration status has been improved to avoid renal complications.

Other practical management strategies include blanketing the horse if ambient conditions are chilly. In hot, humid conditions, blanketing should be avoided. The horse should not be forced to exercise, but as improvement is noted, the animal can be allowed to graze in hand. The owners should be advised to rest the horse for 1 to 2 weeks following a moderate-to-severe myopathy and consult with their veterinarian before resuming training.

Abdominal Pain

The most common types of colic that occur in competition horses are large intestinal impaction and adynamic ileus. Impactions of the large colon or cecum can result from reduced water intake and changes in diet and routine that occur during transport and competition. Adynamic ileus can arise from pathologic alterations in fluid and electrolyte balance, and it most commonly arises after or during strenuous exercise associated with massive sweat losses.

A horse with signs of abdominal pain should be carefully assessed by evaluating mucous membranes, heart rate, abdominal shape, gastrointestinal motility, and findings on rectal examination. A nasogastric tube should be passed, and a siphon should be created to check for gastric reflux. If reflux occurs, the tube is left in place and attempts are made to decompress the stomach every 30 to 60 minutes. Delivering fluid or other treatments must be avoided by this route. If findings on rectal examination are consistent with a lesion that requires surgical correction, or if pain is recurrent or unremitting, the horse should be promptly referred to a veterinary hospital equipped to handle abdominal surgical emergencies. If the treatment veterinarian has the facilities, time, equipment, and personnel, medical colic can be managed on the grounds. If any of these factors are lacking, the horse should be intubated, the condition stabilized, and the horse referred elsewhere.

Mild-to-moderate cases of large bowel impaction can be treated by rehydrating the impacted mass with oral and intravenous fluids. Oral fluid therapy is the most practical approach, but should only be used if the horse has gastrointestinal motility, does not have gastric reflux, and is not showing signs of pain. Mild laxatives such as mineral oil (4–6 L) and psyllium hydrophilic mucilloid (1 pound stirred in 4 L of water for a 450-kg horse) are useful adjuncts. Magnesium sulfate (Epsom salt) acts as a laxative by drawing fluid into the bowel lumen. This laxative should not be used repeatedly or in high doses, and should only be used after the horse has been sufficiently rehydrated. One-quarter pound of magnesium sulfate in 4 L of water for a 500-kg horse is a sufficient dose. Flunixin meglumine (0.5–1.0 mg/kg every 12–24 hours) can be used for analgesia. If the animal's condition is deteriorating or not improving, and if a treatment period of several days is anticipated, referral to a veterinary hospital is the best course of action.

Adynamic ileus is characterized by abdominal pain, elevated heart rate, absent gastrointestinal motility, a variable amount of reflux, and loops of small bowel mildly to moderately distended with fluid detectable on rectal examination. Many horses with adynamic ileus after strenuous exercise respond favorably to restoration of fluids and electrolytes via administration of balanced polyionic fluids such as lactated Ringer's solution given intravenously, analgesia with flunixin meglumine, and gastric decompression until gastrointestinal function returns to normal. Referral to a veterinary hospital for further observation and treatment is indicated once the horse's condition has been stabilized if the condition is not rapidly improving and prolonged therapy is anticipated.

Supplemental Readings

Gowen RR, Lengel JG: Regulatory aspects of drug use in performance horses. Vet Clin North Am Equine Pract 9(3):449–460, 1993.
Hodgson DR: Myopathies in the athletic horse. Compend Contin Ed Pract Vet 7:S551–S555, 1985.
Kohn CW: Veterinarian's role in 3-day eventing. Proc 39th Annu Meet Am Assoc Equine Pract, 1993, pp 173–188.
Rossier Y: Management of exertional rhabdomyolysis syndrome. Compend Contin Ed Pract Vet, 16:381–386, 1994.
Sosa León LA, Davie AJ, Hodgson DR, Rose RJ: The effects of tonicity, glucose concentration and temperature of an oral rehydration solution on its absorption and elimination. Equine Vet J 20[Suppl]:140–146, 1995.
Williamson LW, White S, Maykuth P, Andrews F, Sommerdahl C, Green E: Comparison between two post exercise cooling methods. Equine Vet J 18[Suppl]:337–340, 1995.

Laminitis

GARY M. BAXTER
Fort Collins, Colorado

Laminitis, or acute laminar degeneration, is an inflammation of the laminae within the hoof. The complex interdigitating system of primary and secondary laminae provides a firm bond between the hoof wall and the laminar corium. Damage to the laminae results in breakdown of this interdigitation, and the underlying distal phalanx separates from the hoof wall. Vasoconstriction within the digit, microthrombosis, perivascular edema, arteriovenous shunting of blood at the level of the coronary band, and venoconstriction are all pathophysiologic mechanisms proposed to cause laminitis. All are thought to produce hypoperfusion of the digit leading to ischemia, edema, and necrosis of the laminae. In particular, venoconstriction is thought to increase capillary pressure and hydrostatic movement of fluid into the interstitial space, predisposing to laminar edema and subsequently to poor perfusion. Numerous secondary inflammatory and systemic alterations occur with laminitis, making differentiation between the initiating causes and secondary manifestations extremely difficult.

Numerous factors predispose horses to laminitis (Table 1). Excessive carbohydrate intake is the classic cause of laminitis and has been used to reproduce the syndrome experimentally. However, any systemically ill and potentially endotoxemic horse is at risk for developing laminitis. The risk is even more pronounced if the horse is over-

weight or has been treated with systemic corticosteroids. Sudden changes in diet or overeating of highly digestible high-energy feed such as lush pasture or alfalfa may also induce laminitis. Horses worked excessively on a hard surface may exhibit signs of laminitis from traumatic tearing of the laminae. Support laminitis occurs when one limb has to bear an excessive amount of weight because of severe lameness in the contralateral limb. Direct exposure of the feet to or ingestion of black walnut wood shavings can lead to laminitis, which is usually transient once contact is eliminated.

CLINICAL SIGNS

Laminitis can be broadly classified into acute, subacute, refractory, and chronic stages. The condition is more commonly seen in the front feet but may involve all four feet or a single digit. Lameness associated with laminitis can range from very slight to failure to bear weight to refusal to stand. The gradations of lameness associated with laminitis as described by Obel are as follows: grade 1—the horse lifts its feet repeatedly, often every few seconds; grade 2—the horse moves willingly at a walk, but the gait is characteristic of laminitis, and the horse does not resist lifting of a forefoot; grade 3—the horse moves reluctantly and vigorously resists attempts to lift a forefoot because of pain in the contralateral digit; grade 4—the horse must be forced to move and may be recumbent.

The higher the Obel grade of lameness, the greater the likelihood of permanent damage to the laminae. Unfortunately, acute laminitis in most horses is not recognized by the owners and trainers until the disease has reached grade 3. By this time significant laminar degeneration may have already occurred, reducing the chances of a complete recovery.

Acute Laminitis

The acute form of laminitis should be considered a medical emergency, and aggressive treatment must be initiated promptly. Severe lameness can develop rapidly and is obvious when the horse walks on a hard surface or is forced to turn in a circle. Increased digital pulses and heat over the hoof wall are nearly always present, and pain is elicited when the toe is compressed with hoof testers. Strides are shortened, with each foot placed quickly back on the ground. If the pain is severe, or if all four feet are affected, the horse may be recumbent.

Large overweight horses with primary septic, endotoxemic, or metabolic conditions are prime candidates for distal displacement (sinking) of the distal phalanx. The entire laminar interdigitation becomes detached from the hoof wall, permitting the distal phalanx to drop within the hoof wall. These horses often have all four feet involved and are

---

TABLE 1.   PREDISPOSING FACTORS IN EQUINE LAMINITIS

Carbohydrate overload
  Excess grain intake
  Lush pasture (grass laminitis)
  Feed change to high-energy legume
Endotoxemia, sepsis, infection
  Colitis
  Proximal enteritis
  Small intestinal strangulation/obstructions
  Retained placenta, metritis, abortion
  Septicemia or toxemia from any cause
Excessive unilateral weightbearing (support laminitis)
  Severe lameness
  Rehabilitation of fracture repair
Management
  Ingestion of cold water by overheated horse
  Unconditioned horse worked on hard surface (concussion or road laminitis)
  Overweight horses or ponies
  Trimming the hooves too short
  Black walnut wood shavings used for bedding
Miscellaneous
  Treatment with corticosteroids
  Hypothyroidism
  Diet of plants containing estrogens
  Continuous estrus in mares
  Allergic-type reactions to certain medications

severely lame. Cavitation or depression along the coronary band is often the first clinical sign of sinking. With time, blood or serum may ooze from the coronary band. Sinking may occur alone or in combination with rotation of the distal phalanx. Sinking of a single distal phalanx as a result of severe lameness in the contralateral limb has occurred. These horses are usually not systemically ill, but are often overweight and presumably have overloaded the affected digit.

Subacute Laminitis

Subacute laminitis is a milder degree of acute laminitis. The same clinical signs may be present but are often less pronounced (Obel grades 1 and 2). Horses that have been worked on hard surfaces, have had the hooves trimmed too short, or have been exposed to black walnut wood shavings often exhibit subacute laminitis. Clinical signs often resolve quickly, and permanent laminar damage usually does not occur.

Refractory Laminitis

Frequently, horses with acute laminitis do not respond to aggressive medical therapy. If no improvement is seen within 7 to 10 days, or if an acute exacerbation of the disease occurs after an initial improvement, the laminitis should be considered refractory. Refractory laminitis suggests continued laminar degeneration, inflammation, and edema, or it reflects the severity of the initial laminar damage, both of which indicate a poor prognosis. Rotation or distal displacement of the distal phalanx is inevitable if signs of laminitis cannot be controlled within 10 to 14 days. Severe refractory laminitis can result in complete hoof wall detachment or penetration of the sole by the tip of the distal phalanx.

Chronic Laminitis

Chronic laminitis occurs when rotation or distal displacement of the distal phalanx has occurred and there is no active laminar necrosis or inflammation. Laminar damage results in abnormal hoof growth, which is seen as diverging rings around the hoof wall; these rings are wider at the heel than at the toe. Classically, the toes are long, the heels are overgrown, and the sole has dropped, resulting in a flat or convex appearance to the bottom of the foot. Because of the abnormal horn growth and changes in the digital vasculature of horses with chronic laminitis, subsolar abscessation and recurrent attacks of acute laminitis are common. In addition, the dorsal hoof wall may become detached from the underlying laminae, resulting in a "gas line" visible radiographically, and widening of the white line may occur, predisposing to "seedy toe."

DIAGNOSIS

A horse with increased pulse amplitude in the digital arteries, increased heat within the foot, pain over the toe elicited by hoof testers, and lameness should be suspected of having laminitis. Horses with chronic laminitis exhibit a heel-toe placement of their feet to avoid concussion of their toes. Horses with acute laminitis require an abaxial sesamoid or low palmar-plantar nerve block to alleviate the pain, whereas horses with chronic laminitis may improve significantly with a palmar digital nerve block because of the dropped, bruised sole and secondary abscessation. In some horses with severe acute laminitis it may be very difficult to completely desensitize the digit.

Lateral radiographs of the affected digits should be taken immediately to serve as a baseline for subsequent radiographic comparison and to determine if the horse has had laminitis previously. Serial radiographs are often essential to monitor progression of the disease. Radiographically, laminitis can be divided into five categories: (1) no observable abnormalities (Fig. 1); (2) distal displacement of the distal phalanx (Fig. 2); (3) rotation of the distal phalanx; (4) rotation and sinking of the distal phalanx; and (5) rotation of the distal phalanx with secondary chronic changes. Very early radiographic signs suggestive of laminitis include widening of the area between the distal phalanx and the dorsal hoof wall (see Fig. 1) and roughening along the dorsal aspect of the distal phalanx. The degree of rotation of the distal phalanx can be determined from the radiographs. In general, the greater the rotation, the poorer the prognosis for return to athletic function. However, recently it has been suggested that the severity of lameness was a more reliable means of determining outcome than the severity of rotation or distal displacement of the distal phalanx.

THERAPY

In most situations, it is more rewarding and effective to prevent laminitis than to treat the disease once it has occurred. Preventive measures should be taken with horses at risk for the development of laminitis. Laminitis has been

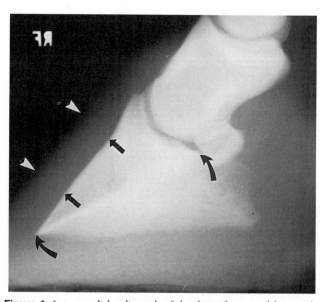

Figure 1. Lateromedial radiograph of the digit of a normal horse. The distance between the dorsal hoof wall (*white arrowheads*) and the distal phalanx (*straight arrows*) should be less than 18 mm or less than 30% of the length of the distal phalanx as measured from the tip of the bone to its articulation with the navicular bone (*curved arrows*). Widening of the distance between the distal phalanx and the dorsal hoof wall may be an early radiographic feature of horses with acute laminitis.

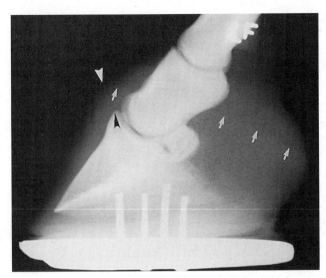

Figure 2. Lateromedial radiograph of a horse with distal displacement of the distal phalanx. Radiographic evidence of sinking includes a soft tissue defect along the coronary band (*white arrows*) or an increased distance between the extensor process of the distal phalanx and the coronary band (*black and white arrowheads*). The soft tissue defect along the coronary band can usually be palpated as a depression or cavitation in this region.

associated with endotoxemia, and therefore the systemic effects of endotoxemia should be minimized. Other therapy includes maintaining hydration, treating septicemia, maintaining frog pressure, ensuring proper feeding and management, and administration of anti-inflammatory drugs and anticoagulants such as acetylsalicylic acid (aspirin)* or heparin.† The use of heparin in horses with laminitis is controversial because it causes red cell agglutination in vitro. Clinical problems associated with agglutination have not been seen. Although heparin has been shown to prevent experimentally induced laminitis in horses, a retrospective study failed to demonstrate a significant benefit of heparin prophylaxis. However, a more recent study evaluating horses with duodenitis and proximal jejunitis found a significant reduction in laminitis in horses receiving heparin prophylaxis.

Despite recent advances in identifying the cause of laminitis, most treatment regimens remain empirical. Because extensive laminar damage can occur within 24 hours of the onset of acute laminitis, aggressive therapy must be given at the first suspicion of the disease. The goals of treatment include (1) correcting the primary illness or removing the causative factor; (2) blocking the pain-hypertension cycle; (3) improving digital blood flow and laminar perfusion; (4) preventing or correcting rotation or sinking of the distal phalanx; and (5) promoting keratinization and healing of sole and hoof defects (Table 2).

When a precipitating factor for laminitis is known, such as lush pasture, excessive grain feeding, or exposure to walnut wood shavings, the horse should be promptly removed from the environment. Mineral oil should be given via nasogastric tube to horses with alimentary disease to

minimize further absorption of endotoxins. Grain and legume hay should probably be eliminated from the diet and the horse fed only grass hay until the signs of acute laminitis have resolved. If the horse or pony is overweight, a weight-reducing diet should be instituted.

In most cases, the primary illness must be treated concurrently with the laminitis. This usually includes intravenous fluids, parenteral antimicrobials, flunixin meglumine,* and possibly hyperimmune plasma or serum. Therapy specifically directed at laminitis includes dimethyl sulfoxide (DMSO),† phenylbutazone, and aspirin. DMSO (0.1 g/kg IV) is a free radical scavenger and anti-inflammatory agent directed primarily at preventing the cellular reperfusion injury that occurs in ischemic tissue. No studies have documented the efficacy of DMSO in laminitis, but clinical impressions dictate its continued use. Likewise, phenylbutazone (4.4 mg/kg) is considered beneficial in the treatment of any form of laminitis, because it is thought to reduce the inflammation, edema, and pain within the digit, thus promoting return of normal foot function and preventing progressive laminar damage. Aspirin (10–20 mg/kg) is used to inhibit platelet aggregation by decreasing thromboxane synthesis, which could predispose to microthrombus formation within the laminae when perfusion is sluggish. This dose of aspirin has minimal anti-inflammatory properties, and the drug can be safely combined with other nonsteroidal anti-inflammatory drugs.

Peripheral vasodilator therapy should be used only in horses with a stable cardiovascular system. The goal is to improve laminar perfusion and to counteract the increased sympathetic tone that often accompanies laminitis. The most commonly used agents include acetylpromazine‡ and isoxsuprine hydrochloride.§ Phenoxybenzamine|| is less readily available and therefore less commonly used (see Table 2). It is unknown if these drugs actually improve circulation to the microvasculature of the laminae. In addition, oral isoxsuprine at 0.6 mg/kg does not cause systemic vasodilation in normal horses. However, horses with acute laminitis appear to benefit from acetylpromazine therapy. Isoxsuprine is used most frequently in horses with chronic laminitis and also as a preventive measure for horses at risk to develop laminitis.

Radical trimming of the feet of horses with acute laminitis should probably be avoided. Shoes should be pulled and if the toes are long, the latter should be shortened. Counterpressure on the frog should be maintained using compressible gauze, cotton, polystyrene, or commercially available frog pads¶ to promote digital circulation and to counteract downward rotation of the distal phalanx. Some horses with distal displacement may actually become more lame with frog and sole pressure. Presumably this occurs because the digital cushion and vascular system are compressed between the solar aspect of the distal phalanx and the horny sole. Therefore, prevention of sinking is difficult because support of the frog and sole by any means may

---

*Acetylsalicylic acid, The Butler Company, Columbus, OH
†Heparin sodium, Elkins-Sinn, Cherry Hill, NJ

*Banamine, Schering, Kenilworth, NJ
†Domoso, Syntex Animal Health, West Des Moines, IA
‡Acepromazine, The Butler Company, Columbus, OH
§Isoxsuprine, Chelsea, Division of Rugby, Rockville Centre, Long Island, NY
||Dibenzyline, SmithKline & French, Philadelphia, PA
¶Lilly Pads, Therapeutic Equine Products, Inc., Indianapolis, IN

TABLE 2. SUMMARY OF TREATMENT OF LAMINITIS

Goal	Techniques
Remove causative factor or correct primary illness	1. Determine potential causes and remove from environment 2. Combat endotoxemia, septicemia, and hemoconcentration a. Systemic antimicrobials b. Flunixin meglumine c. Intravenous fluids d. Mineral oil p.o. e. Hyperimmune plasma or serum 3. Preventive care a. Frog support or pressure b. Well-bedded stall or sand c. Elevated heel shoe? d. Aspirin, phenylbutazone, isoxsuprine, and heparin? (see dosages later)
Block pain-hypertension cycle	1. Local anesthesia of digit: Reserved for animals in severe pain. Not recommended more than once daily. Do not walk horse excessively after desensitization. 2. Analgesics a. Phenylbutazone 4.4 mg/kg b.i.d. IV or p.o. for 3–5 days, then decrease dose gradually b. DMSO 0.1 g/kg diluted to 10% solution IV b.i.d. for 3–5 days 3. Sand stall or heavy bedding; padding of sole and frog 4. Elevated heel shoe?
Improve digital blood flow and laminar perfusion	1. Vasodilators a. Acetylpromazine 0.02–0.06 mg/kg IM 3–4 times daily b. Isoxsuprine hydrochloride 1.2 mg/kg p.o. b.i.d 2. Anticoagulants a. Aspirin 10–20 mg/kg p.o. every other day b. Heparin (?) 40–80 IU/kg IV or SQ 2–3 times daily 3. Maintain frog pressure and support of sole
Prevent further rotation or sinking of distal phalanx	1. Maintain frog pressure with padding or shoes 2. Deep digital flexor tenotomy 3. Hoof trimming: remove excess toe 4. Inferior check ligament desmotomy? 5. Foot casts? 6. Hoof wall resection? 7. Elevated-heel shoes?
Promote keratinization and healing of hoof and sole defects	1. Proper trimming of under-run sole and detached hoof wall 2. Foot soaking and local antiseptics 3. Systemic antimicrobials? 4. Shoeing: Must provide support to frog and sole; variety of methods available 5. Methionine°: 10 g/day 6. Methylsulphonylmethan (MSM)†: 0.5–1.0 g/day 7. Commercially available supplements for hoof growth‡: use as directed 8. Topical hoof dressings
Maintain systemic health in horses with chronic laminitis	1. Prevent and treat pressure sores 2. Ensure adequate feed and water intake, especially if horse is recumbent 3. Prevent impactions of the bowel by use of bran mashes, good-quality feed, and fluids 4. Thyroid hormone replacement?

°D-L-methionine powder, The Butler Company, Columbus, OH
†MSM, Vitality Systems, Gaston, OR
‡Horse Sho-hoof, Manna Pro, Los Angeles, CA

further compress the solar vasculature. Padding and support of the feet can also be achieved by placing the horse on sand, soft ground, or thick bedding. Walking should be avoided in horses with acute laminitis because of the potential to further damage the already compromised laminae. Routine local anesthesia of the digit with subsequent forced exercise is contraindicated. However, periodic desensitization of the affected digits stops the pain-hypertension cycle temporarily and can greatly improve the patient's attitude. Local anesthesia may also cause dilation of the digital vasculature. Warm or cold hydrotherapy or foot soaks can be used but probably do little to alter the course of the disease.

CORRECTIVE TRIMMING AND SHOEING

Treatment of chronic laminitis primarily involves corrective trimming and shoeing and preventing recurrent acute flare-ups. Permanent laminar damage has already occurred, and epidermal hyperplasia results in a wedge of epithelium between the dorsal hoof wall and the distal phalanx. Initial therapy for chronic laminitis often entails removing under-run sole and debriding abscesses. Soaking the feet in a dilute povidone-iodine° and magnesium sulfate† solution

°Betadine, Purdue Frederick, Norwalk, CT
†Epsom salts, Humco, Texarkana, TX

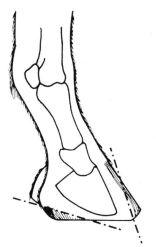

Figure 3. Areas of hoof to be removed during corrective trimming in a horse with chronic laminitis. *(Vertical line)* The amount of hoof wall to be removed so that it parallels the dorsum of the distal phalanx. *(Horizontal line)* The amount of heel areas of hoof to be removed so that the weightbearing surface of the distal phalanx is parallel to the ground. (From Stick JA: Laminitis. *In* Robinson NE (ed): Current Therapy in Equine Medicine, ed 2. Philadelphia, WB Saunders, 1987, p 281. Reproduced by permission.)

may speed resolution of the infection. Systemic antimicrobials may also be used, but their efficacy is questionable. Corrective trimming should attempt to return the distal phalanx to its normal anatomic position and provide a nonpainful weightbearing surface. This usually involves shortening the toes, lowering the heels, and protecting the sole (Fig. 3). Several trimmings at 4- to 6-week intervals are often required to obtain normal alignment in horses with severe distal phalangeal rotation.

Hoof wall resection is usually reserved for horses with chronic laminitis where the hoof wall is unattached (as demonstrated by a gas line on radiographs) or with subsolar abscessation (Fig. 4). However, resection may be used occasionally in acute or refractory cases of laminitis to relieve the pressure from fluid accumulation within the edematous laminae. In addition, hoof wall resection or

stripping has been advocated for horses with sinking of the distal phalanx to remove the pressure-induced ischemia and pain that occur at the dorsal coronary corium. The hoof wall can be removed with a circular sander, electric drill with a burred-tipped drill bit, or hoof rasp. Hoof wall resection can be combined with corrective shoeing to protect the exposed sensitive tissue.

The goals of shoeing horses with laminitis are to (1) protect the painful area of the sole and hoof wall from ground contact; (2) prevent further tissue destruction or rotation of the distal phalanx; (3) provide support to the foot; and (4) enhance healing of the digit. The shoe with or without a pad can be used to lower or elevate the heel, depending on the situation, but should not apply direct pressure to the solar surface or exposed sensitive tissue. Farriers and veterinarians alike have claimed success with nonadjustable heart bar shoes, adjustable heart bar shoes, reverse shoes and pads, wide-web shoes, regular shoes and pads, egg bar shoes with or without a heart bar, and Thera-flex shoe inserts.* Silicone rubber is often used between the pad and sole to further decrease concussion on the sole.

An elevated heel-shoe has been used to treat horses with acute laminitis. The shoe is designed to reduce the pull of the deep digital flexor tendon, thus minimizing rotation of the distal phalanx. An 18° heel wedge has been recommended, but any amount of heel elevation may be beneficial (Fig. 5). The specific shoe can be applied permanently or temporarily with adhesive tape. The type of shoe used to treat horses with laminitis often depends on personal preference, the specific characteristics of the case, and the expertise of the farrier. However, using shoes that do not provide frog or sole support to the feet is thought to increase the likelihood of further rotation or sinking of the distal phalanx. Regardless of the type of shoe used, it is important that the farrier and practitioner work together and understand the principles of shoeing horses with laminitis.

SURGICAL THERAPY

It has been hypothesized that the pull of the deep digital flexor tendon is important in promoting rotation of the

*Thera-Flex, Lawrenceburg, KY

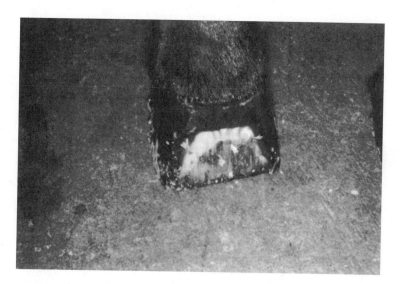

Figure 4. Dorsal hoof wall resection has been performed on a horse with chronic laminitis. The dorsal hoof wall was detached from the underlying laminae, as determined by a gas line visible radiographically, and was removed with a sander.

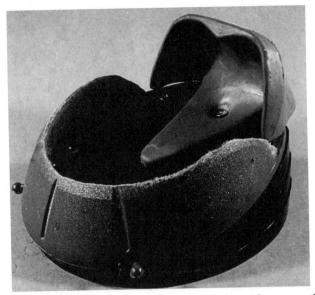

Figure 5. An elevated heel shoe with frog support that can be temporarily attached to the foot of a horse with laminitis. If a good clinical response occurs, an elevated heel shoe can be applied permanently to the foot. The elevated heel shoe can also be used as a preventive measure for horses at risk for laminitis, such as those with severe contralateral limb lameness.

distal phalanx (Fig. 6). Tenotomies of the deep digital flexor tendon can be performed in the palmar-plantar aspect of the pastern or in the mid-metacarpal-metatarsal regions to counteract this rotating force (Fig. 7). Good success has been reported with tenotomy at the midpastern region for treating chronic refractory laminitis with severe rotation of the distal phalanx. Tenotomy at the midcannon bone appears to relieve the pain associated with laminitis but may not alter the ultimate outcome. Only five of 20 horses with acute or chronic laminitis that underwent a tenotomy at the midcannon bone region survived longer than 1 year. Only one of these horses was completely sound. This most likely reflects the severity of the laminitis and does not

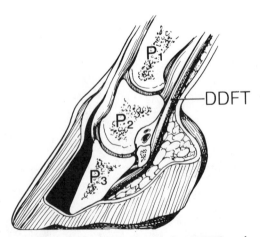

Figure 6. Pull of the deep digital flexor tendon (*DDFT*) on the palmar-plantar aspect of the distal phalanx. Transection of the tendon may prevent further rotation of the distal phalanx and decrease the pain associated with laminitis. P_1 = proximal phalanx, P_2 = middle phalanx, P_3 = distal phalanx. (Courtesy of Dr. Douglas Allen, University of Georgia.)

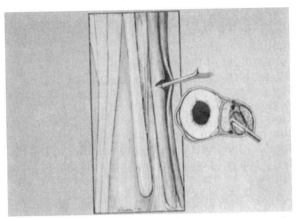

Figure 7. Transection of the deep digital flexor tendon in the midmetacarpus. A guarded bistoury is used to prevent trauma to the palmar vessels and nerves. (Courtesy of Dr. Robert Hunt, University of Georgia.)

mean that tenotomies should not be performed. The location of the tenotomy depends on the health of the horse, degree of rotation of the distal phalanx, financial constraints of the owner, and personal preference. Tenotomy at the midpastern requires general anesthesia, whereas tenotomy at the mid-metacarpus-metatarsus can be performed in the standing animal following a high palmar nerve block and sedation. Either technique should be seriously considered as a salvage procedure when treating refractory or severe chronic laminitis, especially if conventional therapy is failing. However, the author has seen two horses develop severe pain of unknown origin in the palmar heel region after tenotomy of the deep digital flexor tendon in the mid-metacarpus.

PROGNOSIS

The prognosis of a horse with laminitis is guarded. Factors determining the prognosis include (1) the duration of acute laminitis; (2) number of feet affected; (3) amount of distal phalanx rotation; (4) occurrence of sinking; (5) severity of lameness and response to therapy; and (6) occurrence of secondary abscessation and osteomyelitis of the distal phalanx. Horses with less than 5.5° of rotation of the distal phalanx reportedly can return to performance. Horses with subacute or acute laminitis that respond to therapy within 7 to 10 days may also completely recover. Horses with refractory and severe chronic laminitis are unlikely to perform again, and many of these horses are euthanized because of continued pain, lack of response to therapy, and severe permanent laminar and hoof wall changes. In addition, horses in which the distal phalanx sinks or sinks and rotates have a poor prognosis. If they survive, they are likely to be pasture-sound at best.

Supplemental Readings

Allen D, White NA, Foerner JF, Gordon BJ: Surgical management of chronic laminitis in horses: 13 cases (1983–1985). J Am Vet Med Assoc 189:1604–1606, 1986.

Baxter GM: Equine laminitis caused by distal displacement of the distal phalanx: 12 cases (1976–1985). J Am Vet Med Assoc 189:326–329, 1986.

Baxter GM: Acute laminitis. Vet Clin North Am Equine Pract 10(3):627–642, 1994.

Belknap JK, Moore JN: Evaluation of heparin for prophylaxis of equine laminitis: 71 cases (1980–1986). J Am Vet Med Assoc 195:505–507, 1989.

Cohen ND, Parson EM, Seahorn TL, Carter GK: Prevalence and factors associated with laminitis in horses with duodenitis/proximal jejunitis: 33 cases (1985–1991). J Am Vet Med Assoc 204:250–254, 1994.

Goetz TE: Anatomic, hoof, and shoeing considerations for the treatment of laminitis in horses. J Am Vet Med Assoc 190:1323–1332, 1987.

Hunt RJ: A retrospective evaluation of laminitis in horses. Equine Vet J 25:61–64, 1993.

Hunt RJ, Allen D, Baxter GM, Jackman BR, Parks AH: Mid-metacarpal deep digital flexor tenotomy in the management of refractory laminitis in horses. Vet Surg 20:15–20, 1991.

Moore JN, Allen D, Clark ES: Pathophysiology of acute laminitis. Vet Clin North Am Equine Pract 5:67–72, 1989.

O'Grady SE: A practical approach to treating laminitis. Vet Med 88:867–875, 1993.

Stick JS, Jann HW, Scott EA, Robinson NE: Pedal bone rotation as a prognostic sign in laminitis in horses. J Am Vet Med Assoc 180:251–253, 1982.

Yelle M: Clinician's guide to equine laminitis. Equine Vet J 18:156–158, 1986.

Planning for the Care of Horses in Disasters

SEBASTIAN E. HEATH
West Lafayette, Indiana

It is estimated that every year over 10,000 violent thunderstorms, 5000 floods, 800 tornadoes, and several hurricanes and earthquakes disrupt life in the United States. Approximately 15% of the American people live on transitional land, which lies between townships and countryside and has the highest risk of damage from forest fires, floods, and landslides. It is in transitional land where much of the United States horse industry is located. The recent major disasters that have struck the North American continent have resulted in a heightened awareness of the concern for animals and their care providers. This exposure has been associated with increased coverage of animal issues in the news media and a growing societal concern for animal well-being (welfare), including how animals are affected in disasters. The potential for veterinarians to be involved in the coordination of disaster response is very significant.

Historically, the primary concerns of veterinary disaster medicine have been the safety of the human food supply through the health of food-producing animals and their potential to cause or maintain zoonotic and communicable human diseases. However, it has become apparent over the last few years that some of the most important issues that surround animals in disasters arise out of the personal and financial investments that animal owners and care providers have in animals. The same issues apply to horses. In a survey in Kentucky, a large proportion of horse owners indicated that emotions may affect their judgment in disasters. Because of irrational decisions, horse owners may be injured or killed by attempting to rescue their horses from burning or flooded stables and farms. Horses also represent considerable economic and personal value to their owners and care providers, and for several states and many veterinary practices, horses are a vital source of revenue. Appropriate care of horses in disasters should, therefore, be considered an essential component of the care of horses, and an important consideration for the sustainment of all aspects of the horse industries. In this chapter, an overview of the coordination of disaster response is described, and suggestions are made on how veterinarians, horse owners, and managers can prepare themselves for disasters.

THE COORDINATION OF DISASTER RESPONSE

The recommended approach to the coordination of disaster response is a continual cycle of hazard analysis, mitigation, planning, continuing education of disaster response personnel, staging exercises, responding to actual incidents, reviewing the effectiveness of interventions, and public education. Professionally coordinated disaster responses use similar definitions, organizational structures, and allocations of responsibilities.

In the Federal Emergency Management Agency (FEMA), an Emergency Operations Plan (EOP) contains information on the purpose and situations in which the EOP will be activated and deactivated; authority by which it will be implemented; a definition of who is involved; allocation of each group's responsibilities; and integration of each group's personnel and physical resources into the overall operation. This format should form the basic structure of all disaster preparedness programs.

ORGANIZATION OF DISASTER PREPAREDNESS AND RESPONSE

Priorities of Disaster Management

The priorities of disaster response are first to protect and save human life, then to protect human property. Animals have traditionally been viewed by emergency management officials as human property. However, other important issues regarding animals in disasters are restoration of animal-related businesses and catering to the personal relationships between people and animals. Because emergency management officials are not trained to deal with either of these aspects, the involvement of veterinary health professionals in any aspect of disaster management is likely to help both the animals and their owners. It should, however, be remembered that the ultimate decisions on care and responsibility for a horse lie with its owner or designated care provider.

Disaster Declaration

The extent of a disaster usually is the determining factor for whether a disaster is declared. Usually, only large-scale disasters are declared. "Large scale" implies that the incident may be larger than the affected community can deal with alone. A community can be anything from a village to a state. A declaration of a disaster is formally made by the chief elected official of the affected community. A disaster declaration activates the EOP and is often associated with a request for outside assistance and funding. Localized incidents, such as individual house fires and floods, chemical spills, and transport accidents make up the vast majority of disasters, but they are rarely declared. Nevertheless, these local disasters often involve local emergency management officials, such as those from county or city emergency management agencies, and fire or police departments.

Incident Command System

The incident command system (ICS) supplies the logistics of disaster coordination. The ICS provides an organizational tool for coordinating the response to disasters by integrating appropriate agencies into one unified system. Important issues that the ICS addresses are: who is in charge; what are each responder's basic roles and responsibilities; what are the responder's specific tasks; where do the individual responder groups fit into the overall organization; and to whom do responders report. The structure of the ICS is determined in a community's or state's EOP before an incident occurs. This allows the ICS to work within the jurisdictional realities of the community or state.

Emergency operations procedures that follow the directives of FEMA have ICSs that are similar in structure for all types and scales of disasters. Familiarity with the ICS at the local level brings with it the same experience that is needed at the national level. Therefore, it is strongly recommended for veterinarians wanting to become involved in disaster management to learn about the ICS. This is easily done through independent study courses, such as "IS-1 Incident Command Systems" available from the Emergency Management Institute, 16825 South Seton Avenue, Emmitsburg, MD 21727.

Evacuation, Security, and Re-entry

Evacuation is usually under the control of local agencies, because they are invariably the first on site in a disaster. Security is often a joint venture between local law enforcement and military personnel. Re-entry to evacuated sites, however, is usually under the control of the National Guard, whose responsibilities include determining when it is safe for the public to re-enter an area.

A common and major concern in evacuations is animal relocation. Various plans on how to deal with animal reloca-

tion have been proposed. The most notable is the Maryland pet sheltering program, which provides a mechanism by which animal owners can find housing for their cats and dogs in the event of a disaster by phoning a central phone number in Maryland. This program should be seen as a model for other states to follow, as well as for local communities, including individual veterinary practices, and groups of animal owners. Horse evacuations and care present unique problems, but with appropriate planning they can be successful.

Hazard Analysis

Using an "all hazards" identification approach for most communities in the United States, hazard analysis information is generated and maintained by federal, state, and local EMAs. FEMA deals with all hazards by coordinating the resources of 26 federal departments and agencies and the American Red Cross. The activities of these departments are streamlined through 12 emergency support functions (ESFs), which are summarized in the federal response plan. Recognition of the responsibility and contribution for each of these agencies and other volunteer responder groups is achieved through mutual aid agreements, memorandums of understanding, and legislative authority with state or local jurisdictions.

Agencies in Disasters

During federally declared disasters there are two recognized veterinary responder/coordinator groups. These are the United States Army Veterinary Corps and the American Veterinary Medical Association (AVMA) Emergency Response Force. The United States Army Veterinary Corps has the capability to respond to almost any disaster involving animals and to facilitate and coordinate the supply of resources to rebuild affected animal industries. The AVMA is currently organizing veterinary medical assistance teams (VMATs) to function as part of the federal response plan during national-scale disasters. VMATs are activated only at the request of the FEMA via state EMAs, where the care of animals has been incorporated into the EOP. Once on-site, VMATs have relied heavily on the United States Army Veterinary Corps to implement their recommendations. The United States Army Veterinary Corps can be activated by any state EMA or through the Department of Defense.

Other agency personnel with whom veterinary care providers are more likely to interact during federally declared disasters are representatives from the American Red Cross (ARC), Department of Defense (DOD), Department of Health and Human Services (DHHS), Urban Search and Rescue (US and R), and the United States Department of Agriculture (USDA). The major responsibilities for each of these organizations are as follows: The ARC (ESF 6) provides mass care to people; ARC is often the first contact point for disaster victims and therefore a likely first agency that hears about animal owners' needs. The DHHS (ESF 8) is responsible for providing medical care to injured persons during a disaster via the National Medical Defense System. The AVMA veterinary medical assistance teams are included in this ESF to provide care to injured animals and preventive veterinary medicine measures to maintain human health. US and R (ESF 9) has the responsibility to locate and extricate victims trapped in collapsed buildings, primarily those of reinforced concrete construction. The greatest component and cost of US and R relates to construction and use of heavy equipment. Small but important components of some US and R teams are the canine search and rescue teams. These are different from the many amateur canine and equine search and rescue teams that predominantly search for missing and lost persons. The USDA's greatest involvement is fighting forest fires (ESF 4). Other important functions include prevention and control of interstate or international epizootics or widespread zoonotic epidemics (ESF 11).

Hazardous Materials (Hazmat)

It is not uncommon for Hazmat incidents to occur in disasters, because there can be spillage of hazardous materials. The risk of exposure is therefore high. Veterinarians should be aware that Hazmat certification is required to deal with such exposures. Common qualified local responder groups include fire departments, law enforcement agencies, allied medical and health professionals, public works departments, county health agencies, and county agriculture departments. State Hazmat responders often include the highway patrol, state department of transportation, state health departments, and state environmental management agencies. Federal Hazmat responders include the Environmental Protection Agency, Department of Natural Resources, and the United States Coast Guard. Other Hazmat responders often include the responsible party and industry cooperatives.

THE ROLE OF VETERINARIANS IN DISASTERS

Large-scale disasters attract considerable publicity. However, this attention should not distract from the greatest need, which is to deal with the great majority of smaller scale disasters. The most common disasters occur at the local and personal level and are rarely declared or reported. This has important implications for the appropriate level of intervention in disaster reduction by practicing veterinarians. Although large-scale disasters receive most of the attention, it is at the local level where detailed preparedness and response plans need to be worked out. When prior planning has not occurred at the local level, confusion arises over who should provide veterinary care, which animals should receive attention, and how to administer this care at all levels of disaster.

Specific examples of how these problems manifest themselves in the veterinary field include the lack of prior arrangement between neighboring veterinary practices, or between veterinary practices and humane groups, about who will assume which role in a disaster. Poor or nonexistent planning may also be associated with a lack of awareness by emergency management personnel of the high priority that should be given to the restoration of veterinary practices. Experience has shown that whereas the triage and treatment of injured animals can present huge logistic problems, these can be dealt with efficiently through appropriate prior planning, including a prearranged chain of command.

A logical place to put the authority for the capture, rescue, and housing of animals in disasters is with a community's animal control agency; alternatively, communities could form their own networks of care providers. This is probably the best solution for horses, and such a program can be coordinated through veterinary practices.

In the past, the greatest obstacle to veterinarians' becoming involved in disaster reduction programs was the failure to recognize that personal initiative is needed to get a disaster reduction program started in one's community. However, this should not inhibit veterinarians from becoming involved in disaster management. A model that has overcome this reluctance and that can be followed by others is "The Development of the Veterinary Services and Animal Care Annex to the Emergency Operations Plan of Indiana." A detailed description of how appropriate agencies have entered into memorandums of understanding is given. In this disaster preparedness plan, the extent of each veterinary responder group's contributions, credentials, training requirements, liability, and financial support are addressed, as are the means by which these will be coordinated. The plan involved discussions with many stakeholders. Topics include potential hazards, response needs, responsibilities, and credentials. Although this booklet describes a state plan, it is adaptable to all levels and can be expanded to facilitate the collaboration between neighboring states or smaller communities. An example of a local disaster preparedness plan has been described for Los Angeles Area G.

Restoration of Animal Industries

Traditionally, the veterinary profession has been the group with the greatest concern for the restoration of veterinary practices and other animal industries. This is an obvious priority, because veterinarians run small businesses that depend on healthy animal industries in their communities for economic survival. In a business sense, veterinarians are no different from any other small businesses that are affected by disasters and have a commitment to restoring the economic driving force of their community after a disaster. No other animal care provider groups have this broad-based and permanent investment in their community; therefore, veterinarians may be the most objective and dedicated group to coordinate the care of animals in disasters and the restoration of the animal industries.

The long-term recovery phase of a disaster can be very protracted, with substantial adjustments occurring in the disaster-struck community. Restoration of businesses is facilitated through low-interest loans supplied by the Small Business Association and often by local banks. Recovery seems to have been best where affected persons and businesses had appropriate insurance coverage.

LOCAL PREPAREDNESS

There is no better way to cope with disasters than to be prepared for them. Although the large-scale disasters may result in a disaster declaration and may receive considerable publicity, small-scale, local disasters outweigh large-scale disasters by far in frequency and cost. It is not possible to prepare for every disaster, but it is possible to prepare for the most likely ones. The priorities for disaster planning in regard to horses vary to some extent with the use of the horses and the facility where they are kept. In general terms, the greatest priorities (i.e., the most likely disasters to occur with horses) are trailer accidents, floods, fires, power outages due to any cause, and contagious disease outbreaks. Some locations have additional hazards to consider, such as high winds, mud slides, and hazardous materials. For most of these potential problems, expert help is available.

Safety in Equine Transport

Transportation accidents are probably the most common disasters that horse owners encounter. Simple preventive measures include regular inspection of trailers and tow vehicles for safe operation.*

Flooding

Many horse farms are in flood plains. However, many horse owners and stable managers do not know how to interpret the type of flood plain in which they are located. This may lead to a false sense of security. For example, many people do not realize that living in a hundred-year flood plain means that the chance of flooding is calculated as 1% chance of flooding per year, or 30% chance in the lifespan of many mortgages. This indicates that the likelihood of flooding may be actually quite high on some farms. Floods come either rapidly as flash floods or with several days' notice. Horse farms and race tracks may require more time to evacuate in a flood than individual urban households; therefore, horse facilities should have a planned evacuation protocol for flash floods. Owners should adopt the habit of listening to weather reports for potential threats of cresting flooding.

Often the location of a horse farm cannot be changed, but measures to reduce the potential of flooding can be introduced. County area planning offices compile information on flood plains of most properties in their community. The Department of Natural Resources can provide maps and flood-risk assessment information on every property in their state. Owners of horse stables should retrieve this information and critically review the location of their property, as well as the access to their property, because flooding of either of these could leave them stranded. Civil engineers can help in the design and construction of flood-protected farm accesses and make recommendations on suitable locations for stables, paddocks, and high-lying areas that may be used as pasture ground in the event of a flood.

Fire Safety

Barn fires occur much too often, and many precious horses are lost to them. A common time for fires to break out in horse barns is in the winter months when doors are closed and the demand on energy for heating and lighting is at its greatest. Most stables for horses are built of flammable materials, and some even have gas heaters. Simple measures such as keeping fire extinguishers, smoke detectors, and no-smoking policies are often missing or not enforced. Electrical wiring of horse stables is often substandard, when compared with the most basic constructions for humans. These deficiencies can be corrected, and professional advice is available. The state departments of building and fire safety and most local fire departments provide low-cost inspections and recommendations on fire safety for properties. The recommendations are detailed and provide the highest standards by which to prevent fires.

Horse owners should consult with their local fire department on how to fireproof their stables. Local collaboration is a preferred route because it also familiarizes horse owners and local fire fighters with one another. This familiarity is of tremendous help in the event of an emergency. Simple factors like knowing ahead of time where the farm is located, how many horses are there, and where large volumes of water are available can make the difference between a rapid and successful response and a total failure.

Power Supply

Many farms are located in rural areas and may therefore have a low priority for restoration of power following a disaster. This is because the re-establishment of power is usually a priority based on human population density. Many farms are on the periphery of energy grids, and in some cases a farm is the only energy consumer in the area. It is important for owners interested in disaster planning to know the relative priority of their farm for the restoration of power. This important information can make all the difference between expecting to prepare for a few days without power and to be without power, lights, water, heating, and appliance operation for several weeks.

Information on how power is supplied can be obtained from the local electricity supply company. If the priority for restoration of power is low and the anticipated need for power is high, farm owners should consider securing a generator for emergencies. Generators can be secured through contractual agreements with suppliers, but a more reliable solution is for the farm to purchase a unit with sufficient power output. A representative from the electricity company or county cooperative extension agent can advise on the energy requirements to run a farm and the size of generator that is needed to supply the appropriate amount of power, as well as provide information on sources and costs of generators.

Faulty wiring is also a potential cause of fires. Professional electrical contractors should be consulted on how to properly install electrical wiring and power units.

Communications

Dependable communication is fundamental to identifying immediate sources of help where they will be needed most. One goal may be to establish a "buddy system," wherein neighbors and friends determine ahead of time who will be responsible for checking on and helping others and which resources will be shared; such a system can improve their knowledge and sensitivity in horse welfare. An effective method of communication in a disaster is to establish a telephone tree. With such a tree, every person

---

Excellent materials on transport safety are available from the Blue Green Publishing Company, PO Box 1255, Southern Pines, NC 28388. These include "Hawkins' Guide on Equine Emergencies" and "Horse Trailering on the Road." In addition, a videotape on equine trailer rescue is available from the Horse Park of New Jersey, PO Box 548, Allentown, NJ 08501. This video is designed for both horse owners and emergency management personnel to teach them transportation safety for horses.

in an affected area phones two to three other people to see if they need help. These in turn phone two to three others, and so on. Veterinary practices, horse sports groups, local breed associations, and neighborhood groups should take the lead in establishing these trees. Telephone trees should be tested periodically and revised if necessary. A meaningful time to do this is after every severe storm and during floods and droughts.

Veterinary Preparations for a Disaster

Depending on the type of disaster, the most prominent veterinary care issues vary. In high winds, tornadoes, and hurricanes, traumatic injuries predominate; in droughts and in severe winter weather, starvation and dehydration may be problems; and following fires, smoke inhalation and burn wounds are issues with which veterinarians deal. Many disasters also have widespread effects on horses, for example, deposition of debris on pastures many miles from a tornado touchdown and moldy corn following a flood. Therefore, veterinarians should be aware of the widespread ramifications of many disasters, even if they or their clients do not appear to be immediate victims. Many of the medical solutions to these issues are discussed elsewhere in this book.

In disasters, many horses from many different farms may be forced to congregate in a location where the challenge from contagious, yet preventable, disease may be high. Current Coggins tests, vaccinations, and deworming can improve the management and health of horses in disaster areas. Horses coming from many different sources are likely to have been fed a great variety of diets; when they are moved, mixed, and their diets changed they become predisposed to colic, laminitis, and hyperlipidemia. The likelihood of these occurring should be reduced by providing 25% of the dietary energy from oats or sweet feed and the rest from grass hay. Veterinarians can instruct their clients on first-aid for horses and advise on the contents and appropriate use of a first-aid kit.

Relocation

Relocation plans are easy to accomplish when a disaster is not threatening, but may be impossible once many horse owners are threatened by the same incident. Every horse owner should have at least three alternative accommodations arranged for their horses in the event of a disaster. These contacts should be confirmed at least annually. Special sites where large numbers of horses may be congregated include county and state fair grounds, race tracks, and show facilities. Access to these, however, most likely requires prior arrangement and should be addressed by veterinary practices and local horse groups rather than individual owners. Cooperative extension agents often have good relationships with the owners and managers of such facilities, and they may be consulted when trying to identify which facilities are available and who has the authority to allow access to them. Regardless of the facilities chosen, consideration should be given to how large amounts of manure will be disposed of, because manure accumulates rapidly and poses a significant animal and human health problem.

Identification of Horses

In large-scale disasters, when many horses have to be evacuated, identification of the horses and their owners can be difficult. It is not unusual for owners to have lost their horses' and personal identifications in disasters. Ideally, horses should be uniquely and permanently identified, such as by their whorls, with a microchip or tattoo, or by current photographs or other means of identifying the horse. However, when this is not the case (for example, when horses have to be evacuated suddenly) emergency identification methods can be used. These include painting or etching the hooves, body marking with crayon, and neck banding.

Prioritization of Horses

A sad but real side of emergency evacuation and rescue is the need to decide which horses to help first. This is particularly important for large breeding and stable operations, race tracks, and rare breeds farms, where it may not be possible to evacuate or save all of the horses following a sudden-impact incident. Every horse owner and stable owner and manager should have a clear plan to identify those animals they should protect in the event of a sudden disaster, such as a fire, tornado, flash flood, or power outage. This allows a rational approach to rescue in the event of an emergency.

Restoration of Veterinary Practices

Veterinary practices, like any other businesses, may be struck by disasters. Most commonly these are the result of local disasters, such as fires, floods, chemical spills, and tornadoes. It has been estimated that only about 5% of small businesses that are affected by a major disaster ever recover to a functional state. This lack of recovery has been suggested to be primarily the result of inadequate insurance coverage. Many major concerns arise for veterinary practices in disasters. These include personal, client, and patient safety; cash flow; continued income for employees and their families; continued provision of quality care for animals; restoration of a functional practice; changes in community infrastructure; loyalty of clients; and others. Many of these issues can be addressed before a disaster occurs by obtaining adequate insurance coverage for almost all eventualities and by entering into agreements with neighboring practices to share facilities and resources. Small businesses, including veterinary practices, can claim low-interest loans from the Small Business Association (SBA) and banks that have arrangements with the federal government to provide disaster assistance.

TRAINING REQUIREMENTS FOR VOLUNTEERS

The response to disasters is to a large extent provided by volunteers. The main responder groups for animals in recent years have been humane groups, animal control personnel, owners, veterinarians, veterinary technicians, and a large number of ad hoc grassroots organizations. Because many of the individual groups' experiences in disaster preparedness and response are often limited, a variety of perceived training needs has emerged.

Currently, there are no training programs for how to deal with animals in disasters that are recognized by any of the official emergency management groups. However, several motivational orientation sessions are available to the public, which are usually organized by humane groups and attempt to fill this void. In addition, the Emergency Management Institute, the education wing of FEMA, is developing an independent study course for planners and responders to deal with animals in disasters. The current lack of specific training materials related to animals in disasters should not preclude responders for animals from obtaining basic training in emergency management. This basic-level training consolidates and optimizes the response to disasters, and it is highly recommended that anyone wanting to become involved in disaster management attend courses in this area.

Examples of recognized training programs include those organized by volunteer fire departments, military and law enforcement reserves, emergency medical services, the American Red Cross, Hazmat, and EMAs. Volunteers who have attended recognized training sessions can be deployed instantly in disasters, as needed. Trained volunteers know where to report and how to integrate into the incident command system. They should also be familiar with the physical and psychological demands that volunteer work in disasters creates, and how to cope with these. Volunteer groups, such as equine rescue groups, can seek recognition by official emergency management groups. This is most commonly achieved through mutual aid agreements between the EMA and responder groups. Veterinary practices should consider entering into such agreements with their local EMA as an avenue through which they can make significant contributions toward helping animals, their owners, and themselves in disasters.

Liability

During most disasters, many states and communities provide liability coverage for emergency support personnel, including qualified volunteers. This allows a state or smaller community to have large numbers of volunteers on reserve that they be mobilized in the event of a disaster. It is important to realize, however, that only trained and recognized volunteers are covered under these provisions. Therefore, for the protection of the volunteers and the victims with which they will be dealing, additional training through recognized agencies of emergency management is essential.

FINANCIAL ISSUES IN DISASTERS

Disasters are expensive. For example, in California, estimates of annual costs for fire control are between $300 million and $350 million per year. Less than 1% of these costs is ever recovered from people, businesses, and other organizations that are found to have caused fires either illegally or through negligence. These high costs for large-scale disasters, however, should not detract from the fact that most disasters occur locally and are never declared. The national cost to United States citizens for small-scale local disasters, such as hazardous materials spills, individual house floods and fires, severe weather damage, and building collapses exceeds in total the cost of large-scale disasters by several hundred-fold. As for many other disasters, the greatest expense is associated with their repeated nature and the demands during the late recovery phase.

One permanent solution to the source of funding for animals and their owners in disasters is to make the response for animals part of the official local, state, regional, and national emergency management systems. In principle, the AVMA has achieved this for federally declared disasters by defining VMATs and gaining recognition for these as part of the federal response plan. Other examples of integrated EOPs that include animals have been initiated by the VMAs of several states, including Indiana, Kansas, Maryland, and Ohio, and local animal control organizations such as those in Los Angeles. Several local humane groups, veterinary medical associations, and individual veterinary practices, for example, in areas of California, Florida, Indiana, and Ohio, have also been able to achieve this.

Another possible solution to the issue of funding has been the recently established American Veterinary Medical Foundation's Disaster Relief Emergency Fund. This foundation was set up to receive and dispense donations for disaster relief to victims in situations in which animals were involved. Using specific guidelines, funds can be sought to support the following: (1) emergency preparedness, (2) health care for animals, (3) response teams, and (4) grants and loans for veterinarians. The American Veterinary Medical Foundation can also accept and manage funding for specific purposes, such as donations for the support of specific communities or relief agencies. With only a very small operating overhead, this foundation has strong potential to set rational standards for disaster relief for animals and their owners.

Supplemental Readings

American Veterinary Medical Association: AVMA Emergency Preparedness and Response Guide. Schaumburg, IL, 1994.
Auf der Heide E: Disaster response: Principles of preparation and coordination. St. Louis, C. V. Mosby, 1989.
Boge P: Preparing for the worst. Vet Product News 8(2):1, 43, 1996.
Casper J: The Maryland pet-sheltering plan. J Am Vet Med Assoc 203:994–996, 1993.
Heath SE: The development of the Veterinary and Animal Care Annex to the Indiana Emergency Operations Plan. Indiana Veterinary Medical Association, Indianapolis, 1995.
Linnabary RD, New JC, Vogt BM, Griffith-Davies C, Williams L: Emergency evacuation of horses: A Madison County, Kentucky, survey. J Equine Vet Sci 13(3):153–158, 1993.
Proceedings of the First International Conference on Equine Rescue. J Equine Vet Sci 13(5), 1993.
Proceedings of the 2nd International Conference on Equine Rescue. J Equine Vet Sci 15(4), 1995.

Musculoskeletal Injuries in the Eventing Horse

S. ANNE BASKETT
Athens, Georgia

Musculoskeletal injuries occur commonly in eventing horses during training and competition, and they sometimes prove to be career-ending. Fortunately, the catastrophic breakdown injuries and long bone fractures that occasionally occur in Thoroughbred racehorses are rare at combined-training events. One possible reason for the relatively low incidence of serious injuries at these competitions, even at the extremely demanding upper levels, is that the eventing horse must be at least 4 years old to compete in a recognized competition. Consequently, the average eventing horse is more skeletally mature than many Thoroughbred racehorses. Furthermore, the speed of the eventing horse on steeplechase and cross-country events is considerably slower than the 900 to 1000 m/minute required for a competitive Thoroughbred sprint race. As a result of the slower speeds, there is less potential for injury to supporting soft tissue and bony structures.

The majority of the musculoskeletal injuries that occur at 3-day events are "bowed" tendons (most often involving the superficial digital flexor tendon), suspensory ligament desmitis, foot problems associated with losing shoes and bruising, stifle injuries, and limb lacerations. As in most equine sporting events, the majority of these injuries affect the forelimbs. The treatment veterinarian at a combined-training event must be prepared for all eventualities. This section discusses treatment of musculoskeletal injuries at the event site, as well as appropriate therapies that should be instituted before referring a horse with a musculoskeletal injury. The 3-day event organizers should have directions to the nearest referral center available, to save time and minimize confusion.

FRACTURE MANAGEMENT

Management of a fracture on course poses one of the greatest challenges to the treating veterinarian, because the injuries require rapid and effective stabilization and safe removal of the horse from the course. Many cross-country courses are built over extremely variable terrain, sometimes miles from the stabling area. Furthermore, access to parts of the course with a horse ambulance is often difficult. These problems are compounded by the fact that, unlike any other racing or showjumping event, spectators have full access to the cross-country course. Therefore, if an accident occurs on course, measures should be rapidly taken to keep the spectators away from the area. Screens should be available to shield an injured horse from the public during treatment on course. Unless completely unavoidable for humane reasons, euthanasia of a horse should not take place on course. Preferably, the horse's condition should be stabilized and the horse transported to the stable treatment area, and the decision to perform euthanasia made only after the owner or agent and insurance company, if the horse is insured, have been advised of the situation and have granted permission.

Procedure on Course

Initial fracture management is critical to the survival of the horse. Although as little treatment as possible should be done on course, it is crucial to adequately stabilize the limb before loading the horse onto an ambulance. The immediate treatment goals include protection of the surrounding soft tissues to prevent a closed fracture from becoming an open fracture, and limb stabilization to prevent a nondisplaced fracture from becoming a displaced fracture. The way that the horse is holding the injured limb, degree of weightbearing, and deviation of the limb will help identify the affected area and the severity of the injury. Palpation should be done rapidly to assess degree of displacement and whether the fracture is open or closed. If the horse will not bear weight on the limb and no obvious fracture is palpated, the limb should still be adequately protected with a full splint and the horse returned to the treatment area where radiographs and ultrasonography can be performed to determine the extent of the injury. Pain or swelling over a bony area associated with a severe lameness should be treated as a nondisplaced fracture, and the limb should be protected with splints before transport. Horses with a suspected nondisplaced fracture should be referred to a veterinary hospital for further evaluation if radiographs cannot be developed in a reasonable time close to the competition. A displaced fracture should be stabilized and the horse referred to a surgical facility as soon as feasible.

Mild sedation can facilitate assessment, stabilization, and transport of some horses that sustain fractures. Low doses of sedatives and tranquilizers should be used to avoid oversedation and ataxia. The phenothiazine tranquilizers, such as acetylpromazine, should be avoided in anxious horses that are in pain because high levels of circulating catecholamines can exacerbate the hypotensive effects of these drugs. Xylazine (0.3–0.5 mg/kg) or a xylazine/butorphanol combination are the drugs of choice because their hypotensive effects are not as dramatic.

Fractures below the distal third of the radius and the hock are amenable to immobilization using either splints or casts. The application of splints is generally the most rapid and effective method to stabilize a fracture while the horse is on the course. Significant hemorrhage should be managed with pressure wraps and vessel ligation before splinting. A Robert Jones bandage is placed over the limb before application of the splint. Splints should immobilize the joint above and below the fractured bone and should be placed on the limb in a manner that prevents changes in the tension and compression on surfaces of the fractured bone. Ideally, two splints should be placed at 90° to each other. These splints should support the weight of the horse and provide maximum resistance to movement in different planes. On the course, casts are generally useful only for stabilization of the most distal fractures at or below the distal metacarpal/metatarsal bone because applying a cast to more proximal regions requires a great deal of time and possibly general anesthesia.

A splint can be made from various materials. It must be lightweight, yet strong enough to resist bending or breaking if the horse attempts to bear weight. Polyvinylchloride (PVC) pipe is useful because it is readily available, inexpensive, and easily cut to a desired length and width. Pipes of 4- and 6-inch diameters are the most useful for making splints. They can be precut into thirds using a hacksaw or oscillating saw and stored under or behind the seat of the emergency vehicle. Broom handles and 2- × 4-inch lumber can also be modified into splints. Commercial splints are available that stabilize the distal half of the horse's limb. These splints rapidly immobilize fractures involving the distal metacarpus or metatarsus as well as the sesamoids and phalanges, and can be used to stabilize the distal limb subsequent to disruption of the flexor tendons. The Kimzey Leg Saver* is one example of a commercially available splint.

Fractures of the tibia and the proximal radius are difficult to adequately immobilize, but techniques are described for both. Some authorities do not recommend that proximal radial fractures be splinted, because slipping of the bandage can cause further damage by creating a "pendulum effect." If stabilization of a proximal radial fracture is attempted, it is important to remember that limb abduction must be prevented, because this movement can force the bony fragments through the skin on the medial aspect of the radius. Two splints are applied at 90° angles, as for the more distal fractures. However, the lateral splint extends over the shoulder region to the height of the withers to limit abduction. The caudal splint should extend to one joint above the fractured bone, as for more distal fractures. Tibial fractures are more difficult than radial fractures to stabilize, and they readily progress from closed to open fractures on the medial aspect of the limb if the latter is abducted during transport. To prevent abduction, the splint must extend to the level of the tuber coxae, and should be bent to follow the contours of the hindlimb, if possible.

The fractured limb should determine the direction that the horse is loaded for shipping. If the fracture involves a forelimb, the horse should be transported backwards to decrease the pressure on the forelimbs during deceleration. Horses with hindlimb injuries should be shipped facing forward. The body of the horse should be in as confined an area as possible to allow leaning on the bars, and the head and neck should be free enough to be used for balance.

Kimzey Welding Works, Woodland, CA

Procedure at the Stable

At the stable area, the treatment veterinarian can further assess the injury and determine whether referral is necessary and what additional therapy is needed before referral. If referral is the most obvious course of action, unloading and reloading the horse in the stable area should be avoided. An intravenous (IV) catheter can be placed and other necessary treatment initiated with the horse on the trailer if the animal's behavior permits. Intravenous administration of balanced polyionic fluid may be indicated to offset hypovolemia associated with sweating and blood losses. If the fracture is open or involving a joint, broad-spectrum intravenous antibiotics and a tetanus toxoid booster should also be administered. A combination of an aminoglycoside with a cephalosporin or a penicillin offers a good spectrum of coverage until bacterial cultures can be performed.

Table 1 provides a list of drugs and equipment to support treatment at the stable or on the course.

TENDON AND LIGAMENT INJURIES

The most common musculoskeletal injuries encountered by veterinarians at combined-training events involve the tendons and ligaments. Proper management of obvious acute injuries to tendons and ligaments is important, because these injuries can be career-limiting. It is also important to try to identify horses with more subtle fiber

TABLE 1. LIST OF PHARMACEUTICALS AND EQUIPMENT USEFUL FOR EMERGENCY TREATMENT OF MUSCULOSKELETAL INJURIES

Sedatives/tranquilizers
Antibiotics
Antiphlogistine poultice
Local anesthetic
Euthanasia solution
100 L commercially prepared balanced electrolyte solution
Cast padding and felt
3-inch stockinette
4- and 5-inch casting material
Pound cotton
Sheet cottons
Conforming gauze wrap
Elastic wrap
White tape
Gauze squares (sterile and nonsterile)
Roll gauze
Towels
Nonadhering wound pads
Splinting material—polyvinylchloride pipe (4- to 6-inch diameter, cut in thirds)
Hack or oscillating saw
Bucket
Commercial distal limb splint
Ultrasound machine and gel
Suture material
Scalpel blades
Surgical gloves
Field surgical pack (scissors, scalpel handle, forceps, hemostats, needles, needle holders)
Portable light source

disruption, because further exertion before adequate healing has occurred could worsen the injury and consequently the prognosis for future athletic activity. Fatigue, poor footing, conformational weaknesses, poor foot balance, and inadequate conditioning programs all contribute to the development of tendinitis and suspensory desmitis. The superficial digital flexor tendon is most commonly involved in the forelimbs. The hindlimbs are less commonly affected, although suspensory desmitis may occur more frequently than it is definitively diagnosed.

Tendinitis and suspensory desmitis occur most often during the speed and endurance phase of the 3-day event. Examinations and inspections of the horses by the veterinary delegate and ground jury during the 3-day event provide opportunities for the lameness associated with these injuries to be detected and the horse removed from further competition.

Ultrasonography is an invaluable tool for diagnosing distal limb tendon and ligament injuries. Consequently, an ultrasound machine and a competent ultrasonographer should be present at all 3-day events. Ultrasonographic changes in the flexor tendons and suspensory ligament represent the infiltration of blood or edema between tendon fibers, disruption of the fibers, or a combination of these lesions. To adequately evaluate tendons, a scan should be done in both a sagittal and a transverse plane using a 7.5-MHz probe. If doubt exists as to the appearance of a possible lesion, the opposite limb should be scanned for comparison. Deficits can range from a slight decrease in echogenicity, representing mild disruption of collagen fibers and fluid infiltration, to total anechogenicity, representing complete fiber disruption or infiltration of edema or hemorraghic fluid.

Treatment

The initial goals for treatment (see also page 15) of tendinitis and desmitis are to decrease inflammation and pain and minimize further injury. Cold therapy is of the most benefit during the first 48 hours after injury. Regional chilling reduces pain by decreasing blood flow to the site, thereby reducing the release of potentially harmful inflammatory mediators and hydrolytic enzymes in the damaged area. Further, local vasoconstriction decreases fluid accumulation between the tendon fibers, thereby reducing collagen fiber disruption. The affected limb can be treated three to four times daily by placing it in a whirlpool boot or tall bucket filled with water and crushed ice for 20 to 30 minutes. Alternatively, cold hose water, commercially available cold packs, or crushed ice in a plastic bag can be applied to the limb. Between cold therapy sessions, the limb should be wrapped from below the carpus or tarsus to the coronary band with a regular stable bandage over adequate padding (leg quilt or sheet cotton) to help minimize accumulation of fluid in and around the injured tendon or ligament.

Systemic administration of anti-inflammatory agents is indicated to decrease inflammation and provide analgesia; nonsteroidal anti-inflammatory agents are the traditional mainstays of therapy. Phenylbutazone (2.2–4.4 mg/kg p.o. or IV b.i.d.) can be administered for at least the first week after the injury. Medical-grade dimethyl sulfoxide (DMSO; 80–100 ml in 2–3 L 0.9% saline IV s.i.d.) can be administered for 1 to 3 days for its anti-inflammatory and free radical scavenging properties. This route of administration represents extra-label use of the drug.

Topical anti-inflammatory drugs are also used in treating acute tendon injuries. Antiphlogistic poultices and DMSO are the most commonly applied agents, although the efficacy of these compounds is not completely known. Repeated application of DMSO under wraps should be undertaken with caution, because this treatment has been associated with local sloughing of the hair and skin.

TRAUMA TO THE STIFLE AND CARPUS

The cross-country test of a horse trial or 3-day event consists of solid fences built on variable terrain and into water, often involving drops of 6 to 8 feet at the upper levels of competition. Because the fences are solidly built, horses can injure their carpal or radial area or their stifles if they hit the fences. It is particularly common for horses to injure their stifles over the bigger-drop fences. The most common form of stifle injury is soft tissue bruising with or without hematoma formation. This type of injury is rarely severe enough to cause damage to the deeper supporting structures. As the treating veterinarian, it is important to keep in mind that although these horses may be very lame acutely, they may, in some instances, be sound enough to compete the next day.

Treatment

Initial treatment of injuries to the stifle or carpal region should be directed toward decreasing pain and swelling and ruling out fractures or ligamentous damage. Cold therapy, as described previously for tendon and ligament injuries of the distal limbs, is very useful for decreasing inflammation and providing some analgesia. Pressure wraps can be applied if the carpal or radial area is involved. Nonsteroidal anti-inflammatory drugs are also beneficial and are permitted in moderate doses under some rules. However, if the competition is run under FEI rules and there is a possibility that the horse may be sound enough to compete the next day, the latter drugs should not be administered.

Radiographs should be taken shortly after the injury. If bony lesions are not detected, follow-up films should be obtained in 10 to 14 days if the horse's degree of comfort does not dramatically improve and no other cause for the lameness is identified. Ultrasonography may also be useful to help identify damage to tendons or ligaments. In the stifle, damage to the patellar and collateral ligaments and some meniscal injuries can be detected. It is important to note that imaging the meniscal ligaments or cruciate ligaments is difficult in a weightbearing animal. When performing ultrasonography on the carpal area, the extensor carpi radialis and common digital extensor tendon and their sheaths, as well as the lateral collateral ligament, the carpal joint capsule, and the distal articular cartilage of the radius, can be easily imaged. The tendon and tendon sheath of the extensor carpi obliquus, the lateral digital extensor, and the ulnaris lateralis muscle can also be imaged; however, these are not as easily identified.

Supplemental Readings

Bertone AL: Management of orthopedic emergencies. Vet Clin North Am Equine Pract 10(3):603–625, 1994.

Bramlage LR: Current concepts of emergency first aid treatment of equine fracture patients. Compend Contin Ed Pract Vet 10:S568, 1983.

Dyson S: Proximal suspensory desmitis in the hindlimb: 42 cases. Br Vet J 150(3):279–291, 1994.

Dyson SJ: Stifle trauma in the event horse. Equine Vet Ed 6(5):234–240, 1994.

Henninger R: Treatment of superficial digital flexor tendinitis. Vet Clin North Am Equine Pract 10(2):409–424, 1994.

McCullagh KG, Goodship AE, Silver IA: Tendon injuries and their treatment in the horse. Vet Rec 105:54–57, 1979.

Palmer SE, Genovese R, Longo KL, Goodman N, Dyson S: Practical management of superficial digital flexor tendinitis in the performance horse. Vet Clin North Am Equine Pract 10(2):425–481, 1994.

APPENDICES

Appendix 1: Table of Drugs, Approximate Doses

N. EDWARD ROBINSON
East Lansing, Michigan

Name of Drug	Dose	Route
Acepromazine	0.03–0.066 mg/kg for sedation	IM
	0.033–0.055 mg/kg followed by 0.055–0.066 mg/kg butorphanol	IV
	0.04 mg/kg followed by 0.6 mg/kg meperidine	IV
	0.02–0.055 mg/kg t.i.d. for α-adrenoceptor blockade	IM
Acetazolamide	2.2 mg/kg b.i.d.–q.i.d.	p.o.
Acetylcysteine (10%)	2–5 ml/50 kg q.i.d.	Aerosol
Acyclovir	5–10 mg/kg t.i.d.	p.o.
3%	q3–4h	Ophthalmic
Albendazole	25 mg/kg b.i.d. for 5 days for *Dictyocaulus arnfieldi*	p.o.
	50 mg/kg b.i.d. for 2 days for *Strongylus vulvaris* larvae	p.o.
	4–8 mg/kg b.i.d. for 1 month for *Echinococcus*	p.o.
Albuterol	1–2 mcg/kg	Inhalation
Alfaprostol	3 mg/450 kg for luteolysis; 2 doses 14–18 days apart	IM
Allopurinol	5 mg/kg	IV
alpha-tocopherol	1.5–4.4 mg/kg s.i.d.	p.o.
Altrenogest	0.044 mg/kg s.i.d. for 8–12 days; for estrus synchronization follow with luteolytic dose of prostaglandin $F_2\alpha$	p.o.
	0.044 mg/kg to prevent aggression	p.o.
	0.44 mg/kg s.i.d. for pregnancy maintenance	p.o.
Aluminum hydroxide	200–250 ml t.i.d. (antacid)	p.o.
Aluminum hydroxide	60 mg/kg	p.o.
Amikacin	3.5–7.5 mg/kg b.i.d. to q.i.d.	IM or sc
	15–20 mg/kg s.i.d.	IM or sc
	1–10 mg/kg b.i.d. for foals	Slow IV or IM
	75–100 mg	Subconjunctival
	125–250 mg	Intra-articular
	2 g buffered with equal volume of 75% sodium bicarbonate	Intrauterine
Aminocaproic acid	20 mg/kg diluted 1:9 in saline and administered over 30–60 min	IV
Aminophylline	5–10 mg/kg b.i.d.	p.o.
Aminopropazine fumarate	0.5 mg/kg b.i.d.	IM or IV
Aminopyrine	2.5–10 mg/450 kg	IV or IM
Ammonium chloride	20–520 mg/kg s.i.d. (acidifier)	p.o.
	0.3 g/50 kg q.i.d. (expectorant)	p.o.
Amoxicillin	10–22 mg/kg t.i.d.	IM
trihydrate	6–10 mg/kg b.i.d.–t.i.d.	IM
Amphotericin B	0.05 mg/kg q2days for 1 month	IV
	Introduce over 5 days. Dissolve in 1 L 5% dextrose and administer over 1 hour via large-bore catheter	
Ampicillin Na	10–15 mg/kg t.i.d.–q.i.d.	IV or IM
trihydrate	11–22 mg/kg b.i.d. or t.i.d.	IM or p.o.
	50 mg	Subconjunctival

Name of Drug	Dose	Route
Antidiuretic hormone	60 IU q6h for diabetes insipidus	IV
Ascorbic acid	30 mg/kg b.i.d. in IV fluids	IV
Aspirin	10–100 mg/kg b.i.d.	p.o.
Atipamezole	0.05–1.0 mg/kg	IV
Atracurium	0.04–0.07 mg/kg	IV
Atropine	0.01–0.1 mg/kg	IV, IM, or sc
1%	q3–24h	Ophthalmic
Aurothioglucose	1 mg/kg	IM
Azlocillin	25–75 mg/kg q.i.d.	IV
Beclamethasone	3.75 mg b.i.d.	Inhalation
Betamethasone	0.02–0.1 mg/kg	IM or p.o.
	4–10 mg	Intralesional
Bethanecol	0.025–0.1 mg/kg t.i.d. or q.i.d.	sc
	0.3–0.4 mg/kg t.i.d. or q.i.d.	p.o.
Bismuth subsalicylate	0.5–1 ml/kg q4–6h in foals	p.o.
	1–2 L/450 kg b.i.d.	p.o.
Boldenone undecylenate	1 mg/kg repeated at 3-week intervals	IM
Botulinum antitoxin	100–150 IU/ml: 200 ml/foal or 500 ml/adult	IV or IM
Buparvaquone	4–6 mg/kg, single dose	IV
Butorphanol tartrate	0.01–2 mg/kg, see xylazine, detomidine, and acepromazine	IV or IM
Calcium chloride	1–2 g/450 kg, slowly to effect	IV
Calcium gluconate	0.5 ml/kg of 10% solution	Slow IV
Cambendazole	20 mg/kg for *Strongyloides westeri*	p.o.
Captan	3% solution	Topical
Carbenicillin Na indanyl	50–80 mg/kg b.i.d. or t.i.d.	IV or IM
	200 mg	Subconjunctival
	6 g	Intrauterine
Carbon disulfide	24 mg/450 kg	p.o.
Carprofen	0.7 mg/kg s.i.d.	IV
Casein (iodinated)	5 g s.i.d.	p.o.
Cefaclor	20–40 mg/kg t.i.d.	p.o.
Cefadroxil	22 mg/kg b.i.d.	p.o.
	25 mg/kg q4–6h for foals	IV
Cefamandole	10–30 mg/kg q4–8h	IV or IM
Cefazolin Na	15 mg/kg b.i.d. or t.i.d.	IV or IM
	50 mg	Subconjunctival
Cefixime	400 mg/kg t.i.d.	p.o.
Cefonicid	10–15 mg/kg s.i.d.	IV or IM
Cefoperazone	30–50 mg/kg b.i.d. or t.i.d.	IV or IM
Ceforanide	5–10 mg/kg b.i.d.	IV or IM
Cefotaxime Na	15–25 mg/kg b.i.d.–t.i.d.	IV or IM
Cefotetan	15–30 mg/kg b.i.d.	IV or IM
Cefoxitin	30–40 mg/kg t.i.d. or q.i.d.	IM
	20 mg/kg q.i.d.	IV
Ceftazidime	25–50 mg/kg b.i.d.	IV or IM
Ceftiofur	1–5 mg/kg s.i.d.–b.i.d.	IV or IM
	1 g	Intrauterine
Ceftizoxime	25–50 mg/kg b.i.d. or t.i.d.	IV or IM
Ceftriaxone	25–50 mg/kg b.i.d.	IV or IM
Cefuroxime	25–50 mg/kg t.i.d.	IV or IM
axetil	250–500 mg/kg b.i.d.	p.o.
Cephalexin	10–30 mg/kg t.i.d.–q.i.d.	p.o.
Cephalothin Na	20–40 mg/kg t.i.d.–q.i.d.	IV or IM
	100 mg	Subconjunctival
Cephapirin	30 mg/kg q4–6h	IV or IM
Cetizoxime Na	20–30 mg/kg t.i.d.	IV
Charcoal (activated)	1–3 g/kg as slurry (1 g in 5 ml water), repeat if necessary in 8–12 hours	p.o.
Chloral hydrate	60–200 mg/kg for foal restraint	IV
	40–100 mg/kg	p.o.
Chloramphenicol		
palmitate	4–10 mg/kg t.i.d. or q.i.d. (foal)	p.o.
	25–50 mg/kg t.i.d. or q.i.d. (adult)	p.o.
succinate	25 mg/kg t.i.d.–q.i.d.	IV or IM
	50–100 mg	Subconjunctival
Chlorhexidine	0.5–2%	Topical
Chlorpromazine	1 mg/kg	IM
Cimetidine	6.6 mg/kg q4–6h	IV
	18 mg/kg q8h	p.o.
	2.5–4 mg/kg q8h for 2 months for tumor reduction	p.o.
Cisapride	0.1 mg/kg	IM
	0.5–0.8 mg/kg t.i.d. for 7 days	p.o.
Clenbuterol	0.8–3.2 mcg/kg b.i.d.	p.o.
	0.8 mcg/kg b.i.d.	IV
	200 mcg for uterine relaxation	IM or slow IV

Name of Drug	Dose	Route
Clotrimazole	500 mg suspension or cream s.i.d. for 1 week	Intrauterine
Cloxacillin	10–30 mg/kg q.i.d.	IM
Cocaine chloride	1–1.5 ml of 10 mg/ml	Subconjunctival
Colistin	2500 IU/kg q.i.d.	Slow IV
Corticotropin	1 IU/kg	IM
Coumaphos	0.06% wash, 0.1% dust	Topical
Cromolyn sodium	80–300 mg	Insufflated into the pharynx
Cyclosporin 0.2%	q12h	Ophthalmic
Cyproheptadine	0.5 mg/kg b.i.d.	p.o.
D-penicillamine	3–4 mg/kg q6h for 10 days	p.o.
Danthron	15–30 ml/kg	p.o.
Dantrolene Na	10 mg/kg loading dose	p.o.
	2.5 mg/kg q2h, maintenance	p.o.
	2–2.5 mg/kg in saline for acute myopathy	Slow IV
	1–2 mg/kg s.i.d. to prevent myositis	p.o.
Dembrexine	0.3–0.5 mg/kg	p.o.
Demecarium bromide	0.25% b.i.d.	Ophthalmic
Detomidine	0.005–0.02 mg/kg	IV
	0.01–0.02 mg/kg followed by	IV
	0.044–0.066 mg/kg butorphanol	
	0.02–0.04 mg/kg followed by	IV
	2.2 mg/kg ketamine	
Dexamethasone	0.02–0.2 mg/kg s.i.d.	IV, IM, or p.o.
	0.5–2 mg/kg for septic shock	IV
	100 mg/450 kg s.i.d. for 5 days to induce parturition	IV
phosphate	0.1% t.i.d.	Ophthalmic
suspension	0.1% q3–8h	Ophthalmic
Dextran (6% solution)	8 g/kg s.i.d. for up to 3 days	IV
Diazepam	0.03–0.5 mg/kg; repeat in 30 minutes if necessary	Slow IV
Dichlorphenamide	1 mg/kg b.i.d.	p.o.
Dichlorvos	35 mg/kg	p.o.
	0.93% solution	Topical
Dicloxacillin	10 mg/kg q.i.d.	IM
Diethylcarbamazine	1 mg/kg s.i.d. for 21 days for onchocerciasis	p.o.
	50 mg/kg s.i.d. for 10 days for verminous myelitis	p.o.
Digoxin	0.002 mg/kg b.i.d.	IV
	0.01 mg/kg b.i.d.	p.o.
Dihydrostreptomycin	11 mg/kg b.i.d.	IM or sc
Dimercaprol	2.5–5 mg/kg as 10% solution in oil q4h for 2 days, then b.i.d. until recovery	IM
Dimethyl glycine	1–1.6 mg/kg s.i.d.	p.o.
Dimethyl sulfoxide (DMSO)	0.5 mg/kg to 1.0 g/kg (10% solution in 5% dextrose). Repeat lower doses q6–12h	IV
	50% solution	Topical
Dinoprost tromethamine	10 mg/450 kg	IM
Dioctyl sodium sulfosuccinate 5% solution	10–20 mg/kg in 4–8 L water q48h	p.o.
	10 ml in warm water as enema for retained meconium	
Dioxathion	0.15% wash	Topical
Diphenylhydantoin	1–10 mg/kg q2–4h	IV, IM, or p.o.
Dipyrone	5–22 mg/kg	IV or IM
Dobutamine	1–10 mcg/kg per minute (250 mg in 500 ml saline infused at 0.45 ml/kg per hour)	IV
Dolophine HCl	0.2–0.4 mg/kg	IM
Domperidone	0.2 mg/kg	IV
	1.1 mg/kg s.i.d.	p.o.
Dopamine	1–5 mcg/kg per minute (200 mg in 500 ml saline infused at 0.45 ml/kg per hour)	IV
Doxapram	0.5–1.0 mg/kg q5min (do not exceed 2 mg/kg in foals)	IV
	0.02–0.05 mg/kg per minute up to 400 mg total for neonatal foal resuscitation	IV
Doxycycline	3 mg/kg b.i.d.	p.o.
Ecothiophate iodide	0.03% b.i.d.	Ophthalmic
EDTA calcium disodium	75 mg/kg per day in divided doses for lead poisoning	Slow IV
	6.6% solution (1 ml/0.9 kg), q8–12h	IV
Enrofloxacin	2.5 mg/kg b.i.d.	p.o.
Ephedrine sulphate	0.7 mg/kg b.i.d.	p.o.
Epinephrine 1:10,000	0.1–0.2 ml/kg	IM or sc
	1–1.5 ml of 0.33 ng/ml	Subconjunctival
Erythromycin base	0.1 mg/kg per hour to enhance gut motility	IV
estolate or ethylsuccinate	25 mg/kg b.i.d.	p.o.
lactobionate	2.5–5 mg/kg t.i.d. or q.i.d.	IV
	20–40 mg	Subconjunctival
phosphate or stearate	37.5 mg/kg b.i.d.	p.o.
Estradiol	0.004–0.008 mg/kg q2days for urinary incontinence	IM

Table continued on following page

Name of Drug	Dose	Route
Estrone sulfate	0.04 mg/kg s.i.d.	IM
Ethyl alcohol (50%)	5–10 ml/50 kg	Aerosol
Ethylene diamine dihydriodide	0.5–1.5 g/450 kg s.i.d.	p.o.
Famotidine	3.3 mg/kg t.i.d.	p.o.
Febantel	6 mg/kg	p.o.
Fenbendazole	5 mg/kg	p.o.
	10 mg/kg for *Parascaris equorum*	p.o.
	50 mg/kg s.i.d. for 3 days for verminous arteritis	p.o.
	50 mg/kg for *Strongyloides westeri*	p.o.
	50 mg/kg s.i.d. for 5 days for onchocerca	p.o.
Fenoterol	2–4 mcg/kg	Inhalation
Fenprostalene	0.5 mg/450 kg	sc
Ferrous sulfate	2 mg/kg s.i.d.	p.o.
Floxacillin	10 mg/kg q.i.d.	IM
Fluconazole	4 mg/kg s.i.d.	p.o.
Flumazenil	0.5–2.0 mg	Slow IV
Flumethasone	0.002–0.008 mg/kg	p.o.
Flunixin meglumine	0.25–1.1 mg/kg s.i.d.–t.i.d.	p.o., IM, or IV
Fluoroprednisolone acetate	5–20 mg/450 kg	IM
Fluprostenol	250 mcg/450 kg	IM
Flurbiprofen Na 0.03%	t.i.d. or q.i.d.	Ophthalmic
Folic acid	40–75 mg	IM
Folinic acid	50–100 mg	IM
Follicle stimulating hormone	10–50 mg/450 kg	IV, IM, or sc
Furazolidone	4 mg/kg t.i.d.	p.o.
Furosemide	1–3 mg/kg b.i.d.	IV or IM
	250–500 mg 1–4 hours pre-race	IV or IM
Gentamicin	2–4 mg/kg b.i.d.–q.i.d.	IV, IM, or sc
	6.6–8.8 mg/kg s.i.d.	IV, IM, or sc
	10–40 mg	Subconjunctival
	q2–6h	Ophthalmic
	150 mg (unbuffered)	Intra-articular
	1–2 g buffered in equal volume of 75% sodium bicarbonate	Intrauterine
Glucagon	25–50 mg/kg	IV
Glycerin	1 g/kg	p.o.
Glycerol	0.5–2 g/kg for brain edema	IV
Glycerol (5%)	2–5 ml/50 kg	Aerosol
Glycerol guaiacolate	110 mg/kg for convulsions	IV
	0.1–0.2 g/50 kg q.i.d. expectorant	p.o.
Glycopyrolate	0.005–0.01 mg/kg	IV
Glycosaminoglycan polysulfated	250 mg once weekly	Intra-articular
	1 mg/kg q5days	IM
Gonadotropin-releasing hormone	0.05 mg 2 and 0.5 hours prebreeding for low libido	sc
	0.04 mg 6 hours prebreeding to induce ovulation	IM
Griseofulvin	10 g/450 kg s.i.d. for 2 weeks, then 5 g s.i.d. for 7 weeks	p.o.
Guaifenesin (5–10%)	To effect (approx 50–110 mg/kg needed for induction)	Slow IV
	5% with 4.4 mg/kg thiamylal	Rapid IV
Heparin	10 IU/kg loading dose	IV
	15 IU/kg per hour maintenance	Slow IV
	40–100 IU/kg b.i.d. or q.i.d. for acute laminitis	IV
	20–90 IU/kg for peritonitis prevention	sc
Heparin calcium	150 IU/kg loading dose, then 125 IU/kg b.i.d. for 6 doses, then 100 IU/kg	sc
Heparin sodium	40–80 IU/kg	IV
	2 hours later, 40 IU/kg, then 40 IU/kg b.i.d.	sc
Heparin (low-molecular-weight)	50 IU/kg b.i.d.	sc
Human chorionic gonadotrophin	2000 IU to synchronize ovulation	IV
Hyaluronate Na	10–50 mg/joint (see manufacturer's recommendations)	Intra-articular
	500 mg q4days for 7 doses	IM
Hyaluronic acid	20–120 mg locally around inflamed tendon	
	20–50 mg	Intra-articular
Hydralazine	0.5 mg/kg	IV
Hydrochlorothiazide	250 mg/450 kg s.i.d.	p.o.
Hydrocortisone sodium succinate	1–4 mg/kg	IV drip
Hydroxyzine HCl	0.5–1 mg/kg b.i.d.	IM or p.o.
Idoxuridine 0.1%	q2–6h	Ophthalmic
Imidocarb diproprionate	2 mg/kg s.i.d. for 2 days for *Babesia caballi*	IM
	4 mg/kg q3days for 4 treatments for *Babesia equi*	IM
Imipramine	100–600 mg b.i.d. for 2 weeks to improve ejaculation	p.o.
	0.55 mg/kg t.i.d.	IM or IV
	1.5 mg/kg t.i.d.	p.o.
Insulin	0.5 IU/kg	IM or sc
Insulin—protamine zinc	0.15 IU/kg b.i.d.	IM or sc
Iodide Na	20–40 mg/kg s.i.d. for several weeks	p.o.

Name of Drug	Dose	Route
Iodochlorhydroxyquin	10 g/450 kg (repeat for 3–4 days then gradually reduce dose if response is obtained)	p.o.
Ipratropium	2–3 mcg/kg	Inhalation
Iron cacodylate	1 g	IV
Isoflupredone acetate	10–14 mg	IM
Isoniazid	5–20 mg/kg s.i.d.	p.o.
Isoproterenol HCl	0.4 mcg/kg by slow infusion (discontinue when heart rate doubles)	IV
	0.05–1 mcg/kg per minute for foal resuscitation	IV
Isoproterenol (0.05%)	5–10 ml/50 kg q.i.d.	Aerosol
Isoxsuprine HCl	0.4–1.2 mg/kg b.i.d.	IM
Intraconazole	3 mg/kg b.i.d. for up to 2 months	p.o.
Ivermectin	0.2 mg/kg	p.o.
	0.2 mg/kg twice at 4-day intervals for lice and mange	p.o.
Kanamycin	7.5 mg/kg t.i.d.	IV or IM
	1–2 g	Intrauterine
Kaopectate	2–4 qt/450 kg b.i.d.	p.o.
Ketamine	See xylazine and detomidine	
Ketoconazole	30 mg/kg s.i.d. or b.i.d. (dissolve in 0.2 N HCl)	p.o.
Ketoprofen	2.2 mg/kg	IV or IM
Lactulose	0.2 ml/kg b.i.d.	p.o.
Levallorphan tartrate	0.02–0.04 mg/kg	IV
Levamisole	8–11 mg/kg s.i.d.	p.o.
Levothyroxine	10 mg in 70 ml Karo syrup s.i.d.	p.o.
Lidocaine	0.2–0.5 mg/kg bolus q5min up to 1.5 mg/kg total dose	IV
	1.3 mg/kg bolus over 5 minutes, then 0.05 mg/kg per minute for up to 24 hours for treatment of ileus	IV
Lime sulfur	3–5%	Topical
Lindane	3% spray	Topical
Loperamide	0.1–0.2 mg/kg q.i.d.	p.o.
Magnesium hydroxide	200–250 ml t.i.d. (antacid)	p.o.
Magnesium sulfate	0.2–1 g/kg dissolved in 4 L warm water s.i.d.	p.o.
	4 mg/kg boluses q2min up to 50 mg/kg total dose	IV
Malathion	0.5% wash, 5% dust	Topical
Mannitol (20%)	0.25–2.0 g/kg	Slow IV
Mebendazole	8.8 mg/kg	p.o.
	20 mg/kg s.i.d. for 5 days for *Dictyocaulus arnfieldi*	p.o.
	50 mg/kg s.i.d. for 5 days for onchocerciasis	p.o.
Meclofenamic acid	2.2 mg/kg b.i.d.	p.o.
Megestrol acetate	65–85 mg/kg s.i.d.	p.o.
Meperidine	See acepromazine	
Metaclopramide HCl	10 mg/kg	IV
Methadone	0.05–0.2 mg/kg	IV
Methetharimide	10–20 mg/kg	IV
Methicillin	25 mg/kg q4–6h	IM
	100 mg	Subconjunctival
Methionine (DL)	20–50 mg/kg	p.o.
Methocarbamol	5–55 mg/kg q.i.d.	Slow IV
	40–300 mg/kg for convulsions	Slow IV
Methoxychlor	0.5% wash	Topical
Methylcellulose flakes	0.25–0.5 kg/450 kg in 10 L water	p.o.
Methylene blue	8.8 mg/kg as 1% solution	IV
Methylprednisolone		
acetate	0.2–0.7 mg/kg	IM
sodium succinate	2–4 mg/kg	IV
	30 mg/kg, then 5.4 mg/kg per hour for 23 hours for CNS trauma	IV
	20 mg	Subconjunctival
	Up to 100 mg	Intrabursal or intra-articular
Methylsulfonylmethane	30 g/450 kg s.i.d.	p.o.
Methysulfmethoxine	15–20 mg/kg s.i.d.	p.o.
Metoclopramide	0.25 mg/kg t.i.d. or q.i.d.	IV drip or sc
	0.6 mg/kg q4h	p.o.
Metronidazole	15 mg/kg q.i.d.	IV or p.o.
Mezlocillin	25–75 mg/kg q.i.d.	IV
Miconazole (1% IV soln.)	q2–6h	Ophthalmic
Midazolam	0.05–0.2 mg/kg	IV or IM
Mineral oil	10 ml/kg s.i.d.	p.o.
Minocycline	3 mg/kg b.i.d.	p.o.
Misoprostol	1–4 mcg/kg s.i.d.	p.o.
Morphine sulfate	0.2–0.4 mg/kg	IM
	0.25–0.75 mg/kg	IV
Moxalactam	50 mg/kg t.i.d.	IV or IM
Moxidectin	0.4 mg/kg	p.o.
Nafcillin	10 mg/kg q.i.d.	IM
Naloxone	0.01–0.02 mg/kg	IV

Table continued on following page

Name of Drug	Dose	Route
Naproxen	10 mg/kg s.i.d. or b.i.d.	p.o. or IV
Natamycin 5%	q1–2h for 3 days, then reduce frequency	Ophthalmic
Neomycin	1 g/horse q.i.d.	p.o.
	2 g/horse b.i.d.	p.o.
	0.5 g/foal q.i.d.	p.o.
	1.5 g/foal b.i.d.	p.o.
	3–4 g	Intrauterine
	5 mg/kg t.i.d. for 2 days to reduce ammonia production in the bowel	p.o.
Neostigmine	0.004–0.02 mg/kg	sc
Netilmicin	2 mg/kg b.i.d.–t.i.d.	IV or IM
Niclosamide	100 mg/kg	p.o.
Nitrofurantoin	3 mg/kg b.i.d.	IM
Nizatidine	6.6 mg/kg t.i.d.	p.o.
Norepinephrine	0.01 mg/kg	IM
Nystatin	500,000 IU in 30 ml saline s.i.d. for 7–10 days	Intrauterine
Omeprazole	1.5 mg/kg s.i.d.	IV
Ouabain	2.5–3 mg/450 kg q2h until heart rate slows or intoxication develops. Do not exceed 10 g total	IV
Oxacillin	25–50 mg/kg b.i.d. or t.i.d.	IV or IM
Oxfendazole	10 mg/kg	p.o.
Oxibendazole	10–15 mg/kg	p.o.
	15 mg/kg for *Strongyloides westeri*	p.o.
Oxymorphone	0.02–0.03 mg/kg	IM
Oxytetracycline	5–20 mg/kg s.i.d.	IV
Oxytocin	2.5–5 IU/450 kg as bolus q20min	IV
	80–100 IU in 500 ml saline	Slow IV
	10–20 IU/450 kg	IM or IV
	1–3 IU/450 kg for milk letdown	IV
	0.5–10 IU/kg to induce parturition	IV
Pancuronium	0.04–0.066 mg/kg	IV
Paromomycin	100 mg/kg s.i.d.	p.o.
Penicillamine D	3–4 mg/kg q.i.d. for 10 days	p.o.
Penicillin G		
Na	10,000–50,000 IU/kg q.i.d.	IV or IM
K	10,000–50,000 IU/kg q.i.d.	IV or IM
	20,000 IU/kg q.i.d.	p.o.
	5 × 10⁶ IU	Intrauterine
procaine	20–50,000 IU/kg b.i.d. or t.i.d.	IM
benzathine	10,000–40,000 IU/kg q48–72h	IM
Penicillin V	110,000 mg/kg b.i.d.–q.i.d.	p.o.
Pentazocine	0.8 mg/kg	IV
Pentobarbital	2–20 mg/kg for convulsions	IV
Pentosan sulfate	250 mg q7–10days	Intra-articular
Pentoxifylline	8.4 mg/kg b.i.d.	p.o.
Pentylenetetrazol	6–10 mg/kg	IV
Pergolide	1–5 mg/horse s.i.d.	p.o.
Perphenazine	0.3–0.5 mg/kg b.i.d.	p.o.
Phenobarbital	5–25 mg/kg in 30 ml saline for convulsing foals	IV over 30 minutes
	9 mg/kg t.i.d. for maintenance	IV
Phenothiazine	55 mg/kg	p.o.
	27.5 mg/kg with piperazine	p.o.
Phenoxybenzamine HCl	0.7–1 mg/kg in 500 ml saline t.i.d. or q.i.d.	IV
Phenylbutazone	2–4.4 mg/kg b.i.d.	p.o. or IV
Phenylephrine	10%	Ophthalmic
Phenytoin	5–10 mg/kg for convulsing foals	IV
	1–5 mg/kg for maintenance q4h	IV, IM, or p.o.
	10–22 mg/kg b.i.d. for digoxin-induced arrhythmias	p.o.
Physostigmine	0.1–0.6 mg/kg	IM or slow IV
Pilocarpine HCl	4% gel b.i.d.–q.i.d.	Ophthalmic
Piperazine	88–110 mg/kg	p.o.
Pipercillin	15–50 mg/kg b.i.d.–q.i.d.	IV or IM
Pirbuterol	1–2 mcg/kg	Inhalation
Polymixin B or E	5000–10,000 IU/kg q.i.d.	p.o.
	1 × 10⁶ IU	Intrauterine
Potassium chloride	40 g in 4–6 L water b.i.d.	p.o.
	20–40 mEq/L of fluid	IV
Potassium iodide	2–20 g s.i.d.	p.o.
Potassium permanganate	1% solution for mouthwash	
Pralidoxime chloride	20–50 mg/kg	Slow IV or IM
Prednisolone	0.2–4.4 mg/kg s.i.d. or b.i.d.	p.o. or IM
Na succinate	2–5 mg/kg for septic shock	IV
acetate	1% q3–8h	Ophthalmic
Prednisone	0.02–4.4 mg/kg b.i.d.	IM or p.o.
	2 mg/kg s.i.d., immunosuppressive dose	p.o.

Name of Drug	Dose	Route
Primidone	1–2 g/foal b.i.d.–q.i.d.	p.o.
Procainamide	35 mg/kg	p.o.
Progesterone	150 mg s.i.d. to suppress estrus	IM
	300 mg s.i.d. to maintain pregnancy	IM
repositol	1000 mg/450 kg once weekly for abortion prevention	IM
Promazine	0.25–1 mg/kg	IV
	1–2 mg/kg granules	p.o.
Propafenone	0.5–1.0 mg/kg	IV
Propantheline bromide	0.014 mg/kg	IV
Proparacaine	0.5%	Ophthalmic
Propofol	2.4 mg/kg for anesthesia induction in foals, then 0.3 mg/kg per minute for maintenance	IV
Propranolol	0.38–0.78 mg/kg t.i.d.	p.o.
	0.05–0.16 mg/kg b.i.d.	IV
Propylene glycol (5%)	3 ml/50 kg	Aerosol
Prostaglandin $F_2\alpha$	10 mg	IM
Prostalene	2 mg/450 kg, 2 doses 2 weeks apart	sc
Psyllium mucilloid	1 g/kg s.i.d.–q.i.d.	p.o.
Pyrantel		
tartrate	2.64 mg/kg s.i.d. for control of intestinal nematodes	p.o.
pamoate	6.6 mg/kg	p.o.
	13.2 mg/kg for tapeworms	p.o.
Pyrilamine maleate	1 mg/kg	IV, IM, or sc
Pyrimethamine	0.25 mg/kg b.i.d. for 3 days then s.i.d. for 27 days (for equine protozoal myeloencephalitis)	p.o.
Quinidine sulfate	22 mg/kg q2–6h	p.o.
gluconate	2.2 mg/kg q10min until 8–10 mg/kg total	IV
	0.7–3 mg/kg per hour	IV
Ranitidine	6.6 mg/kg t.i.d.	p.o.
	1.5 mg/kg t.i.d.	IV
Reserpine	2–5 mg/kg s.i.d.	p.o.
Rifampin	10–20 mg/kg s.i.d.	p.o.
	3–5 mg/kg b.i.d. with erythromycin for *Rhodococcus equi*	p.o.
Romifidine	0.08–1.0 mg/kg	IV
Ronnel	2.5% spray	Topical
Saline (hypertonic)	7.5%, 4 ml/kg for hypovolemia	IV over 20 minutes
Selenium (Na selenite)	5.5 mg/450 kg	IM
Sodium bicarbonate	30–150 g/day	p.o.
Sodium hypochlorite	0.5%	Topical
Sodium iodide	20–40 mg/kg s.i.d.	p.o.
Sodium sulfate	Up to 3 g/kg dissolved in warm water	p.o.
Sodium thiosulfate (20%)	0.22 ml/kg	Slow IV
Spectinomycin	20 mg/kg t.i.d.	IM
Stanozolol	0.5 mg/kg, up to 4 doses q1–2weeks	IM
Stilbestrol	30 mg/450 kg	IM
Stirofos	1% wash	Topical
Streptomycin	11 mg/kg b.i.d.	IM or sc
Sucralfate	1–4 g b.i.d.–q.i.d.	p.o.
Sulfonamides	100–200 mg/kg on day 1, then 50–100 mg/kg subsequently (check labels on each product)	IV, IM, or sc
Sulfonamides, potentiated	30 mg/kg b.i.d. or t.i.d.	p.o.
Suprofen 1%	b.i.d.–t.i.d.	Ophthalmic
Terbutaline	0.02–0.06 mg/kg b.i.d.	IV, p.o., or inhalation
Tetanus antitoxin	100 IU/kg q3–5days for treatment of tetanus	IM, sc, or IV
Tetracycline	6.6–11 mg/kg b.i.d.	IV
Tetramethrin	0.4% solution, wipe-on	Topical
Theophylline	1 mg/kg q.i.d.	p.o.
Thiabendazole	44 mg/kg	p.o.
	88 mg/kg for *Parascaris equorum*	p.o.
	440 mg/kg s.i.d. for 2 days for verminous arteritis	p.o.
	4% solution in saline or 90% DMSO	Topical
Thiamine HCl	0.5–5 mg/kg	IM
Thiamylal Na	2–4 mg/kg	IV
Thiopental	4–10 mg/kg as 10% solution	IV
Thyroxine L	0.01 mg/kg s.i.d.	p.o.
Ticarcillin	40–80 mg/kg t.i.d.	IV or IM
	6 g	Intrauterine
clavulamate	50 mg/kg t.i.d.–q.i.d.	IV
Ticarcillin/clavulanic acid	6 g/200 mg	Intrauterine
Timolol maleate	0.5% b.i.d.	Ophthalmic
Tobramycin	1–1.7 mg/kg t.i.d. (human dose)	IV or IM
	10–30 mg	Subconjunctival
Tocopherol acetate	6000 IU/250–500 kg s.i.d.	p.o.

Table continued on following page

Name of Drug	Dose	Route
Tolazoline	0.5 mg/kg	IV
Toxaphene	0.5% wash	Topical
Tranexamic acid	1 g	IV
Triamcinolone	0.02–0.1 mg/kg	IM
	(40 mg/ml), 0.25 ml, q2–4days	Subconjunctival
	1–3 mg/site up to 18 mg total	Intralesional
Trichlorfon	40 mg/kg	p.o.
Trichlormethiazide	200 mg/450 kg	p.o.
Trifluorothymidine 1%	q1–2h	Ophthalmic
Triflupromazine	0.2–2.0 mg/kg	IV
Trifluridine 1%	q2–6h	Ophthalmic
Trimethoprim-sulfadiazine	15 mg/kg b.i.d.	IV
	15–30 mg/kg b.i.d.	p.o.
	2.5–5 g s.i.d.	Intrauterine
Tripelennamine HCl	1 mg/kg	IV or IM
Tromethamine	300 mg/kg	IV
Tropicamide	0.5–1%	Ophthalmic
Tylosin	10 mg/kg b.i.d.	IM
Vancomycin	20–40 mg/kg b.i.d.–q.i.d.	IV or p.o.
Verapamil	0.025–0.5 mg/kg q30 min	IV
Vinegar	250 ml/450 kg s.i.d. for enterolith prevention	p.o.
Vitamin C	See Ascorbic acid	
Vitamin E	1500–2000 IU s.i.d. for equine degenerative myeloencephalopathy prophylaxis	p.o.
	6000–9000 IU s.i.d. for treatment of equine degenerative myeloencephalopathy	p.o.
Vitamin K_1	0.5–1 mg/kg q4–6h for warfarin toxicosis	sc
	1–2 mg/kg (divided at several sites) for sweet clover poisoning	sc
	0.5–2 mg/kg for foals	IM
Xylazine	0.2–1.1 mg/kg	IV
	0.33–0.44 mg/kg followed by 0.033–0.066 mg/kg butorphanol	IV
	1.1 mg/kg followed by 1.76–2.2 mg/kg ketamine	IV
	0.6 mg/kg with 0.02 mg/kg acepromazine	IV
	0.66 mg/kg to ejaculate ex-copula	IV
Yohimbine	0.12 mg/kg for xylazine or detomidine antagonism	Slow IV
	0.075 mg/kg to restore intestinal motility	IV

This table was composed from doses recommended by authors in this and previous editions of *Current Therapy in Equine Medicine*. It is recommended that the manufacturer's literature be checked before a drug is used. Many drugs have not been approved for use in horses.

IM = intramuscular; IV = intravenous; p.o. = by mouth; sc = subcutaneous

Appendix 2: Normal Clinical Pathology Data

BRUCE W. PARRY
Werribee, Australia

DUANE F. BROBST
Pullman, Washington

In many clinical cases, evaluation of laboratory tests is a useful adjunct to a carefully collected history and clinical examination. The following laboratory data are derived from the veterinary literature. Clinicians must be aware that these reference values may not be directly applicable to their laboratory data. Differences in reference ("normal") values may arise because of differences in the population of animals studied (e.g., geographic location, age, breed, sex) and the methodology of the test (e.g., reagents, reaction temperatures, equipment). The following data, nevertheless, serve as a guide to results expected in a population of normal animals.

HEMATOLOGY: GENERAL COMMENTS

Horses are usually grouped as hot-blooded or cold-blooded. The former are those of Arabian ancestry, including Arabians, Quarterhorses, Standardbreds, and Thoroughbreds. Cold-blooded horses are draught-type animals, including Clydesdales, Percherons, Shires, and others. The latter group have somewhat lower reference value limits for erythrocyte (RBC) parameters, but similar leukocyte (WBC) data. Warm-blooded horses, such as Hannoverians and Trakeheners and ponies, are more similar to hot-blooded than cold-blooded horses in their hematology values.

Important points to remember about equine hematology are:

1. The equine spleen dramatically alters venous packed cell volume (PCV). For example, excitement and exercise readily cause splenic contraction and a "relative" (physiologic) polycythemia. In contrast, various tranquilizers, such as acepromazine, cause splenic relaxation and an "apparent" anemia.

2. Foals (younger than about 9 months of age) tend to have lower PCV and mean corpuscular volume (MCV) values than adults. Their mean corpuscular hemoglobin concentration is, however, comparable.

3. From a practical viewpoint:

   a. Males and females have virtually the same RBC and WBC parameters.

   b. Hemoglobin concentration, PCV, and RBC count tend to increase during pregnancy.

   c. Seasonal differences, although reported, are not routinely considered in hematologic evaluations.

4. In contrast to many other species, horses do not have circulating reticulocytes under "resting" conditions or in response to an anemia. The bone marrow response to anemia is most easily assessed by measuring PCV at 3- to 5-day intervals. Alternatively, the "new generation" cell counters, which are able to plot a RBC histogram and determine an index of anisocytosis, may assist in the early evaluation of anemias in the horse, because these parameters are likely to be increased in the circulating population of RBC in a regenerative anemia.

HEMATOLOGY—ADULT HOT-BLOODED HORSES

| | Units | Lumsden et al (1980) | | Jain (1986) |
		Thoroughbred Mares	Standardbreds	Hot-blooded Horses
Hb	g/dl	10.9–18.8	11.3–17.9	11.0–19.0
	g/L	109–188	113–179	110–190
PCV	%	29–53	31–48	32–53
	L/L	0.29–0.53	0.31–0.48	0.32–0.53
RCC	×10⁶/µl	6.5–11.6	6.9–10.7	6.8–12.9
	×10¹²/L	6.5–11.6	6.9–10.7	6.8–12.9
MCV	fl	39–49	40–49	37–59
MCHC	g/dl	33.7–38.6	35.0–41.0	31.0–38.6
	g/L	337–386	350–410	310–386
Leukocytes	/µl	5300–11,000	4900–10,000	5400–14,300
	×10⁹/L	5.3–11.0	4.9–10.0	5.4–14.3

Table continued on following page

HEMATOLOGY—ADULT HOT-BLOODED HORSES *Continued*

		Lumsden et al (1980)		Jain (1986)
		Thoroughbred Mares	**Standardbreds**	**Hot-blooded Horses**
Band neutrophils	/μl	0–200	0–400	0–1000
	×10⁹/L	0–0.2	0–0.4	0–1.0
Segmented neutrophils	/μl	2100–6000	2000–5500	2260–8580
	×10⁹/L	2.1–6.0	2.0–5.5	2.3–8.6
Lymphocytes	/μl	1700–5000	1600–4600	1500–7700
	×10⁹/L	1.7–5.0	1.6–4.6	1.5–7.7
Monocytes	/μl	0–600	0–600	0–1000
	×10⁹/L	0–0.6	0–0.6	0–1.0
Eosinophils	/μl	0–800	0–700	0–1000
	×10⁹/L	0–0.8	0–0.7	0–1.0
Basophils	/μl	0–100	0–100	0–290
	×10⁹/L	0–0.1	0–0.1	0–0.3
Platelets	/μl	80,000–397,000	81,000–240,000	100,000–350,000
	×10⁹/L	80–397	81–240	100–350
RBCIA°	fl	16–24		
Refractometer protein	g/dl		5.4–7.5	
	g/L		54–75	
Fibrinogen	mg/dl		150–380	
	g/L		1.5–3.8	

°Weiser (1982): RBC index of anisocytosis (IA).
Hb = hemoglobin; PCV = packed cell volume; RCC = red cell count; MCV = mean corpuscular volume; MCHC = mean corpuscular hemoglobin concentration

HEMATOLOGY—HOT-BLOODED FOALS

		Age			
		1 Day	**1 Week**	**1 Month**	**6 Months**
Hb	g/dl	11.7–16.5	11.8–17.6	10.9–15.6	10.8–14.0
	g/L	117–165	118–176	109–156	108–140
PCV	%	34–46	31–44	28–42	31–41
	L/L	0.34–0.46	0.31–0.44	0.28–0.42	0.31–0.41
RCC	×10⁶/μl	8.8–11.0	7.8–9.6	8.0–10.9	8.6–10.7
	×10¹²/L	8.8–11.0	7.8–9.6	8.0–10.9	8.6–10.7
MCV	fl	37–49	35–42	35–39	32–40
MCHC	g/dl	31–38	35–40	33–39	34–39
	g/L	310–380	350–400	330–390	340–390
Leukocytes	/μl	4500–11,500	7200–13,500	4600–12,900	7400–10,800
	×10⁹/L	4.5–11.5	7.2–13.5	4.6–12.9	7.4–10.8
Neutrophils	/μl	3040–9570	5020–10,720	1720–9740	2890–5560
	×10⁹/L	3.0–9.6	5.0–10.7	1.7–9.7	2.9–5.6
Lymphocytes	/μl	630–2060	1040–3800	1780–9740	3200–6910
	×10⁹/L	0.6–2.1	1.0–3.8	1.8–9.7	3.2–6.9
Monocytes	/μl	50–380	20–430	50–710	40–590
	×10⁹/L	0.05–0.4	0.02–0.4	0.05–0.7	0.04–0.6
Eosinophils	/μl	0–108	0–134	0–540	42–728
	×10⁹/L	0–0.1	0–0.1	0–0.5	0.04–0.7
Basophils	/μl	0–35	0–238	0–129	0–74
	×10⁹/L	0–0.04	0–0.2	0–0.1	0–0.07
Platelets	/μl	125,000–390,000	98,000–385,000	135,000–458,000	187,000–405,000
	×10⁹/L	125–390	98–385	135–458	187–405
Refractometer protein	g/dl	5.1–7.7	5.1–7.5	5.6–7.8	6.2–7.0
	g/L	51–77	51–75	56–78	62–70
Fibrinogen	mg/dl	110–450	160–420	230–710	160–490
	g/L	1.1–4.5	1.6–4.2	2.3–7.1	1.6–4.9

From Harvey JW, Asquith RL, McNulty PK, et al: Haematology of foals up to one year old. Equine Vet J 16:347, 1984.
Hb = hemoglobin, PCV = packed cell volume, RCC = red cell count, MCV = mean corpuscular volume, MCHC = mean corpuscular hemoglobin concentration

Coagulation Tests

Activated Partial Thromboplastin Time (APTT) and Prothrombin Time (PT)

Results for these tests may vary greatly depending on the methodology and reagents used. It is important that the laboratory performing the tests be familiar with results expected for equine specimens. Ideally, an equine control pool specimen will be processed concurrently. APTT has been reported as 47 to 73 seconds (Dorner and Bass, 1974) and 36 to 47 seconds (Meyers et al, 1982). PT has been reported as 9.7 to 11.7 seconds (Dorner and Bass, 1974) and 8.0 to 12.4 seconds (Meyers et al, 1982). An alternative approach to attempt to standardize results is to calculate the ratio of the patient and control pool values. Using such a method, normal APTT and PT are reported as 0.75 to 1.25 (Johnstone and Crane, 1986). Values (ratios) higher than 1.25 are increased (prolonged).

A prolonged APTT with a normal PT indicates a deficiency of one (or more) of the factors in the intrinsic pathway, namely high molecular weight kininogen; prekallikrein; and factors XII, XI, IX, or VIII. A prolonged PT with a normal APTT indicates a deficiency of factor VII (in the extrinsic pathway). A prolonged APTT and PT indicates a deficiency of one (or more) of the factors in the intrinsic and extrinsic pathways or the common pathway. It is most likely to be an "acquired" disorder with several factors decreased in concentration. It may be associated with anticoagulant administration (e.g., heparin) or poisoning (e.g., vitamin K antagonists), or with disseminated intravascular coagulation (DIC).

Antithrombin III (ATIII)

ATIII activity may decrease in animals with a protein-losing glomerulopathy or those with DIC. It has been advocated as a prognostic guide in colic cases. Reference values for ATIII are 75 to 126% (Stephens et al, 1984).

Fibrin Degradation Products (FDP)

FDP concentration increases in cases with DIC. FDP concentration has been advocated as a prognostic guide in colic cases. Reference values for FDP are less than 10 μg/ ml (Meyers et al, 1982) and less than 20 μg/ml (Johnstone and Crane, 1986).

Specific Factors

With the exception of fibrinogen (see later), analysis of specific coagulation factors is seldom undertaken in clinical practice. It is warranted if a congenital coagulopathy is suspected.

Proteins

Serum Protein Electrophoresis

Serum protein electrophoresis is useful in the investigation of cases with marked hypoproteinemia and (especially) hyperproteinemia.

Immunoglobulins

Failure of passive transfer is a common entity in foals. Various methods are available for assessment of immunoglobulin transfer in the neonate (see page 581). Failure of passive transfer is usually regarded as confirmed by a serum immunoglobulin G value less than 200 mg/dl (<2.0 g/L) at 24 hours of age. Adequate passive transfer is considered at a value greater than 800 mg/dl (>8.0 g/L). Colostrum with IgG concentration less than 1000 mg/dl leads to failure of passive transfer.

Specific immunoglobulin concentrations have been reported for foals of various ages and for adult horses. They are infrequently measured in clinical practice.

Fibrinogen

Fibrinogen is the last factor in the coagulation cascade. It is also an "acute phase reactant" protein (one that increases in concentration in response to inflammation). It is often measured to confirm the presence of an inflammatory reaction, especially when the leukogram is equivocal in this regard. It may be assessed in relation to total plasma protein (TPP) concentration.

A TPP/fibrinogen ratio higher than 15:1 suggests that the increase is due to dehydration. A TPP/fibrinogen ratio of 10:1 or less suggests that the increase is due to inflammation.

SERUM PROTEIN ELECTROPHORESIS

		Lumsden et al (1980)			Matthews (1982) 1-year-old or Older
		Thoroughbred Mares	Standardbreds Various Ages	Thoroughbred Foals	
Protein, total	g/dl	5.7–7.4	5.3–7.4	5.0–6.1	5.3–7.9
	g/L	57–74	53–74	50–61	53–79
Albumin	g/dl	2.9–3.6	2.7–3.4	2.6–3.2	2.3–3.7
	g/L	29–36	27–34	26–32	23–37
Globulins, total	g/dl	2.6–4.1	2.2–4.3	2.2–3.2	
	g/L	26–41	22–43	22–32	
Albumin/globulin ratio		0.7–1.2	0.7–1.3	0.8–1.5	
Globulin fractions:					
Alpha-1	g/dl	0.5–1.4	0.7–1.7	0.7–1.2	0.4–0.9
	g/L	5–14	7–17	7–12	4–9
Alpha-2	g/dl				0.3–1.0
	g/L				3–10

Table continued on following page

SERUM PROTEIN ELECTROPHORESIS *Continued*

		Lumsden et al (1980)			Matthews (1982) 1-year-old or Older
		Thoroughbred Mares	Standardbreds Various Ages	Thoroughbred Foals	
Beta-1	g/dl	0.9–1.8	0.6–2.0	0.9–1.2	0.2–1.6
	g/L	9–18	6–20	9–12	2–16
Beta-2	g/dl				0.2–0.9
	g/L				2–9
Gamma-1	g/dl	0.6–1.4	0.8–1.6	0.4–1.0	0.1–0.4
	g/L	6–14	8–16	4–10	1–4
Gamma-2	g/dl				0.3–0.9
	g/L				3–9

Agarose gel electrophoresis.
Foals were 1–6 months old.

GASTROINTESTINAL SYSTEM (INCLUDING THE LIVER)

Liver Function Tests

If a chronic hepatopathy is suspected, it is appropriate to assess liver function before performing a liver biopsy. Such test results are likely to be abnormal when more than 70% of the functional hepatic mass has been lost.

Dye Clearance Studies

Two cholephilic dyes have been used: Bromosulphalein (BSP) and indocyanine green (ICG). They are administered by intravenous injection. Thereafter, at least three blood samples are taken from the contralateral jugular vein, usually between 5 and 12 to 15 minutes. Consult your local laboratory for the protocol used.

Note that prolonged fasting (3 days) may lengthen dye clearance times. Under such circumstances, BSP half time (T 1/2) was 3.7 to 5.9 minutes and ICG T 1/2 was 5.1 to 44.7 minutes (Engelking et al, 1985).

BSP CLEARANCE

Engelking and coworkers (1985) used 4.4 to 5.1 mg/kg body weight (bwt) BSP. The T 1/2 was 2.2 to 4.1 minutes.

ICG CLEARANCE

Engelking and coworkers (1985) used 0.8 to 1.1 mg/kg bwt ICG. The T 1/2 was 5.4 to 13.8 minutes.

Parry and coworkers (1989) used 45 mg ICG/horse (400–500 kg bwt). The T 1/2 was 3.1 to 6.9 minutes.

Bile Acids

Assessment of serum bile acid concentration (and a bile acid tolerance test) may be an alternative to the previously described regimen. Decreased liver function may be associated with increased serum bile acid concentrations. Plasma ammonia concentration may also increase with decreased liver function. However, because the plasma concentration increases after collection, it is probably less useful in clinical practice.

Serum Lipids and Lipoproteins

Watson and coworkers (1991) provide a good introduction to various lipid and lipoprotein reference values for horses and ponies. Values are infrequently measured in clinical practice, but may be useful to confirm hyperlipemia in ponies and hyperlipidemia in horses.

ROUTINE BIOCHEMISTRY TESTS—ADULT HORSES

			Lumsden et al (1980)		Other Studies
			Thoroughbred	Standardbred	
Enzymes					
AP (ALP)	U/L	37°C	26–92	24–67	
AST (SGOT)	U/L	37°C	141–330	123–789	
Amylase	U/L	37°C			14–35°
	Caraway U/L	37°C	120–1400	410–1200	
GGT	U/L	30°C			4–44†
	U/L	37°C			9–29°
LDH	U/L	30°C	81–225	74–206	
	U/L	37°C	137–381	125–349	
Lipase	U/L	37°C			23–87°
Sorbitol (iditol) dehydrogenase	U/L	30°C	<5		
(SDH)	U/L	37°C	<6		3–13†

ROUTINE BIOCHEMISTRY TESTS—ADULT HORSES *Continued*

| | | Lumsden et al (1980) | | |
		Thoroughbred	Standardbred	Others
Nonenzymes				
Ammonia	μg/dl			0–56§
Fasting	μmol/L			0–33
Bile acids	μg/ml			0.2–4.5‖
Fasting	μmol/L			0.5–11.4
Bilirubin				
Total	mg/dl	0.9–2.6	0.9–2.9	
	μmol/L	15–45	15–50	
Unconjugated (U)	mg/dl	0.3–1.7	0.6–2.5	
	μmol/L	5–29	10–43	
Conjugated (C)	mg/dl	0.2–0.8	0.2–0.7	
	μmol/L	3–14	3–12	
U/C ratio	No units	0.7–4.5	0.4–7.5	
Cholesterol	mg/dl	73–138	61–112	
	mmol/L	1.89–3.57	1.58–2.90	
Glucose	mg/dl	69–150	63–101	
	mmol/L	3.8–8.3	3.5–5.6	

°Parry and Crisman (1991)
†Gossett and French (1984)
‡Horney et al (1993)
§Ogilvie et al (1985)
‖Hoffman al (1987)
AP = alkaline phosphatase; AST = aspartate aminotransferase; GGT = gamma glutamyltransferase; LDH = lactate dehydrogenase

ROUTINE BIOCHEMISTRY TESTS—FOALS

| | | Gossett and French (1984) | | | |
		Temp.	0.5–3 days	2–3 wks	5–7 wks
GGT	U/L	30°C	0–94	0–146	0–48
SDH	U/L	RT	0.2–3.8	0–5.3	0–1.5

| | | Schmitz et al (1982) | | | |
		1–2 days	1–2 wks	4–5 wks	6 mo
AP	U/L	30°C	530–2611	347–787	284–734	176–348
	U/L	37°C	1104–5440	723–1640	592–1529	367–725
AST	U/L	30°C	24–123	74–229	101–201	111–178
	U/L	37°C	34–176	106–327	144–287	159–254
Total	mg/dl		0.8–5.8	1.0–3.4	0.6–2.4	0.5–1.7
bilirubin	μmol/L		13–99	17–57	10–41	8–29

| | | Bauer et al (1984) | | | |
		1 day	1 wk	1 mo	6 mo
Unconjugated	mg/dl	0.4–2.8	0.4–1.6	0.2–0.6	0–0.7
bilirubin	μmol/L	7–48	7–27	3–10	0–12
Conjugated	mg/dl	0.2–1.4	0.1–0.9	0–0.7	0–0.7
bilirubin	μmol/L	3–24	2–15	0–12	0–12
Glucose	mg/dl	108–223	126–198	119–205	81–196
	mmol/L	6.0–12.4	7.0–11.0	6.6–11.4	4.5–10.9

AP = alkaline phosphatase; AST = aspartate aminotransferase; GGT = gamma glutamyltransferase; SDH = sorbitol dehydrogenase

ELECTROLYTES AND OSMOLALITY

The commonly measured electrolytes are sodium, potassium, and chloride. Calculation of the fractitional excretion of electrolytes (based on their plasma and urine concentrations) provides a guide to their homeostasis and to renal function.

Equine RBCs contain a high potassium concentration. Therefore, samples should be analyzed as soon as practical after collection, to minimize leakage from RBCs and an apparent (spurious) hyperkalemia. The latter may occur before obvious hemolysis.

Serum or plasma potassium concentration does not reliably reflect intracellular (body) status. Measurement of intraerythrocytic potassium concentration may provide a

better guide (Muylle et al, 1984a,b) and may be a useful adjunct to determining appropriate fluid therapy in horses with diarrhea and other causes of significant electrolyte loss.

A potassium challenge test has been suggested as a diagnostic aid for horses with suspected hyperkalemic periodic paralysis (Speir et al, 1990; Naylor et al, 1993).

Total CO_2 level is a reflection of the acid-base status of an animal. It is about 95% bicarbonate. The anion gap also provides an insight in acid-base balance. It may be calculated as:

$$\text{Anion gap} = ([Na] + [K]) - ([Cl] + [TCO_2])$$

or

$$\text{Anion gap} = ([Na] + [K]) - ([Cl] + [HCO_3])$$

ELECTROLYTES AND OSMOLALITY—ADULTS

		Lumsden et al (1980)		
		Thoroughbreds	Standardbreds	
Serum or Plasma				
Sodium (Na)	mEq/L	134–142	137–143	
	mmol/L	134–142	137–143	
Potassium (K)	mEq/L	2.1–4.2	2.9–4.4	
	mmol/L	2.1–4.2	2.9–4.4	
Na/K ratio		33–66	30–48	
Chloride (Cl)	mEq/L	94–106	96–102	
	mmol/L	94–106	96–102	
Calcium (Ca)	mg/dl	10.7–12.4	10.9–12.9	
	mmol/L	2.67–3.09	2.73–3.23	
Ionized calcium (Ca⁺⁺)	mg/dl			6.01–7.21°
	mmol/L			1.50–1.79
Phosphate (P$_i$)	mg/dl	1.1–4.4	2.2–4.2	
Ca/P$_i$ ratio	mmol/L	0.36–1.42	0.71–1.36	
		2.5–9.3	2–5	
Magnesium (Mg)	mg/dl	1.6–2.3	1.7–2.2	
	mmol/L	0.66–0.95	0.70–0.90	
Total CO_2	mEq/L			27–32†
	mmol/L			27–32
Anion gap	mEq/L			8–13†
	mmol/L			8–13
Osmolality‡	mosm/kg	279–296	281–292	
	mmol/kg	279–296	281–292	
RBC potassium				
High K group	mEq/L			90–104§
	mmol/L			90–104
Low K group	mEq/L			77–90
	mmol/L			77–90

°Kohn and Brooks (1990)
†Gossett and French (1983)
‡Lithium heparin as anticoagulant.
§Muylle et al (1984a). Horses were arbitrarily divided into high K (n = 394) and low K (n = 42) groups, because the data had a bimodal distribution, with a "section point" at 90 mEq/L (90 mmol/L).

ELECTROLYTES AND OSMOLALITY—FOALS

		Bauer et al (1984)			
		1 day	1 wk	1 mo	6 mo
Calcium (Ca)	mg/dl	9.6–13.6	11.2–13.6	11.0–13.4	10.2–13.4
	mmol/L	2.40–3.40	2.80–3.40	2.75–3.35	2.55–3.35
Phosphate (P$_i$)	mg/dl	3.8–7.4	5.4–9.4	4.9–9.3	4.8–7.6
	mmol/L	1.23–2.39	1.75–3.03	1.57–3.01	1.54–2.46
Ca/P$_i$ ratio (mean)		1.6	1.3	1.3	1.5
Sodium (Na)	mEq/L	132–156		Applicable	
	mmol/L	132–156		to all ages	
Potassium (K)	mEq/L	3.5–5.5		Applicable	
	mmol/L	3.5–5.5		to all ages	
Na/K ratio	(mean)	32.0			
Chloride (Cl)	mEq/L	94–114		Applicable	
	mmol/L	94–114		to all ages	
Total CO$_2$ (TCO$_2$)	mEq/L	21–33		Applicable	
	mmol/L	21–33		to all ages	
Anion gap	mEq/L	8–24	9–25	13–25	9–25
	mmol/L	8–24	9–25	13–25	9–25

Anion gap = ([Na] + [K]) − ([Cl] + [TCO$_2$]).

RESTING ACID-BASE AND BLOOD GAS VALUES

The specimen should be collected into a heparinized syringe, taking care to expel any air bubbles before "capping" the end of the needle and then placing the sample on ice (to keep it at 4°C) until it is analyzed (within 1–3 hours).

		Arterial		Venous
		Rose et al (1979)	Grandy et al (1987)	Rose et al (1979)
pH		7.347–7.475	7.387–7.419	7.345–7.433
PCO$_2$	mm Hg	36–46	42–47	38–48
PO$_2$	mm Hg	80–112	100–112	37–56
HCO$_3^-$	mEq/L	22–29		22–29
	mmol/L	22–29		22–29
Base	mEq/L	−2 to 4		−3 to 4
excess	mmol/L	−2 to 4		−3 to 4

With appropriate compensation in acid-base disorders, the following changes are likely to occur (Blackmore and Brobst, 1981; Brobst 1983):

Acute respiratory acidosis: [HCO$_3^-$] increases 1 mEq/L (1 mmol/L) for every 10-mmHg increase in PCO$_2$

Chronic respiratory acidosis: [HCO$_3^-$] increases 3 to 4 mEq/L (3–4 mmol/L) for every 10-mm Hg increase in PCO$_2$

Acute repiratory alkalosis: [HCO$_3^-$] decreases 1 to 3 mEq/L (1–3 mmol/L) for every 10-mm Hg decrease in PCO$_2$

Chronic respiratory alkalosis: [HCO$_3^-$] decreases 5 mEq/L (5 mmol/L) for every 10-mm Hg decrease in PCO$_2$

Metabolic acidosis: PCO$_2$ decreases 1.2 mm Hg for every 1-mEq/L (1-mmol/L) decrease in [HCO$_3^-$]

Metabolic alkalosis: PCO$_2$ increases 0.6 to 1 mm Hg for every 1-mEq/L (1 mmol/L) increase in [HCO$_3^-$]

URINARY SYSTEM

A water deprivation test may be performed to evaluate renal tubular concentrating ability. Horses deprived of water for 60 to 72 hours lost 12 to 16% of their body weight and had maximal urine specific gravities of 1.042 to 1.054, with urine osmolalities ranging from 1359 to 1844 mosm/kg and urine/serum osmolality ratios from 4.4 to 6.2 (Brobst and Bayly, 1982).

Fractional excretion (FE) of electrolytes, such as sodium, potassium, and chloride may be useful in the evaluation of renal function (Morris et al, 1984). Similarly, FE of calcium (Ca) and inorganic phosphate (P$_i$) may be useful guides to their dietary intake (Caple et al, 1982). Mares fed adequate Ca had FECa values greater than 2.5% and FEP$_i$ values less than 4%.

BIOCHEMISTRY

Test		Reference Values		Reference and Comments
		Thoroughbreds	Standardbreds	
Serum or Plasma				
Urea (BUN)	mg/dl	11–24	8–14	Lumsden et al (1980)
	mmol/L	4.0–8.6	2.8–5.0	
Creatinine	mg/dl	0.9–2.1	0.9–1.7	
	μmol/L	80–185	80–150	
Protein				Kohn and Strasser (1986)
Total	mg/kg/day	3.6–22.3		
Albumin	mg/kg/day	0.2–8.8		24-hour urine collection
Globulin	mg/kg/day	3.4–13.6		
Protein/creatinine ratio	No units	0.11–0.60		
	g/mmol	0.013–0.068		
Creatinine clearance	ml/min/kg	1.49–2.74		
Urine output	ml/kg/day	15–25		
Fractional Excretion (FE) Values		Morris et al (1984)	Genetzky et al (1987)	
Sodium (Na)	%	0–0.67	0.004–0.34	
Potassium (K)	%	24.0–53.0	22.7–59.3	
Chloride (Cl)	%	0.53–1.49	0.06–0.73	

Morris et al (1984). All values on 24-hour urine samples.
Morris et al (1984) and Kohn and Strasser (1986) reviewed the literature on creatinine clearance data in horses and ponies and reported clearance data for Na, K, Cl, Ca, and P_i.

URINALYSIS

	Horse	Foal
Gross appearance		
Color	Pale yellow to brown	
Viscosity	Viscous (mucoid)	
Transparency	Slightly turbid (turbidity increased by cooling)	
Specific gravity	1.006–1.050 (usually 1.020–1.050) Should be >1.020 if the blood urea concentration is increased	1.001–1.027
Dipstick-type chemistry values		
pH	7.0–9.0 (usually 7.5–8.5); may be <7.0 in suckling foals)	5.5–8.0
Protein°	None to possibly trace in concentrated urine	Negative to 30 mg/dl
Glucose	None	None
Ketones	None	
Bilirubin	None	
Blood	None	None to 2+
Sediment findings (microscopy)		
Mucus		None to abundant
Casts/LPF	None (possibly rare hyaline cast)	None
RBC/HPF	0–8	None
WBC/HPF	0–8	0–3 (sometimes clumps present)
Epithelial cells/HPF		Squamous cells: None to 2–3 (sometimes clumps present)
Sperm	May be present in stallion urine	
Bacteria	May be noted in free-catch samples, but not in catheterized or cystocentesis ones	Very few may be noted in free-catch samples; none in catheterized samples
Crystals	Usually numerous calcium carbonate crystals	Usually none
	Sometimes "triple phosphate" crystals present	Sometimes abundant calcium oxalate or rare amorphous urate crystals present

"Horse" results are based on a review by Kohn and Chew (1987). Foal results are from Brewer et al (1991).
°Note that false "positive" results for protein may occur on dipstick-type examination of alkaline urine. Such findings should be verified by another method, such as precipitation using sulfosalicylic acid.
HPF = high power field, LPF = low power field

MUSCULOSKELETAL SYSTEM

Equine Exercise Physiology

The biochemical adaptations of the horse to athletic exercise and the alterations that result from various training programs are an important facet of equine sports medicine. Recent international conferences act as an introduction to this field.

Biochemical and histochemical analysis of muscle fiber biopsies has been undertaken, usually from the middle gluteal muscle. Skeletal muscles are a heterogeneous collection of fiber types. Sampling from different areas of the same muscle will consequently yield different results. Therefore, to detect biochemical changes associated with training, several biopsies from the one animal or single samples from several animals are recommended.

ROUTINE BIOCHEMISTRY

Test		Lumsden et al (1980)	
		Thoroughbreds	Standardbreds
Serum or Plasma Enzymes			
AP (ALP)	U/L 37°C	26–92	24–67
AST (GOT)	U/L 37°C	141–330	123–789
CK (CPK)	U/L 37°C	2–147	18–217
LDH	U/L 37°C	137–181	125–349
Serum or Plasma Nonenzymes			
Calcium (Ca)	see Electrolytes		
Phosphate	see Electrolytes		
Lactate	mg/dl	2.5–15.5	4.1–11.0
	mEq/L	0.28–1.72	0.46–1.22
	mmol/L	0.28–1.72	0.46–1.22

Various workers have studied AP, CK, and LDH isoenzymes; however, they are seldom assessed in clinical practice.

AP = alkaline phosphatase; AST = aspartate aminotransferase; CK = creatine kinase; LDH = lactate dehydrogenase

ENDOCRINOLOGY

Endocrinopathies are infrequently evaluated in horses. Reference values vary with the laboratory performing the test. The following references serve as an introduction to the literature in this area:

1. Aldosterone, angiotensin I (plasma renin activity), and arginine vasopressin (antidiuretic hormone): McKeever et al (1992)
2. Cortisol: Dybdal et al (1994)
3. Epinephrine (adrenaline) and norepinephrine (noradrenaline): Yovich et al (1984) and Snow et al (1992)
4. Gastrin: Smyth et al (1989)
5. Oral glucose tolerance test: Jeffcott et al (1986)
6. Insulin: Reimers et al (1982) and Fowden et al (1984)

7. T_3 (triiodothyronine) and T_4 (thyroxine): Duckett et al (1989) and Sojka et al (1993).

CEREBROSPINAL FLUID (CSF)

Cisternal and lumbar taps produce similar values (Mayhew et al, 1977).

Gross appearance in the adult is clear and colorless. In the foal younger than 11 days old, gross appearance is clear to hazy and straw-yellow to colorless. In the foal older than 12 days, CSF is clear and colorless.

Protein

Total protein is usually the only protein measured biochemically. The Pandy test provides a qualitative assessment of immunoglobulin concentration. Results are usually graded as negative to trace.

Enzymes

Creatine kinase is the only enzyme routinely measured in CSF for clinical diagnostic work. Reference values have also been reported for AST (GOT), GGT, and LDH (Mayhew et al, 1977, Rossdale et al, 1982).

CEREBROSPINAL FLUID (CSF)

Test	Units	Adult	Foal
Cytology		Beech (1983)	Furr and Bender (1994)
RBC	/μl		0–320
Total nucleated cell count	/μl	0–48°	0–5
Mononuclear cells			
Small	%	60–94	0–43
Large	%	6–40	0–92
Neutrophils	%	0†	0
Eosinophils	%	0	0
Biochemistry		Mayhew et al (1977)	
CK (CPK)	U/L 37°C	0–8‡	
Glucose	mg/dl	30–75§	
	mmol/L	1.7–4.2	
Total protein	mg/dl	5–105‖	
	g/L	0.05–1.05	

°Mayhew et al (1977) reported that the total nucleated cell count of CSF was 0–6/μl. Many laboratories favor a reference range of 0–10/μl.

†Usually none; 3 animals had "a few" present.

‡Rossdale et al (1982) found somewhat higher CK values of 7–25 U/L for adults. They also measured CSF CK in clinically normal neonatal foals (<40 hours old): CK at 25°C = 4–39 U/L (at 37°C = 9–90 U/L). They found that values declined to within the adult reference range within about 48 hours. Interestingly, 16 premature (induced) foals (also <40 hours old) had CK values within the adult reference range.

§Mayhew et al (1977) reported that CSF glucose concentration was 35–75% of the corresponding blood value. This is lower than the 60–80% ratio that is often accepted for other species. It probably reflects the effect of IV injection of xylazine before sample collection, which results in short-term hyperglycemia.

‖ In addition, Beech (1983) reported total protein of 0–88 mg/dl (0–0.9 g/L). Rossdale et al (1982) reported total protein of 40–170 mg/dl (0.4–1.7 g/L).

PERITONEAL FLUID (PF)

The following adult cytology reference data are based on Bach (1974), Brownlow (1979), and Nelson (1979), and biochemistry reference data are from Nelson (1979) and Parry and Crisman (1991). The foal reference data are from Grindem and coworkers (1990).

Gross appearance (adults and foals) is usually straw-yellow in color, but occasionally is clear to orange. Peritoneal fluid is usually transparent, but occasionally is slightly turbid.

A volume of 5 to 10 ml of fluid can often be collected from normal adult horses within a few minutes. However, sometimes no fluid can be collected, despite repeated attempts at various sites.

PERITONEAL FLUID (PF)

Cytology		Adult	Foal
RBC count	$\times 10^6$/L		100–19,900
	$\times 10^9$/L		0.1–19.9
Total nucleated cell count	/µl	<10,000 (often <5000)	<1400
	$\times 10^9$/L	<10.0 (often <5.0)	<1.4
Neutrophils	%	20–90	2–94
Lymphocytes	%	0–35	0–7 (usually about 1)
Large mononuclear cells	%	5–60°	5–98†
Eosinophils	%	0–5	0–4 (usually 0)
Basophils	%	0–1	0
Total protein	g/dl	<2.5 (usually <1.5)	<2.0
	g/L	<25 (usually <15)	<20

Biochemistry Paired Samples		Adult		Foal	
		Blood	PF	Blood	PF
Amylase‡	IU/L 37°C	14–35	0–14		
Bilirubin (total)	mg/dl	0.8–1.5	0.3–0.8		
	µmol/L	13–25	5–13		
Creatinine	mg/dl	1.5–1.8	1.8–2.7		
	µmol/L	133–156	161–237		
GGT‡	IU/L 37°C	9–29	0–6		
Glucose§	mg/dl	72–100	89–115		
	mmol/L	4.0–5.6	4.9–6.4		
Lactate‡	mg/dl	5.8–15.5	3.8–10.9		
	mmol/L	0.6–1.7	0.4–1.2		
Lipase‖	IU/L 37°C	23–87	0–36		
Urea¶	mg/dl	11–16	13–22	2–14	2–8
	mmol/L	3.9–5.5	4.5–7.8	0.8–4.98	0.83–2.82

°These cells were commonly vacuolated and phagocytic (often of degenerate neutrophils). Occasional mitotic cells were also noted.
†Cells were rarely phagocytic of other cells. On average there were about equal proportions of neutrophils and large mononuclear cells present.
‡Blood value greater than PF value in all horses
§Blood glucose value less than PF value in 95% of horses
‖ Blood lipase value greater than PF value in 95% of horses
¶Plasma urea value less than or equal to PF value in all foals
GGT = gamma glutamyltransferase

PLEURAL FLUID

The following reference data are from Wagner and Bennett (1983). Gross appearance is usually yellow to reddish yellow in color and clear to hazy. Volume is 2 to 8 ml (in 1 of 18 horses, 35 ml was easily collected).

RESPIRATORY SYSTEM CYTOLOGY

Results are influenced by the method of collection and the site sampled. Sites may be the trachea, bronchi, or bronchioles/alveoli, usually by nasopharyngeal or transtra-

PLEURAL FLUID

Parameter	Units	Range	Comments
RBC	×10³/µl	22–540	No erythrophagocytosis
	×10⁹/L	22–540	
Nucleated cell count	/µl	800–12,100	94% of horses tested 800–8000/µl (0.8–8.0 × 10⁹/L)
	×10⁹/L	0.8–12.1	
Neutrophils	%	32–91	
	/µl	450–10,290	
	×10⁹/L	0.5–10.3	
Lymphocytes	%	0–22	94% of horses tested 0–10%
	/µl	0–680	
	×10⁹/L	0–0.7	
Large mononuclear cells	%	5–66	
	/µl	50–2620	
	×10⁹/L	0.1–2.6	
Eosinophils	%	0–9	90% of horses tested 0%, 5% tested 1% and 5% tested
	/µl	0–170	9% (latter horse, result was 170/µl, 0.2 × 10⁹/L)
	×10⁹/L	0–0.2	
Total protein (refractometer)	g/dl	0.2–4.7	90% of horses tested 0.5–3.4 g/dl (5–34 g/L)
	g/L	2–47	

cheal routes. The nasopharyngeal approach may result in contamination with cornified and noncornified squamous epithelial cells and their adherent bacteria.

Tracheobronchial washes have low cellularity and little mucus (Whitwell and Greet, 1984). Total nucleated cell counts are generally 1000/µl (1.0 × 10⁹/L) or less. Many of these cells are ciliated columnar epithelial cells, with some nonciliated columnar cells, goblet cells, and small, often clumped cuboidal cells (also called bronchoalveolar cells). Neutrophils and alveolar macrophages account for many of the remaining cells, but they are also present only in low numbers. Some macrophages may be vacuolated and/or phagocytic of debris, fungal elements, pollen, vegetable fibers, and RBCs; a few other macrophages may contain hemosiderin granules. Lymphocytes are less common and may be difficult to identify. They are usually classified as "mononuclear cells," together with other cells that are not obviously macrophages. Eosinophils are uncommon, whereas basophils and plasma cells are rare.

Washes from the deeper airways may yield somewhat higher cell counts, although this is not invariably the case. Cytology results are often similar to those described earlier.

Some variation in cellularity and cytology may be related to the volume of fluid used in the lavage procedure (Sweeney et al, 1992). Smaller quantities (50 ml) yield more cells per unit volume of fluid recovered with a greater percentage of neutrophils and lymphocytes than larger volumes (300 ml).

Cytology test results of tracheobronchial specimens do not necessarily correlate with those of bronchoalveolar samples, particularly in horses with chronic pulmonary disease (Derksen et al, 1989), and the latter may be more clinically useful.

Tracheobronchial specimens from normal horses are not necessarily sterile. Nonpathogenic and potentially pathogenic bacteria have been isolated from clinically healthy and cytologically normal horses. Fungi may also be seen in some normal animals.

Tracheobronchial aspirates from clinically normal foals may have higher eosinophil and neutrophil percentages than are present in adults (Crane et al, 1989). Thus, as

with any cytology evaluation, results must be interpreted in light of clinical signs.

SYNOVIAL FLUID

The following is based on van Pelt (1962), Persson (1971), Tew (1982, 1983) and Little and coworkers (1990).

Gross Appearance

Synovial fluid is pale yellow in color, clear to occasionally slightly turbid, with a high viscosity. If a drop is allowed to "string" from the end of a needle, it will form a strand about 5 to 10 cm in length. It does not clot, but readily exhibits thixotrophism.

Laboratory Test Results

1. Mucin clot is usually good, but occasionally fair, in character
2. Total RCC: Very few are present (<1400/µl; <1.4 × 10⁹/L)
3. Total nucleated cell count: Usually <500/µl (<0.5 × 10⁹/L); often <200/µl (<0.2 × 10⁹/L)
4. Total protein concentration: 0.5 to 2.2 g/dl (5–22 g/L); often <1.2 g/dl (<12 g/L). Most of the protein present is albumin.
5. Cytology: Usually <10% neutrophils and >90% mononuclear cells. Of the latter, about 50% are lymphoid cells and 50% are large mononuclear cells. Vacuolated (phagocytic) mononuclear cells (macrophages) account for <10% of all nucleated cells.
6. Cartilage fragments: Detectable in 15% or less of "normal" fluid samples. Such fragments are of superficial cartilage (i.e., they lack chondrocytes).
7. Hyaluronate (hyaluronic acid): 19 to 191 mg/dl (0.2–1.9 g/L)
8. Sulfated glycosaminoglycans: <4.5 mg/dl (<0.05 g/L)

References

Bach LG: Exfoliative cytology of peritoneal fluid in the horse. *In* Grunsell CSG, Hill FWG (eds): The Veterinary Annual 1973. Bristol, John Wright, 1974.

			Requirements						
State	Phone	HC	Name of Laboratory	Laboratory Accession #	Date of Test	Temperature Reading of Horse Recorded	Complete Description of Horse	Negative Coggins Test	Additional
Alabama	334-240-7255	Yes						Yes, within 12 mo if 6 mo of age or older	
Alaska	907-745-7200; permit from AK 907-745-3235	Yes	Yes					Yes, within 6 mo if 6 mo or older	If going through Canada, must also abide by Canadian requirements
Arizona	602-255-4293	Yes						No, but indicate results if tested	Yes
Arkansas	501-225-5138	Yes				Yes		Yes, within 12 mo if 6 mo of age or older	
California	916-445-6506	Yes	Yes	Yes				Yes, within 6 mo; nursing foals under 6 mo exempt if accompanying EIA-negative dam	
Colorado	303-239-4161	Yes	Yes					Yes, within 12 mo; nursing foals under 6 mo exempt if accompanying EIA-negative dam	
Connecticut	203-566-4616	Yes	Yes	Yes				Yes, within 12 mo; for sale or auction within 6 mo	
Delaware	302-736-4811	Yes				$\leq$102.0 (within 10 days of entry)		Yes, within 12 mo; for sale or auction within 6 mo	
Florida	904-488-7747	Yes	Yes	Yes	Yes			Yes, within 12 mo if 6 mo of age or older	Test results required on HC
Georgia	404-656-3671; AID 404-656-3667	Yes	Yes	Yes	Yes	$\leq$102.0		Yes, within 12 mo. Foals younger than 6 mo accompanying EIA-negative dam are exempt	Address of laboratory required on HC
Hawaii	808-487-5765	Yes						Yes, within 90 days	Call for complete information. Vaccination no less than 15 days before shipment against EE. No EE within 6 mo. Sponged or sprayed with 5% Malathion or other approved pesticide within 7 days of shipment. Placed on provisional quarantine for 45–60 days after entry
Idaho	208-332-8540	Yes						No	
Illinois	217-782-4944	Yes						Yes, within 12 mo	Persons who consign equidae to IL racetrack and/or IL equine exhibits should contact the officials of the track or exhibit for requirements
Indiana	317-232-1346	Yes	Yes				Yes	Yes, within 12 mo; nursing foals exempt if accompanying EIA-negative dam	
Iowa	515-281-5305	Yes						Yes, within 12 mo if 6 mo of age or older	Name of lab and date of test required
Kansas	913-296-2326	Yes (6 mo & above)						Yes, within 12 mo	
Kentucky	502-564-3956	Yes						Yes, within 6 mo; nursing foals under 6 mo exempt if accompanying EIA-negative dam	For exhibition, racing, trail, or amusement rides, negative EIA within 12 mo. Copy of EIA test with HC

State	Telephone	Entry permit required	Health certificate required	Negative EIA test	Remarks
Louisiana	504-922-1358		Yes	Yes, within 12 mo	
Maine	207-289-3701		Yes	Yes, within 6 mo; nursing foals under 6 mo exempt if accompanying EIA-negative dam	
Maryland	301-841-5810		Yes	Yes, within 12 mo if 9 mo of age or older	
Massachusetts	617-727-3018 (ext. 165)	Yes	Yes	Yes, within 6 mo	
Michigan	517-373-1077		Yes	Yes, within 6 mo	
Minnesota	612-296-5000	Yes	Yes	Yes, within 12 mo. Exceptions to negative EIA test requirements: Rodeo, circus and animal acts, trail rides, exhibition, slaughtering, nursing foal with EIA-negative dam, pending test results if permit is secured	Permit required if EIA test pending, call: 612-295-2967. Address of laboratory required on HC
Mississippi	601-354-6089		Yes	Yes, within 12 mo	Copy of EIA test report with HC
Missouri	314-751-3377	Yes	Yes	Yes, within 12 mo; nursing foals exempt if accompanying EIA-negative dam	Address of laboratory required
Montana	406-444-2043	Yes	Yes	None required from equines from NY	Permit required: 406-444-2976
Nebraska	402-471-2351		Yes	Yes, within 12 mo; foals under 6 mo exempt if accompanying EIA-negative dam	
Nevada	702-688-1180		Yes	Yes, within 6 mo	Copy of EIA test report with HC
New Hampshire	603-271-2404	Yes	Yes	Yes, within 6 mo; nursing foals exempt if accompanying EIA-negative dam	
New Jersey	609-292-3695		Yes	Yes, within 12 mo	Address of laboratory required
New Mexico	505-841-4000	Yes	Yes	Yes, within 12 mo if 6 mo of age or older	
North Carolina	919-733-7601		Yes	Yes, within 12 mo	
North Dakota	701-224-2655		Yes	No for horses from NY and WI	
Ohio	614-866-6361	Yes	Yes	Yes, within 6 mo if 12 mo of age or older	
Oklahoma	405-521-2840	Yes	Yes	Yes, within 12 mo; not required for nursing foals under 6 mo if with dam	Results of tests required on HC
Oregon	503-378-4709	Yes	Yes	Yes, within 6 mo if 6 mo of age or older	Permit required
Pennsylvania	717-783-5301		Yes	Yes, within 12 mo; foals under 6 mo exempt if accompanying EIA-negative dam	
Puerto Rico	908-725-1685		Yes	Yes, within 6 mo	Vaccinated against viral encephalitis with a bivalent vaccine within 6 mo. Negative test for piroplasmosis within 6 mo Rabies vaccination for show, 3 mo and older
Rhode Island	401-277-2781		Yes		
South Carolina	803-788-2260		Yes	Yes, within 6 mo	
South Dakota	605-733-3321		Yes	Yes, within 12 mo	
Tennessee	615-360-0120		Yes	Yes, within 12 mo (or within 6 mo for a sale), if 6 mo of age or older	

Table continued on following page

Requirements *(Continued)*

State	Phone	HC	Name of Laboratory	Laboratory Accession #	Date of Test	Temperature Reading of Horse Recorded	Complete Description of Horse	Negative Coggins Test	Additional
Texas	512-719-0777	Yes	Yes		Yes			Yes, within 12 mo	If going directly to slaughter or consigned to a veterinary clinic for treatment, permit required
Utah	801-538-7160	Yes						Yes, within 12 mo	
Vermont	802-828-2450	Yes						Yes, within 12 mo if 6 mo of age or older	
Virgin Islands	809-772-4781	Yes	Yes		Yes		Yes	Yes, within 6 mo; nursing foals exempt if accompanying EIA-negative dam	All horses are required to be vaccinated for Eastern and Western encephalomyelitis. Date of vaccination
Virginia	804-786-2481	Yes					Yes	Yes, within 12 mo; sales within 6 mo	Horses for research or immediate slaughter require a permit
Washington	206-753-5063	Yes						Yes, within 6 mo if 6 mo of age or older	
West Virginia	304-348-2214	Yes					Yes	Yes, within 6 mo	
Wisconsin	608-266-7145	Yes					Yes	Yes, within 6 mo; nursing foals exempt if accompanying EIA-negative dam	
Wyoming	307-777-7515	Yes	Yes					Yes, within 12 mo; nursing foals exempt if accompanying EIA-negative dam	

EIA = equine infectious anemia; EE = equine encephalitis; HC = health certificate.

Appendix 4: Antidotes for Common Poisons

E. MURL BAILEY, JR.
TAM GARLAND
College Station, Texas

TABLE 1. LOCALLY ACTING ANTIDOTES AGAINST UNABSORBED POISONS

Toxicant	Antidote and Dose or Concentration
Acids, corrosives	Weak alkali—magnesium oxide solution (1:25 warm water) internally. *Never give sodium bicarbonate.* Milk of magnesia: 1–15 ml. Flush externally with water.
Alkali, caustic	Apply paste of sodium bicarbonate. Weak acid, e.g., vinegar (diluted 1:4), 1% acetic acid or lemon juice p.o. Dilute albumin (4 to 6 egg whites to 1 qt. warm water) or give whole milk followed by activated charcoal and then a cathartic, because some compounds are soluble in excess albumin. Local: Flush with copious amounts of water and apply vinegar.
Alkaloids	Potassium permanganate (1:5000–1:10,000) for lavage or p.o. administration. Tannic acid or strong tea (200–500 mg in 30–60 ml of water) except in cases of poisoning by cocaine, nicotine, physostigmine, atropine, and morphine. Purgative should be used for prompt removal of tannates. Activated charcoal may be useful for some alkaloids, although its effectiveness remains to be proved (1 g/kg body weight via stomach tube as a slurry in water).
Arsenic	Sodium thiosulfate, 10% solution p.o. (60–100 gm), followed by lavage. Protein: e.g., evaporated milk, egg whites.
Barium and bismuth salts	Sodium sulfate and magnesium sulfate (20% solution given p.o.). Dosage: 2–25 g.
Carbon tetrachloride	Acacia or gum arabic as mucilage. Empty stomach, give high-protein and high-carbohydrate diet; maintain fluid and electrolyte balance. Hemodialysis is indicated in anuria. Epinephrine is contraindicated (ventricular fibrillation!).
Copper	Albumin: Use as for alkali intoxication. Magnesium oxide: Use as for acid intoxication.
Detergents, anionic (NA$^+$, K$^+$, NH$_4^+$ salts)	Milk or water followed by demulcent (oils, kaolin, acacia, gelatin, starch, egg white).
Detergents, cationic (chlorides, iodides)	Soap (Castile) dissolved in 4 times its bulk of hot water. Albumin: Use as for alkali intoxication.
Fluoride	Calcium (milk, limewater, or powdered chalk mixed with water) p.o.
Formaldehyde	Ammonia water (0.2% p.o.) or ammonium acetate (1% for lavage). Starch: 1 part to 15 parts hot water added gradually. Gelatin soaked in water for ½ hour. Albumin: Use as for alkali intoxication. Sodium thiosulfate: Use as for arsenic intoxication.
Iron	Sodium bicarbonate: 1% for lavage.
Lead	Sodium or magnesium sulfate p.o. See specific antidote. Albumin: Use as for alkali intoxication.
Mercury	Protein: Milk, egg whites (use as for alkali intoxication). Magnesium oxide: Use as for acid intoxication. Sodium formaldehyde sulfoxylate: 5% solution for lavage. Starch: Use as for formaldehyde intoxication. Activated charcoal: Use as for alkaloid intoxication.
Oxalic acid	Calcium: Calcium hydroxide as 0.15% solution. Other alkalis are contraindicated because their salts are more soluble. Chalk or other calcium salts. Magnesium sulfate as cathartic. Maintain diuresis to prevent calcium oxalate deposition in kidney.
Petroleum distillates (aliphatic hydrocarbons)	Olive oil, other vegetable oils, or mineral oil p.o. After ½ hour, sodium sulfate as cathartic. Lavage is contraindicated for ingested volatile solvents, but petroleum distillates are used as carrier agents for more toxic agents.
Phenol and cresols	Soap-and-water or alcohol lavage of skin. Sodium bicarbonate (0.5%) dressings. Activated charcoal and/or mineral oil p.o.
Phosphorus	Copper sulfate (0.2%–0.4% solution) or potassium permanganate (1:5000 solution) for lavage. Activated charcoal. Do not give vegetable oil cathartic. Remove fat from diet.
Silver nitrate	Normal saline for lavage. Albumin: Use as for alkali intoxication.
Unknown (e.g., toxic plants or other materials)	Activated charcoal: Replaces universal antidote; use as for alkaloid intoxication. Follow with a cathartic, and repeat procedure.

TABLE 2.   SPECIFIC SYSTEMIC ANTIDOTES AND DOSAGES

Toxicant	Systemic Antidote	Dosage and Method for Treatment
Amphetamines	Chlorpromazine	1 mg/kg IM, IP, IV; administer only half dose if barbiturates have been given: blocks excitation.
Arsenic, mercury and other heavy metals except cadmium, lead, silver, selenium, and thallium	Dimercaprol (BAL, Hynson; Wescott & Dunning)	10% solution in oil; give 2.5–5.0 mg/kg IM q4h for 2 days, b.i.d. for the next 10 days or until recovery. NOTE. In severe acute poisoning, 5 mg/kg dosage should be given only for the first day.
	D-Penicillamine (Cuprimine; Merck & Co.)	Developed for chronic mercury poisoning, now seems promising. No reports on dosage in horses. Dosage for humans is 250 mg p.o. q6h for 10 days (3–4 mg/kg).
Atropine, belladonna alkaloids	Physostigmine salicylate	0.1–0.6 mg/kg IM (do not overtreat; do not use neostigmine).
Barbiturates	Doxapram	2% solution: 3–5 mg/kg (0.14–0.25 ml/kg) IV only; repeat as necessary.
		NOTE—The above is reliable only when depression is mild. In deeper levels of depression, artificial respiration (and oxygen) is preferable.
Bromides	Chlorides (sodium or ammonium salts)	0.5–1.0 g/day for several days; hasten excretion.
Carbon monoxide	Oxygen	Provide pure oxygen at normal or high pressure, artificial respiration, blood transfusion.
Cholinergic agents	Atropine sulfate	0.02–0.04 mg/kg PRN.
		NOTE—Atropine should be used in horses with extreme care to avoid potentially fatal ileus. A very slow drip is suggested, with constant monitoring of gastrointestinal status. *Avoid atropine toxicosis.*
Cholinesterase inhibitors	Atropine sulfate	0.02 mg/kg, repeated as needed for atropinization. Treat cyanosis (if present) first. Blocks only muscarinic effects. See note, above. *Avoid atropine toxicosis.*
Cholinergic agents and cholinesterase inhibitors (organophosphorus insecticides)	Pralidoxime chloride (2-PAM)	5% solution; five 20–50 mg/kg IM, IV injections (maximum dose is 500 mg/min), repeat as needed. 2-PAM alleviates nicotinic effect and regenerates acetylcholinesterase. Morphine, succinylcholine, and phenothiazines are contraindicated.
Copper	D-Penicillamine (Cuprimine)	See arsenic
Coumarin-derivative anticoagulants	Vitamin K₁ (Aqua-Mephyton, 5-mg capsules, Merck & Co.) (Vitamin K₁, Eschar, 25-mg capsules)	Give 3–5 mg/kg per day with food. Treat for 7 days for warfarin-type, treat for 21 to 30 days for second-generation anticoagulant rodenticides. Oral therapy is more efficacious than IV.
	Whole blood or plasma	Blood transfusion, 25 ml/kg.
Curare	Neostigmine methylsulfate	Solution: 1:5000 or 1:2000. Dose is 0.001 mg/kg SC. Follow with IV injection of atropine (0.04 mg/kg).
	Edrophonium chloride (Tensilon; Roche) Artificial respiration	1% solution: give 0.05–1.0 mg/kg IV.
Cyanide	Methemoglobin (sodium nitrite is used to form methemoglobin)	1% solution of sodium nitrite, dosage is 16 mg/kg IV (1.6 ml/kg).
	Sodium thiosulfate	Follow with: 20% solution at dosage of 30–40 mg/kg (0.15–0.2 ml/kg) IV. If treatment is repeated, use only sodium thiosulfate.
		NOTE—Both of the above may be given simultaneously as follows: 0.5 ml/kg of combination consisting of 10 g sodium nitrite, 15 g sodium thiosulfate in distilled water q. s. 250 ml. Dosage may be repeated once. If further treatment is required, give only 20% solution of sodium thiosulfate at 0.2 ml/kg.
Digitalis glycosides, oleander	Potassium chloride	5–20 g PO in divided doses, or in serious cases as diluted solution given IV by slow drip (ECG monitoring is essential).
	Diphenylhydantoin	25 mg/min IV until control is established.
	Propranolol (β-blocker)	0.5–1.0 mg/kg IV or IM as needed to control cardiac arrhythmias (ECG monitoring is essential).
	Atropine sulfate	0.02–0.04 mg/kg as needed for cholinergic control. See note above. *Avoid atropine toxicosis.*
Fluoride	Calcium borogluconate	3–10 ml of 5%–10% solution.

TABLE 2. SPECIFIC SYSTEMIC ANTIDOTES AND DOSAGES *Continued*

Toxicant	Systemic Antidote	Dosage and Method for Treatment
Fluoracetate (Compound 1080; Sigma)	Glyceryl monoacetin	0.1–0.5 mg/kg IM hourly for several hours (total 2–4 mg/kg), or diluted (0.5%–1.0% IV) (danger of hemolysis). Monoacetin is available only from chemical supply houses.
	Acetamide, pentobarbital	Experimental
	NOTE—All treatments are generally unrewarding.	
Hallucinogens (LSD, phencyclidine [PCP])	Diazepam (Valium; Roche)	PRN. Avoid respiratory depression (2–5 mg/kg).
Heparin	Protamine sulfate	1% solution; give 1.0–1.5 mg by slow IV injection to antagonize each 1 mg of heparin. Reduce dose as time increases between heparin injection and start of treatment (after 30 min, give only 0.5 mg).
Iron salts	Deferoxamine (Desferal; Ciba)	Dose for animals not yet established. Dose for humans is 5 g of 5% solution p.o., then 20 mg/kg IM every 4–6 hours. In case of shock, dose is 40 mg/kg by IV drip over 4-hour period; may be repeated in 6 hours, then 15 mg/kg by drip every 8 hours.
Lead	Calcium disodium edetate, BAL, thiamide	See *Current Therapy in Equine Medicine 3* page 364.
Metaldehyde	Diazepam (Valium; Roche)	2–5 mg/kg IV to control tremors.
	Triflupromazine	0.2–2.0 mg/kg IV.
	Pentobarbital	To effect.
Methanol and ethylene glycol	Ethanol	Give IV, 1.1 g/kg (4.4 ml/kg of 25% solution), then 0.5 g/kg (2.0 ml/kg) q4h for 4 days. To prevent or correct acidosis, use sodium bicarbonate, 0.4 g/kg IV. Activated charcoal: 5 g/kg p.o. if given within 4 hours of ingestion may help (although ability of activated charcoal to bind ethylene glycol is questionable).
Methemoglobinemia-producing agents (nitrites, chlorates)	Methylene blue	1% solution (maximum concentration), give by *slow* IV injection, 8.8 mg/kg (0.9 ml/kg); repeat if necessary. To prevent fall in blood pressure in case of nitrate poisoning, use a sympathomimetic drug (ephedrine or epinephrine).
Morphine and related compounds	Naloxone chloride (Narcan; DuPont)	0.1 mg/kg IV. Do not repeat if respiration is not satisfactory.
	Levallorphan tartrate (Lorfan; Roche)	Give IV, 0.1–0.5 ml of solution containing 1 mg/ml.
	NOTE—Use either of the above antidotes only in acute poisoning. Artificial respiration may be indicated. Activated charcoal is also indicated.	
Oxalates	Calcium	23% solution of calcium gluconate IV. Give 3–20 ml (to control hypocalcemia).
Phenothiazine	Methylamphetamine (Desoxyn; Abbott)	0.1–0.2 mg/kg IV; also transfusion. Only available in tablet form.
	Diphenhydramine HCl	For CNS depression, 2–5 mg/kg IV for extrapyramidal signs.
Phytotoxic lectins (ricin, abrin, robin, crotin) and botulinum neurotoxin	Antitoxins often not available	Specific antitoxins such as botulinum antitoxin.
Red squill	As for digitalis and oleander	
Snake bite (rattlesnake, copperhead, water moccasin)	Antivenin (Wyeth) Trivalent Crotalidae (Fort Dodge)	*Caution*: equine origin. Administer 1–2 vials IV slowly, diluted in 250–500 ml saline or lactated Ringer's only if absolutely necessary to treat systemic effects; otherwise, avoid in horses. Also administer antihistamines. *Corticosteroids are contraindicated.*
Coral snake	(Wyeth antivenin, as above)	*Caution*: equine origin, use only if necessary. May be used as with pit viper antivenin.
Spider bite (black widow)	Antivenin (Merck & Co.)	*Caution*: equine origin. Administer IV undiluted.
	Dantrolene sodium (Dantrium; Norwich-Eaton)	1 mg/kg IV, followed by 1 mg/kg p.o. q4h.
Spider bite (brown recluse)	Dapsone	1 mg/kg b.i.d. for 10 days. Also local treatment of site.
Strontium	Calcium salts	Usual dose of calcium borogluconate.
	Ammonium chloride	0.2–0.5 g p.o. 3–4 times daily.

Table continued on following page

TABLE 2.   SPECIFIC SYSTEMIC ANTIDOTES AND DOSAGES *Continued*

Toxicant	Systemic Antidote	Dosage and Method for Treatment
Strychnine and brucine	Pentobarbital	Give IV to effect. Higher dose is usually required than that required for anesthesia. Place animal in warm, quiet stall.
	Amobarbital	Give by slow IV injection to effect. Duration of sedation usually 4–6 hours.
	Methocarbamol (Robaxin; Robins)	10% solution; average first dose is 149 mg/kg IV (range: 40–300 mg). Repeat half dose as needed.
	Glyceryl guaiacolate (Guaiafenesin; Summit Hill Labs)	110 mg/kg IV as 5% solution. Repeat as necessary.
	Diazepam (Valium; Roche)	2–5 mg/kg to control convulsions. Evacuate stomach, then use other agents.

Note: Page numbers in *italics* refer to illustrations; page numbers followed by t refer to tables.
Page numbers following III refer to pages in *Current Therapy Equine Medicine 3*.

Cushing's disease *(Continued)*
  evaluation of, 500–501
  oral ulceration due to, 156
  ovarian function affected by, 525
  physiology of, 499–500
  treatment of, 501
Cyanide, plants containing, 651
  poisoning due to, 651, 658t
Cyanosis, smoke inhalation causing, 461
Cyathostomes, parasitism due to, 709–710
Cyproheptadine, Cushing's disease treated with, 501
Cystadenoma, ovarian, 529
Cystitis, 482–483
  hematuria due to, 489
  treatment of, 482–483
Cyst(s), dentigerous, 144–145
  endometrial, 522–523
  ovarian, 531
  paranasal sinus with, 421
  pharyngeal, 145
  renal, 492
  uterine, 522–523

Dandruff, 385–386
Dantrolene, rhabdomyolysis therapy with, 119–120
DDS (dioctyl sodium sulfosuccinate), colic treated with, 189–190, 190t
Debridement, foot canker treatment with, 128
Decompression, colic treated with, 185
Dehydration, 200–202
  assessment parameters for, 200t
  colitis with, 200–202, 201t
  fluid therapy for, 200–202, 201t
Dentigerous cysts, 144–145
Deoxypyridinoline, bone marker role of, 113t, 113–114
Depigmentation, 391–393
  acquired, 391t, 391–393
  disorders causing, 391t, 391–393
  genetic factors in, 391t, 391–393
  leukotrichia causing, 391t, 392–393
  vitiligo in, 391–392, 392t
Dermatitis, 377–386
  allergic, 369, 377–380, 383–384
  atopic, 379
  crusting and scaling due to, 367–369, 381–386, 382t
  eosinophilic, III:706–708
  food hypersensitivity causing, 379–380
  history form for, 378
  immune-mediated, 369, 383–384
  insect hypersensitivity causing, 377–379
  pastern affected by, treatment of, 398
  pruritus associated with, 377–381
  seborrheic, 385–386
Dermatophilosis, 367–368, 382–383
  diagnosis of, 382
  treatment of, 382–383
Dermatophytosis, 367–368, 384–385
  clinical signs of, 385
  diagnosis of, 385
  treatment of, 385
Dermoids, eye affected by, 637
Desmitis, 97–99
  accessory ligament (of deep digital flexor tendon) with, 27–29, 28, 29
  collateral tarsocrural, 98–99
  plantar ligament with, 97–98
  sesamoidean, 54–55
    pastern soft tissue disease with, 62t, 63t
  suspensory, 47–48
    limb edema related to, 24t, 27
    metacarpal/metatarsal pain due to, 38–40

Desmitis *(Continued)*
    sesamoid bone affected by, 53–54
Detomidine, 755t
  anesthesia with, 714t, 714–716
  colic treated with, 183, 183t
Dew poisoning, 367, 368, 382–383
Dexamethasone suppression test, 500t
  cortisol levels in, 500t
  protocol for, 500t
Diabetes insipidus, polyuria of, 488
Dialysis, acute kidney failure treated with, 475
Diaphragm, hernia affecting, 465
Diaphyses, hypertrophic osteopathy affecting, 129t, 129–130
Diarrhea, 631–636
  foal with, 631–636
    assessment of, 632–634, 633t
    infectious causes in, 631–634, 633t
    noninfectious causes in, 632
    preventive measures for, 635–636
    treatment for, 634–635
Diastema, 151
Diazepam, anesthesia with, 714t, 714–716
  rhabdomyolysis therapy with, 119
DIC. See *Disseminated intravascular coagulation (DIC).*
Dicoumarol, poisoning with, 666–667
Diet, 675–699. See also *Feeds; Nutrition.*
  bone development role of, III:119–122
  brood mare, 693–695, 694t
  cervical stenosis role of, 306–307, 309
  formulation program for, 677–678, 693–697, 694t, 696t
  pregnancy and, 693–694, 694t
  rhabdomyolysis role of, 115, 119–120
  supplements role in, 675–676, 676t, 688t–690t
  weanlings and, 695, 695t
Digestion, diagnostic testing of, 169
Digital extensor tendon, 16
  rupture of, 15
Digital flexor tendon, 34–38, 43–50
  annular ligament syndrome affecting, 44
  deep, accessory ligament desmitis of, 27–29, 28, 29
    carpal lesions affecting, 18
    hock injury affecting, 98
    inflammation of, 31–33, 32, 62t, 63t, 66, 98
    pastern injury affecting, 62t, 63t, 66
    slipped, 98
  laceration of, 34–38, 35t, 36t, 37t
  limb edema related to, 24t, 26–27
  rupture of, 34–38, 35t, 36t, 37t
  superficial, carpal lesions affecting, 18
    displacement of, 94–95
    hock injury affecting, 93–95
    inflammation of, 62t, 63t, 65–66, 93–95
    metacarpal/metatarsal pain due to, 42
    pastern injury affecting, 62t, 63t, 65–66
  synovitis of, infection causing, 48–50
    noninfectious, 43–44
Digoxin, antiarrhythmia therapy using, 252t, 253
Dimethyl sulfoxide, endotoxemia treated with, 187, 187t
Dimethylglycine, rhabdomyolysis therapy with, 119
Dioctyl sodium sulfosuccinate, colic treated with, 189–190, 190t
Dioxins, poisoning due to, 663
Dipyrone, colic treated with, 182, 183t
  pharmacokinetics of, 724–727, 725t
Disaster response, 743–748
  financial issues of, 748
  planning for, 743–748

Disaster response *(Continued)*
  veterinarian role in, 745
Disseminated intravascular coagulation (DIC), 287–289
  anticoagulant therapy in, 288–289
  clinical signs of, 288
  diagnosis of, 288
  hemolytic anemia in, 282
  prevention of, 289
  treatment of, 288–289
Diuretic agents, heart failure treated with, 254
  kidney failure treated with, 475
DMSO (dimethyl sulfoxide), endotoxemia treated with, 187t, 188
Dobutamide, antiarrhythmia therapy using, 252t, 254
Dog-sitting position, 556
Donkey, anesthesia of, III:101–104
Dopamine, antiarrhythmia therapy using, 251–253, 252t
  cardiac failure therapy using, 254
Doppler studies, cardiographic, 229–231, 230, 231
Dourine, mare with, 513
  stallion with, III:710
DPJ (duodenitis–proximal peritonitis), 190, 212t, III:211–214
Draft horse, III:85–101
  anesthesia of, III:95–101
  lameness in, III:85–91
Drainage, peritoneal, 209–210
Drugs. See also specific drugs and drug types.
  clinical trials of, III:74–75
  colic management with, III:201–206
  dosage tables for, 753t–760t
Dry matter, northeastern forage content of, 681t, 682t
  southern forage content of, 685t, 686t
  United Kingdom feeds content of, 699t–701t
Dry sickness (mal seco). See *Grass sickness.*
Ductus arteriosus (patent), 256–257
  clinical signs in, 256
  diagnosis of, 257
  murmur of, 256
  prognosis in, 257
Ductus deferens, sperm occlusion of, 580
Duodenal ulcer, 191–197
  diagnosis of, 192–194, 193
  drug therapy for, 194–197, 195, 195t, 196
  pathogenesis of, 191–192
Duodenitis–proximal jejunitis (DPJ), 190, 212t, III:211–214
Dust, obstructive pulmonary disease and, 426, 432, 433, 436
Dysautonomia, grass sickness as, 203, 205
Dysphagia, 141–143
  differential diagnosis of, 141–143
  esophageal, 142–143
  grass sickness causing, 204, 205
  pharyngeal, 141–142
  physiologic mechanisms of, 141–143
  systemic diseases causing, 143
  toxic plant causing, 649
Dystocia, 552–559
  anesthesia and restraints for, 553, 553t, 553–555, 554t
  anterior presentation in, 555–557, 556
  approach to diagnosis of, 552
  complications related to, 558t–559t
  manipulations for, 555–559, 556, 557
  posterior presentation in, 557, 557–559
  traction applied in, 559
Dysuria, 482–486

Ear, plaques affecting, 390

ISBN 0-7216-2633-5